AF674772

DIAGNOSTIC CYTOLOGY

DIAGNOSTIC CYTOLOGY

Second Edition

Pranab Dey
MBBS MD MIAC FRCPath

Professor
Department of Cytology
Postgraduate Institute of
Medical Education and Research
Chandigarh, India

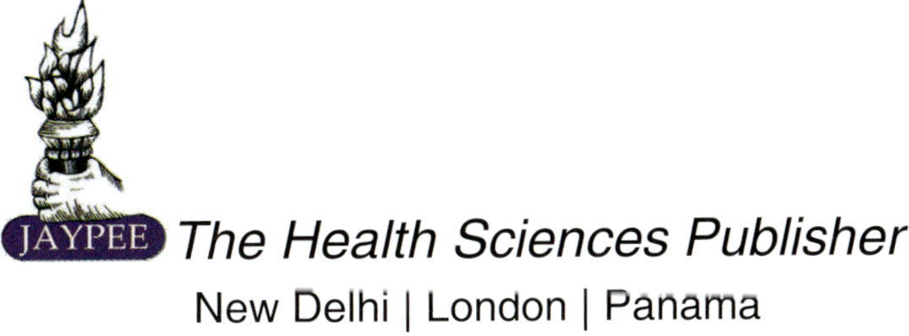

The Health Sciences Publisher
New Delhi | London | Panama

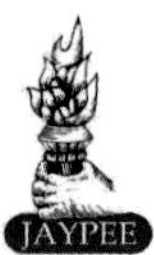

Jaypee Brothers Medical Publishers (P) Ltd

Headquarters

Jaypee Brothers Medical Publishers (P) Ltd
4838/24, Ansari Road, Daryaganj
New Delhi 110 002, India
Phone: +91-11-43574357
Fax: +91-11-43574314
E-mail: jaypee@jaypeebrothers.com

Overseas Offices

JP Medical Ltd
83 Victoria Street, London
SW1H 0HW (UK)
Phone: +44 20 3170 8910
Fax: +44 (0)20 3008 6180
E-mail: info@jpmedpub.com

Jaypee-Highlights Medical Publishers Inc
City of Knowledge, Bld. 235, 2nd Floor, Clayton
Panama City, Panama
Phone: +1 507-301-0496
Fax: +1 507-301-0499
E-mail: cservice@jphmedical.com

Jaypee Brothers Medical Publishers (P) Ltd
17/1-B, Babar Road, Block-B, Shyamoli
Mohammadpur, Dhaka-1207
Bangladesh
Mobile: +08801912003485
E-mail: jaypeedhaka@gmail.com

Jaypee Brothers Medical Publishers (P) Ltd
Bhotahity, Kathmandu, Nepal
Phone: +977-9741283608
E-mail: kathmandu@jaypeebrothers.com

Website: www.jaypeebrothers.com
Website: www.jaypeedigital.com

Inquiries for bulk sales may be solicited at: jaypee@jaypeebrothers.com

Diagnostic Cytology

First Edition: 2014

Second Edition: 2018

ISBN: 978-93-5270-120-9

Printed at: Ajanata Offset & Packagings Ltd., Faridabad, Haryana

Dedicated to

Shree Shree Satyananda Giri
Rini
Madhumanti
and my mother Nisha Dey

Preface to the Second Edition

In this second edition of the book, I have introduced two new chapters on round cell tumors and infections. The newer classifications of diseases and molecular genetics have been provided. In each chapter, I have added review questions along with multiple figures. Many old figures have been either replaced or deleted. Overall, I have changed many chapters. I am sure that this will help the readers significantly.

Pranab Dey

Preface to the First Edition

Cytology is an integral part of pathology curriculum and it is very important to have working knowledge in this area. I designed this book in four sections: general cytology, clinical cytology (exfoliative cytology), laboratory techniques in cytology and fine needle aspiration cytology. I hope that this present book will help immensely all the postgraduate students in pathology, students of cytology (both BSc and MSc), cytology practitioners and all others who are interested in clinical cytology. I have tried to explain various areas of cytology by simple language, tables and illustrations (both line diagrams and microphotographs). All the line diagrams are drawn by me. I hope that these figures are satisfactory. There are multiple boxes in this book which convey the essential and important messages. I will be glad if this book is helpful to the students, teachers and practitioners of cytology.

Pranab Dey

Acknowledgments

I am grateful to Mr Jitendar P Vij (Group Chairman) and Ms Chetna Malhotra Vohra (Associate Director—Content Strategy) of Jaypee Brothers Medical Publishers, for their great support and encouragement in writing the second edition of this book. Mr Subrata Adhikari (Commissioning Editor), Ms Kritika Dua (Development Editor) and the other members of the publishing team also provided me full support and advice during the preparation of the manuscript.

It is my great pleasure to express my thanks to Professor Arvind Rajwanshi, Head, Department of Cytology, Postgraduate Institute of Medical Education and Research, Chandigarh, India. I am also thankful to my departmental colleagues for their routine support. My friend, Dr Suvradeep Mitra helped me to rethink in many aspects of general cytology. I am especially thankful to Dr Manish Rohilla. He thoroughly read the first edition of the book and corrected many chapters and gave me valuable suggestions. My friend, Dr Chandrasekaran Muralidharan taught me the principle of many newer techniques in cytology. My sincere thanks to Mr Ghanashyam Mahato, assistant librarian of Browser library, for helping me to provide many important references.

I am thankful to all my junior residents, senior residents and technical staffs in the Department of Cytology. My wife Rini and daughter Madhumanti provided me constant support and encouragement in writing this book.

Finally, I am grateful to God Almighty for His blessing to make this book successful.

Contents

Section 1: *General Cytology*

Section 3: *Laboratory Techniques*

Abbreviations

AIDS	Acquired immunodeficiency syndrome
ALL	Acute lymphoblastic leukemia
AML	Acute myeloblastic leukemia
ACC	Adenoid cystic carcinoma
APC	Adenomatous polyposis coli
ATP	Adenosine triphosphate
ACC	Adrenocortical carcinomas
APC	Allophycocyanin
AFP	Alpha fetoprotein
ACS	American Cancer Society
APC	Anaphase promoting complex
ALCL	Anaplastic large cell lymphoma
ALK	Anaplastic lymphoma kinase
AR	Androgen receptor
ABC	Aneurysmal bone cyst
AML	Angiomyolipoma
APAF	Apoptosis activating factor
AIF	Apoptosis inducing factor
AGNOR	Argyrophilic nucleolar organizer region
ANN	Artificial neural network
ADH	Atypical ductal hyperplasia
AGC	Atypical glandular cells
AGUS	Atypical glandular cells of undetermined significance
ALT	Atypical lipomatous tumor
ASC	Atypical squamous cell
ASC-H	Atypical squamous cell cannot exclude HSIL
ASC-US	Atypical squamous cell of undetermined significance
ATG	Autophagy related gene
BCG	Bacillus Calmette-Guérin
BE	Barrett's
BCA	Basal cell adenoma
BCC	Basal cell carcinoma
BBN	Bayesian belief network
BTA	Bladder tumor antigen
BAC	Bronchioloalveolar carcinoma
BAL	Bronchoalveolar lavage
BL	Burkitt lymphoma
CEA	Carcinoembryonic antigen
CKI	CDK inhibitor
CSF	Cerebrospinal fluid
CIN	Cervical intraepithelial neoplasia
CHS	Chondrosarcoma
CIN	Chromosomal instability
CLL	Chronic lymphocytic leukemia
CML	Chronic myeloid leukemia
CCSK	Clear cell sarcoma of kidney
CLIA	Clinical Laboratory Improvement Amendments
CDK	Cluster of differentiation
CGH	Comparative genomic hybridization
CT	Computerized tomography
CP	Conditional probability
CP	Conventional preparation
CIMP	CpG island methylator phenotype
CDK	Cyclin dependent kinases
CKI	Cytokeratin
CMV	Cytomegalovirus
CP	Cystosarcoma phyllodes
DFC	Dense fibrillar component
DNA	Deoxyribonucleic acid
DSRCT	Desmoplastic small round cell tumor
DLBCL	Diffuse large B cell lymphoma
DPAM	Disseminated peritoneal adenomucinosis
Dnmt	DNA methyl transferases
DCIS	Ductal crcinoma in situ
EST	Endodermal sinus tumor
ER	Endoplasmic reticulum
ERCP	Endoscopic retrograde cholangiopancreatography
EUG FNAC	Endoscopic ultrasound guided FNAC
EGF	Epithelial growth factor
EMA	Epithelial membrane antigen
EMT	Epithelial mesenchymal transition
EST	Epithelioid sarcoma
EBV	Epstein-Barr virus
ER	Estrogen receptor
EWS	Ewing's sarcoma
FADD	Fas-associated death domain
FC	Fibrillar center
FDP	Fibrin degradation product
Fad	Fibroadenoma
FGF	Fibroblast growth factor
FD	Fibrocystic diseases
FNAB	Fine needle aspiration biopsy

FNAC	Fine needle aspiration cytology
FNS	Fine needle sampling
FCM	Flow cytometry
FCI	Flow cytometry immunophenotyping
FITC	fluorescein isothiocyanate
FISH	Fluorescence in situ hybridization
FNH	Focal nodular hyperplasia
FA	Follicular adenoma
FC	Follicular carcinoma
FCC	Follicular centre cell lymphoma
FL	Follicular lymphoma
FN	Follicular neoplasm
FVPTC	Follicular variant of papillary carcinoma of thyroid
FDA	Food and Drug Administration
GIST	Gastrointestinal stromal tumor
GIT	Gastrointestinal tract
GCT	Giant cell tumor
GCTTS	Giant cell tumor of tendon sheath
GFAP	Glial fibrillary acidic protein
GLUT-1	Glucose-transport protein 1
GC	Golgi complex
GPCR	G-protein-coupled receptors
GC	Granular components
GM	Granulomatous mastitis
GTP	Guanosine triphosphate
GDP	Gunasonsine diphosphate
HCC	Hepatocellular carcinoma
HSV	Herpes simplex virus
HP	Heterochromatin protein
HSIL	High grade squamous intraepithelial lesion
HMGB1	High mobility group box 1
HP	High power
HDAC	Histone deacetylases
HMTase	Histone methyltransferases
HL	Hodgkin lymphoma
HL	Hodgkin's lymphoma
HSR	Homogenously staining region
HCG	Human chorionic gonadotropin
HHV	human herpes virus
HIV	Human immunodeficiency virus
HPV	Human papilloma virus
HA	Hyaluronic acid
HC	Hybrid capture
ICM	Image cytometry
IDC	Infiltrating duct carcinoma
INM	Inner nuclear membrane
IC	Insular carcinoma
IQC	Internal quality control
ISUP	International Society of Urologic Pathologists
INI	Intranuclear pseudoinclusions
IUCD	Intrauterine contraceptive devices
ILC	Invasive lobular carcinoma
LDH	Lactate dehydrogenase
LBR	Lamin B receptor
LAP	Lamina associated polypeptide
LCH	Langerhans cell histiocytosis
LCC	Large cell carcinoma
LSC	Laser scanning cytometry
LMS	Leiomyosarcomas
LPS	Liposarcoma
LBC	Liquid based cytology
LOH	Loss of heterozygosity
LSIL	Low grade squamous intraepithelial
LP	Low power
LE	Lupus erythematous
LBL	Lymphoblastic lymphoma
L & H	lymphocytic and/or histiocytic
LESA	Lymphoepithelial sialadenitis
LG	Lymphoglandular body
LPL	Lymphoplasmacytic lymphoma
MFH	Malignant fibrous histiocytoma
MM	Malignant mesothelioma
MPNST	Malignant peripheral nerve sheath tumor
MRCT	Malignant round cell tumor
MCL	Mantle cell lymphoma
MZL	Marginal zone lymphoma
MAR	Matrix attachment region
MGG	May Grunwald Giemsa
MDC1	Mediator of DNA damage checkpoint 1
MP	Medium power
MCL	Medullary carcinoma
m-RNA	Messenger RNA
miRNA	Micro RNA
MN	Micronucleus
MSI	Microsatellite instability
MT	Mitochondria
MCN	Mucinous cystic neoplasia
MEC	Mucoepidermoid carcinoma
MALT	Mucosa associated lymphoma
M-FISH	Multicolor FISH
MEN	Multiple endocrine neoplasia
MLS	Myxoid liposarcoma
NPC	Nasopharyngeal carcinoma
NHS UK	National Health Service, United Kingdom
NKT	Natural killer T
NILM	Negative for intraepithelial lesion or malignancy
NB	Neuroblastoma
NSE	Neuron specific enolase

NLPHL	Nodular lymphocytic predominant HL
NHL	Non-Hodgkin lymphoma
NTM	Non-tuberculous mycobacteria
NMP	Nuclear matrix proteins
NPC	Nuclear pore complex
N/C	Nucleocytoplasmic
NOR	Nucleolar organizing regions
NA	Numerical aperture
OI	Oil immersion
ORF	Open reading frames
OCP	Oral contraceptive pill
OG	Orange G
ORC	Origin recognition complex
ONM	Outer nuclear membrane
53BP1	p53 binding protein 1
PET	Pancreatic endocrine tumor
PUNLMP	Papillary neoplasia of low malignant potential
PTC	Papillary thyroid carcinoma
PAS	Periodic Acid Schiff's
PNET	Peripheral neuroectodermal tumor
PTCL	Peripheral T cell lymphoma
PMCA	Peritoneal mucinous carcinomatosis
PI3P	Phosphatidylinositol 3-phosphate
PtdSer	Phosphatidylserine
PE	Phycoerythrin
PT	Phyllodes tumor
PLAP	Placental alkaline phosphatase
PCM	Plasma cell myeloma
PDGF	Platelet derived growth factor
PA	Pleomorphic adenoma
p-CEA	Polyclonal carcinoembryonic antigen
PCR	Polymerase chain reaction
PLGA	Polymorphous low grade adenocarcinoma
pre-RC	pre replicative
pre-miRNA	Precursor miRNA
PEL	Primary effusion lymphoma
PMLBCL	Primary mediastinal large B-cell lymphoma
pri-miRNA	Primary miRNA
PNET	Primitive neuroectodermal tumor
PR	Progesterone receptor
PCD	Programmed cell death
PCNA	Proliferating cell nuclear antigen
PBD	Proliferative breast disease
PSA	Prostate specific antigen
PB	Psammoma bodies
RMS	Rhabdomyosarcoma
RLH	Reactive lymphoid hyperplasia
RS	Reed-Sternberg's
RCC	Renal cell carcinoma
RLF	Replication licensing factors
Rb	Retinoblastoma
RT-PCR	Reverse transcriptase PCR
RM	Rhabdomyoma
RMS	Rhabdomyosarcoma
RNA	Ribonucleic acid
rRNA	Ribosomal RNA
RFBP	Ring finger binding protein
RER	Rough endoplasmic reticulum
SR	Scavenger receptors
SC	Sebaceous carcinoma
SSCP	Single strand conformation polymorphism
SHML	Sinus histiocytosis with massive lymphadenopathy
SCC	Small cell carcinoma
SLL	Small lymphocytic lymphoma
SER	Smooth endoplasmic reticulum
STS	Soft tissue sarcoma
SCPN	Solid and cystic papillary neoplasm
SKY	Spectral karyotyping
SAC	Spindle assembly check point
SQC	Squamous cell carcinomas
SIL	Squamous intraepithelial lesion
SOP	Standard operating protocol
SS	Synovial sarcoma
SCAP	Syringocystadenoma papilliferum
SLE	Systemic lupus erythematosus
TBP	TATA binding protein
TRAP	Telomeric repeat amplification protocol
TUNEL	Terminal deoxynucleotidyl transferase mediated dUTP Nick End Labeling
TBS	The Bethesda System
TSH	Thyroid stimulating hormone
TSI	Thyroid stimulating immunoglobulin
TTF	Thyroid transcription factor
TBNA	Transbronchial fine needle aspiration cytology
tRNA	Transfer RNA
TCC	Transitional cell carcinoma
TV	Trichomonas vaginalis
TNF-receptors	Tumor necrosis factor-receptors
USG	Ultrasonography
URR	Upstream regulatory region
UC	Urothelial carcinoma
VEGF	Vascular endothelial growth factor
VPF	Vascular permeability factor
VIA	Visual inspection of cervix with acetic acid
WT	Wilms' tumor
WHO	World Health Organization

Section 1

General Cytology

Chapter Outline

1. Cell
2. Cell Cycle and Cell Proliferation
3. Cellular Reaction to Injury and Cell Death
4. Molecular Genetics: Basic Principles and Clinical Applications
5. Neoplasm
6. Tissue and Cell Organization

CHAPTER 1

Cell

INTRODUCTION

Cell is the structural and functional unit of life. Human body is made of various types of cells. The fundamental characteristics of these cells are essentially same. However, during the process of differentiation, the cell acquires many unique morphological and functional properties.

EUKARYOTIC VERSUS PROKARYOTIC CELLS

The cells are mainly classified as prokaryotic and eukaryotic cell (Table 1.1). The cells of bacterial and other lower organisms are known as prokaryotic cell. The higher animals are made of eukaryotic cells. In prokaryotic cell, deoxyribonucleic acid (DNA) is present within the cytoplasm without any distinct nucleus. The main distinguishing features of eukaryotic cells are:

- Deoxyribonucleic acid is enclosed by membrane.
- The cell contains mitochondria and other membrane bound vesicles (Table 1.1).
- Deoxyribonucleic acid is double stranded compared to circular DNA in prokaryotic cells.

Unlike histology, in cytological examination detailed cell-to-cell relation is often lost.

Table 1.1: Differences between prokaryotic and eukaryotic cells.

Features	*Eukaryotic cell*	*Prokaryotic cell*
Nucleus	True nucleus with nuclear membrane	No true nucleus and no membrane bound nucleus
DNA	Circular DNA	Linear DNA
Ribosomes	Complex, five kinds of rRNA	Relatively simple, three kinds of rRNA
Membrane bound organelles	Present	Absent
Cell type	Multicellular	Unicellular
Mitochondria	Present	Absent

Cytologist studies cluster of cells or single cell for diagnosis. It is essential to know the detailed morphology and function of the cell to understand the alteration of its constituents in reaction to various external and internal stimuli. The various morphological constituents of a cell are highlighted in Box 1.1 and demonstrated in Figure 1.1. Electron microscopic features of the cell are shown in Figure 1.2. The constituents of the cell can be divided into cytoplasmic organelles and nucleus.

Box 1.1: Cell.

- *Cytoplasm*
  - Plasma membrane
  - Golgi bodies
  - Endoplasmic reticulum: Rough and smooth
  - Mitochondria
  - Centrioles
  - Lysosomes
  - Ribosomes
  - Vacuoles
  - Cytoskeleton
- *Nucleus*
  - Nuclear membrane
  - Nucleoli
  - Chromatin
  - Nuclear matrix

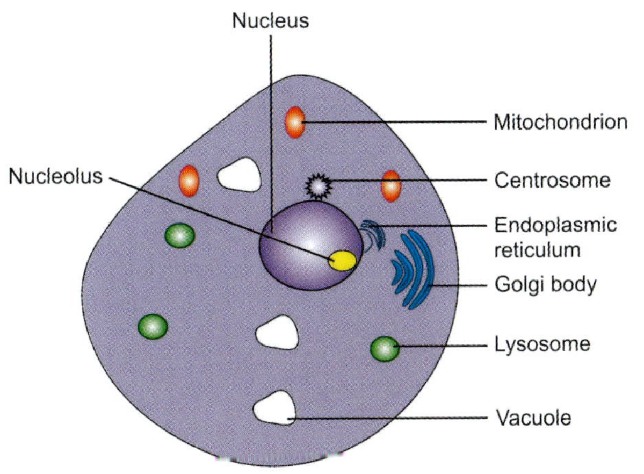

Fig. 1.1: Schematic diagram of eukaryotic cell.

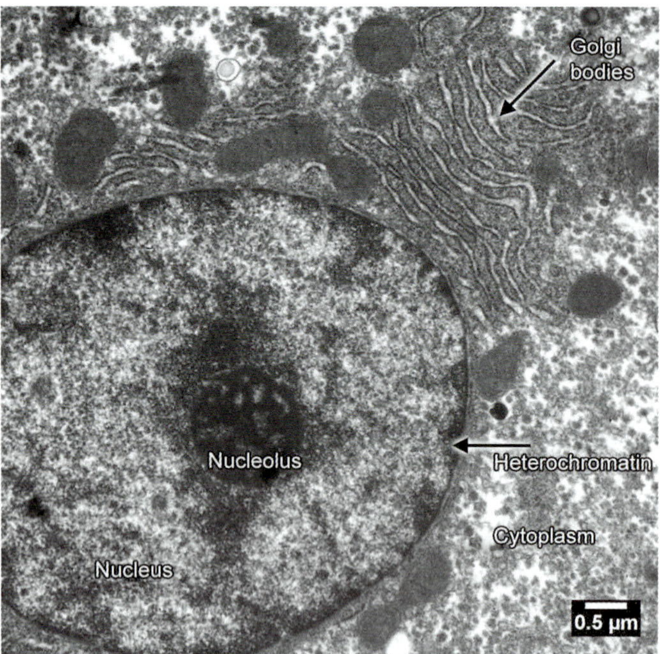

Fig. 1.2: Electron microscopic picture of a cell.
Courtesy: Dr Charan Singh Rayat.

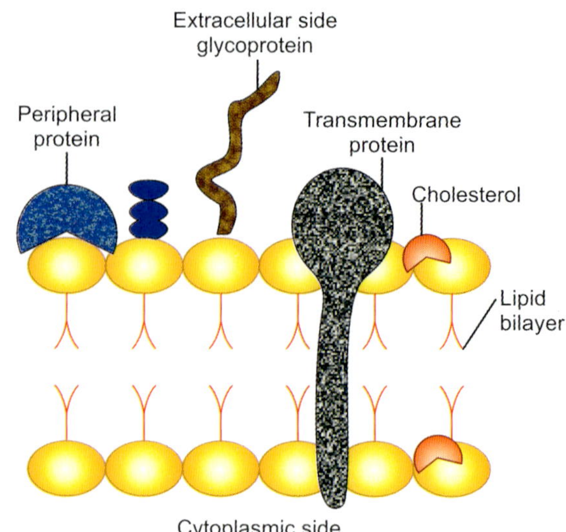

Fig. 1.3: Schematic diagram of lipid bilayer cell membrane.

Cell Membrane (Fig. 1.3)

Cell membrane is a selectively permeable biological membrane that separates the cell from its interior and the external environment.

Singer SJ and Nicolson GL[1] first proposed the "fluid mosaic model". They said that the plasma membrane is just like fluid. The membrane proteins are floating on discontinuous fluid like lipid bilayers. The proteins of the membrane are a set of heterogeneous globular molecules. The highly polar groups are protruding out of the membrane and the nonpolar groups are within the interior portion of the phospholipid membrane. The membrane is described as "mosaic" because it is composed of different types of molecules such as phospholipids, glycolipids, cholesterol and proteins.

Composition and Structure (Box 1.2)

Box 1.2: Cell membrane: Composition.

- *Lipids: Phospholipids, cholesterol, and glycolipids*
  - Double layer, hydrophilic ends outer side and hydrophobic ends facing each other.
- *Carbohydrates*: Glycoproteins and glycolipids.
- *Proteins*:
  - *Integral protein*: Incorporated within the membrane.
  - *Transmembrane protein*: Present through complete breadth.
  - *Peripheral membrane protein*: Present in the inner and outer parts of the membrane.

The cell membrane is composed predominantly of bilayered phospholipid molecules, proteins, and carbohydrates.

Lipids: There are three classes of lipids: (1) phospholipid, (2) cholesterol, and (3) glycolipid. The phospholipids are the predominant type of lipids noted in the cell membrane. There are four varieties of lipids: (1) phosphatidylcholine, (2) phosphatidylethanolamine, (3) phosphatidylserine, and (4) sphingomyelin. Phospholipids have the hydrophilic or polar ends and hydrophobic or nonpolar ends. In the hydrophilic ends usually the glycerol molecules combine with serine, choline or ethanolamine, whereas, in the hydrophobic ends the glycerol molecule is attached with the long chain fatty acids.

Hydrophobic ends of the molecules are facing each other and they are away from the cytosol or external environment. Whereas the hydrophilic ends are facing toward the cytosol. At low temperature, the bilayered lipid is just like gel. However, in body temperature, the lipid bilayer is fluid and moving and can exchange their places.

Good amount of cholesterol molecules are also present in the plasma membrane and one cholesterol molecule is present for one phospholipid molecule. The cholesterol molecules are embedded within the phospholipid layers. They prevent the mobility of the first few hydrocarbon molecules of the phospholipid and also prevent the crystallization of the hydrocarbon. Thus, cholesterol maintains the fluidity and stability of the membrane.

Carbohydrate: Carbohydrates are present in the form of glycoprotein and glycolipids. Glycoprotein is the predominant type of carbohydrate and is generally noted on both sides of the membrane. They are involved with cell recognition and protection of the membrane.

Proteins: Proteins are the 50% constituents of the membrane and depending of their positions they may be labeled as:

- *Integral protein*: Integral proteins are incorporated within the membrane (Fig. 1.3). Transmembrane proteins are the type of integral proteins that traverse through the complete breadth of the membrane.
- *Peripheral membrane protein*: These proteins remain only on the inner or outer surface of the membrane.

Functions of Plasma Membrane (Box 1.3)

The plasma membrane is biologically active semi-permeable membrane with many important functions.

- *Cell identity*: Plasma membrane encircles the essential component of the cell and acts as a physical barrier between the cell and its surroundings.
- *Transport*: Plasma membrane is selectively permeable to various substances. As the membrane is hydrophobic in its interior so it is impermeable to most polar molecules such as Na^+, H^+ and Cl^-. However, the lipid bilayer is permeable to small non polar molecules such as CO_2 and O_2. There are two types of transport through the membrane:
  1. *Active transport*: Energy is needed for this type of transport.
  2. *Passive transport*: No additional energy is needed. This can be channel or transporter protein mediated facilitated diffusion or by osmosis. In osmosis passive transport occurs across the concentration gradient. In case of facilitated diffusion, two types of protein take part in action:
     i. *Transporter proteins*: This type of protein alters the conformation of the solutes to be transported and sequentially transport the solute through the lipid bilayer.
     ii. *Channel protein*: This protein forms an aqueous pore across the membrane.
- *Signal transduction*: Plasma membrane contains many membrane-bound receptors. These receptors bind with signaling molecules and transport the information via the intracellular signaling proteins. The signaling molecules may be soluble, attached with the other cell or may be bound to the extracellular matrix. The three major classes of plasma membrane receptor proteins are involved in signal induction (Fig. 1.4):
  1. *Ion-channel-coupled receptors*: These receptor proteins are involved in transient opening and closing the ion channel after binding with the signaling molecules.
  2. *G-protein-coupled receptors (GPCR)*:[2] The GPCRs mediate their actions by transiently binding with a trimeric GTP (Guanosine triphosphate)-binding protein (G protein) (Fig. 1.4). The binding of G-protein coupled receptors and G-protein further activates an enzyme or changes the ion permeability of

Box 1.3: Cell membrane: Functions.

- *Cell identity*: Maintains cell identity
- *Transport*: Selectively permeable to various substances
- *Signal transduction*: Plasma membrane contains many receptors that transport the information via the intracellular signaling proteins
- *Cell polarity*: Membrane protein complexes are responsible for the polarity of the epithelial cells
- *Cell-to-cell recognition*
- *Intercellular joining*
- *Attachment* of cytoskeleton and extracellular matrix

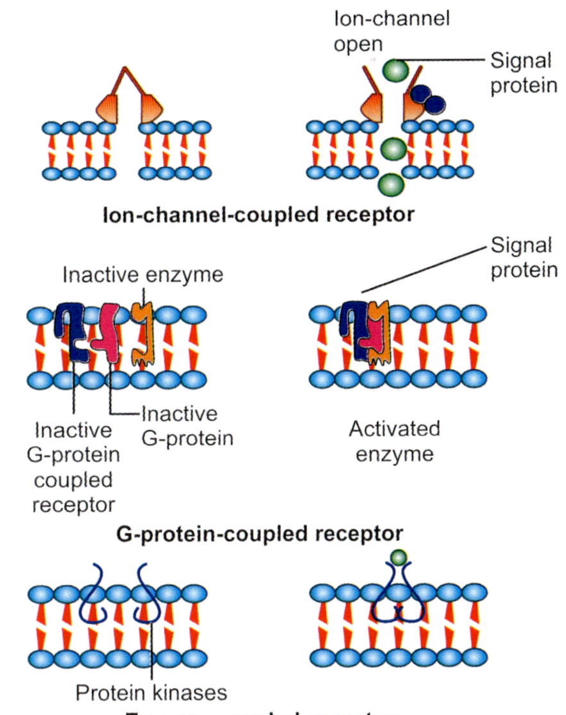

Fig. 1.4: Three types of plasma membrane receptors have been highlighted: Ion channel-coupled receptors, G-protein-coupled receptors and enzyme-coupled receptors.

the plasma membrane. The receptor site of GPCR is located toward the extracellular space and the other long chain portion coils the plasma membrane several times.

3. *Enzyme-coupled receptors*: These receptor proteins are predominantly protein kinases. In their activated form they phosphorylate the specific types of proteins.

- *Cell polarity (Box 1.4):* Most of the cells in human body are polarized. Cell polarization is studied in the epithelial cell. The epithelial cells have distinct polar distribution such as luminal surface and basolateral surface facing towards the basement membrane and side of the cell. Various membrane protein complexes are responsible for the polarity of the epithelial cells. Three types of polarity complex proteins are described in the membrane of the epithelial cells: (1) PAR (CDC42–PAR3–PAR6–aPKC), (2) Crumbs (Crb–PALS–PATJ), and (3) Scribbles (Scrib–Dlg–Lgl). PAR and Crumbs complexes are involved in the apical polarization and Scribbles complexes are responsible for basolateral polarization of the epithelial cells. They are also involved in the asymmetric cell division, cell proliferation and cell migration.[3] Asymmetric cell division suppresses cell proliferation. Disruption of the polarity complexes is related with cell proliferation. It is noted that the loss of epithelial cell polarity complexes is related with tumor, progression and invasion.[4] So, in fact, the membrane polarity complexes behave as tumor suppressor elements.

Box 1.4: Cell polarity.

- PAR (CDC42–PAR3–PAR6–aPKC), Crumbs (Crb–PALS–PATJ) and Scribbles (Scrib–Dlg–Lgl) are three major polarity complex proteins.
- PAR and Crumbs for apical polarity.
- Scribbles for basolateral polarity.
- Many polarity complex proteins are mutated in cancer.
- PAR, Crumbs and Scribbles are indirectly related with asymmetric cell division, cell proliferation and migration.
- Cell polarity protein complexes are related with EMT, tumor progression and invasion.

Box 1.5: Epithelial mesenchymal transition.

- The epithelial cells lose their characteristics and gain the properties of the mesenchymal cells.
- Key steps of embryonic development, chronic degenerative fibrosis and cancer metastasis.
- In EMT:
  - Loss of polarity of the epithelial cells
  - Separation of the individual cells from the basement membrane
  - Cells gain mobility
- The transformed epithelial cells show augmented expression of: N-cadherin, Snail 1 and Snail 2, vimentin, catenin, and matrix metalloproteinase.

Epithelial Mesenchymal Transition and Cell Polarity (Box 1.5)

Epithelial mesenchymal transition (EMT) is an orchestrated series of events in which the epithelial cells changes by shedding out some characteristics properties and acquiring many typical properties of the mesenchymal cells. It is one of the key steps during embryonic development, chronic degenerative fibrosis, and cancer metastasis.[5] During the process of EMT in vitro, the following steps happens (Fig. 1.5):

- The epithelial cells lose polarity
- Separation of the individual cells, and
- Gaining of cell motility followed by subsequently dispersion of the cells.[6]

During intravasation, tumor cells pass through the endothelial membrane of the vascular channels and come into the systemic circulation. In extravasation the tumor cells attach to the blood vessels and leave the bloodstream.[7] Finally the tumor cells make new colony in the new host environment. It is very much essential to understand the initial steps of metastasis because this knowledge may help to develop strategies to prevent metastasis of tumor cells. EMT plays significant role in tumor metastasis.

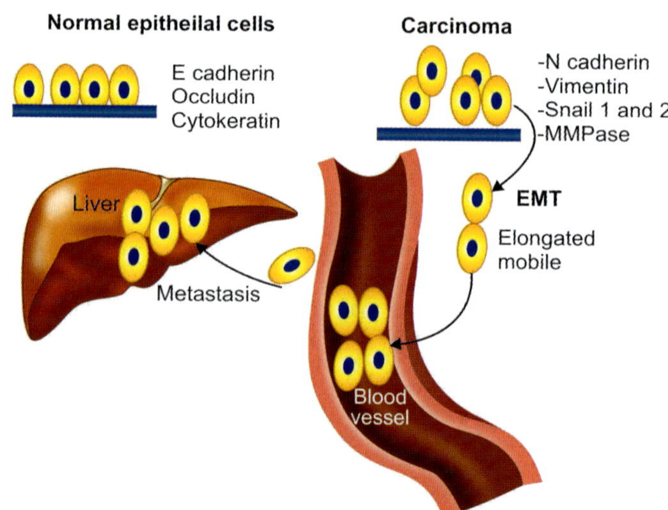

Fig. 1.5: Schematic diagram showing epithelial mesenchymal transition related with metastasis.
(MMPase: Matrix metalloproteinase).

As mentioned before, the typical epithelium is sheet of cells where the cells are attached with the basal basement membrane and laterally with other by cell junctions. These cell junctions prevent the movement of the individual cells. Mesenchymal cells are usually more elongated and they show front to back polarity rather than apicobasal polarity. In EMT apical/basolateral polarity of the epithelial cells are lost due to decreased expression of cell polarity proteins.[7] Intracellular architecture of the epithelial cells is also lost so that the cells gain mobility.

E-cadherin, a transmembrane protein, helps to maintain the adherens junctions. E-cadherin molecules bind cytosolic catenin with the help of its intracellular domain and make a link with actin cytoskeleton. The extracellular domain of this molecule helps in the interaction with other neighboring cells. The epithelial cells become loose in attachment and become movable when they lose E-cadherin from their membrane.

In EMT, the transformed epithelial cells show increased expression of:

- N-cadherin
- Vimentin
- Catenin
- Matrix metalloproteinases.[8]

N-cadherin is usually present in the mesenchymal and is not normally expressed in the epithelial tissue. The increased expression of N-cadherin in the epithelial cells facilitates their movement within the stromal tissue.[8] The transformed cells in EMT also produce increased amount of transcription factors such as Snail 1 and Snail 2, vimentin, catenin and matrix metaloproteinase.[8] Overall, due to EMT the transformed cells acquire the properties of increased migration, invasion and scattering.

Box 1.6: "Cilia" and "Brush" border.

Cilia
- Cilia and flagella are the extension from the surface of the cytoplasm.
- Cilia are present on the lining epithelium of the upper respiratory tract and fallopian tube.
- Basal body is present in the base of cilia.
- Axoneme is the central elongated part of cilia.
- *The shaft of the axoneme*: Nine peripheral doublet microtubules and two central singlet microtubules.

Function: Movement of the particles or organism in one direction.

Brush border
- Regular finger-like projections on the cell surface of certain specialized epithelial cells
- Commonly seen on the intestinal epithelium and proximal tubular epithelial cells of kidney.

Function: The brush border helps in better absorption of the substances from the large surface area.

- *Cell-to-cell recognition*: Glycolipids and glycoproteins are responsible for mutual cell-to-cell recognition.
- *Intercellular joining*: One of the important functions of the plasma membrane is connection between two cells. This is discussed below.
- Attachment to the cytoskeleton and extracellular matrix.

Cilia and Flagella

Cilia and flagella are the mobile extension from the surface of the cytoplasm (Box 1.6). Cilia are the small, regular and multiple in number, whereas, the flagellum is single slender structure. Cilia are seen on the lining epithelium of the upper respiratory tract and fallopian tube. Each cilium is attached with the thick terminal plate near the apical surface of the cell. The ciliated cells are usually polar and are attached with the basement membrane. The central elongated portion of the cilium is known as axoneme. At the base of the cilium or flagellum is a basal body. The basal body is composed of microtubules. There are total 11 microtubules. In the center there are two singlet microtubules surrounded by nine triplet microtubules (Fig. 1.6). The outer peripheral doublet microtubules in the axoneme have a pair of dynein arms that are extended to the adjacent microtubules. These dynein arms help in the movement of the cilium and flagellum. Cilia are usually lost in the cancer cell originated from the bronchial epithelium. Therefore, the presence of cilia on the cell almost safely excludes the possibility of malignancy.

Function: Cilia help in the movement of the particles or organism in one direction.

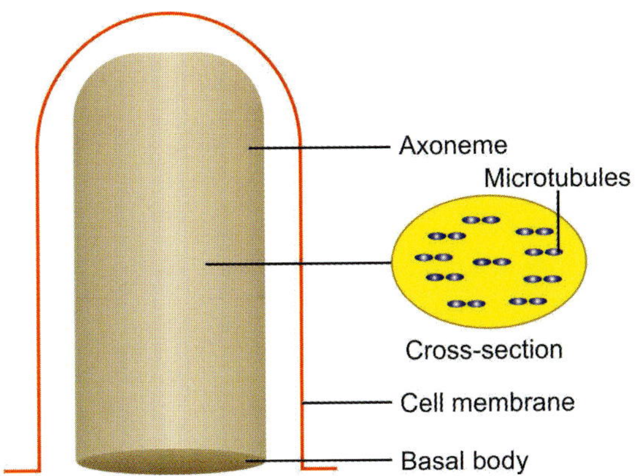

Fig. 1.6: The structure of cilia is shown. The long shaft of axoneme is originated from the basal body. The cross-section of axoneme shows 9 doublet microtubules and two central singlet tubules.

Brush Border

The surface of the certain specialized epithelial cells covered with multiple microvilli is known as brush border (Box 1.6). They are regular finger-like projections on the cell surface about 1 micron in length. Microvilli are commonly seen on the luminal surface of the intestinal epithelium (Fig. 1.7) and also on the proximal tubular epithelial cells of kidney. On light microscopy the microvilli are seen as fuzzy appearance.

Function: The brush border increases the surface area of the cell and helps in better absorption of the substances from the large surface area.

Cell Junction

Cell junction can be classified by depending on localization of the junction (Fig. 1.8):

- Cell to cell:
  - Tight junction
  - Adherens junction
  - Desmosomes
  - Gap junction
- *Cell to matrix*: Hemidesmosomes
- *Tight junction*: This is located in the apical region of the epithelial cells and almost completely seals the gap between the two epithelial cells toward the luminal site. The sealing strands of transmembrane adhesion proteins encircle the apical part of the cell membrane of the two cells and hold them tightly. Claudins and occludins are two major transmembrane adhesion proteins.
  - *Function*: There are two "major functions" of the tight junctions: (1) Tight junction closes the gap between luminal side and the intercellular space. This helps in effective transport of substances from luminal side of the cell to extracellular fluid compartment. (2) It prevents the drift of the apical membrane proteins to the basal region and vice versa.
- *Adherens junction*: The adherens junction holds the two cells together and confers mechanical strength. Adherens junction is made of cadherin, catenin and intracytoplasmic actin filaments. Altogether they form adhesion belt like structure.
  - *Function*: To provide cell-to-cell adhesion and mechanical strength.
- *Desmosomes*: These are button like spots which connect the plasma membrane of two cells together. Desmosomes are linked to the intermediate filaments. The type of intermediate filament depends on type of the cell.
  - *Function*: The desmosomal junction provides tensile strength and rigidity of the tissue.
- *Gap junctions:* These are intercellular channels that connect two adjacent cells. In gap junctions, the two plasma membranes are connected by the transmembrane proteins known as connexins.
  - *Function*: There are continuous channels between the two adjacent cells and therefore the cells can rapidly share small molecules and ions. With the help of the gap junctions the action potential can rapidly travel among a group of cells without any neurotransmitter.

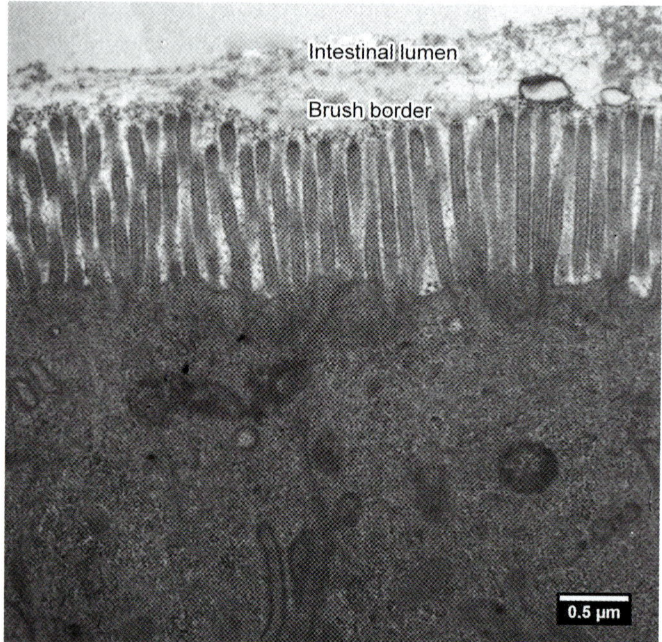

Fig. 1.7: Electron microscopic picture of brush border of intestinal cell. *Courtesy*: Dr Charan Singh Rayat, Department of Histopathology, PGIMER, Chandigarh, India.

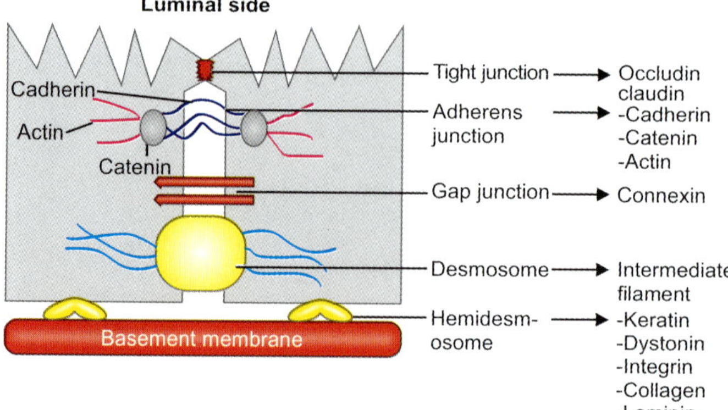

Fig. 1.8: Schematic diagram showing various types of cell junctions.

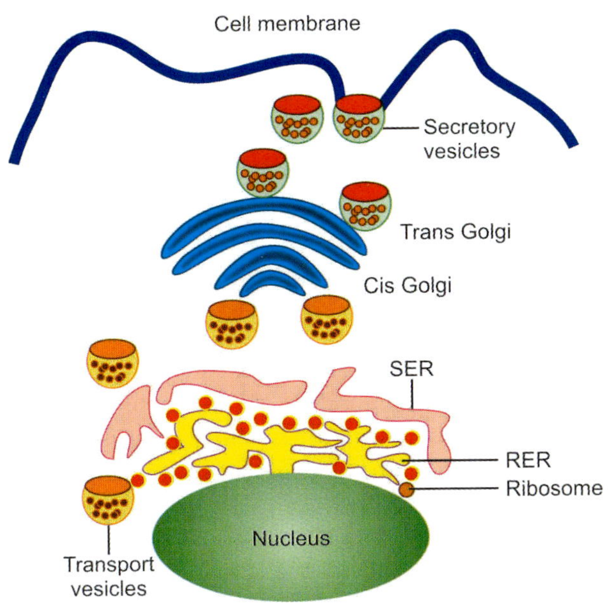

Fig. 1.9: Rough endoplasmic reticulum (RER) is studded with ribosomes. The membrane of RER is continuous with outer layer of nuclear membrane. Golgi complex has cis, trans, endo and medial parts. Cis Golgi faces toward the nucleus and trans Golgi toward the cell membrane.

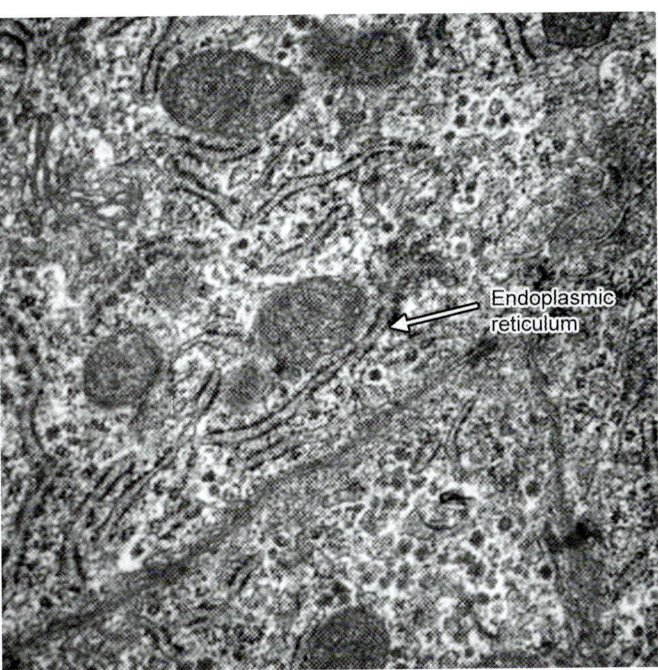

Fig. 1.10: Electron microscopic picture of rough endoplasmic reticulum.
Courtesy: Dr Uma Nahar Saikia, Professor, Department of Histopathology, PGIMER, Chandigarh, India.

- *Hemidesmosomes*: Hemidesmosomes connect the cell with the basal lamina. Hemidesmosomes are composed of keratin filaments, dystonin, plectin, integrin, collagen XVII and laminin. In hemidesmosome, integrin binds with keratin in cytoplasmic side by dystonin and plectin. It also binds with collagen XVII and laminin toward basal lamina side.
  - *Function*: It attaches cell with the basal lamina.

Cytoplasmic Organelles

Endoplasmic Reticulum (Figs. 1.9 and 1.10)[9]

These are tubular and cistern like spaces and vesicular structures folded within the cytoplasm. Endoplasmic reticulum (ER) is generally connected with cell membrane to nuclear membrane (Box 1.7). The cisterns are membrane like long flat spaces which are straight, whereas tubules are irregularly branched structures. The ER contains fluid with many enzymes and proteins. Two types of ER are present:

1. Rough endoplasmic reticulum (RER), and
2. Smooth endoplasmic reticulum (SER).

Rough endoplasmic reticulum: They are tightly packed parallel bundles of cistern like spaces which are beaded in appearance due to ribosome particles attached to the surface of RER. The ribosomes are bound with RER by a receptor known as "Rhiboporin".

Function: It is the site of synthesis of secretory protein and lysosomal enzymes.

Smooth endoplasmic reticulum: The SER predominantly contains tubules and vesicles. SER is connected with Golgi apparatus and plasma membrane.

Function: Synthesis of lipids.

Box 1.7: Endoplasmic reticulum.

- Tubular and cistern like spaces and vesicular structures folded within the cytoplasm.

Rough endoplasmic reticulum:
- Membrane of RER is in continuation with the nuclear membrane.
- Beaded in appearance due to ribosome particles attached to the surface.

Function: Synthesis of secretory protein and lysosomal enzymes.

Smooth endoplasmic reticulum
- Connected with Golgi apparatus and plasma membrane

Function: Synthesis of lipids

(RER: Rough endoplasmic reticulum).

Golgi Complex (Box 1.8)

Golgi apparatus are stacks of membrane bound cistern like spaces within the cytoplasm arranged in polarized fashion. Each stack of Golgi complex (GC) has four parts (Fig. 1.9):

1. *Cis-Golgi network*: Cis-Golgi network is the concave surface of the stack of GC that faces toward the RER and small transfer vesicles. Cis-Golgi network receives the initial protein from ER.
2. and 3. *Endo-Golgi and Medial-Golgi network*: These are the middle parts of GC and most of the proteins are modified here.
4. *Trans-Golgi network*: This is the convex surface of the stack of the GC. Trans-Golgi network is associated with large secretory vesicles and final transport of the protein.

Function: The main function of the GC is chemical processing of the protein received from RER followed by packaging and transfer. Along with classical "protein trafficking", there are many other novel functions of GC such as entry of the cell to mitotic check point, calcium homeostasis and cytoskeletal organization.[10]

Protein modification: N-linked and O-linked glycosylation of protein and lipids occur in the GC.

Protein transport: Golgi complex receives the neosynthesized protein from the ER and transport to their respective destination. The cargo proteins are first modified, and then they are transported by GC. The mechanism of the transport of cargo proteins is not exactly known. However, there are two theories:

1. *Vesicular transport model theory*: The cargo protein is transported by an anterograde way with the help of vesicles that bud from one cisterna and then fuse to the next one.
2. *Cisterna maturation model*: In this model, it is assumed that the Golgi cisterns are formed de novo, progressively mature and finally dissipate.[11]

Box 1.8: Golgi complex.

- Membrane bound cistern like spaces arranged in polarized fashion.
- *Types*: Cis-Golgi network, Endo-Golgi and Medial-Golgi and Trans-Golgi network.

- *Functions*:
  - *Processing of the protein* received from RER. N-linked and O-linked glycosylation of protein and lipids
  - *Calcium storage*
  - *Platform of various cell signaling*

Calcium storage: Golgi complex is the most important site of intracellular calcium storage and can also release Ca^{2+} in case of agonistic stimulation.

Platform of different cells signaling: Golgi complex acts as the platform of different signaling events within the cell. In addition to the receiving initial signal, GC can also induce a cascade of signal transduction.

Mitochondria

These are 0.5–1 μ diameter organelle considered as the power house of the cell as they are the major source of energy (Box 1.9). Mitochondria (MT) are richly localized in that part of the cells that requires energy such as interfibrillar space in the striated muscle and in the middle part of the sperm. Other than nuclear DNA, mitochondria have its own independent DNA and this is the unique feature of MT.

Structure

Mitochondria are double membrane-bound structures, which consist of following parts (Figs. 1.11 and 1.12).

- Outer membrane
- Inner membrane
- Intermembranous space
- Cristae
- Mitochondrial matrix

Box 1.9: Mitochondria.

- Power house of the cell.
- Mitochondria are double membrane bound structures.
- *Parts*: Outer membrane, inner membrane, intermembranous space, cristae, and mitochondrial matrix.

- *Outer membrane*
  - Rich in porin
  - Small ions and proteins can pass
  - Connected with ER.

- *Inner membrane*
  - Rich in cardiolipin
  - Impermeable to proton, ion and electrons
  - Rich in (1) ATP synthase (2) respiratory chain protein, complexes, e.g. NADH dehydrogenase complexes, cytochrome $b\text{-}c_1$ and cytochrome oxidase and (3) transport protein complexes.
- *Matrix*: Rich in enzymes of citric acid cycle and mitochondrial DNA.

Functions: Main function of MT is energy production in the form of ATP synthesis.

- *Citric acid cycle*: Main reactions of citric acid cycle occur in MT.
- *Electron transport*: During oxidative phosphorylation, a series of electron transport reactions occur.
- *Calcium storage*: Play important role in calcium homeostasis.
- *Cell cycle*: Signaling platform for cell cycle progression.
- *Apoptotic death*: Play key role in apoptosis by activating proapoptotic enzymes.

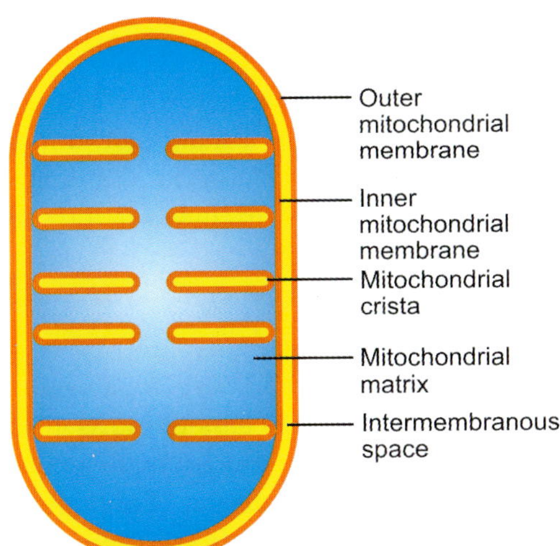

Fig. 1.11: Double membrane-bound structure of mitochondrion with outer and inner membranes.

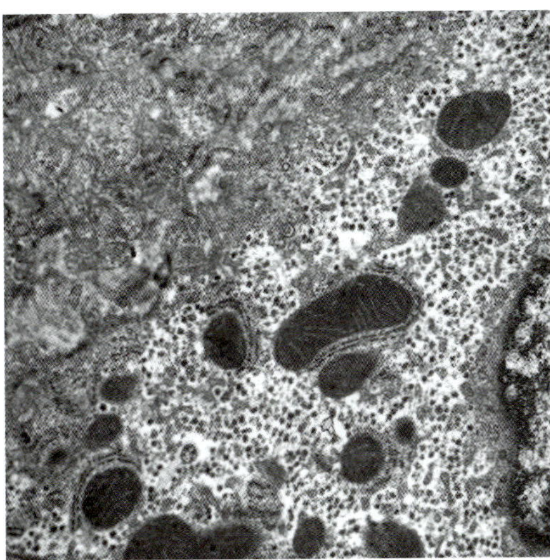

Fig. 1.12: Electron microscopic picture of mitochondria. *Courtesy*: Dr Uma Nahar, Saikia, Professor, Department of Histopathology, PGIMER, Chandigarh, India.

Outer membrane: This is composed of phospholipid bilayers. The outer membrane of MT is rich in porin, a variety of integral proteins. This forms a through and through aqueous channel in the outer membrane. Therefore, the small ions and proteins can easily cross the outer membrane. MT associated endoplasmic reticulum connects the ER and outer membrane of MT.

Inner membrane: This is the inner phospholipid bilayer of the MT. The inner membrane is rich in double phospholipid known as cardiolipin. The cardiolipin possesses four fatty acids rather than two, and the presence of the cardiolipin makes the inner membrane impermeable to proton, ion and electrons. In certain regions the outer and inner membrane joins together known as contact sites and makes a passage of the proteins and small molecules from the cytoplasm to the matrix space. The inner membrane contains the large number of lollypop like structure with small stalk attached to the inner membrane and globular region in the matrix. These globular regions contain protein complex of ATP (adenosine triphosphate) synthase. The inner membrane contains three types of enzyme: (1) ATP synthase, (2) the respiratory chain protein complexes such as NADH dehydrogenase complexes, cytochrome b-c_1 and cytochrome oxidase, and (3) transport protein complexes.

Intermembranous space: This is the tiny space bounded by two membranes of the MT. The concentration of small molecules is same in both cytoplasm and intermembranous space.

Cristae: this is the small shelf like folds of the inner membrane. This makes the larger space in the inner membrane to retain more enzymes.

Matrix: It is the innermost space of MT encircled by the inner membrane. The matrix consists of dense fluid that is rich in viscosity. Matrix is rich in enzymes of citric acid cycle and also contains mitochondrial DNA.

Functions

Main function of MT is energy production in the form of ATP synthesis. However, it is also involved in other important functions such as calcium storage, cell death, etc.[12]

- *Citric acid cycle*: The essential enzymes in citric acid cycles are located in the mitochondrial matrix, and the main reactions of citric acid cycle happen in the mitochondrial matrix. Initial oxidative breakdown of glucose occurs in the cytoplasm by the process known as glycolysis.
- *Electron transport*: During the oxidative phosphorylation, a series of electron transport reaction occurs in the inner mitochondrial membrane. The energy released in these reactions is used to generate ATP from ADP.
- *Calcium storage*: Mitochondria can store calcium and play an important role in calcium homeostasis.
- *Cell cycle*: Various signaling reactions of cell cycle occur in the MT.[13]
- *Apoptotic death*: Mitochondria play key role in apoptosis.[14] This has been discussed in detail in Chapter 3.

Mitochondrial Deoxyribonucleic Acid

Mitochondrial DNA is unique to MT and it is considered as separately developed during evolution (Box 1.10). In sexual reproduction, MT is exclusively inherited from mother and so MT DNA is of maternal origin. MT DNA is organized in nucleoid. The nucleoid is the combination of MT DNA and proteins. The nucleoid is also known as DNA-protein complex (DNP). MT DNA is 16.6 KB circular DNA molecule that encodes only 37 genes. It is responsible for the production of selected MT protein, ribosomal RNA (rRNA) and transfer RNA (tRNA). The remaining 99% proteins in the MT are produced by nuclear MT gene. Therefore two parallel encoding of proteins in MT are going on (1) by MT DNA and (2) Nuclear mitochondrial DNA. Replication of mitochondrial DNA is dependent with the cell cycle.

Mitochondrial dysfunction may occur due to defects in MT DNA or nuclear mitochondrial DNA (nDNA). Interestingly, mutations in the MT DNA are heteroplasmic that means both mutant and wild type molecules remain in the same cell in varying proportion. The cell can tolerate a threshold of defective proteins and after that behaves abnormally. In course of time all MT DNA may be of same genomic type. This is known as homoplasmy. Two types of mutation may occur in MT DNA: (1) point mutation, (2) deletion.[15]

Point mutation: Almost all the genes of MT DNA are affected by point mutation. This is maternally transmitted. The mother may be unaffected due to less than critical threshold to produce the disease. However, the child may be affected by the disease. The patient may have *M*itochondrial *E*ncephalopathy, *L*actic *A*cidosis and *S*troke (MELAS).

Single large scale deletion of MT DNA: The deletion of MT DNA is usually sporadic and occurs de novo. It involves several genes. The diseases produced by deletion of MT DNA include progressive external ophthalmoplegia, Pearson syndrome and Kearns Sayre syndrome.[16]

Nuclear DNA mutation causing mitochondrial disease: These diseases follow Mendelian inheritance and they are X-linked (both dominant and recessive). De novo mutation may also occur. The mutation of nDNA genes may cause:

- Defects in structural subunit of oxidative phosphorylation complexes
- Defects in mitochondrial import (dilated cardiomyopathy, spastic paraplegia, etc.)
- Defects in mitochondrial fusion (Charcot-Marie-Tooth disease)
- Defects in mitochondrial translation
- Defects in mitochondrial maintenance (myopathy, encephalomyopathy, etc.)
- Coenzyme Q_{10} deficiency
- Defects in F-S clusters (Friedreich-ataxia syndrome, multiple mitochondrial dysfunction syndrome).

Box 1.10: Mitochondrial DNA.

- Mitochondrial DNA (MT DNA) is of maternal origin
- It is 16.6 KB circular DNA molecule
- It encodes only 37 genes
- Approximately 99% proteins in the MT is produced by nuclear MT gene
- Replication of mitochondrial DNA is cell cycle independent and may occur in any phase of the cell cycle
- Two types of mutation may occur in MT DNA: (1) point mutation, (2) deletion
- *Point mutation*:
  - Maternally transmitted.
  - *M*itochondrial *E*ncephalopathy, *L*actic *A*cidosis and *S*troke (MELAS).
- *Single large scale deletion of MT DNA*
  - Sporadic and occurs de novo
  - Several genes are involved
  - Progressive external ophthalmoplegia, Pearson syndrome and Kearns-Sayre syndrome
- *Nuclear DNA mutation causing mitochondrial disease*
  - X-linked (both dominant and recessive)
  - Defects in structural subunit of oxidative phosphorylation complexes, mitochondrial import (dilated cardiomyopathy, spastic paraplegia, etc.), mitochondrial fusion (Charcot-Marie-Tooth disease), mitochondrial translation, mitochondrial maintenance (myopathy, encephalomyopathy, etc. F-S clusters (Friedreich-ataxia syndrome, multiple mitochondrial dysfunction syndrome).

Ribosomes

Ribosome is the sites of protein synthesis (Box 1.11).

Box 1.11: Ribosomes.

- Sites of protein synthesis
- Present as free ribosomes in cytosol and membrane bound form attached with ER
- Made up of r-RNA and proteins
- Classified according to the sedimentation coefficient in ultracentrifugation
- It has two units: (1) a smaller 40s and (2) larger 60s.
- Small subunit has the binding site for mRNA and t-RNA
- rRNA of the larger subunit has enzymatic activity to catalyze the peptide bond.

Function: Decode the information from mRNA and help the molecules of tRNA to assemble the particular amino acids to make a protein.

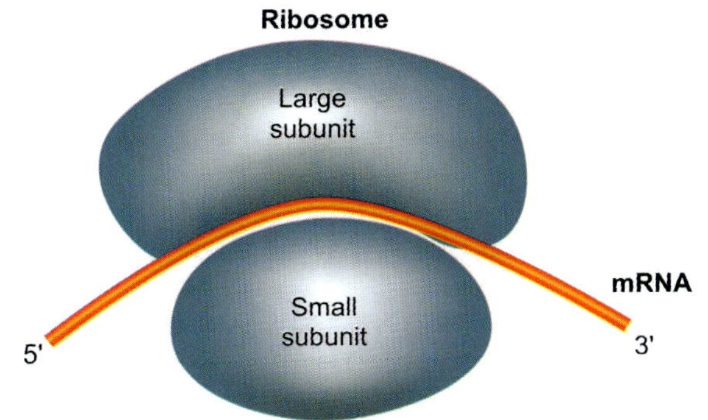

Fig. 1.13: Schematic diagrams of two subunits of a ribosome.

Structure (Fig. 1.13)

Ribosomes are small 25–30 nanometer particles present in the cytoplasm. They are present both as free ribosomes in cytosol and also in the membrane-bound form attached with ER and thus forming rough endoplasmic reticulum. The ribosome is made up of r-RNA and proteins. The ribosome is classified according to the sedimentation coefficient in ultracentrifugation. The eukaryotic ribosome has two units a smaller 40s and a larger 60s subunit. In its inactivated form the two subunits are detached however when the ribosome is engaged in protein synthesis both the units are attached together. Small subunit has the binding sites for mRNA and t-RNA. Some rRNA of the larger subunit has enzymatic activity to catalyze the peptide bond. These rRNA are known as the ribozyme.

Function

Ribosomes take part vital role in protein synthesis by decoding information from mRNA and then help molecules of tRNA to assemble particular amino acids to make a protein.

Lysosomes

These are 0.2–0.4 μ small membrane-bound vesicles present in the cytoplasm (Box 1.12). They contain near about 40 acid hydrolytic enzymes. Lysosomal enzymes are produced in the endoplasmic reticulum and carried over in Golgi complex. The lysosomal enzymes and membrane of the lysosome are finally synthesized in the trans-Golgi network and are carried to the endosome by clathrin coated transport vesicles. The final lysosomal vesicles are synthesized in the late endosomal intermediate (also known as "endolysosome").

Box 1.12: Lysosome.

- Lysosomal enzymes are produced in the endoplasmic reticulum.
- *Primary lysosome*: No morphological sign of hydrolytic enzymes.
- *Secondary lysosomes*: Lysosome fuses with other phagocytic vesicles or organism and shows enzymatic activities.

Functions:

- Lysosome contains acid hydrolytic enzymes such as (1) lipase, (2) amylase, (3) protease, (4) nuclease. Lysosomal enzymes degrade the protein and carbohydrate components of the organism.

There are two types of lysosome: (1) Primary lysosome: No morphological sign of hydrolytic enzymes, and (2) Secondary lysosomes: When lysosome fuses with other phagocytic vesicles of an organism it shows enzymatic activities and this lysosome is known as "secondary lysosomes".

Functions

Lysosome contains acid hydrolytic enzymes such as (1) lipase, (2) amylase, (3) protease, and (4) nuclease. These enzymes are activated in the acid environment. The lysosomal enzymes digest the macromolecules, destroy the microbes and remove the other cytoplasmic organelle such as mitochondria. The foreign organisms enter the cytoplasm as phagocytic vesicles. Lysosome fuses with the phagosome and release acid hydrolytic enzymes, which degrade the protein and carbohydrate components of the organism. The lipid component is more resistant to digestion and may remain as the residual body. At times, lysosome fuses with the nonfunctioning MT or fragments of RER to clear these substances from the "autophagic" vacuoles in the cytoplasm. When these autophagic vacuoles remain persistently in the cytoplasm, they accumulate pigment known as "Lipofuscin".

Peroxisome

These are tiny vesicles of 0.2–1 μ in size. They are synthesized from RER. Peroxisomes contain many oxidative enzymes. The enzymes in the peroxisome break down fatty acid by beta oxidation and generate acetyl coenzyme A and H_2O_2. Acetyl coenzyme A is involved in various energy producing metabolic processes. The hydrogen peroxide helps to kill the various organisms. Excess hydrogen peroxide is further degraded by catalase enzyme of peroxisome into water and oxygen.

Box 1.13: Cytoskeleton.

Three types: Microfilament, microtubules, intermediate filaments

1. *Microfilament (actin filament)*:
   - Fine network of thin actin filament within the cytoplasm
   - Globular G-actin which is polymerized and forms a long chain of F-actin.
   - Forms a robust supporting meshwork just underneath the plasma membrane known as "cell cortex".

Functions: Maintains shape of the cell, cell contraction, cell movement, phagocytosis, and transport of vesicles in the cytoplasm.

2. *Microtubules*:
   - The basic constituents: α- and β-tubulin.
   - α- and β-tubulin are arranged alternatively to form a protofilament.
   - The protofilament of tubulin is polar as one end is formed by β-tubulin and other end is formed by α-tubulin.

Functions: Intracellular transport, mitotic spindle movement, movements of cilia and flagella.

3. *Intermediate filament*:
   - The diameter of intermediate filaments is in between the microfilament (7 nanometers) and microtubules (25 nanometers).
   - The polypeptide is alpha helix with 310–350 amino acids.
   - Two such alpha helix monomer coils to form a dimer and the two dimmers coil in a staggered antiparallel fashion to form a tetramer. Eight such tetramers form an intermediate filament.
   - *Types of intermediate filaments*: Acidic and neutral basic keratin, vimentin, desmin, glial fibrillary acidic protein, peripherin, neurofilaments, lamin and nestin

Functions: Support of the cytoskeletal structure, chromatin organization of the nucleus.

Cytoskeleton (Box 1.13)

Cytoskeleton is the meshwork of protein filaments within the cytoplasm that maintains the shape of the cell along with other important functions such as cell movement, cell contraction and maintaining cell polarity. There are three components of the cytoskeleton:

1. Microfilament
2. Microtubules
3. Intermediate filaments

Microfilament

It is also known as "actin filament". These are the thinnest filaments and present either as a bundle form or as fine network within the cytoplasm. The actin filament is composed of globular G-actin which is polymerized and forms a long chain of F-actin (Fig. 1.14). Most of the G-actin is bound with small proteins such as profilin and thymosin. Binding of these small proteins prevents the polymerization of G-actin. Actin filament binds with filamin and makes a robust supporting meshwork just underneath the plasma membrane known as "cell cortex". There are three types of actin: (1) Alpha actin, (2) Beta actin, and (3) Gamma actin. Alpha actin is present in muscle and other two forms of actin are present in nonmuscular cells.

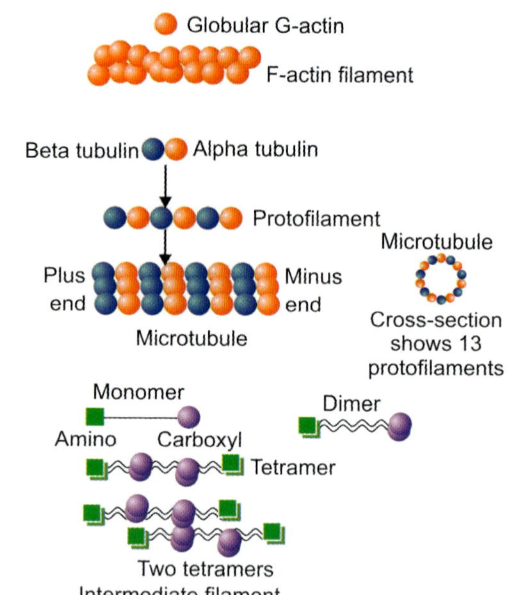

Fig. 1.14: Three types of cytoskeletal structures: Actin filament, microtubules and intermediate filament.

Functions

- Actin maintains shape of the cell.
- Actin binds to the myosin and helps in contraction of muscle fibers.
- Actin can shorten its length and helps in the movement of the cell.
- Phagocytosis or pinocytosis is helped by actin.
- Actin helps in the transport of various vesicles within the cytoplasm.

Microtubules

Microtubule is long, straight, hollow rigid tubules of 25 nanometers in diameter. These are dynamic fibers that mean they are always in the process of assembling and disassembling. The microtubules constitute mitotic spindles, centrioles, cilia and flagella. The basic constituents of the microtubules are α- and β-tubulin.

These tubulins are arranged alternatively to form a protofilament (Fig. 1.14). GTP is tightly bound with α tubulin and resistant to hydrolysis whereas it is loosely bound with β tubulin and can be separable by hydrolysis. The protofilament of tubulin is polar as one end, is formed by β tubulin and other end is formed by α tubulin. The β end of the tubulin protofilament is plus end as the growth and shrinkage of this end is rapid. The opposite α tubulin end is known as the minus end. In each microfilament, there are 13 total protofilament attached parallel with each other with a central hollow structure. All the plus ends or growing ends of the protofilaments are in one direction.

Functions: The main functions of the microtubule are:

- *Intracellular transport*: Microtubules help in the transport of the vesicles containing proteins from the Golgi complex to plasma membrane.
- *Mitotic spindle movement*: The mitotic spindles are formed by microtubules. The chromatids are separated and pulled to each daughter cell nucleus by the mitotic spindles formed by microtubules.
- *Movements*: Movements of cilia and flagella are done by the microtubules.

Centrosome

It is small round body located near the nucleus in the interphase cell. This is also known as microtubule organizing center. The microtubules are attached with the centrosome by their minus ends, and they radiate from the centrosome like a star-shaped manner. Centrosome consists of a pair of centrioles arranged in L-shaped manner surrounded by the amorphous matrix material known as centrosome matrix or pericentriolar material. Centrosome matrix material takes the main role in the development of the microtubule. Centrioles are the basal bodies of cilia or flagella. During mitosis, the centrosome duplicates and each one contains one pair of centrioles. From each of the centrosomes, microtubules radiate and form a complete mitotic spindle.

Intermediate Filament

Intermediate filaments have average diameter 10 nanometers. The name of the intermediate filaments is such because the diameter of intermediate filaments is in between the microfilament (7 nanometers) and microtubules (25 nanometers). The intermediate filaments are made of individual polypeptides. These are alpha helix structures that contain 310–350 amino acids. It has N and C terminals. Two alpha helix monomer coils with each other to form a dimer. Both the N and C terminals are in same direction in this monomer. Two dimmers then coil in a staggered anti-parallel fashion to form a tetramer. Eight such tetramers twist in a rope like manner to form an intermediate filament. Therefore, in a cross-section of intermediate filament there are 32 alpha helix coils.

Types of intermediate filament:[17] There are a total six types of intermediate filament (Table 1.2).

- Type I (acidic) and type II (basic): Present in epithelial and hair keratins.
- Type III:
    - *Vimentin*: Vimentin is expressed predominantly in mesenchymal cells and also in leukocytes, vascular endothelial cells and some epithelial cells.
    - *Desmin*: Present in the skeletal and cardiac muscles.

Table 1.2: Intermediate filaments.

Type	*Varieties*	*Location*	*Molecular weight (Da)*	*Function*
I	Acidic keratin (11 epithelial keratin, four hair keratin)	Epithelial cells	40,000–70,000	Tensile strength
II	Basic keratin (8 epithelial keratin and 4 hair keratin)	Cells of hair and nail	40,000–70,000	Tensile strength
III	a. Vimentin b. Desmin c. Glial fibrillary acidic protein d. Peripherin	a. Mesenchymal cells, leukocytes, vascular endothelial cells and some epithelial cells b. Skeletal and cardiac muscle fibers c. Astrocytes and other glial cells. d. Neurons of the dorsal root ganglia, sympathetic ganglia and cranial nerves	a. 54,000 b. 53,000 c. 50,000 d. 56,000	a. Support the cytoplasmic membrane and helps in holding the various organelles in proper position. b. Helps in stabilizing sarcomeres of the contracting muscle cells c. Supports the glial cells d. Supports the neurons
IV	Neurofilaments (NF) a. NF-Light b. NF-Medium c. NF-High	Mature neurons	a. 62,000 b. 102,000 c. 110,000	They form the cytoskeleton of dendrites and axons.
V	Lamins A, B and C	Nuclear envelope	65,000–75,000	Control of assembly of the nuclear envelope during mitotic event and chromatin organization
VI	Nestin	Stem cells of the central nervous system	200,000	

- *Glial fibrillary acidic protein (GFAP)*: Present in astrocytes and other glial cells.
- *Peripherin*: It is present in the peripheral neurons and cranial nerves.
- Type IV: Neurofilaments: Neurofilaments are expressed in the mature neurons.
    - *Alpha internexin*: They are present in developing central nervous system.
- Type V: Lamin: They are present underneath the nuclear membrane (Lamin A, Lamin B and Lamin C). Lamin helps in chromatin organization and gene expression.
- Type VI: Nestin: Nestin is present in stem cells of the central nervous system and in developing striated muscle.

Unclassified

Filensin: It is present in the epithelial cells of the lens at the time of differentiation.

Functions of the Intermediate Filaments

- *Supporting the cytoskeleton structure*: Intermediate filaments are more stable than microtubules and microfilaments and provide good support and tensile strength of the cytoskeleton of the cell. Desmin links myofibrils of the striated muscles. GFAP supports the glial structure, and neurofilaments support the cytoskeleton of the axons and dendrites.
- *Chromatin organization*: Nuclear lamin takes part and plays an important role in chromatin organization of the nucleus. Lamin also controls the assembly of the nuclear envelope at the time of mitosis.

Nucleus

Nucleus is the central processing unit of the cell and act as the controlling center of the cell (Box 1.14). The important components of the nucleus are:

Box 1.14: Nuclear membrane.

- *Nuclear membrane*:
    - Outer nuclear membrane (ONM)
    - Inner nuclear membrane (INM)
    - Perinuclear space
    - *The nuclear lamina*: location: nuclear side of the INM.
    - ONM: continuous with the ER.
    - INM
- Contains lamin B receptor, lamina-associated polypeptide, emerin, and ring finger binding protein (RFBP).

Functions

- Physical barrier between cytoplasm and nucleus
- Helps in chromatin remodeling and gene expression.

- Nuclear envelope and pore
- Nuclear matrix
- Nuclear chromatin
- Nucleoli.

Nuclear Envelope

Nuclear envelope is the barrier between the nucleus and cytoplasm. It has three parts:

1. Nuclear membrane
2. Nuclear pore
3. Nuclear lamina.

Nuclear Membrane (Figs. 1.15 and 1.16)

The nuclear membrane is further divided into (a) outer nuclear membrane (ONM), (b) inner nuclear membrane (INM) and (c) perinuclear space.

The ONM is the most outer part of the nuclear membrane, and it is 6 nm thick. ONM is continuous with the ER. The ONM is usually studded with multiple ribosomes on its cytoplasmic side that are involved in protein synthesis. The INM is parallel to ONM and is directly attached to the nuclear lamina. The space in between the ONM and INM is known as perinuclear space. The width of this space is 50 nm. Both the ONM and INM are perforated by multiple nuclear pores.

The nuclear lamina is situated in the inner side of the INM. It is made up of nuclear lamin that is intimately related to the cytoplasmic intermediate filaments. The INM contains lamin B receptor (LBR), lamina associated polypeptide (LAP), MAN 1, emerin, nurim and ring finger binding protein (RFBP).[18]

Functions

- Acts as a physical barrier between the cytoplasm and nucleus

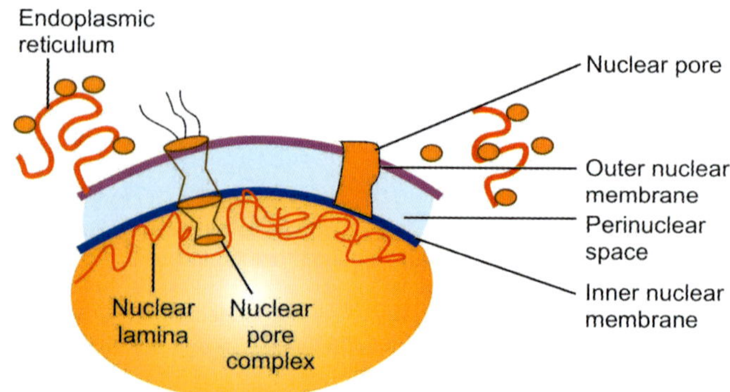

Fig. 1.15: Double layered nuclear membrane is perforated by multiple nuclear pores.

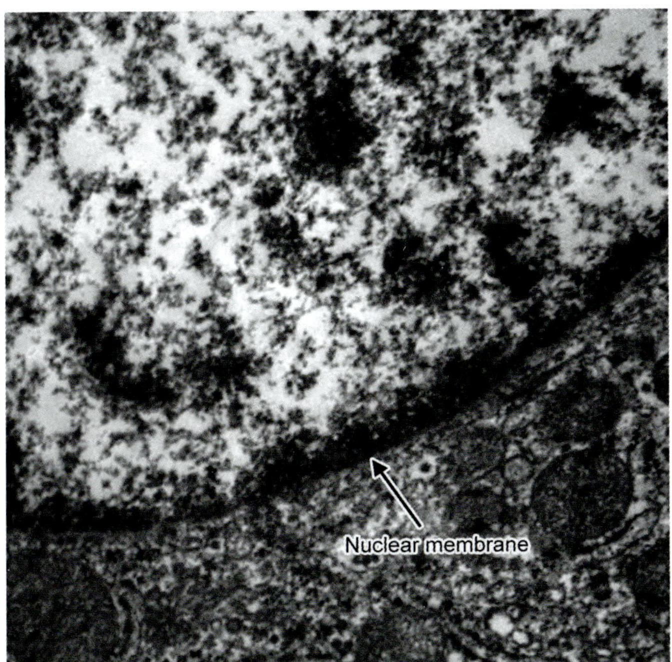

Fig. 1.16: Electron microscopic picture of nucleus and its membrane. *Courtesy*: Dr Uma Nahar Saikia, Professor, Department of Histopathology, PGIMER, Chandigarh, India.

- Various integral proteins such as LBR, LAP, RFBP help in chromatin remodeling and gene expression. LAP and lamin A/C bind with Rb-protein that further recruits histone deacetylases (HDAC), DNA methyl transferases (Dnmt 1), histone methyltransferases (HMTase) and heterochromatin protein 1 (HP1). The action of these enzymes changes the higher-order conformation of chromatin, and ultimately causes gene silencing by inhibiting transcriptional activation of E2F.[19]

Nuclear Pore

At certain positions: the ONM and INM fuse with each other and, therefore, make the pore on the nuclear membrane that makes the direct connection site between the nucleus and cytoplasm. The diameter of each nuclear pore is about 100 nanometer. The number of nuclear pore varies from few 100s to 1,000s depending on the metabolic activity of the cell. The nuclear pore complex (NPC) is the gateway of the nucleus across the double membrane nuclear envelope (Fig. 1.16) that selectively allows the passage of various macromolecules across the nucleus.[19]

Nuclear pore complex consists of a cytoplasmic ring, a nuclear ring and a distal ring connected by nuclear basket (Fig. 1.15).[20]

Function: The main function of the nuclear pore is the facilitation of the cytoplasmic to nuclear traffic and vice versa.

Nuclear Matrix

It is the internal skeleton of the nucleus and consists of an RNA network, protein complexes, peripheral nuclear lamin and residual nucleoli. Nuclear matrix is the remaining part of the nucleus after removal of chromatin, nuclear membrane and the other soluble components of the nucleus. Its composition is dynamic and varies with nuclear activities. In fact, nuclear matrix protein (NMP) may be just a processional artifact only as its demonstration depends on the selected conditions on removing the chromatin and lamin. The NMP is tissue specific and it differs from normal and neoplastic tissue of the same type. NMP is interlinked with the intermediate filaments of the cell cytoplasm and provides the overall support of the nucleus. Nuclear matrix contains both proteinaceous substances, nuclear mitotic apparatus protein, actin and RNA.[21] The chromatin forms a loop and the base of the loop is attached with nuclear matrix. The strings of DNA attached with the nuclear matrix is labeled as matrix attachment region (MAR) and the corresponding nuclear matrix is called MAR-binding proteins. Active sites of genes are usually located in MAR sites than the loop areas. Other than gene transcription, NMP also participates in gene translation.

Nuclear Chromatin

Chromatin Structure

Chromatin represents the uncoiled chromosome of the interphase nucleus (Box 1.15). It is composed of DNA, histone and nonhistone proteins.[22] In the interphase, the individual chromosomes are present in the specific region of the nucleus which is known as chromosomal territories. The channels that separate the chromosomes are known as interchromosomal domains.

Chromatin can be classified as heterochromatin and euchromatin (Table 1.3).

Heterochromatin

Heterochromatin is located on the nuclear membrane (Fig. 1.2). It is the condensed part of chromatin and contains inactive genes. Heterochromatin is further divided into facultative heterochromatin and constitutive

Box 1.15: Chromatin.

- *Chromatin*: The uncoiled chromosome of the interphase nucleus.
- Composed of:
  - DNA
  - Histone
  - Nonhistone proteins.
- Types
  - Inactive heterochromatin
  - Active euchromatin.
- *Nucleosome*:
  - The basic unit of chromatin
  - DNA encircles around a central octameric protein core containing two copies each of histone H2A, H2B, H3, and H4.
  - Strings of nucleosomes are twisted and folded to form the complex three dimensional organization of chromatin.

Table 1.3: Differences between euchromatin and heterochromatin.

Features	*Euchromatin*	*Heterochromatin*
Condensation	Less condensed	More condensed
Position	Central part of nucleus	Peripheral part of nucleus
Transcription	Transcriptionally active	Transcriptionally inactive
Occurrence	Both prokaryote and eukaryotic cell	Only in eukaryotic cells

heterochromatin. The facultative heterochromatin contains inactive genes in certain stages of development of the cells. The constitutive heterochromatin is made of inactive genes that are the structural components of the chromosomes, e.g. telomeres and centromeres.

Euchromatin

It is located in the interior of the nucleus. In comparison to heterochromatin, euchromatin is less condensed and consists of the actively transcribed genes.

Nucleosome—the Basic Unit of Chromatin

Nucleosome is the basic unit of chromatin. It is made of approximately 146 bp of DNA. This DNA encircles in two turns around a central octameric protein core. This core histone complex is composed of two copies each of histone H2A, H2B, H3, and H4 (Fig. 1.17). Two copies of H3 and H4 remains in the center as tetramer and two H2A-H2B dimmers located on either side of the tetramer. Therefore, the linear arrangement of these four histones is: (H2A/H2B)-(H4/H3)-(H3/H4)-(H2B/H2A). The DNA chain in between the two nucleosomes is the linker DNA. The linker histone (Histone H1) binds the linker DNA chain

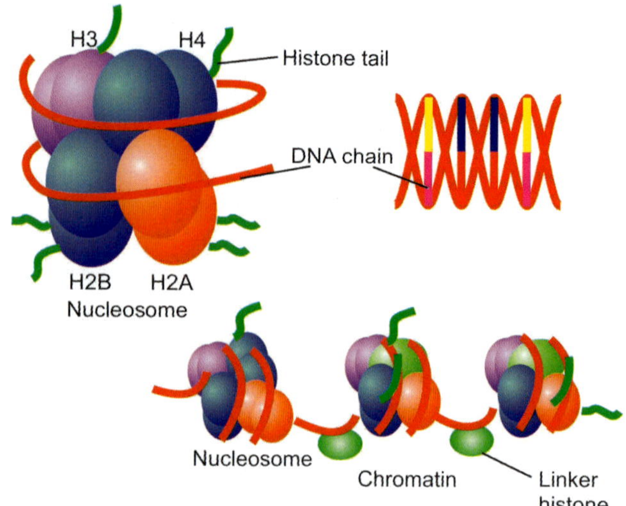

Fig. 1.17: Schematic diagram of nucleosomes and chromatin.

and the core histone. The strings of linked nucleosomes are repeatedly twisted to form the more complex three-dimensional organization of chromatin.

Histone Modification

The core histones are the dynamic structures and are continuously modified (Fig. 1.18). The tail parts of histone are projected out of the nucleosomes. The various histone modifiers act on the amino terminal ends of these histone tails and control the remodeling of the chromatin structure. The unwound remodeled chromatin facilitates the transcriptional proteins to interact with promoter sequence of DNA and thereby helps in DNA transcription.

Histone Tails Modification[22]

Acetylation: Lysine side chain of H3 and H4 are acetylated with the help of histone acetyltransferases (HATs) enzyme. This acetylation neutralizes the charge between lysine (positively charged) and DNA (negatively charged). The chromatin becomes opened up to recruit various transcription factors for transcriptional activation.

Histone deacetylase (HDAC): HDAC enzyme helps in deacetylation of histone tails that causes chromosomal recondensation and subsequently repression of DNA transcription.

Histone methylation: Histone methyltransferases (HMT) enzymes help in the methylation of lysine or arginine residues of histone H3 and H4.

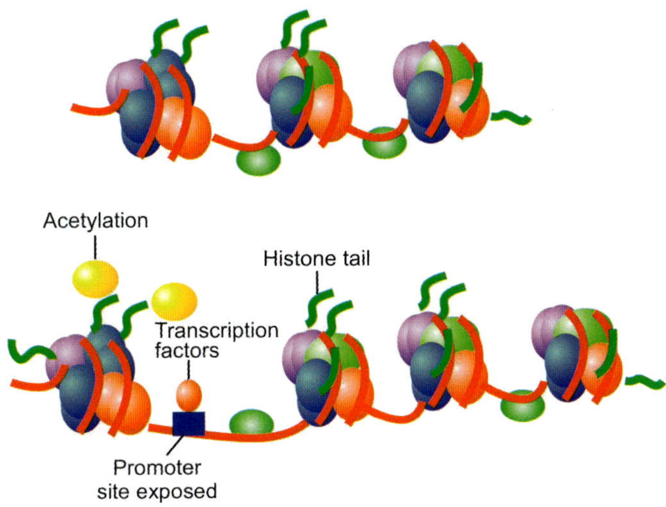

Fig. 1.18: Schematic diagram showing histone modification.

Phosphorylation: Aurora A, B and C phosphokinase help in mitotic phosphorylation of histone H3 and take important role in transcription, DNA repair and apoptosis.

In addition, histones are also modified by ubiquitylation and sumoylation.

Histone code: Histone code is a hypothesis that says that DNA transcription is regulated by the modification of histone proteins. It hypothesizes that there may be a particular set of combination of modification of histone tail. This pattern may produce the code which is read by the particular histone modifiers. There may be bromodomain that binds to acetylated lysine causing gene transcription. Whereas, chromodomain specifically binds with methylated lysine causing transcriptional repression.[23]

Nucleoli

Nucleolus is the subnuclear round to oval small structure within the nucleus and about 1 μ in diameter (Box 1.16). It is not a membrane bound structure. Nucleolus is usually situated in the center of the nucleus; however, the position of the nucleolus may vary. The number of nucleolus may vary from 1 to 3. The size of the nucleolus depends upon the requirement of ribosome and protein synthesis. So it is expected that metabolically active cell with higher amount of protein synthesis will have larger nucleoli. Nucleolus is easily recognizable by light microscopic examination. It looks like eosinophilic round body in H & E smear and light blue colored structure in MGG stain.

Box 1.16: Nucleoli.

- Subnuclear, nonmembrane bound.
- Round to oval small structure, about 1 μ in diameter.
- Size of the nucleolus depends upon the requirement of ribosome and protein synthesis.
- *Contains*: Protein and ribosomal RNA.
- *Formation*: At the end of the mitosis around ribosomal DNA (rDNA) genes.
- *Nucleolar organizing regions (NOR)*: Seen in homologous chromosomes of 13, 14, 15, 21, and 22.
- *Functions:*
  - The site of rRNA transcription, processing and ribosomal assembly.

The nucleoli are formed at the end of the mitosis (Fig. 1.19A). The specific genetic loci of the origin of nucleoli are known as "nucleolar organizing regions (NORs)". The nucleolar organizer loci are seen in homologous chromosomes of 13, 14, 15, 21, and 22. Therefore at the end of mitosis, tiny 10 nucleoli appear to from the NOR of the five pair of chromosomes (total 10 chromosomes). These small nucleoli conglomerate to form a single larger nucleolus. The nucleolus contains protein and ribosomal RNA. The protein and r-RNA are surrounded by chromosomal DNA of the nucleolus.

Structure

On electron microscopy, the nucleoli show three major subregions[24] (Fig. 1.19B).

1. *Fibrillar center (FC)*: Round structures with different size having very low electron opacity.
2. *Dense fibrillar component (DFC)*: It is made of densely aggregated fibrils and is located in the peripheral rim of FC.
3. *Granular components (GC)*: This is the outermost region and is composed of granules.

These different regions of nucleoli probably indicate the stages of RNA transcription and ribosomal assembly.

Function

The nucleolus is the site of rRNA transcription, processing and ribosomal assembly.

1. *rRNA transcription*: Active rRNA genes are situated in the FCs and DFCs. RNA polymerase I enzyme helps in the transcription of rRNA genes. The primary transcript of the ribosomal DNA is pre-rRNA. Subsequently, the preribosomal RNA transcripts are handled in the DFC with the help of small nucleolar RNA and other protein

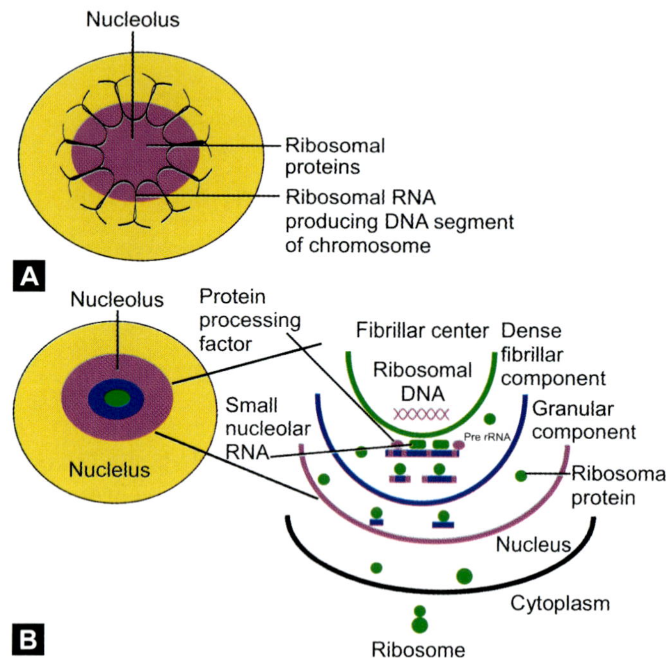

Figs. 1.19A and B: (A) Organization of nucleoli. Five pairs of chromosomal parts that produce ribosomal DNA with ribosomal proteins make nucleoli; (B) Nucleolar structure and functions are highlighted.

processing factors. A series of cleavages occur during the processing of preribosomal RNA to mature rRNA. In addition, considerable amount of methylation of the bases and ribose residues also happens. The various proteins in the nucleolar organizing regions (AgNOR) are demonstrated by the silver precipitation technique.[25]

2. *Ribosomal synthesis (Fig. 1.19B)*: Outside the nucleus, the genes of the ribosomal proteins are transcribed and from the cytoplasm these proteins are transported to the nucleolus. With the help of rRNA these ribosomal proteins are assembled within the nucleolus to form preribosome. The preribosome is transported back to the cytoplasm for final maturation.

Deoxyribonucleic Acid

Deoxyribonucleic acid, the nucleic acid, carries the vital genetic information of the cell (Box 1.17).

The portion of DNA that carries the genetic information is known as "gene". Within the nucleus DNA is coiled and supercoiled to make a thread like structure known as chromosome. During cell division the chromosomes are visible by light microscopy as a distinct entity and in interphase nucleus the chromosome remain as partly condensed and partly extended form and not possible to locate as a separate entity. There are 23 pairs of chromosomes and out of which 22 pairs are autosomes and one pair is sex chromosome. Sex chromosomes in the male are X and Y chromosomes and in the female are X and X chromosomes. The chromosomes are different from chromatin and the differences are highlighted in Table 1.4.

Box 1.17: Deoxyribonucleic acid.

- *Double helical strands* containing a sugar phosphate backbone and bases attached with the sugar molecule.
- *Sugar molecule*: a pentose sugar attached with the phosphate by 3rd and 5th carbon atom alternatively.
- *Four base pairs*: Adenine, cytosine, guanine and thymine
- Adenine joins only with thymine and cytosine joins only with guanine.
- *Nucleotides*: The unit of pentose sugar, phosphate and nucleobase.
- *Gene*: The specific portion of DNA with particular arrangement of nucleobases that carries the genetic information.

Table 1.4: Differences between chromatin and chromosome.

Chromatin	*Chromosome*
Loosely packed DNA	Tightly packed DNA
It is seen in interphase nuclei	Noted in cell division
Composed of histone and DNA chain	DNA chain only

Structure (Fig. 1.20)

Deoxyribonucleic acid is made of double helical strands containing a sugar phosphate backbone and bases attached with the sugar molecule.[26] Each strand of DNA is made up of alternate sugar and phosphate molecules. The sugar molecule is a pentose sugar and it is attached with the phosphate by third and fifth carbon atom alternatively. The nucleobase is attached with each sugar molecule and then links with the other base of the opposite strand by a weak hydrogen bond. There are four base pairs: (1) adenine (A), (2) cytosine (C), (3) guanine (G), and (4) thymine (T). Adenine and guanine are purine bases. Cytosine and thymine are pyrimidine bases. Adenine joins only with thymine, and cytosine joins only with guanine. This is known as complementary base pairing. There is another pyrimidine base known as "uracil" that is found in RNA.

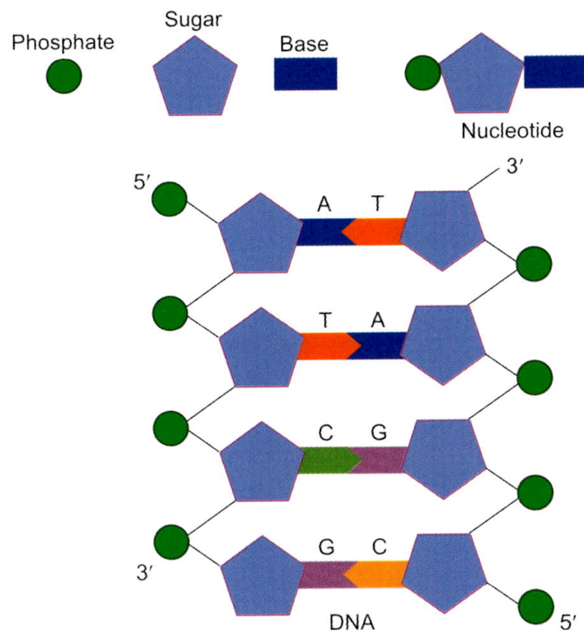

Fig. 1.20: Nuclear chromatin and DNA structure. Double helix DNA structure is made of sugar, phosphate back bone and four bases Adenine (A), Guanine (G), Cytosine (C), and Thymine (T).

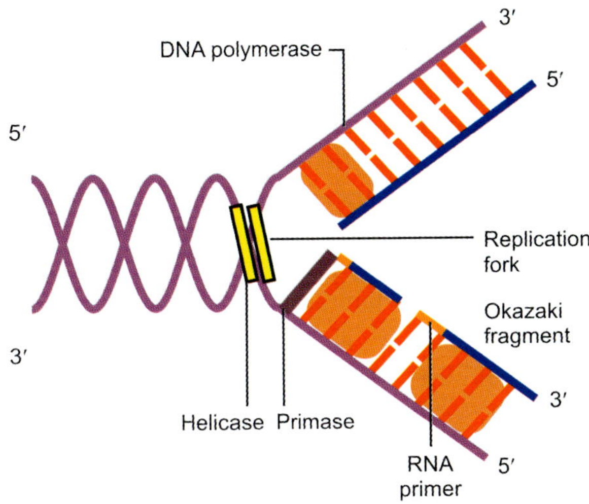

Fig. 1.21: DNA replication steps are highlighted in this schematic diagram. Helicase enzyme breaks the double-stranded DNA and a replication fork is formed. With the help of DNA polymerase enzyme DNA strand is made. In the leading strand DNA is synthesized in continuous manner at the direction of replication fork whereas in lagging strand DNA is synthesized in opposite direction as small segments. These small segments are known as Osazaki segments.

Nucleotide

Nucleotide is the basic structural unit of DNA. It consists of a pentose sugar, phosphate and nucleobase (adenine, cytosine, guanine or thymine). Nucleobase and sugar molecule form a nucleoside.

Gene

Gene is the specific portion of DNA with particular arrangement of nucleobases that carries the genetic information for making a particular protein. It is the sequence of A, T, C and G that determine the genetic information. Triplet of three consecutive bases of DNA is known as "codon" and each codon is specific for a particular amino acid. This specifies the sequence of amino acids and subsequently the protein formation. Only the certain parts of the DNA are involved in genetic information to carry and the "in-between part" of the DNA, is commonly known as "noncoding DNA" or "junk DNA". Near about 98% of human DNA is noncoding and is not involved in protein synthesis. However, it has been noted that the major parts (80%) of DNA are involved in different biochemical activities and therefore are active and are not really junk.[27] The exact biological function of the noncoding DNA is not known. Evidences suggest that noncoding DNA interacts with microRNA and thereby controls transcriptional and translation of protein coding sequences.[28]

Deoxyribonucleic Acid Replication (Fig. 1.21)

Deoxyribonucleic acid replication is a semi-conservative process by which genetic inheritance is maintained. When a cell divides, DNA replication process happens. Here each strand of DNA serves as a template and an identical complementary daughter DNA strand is formed. Each of the newly formed daughter cell contains DNA made up of one original strand and one freshly made strand. Therefore, the DNA double helix replication is a semi-conservative process. This replication process is well controlled and free of mistakes because of stringent proofreading and error checking mechanisms.

Deoxyribonucleic acid replication process needs following enzymes:

Deoxyribonucleic Acid Polymerases

These are the major enzymes in DNA replication process. These enzymes help in the polymerization of deoxyribonucleotides into the DNA strand. The DNA polymerase enzyme reads the intact template DNA strand to make the complementary DNA strand. On the basis of sequence homology and structural similarities DNA polymerases are classified into five major families:[29] A, B, C, X and Y. The three major varieties of eukaryotic DNA polymerases α, δ and ε belong to family B. The mitochondrial DNA polymerase γ belongs to family A. There are two important and fundamental properties of DNA polymerases:

1. They only can add free nucleotides in the 5′ to 3′ direction.
2. They need a preformed primer strand which is attached to the template DNA by hydrogen bonding. DNA polymerase adds a deoxyribonucleoside 5′ triphosphate to the 3′ OH group of the primers strand.

DNA replication is the coordinated activities of various enzymatic processes. The basic mechanisms of DNA replication process is evolutionary preserved. DNA replication events are initiated in many hundreds of points in chromosomes. This initiation point of the segment of DNA is known as "origin". The protein complex that acts on the origin as initiator of the DNA replication is known as "origin recognition complex (ORC)". The human ORC is site nonspecific. However, it is suggested that in somatic differentiated cells human ORC binds to genomic DNA with certain specificity.[30] DNA is replicated in S phase of the cell cycle. Total time of replication of DNA is usually fixed.

For the purpose of description the replication process can be divided by series of steps:

Steps of Deoxyribonucleic Acid Replication[31] (Box 1.18)

- *At first two strands of DNA is separated in particular point known as origin*: Here the initiator protein along with other associated protein forms a prereplication complex that separates the two strands of DNA. Therefore, a fork like structure is formed known as "replication fork". Helicases enzymes break the hydrogen bonds in between the bases and the unwound DNA strands are stabilized by single-stranded DNA binding proteins.
- *The binding of RNA primase in the initiation point of the 3′–5′ parent chain*: There is extension of the RNA primers by DNA polymerase that binds to the DNA nucleotides of the 3′–5′ strand due to the hydrogen bonds between the bases.

Box 1.18: Deoxyribonucleic acid replication.

- Semi-conservative process
- DNA replication needs:
  - DNA template
  - Helicase enzymes
  - DNA polymerases and other associated factors.

Steps:

- The initiator protein along with other associated protein forms a prereplication complex.
- *Helicases* enzymes break the hydrogen bonds in-between the bases
- *Replication* fork is formed
- Extension of the RNA primers by DNA polymerase
- *DNA polymerase adds the matching loose nucleotide*
- In *leading strand* DNA is synthesized in continuous manner and starts from 3′ end of the parent strand toward the replication fork.
- In *lagging strand*, the process of DNA synthesis occurs in discontinuous manner opposite the direction of the replication fork.
- *Okazaki fragments*: The multiple small pieces of DNA in lagging strand.
- The lagging strands are joined by DNA ligase.

- *DNA polymerase adds the matching loose nucleotide*: DNA polymerase can act only from 5′ to 3′ direction. Therefore, DNA replication is different in two strands of DNA. Original 5′ to 3′ strand of DNA replication starts from 3′ end and proceeds to the direction of the breakage of the replication fork. The strand of DNA here is known as "leading strand". In leading strand DNA is synthesized in continuous manner. In other strand of DNA, known as "lagging strand", the process of DNA synthesis is in discontinuous manner opposite the direction of the replication fork. This occurs in the multiple areas of the DNA strand. Therefore the multiple small pieces of DNA are synthesized known as "Okazaki fragments".
- *Joining of intact lagging strand*: The RNA strands are removed by the action of "RNase enzyme" and "DNA Pol I-exonuclease". The lagging strands are joined by DNA ligase.

Ultimately the DNA replication is terminated. Each double helix DNA contains one old template strand and one newly synthesized fresh strand.

Deoxyribonucleic Acid Transcription and Protein Synthesis (Box 1.19)

The principle key factor of protein synthesis remains in the DNA sequence of the nucleus. At first the portion of DNA template is copied into the messenger RNA (mRNA). This mRNA is processed within the nucleus and finally comes out from the nucleus to the cytoplasm through

Box 1.19: Deoxyribonucleic acid transcription.

- The information of DNA is transferred to the corresponding m-RNA.
- The m-RNA synthesis needs:
  - A DNA chain
  - Transcription factors
  - RNA polymerase II
- TATA binding protein (TBP) binds with TATA Box of DNA
- The transcription factors complex help in binding RNA polymerase to DNA.
- *Helicases* enzyme of TFIIH unwinds DNA.
- RNA polymerase now moves from the promoter and synthesis of m-RNA from the DNA strand starts.
- The terminal codon of DNA stops the m-RNA synthesis by RNA polymerase.

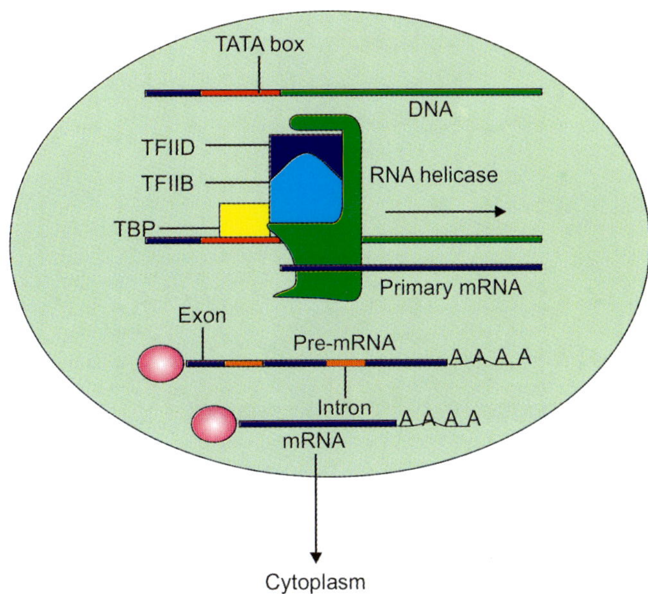

Fig. 1.22: Schematic diagram showing mRNA transcription from DNA. Intron regions are sliced out and ultimately mRNA is formed from pre-mRNA.

nuclear pore. Within the cytoplasm on the small subunit of ribosome attached with RER the mRNA is decoded and protein is synthesized with the help of t-RNA.

The two major steps of the protein synthesis are:

1. *Transcription*: It is the process of making mRNA (messenger RNA) from DNA.
2. *Translation*: The process of synthesizing protein from the mRNA code is known as translation.

Transcription (Fig. 1.22)

In this process, m-RNA is formed from the particular sequence of nucleotides of DNA carrying the genetic information to make a particular protein. Therefore, in this step the information of DNA is transferred to the corresponding m-RNA. The basic information of DNA remains same so the process is known as transcription. RNA is essentially same as DNA in structure except in certain points: (a) This is a liner polymer of nucleotides, (b) here the sugar moiety is ribose, and (c) RNA contains the base uracil (U) instead of thymine (T).

There are three important steps of transcription: (a) initiation, (b) elongation, and (c) termination.

- *Initiation*: Initiation of the m-RNA synthesis needs a DNA chain, transcription factors and RNA polymerase II. At first TATA binding protein (TBP) binds with TATA box of DNA. TBP is a part of general transcription factor called TFIID. The binding of TFIID promotes the binding of another protein known as TFIIB. This complex helps in binding RNA polymerase to DNA. After the recruitment of RNA polymerase another two transcription factors TFIIE and TFIIH binds with this complex and initiation complex is completed.
- *Elongation*: The helicases enzyme of TFIIH unwinds DNA and the RNA polymerase starts synthesis of m-RNA from the DNA strand. RNA polymerase now moves from the promoter and elongation phase starts. The DNA strand is read from 3′ to 5′ direction and subsequently RNA strand is made from 5′ to 3′ direction.
- *Termination*: When the RNA polymerase reaches to the terminal codon of DNA the m-RNA synthesis is stopped.

Translation (Fig. 1.23)

In translation phase, "information" of m-RNA is decoded and the protein is synthesized. The newly formed mRNA passes through the nuclear pore and binds properly with the small unit of ribosome. Ribosome contains many proteins and ribosomal RNA (rRNA). There are four nucleotides (adenine, guanine, cytosine and uracil) in RNA and each group of three consecutive nucleotides of m-RNA is called a "codon" (Box 1.20). Each codon indicates one specific amino acid. More than one codon may also specify a particular amino acid. Now for each codon of m-RNA there is a specific (transfer RNA) tRNA carrying the complementary codon nucleotide sequence called "anticodon". Each such tRNA molecule is linked with a particular amino acid. The recognition and attachment of the specific amino acid with this tRNA is dependent on enzymes known as aminoacyl-tRNA synthetase.

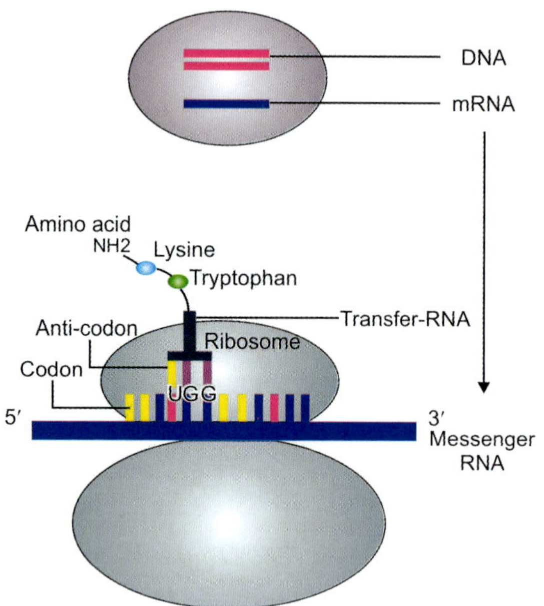

Fig. 1.23: Translation of mRNA to protein synthesis in ribosomal surface is highlighted. Information of mRNA is decoded and tRNA with complementary anti-codon brings a specific amino acid to form a protein.

Box 1.20: Translation of mRNA code.

- Information in m-RNA is decoded to synthesize protein.
- Codon:
- A group of three consecutive nucleotides of m-RNA.
- Each codon indicates one specific amino acid.
- Anticodon:
  - A specific tRNA carrying the complementary codon nucleotide sequence.
  - Each tRNA molecule is linked with a particular amino acid.

Steps:

- mRNA is attached with the surface of ribosome.
- The specific tRNA with amino acid is attached with the start codon of the mRNA.
- Ribosome moves from 5' to 3' direction of mRNA and then a new tRNA with another particular amino acid is attached.
- A complete chain of amino acid of protein is formed.

At first mRNA is attached with the surface of ribosome. Then specific tRNA is attached with the start codon of the mRNA carrying a particular amino acid. Ribosome moves from 5' to 3' direction of mRNA and then a new tRNA with another particular amino acid is attached next to the previous one. The former tRNA is released from the mRNA. This process continues till the end of the tRNA meets the stop codon and ribosome stops translation. The complete protein is synthesized and comes to the cytoplasm.

REFERENCES

1. Singer SJ, Nicolson GL. The Fluid Mosaic Model of the Structure of Cell Membranes. Science. 1972;175(4023):720-31.
2. Tuteja N. Signaling through G protein coupled receptors. Plant Signal Behav. 2009;4(10):942-7.
3. Macara IG. Parsing the polarity code. Nature Rev Mol Cell Biol. 2004;5:220-31.
4. Martin-Belmonte F, Perez-Moreno M. Epithelial cell polarity, stem cells and cancer. Nat Rev Cancer. 2012;12:23-38.
5. Hugo H, Ackland ML, Blick T, et al. Epithelial-mesenchymal and mesenchymal-Epithelial transitions in carcinoma progression. J Cell Physiol. 2007;213:374-83.
6. Wu Y, Zhou BP. New insights of epithelial-mesenchymal transition in cancer metastasis. Acta Biochim Biophys Sin. 2008;40:643-50.
7. Royer C, Lu X. Epithelial cell polarity: a major gatekeeper against cancer? Cell Death Differentiation. 2011;18:1470-7.
8. Hazan RB, Kang L, Whooley BP, et al. N-cadherin promotes adhesion between invasive breast cancer cells and the stroma. Cell Adhes Commun. 1997;4(6):399-411.
9. Ellgaard L, Helenius A. ER quality control: towards an understanding at the molecular level. Curr Opin Cell Biol. 2001;13(4):431-7.
10. Wilson C, Venditti R, Rega LR, et al. The Golgi apparatus: an organelle with multiple complex functions. Biochem J. 2011;433(1):1-9.
11. Glick BS, Malhotra V. The curious status of the Golgi apparatus. Cell. 1998;95:883-9.
12. McBride HM, Neuspiel M, Wasiak S. Mitochondria: more than just a powerhouse. Curr Biol. 2006;16(14):R551-60.
13. Harris SL, Levine AJ. The p53 pathway: positive and negative feedback loops. Oncogene. 2005;24:2899-908.
14. Jurgensmeier JM, Xie Z, Deve raux Q, et al. Bax directly induces release of cytochrome c from isolated mitochondria. Proc Natl Acad Sci USA. 1998;95:4997-5002.
15. Alston CL, Rocha MC, Lax NZ, et al. The genetics and pathology of mitochondrial disease. J Pathol. 2016.
16. Mancuso M, Orsucci D, Angelini C, et al. Redefining phenotypes associated with mitochondrial DNA single deletion. J Neurol. 2015;262:1301-9.
17. Fuchs E, Weber K. Intermediate filaments: Structure, dynamics, function, and disease. Annu Rev Biochem. 1994;63:345-82.
18. Foisner R, Gerace L. Integral membrane proteins of the nuclear envelope interact with lamins and chromosomes, and binding is modulated by mitotic phosphorylation. Cell. 1993;73:1267-79.
19. Dey P. Nuclear margin irregularity and cancer: a review. Anal Quant Cytol Histol. 2009;31(5):345-52.
20. Beck M, Lucic V, Forster F, et al. Snapshots of nuclear pore complexes in action captured by cryoelectron tomography. Nature. 2007;449:611-5.
21. Tsutsui KM, Sano K, Tsutsui K. Dynamic view of the nuclear matrix. Acta Med Okayama. 2005;59(4):113-20.

22. Dey P. Chromatin remodeling, cancer and chemotherapy. Curr Med Chem. 2006;13(24):2909-19.
23. Jenuwein T, Allis CD. Translating the histone code. Science. 2001;293(5532):1074-80.
24. Boisvert FM, Koningsbruggen SV, Navascues J, et al. The multifunctional nucleolus. Nat Rev Mol Cell Biol. 2007;8:574-85.
25. Sirri V, Roussel P, Hernandez-Verdun D. The AgNOR proteins: qualitative and quantitative changes during the cell cycle. Micron. 2000;31:121-6.
26. Watson JD, Crick FHC. A structure for deoxyribose nucleic acid. Nature. 1953;171(4356):737-8.
27. An integrated encyclopedia of DNA elements in the human genome. ENCODE Project Consortium. Nature. 2012;489(7414):57-74.
28. Elgar G, Vavouri T. Tuning into the signals: noncoding sequence conservation in vertebrate genomes. Trends Genet. 2008;24(7):344-52.
29. Ohmori H, Friedberg EC, Fuchs RP, et al. The Y-family of DNA polymerases. Mol Cell. 2001;8(1):7-8.
30. Vashee S, Cvetic C, Lu W, et al. Sequence-independent DNA binding and replication initiation by the human origin recognition complex. Genes Dev. 2003;17:1894-908.
31. Bell SP, Dutta A. DNA replication in eukaryotic cells. Annu Rev Biochem. 2002;71:333-74.

Review Questions

1. Increased expression of all these molecules is responsible for epithelial mesenchymal transition of epithelial cells except:
   a. E-cadherin
   b. N-cadherin
   c. Snail 1
   d. Vimentin

2. The junction that connects the cell with the basal lamina:
   a. Adherens junction
   b. Tight junction
   c. Desmosomes
   d. Hemidesmosomes

3. The most important site of intracellular calcium storage:
   a. Smooth endoplasmic reticulum
   b. Golgi complex
   c. Lysosome
   d. Ribosome

4. During oxidative phosphorylation, a series of electron transport reactions occur in this cytoplasmic organelle:
   a. Smooth endoplasmic reticulum
   b. Golgi complex
   c. Mitochondria
   d. Ribosome

5. Which one is not an intermediate filament?
   a. Actin
   b. Lamin
   c. Glial fibrillary acidic protein
   d. Desmin

6. This enzyme breaks the hydrogen bonds in between the bases of DNA:
   a. DNA polymerase
   b. RNase
   c. Helicase
   d. DNA Pol I-exonuclease

7. The main reactions of citric acid cycle happen in the:
   a. Mitochondrial matrix
   b. Mitochohndrial inner membrane
   c. Mitochohndrial outer membrane
   d. Golgi complex

Identify True/False

8. Prokaryotic cells do not have any true nucleus and no membrane bound nucleus. *(True/False)*

9. The loss of E-cadherin in epithelial cells enables them to detach easily and facilitates dispersion of carcinoma cells. *(True/False)*

10. Rough endoplasmic reticulum is related with lipid synthesis. *(True/False)*

11. Mitochondrial DNA is exclusively inherited from mother. *(True/False)*

12. Glial fibrillary acidic protein is not an intermediate filament. *(True/False)*

13. Euchromatin is the condensed portion of chromatin where genes are usually inactive. *(True/False)*

14. Histone deacetylase causes chromosomal recondensation and subsequently repression of DNA transcription. *(True/False)*

15. Chromodomain binds to acetylated lysine causing gene transcription. *(True/False)*

Answers

1. a. E-cadherin
2. d. Hemidesmosomes
3. b. Golgi complex
4. c. Mitochondria
5. a. Actin
6. c. Helicase
7. a. Mitochondrial matrix
8. True
9. True
10. False
11. True
12. False
13. False
14. True
15. False

CHAPTER

2

Cell Cycle and Cell Proliferation

INTRODUCTION

The cell division is the process where one cell divides into two or more daughter cells. This is the fundamental process that helps in the development of the organ, replacement of damaged cells and maintenance of tissue in its steady state. The three key steps in cell division are:

1. Replication of DNA
2. Production of the cellular constituents
3. Successful equal division of these elements in two daughter cells.

CELL CYCLE

Cell cycle is a continuous successive process that leads to a cell division.

Somatic cells divide into two daughter cells by mitosis. The cell continuously goes through mitosis and the preparatory phase before mitosis. This preparatory phase is also known as "interphase", which is the combination of resting phase and DNA synthesizing phase. The cell cycle of eukaryotic cell undergoes into four main successive events: G_1, S, G_2 and M phase (Fig. 2.1 and Box 2.1).

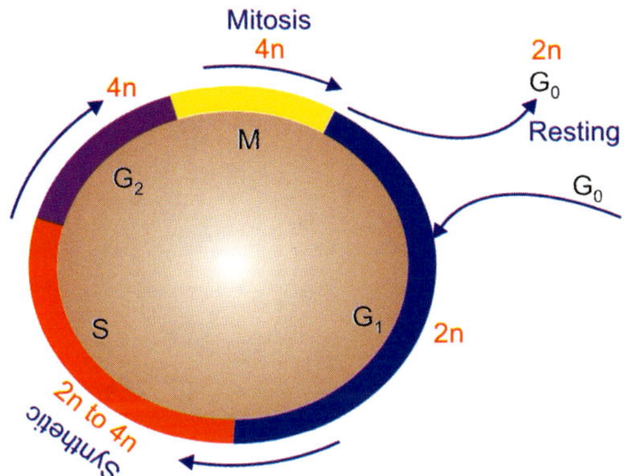

Fig. 2.1: Schematic diagram of cell cycle. The cell in cell cycle passes through G_1, S, G_2 and M phase. G_0 is the resting phase of the cell.

Synthetic (S) phase: In S phase, the cell synthesizes DNA and duplicates the chromosome. The time taken for S phase is usually 10–12 hours and this phase occupies half the time of cell cycle. S phase contains variable amount of DNA from 2n to 4n (here *n* denotes the haploid DNA content).

Mitotic or M phase: After the completion of chromosomal duplication, the chromosomes segregate and the cell enters into the mitotic phase. Here each cell divides and the chromosomal material is divided equally in these two daughter cells. This phase contains 4n DNA. When the daughter cells are generated each one contains 2n DNA.

Gap 2 or G_2 phase: This is the gap between the S phase and mitosis. In G_2 phase the cell dividing cell takes time to grow and prepare prior to mitosis.

Gap 1 or G_1 phase: After the completion of the mitotic phase the cell takes some time to grow before undergoing S phase. This is known as G_1 phase. In this period the cell grows and generates more cellular organelles. The total amount of DNA is diploid (2n). The cell remains in this phase till it enters to S phase for the next round of cell division.

Box 2.1: Cell cycle.

G_0 phase
- The cell does not divide and does not undergo cell cycle
- Diploid (2n) DNA (here *n* denotes the haploid DNA content)

Gap 1 or G_1 phase
- This is in between the mitotic and synthetic phase
- Diploid (2n) DNA content

Synthetic or S phase
- It contains variable amount of DNA from 2n to 4n
- DNA is synthesized

Gap 2 or G_2 phase
- This is in between the S and M phase.
- The dividing cell grow and prepare prior to mitosis
- The cell contains tetraploid (4n) DNA

Mitotic or M phase
- Each cell divides and the chromosomal material is divided into equally in these two daughter cells
- The cell contains tetraploid (4n) DNA

There is another phase of cell cycle when a cell does not divide and does not undergo cell cycle. This phase is known as "G_0 phase". The cell may remain in this phase for days to years till it receives stimulation for cell division.

Duration of each phase of cell cycle varies widely. However, the major bulk of cell cycle time is taken in G_1 and S phase. In 24 hour duration of cell cycle, G_1 and S phase take near about 19 hours, whereas M phase takes only 1 hour time. Depending on the period of staying in G_0 phase, the cells may be divided into three types:

1. *Labile cell*: The cells of this type remain short period in G_0 phase and quickly enter into the cell cycle. The labile cells are rapidly proliferating population of cells. Intestinal epithelial cells are the example of labile cells.
2. *Stable cells*: This type of cells remains in G_0 phase for long time until there is stimulation to divide. Liver cells, lining of kidney tubular cells and pancreatic cells are stable cells. They usually do not divide until a fraction of them are destroyed by injury or inflammation.
3. *Permanent cell*: Some cells remain permanently in G_0 phase and never undergo cell division such as neuronal cell. These cells are known as permanent cell.

CELL DIVISION

There are two types of cell division—mitosis and meiosis.

Mitosis

In mitosis phase the parent cell divides into two identical cells with identical chromosomal material in each nucleus (Box 2.2). Figure 2.2 shows typical mitotic figure in cytology smear. There are four stages of mitosis: (1) prophase (sometimes divided into early prophase and prometaphase), (2) metaphase, (3) anaphase and (4) telophase (Fig. 2.3).

Prophase

It is the preparatory phase of mitosis proper. The following changes are seen:

- The nucleoli and nuclear membrane both disappear.
- The duplicated chromosomes in G_2 phase condense and form two identical chromatids. These sister

Box 2.2: Mitosis.

Prophase
- The nucleoli and nuclear membrane both disappear
- The chromosomal pair condenses and forms two identical chromatids
- The centrioles replicates and two pair of centrioles form that travel to the opposite poles
- Microtubules polymerize and the mitotic spindle is formed

Prometaphase
- Mitotic spindle formation completes
- The kinetochore of each sister chromatids attaches with the microtubules of the mitotic spindle

Metaphase
- All the chromatids are arranged to the equatorial plane of the mitotic spindle

Anaphase
- The two sister chromatids are separated
- The chromatids move toward the opposite pole and two identical set of chromosomes reach to each pole

Telophase
- The remnants of the mitotic spindle disappear
- The nuclear membrane and new nucleoli are formed

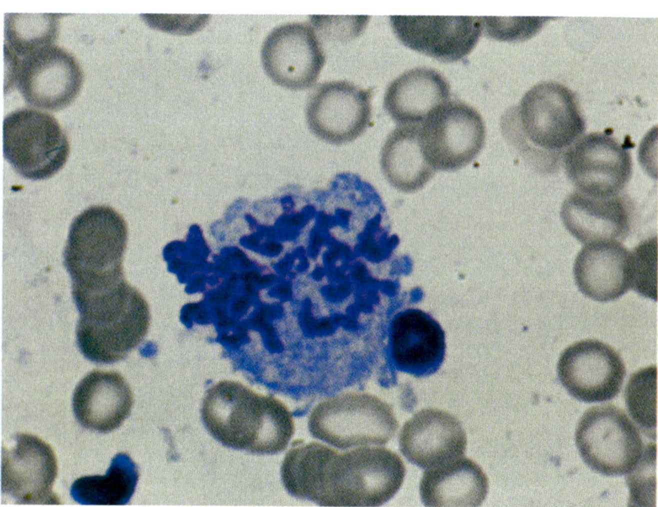

Fig. 2.2: Mitotic figure in cytology smear (Papanicolaou's stain X OI).

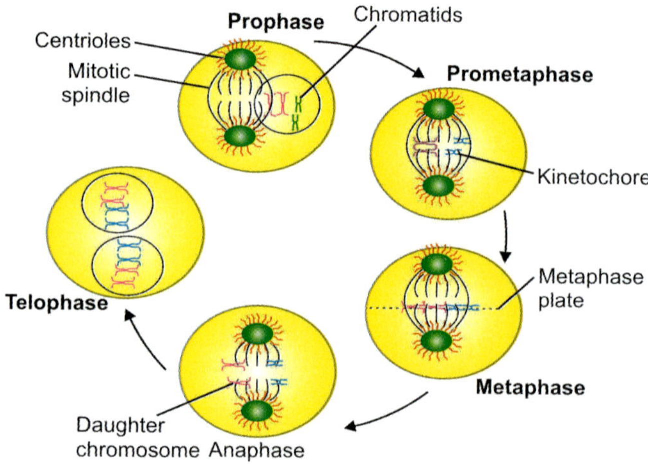

Fig. 2.3: Schematic diagram of different phases of mitosis.

chromatids are joined together in centromeres by a special protein known as cohesin. Centromere is a DNA sequence to which proteins are attached to form a kinetochore, the complex protein structure.

- The pair of original centrioles replicates and two pair of centrioles are formed that travel to the opposite poles.
- The microtubules start to polymerize to generate mitotic spindle.

Prometaphase

This is the transition phase between prophase and metaphase. In this phase microtubules completes the formation of the mitotic spindle. Some microtubules are extended from the pole to the equatorial plane and others are extended from one pole to the other pole. Here the kinetochore of each sister chromatids attaches with the microtubules of the mitotic spindle. Each kinetochore attaches with the microtubules called kinetochore microtubules that emanates from the opposite pole of the spindle.

Metaphase

In metaphase all the chromatids are well arranged to the equatorial plane of the mitotic spindle and journey of the chromatids toward the each pole is set. Every kinetochore should be properly attached to the kinetochore microtubule of the mitotic spindle as this is mandatory for the proper distribution of the chromosome to the daughter cell and to avoid aneuploidy. Any unattached kinetochore generates signal to halt the mitosis in this phase and this is known as mitotic spindle checkpoint.

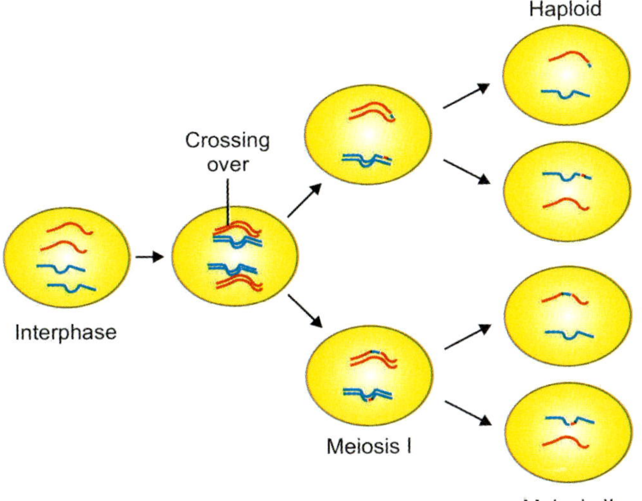

Fig. 2.4: Schematic diagram of different phases of meiosis.

Anaphase

Here at first the two sister chromatids are separated and become separate daughter chromosomes. Now the kinetochore microtubules shorten and spindle tubules elongate. The two poles go apart and simultaneously pull the chromosomes pair toward the pole. The pair of each chromosomes move to the opposite pole at the same speed.

Telophase

This is just the reversal of prophase and metaphase. Here the remnants of the mitotic spindle disappear; nuclear membrane and new nucleoli are formed.

Cytokinesis

In the late anaphase, the process of cytokinesis starts and a constriction of cytoplasm develops in the equatorial plane of the original mitotic spindle. The process of cytokinesis continues till the end of the telophase.

Meiosis

Meiosis occurs in the gamete producing cells. In this process of cell division the single diploid cell divides into four daughter cells and each contains half of the parental chromosomes (Fig. 2.4, Box 2.3). The cells with haploid chromosome need to maintain the diploid number of chromosomes in the fertilized cell. Meiosis occurs in the process of gametogenesis to produce sperm or ovum.

Meiosis is divided into two parts: (1) "First meiotic division (Meiosis I or reductional division)," and (2) "Second meiotic division (Meiosis II)".

The first meiotic division is known as reductional division because in this phase, the each member of the homologous chromosome goes to one each cell and the each one daughter cell contains haploid chromosome. During the S phase prior to first meiotic I the DNA replicates and each chromosome produces two identical sister chromatids. The non-sister chromatids exchange their genetic material that is known as "cross over" (Box 2.4). Unlike mitosis, both

Box 2.3: Meiosis.

- *Meiosis I or reductional division:* Each member of the homologous chromosome goes to one each cell
- *Meiosis I*
  - Prophase of the meiosis is divided into five phases: Leptotene, zygotene, pachytene, diplotene and diakinesis
  - *Synapsis occurs in zygotene phase*
  - Cross over occurs in pachytene phase.
- *Meiosis II:* Mechanically same as mitosis

Box 2.4: Cross over.

a. Overlapping of homologous region of the matching chromosome of nonsister chromatids in Pachytene phase of prophase I
b. The double stranded DNA breaks into single strand
c. In the cross over region DNA breaks in both the non-sister chromatids
d. Exchange of genetic information occurs in cross over region
e. Paternal DNA exchanges information with maternal DNA
f. Maintains genetic diversity

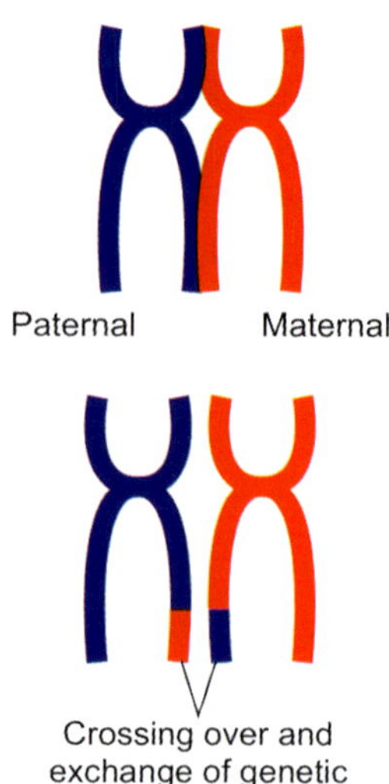

Fig. 2.5: Schematic diagram of crossing over with exchange of genetic material. Genetic diversity is maintained with the help of crossing over.

the sister chromatids of the homologous chromosome go to one each nucleus. The meiosis I is subsequently followed by the second meiotic division, meiosis II that is mechanically same as mitosis. After the completion of the meiosis II a parent cell generates total four daughter cells with haploid chromosome.

Meiosis I

Prophase of the meiosis is divided into five phases: (1) leptotene, (2) zygotene, (3) pachytene, (4) diplotene, and (5) diakinesis.

Leptotene: Progressive condensation and coiling of the chromosome occur in this phase. The chromosome looks like long convoluted thread.

Zygotene: In this phase both the homologous chromosomes are closely associated and aligned completely with each other point by point in their entire length. This is known as "synapsis". This paired homologous chromosomes in synapsis known as bivalent chromosome.

Pachytene: In this phase the chromosomes become more condensed and thick. The homologous chromosomes begin to move away but in certain regions they are overlapping like a cross. In those overlapping zones of non-sister chromatids of the homologous chromosome exchange of genetic information takes place (Fig. 2.5). This is known as "cross over (chiasmata)". This is a very important event as exchange of genetic information occurs in cross over region and this gives rise to genetic heterogeneity in the gametes.

Diplotene: In this phase homologous chromosome separates completely except in the points of cross over regions.

Diakinesis: This is the end stage of the prophase I where the chromosome condenses fully and the four tetrad chromatids are visible. Mitotic spindle starts forming in this phase. The nuclear membrane and nucleoli dissolves.

Metaphase I

The homologous chromosome with two sister chromatids attach to the kinetochore microtubules and align to the equatorial plane of the mitotic spindle.

Anaphase I

The kinetochore microtubules begin to contract and the whole homologous chromosome with sister chromatids move to one pole of the mitotic spindle. Unlike mitosis there is no such disjunction of the sister chromatids in meiosis and the centromeres remain intact.

Telophase I

The chromosomes reach to the each pole and each daughter cell receives haploid number of chromosome. Mitotic spindle dissolves, nuclear membrane and nucleoli appear and cytokinesis starts.

Meiosis II

It is mechanically similar to mitosis and can be divided into prophase II, metaphase II, anaphase II and telophase II. In the anaphase II there is disjunction of the sister chromatids and breakage of centromeres. The sister chromatids, that means chromosome, move towards the opposite pole.

Meiosis occurs in ovary and testis to produce gamete. Each gamete contains haploid chromosome. During fertilization of ovum with sperm a complete diploid cell is generated from the fusion of the two haploid cells. Sperms contain either 23Y or 23X chromosome and ovum has 23X chromosome. Fertilization of ovum by the sperm containing 23Y generates male embryo whereas fertilization of the ovum by the sperm containing 23X generates female embryo.

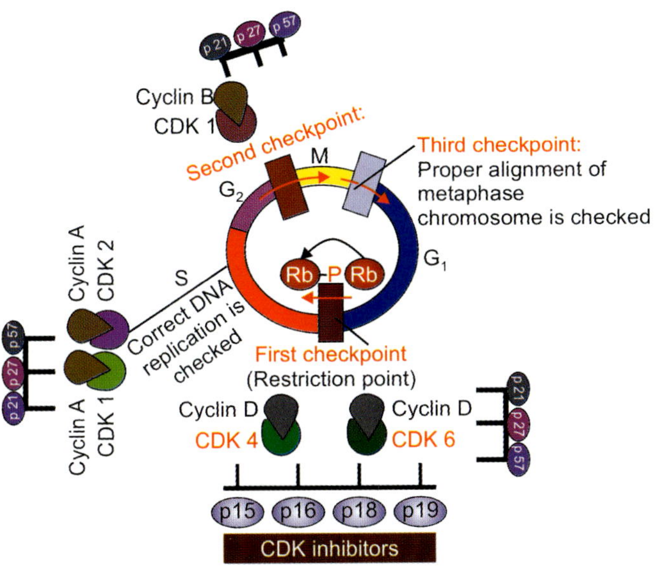

Fig. 2.6: Three different points of cell cycle restriction is highlighted in this schematic diagram.

Box 2.5: Cyclin-dependent kinases (CDK).

- CDK is activated by binding with specific cyclin
- Activated CDK phosphorylates the enzymatic proteins
- Phosphorylated active enzymes act on specific genes involved in DNA synthesis and replication
- CDK level is constant in a cell
- Cyclin level oscillates in different phase of cell cycle

Table 2.1: Cell cycle checkpoints and cyclins, cyclin-dependent kinase and their inhibitors.

Cell cycle checkpoint	*Cyclin*	*Cyclin-dependent kinase (CDK)*	*CDK inhibitors*
First: G_1-S (restriction point)	Cyclin D, Cyclin E	1. Cyclin D binds CDK 4, CDK 6 2. Cyclin E binds CDK 2	1. INK4 proteins: p15, p16, p18, p19 2. Cip/Kip protein: p21, 27, 57. Inhibits Cyclin E-CDK2 and also Cyclin D-CDK 4/6
Second: Junction of G_2 and M phase	Cyclin A	CDK 2, CDK 1	Cip/Kip protein: p21, 27, 57

CELL CYCLE CHECKPOINT

Proper control of the cell cycle is needed for the growth of the body. For the last billion years the mechanism of cell cycle control is almost same. The important features of cell cycle control system are:

- It is very robust
- It is adaptive
- The control switches or restriction points are binary off and on that means once initiated they are usually irreversible.[1]

The "control points or cell cycle restrict points" are located (Fig. 2.6):

- *Near the end point of G_1 phase*: The checkpoint near the end of G_1 phase of the cell cycle is called "restriction point". Here the environment is assessed and if the surrounding environment is favorable then the cell is allowed to enter into the S phase.
- *At the junction of G_2 and M phase*: In the G_2/M checkpoint two fundamental factors are assessed: whether all DNA properly replicated or not and the environment is favorable for proliferation or not?
- *In the M phase at the junction of metaphase and anaphase*: When every chromosome is correctly aligned and attached to the kinetochore microtubules in the equatorial region of the mitotic spindle then the cell is allowed to go to metaphase to anaphase. Therefore, this checkpoint is also known as spindle assembly checkpoint.

CELL CYCLE REGULATOR PROTEINS

The journey through the cell cycle checkpoint requires the activity of group of protein kinase enzymes known as "cyclin-dependent kinases (CDKs)".[2] These enzymes are structurally related to each other and are activated when they combine with another group of proteins known as "cyclin" (Box 2.5). A specific CDK can combine with many different cyclins, and similarly a particular cyclin can also interact with different CDKs.[3]

Activated CDKs play key role in cell cycle control by "phosphorylation" of various protein enzymes essential for activating the genes involved in DNA synthesis and replication (Fig. 2.8). They also control nutrient uptake, breakdown of nuclear membrane, formation of mitotic spindle and chromosomal condensation. The level of CDKs in the cell is constant; however the cyclin level oscillates in various phases of cell cycle. The increased amount of cyclin-CDK complex (activated CDKs) triggers various cell cycle events. Depending on the binding of the CDKs in different stages of the cell cycle, cyclins are classified in three major classes (Table 2.1):

1. Cyclins acting on G_1/S transition (G_1/S cyclin): Cyclin D and E
2. Cyclins acting on S phase (S cyclin): Cyclin A, Cyclin E
3. Cyclins acting on M phase (M cyclin): Cyclin B and Cyclin A.

In a resting cell that comes out from the mitotic phase, retinoblastoma protein (Rb) is tightly bound with

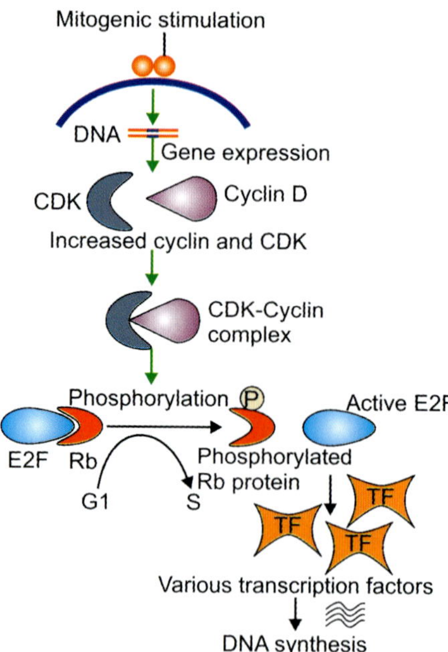

Fig. 2.7: External mitogenic stimulation activates gene to produce cyclin D. Cyclin-CDK complex phosphorylates retinoblastoma (Rb) protein and liberates E2F. E2F, the transcription factor, stimulates DNA to produce various cell cycle enzymes such as cyclin E and A that help in DNA replication. (CDK: Cyclin-dependent kinese; DNA: Deoxyribonucleic acid).

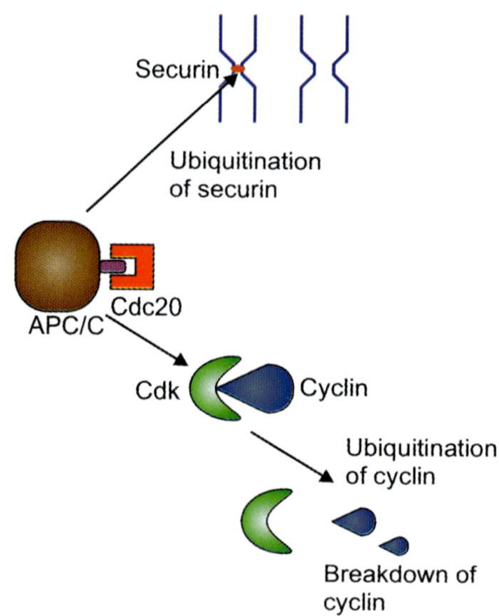

Fig. 2.8: Schematic diagram shows the mechanisms to control metaphase-anaphase transition.

E2F transcription factors. The cells cannot go into the proliferation phase due to unavailability of E2Fs (Fig. 2.7). The stimulation of the cell by external mitogenic factors increases the level of cyclin D, which combines with respective CDKs (CDK4 and CDK6).

The activated CDKs then phosphorylate Rb protein and release E2F transcription factors. Released E2F stimulates cyclin E and cyclin A and other large set of factors essential for DNA replication. Cyclin E-CDK complex can also phosphorylate Rb protein by itself and therefore behaves as a positive feedback loop to inactivate Rb protein and S phase entry of the cell. Therefore, phosphorylation of Rb protein by activated CDKs play important role in cell cycle initiation.[4]

M cyclin (Cyclin B) functions during mitosis by activating CDK1. Cyclin B-CDK 1 complex controls the entry of the cell in mitotic phase by controlling G2-M checkpoint. It phosphorylates the various proteins leading to the breakdown of the nuclear membrane, assembly of mitotic spindle and attachment of the chromatids with the spindle.

The specific Cyclin-CDK complex acts mainly in the G_1/S and G_2/M checkpoint by phosphorylation of proteins. However, the progress from metaphase to anaphase is regulated by protein destruction. Anaphase promoting complex (APC) is activated by the Cdc20. This activated APC catalyzes the ubiquitylation and destruction of securing protein (Fig. 2.8).[5] This securing protein is responsible for holding the two sister chromatids. Therefore destruction of securing separates the sister chromatids and promotes the cell cycle progression from metaphase to anaphase. APC/C also destroys S and M cyclins and therefore inactivates CDKs within the cell (Fig. 2.8).

CDK Inhibitors: INK 4 Family Members

Till now four known members of INK 4 protein family have been described[6]: (1) $p16^{INK4a}$, (2) $p15^{INK4b}$, (3) $p18^{INK4c}$, and (4) $p19^{INK4d}$. These proteins specifically bind with CDK 4 and CDK 6 and inhibit their kinase activity and subsequently block cyclin D activity. INK4a and INK4b genes are located in short arm of chromosome 9, and INK 4c and INK 4d are located in chromosome 1 and 19. INK4 proteins functions depend upon the presence of functional Rb proteins. These INK 4 proteins inhibit cyclin D-CDK and thereby accumulate hypophosphorylated Rb that inhibits the entry of G_1 phase cell to S phase cell cycle. The loss of INK 4a function has been described in several cancers. INK 4a mutation or deletions are noted in gliomas, nasopharyngeal carcinoma, sarcoma, ovarian carcinoma and non-small cell lung carcinomas.[7]

CDK Inhibitors: The Cip/Kip Family

Cyclin E-CDK2 complex is activated in G_1-S phase restriction point. The action of this complex is mitogen independent and it helps in phosphorylation of Rb protein. The activity of CDK 1, 2, and 3 is inhibited by the Cip/Kip group of inhibitors: $p21^{Cip1}$, $p27^{Kip1}$, and $p57^{Kip2}$. They also inhibit Cyclin D-CDK 4/6 complexes.

CELL CYCLE CONTROL AND CANCER

Uncontrolled cell proliferation due to deregulation of cell cycle engine is responsible for cancer. One or more cell cycle checkpoints are disrupted in cancer (Box 2.6).[8]

Entrance to G_1 Checkpoint and Cancer

"Mitogenic stimulation-active G_1-CDK-pRB phosphorylation-active G_1-S cyclin" pathway may be altered by number of ways that may liberate E2F continuously leading to uncontrolled cell proliferation. This may happen by:

Box 2.6: Cell cycle checkpoint and cancer.

- *G_1 entry checkpoint and cancer*
  - *Rb gene inactivation* due to mutation or hypermethylation
  - Cyclin D1 and CDK4 gene amplification
  - HER-2 gene amplification
- *DNA replication license and cancer*
  - Deregulation of the pre-replicative (pre-RC) complex system
- *DNA damage, repair and cancer*
  - Mutation of p21, p53 and BRCA1

- In cancer, Rb gene may be inactivated due to mutation or hypermethylation[9]
- Cyclin D1 and CDK4 gene amplification
- HER-2 gene amplification.

There may be incessant activity of CDK-cyclin complex because of inactivation of CDKIs gene.

DNA Replication License and Cancer

DNA synthesis is tightly controlled by replication licensing system. At the time of end of mitosis and early G_1 phase, licensing proteins origin recognition complex (ORC), Cdc6, Cdt1 and Mcm2–7 accumulate into pre-replicative (pre-RC) complexes and license the "origin" for DNA synthesis in S phase (Fig. 2.9). This licensing system is shut down when the cell enters into S phase. This prevents the reinitiation of the DNA replication. Disruption of the licensing system may be responsible for oncogenesis.[10]

DNA Damage, Repair and Cancer

There are checkpoints in S phase and G_2-M phase to prevent the cell cycle progression in case of DNA damage. The steps are:

- Breaking of double stranded DNA is quickly recognized by two proteins ataxia telangiectasia mutated (ATM) and ataxia telangiectasia mutated and Rad 3 related (ATR) proteins (Fig. 2.10).[11]
- The activated ATM/ATR kinase subsequently activate two other proteins checkpoint kinase (CHK) 1 and CHK 2.

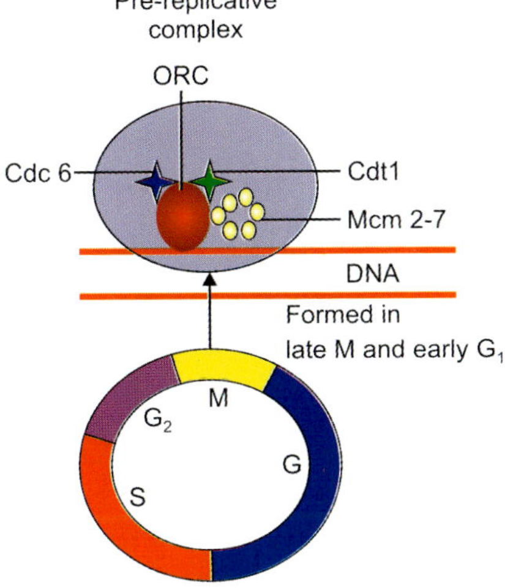

Fig. 2.9: Schematic diagram shows pre-replicative (pre-RC) complex formation by origin recognition complex (ORC), Cdc6, Cdt1 and Mcm.[2-7]

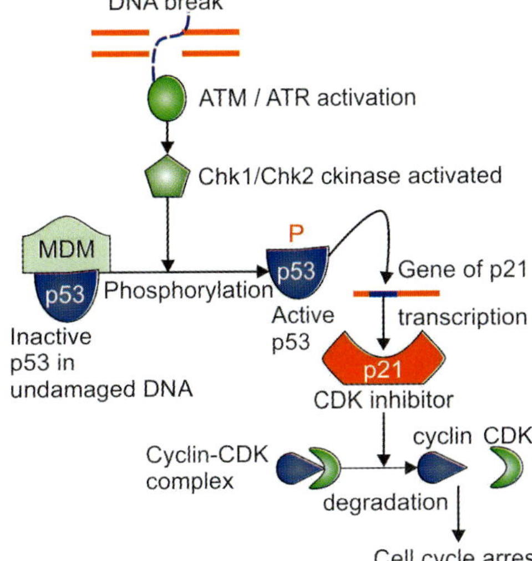

Fig. 2.10: Schematic diagram shows DNA damage checkpoint.

- These two kinases CHK 1 and CHK 2 phosphorylate various target proteins that help in cell cycle arrest and p53 is one such proteins.
- Ordinarily in the cell with undamaged DNA, p53 binds with Mdm 2, a negative regulator (inhibitor) of p53. Mdm 2 is an ubiquitin ligase and destroys its target p53.
- Phosphorylation of p53 reduces its binding with Mdm 2.
- Marked increase concentration of p53 enhances its ability of stimulation of gene transcription of p21, a CDK inhibitor.
- Broken down Cyclin-CDK complex (G_1-/S-CDK and S-CDK) finally are responsible for cell cycle arrest.

CELL PROLIFERATION MARKERS

Assessment of cell proliferation is considered an important biological marker of predicting tumor behavior. There are many cell proliferative markers.[12] The counting of mitosis is the oldest and one of the most reliable methods of assessment of cell proliferation activity. The other methods to measure the cell proliferation activity include DNA flow cytometry (FCM) to assess the S phase, bromodeoxyuridine incorporation techniques, immunocytochemistry of various cell proliferation related antigens, nucleolar organizer regions (NORs) counting, etc. These techniques are compared in Table 2.2.

Mitotic Index

Mitosis is visible by light microscope in simple routine stain (*see* Fig. 2.3) and it can be measured easily.[13] The ideal mitotic figures have the following morphology:

- No nuclear membrane
- No clear zone in the center

Table 2.2: Different techniques to assess cell proliferation.

Technique	*Principle*	*Cell cycle*	*Advantages*	*Disadvantages*
Mitotic count	Estimation of mitotic figures on light microscopy	M phase cells	1. Easy 2. Reproducible 3. Possible on archival material and routine smear or section	1. Mitotic count may vary depending on tissue fixation 2. Mitotic score may vary subjectively 3. Many other things such as apoptotic body and mast cells may simulate mitotic figures
AgNOR	NOR related associated proteins are argyrophilic and can be stained with silver. AgNOR is closely related with cell proliferation	All proliferating cells	1. Easy 2. Can be done on archival tissue	1. Counting is too some extent subjective 2. Difficult in daily routine practice
Flow cytometry	DNA stoichiometric dye stains DNA of single cells and relative DNA content is measured when the cells are in flow	Measure G_0/G_1, S and G_2/M phase cells separately	1. Rapid 2. Large number of cells can be analyzed 3. Reproducible	1. Sophisticated technique 2. Target cells cannot be visualized
Image cytometry	DNA stoichiometric dye stains DNA and relative DNA content is measured on smear or section	Measure G_0/G_1, S and G_2/M phase cells separately	1. Target cells can be visualized by light microscopy and manual selection can be done	1. Slow 2. Low resolution of the histogram
Ki67 scoring	Ki67 antigen is expressed in proliferating cells	G_1, S and G_2 phase	1. Easy 2. Reproducible 3. Short half-life of the antigen, so accurate	1. Strict measuring criteria are needed
MCM	Initiating protein complex of DNA replication that binds with origin of replication	Proliferating cells	1. Easy 2. Reliable marker as the protein is stable throughout the cell proliferation 3. Better than Ki67	1. No major disadvantage
DNA precursor base incorporation: BrDU incorporation	BrDu is picked up by proliferating cells in S phase and later can be stained by immunohistochemistry	S phase cell is measured	1. Gold standard. As it is very accurate and reliable	1. Not possible in routine life to apply in clinical cases

(BrDU: Bromodeoxyuridine; AgNOR: Silver stained nucleolar organizer region count).

- Hairy extension from the side
- Surrounding basophilic cytoplasm instead of eosinophilia.

Mitosis count is more predictable and reliable on histology section than cytology smear. Mitosis in tumor can be counted as number of mitotic figures per 10 high power fields. However, the field of vision may vary from microscope to microscopes. Therefore, it is better to express the mitosis count as number of mitotic figures per 1,000 cells (mitotic index).

Advantage

- Easy and more or less reliable.

Disadvantages

- Mitotic activity may vary depending on the fixation of the tissue. If the tissue is not fixed immediately then the cell may complete its mitosis and the mitotic count may be low.
- Many other things may simulate mitotic figures such as apoptotic cell, mast cells, degenerated lymphocytes, etc. and mitotic count should be done carefully.

Incorporation Technique

This is based on the incorporation of the labeled nucleotide analogs (tritiated thymidine or bromodeoxyuridine).[14] The proliferating cells incorporate the labeled nucleotide analog during DNA synthesis. This can be demonstrated by autoradiography in case of radioactive thymidine and immunohistochemistry in case of bromodeoxyuridine.[15]

Disadvantages

Clinical utility of incorporation techniques is limited. Radioactive thymidine has radioactive hazards. However, presently radioactive thymidine is totally replaced by bromodeoxyuridine which can be stained by immunohistochemistry.

DNA Flow Cytometry and Image Cytometry

DNA histogram in DNA FCM helps in the identification of the population of G_0/G_1, S phase and G_2/M phase cells.[16] Similarly, image cytometry (ICM) also produces histogram that can help to assess the different population of cells in cell cycle.[17] In case of DNA FCM and ICM, a stoichiometric dye is used which binds with DNA depending on its amount. The amount of staining is measured, which indicates relative DNA content of the nucleus. The cells in G_0/G_1 phases contain diploid amount (2n) of DNA and cells in G_2/M phases contain tetraploid (4n) amount of DNA. S phase cells contain diploid to tetraploid amount of DNA (2n to 4n).

Advantages

DNA flow cytometry can rapidly analyze large population of cells and therefore gives better resolution of the histogram and reliable result.

Disadvantages

- The specific population of tumor cell is not visible in DNA FCM and therefore it gives the result of all cells including vascular endothelial cells and stromal cells.
- This is more sophisticated and costly technique.

Immunohistochemistry

There are various proliferation related antigens to measure cell proliferation.

Proliferating Cell Nuclear Antigen

Proliferating cell nuclear antigen (PCNA) was once popular cell proliferation marker. PCNA is related with the initiation of DNA replication and cell proliferation.[18] Its concentration within the cell is transcriptionally regulated and the concentration of PCNA increases from resting cell to proliferating cell. There is progressive increase of PCNA in advanced G_1 and S phase cells. This is followed by decreased level of PCNA in G_2 and M phase of cells. There is prolonged half-life of PCNA and therefore it may be demonstrated even the cells in G_0 phase.[19] PCNA has three important functions:

1. *DNA replication:* It coordinates the synthesis of leading and lagging strand of DNA and also recruits various DNA replicating enzymes.
2. *DNA repair:* PCNA helps in nucleotide excision repair (NER) and mismatch repair (MMR) of DNA.
3. *Cell cycle control:* PCNA binds with S phase specific cyclin-CDK complex and promotes the cell to proliferate.

Advantage

Prolifteration cell nuclear antigen (PCNA) immunostain can be done in paraffin embedded material.

Disadvantages

- The correlation between PCNA score and Ki67 labeling index is poor.[20]
- PCNA is not cell proliferation specific and is involved in DNA repair as mentioned earlier.[21] It is better to avoid PCNA as cell proliferation marker in cytology/histology.

Ki67

The name Ki67 is derived from Kiel University, Germany, and the number 67 refers to the clone number on the 96-well plate.[22] Ki67 antigen is the most potent antigen to detect proliferating cells. The gene of Ki67 antigen is present in chromosome 10. The Ki67 is expressed in proliferating cells in G_1, S and G_2 phase of the cell cycle. Ki67 is specifically not expressed in G_0 and early G1 phase. The exact function of Ki67 is still unknown. It probably helps in ribosomal RNA (rRNA) synthesis and also maintenance of the mitotic spindle.

Originally Ki67 immunostaining was only possible in frozen sections; however, at present days, other Ki67 monoclonal antibody (MIB-1) works on formalin fixed paraffin section and is reproducible and reliable (Fig. 2.11).

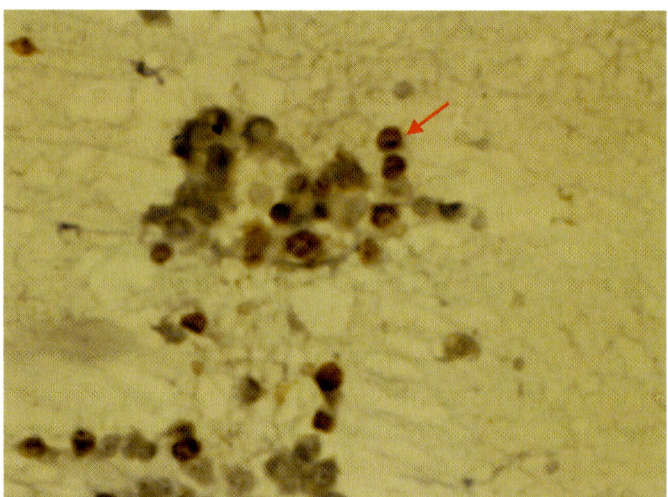

Fig. 2.11: Ki67 immunostaining on cytology cell block section. Red arrow indicates Ki67 positive cell (Ki67 immunostain × MP).

Advantages

- Ki67 is considered as the best proliferation markers for application in routine use.
- It is an important prognostic marker of various malignancies. Ki67 level above 10–14% indicates high-risk group in term of prognosis.

Disadvantage

Proper Ki67 scoring (percentage of Ki67 positive cell) is important for exact evaluation of cell proliferation.

MCM 2–7

MCM proteins are group of proteins that are responsible for maintenance of minichromosome. MCM proteins are important in the initiation of DNA replication and elongation of replication. In this MCM family there are total six proteins MCM 2 to MCM 7. They combine with each other and make a heterohexameric structure. As mentioned earlier, MCM proteins along with ORC, Cdt1 and Cdc6 make a complex structure in the origin of replication of DNA. This complex gives license to initiation of DNA replication.

Advantages

- The MCM 2–7 proteins are the reliable markers of proliferating cells because the quiescent cells do not express this marker.
- MCM is a good prognostic marker and well correlated with histological grade and lymph node metastasis of cancer.

Nucleolar Organizing Regions

Nucleolar organizing regions (NORs) are the segments of DNA on the short arm of acrocentric chromosomes 13, 14, 15, 21 and 22. NOR encode genes for r-RNA, and various proteins for cell proliferation.[23]

The transcriptionally active NORs have argyrophilic proteins and therefore can be demonstrated by silver (Ag) staining technique. So the term AgNOR has been developed. AgNOR assessment is intimately related with rate of cell proliferation.

Advantage

Easy technique to measure cell proliferation.

Disadvantages

- Noncycling cell may also synthesize protein and may show AgNORs. Therefore baseline AgNOR score measurement is needed.
- AgNOR scoring may vary depending on thickness of the section.

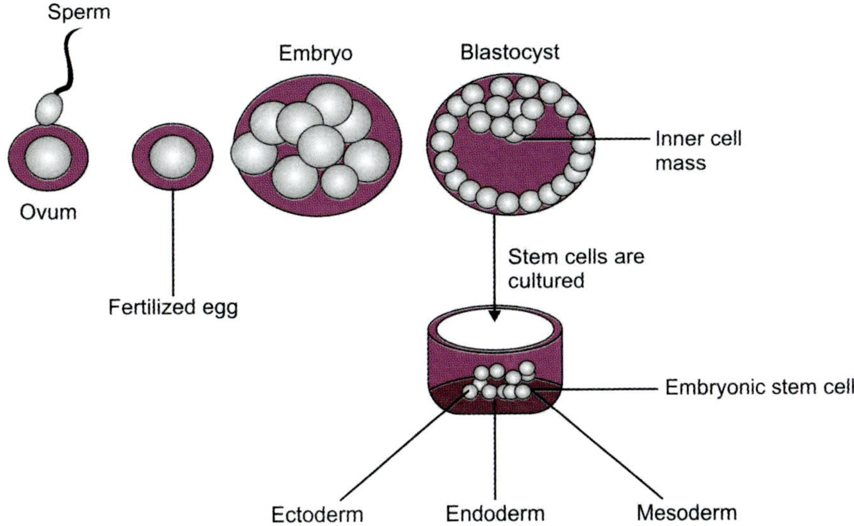

Fig. 2.12: Schematic diagram of embryonic stem cells derived from the inner cell mass of the blastocyst.

STEM CELL

Stem cells are reserve cell population that give rise to various differentiated cells and also maintain the damaged cell population. The body maintains a homoeostasis between the stem cell and the differentiated cells and therefore these cells are essential for the tissue regeneration and repair. Stem cells are specialized cells characterized by three unique properties:[24]

1. *Asymmetric cell division*: Here the cell divides into two daughter cells and one of them goes to the stem cell pool and the other one is differentiated.
2. *Self-renewal*: The cell divides and maintains the overall number.
3. *Differentiation to more specialized cells*: The stem cells have the capability to differentiate into more differentiated cell with specific function.

Stem cells may be classified as:

- Embryonic stem cells (ESC)
- Non-embryonic stem cells: Adult stem cells.

Embryonic Stem Cells

Embryonic stem cells are the pluripotent stem cells (Fig. 2.12). The inner cell mass of the blastocyst produces ESC. The inner cell mass can be removed from the blastocyst and the cells can be grown in the laboratory. ESC gives rise to all embryonic germ layers: ectoderm, endoderm and mesoderm.

Table 2.3: Embryonic stem cell markers.

Type of markers	*Markers proper*
Cell surface markers	CD117 (c-KIT, SCFR), CD 324 (E-Cadherin), CD29 (β1 integrin), CD 31
Transcription factors	Oct-3/4, Sox2, Nanog
Signal pathway-related intracellular markers	SMAD1/5/8, SMAD4, β-catenin
Enzymatic markers	Alkaline phosphatase and telomerase

Somatic cell nuclear transfer (SCNT): It is an alternative method to develop ESC. The transfer of the postmitotic cell into an unfertilized, enucleated oocyte may develop ESC.

The markers of the embryonic stem cell (Table 2.3): The markers of embryonic stem cell include:

- Isozyme of alkaline phosphatase
- Transcription factor Oct4, nanog
- High telomerase activity
- A variety of cell-surface markers recognized by monoclonal antibodies to stage-specific embryonic antigens.[25]

Non-embryonic Stem Cell: Adult Stem Cell

Adult stem cells are found in the adult organ and they are in close association with differentiated cells. The cells are usually committed and give rise to more specialized, differentiated cells. Adult stem cells are mainly hematopoietic stem cells (HSC) and mesenchymal stem cells (MSC). They are also found in liver, skin, muscle, and brain.

Different Types of Adult Stem Cell

- *Hematopoietic stem cells*: HSCs are present in the hematopoietic organs. They have the capacity of self-renewal and also to differentiate into adult blood cell. These cells are round with enlarged nuclei and morphologically difficult to distinguish from lymphocytes. The cells are positive for CD34, CD133, aldehyde dehydrogenase, low positive for Thy 1, and c-kit and negative for CD33, CD38, B and T cell markers.
- *Mesenchymal stem cells*: MSCs are non-hematopoietic stromal cells. They can differentiate into various mesenchymal tissues such as muscle, cartilage, bone and adipose tissue. The cells express CD105, CD106, CD44, CD71, CD73, CD90 and do not express the hematopoietic markers like CD45, CD13, CD11 or CD14.

Implications of Stem Cells

- *Hematological diseases*: Stem cells are used both in nonmalignant and malignant hematological diseases to replace the bone marrow by healthy cells. Stem cell therapy may be used in—(a) hematological malignancies such as acute leukemia, plasma cell disorder and myelodysplastic syndrome; (b) inherited metabolic disorders such as metachromatic leukodystrophy, osteopetrosis; (c) inherited red cell disorders such as pure red cell aplasia, sickle cell disease, thalassemia, etc.; (d) bone marrow failure syndrome such as aplastic anemia.
- *Clinical trial*: Stem cell therapy may be used in ischemic heart disease, nonunion of fractured bone, Parkinson disease, spinal cord lesions, etc.
- *Other uses*: Generation of disease model and preserving endangered animals.

REFERENCES

1. Orlando DA, Lin CY, Bernard A, et al. Global control of cell-cycle transcription by coupled CDK and network oscillators. Nature. 2008;453(7197):944-7.
2. Morgan DO. Principles of CDK regulation. Nature. 1995;374:131-4.
3. Pines J. Cyclins and cyclin-dependent kinases: a biochemical view. Biochem J. 1995;308:697-711.
4. Murray AW. Recycling the cell cycle: cyclins revisited. Cell. 2004;116:221-34.
5. Musacchio A, Salmon ED. The spindle-assembly checkpoint in space and time. Nat Rev Mol Cell Biol. 2007;8(5):379-93.
6. Hirai H, Roussel MF, Kato J, et al. Novel INK4 proteins, p19 and p18, are specific inhibitors of the cyclin D-dependent kinases CDK4 and CDK6. Mol Cell Biol. 1995;15:2672-81.
7. Sherr CJ. Cancer cell cycles. Science (Washington DC). 1996;274:1672-7.
8. Williams GH, Stoeber K. The cell cycle and cancer. J Pathol. 2012;226:352-64.
9. Malumbres M, Barbacid M. Milestones in cell division: to cycle or not to cycle: a critical decision in cancer. Nat Rev Cancer. 2001;1(3):222-31.
10. Honeycutt KA, Chen Z, Koster MI, et al. Deregulated minichromosomal maintenance protein MCM7 contributes to oncogene driven tumorigenesis. Oncogene. 2006;25:4027-32.
11. Bakkenist CJ, Kastan MB. DNA damage activates ATM through intermolecular autophosphorylation and dimer dissociation. Nature. 2003;421:499-506.
12. Juríková M, Danihel Ľ, Polák Š, et al. Ki67, PCNA, and MCM proteins: Markers of proliferation in the diagnosis of breast cancer. Acta Histochem. 2016;118(5):544-52.
13. Baak JP. Mitosis counting in tumors. Hum Pathol. 1990; 21:683-5.
14. Taylor JH. Chromosome reproduction. Int Rev Cytol. 1962; 13:39-44.
15. Meyer JS, Nauert J, Kohem S, et al. Cell kinetics of human tumors by in vitro bromodeoxyuridine labeling. J Histochem Cytochem. 1989;37:1449-54.
16. Dey P. Flow cytometry review. J Cytol. 2003;20(1):10-4.
17. Dey P, Luthra UK, Sheikh ZA, et al. Cytological grading and DNA Image cytometry of breast carcinomas on fine needle aspiration cytology smears. Anal Quant Cytol Histol. 1999;21:17-20.
18. Garcia JE, Celis A. Cell-cycle dependent variations in the distribution of the nuclear protein cyclin proliferating cell nuclear antigen in cultured cells: subdivision in S-phase. Proc Nad Acad Sci USA. 1985;82:3262-6.
19. Bravo R, MacDonald-Bravo H. Existence of two populations of cyclin/proliferation cell nuclear antigen during the cell cycle: association with DNA replication sites. J Cell Biol. 1987;105:1549-54.
20. Leonardi E, Girlando S, Serio G, et al. PCNA and Ki67 expression in breast carcinoma: correlations with clinical and biological variables. J Clin Pathol. 1992;45(5):416-9.
21. Hall PA, Levison DA, Woods AL, et al. Proliferating cell nuclear antigen (PCNA) immunolocalization in paraffin sections: an index of cell proliferation with evidence of deregulated expression in some neoplasms. J Pathol. 1990;162:285-94.
22. Gerdes J, Schwab U, Lemke H, et al. Production of a mouse monoclonal antibody reactive with a human nuclear antigen associated with cell proliferation. Int J Cancer. 1983;31:13-20.
23. Mourad WA, Connelly JH, Sembera DL, et al. The comparison of two argyrophilic nucleolar organizer region counting methods with bromodeoxyuridine labeling index: a study of metastatic tumors of the brain. Hum Pathol 1993;24:206-10.
24. Blau HM, Brazelton TR, Weimann JM. The evolving concept of a stem cell: entity or function? Cell. 2001;105(7):829-41.
25. Zhao W, Ji X, Zhang F, et al. Embryonic stem cell markers. Molecules. 2012;17(6):6196-236.

Review Questions

1. **All are true for crossing over except:**
   a. The double stranded DNA breaks into single strand
   b. In the cross over region DNA breaks in both the non-sister chromatids
   c. Exchange of genetic information occurs
   d. It happens in zygotene phase of meiosis I
2. **All are true about the location of the cell cycle restriction points except:**
   a. At the beginning of S phase
   b. Near the end point of G_1 phase
   c. At the junction of G_2 and M phase
   d. In the M phase at the junction of metaphase and anaphase
3. **Which one is the most reliable cell proliferation marker?**
   a. Ki67
   b. PCNA
   c. AgNOR
   d. Image cytometry
4. **Which one is not the marker of stem cell?**
   a. CD117
   b. Sox2
   c. Nanog
   d. MCM 2–7
5. **The most important characteristic of stem cell is:**
   a. Self-renewal
   b. Symmetric cell division
   c. Unable to differentiate further
   d. Stem cells are not seen in adult organ

Identify True/False

6. **S phase contains variable amount of DNA from 2n to 4n.** *(True/False)*
7. **In mitosis the two sister chromatids are separated in telophase.** *(True/False)*
8. **Cross over occurs in Zygotene phase of Meiosis I.** *(True/False)*
9. **INK 4 proteins inhibit cyclin D-CDK and thereby accumulate hypophosphorylated Rb.** *(True/False)*
10. **Mdm2, the ubiquitin ligase, destroys its target pRb protein.** *(True/False)*

Answers

1. d. It happens in Zygotene phase of meiosis I
2. d. In the M phase at the junction of metaphase and anaphase
3. a. Ki 67
4. d. MCM 2-7
5. a. Self-renewal
6. True
7. False
8. False
9. True
10. False

CHAPTER

3 Cellular Reaction to Injury and Cell Death

INTRODUCTION

Various external and internal stimuli can cause cell injury. These injurious stimuli may be gross external or from intricate molecular level. The different causes of cell injury have been highlighted in Box 3.1.

In response to various stresses individual cell responses variedly. The exact cellular responses to stress are determined by: type of stress, intensity, and duration of injury or stress (Fig. 3.1). The cell initially tries to maintain a steady state called homeostasis. If the stress or injury to the cell is more, the cell takes an adaptive state such as the number of the cells may be increased or decreased or the cell may change its type. If the cells fail to adapt to the increased stress or if there is acute internal or external stimuli, the cells undergo injury. Cellular injury may be reversible or irreversible. In case of irreversible injury, the cell dies which is the ultimate fate of any cell.

CELLULAR ADAPTATION

The various types of cellular adaptations are (Fig. 3.1):

- Hyperplasia
- Hypertrophy
- Atrophy
- Metaplasia.

Box 3.1: Different causes of cell injury.

- *Inherited stress*:
  - *Genetic defects*: Inborn errors of metabolism, chromosomal abnormalities, etc.
- *Acquired stress*:
  - *Hypoxia*: Loss of vascular supply or less oxygen carrying capacity of blood
  - *Physical agents*: Heat, cold, electrical injury, radiation effect, pressure effect
  - *Chemical agents and drugs*: Different chemical poisons, insecticides, drugs, etc.
  - *Nutritional causes*: Nutritional imbalances, such as protein calorie malnutrition, hyperlipidemia, vitamin deficiency, etc.
  - *Infectious agents*: Virus, bacteria, parasites, etc.
  - *Immunological diseases*: Autoimmune diseases, inborn immune disorder

Hyperplasia

The term "hyperplasia" indicates increase in number of cells in a tissue or organ. This causes an overall increase of volume or weight of the tissue due to cell proliferation. Hyperplasia occurs when the cells are capable of synthesizing their deoxyribonucleic acid (DNA) and are able to replicate. Hyperplasia is usually caused due to: (a) increased growth factors, (b) increased growth factor receptors, or (c) increased intracellular signaling (Fig. 3.1). At times, the stem cells may also proliferate to take part in hyperplasia.

Hyperplasia often gives rise to neoplastic proliferation, particularly in case of atypical hyperplasia.

- *Physiological hyperplasia*: This type of hyperplasia occurs due to hormonal or growth factor stimulation.

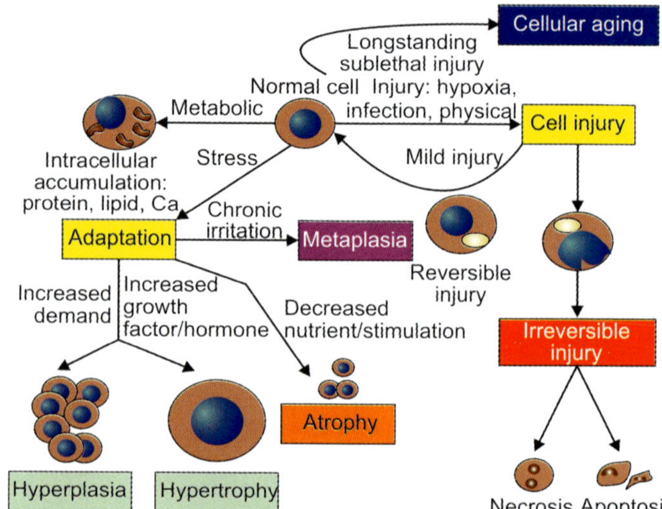

Fig. 3.1: Schematic diagram showing different types of cell responses to injury.

The physiological hyperplasia is seen in breast enlargement in puberty or progenitors of red cell hyperplasia in acute blood loss.

- *Pathological hyperplasia*: This may occur due to the excessive hormonal stimulation or growth factors in pathological condition. The pathological hyperplasia is seen in endometrial hyperplasia due to excessive estrogen. The cases of pathological hyperplasia may undergo neoplastic changes.

Hypertrophy

The term "hypertrophy" indicates increase in volume of the cell leading to increase in organ size. No cellular proliferation occurs in case of hypertrophy. The individual cells may be larger in size with enlarged nuclei. Hypertrophy occurs due to following factors: (1) increased growth factors, e.g. fibroblast growth factor, (2) increased vasoactive agents such as endothelin-1, angiotensin-II, and (3) mechanical stretch due to increased workload.

Hypertrophy is difficult to assess by light microscopy on cytology smears.

Atrophy

Atrophy means reduction of the number of cells leading to shrinkage of tissue or organ. The causes of atrophy may be variable such as inadequate nutrition, loss of endocrine stimulation, loss of innervations, decreased workload, pressure effect or aging. By light microscopy, epithelial atrophy can be recognized on a cytology smear such as atrophic cellular pattern on cervical cytology.

Metaplasia

Metaplasia is a reversible change characterized by the change of one type of mature cell type to another mature cell type. This replaced epithelium may better resist the adverse circumstances. The most common epithelial metaplasia is columnar to squamous metaplasia. This may be noted in the squamocolumnar junction of the cervix or in endocervical glands (Fig. 3.2), in the bronchial respiratory lining epithelium, in the salivary excretory duct. Metaplasia from squamous to columnar epithelium may occur in Barrett's esophagus which is a known precancerous condition.

In case of metaplasia, the stem cell is reprogrammed to develop a different type of tissue rather than the change of phenotypic expression of the mature epithelium. Possibly one tissue-specific gene becomes off and the other tissue-specific gene becomes on.

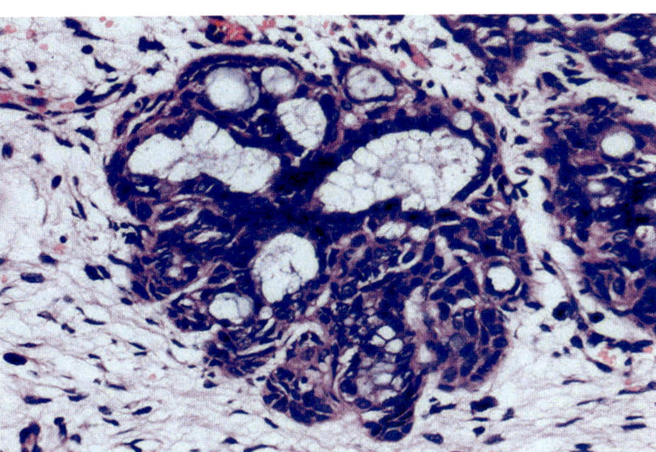

Fig. 3.2: Squamous metaplasia of endocervical glands (hematoxylin and Eosin X MP).

REVERSIBLE CELL INJURY

When a cell faces stress or acute stimulation, which is beyond the limit of adaption, the cell suffers injury. If the acute assault is withdrawn in a short period of time then the cell restores its structure and function. However, it is still unknown at which point reversible injury will go to "the point of no return" or irreversible pathway.

Morphological Changes of Reversible Injury

The morphological changes of reversible injury are difficult to recognize by light microscope. However the following changes may be visible:

- *Cytoplasmic vacuoles*: Single to multiple small vacuoles may be seen within the cytoplasm. These vacuoles are the distended part of endoplasmic reticulum
- Increased eosinophilic cytoplasm.

By electron microscopy, the following changes are seen:

- Blunting, distortion, and loss of microvilli of plasma membrane
- Dilatation of endoplasmic reticulum
- Swelling of mitochondria
- Disaggregation of fibrillar and granular components of the nucleolus.

IRREVERSIBLE CELL INJURY

The ultimate fate of all cells is death. The cell death can be divided into two basic forms: (1) programmed cell death

(PCD) and (2) accidental cell death by necrosis. The PCD is now classified as type I (apoptosis), type II (autophagy), and type III (programmed necrosis).[1]

For a long time, the term "apoptosis" was used as a general term to describe PCD and the concept of non-apoptotic PCD was deliberately ignored. Due to the advancement of molecular technology, other forms of non-apoptotic PCD is getting increased attention.

- Type I PCD or apoptosis is critically important for the developmental morphogenesis, tissue homeostasis, and defense against pathogens. It is a highly conserved phenomenon both genetically and also biochemically.
- Type II PCD (autophagic cell death) is a major cellular catabolic pathway. It helps to degrade proteins and cytoplasmic organelles. Thus autophagic PCD helps in maintenance of proteins and cytoplasmic organelles and enhances cell survival. It occurs in tissue and cell remodeling, starvation, and cell death.
- Type III PCD (programmed necrosis) is a passive process that affects the cells by combined use of selected effectors along with other cell death factors. It is called as programmed necrotic death because the cellular signaling pathways lead to necrosis in response to specific effectors rather than by simple accident.

Apoptosis or Type I Programmed Cell Death

The word "apoptosis" is taken from the Greek language. "Apo" means from and "ptosis" means fall. So "apoptosis" indicates "leaves falling from a tree". Apoptosis is a type of suicidal death and it is distinctly different than necrosis (Table 3.1). The predominant biochemical events in apoptosis are activation of intracellular proteases and step ladder type of fragmentation of internucleosomal DNA. The various cell surface molecules are altered in the apoptotic cells resulting in instant identification and phagocytosis of them by neighboring cells. This orderly elimination of the apoptotic cells prevents any inflammatory reaction.

Morphology of Apoptosis

Apoptosis typically occurs in individual cells without any surrounding inflammatory reactions. The following morphologic changes are noted in apoptotic cells[2] (Box 3.2).

Nucleus (Figs. 3.3 and 3.4)

- The chromatin becomes pyknotic. It condenses and aggregates in the inner surface of the nuclear envelope. This often gives half-moon or sickle-like appearance of the chromatin.
- In most of the cases, nuclear outline becomes convoluted.
- Severe nuclear convolution causes multiple budding and nuclear fragments of different sizes (budding phenomenon).

Box 3.2: Morphological changes of apoptosis.

- Nuclear changes:
  - Chromatin condensation and aggregation
  - Nuclear convolution and multiple budding
  - Nuclear fragments are covered by double layer of membrane
- Cytoplasmic changes:
  - Cytoplasm condenses
  - Extensive protrusion of the cell surface
  - The protuberance of the cell surface is separated and sealed by the plasma membrane

Table 3.1: Distinguishing points between apoptosis and necrosis.

Features	*Apoptosis*	*Necrosis*
Energy	Active process and energy is required	Passive process and no ATP is required
Nucleus	Condensed peripheral chromatin	Fragmented chromatin
Cell size	Cell shrinkage	Cell swollen
Death pattern	Single cell death	Group of cells dye
Inflammatory response	No inflammation	Inflammation
DNA fragmentation	Regular internucleosomal 180 bp length	Irregular fragments
Cell membrane	Preserved membrane	Fragmented membrane

(DNA: Deoxyribonucleic acid; bp: Base pairs; ATP: Adenosine triphosphate).

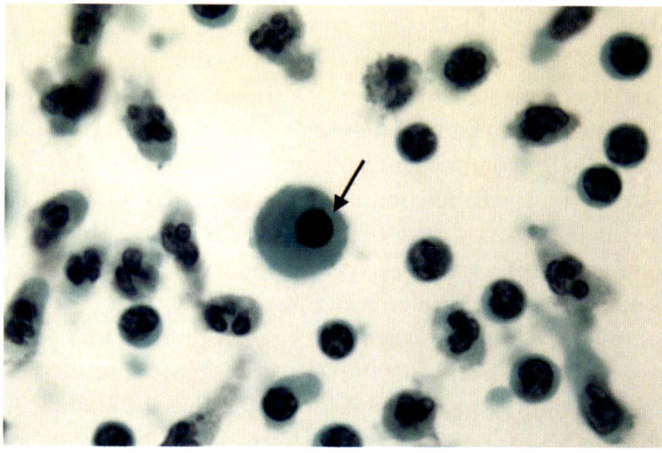

Fig. 3.3: Cell with moderate amount of cytoplasm and dense nucleus in case of an apoptotic cell (*see* arrow) (Papanicolaou's stain × HP).

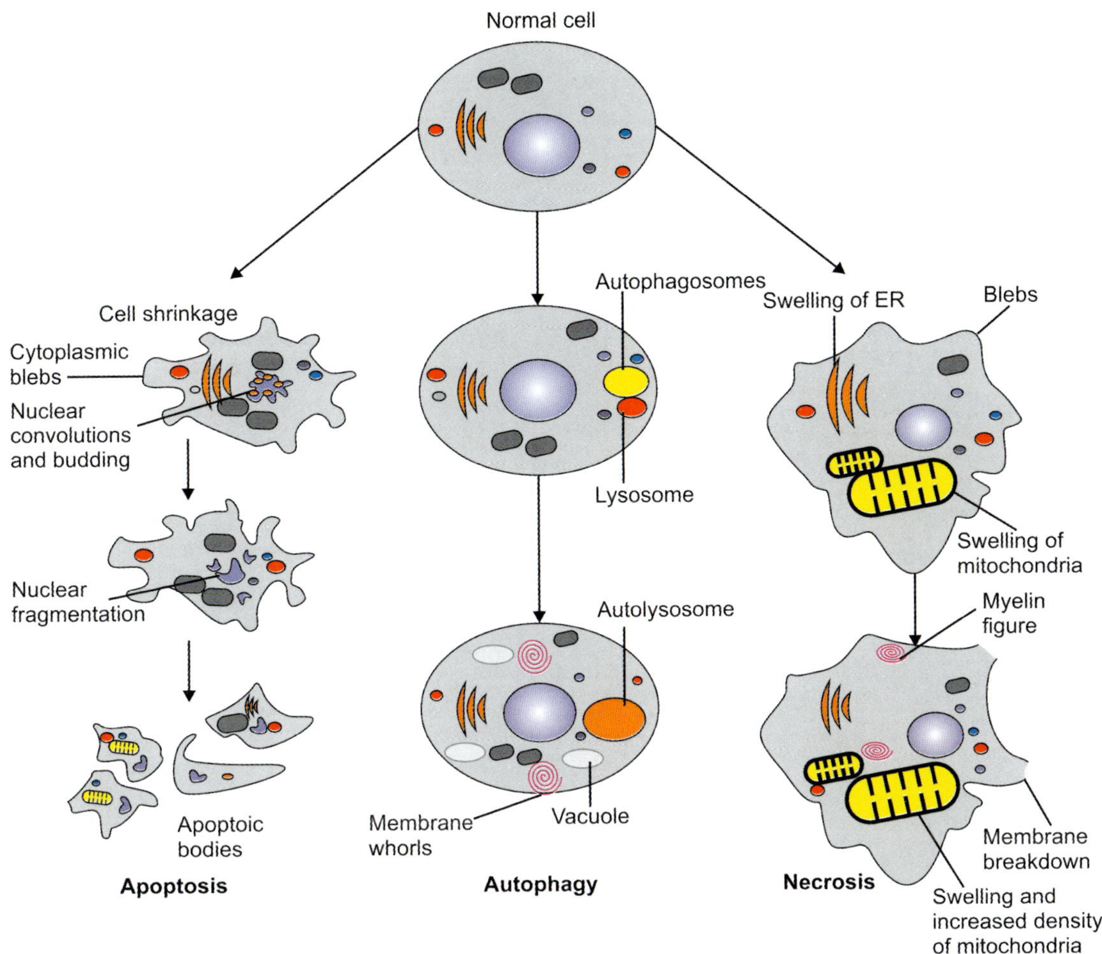

Fig. 3.4: Schematic diagram showing morphological changes in apoptosis, autophagy, and necrosis.

- Each nuclear fragment is covered by a double layer of membrane.

Cytoplasm

- Cytoplasm condenses and extensive protrusion or blebbing appears on the cell surface.
- Numerous clear vacuoles appear in the cytoplasm.
- The protuberance on the cell surface is separated and sealed by the plasma membrane forming multiple membrane-bound apoptotic bodies.
- There is no swelling of mitochondria.

The macrophages instantly phagocytose and destroy the apoptotic bodies. During the process of degradation the apoptotic bodies can be visualized if the cell contains remarkable condensed chromatin. Overall tissue architecture is not disturbed in the apoptotic process as there is death of single isolated cells.

Molecular Pathways of Apoptosis[3] *(Box 3.3)*

The molecular pathways of apoptosis are:

- Death receptor pathway
- Mitochondrial pathway.

These pathways are activated in different conditions and they may also intersect with each other.

- *Death receptor pathway (Fig. 3.5)*: Death receptors receive the various extracellular death signals and then switch on the apoptotic pathway of cell death. Death receptors are the members of tumor necrosis factor (TNF) receptors (TNFRs) gene superfamily and are located on the cell surface. There are two parts of death receptor, an intracytoplasmic domain known as "death domain" and cysteine-rich extracellular domain. The "death domain" plays an important role to trigger intracellular apoptotic machinery. The most well-known death receptors are CD95 [also called Fas or Apo-1 (apoptosis antigen 1)], type 1 TNFR (TNFR1), TRAIL1, and TRAIL 2. The ligands that activate these receptors are structurally related molecules. CD95 ligand (CD95L) binds to CD95; TNF and lymphotoxin alpha bind to TNFR1. When Fas ligand binds with the Fas receptors then several molecules of Fas cluster in that particular site and they recruit the adaptor protein FAS-associated death domain (FADD). This FADD protein further activates caspase 8 and this subsequently activates the caspase 3, the main executioner enzyme. This activated caspase 3 cleaves the various substrates.

- *Mitochondrial pathway*[4] *(Fig. 3.5)*: BCL-2 group of proteins have important role in the mitochondrial pathway of apoptosis. Increased intracellular reactive oxygen species, DNA damage or other intracellular factors initiate this pathway by inhibiting anti-apoptotic proteins BCL-2/BCl-x. The decrease level of BCL-2/BCl-x is replaced by proapoptotic proteins Bak, Bax, and Bim. The multiple stimuli such as proapoptotic proteins (Bak, Bax, and Bim), Ca^{++} overload, oxidants, and active caspases increase mitochondrial membrane permeability and release caspase activation protein cytochrome c (CytoC) and apoptosis inducing factor (AIF) from the mitochondria to the cytoplasm. CytoC binds with apoptosis activating factor (APAF-1) that further helps in activation of caspase 9 and initiates the proteolytic cascade resulting to apoptosis.[4]

Box 3.3: Molecular pathway of apoptosis.

Death receptor pathway:
- Death receptor:
  - Intracytoplasmic domain (death domain)
  - Cysteine-rich extracellular domain
  - Cluster of differentiation 95 (CD95) [FAS or Apo-1 (apoptosis antigen 1)]
  - Type 1 tumor necrosis factor (TNF) receptor (TNFR1)
- CD95 ligand binds to CD95; TNF binds to TNFR1
- Binding of death receptor with the ligand recruits the adaptor protein FADD (FAS-associated death domain)
- FADD protein further recruits caspase 8 and this subsequently activates the caspase 3

Mitochondrial pathway:
- Increased intracellular reactive oxygen species, DNA damage or other intracellular factors inhibit anti-apoptotic proteins B-cell lymphoma 2 (BCL-2)/BCl-x
- Increased proapoptotic proteins Bak, Bax, and Bim.
- Increased mitochondrial membrane permeability releases cytochrome c.
- Activation of caspase 9.

Final phase:
- Caspase 8 and caspase 9 subsequently activate the caspase 3 which act as executioner enzyme.

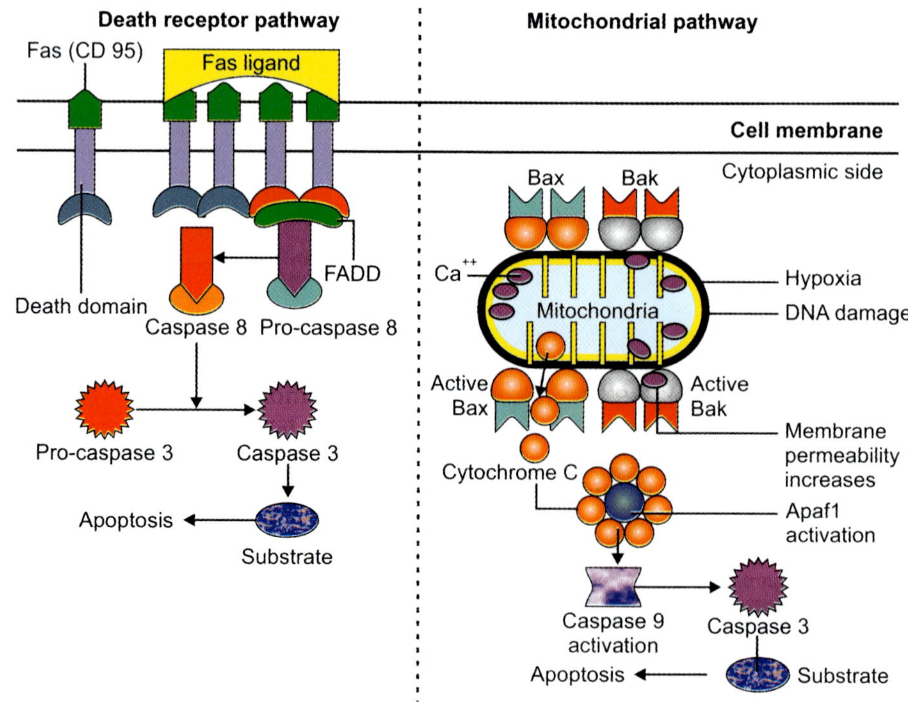

Fig. 3.5: Schematic diagram showing mechanism of death receptor pathway of apoptosis and mitochondrial pathway of apoptosis.

Table 3.2: BCL-2 family of proteins.

Type	*Proteins*	*Function*
Anti-apoptotic	BCL-2, BCL-XL, BCLW, MCL1, A1/BFL 1, BOO/DIVA	Maintain the permeability of outer mitochondrial membrane
Proapoptotic	BaX, BaK, BOK/MTD, BCL-X_S	Following death stimulation the monomeric protein dimerize and open the mitochondrial channel to release death induced protein cytochrome-C
BH 3 only (sensors)	BID, BAD, BIM, BLK, NIP 3, HRK, NIX	These sensor proteins recognize the cellular stress and DNA damage. They balance anti- and proapoptotic proteins

BCL-2 Family[5] (Table 3.2)

The mitochondrial pathway is mainly controlled by BCL-2 family of proteins. The gene of BCL-2 was identified in follicular lymphoma where it inhibits apoptosis of lymphoid cells. The family of BCL-2 has both proapoptotic and anti-apoptotic members.

Prosurvival (anti-apoptotic) members: These groups of proteins contain four BCL-2 homology (BH) domains. BCL-2, BCL-XL, BCLW, MCL1, A1, and BOO/DIVA are six prosurvival members of BCL-2 family. These proteins remain in the outer mitochondrial membrane and also other membrane such as endoplasmic reticulum. They combine with the proapoptotic proteins to prevent death. These six proteins maintain the permeability of the outer mitochondrial membrane and thereby prevent the leakage of the CytoC and other death induced proteins.

Proapoptotic members: Bax and Bak are the two principal proapoptotic proteins. After activation by death signal, these proteins oligomerize and make a channel in the outer mitochondrial membrane. The increased permeability of the membrane releases death promoter factors (CytoC, Ca^{++}) from the mitochondria to cytoplasm.

BH3 only (sensors): These groups of proteins contain only one BH domain (BH 3). The members of this group are BID, BAD, BIM, BLK, NIP 3, etc. These proteins act as sensors of stress or DNA damage in the cell and maintain delicate balance between the pro- and anti-apoptotic proteins.

Final Phase and Biochemical Changes (Box 3.4)

Activated caspase 8 generated from the death receptor pathway and activated caspase 9 generated from the mitochondrial pathway both ultimately mobilize caspase 3, 6 and 7 proteases.[3] These executioner caspases act on numerous cellular components.

Box 3.4: Biochemical pathway of apoptosis.

Proteins breakdown:
- Activated caspases (particularly caspase 3) cleave:
  - Cytoskeletal proteins
  - Nuclear matrix proteins
  - Proteins involved in DNA transcription, replication and repair

DNA breaks down:
- Caspase 3 activates the cytoplasmic DNase and breaks internucleosomal DNA into segments into multiples of 185 bp.

Phagocytosis:
- The caspase produces the loss of phospholipid asymmetry and the exposure of phosphatidylserine (PtdSer) on the plasma membrane
- PtdSer acts as a ligand for the scavenger receptors (SR) of macrophages
- The interaction between SR and PtdSer helps in phagocytosis

Protein breakdown: Activated caspases (particularly caspase 3) cleave various proteins such as cytoskeletal proteins, nuclear matrix proteins and proteins involved in DNA transcription, replication and repair.

DNA breakdown: Caspase 3 activates the cytoplasmic DNase which characteristically breaks internucleosomal DNA into segments that are multiples of approximately 185 bp (base pairs). This step ladder type of fragments of DNA can be demonstrated by gel electrophoresis.

Removal of the apoptotic bodies: The macrophages readily phagocytose the apoptotic bodies to prevent the release of potentially noxious or immunogenic materials from the apoptotic cells and initiation of inflammation. The apoptotic cells express certain unique signals to the phagocytes so that the phagocytes recognize the apoptotic bodies. The caspase activity in the apoptotic process causes certain changes in the plasma membrane such as the loss of phospholipid asymmetry and the exposure of phosphatidylserine (PtdSer) on the outer surface of the plasma membrane.[6] PtdSer acts as a ligand for the scavenger receptors (SR) of macrophages and the interaction between SR and PtdSer helps in phagocytosis of the apoptotic body. The phagocytosed apoptotic bodies are digested further by lysosomal enzymes of the phagocytes.

Apoptosis in Physiological Conditions

The apoptosis occurs in various physiological conditions:

- *Embryogenesis*: Apoptosis takes part key role in embryogenesis by the programmed death of specific cell type during the time and spatial level.

- *Homeostasis of the cell population*: Apoptosis maintains the total amount of viable functioning cells by deletion of the cells.
- *Hormone-dependent involution*: Apoptosis plays key role in the hormone-dependent regression in various organs such as regression of ovarian follicles, prostate shrinkage after testicular removal, etc.
- *Cell death in infection*: Apoptosis occurs as a defense mechanism by cytotoxic T cells during viral infection.
- *Prevention of autoimmunity*: With the help of apoptosis, the autoreactive lymphocytes are eliminated from the body.

Apoptosis in Diseases (Box 3.5)

There are widespread clinical implications of apoptosis as too little or too much apoptosis, both cause diseases.

Diseases associated with less apoptosis and increased cell survival:

- *Apoptosis and cancer*: Death by apoptosis plays significant defense mechanism against malignant transformation.[7] The failure of apoptosis causes uncontrolled proliferation of the cells and therefore produces the ideal environment of genetic instability and mutation. The majority of cancers, such as follicular lymphoma, breast cancer, and prostate cancer, have defects in apoptosis. The predominant defects are the overexpression of anti-apoptotic protein BCL-2 and mutation of tumor suppressor gene p53. The mutation of p53 gene causes defective p53 protein production and failure of apoptosis during DNA damage.[8]

Box 3.5: Apoptosis in diseases.

Diseases associated with less apoptosis and increased cell survival:
- *Apoptosis and cancer*: Follicular lymphoma, ovarian cancer, breast cancer, prostate cancer, etc.
- *Immunological disorders*: Autoimmunity, such as SLE, immune-mediated glomerulonephritis
- *Apoptosis in viral infection*: Herpes virus, adenovirus, etc. Virus-infected cells do not undergo apoptosis

Diseases associated with more apoptosis and decreased cell survival:
- *Virus-induced lymphocyte depletion*: In HIV infection
- *Apoptosis in neurodegenerative disorders*: Parkinson's disease, Alzheimer's disease, spinal muscular atrophy, retinitis pigmentosa, and amyotrophic lateral sclerosis
- *Apoptosis in hematological disorders*: Aplastic anemia, myelodysplastic syndromes, anemia associated with chronic disease and chronic neutropenia

(SLE: Systemic lupus erythematosus; HIV: Human immunodeficiency virus).

- *Immunological disorders*: Apoptosis removes the potentially autoreactive T and B lymphocytes during the development and also excess cells after finishing the immune response. Failure of deletion of such cells may increase the susceptibility of autoimmunity, such as systemic lupus erythematosus (SLE), immune-mediated glomerulonephritis, etc.[8]
- *Apoptosis in viral infection (herpes, adenovirus, and pox virus infection)*: Virus-infected cells undergo apoptosis and thus prevent the spread of the infection. To combat the host's defensive mechanism many viruses have developed ways to disrupt the apoptotic machinery within the infected cell.[8]

Diseases associated with more apoptosis and decreased cell survival: The various genetic and acquired conditions may cause excessive cell death by enhancing the signal for induction of apoptosis, or by decreasing the threshold of induction of apoptosis.

- *Virus-induced lymphocyte depletion*: In acquired immunodeficiency syndrome (AIDS), the human immunodeficiency virus (HIV) infection causes selective destruction of CD4+ T lymphocytes by inducing apoptosis and destruction of the host's body defense.[9]
- *Apoptosis in neurodegenerative disorders*: The gradual loss of a specific set of neurons by apoptosis occurs in large numbers of neurodegenerative disorders, such as Parkinson's disease, Alzheimer's disease, spinal muscular atrophy, retinitis pigmentosa, and amyotrophic lateral sclerosis.[8]
- *Apoptosis in hematological disorders*: Increased apoptosis and cell destruction are related to a wide number of hematological disorders, such as aplastic anemia, myelodysplastic syndromes, anemia associated with chronic disease and chronic neutropenia.[10]

Detection of Apoptosis

There are various ways to detect apoptosis[11] (Table 3.3):

- *Light microscopy*: The apoptotic cells can be identified in light microscopy on routine Hematoxylin and Eosin stain smears or on histology sections. The apoptotic cells are small round with small condensed chromatin (*see* Fig. 3.5). No inflammatory response is seen around the apoptotic cells.
- *Electron microscopy*: The apoptotic cells are better visualized by transmission electron microscopy. The cells show extensive blebbing of plasma membrane. Subsequently small apoptotic bodies are formed with cytoplasm, condensed nuclear fragment, and cytoplasmic organelles.

Table 3.3: Different markers of apoptosis.

Name	*Principle*	*Advantage*	*Disadvantage*
Light microscopy	Morphologic visualization	Reliable and inexpensive	Quantitative measurement is less objective and nonreproducible
Electron microscopy	Detailed morphologic changes seen	• Provides extensive detailed information • Useful in biochemical and molecular studies	Very tedious and time consuming
Gel electrophoresis	DNA breaks in single and double strands in small fragments and step ladder-like pattern is characteristic	Sensitive and reliable. Comet assay gives information of individual cells	Tedious process. Cell morphology is not demonstrable
Flow cytometry (FCM)	DNA dye propidium iodide if used then a sub-diploid peak is formed by apoptotic cell	Easy and rapid. FCM gives accurate quantitation of the apoptotic cells.	Costly technique
TUNEL	The 3' OH ends of the small DNA fragments are coupled with labeled biotinylated deoxynucleotides by using DNA polymerase I or terminal deoxynucleotidyl transferase as catalyst	• Early apoptotic cells can be detected • Apoptotic cells are identified in the molecular level	Sensitivity and specificity may vary depending on fixative and concentration of terminal transferase enzyme
Immunohistochemistry	• Caspase 3 and annexin V are related with the pathogenesis of apoptosis • M30 is the neoepitope that is developed due to caspase activity	Easy to do, reliable and specific	• M30 detects only apoptotic epithelial cell. • Annexin V cannot distinguish apoptotic and necrotic cell

- *Gel electrophoresis*: In case of apoptosis, initially high molecular weight (HMW) DNA fragmentation (~300 kb) occurs. This DNA is extracted from the apoptotic cells in culture. On gel electrophoresis, step ladder-like pattern is seen in apoptosis due to internucleosomal DNA fragmentation. This pattern is not very specific for apoptosis.
  - *Conventional gel electrophoresis*: In this conventional technique, characteristic step ladder-like pattern of discontinuous DNA fragments are seen.
  - *Pulse field gel electrophoresis*: Here, alternating electric field is used to separate DNA molecules of higher range of fragment (50 kb to several Mbp).
  - *Field-inversion gel electrophoresis (FIGE)*: In this technique, periodic inversion of the electric field is used to develop higher voltage in one direction. It has the special advantage to separate DNA in different size range (100 kb to 2 Mbp).
  - *Single cell gel electrophoresis (SCGE)*: SCGE is more sophisticated and delicate technique by which one can visualize DNA damage of a single cell. This is also known as comet assay as the apoptotic cell shows a small head with extended tail. In comparison, the necrotic cell shows large nuclear head with nearly invisible tail.
- *Terminal deoxynucleotidyl transferase mediated dUTP nick end labeling (TUNEL)*: In this technique, the 3′ OH ends of the small DNA fragments are coupled with labeled biotinylated deoxynucleotides by using DNA polymerase I or terminal deoxynucleotidyl transferase as catalyst. Only the apoptotic cells incorporate the biotinylated deoxynucleotides into their DNA fragments and then are demonstrated by simple immunohistochemistry on light microscopy.[12] This technique can be done on histology section or cytology smear and the exact quantification of the apoptotic cells are possible in clinical samples.
- *Flow cytometry (FCM)*: DNA fluorochrome dye is used to stain DNA stoichiometrically. The relative DNA content of the cells is measured. The apoptotic cells contain less amount of DNA and are readily identified by FCM as hypodiploid peak or so called "sub-G1" peak in DNA histogram. Apoptotic cells take less propidium iodide (PI) dye than viable cell and they take more Hoechst 33342 dye than viable cells. Therefore, simultaneous uses of these two dyes help in the identification of apoptotic cell.

Immunohistochemistry: The apoptotic cell can be detected with the help of antibody against some specific markers of apoptosis.

Caspase 3: Caspase 3 is an important player of apoptosis. The demonstration of activated caspase 3 by immunohistochemistry is a simple and reliable marker of apoptosis.

Annexin V: Annexin V is a membrane bound protein that combines with phosphatidylserine (PS) of the membrane in calcium-dependent manner. In early part of apoptosis,

PS migrates from the inner side to outer side of the plasma membrane. Annexin V attached with this PS and can be detected in the early apoptotic cell with the help of immunohistochemistry. One important fact is to note that the annexin V preferably binds with membrane of the apoptotic cells and even the cells undergo necrosis; they are positive for annexin V. This problem can be solved by simultaneous staining of annexin V with a viable dye such as PI. Viable cells and early apoptotic cells exclude PI; however, necrotic cells retain the dye.

Healthy cell: Negative for both annexin V and PI.

Early apoptotic cell: Positive for annexin V and negative for PI.

Late apoptotic/necrotic cell: Positive for both annexin V and PI.

M30: M30 is a neoepitope of cytokeratin 18 and it appears due to caspase cleavage of the epithelial cells. M30 antibody can demonstrate epithelial apoptotic cells even in the paraffin-embedded tissue.

AUTOPHAGY (BOX 3.6)

The "Autophagy" is a Greek word. The term "Auto" means self and "phagy" means "to eat". Autophagy is a PCD by which cells recycle their own, redundant or damaged organelles.[13] This is the active physiological process by which the cells actually regain the essential substances, e.g. amino acids and fatty acids.

Box 3.6: Autophagy.

Definition: The programmed cell death by which cells recycle their own nonessential, redundant or damaged organelles.

Microautophagy: Lysosomal membrane directly engulfs cargo proteins.

Chaperone-mediated autophagy: Chaperones are utilized to capture the specific proteins to be destroyed and these proteins are transferred to lysosome.

Macroautophagy: De novo membrane bound vesicle known as "autophagosome" is formed. This fuses with lysosome to form autolysosome.

Morphological changes in autophagic death:
- *Autophagosomes formation*: Double membrane vesicles containing engulfed cytoplasmic organelles
- *Autolysosome*: Fusion of autophagosome and lysosome
- Loss of organelles and cytoplasmic vacuoles
- Nuclear chromatin condensation and destruction of nucleus.

Molecular pathway:
- Controlled by a group of autophagy-related genes.
- Class III PI3-kinase is the major lipid signal that generates. Phosphatidylinositol 3-phosphate (PI3-P).
- PI3-P helps in the autophagic vesicle formation.

Clinical implications of autophagy:
- Autophagy plays an important role in:
  - Infection
  - Cardiovascular disease
  - *Neurodegenerative disorders*: Parkinson's disease, Huntington's disease, Alzheimer's disease, etc.
  - Cancers

These are further used for protein synthesis or adenosine triphosphate (ATP) production. Thus, autophagy maintains an adequate nutrient level at the time of stress or starvation. Cell death by autophagy is caspase independent programmed death. Table 3.4 shows the differentiating points between autophagy and apoptosis.

Types of Autophagy

There are three types of autophagy[14] (Fig. 3.6) as described next.

Microautophagy

In case of microautophagy, the cargo elements (substrates and cytoplasmic organelles) directly come in contact with

Table 3.4: Comparison of apoptosis and autophagy.

Features	*Apoptosis*	*Autophagy*
Programmed death	Yes	Yes
Role of caspase	Yes	No
Cytoskeletal breakdown	Early part	Later or terminal part
Organelles	Not destroyed in early part	Destroyed in early part
Light microscopy	Visible	Not visible, only demonstrable in electron microscopy
Role	Direct role in neoplasia. Too less apoptosis causes cancer	Autophagy plays dual role in tumorigenesis

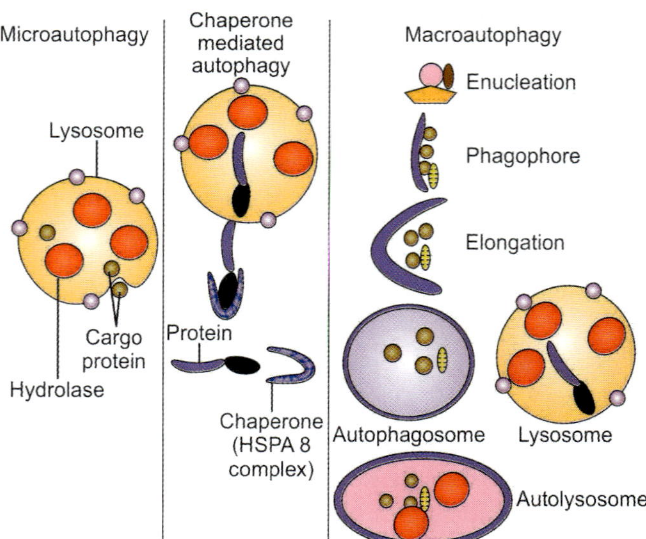

Fig. 3.6: Schematic diagram showing different types of autophagy and pathways of formation of autophagy.

the lysosomal membrane for degradation and recycling. Very little is known on this type of autophagy.

Chaperone-mediated Autophagy

Chaperone-mediated autophagy (CMA) is a unique type of autophagy. Unlike micro- or macroautophagy, CMA is directed to specific cargo proteins. In case of CMA, chaperones are appointed to recognize and translocate the cargo proteins individually to the lysosomal membrane. All the cargo proteins have a specific pentapeptide targeting motif (KFERQ). This KFERQ motif is identified by the heat shock protein *HSPA8*, a chaperone. Subsequently the cargo proteins are delivered individually to lysosomal membrane for degradation.

Macroautophagy

This is most well studied and described in detail. The unique feature of macroautophagy is the de novo generation of membrane bound vesicles (autophagosome). The vesicle sequesters the cytoplasmic organelles and transports the cargo to the lysosomal vesicle. Autophagosome fuses with the lysosome to form autolysosome and the cytoplasmic organelles are destroyed.

Stages of Macroautophagy with Molecular Mechanism

Induction

At first, the nucleation of the phagophore occurs de novo in the cytoplasm. This is induced by the ULK1/2 complex which is made up of ATG13, ATG 101, ULK 1 and RB1 CC1.

Nucleation

After the induction, the next step is the nucleation which is formed by the ATG14-containing class III phosphatidylinositol 3-kinase (PtdIns3K) complex. The membrane begins to enlarge in this stage and forms phagophore assembly site (PAS). The sources of the membrane are possibly from plasma membrane, endoplasmic reticulum, Golgi complex and mitochondria.

Elongation

In this step, the membrane of the phagophore is further elongated with the help of ATG12-ATG5-ATG16 complex, the class III PtdIns3K complex, ATG8, and ATG9.

Completion of Autophagosome Formation

The membrane completely encircles the cargo to form autophagosome.

Fusion of Autophagosome with Lysosome

Eventually the autophagosome fuses with lysosome and autolysosome is formed. The cytoplasmic organelles are degraded and then finally transported to the cytoplasm for recycling.

Molecular Basis of Autophagy

The molecular pathway of autophagy is initially discovered in yeast and it is still evolutionally conserved in human. The autophagy is regulated by a group of autophagy-related genes (ATG genes) which are almost similar to that of yeast. These genes produce at least 27 proteins that are involved in the execution of autophagy, such as vesicle enucleation, autophagic vesicle fusion to late lysosome, and cargo degradation.

Autophagy is also related with class III PI3 kinase types I and III. Class III PI3-kinase is the major lipid signal that generates phosphatidylinositol 3-phosphate (PI3-P). This PI3-P plays key role in the autophagic vesicle formation (Fig. 3.7). A protein complex consisting of Atg6 (Vps30 or Beclin-1 in mammalians) regulates the activity of the class III PI3-kinase (Fig. 3.7).[15] Growth factor particularly insulin activates PI3 kinase type I, whereas mammalian target of rapamycin (mTOR) inhibits autophagy.

Class III PI3 kinase makes a complex with ATG6 and promotes nucleation of the membrane. Subsequently two other pathways to autophagy take part:

1. *ATG12 pathway involving ATG5, ATG7 and ATG10*: ATG12 binds with ATG5 with the help of ATG7 and ATG10. Following conjugation of ATG12-ATG5, further dimerization of the molecule occurs with the help of ATG6.
2. *ATG8 pathway involving ATG7, ATG3 and ATG4*: In this pathway, ATG8 acts along with ATG7, ATG3, and ATG4. ATG8 conjugates with a lipid molecule, phosphatidylethanolamine (PE) and several such binding help in the expansion of the membrane of the autophagosome.

Control of Autophagy

Macroautophagy is stimulated by deprivation of nutrients, hypoxia, absence of growth factors and insulin. There are three kinases that are involved in the control of macroautophagy (Fig. 3.8):

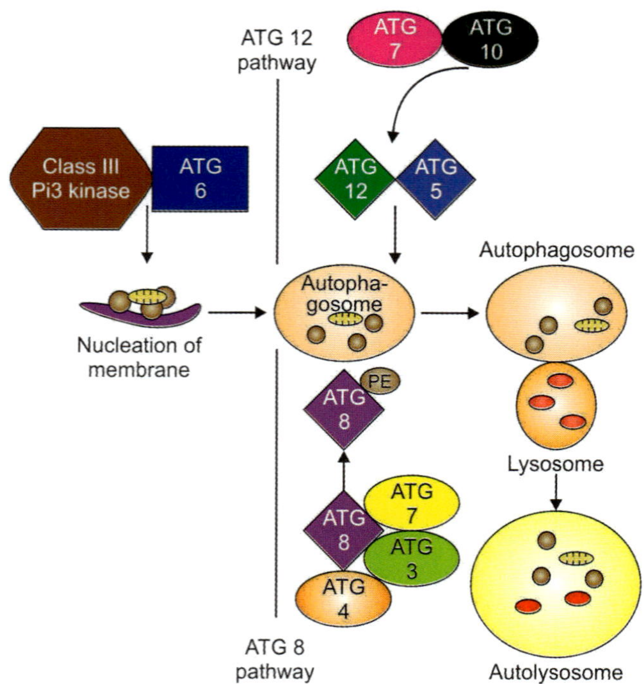

Fig. 3.7: Schematic diagram showing molecular mechanism of autophagic cell death.

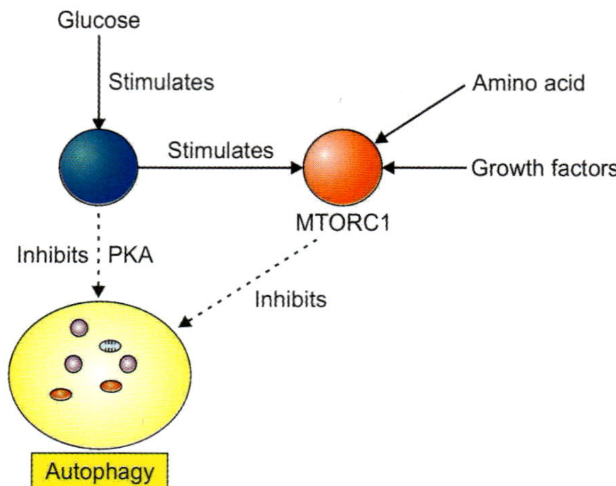

Fig. 3.8: Schematic diagram showing controlling factors of autophagy.

1. *cAMP-dependent protein kinase A (PKA)*: PKA is stimulated by glucose. PKA directly inhibits autophagy and it stimulates MTORC1.
2. *AMP-activated protein kinase (AMPK)*: AMPK, the energy sensing kinase, inhibits MTORC1.
3. *Mechanistic target of rapamycin complex 1 (MTORC1)*: MTORC1 is activated by growth factor, amino acid and oxygen. MTORC1 is known to inhibit macroautophagy.

Selective Autophagy

Macroautophagy may be also selective in action, such as selective degradation of ubiquitinated proteins peroxisome, mitochondria, etc.

Pexophagy

Selective destruction of peroxisome by macroautophagy is called as pexophagy. This occurs in normal physiological condition. Pexophagy is stimulated by starvation. Excessive pexophagy may have negative influence on health.

Mitophagy[14]

The term "mitophagy" indicates selective destruction of mitochondria by macroautophagy. It is important for steady turnover and removal of damaged mitochondria. Mitophagy is also helpful in the development of certain cells such as removal of mitochondria is required in immature red blood cell (RBC) to transform into mature RBC.

Mechanism of mitophagy: In case of mitophagy, the mitochondrial outer membrane enzyme PTEN-induced putative kinase 1 (PINK1) kinase appoints PARK2/Parkin. This combined PINK1-PARK2 enzyme complex ubiquitinates the other mitochondrial proteins and ultimately the damaged mitochondria are degraded. PINK1 and PARK2 genes are mutated in case of recessive Parkinson's disease.

Clinical Implications of Autophagy

Autophagy plays an important role in the cellular homeostasis. The derangement of autophagy may cause various diseases.

- *Infection*: Autophagy helps in the removal of various intracellular organisms. Bacteria may inhibit or induce autophagy for their survival benefit.
- *Autophagy in neurodegenerative diseases*: The different steps of autophagic process is impaired in neurodegenerative diseases such Parkinson's disease, Huntington's disease, Alzheimer's disease, and amyotrophic lateral sclerosis.
- *Cardiovascular disease*: Decreased autophagy is noted in various vascular and heart diseases.
- *Malignancy*: Autophagy probably plays double role in tumorigenesis because in one hand it helps to keep normal function of the cell and in other hand it helps the tumor cell survival. Mutations and deletions of various autophagic genes have been demonstrated in breast,

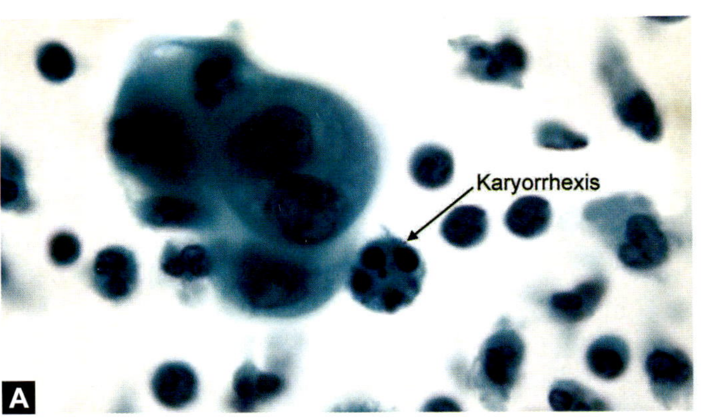

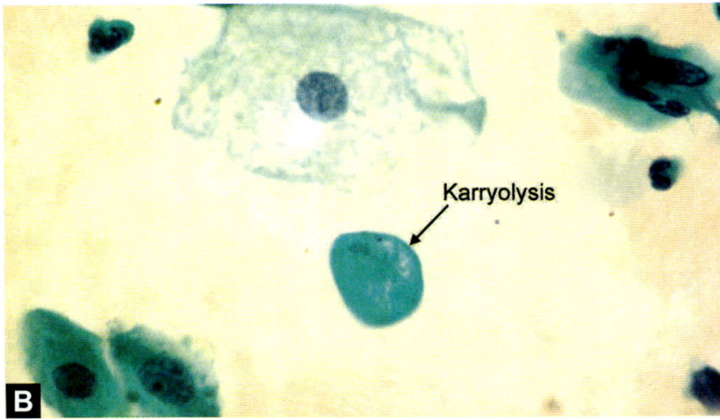

Figs. 3.9A and B: Cytology smear showing typical karyorrhexis (A) and karyolysis (B) of the nuclei (Papanicolaou's stain X HP).

ovary, prostate, gastrointestinal, and liver carcinomas. Tumor suppressor role of autophagy has also been described, however, the exact mechanism of which is unknown. Probably loss of autophagy causes accumulation of free radical in the cells leading to tumorigenesis.

NECROSIS

The word "necrosis" is derived from the Greek word "nekros", for corpse. It usually occurs due to ischemia or hypoxia such as in myocardial infarction. In neoplasm, necrosis occurs when the cells proliferate rapidly without adequate angiogenesis.

Morphological Changes in Necrosis

Morphological changes in necrosis include:

- *Cytoplasmic changes*: Cytoplasm of the necrotic cells shows extensive vacuolization and intense eosinophilia on hematoxylin and eosin-stained smears.
- *Nucleus*: Nucleus of the necrotic cell shows following changes:
  - *Pyknosis*: Nucleus becomes small and deeply basophilic with clumped chromatin.
  - *Karyorrhexis (Fig. 3.9A)*: Nucleus undergoes fragmentation and smaller fragments scattered within the cytoplasm.
  - *Karyolysis (Fig. 3.9B)*: There is progressive loss of chromatin staining and basophilia of the nucleus fades out.

The ultrastructurally necrotic cell shows early swelling of intracellular organelles such as mitochondria, endoplasmic reticulum, and Golgi apparatus, aggregated cytoskeletal elements and loss of plasma membrane integrity.

PROGRAMMED NECROSIS

In certain conditions, the necrosis is programmed. In programmed necrosis, the cell death occurs in sequential events due to the effect of multiple signaling pathways rather than a single well-described signaling cascade. Unlike apoptosis and autophagy, in programmed necrosis there is no involvement of caspase or lysosomal enzyme. The cells show loss of mitochondria, collection of reactive oxygen species, depletion of ATP and proteolysis. During cell destruction by necrosis, high mobility group box 1 (HMGB1) protein is released from the nucleus. This HMGB1 protein promotes inflammatory response. The programmed necrosis is regulated by different proteins, such as TRAIL, TRADD, TRAF2, JNK1, RIP1, XRCC1, AIF, calpains, Bax, or Drp1.[16]

INFLAMMATION

Inflammation is the response of tissue reaction to exogenous or endogenous stimuli in vascularized tissue. It is fundamentally a protective response of the body to get rid of the pathogenic insult and to remove the injured dead tissue so that healing can occur. Specific cells accumulate in the site of insult to fight with the infective agents. Vasodilatation and increased vascular permeability produce excess fluid in the site of inflammation and dilute the causative agents. Neutrophils and macrophages remove the dead cells and help in healing.

Inflammation is classified as:

- Acute inflammation
- Chronic inflammation
- Granulomatous inflammation.

Acute Inflammation

It is characterized by direct injury to tissue leading to necrosis, damage of larger vessels and infiltration by polymorphonuclear leukocytes. In acute inflammation series of changes occur: (1) transient and rapid constriction and dilatation of blood vessels, (2) increased vascular permeability leading to local edema in the tissue, (3) release of soluble mediators (histamine, serotonin, prostaglandin, nitric oxide) in the site of inflammation, and (4) infiltration of neutrophils. In most of the time acute inflammation heals, however, the other outcomes of acute inflammation are scar, abscess formation and transition to chronic inflammation.

Chronic Inflammation

Chronic inflammation is always of prolonged duration, and is associated with acute inflammation and tissue damage. In case of chronic inflammation, the predominant inflammatory cells are mononuclear cells such as lymphocytes, plasma cells, and macrophages. Tissue destruction continues with persistent action of the causative agents. There is usually disordered attempt to restore the tissue architecture by angiogenesis and fibrosis.

Granulomatous Inflammation

Granulomatous inflammation is characterized by focal collection of activated macrophages resembling epithelial cells (known as epithelioid cells). In fact, granulomatous inflammation is the protective response to chronic inflammation by which the persistent causative agent is removed to protect the host.

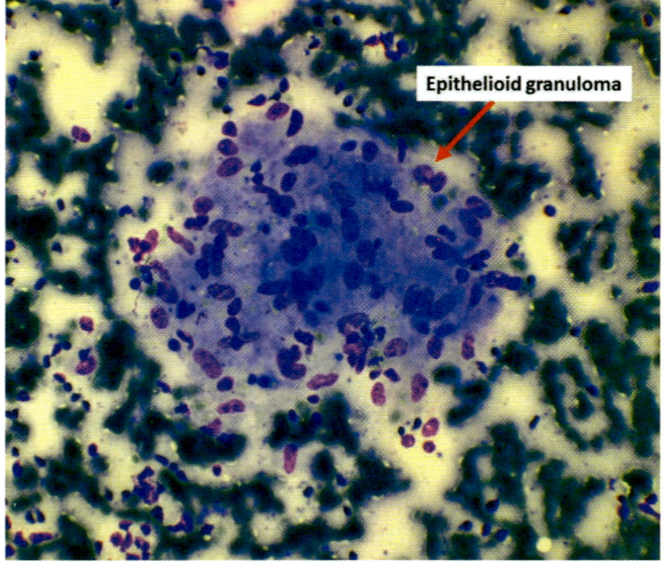

Fig. 3.10: Epithelioid cell granuloma in a case of granulomatous inflammation (May-Grünwald-Giemsa stain X MP).

Morphology

The hallmark of granulomatous inflammation is epithelioid cell granuloma (Fig. 3.10). This is a well-circumscribed nodular lesion formed by epithelioid cells, lymphocytes, and plasma cells. Epithelioid cells have abundant cytoplasm with indistinct cytoplasmic margin. The nucleus is oval to elongated with blunt ended having fine chromatin and inconspicuous nucleoli. Epithelioid cells may often fuse together to form multinucleated giant cells. These giant cells are large 40–50 μ in diameter with 15–20 nuclei. The nuclei may be arranged haphazardly in the cell as we see in foreign body granuloma or they may be arranged around the periphery of the cell in a horse shoe-shaped manner giving rise to the typical appearance of Langhans type of giant cell.

Granuloma may be further classified as described next.

Granuloma with necrosis: Here, necrosis is often seen in association with the epithelioid cell granulomas. This is typically seen mycobacterium infection.

Granuloma without necrosis: Here, no necrosis is seen in association with granulomas. This type of reaction is typically seen in sarcoidosis.

Causes of Granulomas

Box 3.7 highlights the various causes of granulomatous reaction in the body.[17]

Morphologically it is difficult to identify the exact causes of granulomatous reaction. However, the presence of foreign bodies within the giant cells may indicate foreign body granulomas. At times, special stain may help to identify the bacteria or fungi.

Box 3.7: Causes of granulomatous reaction.

- Infective agents:
  - Bacterial:
    - *Mycobacterium tuberculosis*
    - *Mycobacterium leprae*
  - Spirochetes:
    - *Treponema pallidum*
  - Fungus: *Histoplasma capsulatum*, Aspergillus, Cryptococcus, etc.
- Autoimmune diseases:
  - Rheumatoid arthritis, giant cell arteritis, etc.
- *Foreign body granulomas*: Different type of foreign bodies such as suture material, talcum powder, etc.
- Granuloma of unknown etiology:
  - Sarcoidosis

REFERENCES

1. Edinger AL, Thompson CB. Death by design: apoptosis, necrosis and autophagy. Curr Opin Cell Biol. 2004;16(6):663-9.
2. Majno G, Joris I. Apoptosis, oncosis, and necrosis. An overview of cell death. Am J Pathol. 1995;146(1):3-15.
3. Hotchkiss RS, Strasser A, McDunn JE, et al. Cell death. N Engl J Med. 2009;361(16):1570-83.
4. Green DR, Reed JC. Mitochondria and apoptosis. Science. 1998;281(5381):1309-12.
5. Gross A, McDonnell JM, Korsmeyer SJ. BCL-2 family members and the mitochondria in apoptosis. Genes Dev. 1999;13(15):1899-911.
6. Zwaal RF, Schroit AJ. Pathophysiologic implications of membrane phospholipid asymmetry in blood cells. Blood. 1997;89(4):1121-32.
7. Sun Y, Peng ZL. Programmed cell death and cancer. Postgrad Med J. 2009;85(1001):134-40.
8. Thompson CB. Apoptosis in the pathogenesis and treatment of disease. Science. 1995;267(5203):1456-62.
9. Meyaard L, Otto SA, Jonker RR, et al. Programmed death of T cells in HIV-1 infection. Science. 1992;257(5067):217-9.
10. Yoshida Y. Hypothesis: apoptosis may be the mechanism responsible for the premature intramedullary cell death in the myelodysplastic syndrome. Leukemia. 1993;7(1):144-6.
11. Archana M, Bastian, Yogesh TL, et al. Various methods available for detection of apoptotic cells—a review. Indian J Cancer. 2013;50(3):274-83.
12. Dey P, Luthra UK, George SS, et al. Terminal uridine nick end labelling and mitosis in carcinoma of breast. Correlation with tumor grade and p53 overexpression. Anal Quant Cytol Histol. 2001;23(1):27-30.
13. Lippai M, Szatmári Z. Autophagy-from molecular mechanisms to clinical relevance. Cell Biol Toxicol. 2017;33(2): 145-68.
14. Parzych KR, Klionsky DJ. An overview of autophagy: morphology, mechanism, and regulation. Antioxid Redox Signal. 2014;20(3):460-73.
15. Stack JH, DeWald DB, Takegawa K, et al. Vesicle-mediated protein transport: Regulatory interactions between the Vps15 protein kinase and the Vps34 PtdIns 3-kinase essential for protein sorting to the vacuole in yeast. J Cell Biol. 1995;129(2):321-34.
16. Vanden Berghe T, Van Loo G, Saelens X, et al. Differential signaling to apoptotic and necrotic cell death by Fas-associated death domain protein FADD. J Biol Chem. 2004;279(9):7925-33.
17. Adams DO. The granulomatous inflammatory response. A review. Am J Pathol. 1976;84(1):164-92.

Review Questions

1. Step ladder type of fragmentation of internucleosomal DNA is noted in:
   a. Autophagy
   b. Necrosis
   c. Apoptosis
   d. Fatty degeneration

2. Final execution of apoptosis is caused by:
   a. Caspases 8 and 9
   b. CD95 ligand binds to CD95
   c. TNF binds to TNFR1
   d. Caspase 3

3. Which one is a proapoptotic protein?
   a. BaX
   b. BCL-2
   c. BCL-XL
   d. MCL1

4. Which one is not a marker of apoptosis?
   a. M30
   b. Annexin V
   c. Caspase 3
   d. BCL-2

5. "Autophagosome" is formed in:
   a. Microautophagy
   b. Macroautophagy
   c. Chaperone-mediated autophagy
   d. Early apoptosis

6. Granuloma without necrosis is typically seen in:
   a Sarcoidosis
   b. Tuberculosis
   c. Cryptococcal infection
   d. *Mycobacterium leprae*

Identify True/False

7. Apoptosis is an active process and energy is required. *(True/False)*

8. BaX and BaK are the two principal proapoptotic proteins. *(True/False)*

9. The demonstration of activated caspase 3 by immunohistochemistry is a reliable method for the detection of apoptosis. *(True/False)*

10. De novo membrane bound veside lenowa as " autophagosome" is formed in microcutophagy. *(True/False)*

Answers

1. c. Apoptosis
2. d. Caspase 3
3. a. BaX
4. d. BCL 2
5. b. Macroautophagy
6. a. Sarcoidosis
7. True
8. True
9. True
10. False

CHAPTER

4

Molecular Genetics: Basic Principles and Clinical Applications

CHROMOSOME

The chromatin of the nucleus is more condensed in the mitotic phase and is known as chromosome. So, chromosome is the coiled and super-coiled DNA chain along with other proteins within the nucleus. DNA chain takes two complete rounds along the octameric core histone and thus forms a nucleosome. The string of linked nucleosome is repeatedly twisted to form the more complex three-dimensional organization of chromatin.

CHROMOSOMAL NUMBER

There are total 46 chromosomes (arranged in 23 pairs) in every somatic cell of our body. In each set of pair, one chromosome is derived from ovum and other one is derived from the sperm. The number of chromosome is given according to its length from the longest to shortest. The first 22 pairs of chromosomes are labeled as autosomes and the last pair is known as sex chromosome. Sex chromosomes in the normal human may have two X chromosomes (female) or one X and one Y chromosome (male).

Box 4.1: Human chromosome.

- Total number 46
- Autosomes: 22 pairs
- Sex chromosomes: One pair (X and Y)
- Male: XY, Female: XX
- Each chromosome has a short (p) and a long arm (q).
- Centromere: The constricted part between short and long arm.
- Chromosomal bands are labeled from nearer to far from the centromere.
- *Telomere*:
  - The repetitive nucleotide sequences at the end of the chromosome
  - It protects the end sequences of DNA
  - Shortens in the process of DNA replication
- *Kinetochores*:
  - Help in the attachment of the centromere with the mitotic spindle fibers.
  - Verification of the anchoring of the centromeres to the mitotic spindle.

CHROMOSOMAL STRUCTURE

The chromosome has a short arm and a long arm that are labeled as p (petit) and q (named as the next letter after p), respectively (Box 4.1). When chromosomes are arranged for karyotyping the p arm should always be kept in top. These two arms are divided by a constricted point known as centromere (Fig. 4.1). As described earlier, the centromere is attached to the mitotic spindle at the time of cell division. Kinetochores are the complexes of proteins that help in the attachment of the centromeres with the mitotic spindle fibers. Kinetochores also help in the verification of the anchoring of the centromeres to the mitotic spindle, activation of the spindle checkpoint and movement of chromatids during cell division. Each chromosome is protected by the cap of *telomere* in its two ends. The term telomere name is derived from the Greek word "telos" means end and "meros" means part. Telomere is the repetitive nucleotide sequences at the

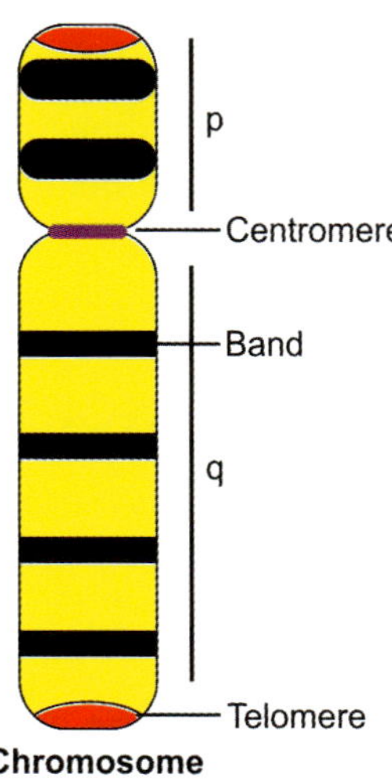

Fig. 4.1: Schematic diagram of a chromosome. Short arm of the chromosome is indicated by "p" and the long arm is represented by "q".

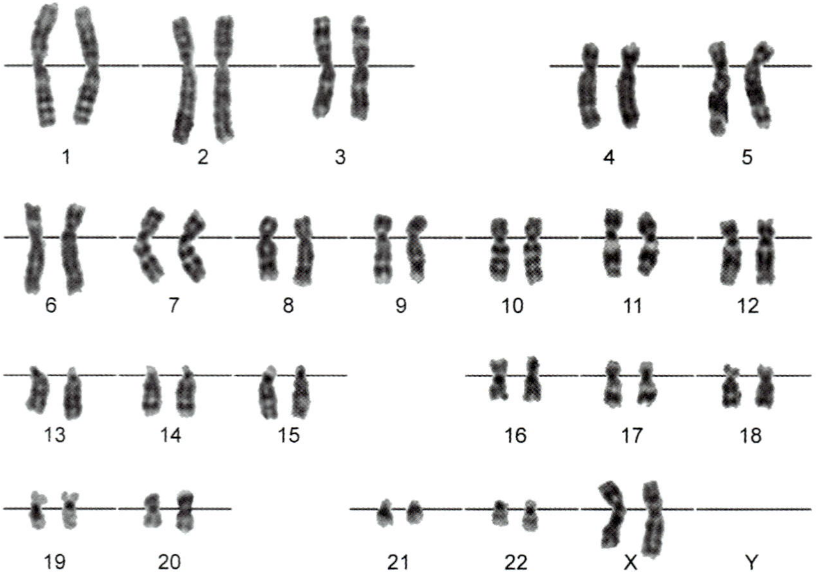

Fig. 4.2: Normal karyotype in a female: 46, XX.
Source: Dr Neelam Verma, Professor and Head, Department of Hematology, PGIMER, Chandigarh, India.

end of the chromosome. During replication of DNA, the enzyme DNA polymerase is unable to replicate the DNA sequence of the ends of the chromosomes and the important genetic information may be lost. The telomeres protect the end sequences of DNA and they themselves become shortened in the process of DNA replication. In each cell cycle, telomere becomes more and more shortened. Therefore, the length of the telomere indicates the age of a cell. The telomere also prevents the fusion of the two ends of the chromosomes.

Chromosomes should be stained for visualization under the light microscope. The stained chromosomes look like strings with multiple dark and light horizontal bands that are numbered according to their location from the centromere. The higher number of the band indicates that the band is far away from the centromere. Figure 4.2 shows the complete set of human chromosome.

CHROMOSOMAL ABNORMALITIES

There may be two types of chromosomal abnormalities: Numerical abnormalities and structural abnormalities (Box 4.2).

Box 4.2: Chromosomal abnormalities.

Numerical abnormalities: Gain or lose of whole chromosome.
Structural alteration:
- *Deletion*: A segment of chromosome is deleted completely
- *Chromosomal duplication*: Part of the chromosome is duplicated
- *Inversion*: Broken part of chromosome is attached upside down.
- *Translocation*:
  - *Reciprocal translocation*: Segments of chromosome from two different nonhomologous chromosomes are broken and then attached to each other reciprocally.
  - *Robertsonian translocation*: One entire acrocentric chromosome attaches with the other chromosome in the centromeric region.
  - *Ring chromosome*: A ring is formed from the broken chromosome.

Numerical Abnormalities

Here a whole chromosome may be missing from the pair or there may be gain of one more chromosome. In monosomy, there is loss of one chromosome. This is seen in Turner's syndrome where one X chromosome is less. Gain of one chromosome is seen in Down's syndrome. In this disease, there are three copies of chromosome 21.

The common cause of numerical chromosome is nondisjunction of the sister chromatids during migration at the polar ends of the spindle.

Structural Alteration

In case of structural alteration, there is a change of chromosomal DNA arrangement. The chromosomal alteration may be balanced or unbalanced. In balanced alteration, there is neither loss nor gain of genetic material. However, in unbalanced chromosomal structural alteration there is either addition or deletion of genetic material. This type of unbalanced chromosomal defects is commonly associated with disease.

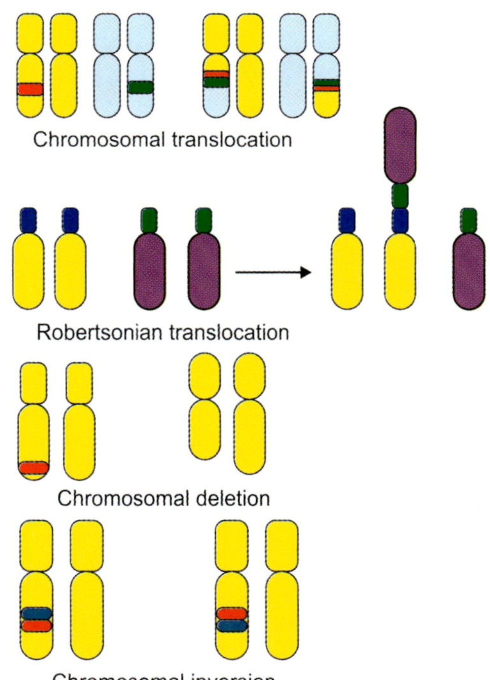

Fig. 4.3: Schematic diagram showing different types of chromosomal changes.

Deletion

A segment of chromosome is deleted completely and the impact of deletion depends on the number of the affected genes in that segment of chromosome (Fig. 4.3).

Chromosomal Duplication

Here the particular segment of the chromosome is duplicated and therefore there are three copies of particular segment of DNA within the nucleus.

Inversion

A segment of chromosome is broken and again attached in the chromosome with upside down (Fig. 4.3).

Translocation

In case of translocation, a segment of chromosome is broken and then transferred to any other chromosome. There may be two types of translocation:

1. *Reciprocal translocation*: The part of chromosomes are broken from two different nonhomologous chromosomes and then attached to each other reciprocally. Therefore, the total amount of genetic material remains constant.

Box 4.3: Chromosomal changes in malignancies.

Chromosomal rearrangement
- *Chimeric fusion gene with new activity*
  - *Aberrant or enhance tyrosine kinase activity*: Philadelphia chromosome in chronic myeloid leukemia t(9;22)(q34.1;q11.23)
  - *Aberrant or enhance enhanced transcriptional activity*: Acute promyelocytic leukemia t(8;21)(q22;q22.3)
- *Enhance the activity of the proto-oncogene*: Juxtaposition of the proto-oncogene coding sequence near a normal tissue regulatory element may enhance the activity of the proto-oncogene.
- *Chromosomal gain or loss*:
  - *Chromosomal gain*:
    - » Complete or partial trisomy
    - » Intrachromosomal amplification of genes
    - » Extrachromosomal amplification of genes
    - » Certain gene activity enhances leading to tumor initiation or progression.
  - *Chromosomal loss*: Portion of gene is lost.

2. *Robertsonian translocation*: One entire chromosome is fused with another chromosome in the centromeres region to form a single chromosome (Fig. 4.3).

Ring

A segment of chromosome is broken and forms a circle of ring.

CHROMOSOMAL ABNORMALITIES IN MALIGNANCIES (BOX 4.3)

Cancer is believed to develop from progressive series of multiple genetic abnormalities in a clone of cells.[1] The chromosomal abnormalities are present in large number of cancer.[2] These cytogenetic abnormalities are considered as diagnostic and prognostic markers in hematologic and solid malignancies. Moreover, the knowledge on chromosomal abnormalities helped us to understand the mechanisms of carcinogenesis.

The chromosomal changes in cancer may be due to: (1) *Primary chromosomal changes* that are mainly responsible for the initiation of the tumor and (2) *Secondary or tumor-associated changes* that are associated with tumor growth and progression.

Chromosomal Rearrangement

Chromosomal rearrangement occurs in reciprocal translocation, inversion and insertion. Reciprocal translocation is the characteristic cytogenetic hallmark of leukemia and lymphoma. Specific chromosomal translocation of *BCR-ABL1* fusion gene may be used as an indicator in

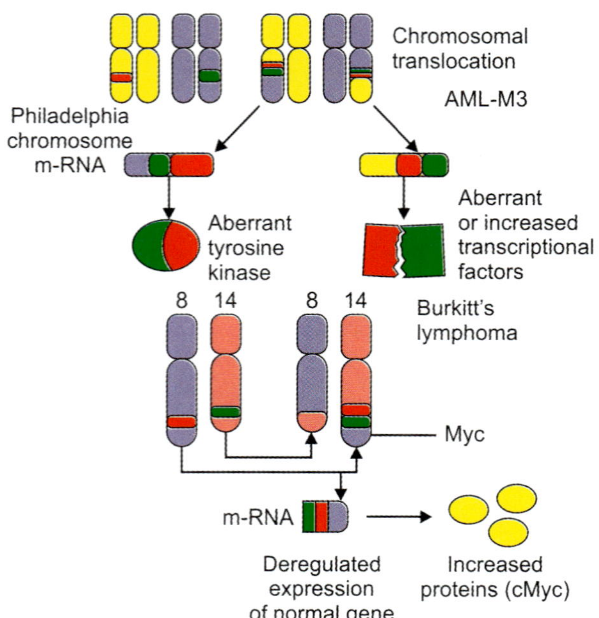

Fig. 4.4: Schematic diagram showing effects of chromosomal translocations in tumor development.

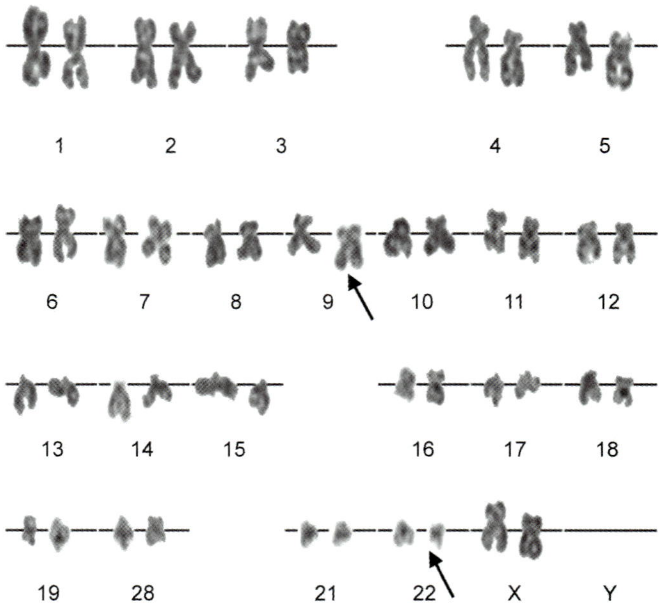

Fig. 4.5: Philadelphia chromosome in a female patient with chronic myelogenous leukemia (CML): 46, XX, t(9;22).
Source: Dr Neelam Verma, Professor and Head, Department of Hematology, PGIMER, Chandigarh, India.

the assessment of response to chemotherapy in chronic myeloid leukemia.[3] Due to chromosomal rearrangement, two things may happen: (1) a fusion gene (chimeric gene) with new functions, (2) excessive expression of normal gene.

1. *Chimeric fusion gene (Fig. 4.4)*: The majority of the chromosomal rearrangement causes fusion of two genes and therefore produces a chimeric gene. These chimeric genes may produce:
   (a) Aberrant or enhance tyrosine kinase or, (b) Aberrant or enhance enhanced transcriptional activity.
   - *Aberrant or enhance tyrosine kinase*: The best example of reciprocal translocation involving tyrosine kinase gene is Philadelphia chromosome in chronic myeloid leukemia. There is reciprocal translocation, t(9;22)(q34.1;q11.23) in Philadelphia chromosome (Fig. 4.5). The *BCR* gene on band 22q11.23 is broken and then joined with the *ABL1 tyrosine kinase* gene located on band 9q34.1. This causes production of a chimeric protein, BCR-ABL1 that has aberrant tyrosine kinase activity.[4] The chimeric tyrosine kinase gene formation is also present in various other malignancies such as nonsmall cell lung carcinoma, anaplastic large cell lymphoma, etc. (Table 4.1).
   - *Aberrant or enhance enhanced transcriptional activity*: Chromosomal translocation may generate chimeric fusion gene that produces aberrant or increased transcription factors (Table 4.1). In case of acute promyelocytic leukemia there, is t(8;21)(q22;q22.3). This produces a fusion gene *RUNX1-RUNX1T1*. This chimeric gene generates a transcription factor. The binding of the abnormal transcription factors (chimeric) with its target gene inhibits normal myeloid differentiation and thereby causing increased number of immature myeloid cells in acute myeloid leukemia.[5]
2. *Deregulation of normal gene (Fig. 4.4)*: Chromosomal translocation may help to juxtapose the proto-oncogene coding sequence near a normal tissue regulatory element and may enhance the activity of the proto-oncogene. In Burkitt's lymphoma, there is translocation of t(8;14)(q24.21;q32.33). This translocation causes juxtaposition of c-MYC and immunoglobulin heavy chain gene which is responsible for deregulation of c-MYC transcription.[6]

Chromosomal Gain or Loss

Chromosomal loss may occur due to deletion of the segment of gene (Fig. 4.6). This deletion of genetic material

Table 4.1: Chromosomal translocation in hematological and lymphoid malignancies.

Disease	*Rearrangement*	*Gene involved*
Gene fusion		
Chronic myeloid leukemia, acute lymphoblastic leukemia, acute myeloid leukemia	t(9;22)(q34.1;q11.23)	*BCR-ABL1*
Anaplastic large-cell lymphoma	t(2;5)(p23;q35)	*ALK-NPM1*
Multiple myeloma	t(4;14)(p16.3;q32.33)	*WHSC1-IGHG1*
Acute myeloid leukemia	t(8;21)(q22;q22.3)	*RUNX1-RUNX1T1*
Acute myeloid leukemia	t(9;11)(p22;q23)	*MLL-MLLT3*
Acute megakaryoblastic leukemia	t(1;22)(p13;q13)	*RBM15-MKL1*
Acute promyelocytic leukemia	t(15;17)(q22;q21)	*PML-RARA*
Burkitt's lymphoma	t(8;14)(q24.21;q32.33)	*MYC-IGHG1*
Follicular lymphoma	t(14;18)(q32.33;q21.3)	*IGHG1-BCL2*
Mantle-cell lymphoma	t(11;14)(q13;q32.33)	*CCND1-IGHG1*
Gene nonfusion		
T-Acute lymphoblastic leukemia	t(8;22)(q24;q11)	*c-MYC(8q24)*
B-Chronic lymphocytic leukemia (CLL)	t(8;12)(q24;q22)	*c-MYC(8q24)*
T-Acute lymphoblastic leukemia (ALL)	t(7;19)(q35;p13)	*LYL1(19p13)*
Diffuse large B-cell lymphoma (DLBCL)	t(3;14)(q27;q32)	*Laz3/BCL-6(3q27)*
B-non-Hodgkin lymphoma (NHL)	t(10;14)(q24;q32)	*Lyt-10(10q24)*

causes initiation or progression of malignancies (Table 4.1). The chromosomal deletions may be specific to a particular tumor such as Wilms' tumor shows 11p13 deletions. Gene deletion may occur in multiple chromosomes in a particular cancer. Therefore, it may be difficult to decide the role of particular gene/s in tumorigenesis.

In case of chromosomal gain, certain gene activity enhances leading to tumor initiation or progression. Genomic gains commonly occur due to complete or partial trisomy, intrachromosomal and extrachromosomal amplification of genes. In large-scale genomic gain, there is gain of large segment of chromosome affecting multiple genes. Trisomy of chromosome number 8 is the example of large genomic gain that is commonly seen in many hematological malignancies. In case of solid tumors, triosomy of chromosome 7 is noted in malignant neurogenic tumor.[7] Chromosomal gains of small segment of the genomic regions or single gene amplification are infrequent. Homogeneously staining region (HSR) indicates focal amplification of small number of genes (Fig. 4.6).[8]

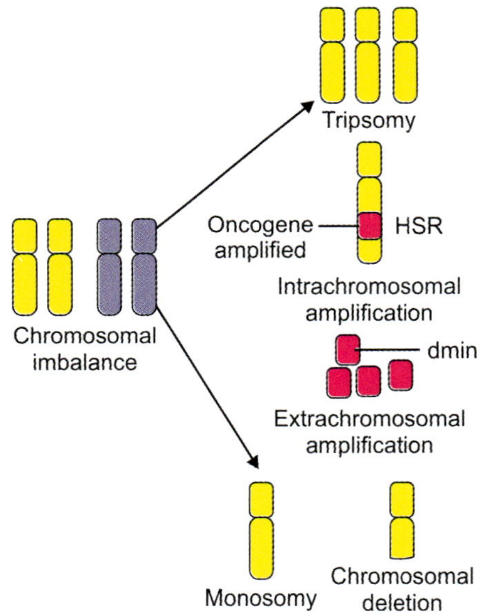

Fig. 4.6: Schematic diagram showing effects of chromosomal imbalance in tumorogenesis.

The HSR does not show any typical banding pattern. Gene amplification is specifically seen in some solid tumors with poorer prognosis.[9] Extrachromosomal DNA amplification is seen as double-minute chromosomes (dmin) (Fig. 4.6). These circular-shaped dmin automatically replicate the DNA strands. This single gene amplification is detected by comparative genomic hybridization and single-nucleotide polymorphism genotyping.[10]

CYTOGENETICS

The study of chromosomes under microscope is known as cytogenetics. The cytogenetics may be of two types: Conventional cytogenetics and molecular cytogenetics.

Conventional Cytogenetics

This is the traditional method of chromosomal analysis. *Karyotype* is the study of the number and appearance of chromosome in the cell. Conventional cytogenetics is also known as karyotyping.

In case of the conventional cytogenetics, the essential steps include:

- Culture of the collected cells,
- Mitotic phase arrest of these cells by using colchicine
- Treatment of these cells by hypotonic solution to have chromosome in metaphase,
- Chromosome banding,
- Study of the chromosome under microscope.

The chromosomes are studied according to length, position of centromeres, banding pattern and other physical appearances. The different types of staining or banding techniques for visualization of chromosomes include G banding, Q banding, C banding, and R banding (Box 4.4). The other types of techniques include *digital karyotyping* and *Spectral karyotyping*. *Digital karyotyping* helps in quantitative analysis of DNA copy number. The multiple short sequences of DNA all over the genome are isolated and enumerated. In *spectral karyotyping,* all the chromosomes are stained by chromosome-specific DNA labeled with different fluorochrome.

Chromosomal abnormalities detected:

- *Aneuploidy*: Trisomy, monosomy, etc.
- *Translocations*: Robertsonian translocation, reciprocal translocation, insertional translocation, etc.
- Deletions
- Isochromosomes
- Ring chromosomes.

Advantages of Conventional Cytogenetics

Relatively easy, low cost and low-resource technology.

Disadvantages

- Low sensitivity and only those chromosomal abnormalities are detected that are visualized by light microscopy. The submicroscopic chromosomal abnormalities such as mutations are missed.
- It requires good number of proliferating cells.
- Many molecular changes are impossible to detect.
- At times, cell culture is difficult.

Molecular Cytogenetic Techniques

In last few decades, there is massive development of cytogenetic techniques. These techniques are more sophisticated, sensitive, and can be done on archival material bypassing the cell culture. The comparison of different techniques has been done in Table 4.2.

Fluorescent in situ Hybridization Technique

In this technique, specific DNA probes tagged with fluorescent dyes are used to detect any genetic change in the chromosome. Fluorescence in situ hybridization (FISH) is also known as "interphase cytogenetics" and it can be done in the cytology smear or paraffin embedded histology sections.

Box 4.4: Conventional cytogenetics.

Karyotype: The study of the number and appearance of chromosome in the cell

- Chromosomes are extracted and the photographs of chromosomes are taken
- Chromosomes are arranged according to length, band pattern and position of centromeres

Types of banding technique

- *G banding*:
  - Giemsa staining of the chromosome is done
  - Alternate dark and light band
  - Dark band adenine and thymine (AT) rich, light band guanine and cytosine (GC) rich
- *C banding*:
  - Specially stains the centromeric or constitutive heterochromatin region of the chromosome
- *Q banding*:
  - Stained by fluorescent dye, quinacrine dihydrochloride
  - Visualized by fluorescent microscope
  - Resolution of the bands is better
- *R banding*:
  - Reverse of the G banding
  - Dark region GC rich, light region AT rich

Spectral karyotyping:

- DNA probes are labeled by five fluorochrome dyes and fluorescence in situ hybridization is done
- Used as screening method for complex chromosomal rearrangements

Digital karyotyping:

- Multiple short sequences of DNA are isolated and enumerated

Advantages: Relatively easy, low-cost and low-resource technology

Disadvantages: (1) Low sensitivity; (2) Proliferating cells are needed; (3) Many molecular changes are impossible to detect; (4) The cell culture is difficult at times

Table 4.2: Comparison of different cytogenetic technique.

Technique	*Basic principles*	*Advantages*	*Limitations*	*Comments*
Traditional cytogenetic by band technique	Cells are cultured, and chromosome is stained with dye	1. Easy and simple 2. Low cost 3. Robust	1. Poor resolution 2. Cell culture is needed	It is a traditional old technique to detect structural and numerical chromosomal abnormalities
Fluorescence in situ hybridization (FISH) technique	The double helix DNA is made into single stranded DNA and a probe of complementary DNA is hybridized with the target DNA segment and visualized	1. High resolution 2. It can be done in interphase cell and do not need cell culture 3. Archival material can be used 4. It correlates the cytogenetic alteration to morphological detail	1. Only the known abnormality is detected with selected available probes 2. As cytogenetic data of currently used probe is only available, so it is not a good screening test	Chromosomal translocation and amplification is well visualized
Comparative genomic hybridization (CGH)	Tumor DNA and normal reference DNA is differentially labeled and then hybridized with metaphase spread of chromosome. The relative fluorescence level of tumor and normal DNA is measured	1. Good screening test 2. Genome-wise screening is possible	1. Low resolution 2. Balanced rearrangement is undetected. 3. Exact structural change in the chromosomal gain or loss	Chromosomal amplification and deletion can be demonstrated

Principle (Fig. 4.7)

The principles of FISH are:

- The double-helix DNA is made into single stranded DNA by heat denaturation.
- A suitable complementary fluorescent dye labeled DNA probe is used for target DNA.
- The DNA-specific complementary probe binds with the target DNA and forms a new DNA duplex.
- The hybridized DNA probe with target DNA is then visualized by fluorochrome dye.

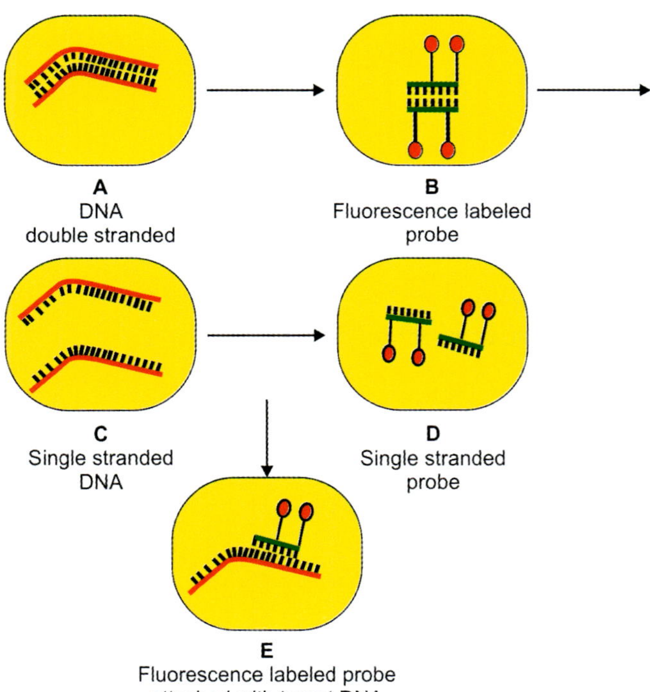

Fig. 4.7: Basic principles of fluorescence in situ hybridization (FISH) technique are highlighted in the schematic diagram.

Probes Used in Fluorescence in situ Hybridization

Predominantly three types of probes are applied in FISH:

1. *Centromeric probes (chromosome enumeration probes)*: These types of probes are used to identify the centromeric region of DNA and are made up of alpha satellite DNA. The centromeric probes are used against multiple repetitive sequences in the centromeric region of the chromosome.[11] They give very strong detectable signals. These probes are generally used for gain or loss of chromosome.
2. *Whole chromosome probes (chromosome painting)*: These are multiple complex mixtures of probes labeled with the single fluorochrome. These probes are made for the whole length of the chromosome and hybridize with the corresponding DNA sequence of the specific chromosome. Whole chromosome probes are useful to detect any structural derangement such as translocation or deletion. This is suitable for the analysis of metaphase nucleus only as the interphase nucleus is spread throughout the nucleus and gives only diffuse staining pattern.

3. *Locus-specific probes (locus-specific identifier)*: These probes are used to identify the specific genes of interest. These probes are used to mapping of genes on the chromosome and detection of any structural rearrangement such as translocation or deletion.

Three-dimensional Fluorescence in situ Hybridization

In case, three-dimensional (3D) FISH with the help of suitable image acquisition technology, the series of images collected from the multiple planes of the nucleus are reconstructed and a 3D image is made. 3D FISH helps to study the higher order chromatin structure.[12]

Living Cell Cytogenetic (Four-dimensional Fluorescence in situ Hybridization)

Here fluorescent-tagged nucleotides are incorporated into DNA during the S phase of the cell cycle. This helps in the visualizing of DNA and proteins within the living cells.[13]

Advantages of Fluorescence in situ Hybridization

Fluorescence in situ hybridization technique has several advantages such as:

- High-resolution capability
- Fluorescence in situ hybridization helps to demonstrate the specific location of DNA sequence directly in the chromosome. It is helpful to correlate the cytogenetic alteration to morphological detail.
- It can be done on archival material.
- No cell culture technique is needed for FISH technique and it can be done in interphase state of cells. Therefore, FISH is greatly helpful in cytogenetic of solid tumors.
- Fluorescent tags are safer, simpler and easy to store for indefinite period of time.

Disadvantages/Limitations of Fluorescence in situ Hybridization

- Fluorescence in situ hybridization only gives specific information of the particular chromosomal region of interest that are visualized by the probes used, whereas the conventional cytogenetic provides global information. Therefore, FISH may be a supplement to conventional cytogenetic study.
- In case of detection of minimal residual disease, one needs at least 5–10% positive cells among the total number of cells to distinguish true positive from the background false signal. Therefore, in case of small number of positive cells, reverse transcription-polymerase chain reaction (RT-PCR) is much better technique than FISH.
- Fluorescence in situ hybridization does not give any allele specific information that means it does not provide any information between maternal or paternal alleles.

Variants of Fluorescence in situ Hybridization

Multiplex FISH/Spectral karyotyping (SKY): In multiplex FISH (M-FISH)/SKY, multiple (24) chromosome probes are used with multiple fluorochrome dyes in different combination. With the help of a digital microscope, color charged device camera (CCD) and appropriate software, all the human chromosome can be visualized by using different color probes. This is helpful to detect complex structural abnormalities (translocation) and numerical disorders. However, deletion, duplication and inversion cannot be detected.

Comparative Genomic Hybridization

Comparative genomic hybridization (CGH) is the genome-wide screening by which one can detect the change of chromosomal copy number without performing any cell culture.[14]

Basic Principles

In this technique, the tumor DNA from the sample and normal DNA from the control are extracted, fragmented and differentially labeled (green color for tumor and red color for normal) followed by hybridization with a normal human metaphase spread of chromosome. The tumor DNA (green labeled) and normal DNA (red labeled) fragments compete and hybridize to their matching locus in the chromosome. With the help of a digital computer, the green to red fluorescence ratio is measured along the entire length of the chromosome. Chromosomal region deleted in the tumor will show excess green (ratio > 1), whereas gain of the chromosomal region will show excess red (ratio < 1).

Basic Steps of Comparative Genomic Hybridization

Basic steps of CGH (Fig. 4.8) are:

- *Tumor DNA labeling by green fluorochrome*: At first, DNA is extracted from the tumor sample and labeled with green fluorophore fluorescein isothiocyanate (FITC).

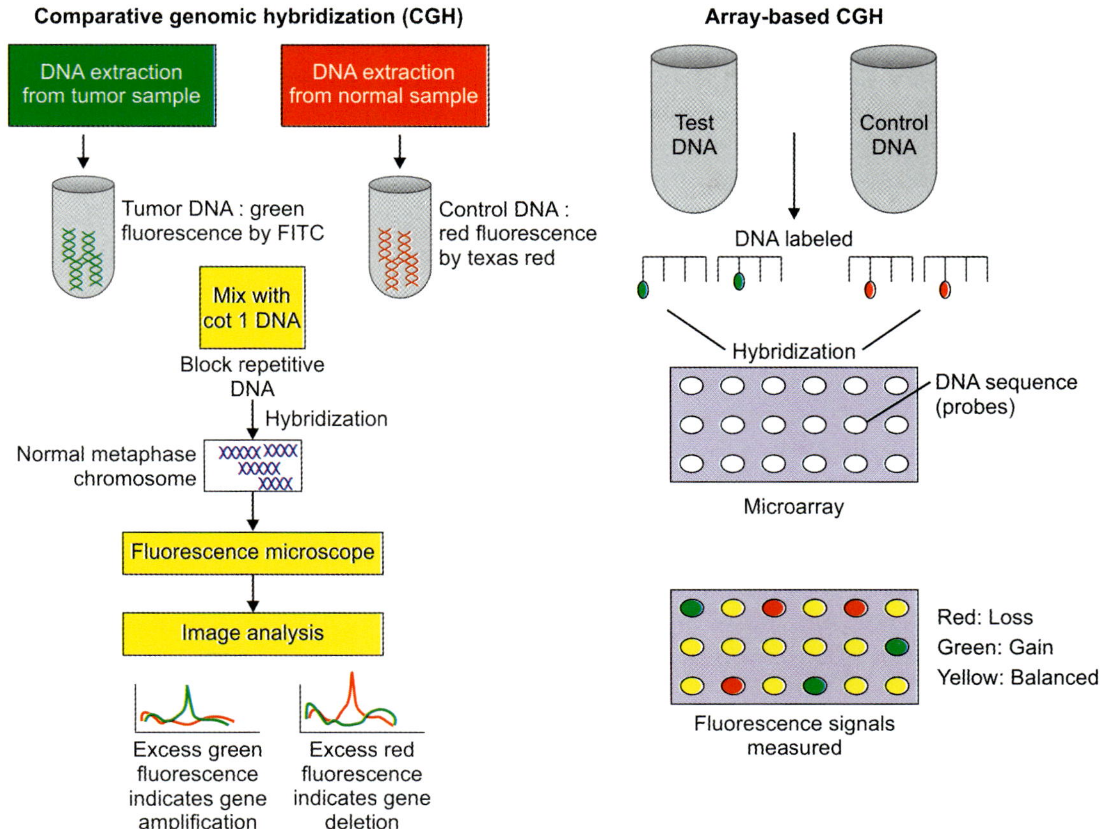

Fig. 4.8: Schematic diagram showing basic principles of comparative genomic hybridization (CGH) and array-based CGH.

- *Control normal DNA labeling by red fluorochrome*: DNA from the normal reference sample is also similarly extracted, fragmented and labeled with red fluorophore Texas Red.
- *Blocking repetitive DNA sequence*: Next, equal amount of tumor DNA and control normal DNA are coprecipitated along with Cot-1 DNA to block the repetitive sequence.
- *Hybridization with metaphase spread chromosome*: Subsequently this DNA mixture is hybridized with normal metaphase spreads DNA.
- *Observation by a fluorescence microscope*: The tumor DNA and normal DNA will compete for the homologous sites for hybridization with the normal metaphase chromosome. After proper washing, the metaphase spreads are studied by a fluorescence microscope and the images are analyzed by an image analyzer.
- *Analysis of color balance by image analyzer*: Green to red ratio of the fluorescence color along the chromosomal axis is measured by the software.
- *Result*:
    - Green: Red > 1, indicates chromosomal gain or amplification
    - Green: Red < 1, indicates chromosomal loss
    - Green: Red = 1, produces yellow color, balanced chromosome.

Advantages of Comparative Genomic Hybridization

- Comparative genomic hybridization technique does not require any prior information of the chromosome imbalance in tumor DNA.
- Comparative genomic hybridization can be done on the small amount of microdissected cells.

Disadvantages to Comparative Genomic Hybridization

- Time consuming and complicated technique
- Comparative genomic hybridization has limited use if the chromosomal rearrangement does not cause any genomic imbalance.

- It does not give any information about the exact structural change in the chromosomal gain or loss.
- Less sensitive than PCR-based technique and the sensitivity may be affected by contamination with normal cell and tumor cells.

Array-based Comparative Genomic Hybridization[15]

Comparative genomic hybridization does not have significantly better resolution than conventional G band karyotyping. Newer array-based CGH (aCGH) provides better resolution. In this aCGH, the metaphase chromosome is replaced by specific target DNA sequence [genomic bacterial artificial chromosome (BAC), P1, cosmid or cDNA] in arrays. The basic principle of CGH and array CGH is same. However, array CGH provides better resolution and more information on genomic gain or loss. The steps of array CGH are (Fig. 4.8):

- Tumor DNA is isolated and labeled with green fluorochrome dye
- Control DNA from healthy volunteer is isolated and labeled with red fluorochrome dye
- Hybridization of the probe in the array of DNA sequence
- Measurement of the color by image analyzer.

Advantages of Array-Comparative Genomic Hybridization

- Higher resolution
- Shorter sequence of DNA can be used as target such as very small cDNA fragments and PCR products.
- Cohybridization of tumor DNA and control DNA is not required as tumor DNA can directly hybridize with target DNA sequence in the array.
- *Studying specific regions of chromosome*: aCGH are used to study subtelomeric and also pericentromeric arrangements in the chromosome. It has unrevealed various complex arrangements in these regions.

Clinical Applications of Cytogenetics

The old traditional and newer molecular cytogenetics have great impact on diagnosis, screening of diseases and prognostic assessment of cancer. Chromosomal abnormalities are specific for diagnosis of many solid tumors (Tables 4.3 and 4.4).

Table 4.3: Chromosomal translocation in solid cancer.

Disease	*Rearrangement*	*Gene involved*
Non-small-cell lung cancer	inv(2)(p22-p21p23)	*EML4-ALK*
Papillary thyroid cancer	inv(10)(q11.2q11.2)	*RET-NCOA4*
Papillary thyroid cancer	inv(10)(q11.2q21)	*RET-CCDC6*
Follicular thyroid cancer	t(2;3)(q12-q14;p25)	*PAX8-PPARG*
Ewing's sarcoma	t(11;22)(q24.1-q24.3;q12.2)	*FLI1-EWSR1*
Ewing's sarcoma	t(21;22)(q22.3;q12.2)	*ERG-EWSR1*
Synovial sarcoma	t(x;18)(p11.2;q11.2)	Not identified
Melanoma of soft parts	t(12;22)(q13;q12)	*ATF 1(12q13)* *EWS(22q12)*
Liposarcoma	t(12;16)(q13;p11)	*CHOP(12q13)* *FUS(16p11)*
Rhabdomyosarcoma	t(2;13)(q35;q14)	*PAX3(2q35)* *FKHR(13q14)*

Table 4.4: Chromosomal deletion and gain in solid tumors.

Tumor	*Deleted chromosome*	*Gene involved*
Neuroblastoma, medullary thyroid carcinoma, pheochromocytoma, multiple endocrine neoplasia type 2 (MEN-2), melanoma	1p	ND
Breast carcinoma	1p, 2q	ND
Leiomyosarcoma	3q	ND
Anaplastic oligodendroglioma	19q	ND
Melanoma	7q	ND
Colorectal carcinoma	17p, 18q, 11p13	ND
MEN-1	11q	ND
Renal cell cancer	del(3p26-p25)	*VHL* gene involved
Colon cancer	del(4)(q12)	*REST* gene involved
Colon cancer	del(5)(q21-q22)	*APC*
Retinoblastoma	del(13)(q14.2)	*RB1*
Wilms' tumor	del(X)(q11.1)	*FAM123B*
Testicular tumors	12q	ND
Uterine cancers	del(10)(q23.3)	*PTEN*
Chromosomal gain by amplification		
Breast cancer	amp(1)(q32.1)	*IKBKE*
Breast cancer	amp(6)(q25.1)	*ESR1*
Neuroblastoma	amp(2)(p24.1)	*MYCN*
Hepatocellular carcinoma	amp(11)(q13-q22)	*YAP1, BIRC2*
Malignant melanoma	amp(3)(p14.2-p14.1)	*MITF*
Non-small-cell lung cancer	amp(14)(q13)	*NKX2-1*

Note: ND= Not detected.

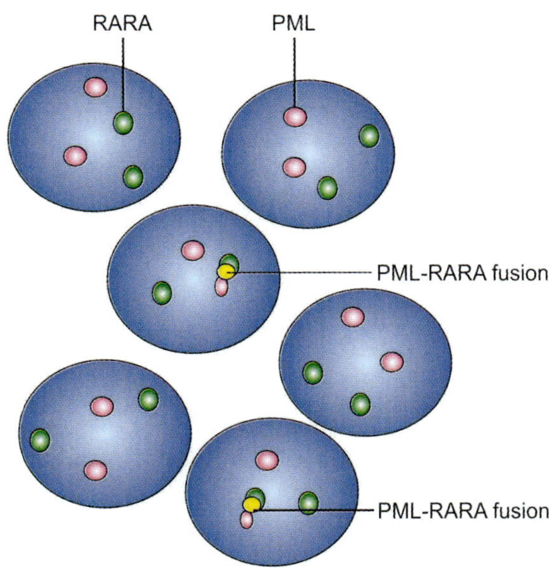

Fig. 4.9: Schematic diagram showing *PML* (red) and *RARA* (green) gene and chromosomal translocation (yellow) in case of acute promyelocytic leukemia.

- *Diagnosis and subclassification*: The demonstration of specific chromosomal abnormalities is one of the diagnostic features of many hematological malignancies and solid tumors.
  - The detection of t(14;18) is a marker of follicular lymphoma (FL).[16]
  - The demonstration of reciprocal translocation t(11;14) by FISH is essential in diagnosing mantle cell lymphoma.[17]
  - Demonstration of Philadelphia chromosome [chromosomal translocation of t(9;22)] is the important diagnostic marker of chronic myeloid leukemia (CML).
  - Acute myeloid leukemia (AML)–M3 is characterized by t(15:17) (Fig. 4.9).
  - Chromosomal abnormalities are also specific for diagnosis of many solid tumors (Ewing's sarcoma, synovial sarcoma, etc.) (Tables 4.3 and 4.4).
- *Target therapy*: *HER-2* gene amplification in breast cancer patients need target therapy with trastuzumab.
- *Prognosis of the patient*: Certain chromosomal abnormalities are related with prognosis of the patients such as:
  - Amplification of c-erb-B-2 is related with bad prognosis of breast cancer.
  - Gains of chromosomes 7 and 8 are associated with poor prognosis and potential markers for tumor aggressiveness in prostate cancer.[18]
- *Detection of recurrence of malignancy*: The demonstration of certain chromosomal abnormalities indicates early recurrence such as in:
  - Bladder cancer
  - Detection of malignancy in cerebrospinal fluid (CSF)
- *Monitoring therapy*: The demonstration of the cytogenetic markers during the time of chemotherapy or after treatment may be helpful to monitor the response of the treatment. Significant reduction of Philadelphia chromosome in CML patients indicates sustained chronic phase and better survival. Therefore, the demonstration of Philadelphia chromosome may help in monitoring response to interferon in CML therapy.
- *Monitoring of surgical margins in head and neck carcinomas*: The identification of chromosomal abnormalities in the surgical margins of the head and neck cancer patient may be helpful to assess the tumor free resection margin.[19]

Specific Applications of Molecular Techniques in Cytology Samples

As mentioned before FISH is used to detect:
- Abnormality in the chromosome number
- Deletion
- Chromosomal translocation, and
- Amplification.

Presently the major applications of FISH in cytology include:

Lung Carcinoma

Specimen: Bronchial wash/brush.

Sample: Alcohol fixed smear or sample may be collected in saline solution or fixatives of liquid-based cytology.

Various chromosomal abnormalities in bronchial washing and brushing specimen can be used to detect lung cancer.[20]

The common probes used to diagnose lung carcinoma include:
- Locus-specific probes to 5p15: Labeled spectrum green
- 8q24 (containing *C-MYC* gene): Labeled spectrum gold
- 7p12 (containing *EGFR* gene): Labeled spectrum red
- Centromeric probe to chromosome 6: Labeled spectrum aqua.

These probes are available commercially by multicolor probe set LAVysion (Vysis, Downers Grove, IL).

Interpretation: Normal cells of the respiratory tract show two aqua, two green, two red, and two gold signals in the multicolor FISH analysis probe. In case of deletion, one of the pair of the colored signal will be absent. In case of amplification, the number of colored signals increases, e.g. number of gold color signal (represent 8q24, myc gene) will increase in myc amplification.

As cytology diagnosis is highly specific and cheap, so FISH should be applied in cases of equivocal cytology or cytology negative but clinically suspected cases.

Bladder Carcinoma

Sample: Voided urine (alternatively, one can use bladder washings, upper tract washings or previously stained ThinPrep slides).

Urothelial carcinomas show various cytogenetic abnormalities related with chromosomes 1, 3, 4, 7, 8, 9, 11, 17. The chromosomal abnormalities can be demonstrated to detect urothelial carcinoma in urine cytology sample by applying commercially available probes produced by UroVysion (Abbott Molecular Inc, Des Plaines, IL). Two types of probes are used:

1. Chromosome enumeration probes:
   - Chromosome 3: Red
   - Chromosome 7: Green
   - Chromosome 17: Aqua
2. Locus-specific indicator:
   - 9p21: Gold

After counterstaining, the smears are interpreted under fluorescent microscope.

Interpretation:

Positive smear:

- More than five urothelial cells with gains of two or more chromosomes or more than 10 urothelial cells with gain of a single chromosome.
- Homozygous detection of 9p21 locus more than 20% of epithelial cells.

Fluorescence in situ hybridization is more sensitive (86%) but slightly less specific (93%) than cytology.

Gastrointestinal Tract

Fluorescence in situ hybridization helps to detect dysplasia and adenocarcinoma in Barrett's esophagus by using the chromosomal probes.[21] The commonly used probes are:

- 9p21
- 17q11
- 8q24
- 20q13.

Biliary Tract Malignancy

Fluorescence in situ hybridization can be used to diagnose malignancy in biliary tract brushing. Trisomy and polysomy in biliary brushing may indicate malignancy in cytology specimen. The same set of probes that are used in urinary tract can also be used in biliary tract brushing to detect malignancy.[22]

REFERENCES

1. Armitage P, Doll R. The age distribution of cancer and a multi-stage theory of carcinogenesis. Br J Cancer. 1954; 8(1):1-12.
2. Fröhling S, Döhner H. Chromosomal abnormalities in cancer. N Engl J Med. 2008;359(7):722-34.
3. Hughes T, Deininger M, Hochhaus A, et al. Monitoring CML patients responding to treatment with tyrosine kinase inhibitors: review and recommendations for harmonizing current methodology for detecting BCR-ABL transcripts and kinase domain mutations and for expressing results. Blood. 2006;108:28-37.
4. Rowley JD. A new consistent chromosomal abnormality in chronic myelogenous leukaemia identified by quinacrine fluorescence and Giemsa staining. Nature. 1973;243:290-3.
5. Licht JD, Sternberg DW. The molecular pathology of acute myeloid leukemia. Hematology Am Soc Hematol Educ Program. 2005:137-42.
6. Küppers R. Mechanisms of B-cell lymphoma pathogenesis. Nat Rev Cancer. 2005;5:251-62.
7. Mitelman F, Kaneko Y, Trent JM. Report of the committee on chromosome changes in neoplasia. Cytogent Cell Genat. 1990;55:358-86.
8. Storlazzi CT, Lonoce A, Guastadisegni MC, et al. Gene amplification as double minutes or homogeneously staining regions in solid tumors: origin and structure. Genome Res. 2010;20(9):1198-206.
9. Myllykangas S, Böhling T, Knuutila S. Specificity, selection and significance of gene amplifications in cancer. Semin Cancer Biol. 2007;17(1):42-55.
10. Dutt A, Beroukhim R. Single nucleotide polymorphism array analysis of cancer. Curr Opin Oncol. 2007;19:43-9.
11. Greig GM, England SB, Bedford HM, et al. Chromosome-specific alpha satellite DNA from the centromere of human chromosome 16. Am J Hum Genet. 1989;45:862-72.
12. Bolzer A, Kreth G, Solovei I, et al. Three-dimensional maps of all chromosome positions indicate a probabilistic order in human male fibroblast nuclei and prometaphase rosettes. PLoS Biol. 2005;3(5):e157.
13. Belmont A. Dynamics of chromatin, proteins, and bodies within the cell nucleus. Curr Opin Cell Biol. 2003;15:304-10.
14. Weiss MM, Hermsen MA, Meijer GA, et al. Comparative genomic hybridisation. Mol Pathol. 1999;52(5):243-51.
15. Lucito R, Healy J, Alexander J, et al. Representational oligonucleotide microarray analysis: a high-resolution method to detect genome copy number variation. Genome Res. 2003;13(10):2291-305.

16. Gong Y, Caraway N, Gu J, et al. Evaluation of interphase fluorescence in situ hybridization for the t(14;18)(q32;q21) translocation in the diagnosis of follicular lymphoma on fine-needle aspirates: a comparison with flow cytometry immunophenotyping. Cancer. 2003;99(6):385-93.
17. Remstein ED, Kurtin PJ, Buño I, et al. Diagnostic utility of fluorescence in situ hybridization in mantle-cell lymphoma. Br J Haematol. 2000;110:856-62.
18. Barranco MA, Alcaraz A, Corral JM, et al. Numeric alterations in chromosomes 7 and 8 detected by fluorescent in situ hybridization correlate with high-grade localized prostate cancer. Eur Urol. 1998;34:419-25.
19. Barrera JE, Ai H, Pan Z, et al. Malignancy detection by molecular cytogenetics in clinically normal mucosa adjacent to head and neck tumors. Arch Otolaryngol Head Neck Surg. 1998;124:847-51.
20. Sokolova IA, Bubendorf L, O'Hare A, et al. A fluorescence in situ hybridization–based assay for improved detection of lung cancer cells in bronchial washing specimens. Cancer. 2002;96:306-15.
21. Brankley SM, Wang KK, Harwood AR, et al. The development of a fluorescence in situ hybridization assay for the detection of dysplasia and adenocarcinoma in Barrett's esophagus. J Mol Diagn. 2006;8:260-7.
22. Moreno Luna LE, Kipp B, Halling KC, et al. Advanced cytologic techniques for the detection of malignant pancreatobiliary strictures. Gastroenterology. 2006;131:1064-72.

Review Questions

1. One entire chromosome is fused with another chromosome in the centromeres region to form a single chromosome is known as:
   a. Ring chromosome
   b. Robertsonian translocation
   c. Reciprocal translocation
   d. Chromosomal duplication

2. Philadelphia chromosome is an example of:
   a. Reciprocal translocation
   b. Chromosomal duplication
   c. Robertsonian translocation
   d. Deletion

3. The characteristic chromosomal translocation of follicular lymphoma is:
   a. t(9;22)(q34.1;q11.23)
   b. t(8;14)(q24.21;q32.33)
   c. t(14;18)(q32.33;q21.3)
   d. t(2;5)(p23;q35)

4. ALK-NPM1 gene fusion occurs in translocation of:
   a. t(2;5)(p23;q35)
   b. t(8;14)(q24.21;q32.33)
   c. t(11;14)(q13;q32.33)
   d. t(8;21)(q22;q22.3)

5. All are true for comparative genomic hybridization *except*:
   a. Balanced rearrangement is detected
   b. Genome-wise screening is possible
   c. Chromosomal amplification and deletion can be demonstrated
   d. The relative fluorescence level of tumor and normal DNA is measured

6. All are true for FISH technique *except*:
   a. No cell culture technique is needed
   b. It can be done on archival material
   c. It demonstrates the specific location of DNA sequence directly in the chromosome
   d. It provides specific information between maternal or paternal alleles

7. Repetitive nucleotide sequences at the end of the chromosome are known as:
   a. Amplification
   b. Telomere
   c. Centromere
   d. Microsatellite instability

8. The characteristic chromosomal translocation in synovial sarcoma is:
   a. t(11;22)(q24.1-q24.3;q12.2)
   b. t(12;16)(q13;p11)
   c. t(2;13)(q35;q14)
   d. t(x;18)(p11.2;q11.2)

Identify True/False

9. Whole chromosome probes are useful to detect chromosomal translocation or deletion. *(True/False)*

10. Comparative genomic hybridization (CGH) has limited use if the chromosomal rearrangement does not cause any genomic imbalance. *(True/False)*

11. Polymerase chain reaction (PCR) products can be used in array-based comparative genomic hybridization *(True/False)***.**

Answers

1. b. Robertsonian translocation
2. a. Reciprocal translocation
3. c. t(14;18)(q32.33;q21.3)
4. a. t(2;5)(p23;q35)
5. a. Balanced rearrangement is detected
6. d. It provides specific information between maternal or paternal alleles
7. b. Telomere
8. d. t(x;18)(p11.2;q11.2)
9. True
10. True
11. True

CHAPTER 5

Neoplasm

INTRODUCTION

The term neoplasm means new growth. The word "neoplasm" is originated from the Greek word "neo" means new and "plasia" means molding. The term "tumor" is originally derived from the Latin word for swelling. However, presently the word tumor is now used as synonymous to neoplasm. It is difficult to exactly define neoplasm. The British oncologist Willis defined neoplasm as "a neoplasm is an abnormal mass of tissue, the growth of which exceeds and is uncoordinated with that of the normal tissues, and persists in the same excessive manner after cessation of the stimulus which evoked the change."[1] This definition is true for most of the neoplasm in our body.

Neoplasm can be divided into two types: (1) benign and (2) malignant.

Benign Neoplasm

Benign tumors have certain important characteristics:

- They have restricted growth rate
- They are usually well encapsulated and not invasive to the surrounding tissue
- They are well differentiated
- They do not metastasize.

Benign tumors are usually classified based on the cells of origin. Tumors arising from the specific type of tissue resemble their cell of origin such as a tumor that arises from the gland will show glandular differentiation. In general, the suffix "oma" is attached to the cell of origin of benign tumors. For example, the tumor of fat is known as "lipoma"; tumor of osteoblast is known as osteoma, tumor of chondroid element is known as "chondroma". Tumor of the endodermal glandular epithelium is known as adenoma, whereas the tumor of epithelial origin is known as papilloma (Table 5.1).

Malignant Tumor

A malignant tumor is rapidly growing and aggressive in nature. They often show poor resemblance with its cell of origin, locally invasive and metastasize to the distant organ. Cancer is a general term for any types of malignant tumor. The word "cancer" probably came from Latin which means crab. This is because the cancer in any tissue clings with it firmly.

The nomenclature of malignant tumor is almost same as that of benign tumor. Malignant tumors originating

Table 5.1: Classification of neoplasm.

Tissue of origin	*Benign*	*Malignant*
Epithelial		
Stratified squamous, Basal cells of skin or adnexa	Squamous cell papilloma	Squamous cell carcinoma
Columnar epithelium	Adenoma	Adenocarcinoma
Respiratory epithelium	Bronchial adenoma	Bronchogenic carcinoma
Renal epithelium	Renal adenoma	Renal cell carcinoma
Urinary tract epithelium	Transitional cell papilloma	Transitional call carcinoma
Mesenchymal tissue		
Blood vessels and lymphatic tissue	Hemangioma Lymphangioma	Angiosarcoma, Kaposi's sarcoma
Mesothelial cells	Mesothelioma	Malignant mesothelioma
Fat	Lipoma	Liposarcoma
Striated muscle	Rhabdomyoma	Rhabdomyosarcoma
Smooth muscle	Leiomyoma	Leiomyosarcoma
Fibrous tissue	Fibroma	Fibrosarcoma
Bone	Osteoma	Osteosarcoma
Cartilage	Chondroma	Chondrosarcoma
Trophoblast	Hydatidiform mole	Choriocarcinoma
Germ cell	Mature teratoma	Malignant teratoma, seminoma, dysgerminoma

from the epithelial cell are labeled as carcinoma. Carcinoma is further classified depending on the precise cell of origin such as carcinoma developed from the glandular epithelium labeled as adenocarcinoma whereas the carcinoma developed from the squamous epithelium is labeled as squamous cell carcinoma (*see* Table 5.1). Malignant tumors developing from connective tissues are labeled as sarcoma. For example, malignant tumor of bone, fibrous tissue or fat cells are labeled as osteosarcoma, fibrosarcoma and liposarcoma, respectively.

The tumor may undergo divergent differentiation of the parenchymal tissue into mesenchymal tissue and this is known as a mixed tumor such as pleomorphic adenoma of salivary gland or adenofibroma of the uterus. The certain tumors develop from totipotent germ cells and are labeled as teratoma. The teratoma may show different types of epithelial and mesenchymal tissue simultaneously, such as mature cystic teratoma of the ovary often shows squamous epithelium, glands, sebaceous cells, cartilage or bone. Tumors developed from germ cells are known as dysgerminoma/seminoma.

Misnomers: The suffix "oma" is attached with the name of some tumors and they wrongly give an impression of benign tumors such as—seminoma: a malignant germ cell tumor of testis; hepatoma: malignant tumor of hepatocytes, and lymphoma: malignant tumor of the lymphoid cells, etc.

BIOLOGICAL CHARACTERISTICS OF MALIGNANT TUMOR OR CANCER

A malignant tumor is always aggressive in behavior and sooner or later kills its host. The principal differences of a benign and malignant neoplasm are highlighted in Table 5.2.

Table 5.2: Differentiating features of benign and malignant tumor.

Feature	*Benign*	*Malignant*
Growth	Slow	Rapid
Proliferative activity	Low mitotic rate	High mitotic rate and low cell death or apoptosis
Capsule	Usually well encapsulated	Un-encapsulated, poorly defined border
Local invasion	Absent	Locally invasive
Metastasis	Absent	Distant metastasis
Differentiation	Resembles the tissue of origin	Poor differentiation
Behavior	Modest, usually does not kill the patient	Aggressive and ultimately kills its host

HALLMARKS OF CANCER

There are certain "important hallmarks of cancer".[2] These are (Fig. 5.1):

- Sustained proliferation without any growth signal
- Insensitivity to antigrowth signal (evading growth suppressor)
- Resisting cell death or evading apoptosis
- Unlimited replicative potential
- Sustained angiogenesis
- Invasion and metastasis
- Altered cellular metabolism
- Genomic instability and mutation
- Promoting inflammation
- Bypassing immune destruction.

Sustained Proliferation (Fig. 5.2)

The cancer cells have the great capability to grow or proliferate by their own without any exogenous growth stimulation. They can achieve this by:

- Generating own growth factor ligands
- Stimulating the tumor associated normal cells for the production of growth factor
- Altering the cell surface receptors or intracellular receptor pathways.

Insensitivity to Antigrowth Signal (Evading Growth Suppressor)

Cancer cells acquire the immense capability to overcome the antigrowth signals that normally operate in the system to maintain tissue homeostasis and cellular quiescence.

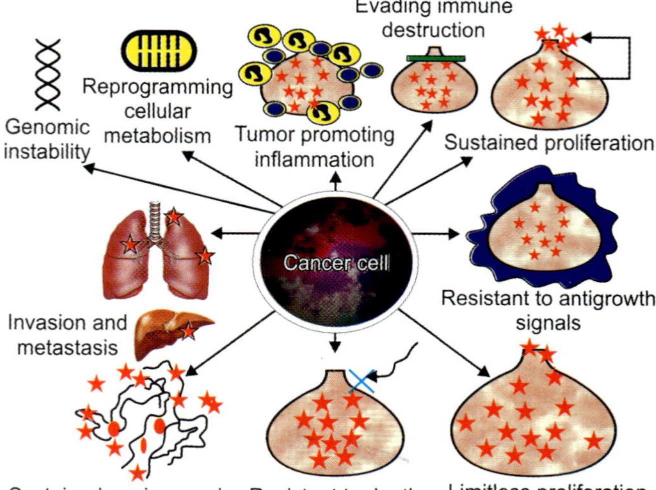

Fig. 5.1: Schematic diagram shows various hallmarks of cancer.

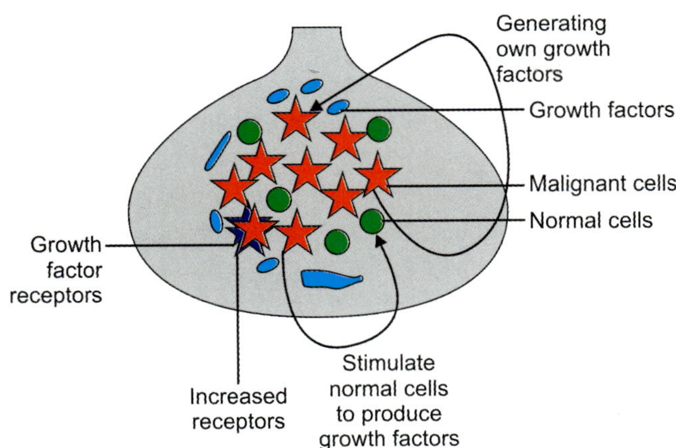

Fig. 5.2: Schematic diagram shows mechanisms of sustained proliferation of cells in cancer. Tumor cells generate their own growth factor ligands, stimulate the tumor associated normal cells for production of growth factor and alter the intracellular pathways of receptors.

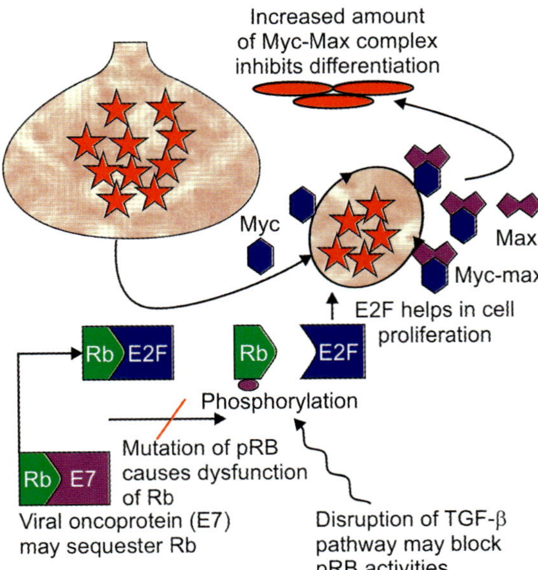

Fig. 5.3: Diagram shows how the cancer cells evade the influence of antigrowth signals. Retinoblastoma and p53 pathway of the cell cycle inhibition is disrupted due to the mutation of p53 or Rb gene. Rb and p53 gene products may also be sequestered by viral oncoproteins. There may be mutation, dysfunction and down regulation of TGF-β receptors causing disruption of inhibitory pathway of Rb protein. Excess Myc protein may bind with Max and Myc-Max complex may have inhibitory effect on cell differentiation.

The evasion from growth suppression can be done by (Fig. 5.3):

- *Disruption of pRB and p53 pathways*: Cancer cell continuously recruits the cells in the cell cycle by disruption of pRB and p53 pathway due to mutation of Rb and p53 gene. Functional activity of pRB may also be lost due to sequestration of pRB by viral oncoprotein (such as E7).[3]
- *Disruption of TGF-β pathway that originally blocks pRb activity*: This may occur by mutation, dysfunction and downregulation of TGF-β receptors.[4]
- *Avoiding terminal differentiation of cells*: In normal condition, the certain fraction of proliferating cells goes to the terminal differentiation and leaves the cell cycle forever. By this process, the normal tissue checks the cell proliferation. However, the cancer cells take various strategies to avoid terminal differentiation. Cancer cells often overexpress c-Myc oncogene and produce increased c-Myc proteins. This c-Myc protein binds with Max and increased Myc-Max complex impairs differentiation and enhances cell proliferation.

Resisting Cell Death or Evading Apoptosis

Cancer cell has the ability to resist apoptosis. This capability is achieved by a variety of strategies (Fig. 5.4).

- In the vast majority of the malignant tumor, the cancer cell blocks the functional activity of p53 protein by mutation of p53 gene that normally acts as proapoptotic.
- Cancer cells may also resist apoptosis by enhancing the expression of the anti-apoptotic signals such as BCL2 or by downregulating proapoptotic signals (Bax).

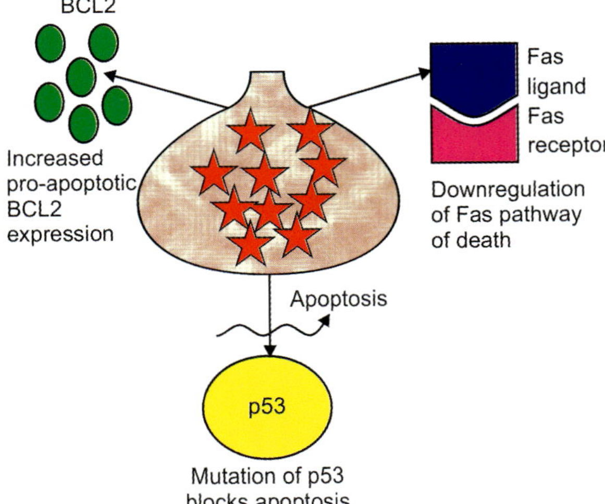

Fig. 5.4: Schematic diagram shows the mechanisms of blockage of apoptosis. This blockage of apoptosis may be done by downregulation of Fas receptor pathway, mutation of p53 and increased production of proapoptotic protein BCL2.

- Death ligand Fas binds to the death receptor and causes apoptosis. Cancer cell deregulates this Fas death receptor pathway.[5]

Unlimited Replicative Potential (Fig. 5.5)

The cancer cell acquires the limitless potential to replicate. The normal cells have limited number of cell division and proliferation. After a certain number of proliferative cycles the normal cells have to cross two distinct barriers of proliferation, senescence and crisis phase. Senescence is the irreversible nonproliferative but viable state. The certain fraction of cell undergoes to the crisis phase and dies. This replicative barrier or check point is maintained by telomeres of the chromosome. Telomeres are the multiple repeats of hexanucleotide sequence that protect the ends of the chromosomal DNA. There is progressive loss of telomere at the end of each cell cycle. After the end of certain number of cell cycles the telomere shortens significantly and triggers the cell to enter into crisis phase of death.[6] Unlike the normal cell, the tumor cells upregulate the expression of the telomerase enzyme and preserve the length of the telomere by adding the repetitive nucleotide sequence onto the end of the telomeric DNA. This prevents the cancer cells to enter into senescence phase and keep them in the continuous replicative phase.

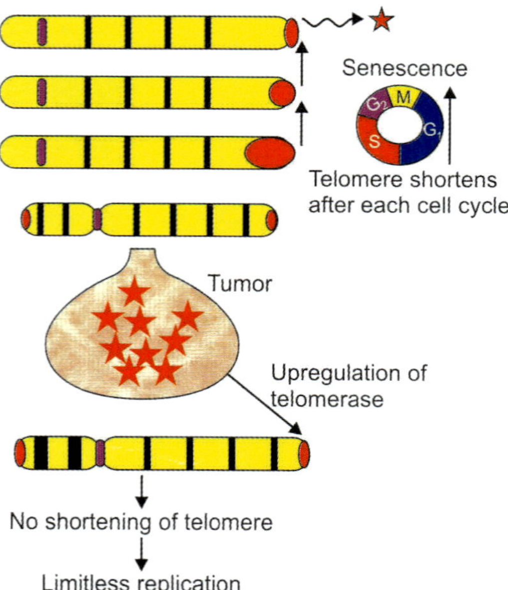

Fig. 5.5: Schematic diagram shows how the tumor cells gain limitless replicative potential. At the time of each cell cycle, the telomere portion of DNA shortens. The cell undergoes senescence when the telomere reaches to a critical length. Tumor cells produce telomerase enzyme that prevents the reduction of telomere length. Therefore the cells do not enter in senescence phase and gain limitless replicative potential.

Sustained Angiogenesis

The cancer cells try to maintain continuous supply of oxygen and nutrients by the sustained angiogenesis. They activate the angiogenic switch by over production of angiogenic factors such as vascular endothelial cell growth factor (VEGF) and fibroblast growth factor (FGF) and downregulating the antiangiogenic factors such as thrombospondin-1 and β-interferon.[7] However the neoangiogenesis in cancer is aberrant and is characterized by precocious capillaries, excessive branching of the blood vessels, microhemorrhage and distorted vessels with erratic blood flow.

Tissue Invasion and Metastasis

Invasion to the local tissue and distant metastasis are two unique characteristics of the cancer cell. Both local invasion and metastasis are well related events. Metastasis of cancer cell is achieved by (Fig. 5.6):

- *Downregulation or mutational inactivation of E-cadherin*: E-cadherin is a cell to cell adhesion molecule. It helps to form sheets of epithelial cells by adhering two cells together and prevents metastasis. In majority of cancer the function of E-cadherin is lost and metastasis occurs.[8]
- *Changing the type of integrin expression*: Cancer cell produces different spectrum of integrins (integrin α and β) that best fit with the tissue matrix of the metastatic site.

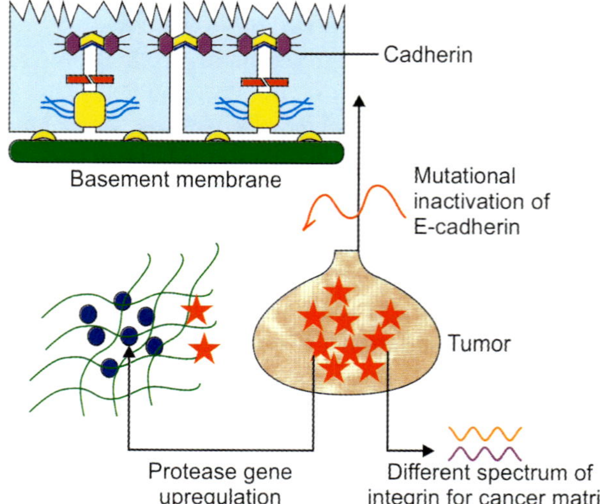

Fig. 5.6: The schematic diagram shows the mechanisms of invasion of cancer cells. E-cadherin maintains cell to cell adhesion. Mutation of E-cadherin in cancer cell causes disaggregation of the tumor cells. Simultaneously increased amount of protease or downregulation of the protease inhibitors helps in tissue invasion by cancer cell. Cancer cells also produce different types of integrin that make cancer specific tissue matrix.

- *Liberation of protease*: Proteases genes are upregulated and inhibitor of proteases are downregulated by cancer cell. The increased protease activity helps in tissue invasion and metastasis.[9]

Reprogramming Cellular Metabolism

Cancer cells alter the glucose metabolism and gets energy from glucose by glycolysis even in the presence of oxygen.

Genomic Instability

Negrini et al. considered that genomic instability is an emerging hallmark of cancer cell.[10] Chromosomal instability (CIN) is one important form of genomic instability by which chromosome number and structure are changed in course of tumor development. Microsatellite instability (MIN) is another cause of genomic instability. In case of MIN there is change of the number of oligonucleotide repeats in microsatellite sequences. Genomic instability causes increased spontaneous mutation rate in cancer cells and makes the cancer cell more aggressive.[11]

Tumor Promoting Inflammation

Inflammation contributes to the progression of tumor by supplying various bioactive molecules, growth factors, angiogenic factors and enzymes that breakdown the matrix. Tumor promoting inflammation is considered as one of the emerging hallmarks of cancer.

Evading Immune Destruction

Normal human immune system makes significant barrier in the progression of tumor. Cancer cell evades the immune mechanism of the body by secreting TGF-β or other immunosuppressive factors and also by recruiting immunosuppressive T regulatory cell.[12]

CANCER STEM CELLS

The malignant cells in the tumor have immense potential to replicate. A subset of cancer cells has the ability to generate new tumor on transplantation. Therefore one can assume that the subset of malignant cells has the functional properties of stem cell and these cells are called "cancer stem cell (CSC)". Cancer stem cells like normal stem cells have immense self-renewal capacity, long life span, and ability to resist apoptosis (Box 5.1). Like somatic stem cells they can also migrate to distant tissue. Somatic stem cells generate specific tissue in highly regulated way, whereas CSCs are the source of tumor production in aberrant poorly regulated way. Most probably the somatic stem cell of the tissue undergoes molecular damage due to viral infection, chemicals or inherited mutation. The somatic stem cell is converted to CSC that may produce both proliferating cell and also terminally differentiated cell. Unlike normal tissue renewal, the cells in tumor do not differentiate further and only accumulate in an unrestricted manner.

Evidence of Cancer Stem Cell

- In case of in vitro colony-forming assays of mouse myeloma cells only a few cancer cells are able to form colonies.
- Similarly, only a minor population of cells is clonogenic in solid cancers.

Significance of Cancer Stem Cell

Significance of the CSC is related with the failures of cancer treatment because if the drug is used only against cancer cells then the tumor may recur from the CSC. Therefore, cancer therapy should be specifically targeted to CSC for its success.

MOLECULAR BASIS OF CANCER

Multistep Process of Carcinogenesis (Box 5.2)

The carcinogenesis is a multistep process, which consists of cumulative changes of genetic abnormalities in the tumor cell. The genetic abnormalities may be in two ways:

Box 5.1: Cancer stem cell.

- A malignant cell with many functional properties of stem cell
- *Characteristics*
  - Poorly regulated self-renewal
  - Unlimited proliferative capacity (resistant to apoptosis)
  - Differentiates to produce tumor
  - Long life span
- *Stem cell model of cancer*: Only specific stem cells undergo mutation to produce tumor rather than differentiated cell
- *Therapeutic significance*: Cancer stem cells are slowly growing and difficult to eradicate

Box 5.2: Multistep process of carcinogenesis.

- Cumulative changes of genetic abnormalities in the tumor cell
- Two types of abnormalities
  - DNA sequence change
  - Epigenetic change causing gene silencing
- Each mutation or genetic changes provides additional advantages of the tumor cell
- Best studied in colonic carcinoma

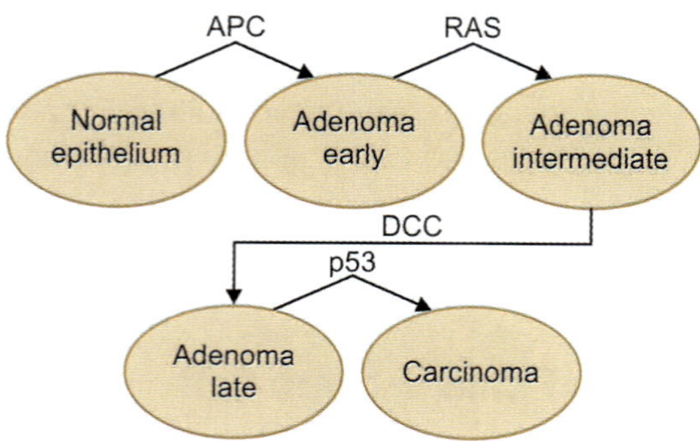

Fig. 5.7: The schematic diagram shows the process of multistep carcinogenesis in colonic adenoma to carcinoma. The various crucial genetic mutations happen in each step. Mutation of adenomatous polyposis coli (APC) gene is the rate-limiting step of the carcinogenesis. After this mutation, the tumor subsequently undergoes various other genetic mutations.

1. DNA sequence change
2. Epigenetic change causing gene silencing.

Kinetic analyses showed that the cancer cell undergoes at least six rate-limiting mutations before it becomes clinically evident.[13] Each mutation or genetic change provides additional advantages of the tumor cell. In addition, the loss of the normal control of the mutation may probably help in stable mutations of the affected cells. The normal cells transform into a cancer cell when some "critical transformation associated target genes" are damaged. This multistep process is well illustrated in colonic carcinoma which typically develops over decades and passes through adenoma to carcinoma sequences. During this transformation there are at least 6–7 mutational changes happen that take vital role in neoplastic transformation. Mutation of adenomatous polyposis coli (APC) gene is the rate-limiting step that initiates the tumorigenesis of normal colonic epithelial cells. This is followed by successive mutation of K-RAS, DCC and p53 genes (Fig. 5.7).[14]

The precise nature and the sequence of the genetic or epigenetic abnormalities in other malignancies are not known. It is possible that each tumor has its own sequence of genetic or epigenetic changes and there may be immense complexities in the sequence of genetic changes.

Clonal Evolution of Cancer

Few decades ago, Nowel first time proposed the clonal origin of cancer.[15] Today, it is of beyond doubt that cancer evolves as clonal proliferation and selection of group of cells that are originated from single precursor cell (Fig. 5.8). The evolution and progression of cancer is just like a complex Darwinian adaptive system.[16]

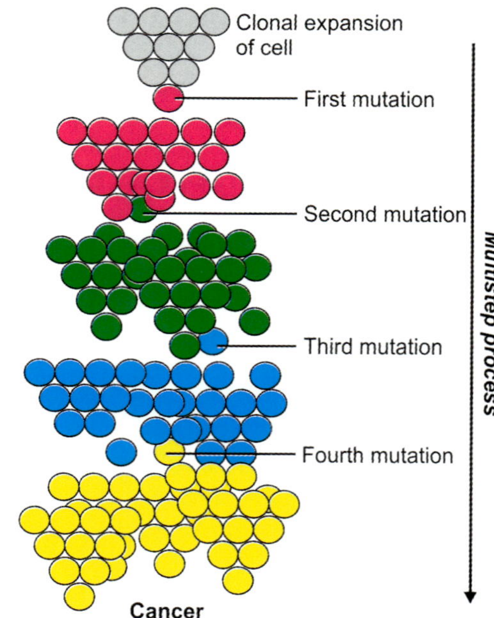

Fig. 5.8: The schematic diagram shows the clonal evolution of cancer. In each successive mutation the cancer cells gain certain unique properties and become more and more aggressive.

In earth, evolution of the habitat took place in the ecosystem whereas in tumorigenesis the evolution of the cancer cell happens in the microenvironment of the tissue. The evolving cancer cell tries to fit itself for space and nutrient. Possibly blind and purposeless multiple mutations of the DNA sequence occur in the evolving cancer cells. In course of time, the cancer clone emerges through the selective advantageous mutations that help in limitless proliferation, self-renewal, insensitive to antigrowth factors, evasion of apoptosis, angiogenesis and metastasis. The exact kinetics of the clonal evolution of cancer largely depends on mutation rate (and also epigenetic changes) and clonal expansion. The rate of epigenetic changes is much more than mutational changes.

ONCOGENES AND CANCER

Oncogenes are certain group of genes that control many intracellular signaling pathways and promote autonomous cell growth of cancer cells. The proto-oncogenes are normally present in the cell. They are the normal cellular counterpart of oncogenes in healthy cell. Proto-oncogene encodes various proteins that help in normal physiological cell growth and proliferation. Products of proto-oncogene are under direct regulatory control of the cell whereas the oncoproteins encoded by oncogenes are autonomous.

Table 5.3: Oncogenes: Position, function and related with diseases.

Oncogene	Chromosome	Position	Mode of activation	Function	Disease
H-RAS	11	Membrane	Point mutation	Signal transduction	Colon, lung, pancreas
K-RAS	12	Membrane	Point mutation	Signal transduction	AML, thyroid carcinoma
ERB-B2	7	Membrane	Amplification	Growth factor receptors	Breast and ovarian cancer
RET	10	Membrane	Point mutation	Growth factor receptors	Multiple endocrine neoplasia 2A, 2B
SIS	20	Membrane	Overexpression	Growth factor	Osteosarcoma
C-MYC	8	Nucleus	Translocation	Transcriptional activator	Burkitt's Lymphoma
N-MYC	8	Nucleus	Amplification	Transcriptional activator	Neuroblastoma

Oncogene acts in dominant way that means if one of the two alleles of the genes is altered then the oncogene will show its biological action. A wide variety of oncogenes have been described so far (Table 5.3). These oncogenes are also localized in different parts of a cell such as cell membrane, cytoplasm and nucleus to do wide range of functions.

Activation of Oncogenes

Oncogenes are activated by various ways (Fig. 5.9):

- Chromosomal translocation
- Mutation
- Gene amplification.

Chromosomal Translocation

- *Fusion gene*: Chromosomal translocation may cause formation of chimeric fusion gene and thereby produces chimeric protein with excessive tyrosine kinase activity or involving transcription factors.
  - *Tyrosine kinase activity*: BCR-ABL1 fusion gene in Philadelphia chromosome is the classic example of chimeric fusion gene causing excessive tyrosine kinase activity.
  - ALK-NPM1 fusion oncogene is generated by t(2;5)(p23;q35) in case of anaplastic large cell lymphoma.
  - *Transcription factors*: Chromosomal translocation can cause fusion protein with aberrant transcriptional activities. In Ewing's sarcoma there is t(11:22)(q24:q12) translocation that produces ERG-EWSR1 fusion gene with excessive transcription factors activity.
- *Deregulated expression of structurally normal genes*: Chromosomal translocation may often bring the proto-oncogene into a new position which is under the influence of gene promoter or enhancer sequence of the other normal tissue regulatory element. Therefore, there may be excessive expression of the proto-oncogene. In case of Burkitt's lymphoma C-MYC oncogene is transferred near the heavy chain gene onto chromosome 14 and is upregulated by the neighboring promoter.

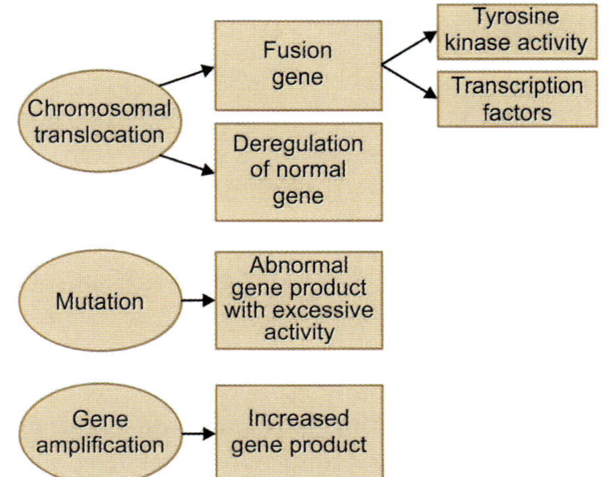

Fig. 5.9: The schematic diagram shows the various mechanisms of activation of oncogene and their effects. The three major ways of oncogene activation are chromosomal translocations, mutation and gene amplifications.

Gene Amplification

Gene amplification is seen in many advanced cancers and multiple copies of the gene are noted in the cancer cells. Several hundred kilobases of DNA segment is usually amplified that contains many genes. Usually oncogene families of MYC, EGFR, RAS and cyclin D1 are amplified. Amplification of ERB-B2 is usually seen in breast cancer and its increased expression correlates with poor prognosis.[17] MYC is amplified in small cell lung cancer, cervical cancer, breast and esophageal cancer.[18]

Mutation

Mutation of the oncogene may cause abnormal gene product with excessive activity, such as point mutation in RAS gene encodes a protein that remains continuously in active state and incessantly produces growth promoting signals to the nucleus.[19] Point mutations of BRAF gene encodes a protein with change of valine residue at position 599 to glutamic acid in the kinase domain. This aberrant BRAF protein continuously stimulates MAP kinase cascades resulting incessant cell proliferation.[20]

Functional Properties of Oncogene

Oncogenes perform their function by the production of oncoproteins that can be classified as: (1) Growth factors, (2) Growth factor receptors, (3) Signal transducers, (4) Transcription factors, (5) Chromatin remodelers, and (6) Apoptosis regulators (Box 5.3).

Growth Factors

Cancer cells often overexpresses various growth factor genes that produce growth factors. SIS oncogene is overexpressed in osteosarcoma and low-grade astrocytoma[21] resulting in excessive production of platelet derived growth factor (PDGF-β) that causes unrestricted cell proliferation. HST-1 and INT-2 genes are overexpressed in stomach, breast and bladder carcinoma and produce the oncoproteins, FGF, etc.

Growth Factor Receptors

Growth factor receptor has three parts: (1) external ligand binding domain, (2) membranous domain, and (3) cytoplasmic domain. Normally when the ligand binds with external ligand binding domain of the growth factor receptors there is transient activation of tyrosine kinase enzyme by dimerization followed by phosphorylation of various substrates. Oncogenes may produce the growth factor receptors that are persistently activated without any binding with its ligand (Fig. 5.10). In multiple endocrine neoplasia (MEN) 2A and 2B there is point mutation of RET gene resulting encoding of the oncoproteins that has persistent activity of cytoplasmic domain of the tyrosine kinase receptors.

ERB-B2 gene is amplified in breast and ovarian cancer causing excessive production of epithelial growth factor (EGF) receptors which is responsible for cell proliferation. In large number of squamous cell carcinomas, ERB-B1 oncogene is over expressed resulting in excessive production of EGF receptor.

Box 5.3: Functional activity of oncogene.

- *Growth factors*: Overexpression of various growth factor genes, e.g. SIS oncogene in osteosarcoma, HST-1 and INT-2 genes in stomach, breast and bladder carcinoma
- *Growth factor receptors*:
  - Oncogenes produce abnormal growth factor receptors: *Activated without any binding* with its ligand
  - *Amplification of receptors*: For example ERB-B2 gene is amplified in breast and ovarian cancer with excess EGF receptors
- *Signal transducers*: Cytoplasmic signal transducing proteins with *persistent activity*, e.g. point mutation of RAS oncogene generates persistent activated RAS protein
- *Transcription factors*: Chimeric fusion gene with aberrant activity of transcription factor
- *Chromatin remodelers*: Oncogene plays critical role in chromatin remodeling by modification of histones of the nucleosomes

Signal Transducers

Oncogenes may produce oncoproteins that mimic cytoplasmic signal transducing proteins with persistent activity. RAS, the signal transducing molecule, is present

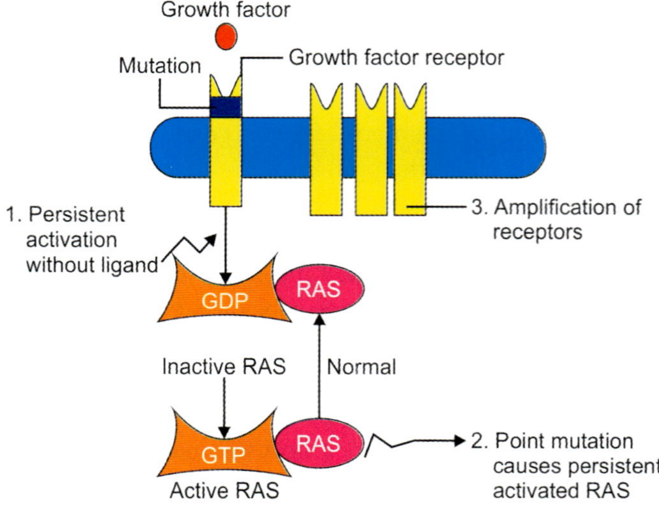

Fig. 5.10: The schematic diagram shows the mechanism of persistent signal transduction in cancer cell. Normally after binding the growth factor and its receptor the cytoplasmic domain of the receptor converts inactive guanosine diphosphate (GDP) bound RAS to active guanosine triphosphate (GTP) bound RAS. This active RAS becomes inactive again when GTP is hydrolyzed to GDP. In case of cancer, there may be mutation of—(1) growth factor receptors, or (2) mutation of RAS causing persistent activation of RAS, (3) growth factor receptor may also be amplified.

in the inner surface of the cell membrane as Guanosine diphosphate (GDP) bound inactive form. When a normal cell is stimulated through a growth factor receptor the inactive GDP bound RAS, becomes active Guanosine triphosphate (GTP) bound RAS. This is done by transforming GDP to GTP. After the stimulation, there is rapid hydrolysis of GTP to GDP and active RAS again reverts to inactive RAS. The point mutation of RAS oncogene generates persistently activated RAS protein as it is resistant to hydrolyze GTP to GDP. This is responsible for persistent stimulation of the receptor pathway without any external factors (Fig. 5.10).

Oncogenes encode oncoproteins that simulate both non-receptor protein kinases and guanosine-triphosphate-binding proteins. The nonreceptor protein kinases are—(1) tyrosine kinases, and (2) serine and (3) threonine kinases.[22]

Transcription Factor

As mentioned earlier, chromosomal translocation often produces chimeric fusion gene with aberrant activity of transcription factor. In Ewing's sarcoma there is t(11:22)(q24:q12) that produces ERG-EWSR1 fusion gene with excessive transcription factors activity. In carcinoma of lung and neuroblastoma there is N-MYC amplification causing excessive production of transcription factor resulting in cell proliferation.

Chromatin Remodelers

When a portion of chromatin opens up, the transcription factors get a chance to interact with promoter regions of DNA. Therefore, chromatin remodeling is important in the control of gene expression. Oncogene plays critical role in chromatin remodeling. There are two kinds of enzymes that regulate chromatin remodeling: (1) ATP dependent enzymes, and (2) histone modifiers.[23] In case of acute lymphatic leukemia and acute myeloid leukemia, chromosomal translocation of 11q23 produces chimeric fusion oncogene ALL1 (MLL). The fusion protein of ALL1 is involved with chromatin remodeling by modification of histones of the nucleosomes.[24]

MICRO-RNA AND CANCER

Micro-RNAs (miRNA) are evolutionarily conserved, non-protein-coding, endogenous, small RNAs molecules. They inhibit gene expression at the post-transcriptional level (Box 5.4). miRNAs do not code any proteins, however, they transcriptionally control protein formation of genes by cleaving the mRNA, decaying mRNA and translational repression.

Box 5.4: Micro-RNA.

- *Definition*: Micro-RNAs (miRNA) are evolutionarily conserved, short, single-stranded RNA molecules
- *Main function*: Anneals to the complementary strand of messenger RNA and causes translational repression and/or degradation
- *Physiologic function*
  - Cellular differentiation
  - Cell proliferation
  - Apoptosis
  - Stem cell maintenance miRNA in cancer
- Dysregulation of oncogene or tumor suppressor gene
- *Mutation or epigenetic changes of miRNA*
- *Antiapoptosis*: The loss of miRNA causes unopposed expression of BCL2
- Regulation of cell adhesion, angiogenesis, and cell matrix digestion

Clinical application:
- Diagnostic marker
- Primary site detection of tumor
- Subtyping of cancer
- Prediction of clinical outcome
- Possible therapy in cancer by modulating miRNA

Biogenesis of miRNA[25] (Fig. 5.11)

Primary miRNA Formation

Micro-RNA genes may be located in the intronic coding, intronic non-coding region and exonic noncoding region. The miRNA genes are transcribed by RNA polymerase II and primary miRNAs (pri-miRNA) are formed.

Pre-miRNA

The nascent pri-miRNA is like hair pin loop like structure and is cleaved by RNase III endonuclease Drosha to precursor miRNA (pre-miRNA).

Transport to nucleus: The pre-miRNA is carried from nucleus to cytoplasm by "exportin 5".

Mature miRNA

In the cytoplasm, the enzyme RNase III endonuclease Dicer cleaves the pri-miRNA into small, imperfect dsRNA duplex miRNA-miRNA. This complex consists of mature miRNA strand and its complementary strand (miRNA). The enzyme Dicer also transforms long dsRNA molecules into small interfering RNA (siRNA) duplexes.

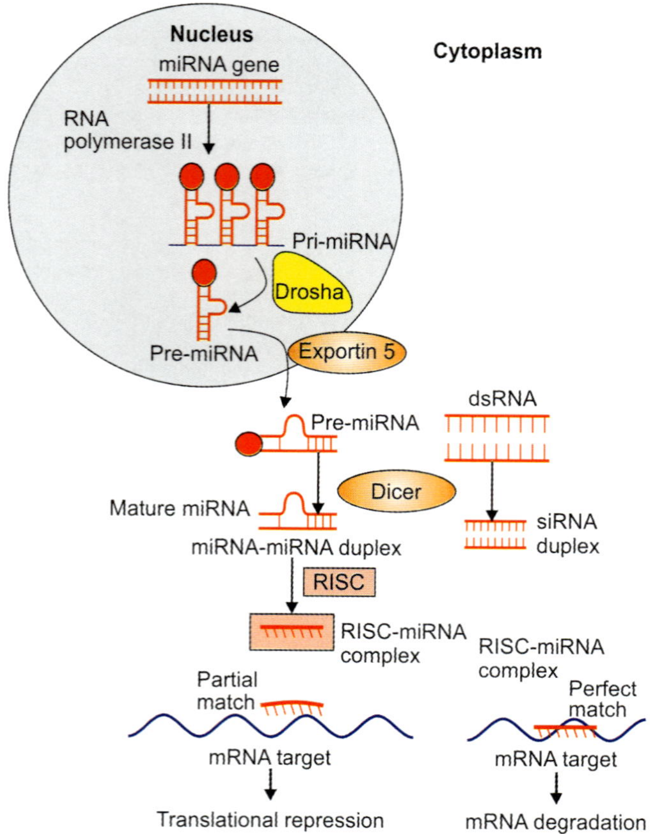

Fig. 5.11: The schematic diagram shows micro-RNA formation and its function. At first primary micro-RNA (pri-microRNA) is formed followed by pre-micro-RNA and mature micro-RNA. This mature miRNA combines with mRNA at specific sites and blocks its action.

Combination with RNA-induced Silencing Complex

Only one strand of miRNA or siRNA duplex selectively combines with RNA-induced silencing complex (RISC).

Terminal activity: The Complex RISC with miRNA/siRNA binds with target mRNA and then depending on complementarity—(1) degrades the target mRNA, or (2) repress the translation of target mRNA.

Functions of miRNA

Micro-RNA molecule anneals to the complementary strand of messenger RNA leading to

- *Translational repression*: When there is partial complementarity with the target mRNA, or
- *Degradation*: When there is perfect match with the target mRNA.[25]

By combining with mRNA, the miRNA controls the ultimate expression of genes and therefore takes part in various important physiological functions. As miRNA works on partial complementarity basis with mRNA so a single miRNA is able to inhibit many mRNA and similarly many miRNA can block a particular mRNA. The known functions of miRNA include:

- Cellular differentiation
- Cell proliferation
- Apoptosis
- Stem cell maintenance.

miRNA and Cancer[26]

The genes of miRNAs play important role in cellular transformation and carcinogenesis. miRNA is dysregulated in various solid and hematological tumors, such as colorectal cancer, breast and lung cancer, and lymphoma tumors. The possible ways of carcinogenesis by miRNA are:

- *Altering the cell growth and apoptosis*: miRNA interacts with apoptotic gene and the antiapoptotic function promotes tumorigenesis. The miR-15 and miR-16 induce apoptosis by reacting with BCL2 gene produced mRNA in lymphoma.
- *Dysregulation of oncogene or tumor suppressor gene*: Excess miRNA may block the tumor suppressor gene proteins and may promote tumorigenesis. Similarly reduced expression of miRNA may promote the oncogene.
- *Mutation or epigenetic changes of miRNA*: Germ line or somatic mutation of miRNA or epigenetic changes by methylation may affect its normal inhibitory function leading to malignancy.
- *Others*: Various miRNAs regulate the cell adhesion, angiogenesis, and cell matrix digestion and cell signaling pathway and promote tumor invasion and metastasis.

Clinical Applications of miRNA

The clinical applications of miRNA include:

- *Diagnostic markers*: miRNA expression profiles may help—(1) to distinguish malignant cells from benign cells, (2) to identify the primary site of the tumor in case of metastatic poorly differentiated tumor, and (3) to subclassify the tumors.
- *Clinical outcome and prognosis*: The expression profile of miRNA in tumor may help in the prediction of relapse and metastasis.
- *Therapeutic effect*: In future, the miRNA can be modulated in different ways to battle with cancer. The production of tumor promoting proteins can be inhibited by applying synthetically prepared miRNA against the

respective mRNA. Researchers have also blocked the expression of oncogenic miRNA for cancer therapy.

GENOMIC INSTABILITY

Genomic instability is considered as one of the important causes of tumorigenesis. The genomic instability may occur by various ways:

- Chromosomal instability (CIN)
- Microsatellite instability (MSI)
- CpG island methylator phenotype (CIMP)
- In addition potentially other, presently not yet identified mechanism may be present.

Chromosomal Instability

It is one of the important ways to develop genomic instability. Chromosomal instability is defined as "a persistently high rate of loss and gain of whole chromosomes or part of the chromosome".[27] The result of CIN is the loss of heterozygosity (LOH) or imbalance of the number of chromosome (aneuploidy).

In case of CIN there is defect in proper segregation of chromosome in the mitotic phase. This may be due to—(1) cohesion defects, (2) spindle assembly check point (SAC) defects, (3) supernumerary centrosomes, (4) defects in Kinetochore-Microtubule attachment, and (5) defects in Cell-Cycle regulation (Box 5.5).

Cohesion Defects

Certain proteins are responsible for cohesion of sister chromatids. Acute depletion of such proteins elevates the number of tetraploid cells.[28] Similarly, overexpression of separase also increases the incidence of tetraploid cells.[29]

Spindle Assembly Check Point Defects

This check point regulates the proper alignment of the chromosome in the equatorial plate in anaphase and successful delivery of a correct chromosome set to each daughter cell. Defects in the spindle assembly check (SAC) point may cause aberration in anaphase leading to chromosome missegregation and aneuploidy. The proteins encoded by hBUB1 and MAD2 are two important regulatory molecules of the spindle assembly check point.[30]

Mutations of SAC genes may be present in breast, colon and gastric cancer cell lines.[31] However, the role of SAC to the occurrence of CIN in clinical cancer is still a matter of debate.

Box 5.5: Chromosomal instability (CIN).

Definition: Persistently increased rate of loss and gain of whole chromosomes or part of the chromosome

Result

- Loss of heterozygosity (LOH) or
- Imbalance of the number of chromosome (aneuploidy)

Mechanisms

- *Cohesion defects*: Depletion of proteins responsible for cohesion of sister chromatids
- *Spindle assembly check point defects*: Regulates the proper alignment of the chromosome in the equatorial plate in anaphase
- *Supernumerary centrosomes*: Centrosome amplification due to over expression of Aurora A kinase
- *Defects in Kinetochore-Microtubule Attachment*: Excessive stabilization of microtubule-kinetochore attachment
- *Defects in Cell-Cycle Regulation*: Mutation of cell cycle regulator genes such as BRCA1, BRCA2, Rb, p53, Mdm2, etc.

Supernumerary Centrosomes

The centrosome amplification is seen due to overexpression of Aurora A kinase.[32] Extra centrosomes may produce multiple spindle formation leading to tetraploidy. The tetraploid cells are prone to have CIN.

Defects in Kinetochore-Microtubule Attachment

Microtubule is reversibly attached to kinetochore. There is a dynamic relation in kinetochore-microtubule attachment and this is generated by repeated attachment and detachment of the microtubule and kinetochore. This is helpful in error correction of microtubule attachment. Excessive stabilization of microtubule-kinetochore attachment causes defect in the kinetochore attachment leading to aneuploidy. Aurora B kinase is central to this control system. However, perturbation of other proteins such as MCAK, CNEP-E and APC, etc. are also involved in defective microtubule-kinetochore attachment.[33]

Defects in Cell-Cycle Regulation

A large numbers of cell cycle regulator genes are also involved in CIN such as BRCA1, BRCA2, Rb, p53, Mdm2, etc.[34] These cell cycle regulatory genes possibly promote CIN by, chromosome missegregation, centrosome duplication during S phase or allowing defective chromosome to undergo mitosis.

Microsatellite Instability (Box 5.6)

What are Microsatellites?

Microsatellites are stable inherent, short repetitive sequence of 1–6 base pair of DNA that are unique to each

Box 5.6: Microsatellite instability.

- Microsatellites:
  - Stabile, inherent
  - Short repetitive sequence of DNA
  - Unique to each individual
- Microsatellite instability (MSI): Alteration of the pattern of polymorphic short tandem repeat segments of DNA
- Genes commonly mutated in MIN: hMSH2, hMSH6, hMSH3, hMLH1, hPMS1 and hPMS2
- MSI is responsible for multiple mutations of cancer-related genes
- A marker of genomic instability
- MSI: Noted in colonic, gastric, esophageal and endometrial cancer
- MSI is measured by PCR

individual and have very low inherent mutational rate. The repetitive unit may be mono-, di-, tri-, tetra-, penta- or hexanucleotides. This is unique for each individual. Microsatellites are distributed in the entire genome including both the coding and noncoding genomic region.

Microsatellite instability means alteration of the pattern of polymorphic short tandem repeat segments of DNA. Normally, during replication of DNA there may be mutation of microsatellite. However, the rate of microsatellites mutation is very low. The replication errors of microsatellite are normally repaired by the mismatch repair system (MMR). To date six DNA mismatch repair genes are identified: hMSH2, hMSH6, hMSH3, hMLH1, hPMS1 and hPMS2[35] (Fig. 5.12). Loss of action of these DNA mismatch repair genes may cause increased replication error of microsatellite which is represented by high MSI. MSI can be demonstrated by PCR amplification of genetic loci of microsatellite.

MSI in Human Cancer

Microsatellite instability (MSI) reflects mutation of MMR and mutation of the mismatch repair genes. The defect in MMR may cause mutation of various other cancer promoting genes. Increased mutations in microsatellite sequences are present in colonic carcinoma and other human solid tumors such as endometrial carcinomas, esophageal, and gastric carcinomas.[35] Approximately 15% of colorectal carcinoma (CRC) shows high MSI and out of which 3% cases are related with Lynch syndrome and the rest 12% are caused by MLH1 gene hypermethylation. CRCs with MSI are unique and show several distinctive features such as occurrence in younger age, frequent involvement of the proximal colon, involvement of right colon, mucinous or signet ring morphology, poorly differentiated, and have better prognosis.

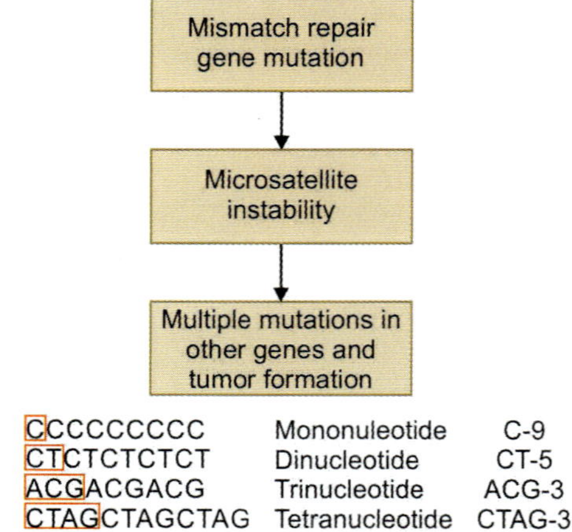

Fig. 5.12: The schematic diagram shows that mismatch repair genes are responsible for microsatellite instability (MSI) and subsequently tumor formation. Microsatellite may be formed due to repetition of one, two, three or more nucleotides.

Diagnostic Criteria of MSI

The tumor that shows mutation of two or more of the five microsatellite sequences (enlisted by the National Cancer Institute) is labeled as MSI-high. MSI-low tumor shows mutation of one of the microsatellite sequences.

Microsatellite stable tumor does not show any mutation in the enlisted microsatellite panel.

CpG Island Methylator Phenotype

So far we have discussed various genetic changes in cancer. However, now we know that many epigenetic changes are also responsible for carcinogenesis.

WHAT IS EPIGENETICS?

The term epigenetics indicates the heritable changes of the expression of gene without any change of the original DNA sequence in gene. The epigenetic changes occur in the following ways:

- Methylation of cytosine at the CpG islands of DNA
- Post-translation modification of histone
- Nucleosome remodeling by ATP dependent chromatin complexes
- miRNA modification.

Methylation of DNA

This occurs by addition of a methyl group to the carbon-5 position of cytosine with the help of DNA methyltransferase enzymes. Specific DNA methylation in the promoter region of DNA causes silencing of the respective gene (Fig. 5.13). CpG dinucleotides are unevenly distributed in the DNA and are concentrated in the CpG-rich DNA stretches that are labeled as CpG islands. Normally majority of the CpG islands are unmethylated. However, methylation of CpG island in the promoter region may cause silencing of the gene. Therefore the genes responsible for cell cycle control or DNA repair or apoptosis may be inactivated by DNA hypermethylation.[36] There is no doubt that DNA hypermethylation is a significant epigenetic changes in carcinogenesis. However, the initial triggering factor of hypermethylation is unknown. Possibly this occur as an early events in carcinogenesis affecting the tumor suppressor genes.

Post-translation Modification of Histone[37]

Histone proteins form the core nucleosome around which DNA chain winds two and half turn. The histone has C-terminal domain and N-terminal tail. This N-terminal tails may undergo various types of post-translation modification such as acetylation, methylation, phosphorylation, etc. The histone modification probably works by changing the conformation of chromatin and thereby modifying the accessibility of the various nonhistone recruiting proteins that are needed for gene transcription. The specific action of gene activation or repression depends on the exact type of modification and the specific amino acid residue to be modified. For example acetylation of lysine causes gene activation, whereas, methylation of the lysine may cause either gene activation or repression depending on which lysine residue is methylated on which type of histone. Therefore the histone modification may take active role in tumorigenesis by activation the oncogene or suppressing the tumor suppressor genes. This may also regulate cellular transcription, translation and DNA repair process significantly.

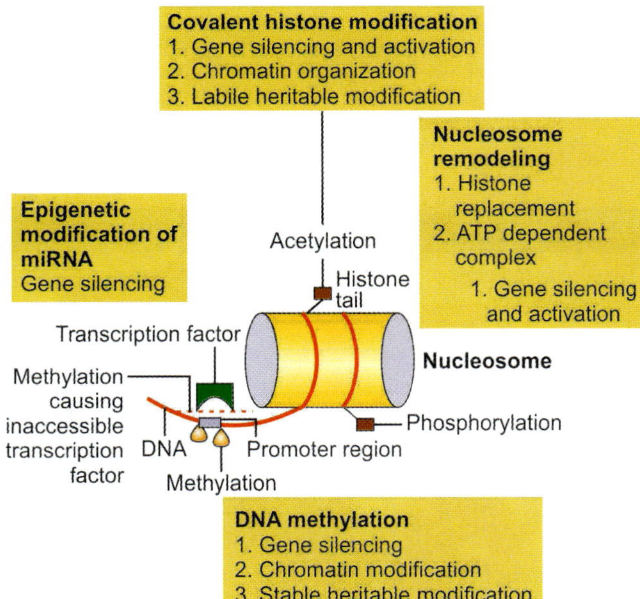

Fig. 5.13: The schematic diagram shows various mechanism of DNA silencing. Methylation of cytosine at the CpG islands of DNA promoter sites causes silencing of the respective gene. In addition, acetylation of histone tail may cause gene activation, whereas deacetylation may be responsible for gene silencing.

Nucleosome Remodeling

Nucleosome may be remodeled by the replacement of one type of histone with the more specific histone proteins and also by ATP-dependent chromatin-remodeling complexes. The nucleosome modification open the access of the gene promoter sites to the various transcription factors and paly the vital role in gene expression.

Modification of miRNA

As mentioned earlier, miRNA regulates protein synthesis by degrading or silencing mRNA. The expression of miRNA genes may also be regulated by epigenetic mechanism.[38]

TUMOR SUPPRESSOR GENES

Tumor suppressor genes are normally present in the cell and regulate the physiological cell division and growth. These genes function as a negative regulator of oncogenes and cell cycle check points and protect the body against tumor development. Tumor suppressor gene is recessive and therefore, both alleles must be mutated to get the adverse biological consequence.

Knudson's Two Hit Hypothesis

In relation to tumor suppressor gene, it is important to mention two hit hypothesis theory proposed by Knudosn AG. He suggested that in children with early onset retinoblastoma, there is an inherited mutation in retinoblastoma gene which is present in all the somatic cells and a second or additional somatic mutation (second hit) in other allele may lead to retinoblastoma. In case of late onset retinoblastoma (sporadic cases) of the children, two somatic mutations occur in the single retinal cell and tumor develops (Fig. 5.14). This important hypothesis explains the presence and nature of the tumor suppressor genes.

Table 5.4 shows the location and functions of some essential tumor suppressor genes.

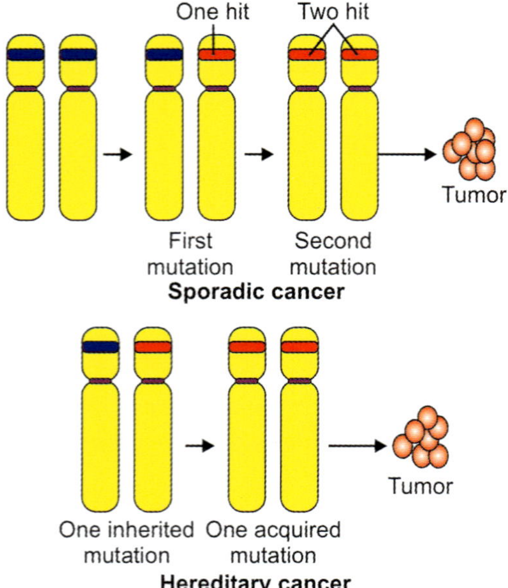

Fig. 5.14: The schematic diagram shows Knudson's two hit hypothesis of carcinogenesis. In case of sporadic cancer two mutations occur in the somatic cells. The tumor develops when both the alleles undergo mutation. In hereditary cancer, there is an inherited mutation in one of the genes followed by another mutation of the allele.

p53, Policeman of the Genome (Box 5.7)

This is the most widely studied tumor suppressor gene so far. This gene is located in Chromosome 17p13.1. The other family members of p53 tumor suppressor include p63 and p73.[39] These proteins are functionally related with p53 and has clear role in normal development. Wild type p53 controls cell cycle and apoptosis. It is capable of suppressing the growth of the tumor. Loss of heterozygosity of the wild type p53 may cause cancer. It is a commonly mutated gene and more than 50% of the human cancer shows p53 mutation. Mutant form of p53 has prolonged half-life than wild type. However, mutant p53 protein is devoid of any functional activity.

Box 5.7: p53, the tumor suppressor gene.

- *Location*: Chromosome 17p13.1
- Wild type p53 takes important role in *cell cycle control* and *apoptosis*
- Mutant p53 protein is devoid of any functional activity
- Mutant form of p53 has increased half-life than wild type
- The most commonly mutated gene in cancer

Mechanism of loss of function

- Mutation
- Loss of heterozygosity
- Deranged function due to inactivation by binding with other proteins
- Mutations of regulators of p53

Functions of p53

- *Cell cycle arrest*: Activated p53 protein produces p21 that inhibits CDK and prevents phosphorylation of pRB
- *Repair of DNA damage*: p53 activates GADD45 gene that encodes a protein related with DNA repair
- *Apoptosis*: Excess BAX protein and cell surface death receptors such as DR5 and FAS are produced

Table 5.4: Tumor suppressor genes.

Gene	*Chromosome*	*Location of encoded protein within cell*	*Protein function*	*Familial cancer association*	*Tumor associated with somatic mutation*
p53	17	Nucleus	Cell cycle arrest and apoptosis	Li-Fraumeni syndrome	Many human cancers (over 50%)
Rb	13	Nucleus	Cell cycle control	Retinoblastoma	Retinoblastoma, osteosarcoma, breast, lung and bladder carcinoma
APC	5	Cytoplasm	Binds and degrades β catenin, inhibition of signal transduction	Familial adenomatous polyposis	Colorectal cancer
WT1	11	Nucleus	Transcriptional regulation	Wilms' tumor	Wilms' tumor
PTEN	10	Cytoplasm		Cowden syndrome	Endometrial carcinoma, thyroid and prostate cancer
BRCA1, BRCA2	17/13	Nucleus	DNA damage repair	Familial breast and ovarian cancers	Not known
p16(INK4A)	9	Nucleus	CDK inhibitor	Melanoma	Breast, esophagus and pancreatic cancer

Mechanism of Loss of Function of p53

The function of p53 may be lost in various ways:

- *Mutation*: Usually missense point mutation occurs in the central sequence specific DNA binding domain of p53.This mutation changes the conformation of the sequence specific DNA-binding domain of p53 and the transcriptional activity of p53 protein is lost. The mutant p53 protein is relatively stable with prolonged half-life than wild-type p53, and is present at higher level in the tumor cell. In addition the mutant form of p53 has oncogenic potential and can act as dominant negative inhibitor toward wild type p53.[40]
- *Loss of heterozygosis*: LOH of wild type p53 has also been noted in many human cancers leading to the loss of function of p53.
- *Deranged function due to inactivation by binding with other proteins*: Various virally derived proteins such as SV40 large T antigen, the HPV E6 ORF, hepatitis B X antigen, and adenovirus E1a bind with wild type p53 protein and inactivate its function.[41]
- *Mutations of regulators of p53*: Mutation of the regulators or stabilizers of p53 protein may cause loss of p53 function. MDM2 protein activates and stabilizes p53 protein. Therefore, any defect in this pathway due to mutation of MDM2 may derange the function of p53.[42]

Functions of p53 and Carcinogenesis

p53 interacts with various target genes or proteins to perform its function (Fig. 5.15). It binds with the DNA sequence of the regulator of the target genes and either activates or represses the genes. p53 also acts as non-transcriptional activator of apoptosis, signal transduction and replication factor. It also interacts directly with many cellular proteins and several viral proteins.

Cell cycle arrest: The main function of p53 is cell cycle arrest, DNA damage repair and apoptosis. Initially p53 is stimulated by various types of cellular stresses, e.g. DNA damage, telomere erosion, hypoxia, metabolic changes, cytokines or activated oncogenes. The activated p53 protein binds with the specific DNA sequence of several target genes and stimulates their transcription. Predominantly p21, a CDK inhibitor and GADD45 are produced. Increased level of p21 prevents CDK to phosphorylate Rb protein resulting to cell cycle arrest in G1 phase.[43] In case of

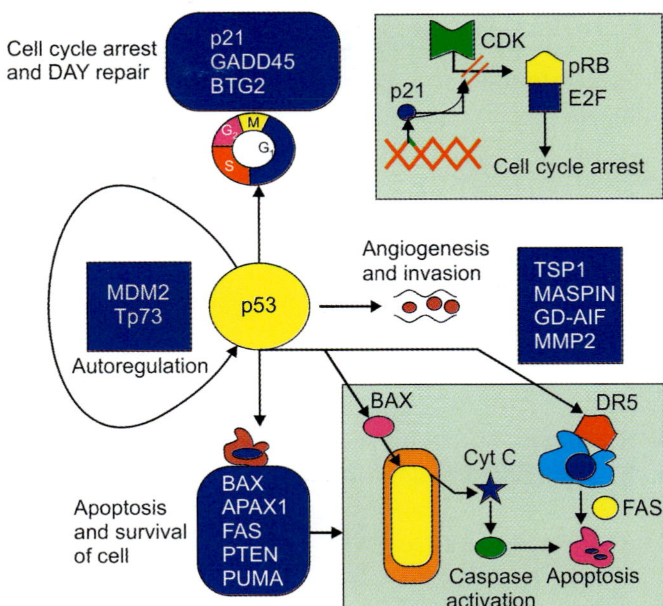

Fig. 5.15: The schematic diagram shows various target genes of p53. p53 is normally involved in cell-cycle control, apoptosis and DNA repair.

tumor, after DNA damage, the mutant p53 fails to block the cell cycle by p21 transcription. Therefore, the tumor cells proliferate with damaged DNA leading to genetic instability and multiple mutations.

Repair of DNA damage: When there is any damage in DNA, p53 activates GADD45 gene that encodes a protein related with DNA repair. If the damaged DNA is not repaired successfully, then p53 stimulates the apoptosis induced genes and induces apoptotic cell death.

Apoptosis: p53 induces apoptosis if the cell fails to repair its damaged DNA or fails to adapt up with stress. It induces various genes responsible for mitochondrial pathway of apoptosis. Induction of BAX gene by p53 protein causes excess BAX protein in mitochondrial membrane leading to increased mitochondrial permeability. This subsequently releases cytochrome C from the mitochondria to cytoplasm. This further activates caspase cascades resulting in apoptosis. p53 may also activate the other transcriptional targets related with cell surface death receptors such as DR5 and FAS. These receptors when bind with the respective ligands, activates the caspase pathway to initiate apoptosis.[44] Mutant p53 not only fails to initiate apoptosis and to promote tumorigenesis, but also enhances tumor cell resistance to death.[45]

Retinoblastoma Gene

Retinoblastoma gene is a recessive gene and both the gene should be inactivated before derangement of their function.

Inactivation of Rb Gene

The gene is located in 13q14 location. The gene may be inactivated by mutation or deletion. Rb gene produces Rb protein and this can be inactivated by binding with the viral products.

Functions of Rb Protein (Box 5.8) [45]

- Cell cycle checkpoint in G1 to S phase
- Cellular differentiation
- Cell survival
- Cellular senescence
- Genomic instability.

Cell cycle control: pRB interacts with various cellular and viral proteins. Hypophosphorylated pRB protein combines with the sequence specific DNA binding E2F transcription factor, the product of E2F transcription gene.[45] Cyclin-cyclin dependent kinase complex phosphorylates pRB and releases E2F from the pRB-E2F complex. E2F helps in transcription of many essential genes responsible for cell cycle progression (Fig. 5.16). Thus normally by blocking the action of E2F, pRb regulates the entry of the cell in the cell cycle. Inactivation of pRb by mutation or deletion may cause uncontrolled cell proliferation and cancer. The function of retinoblastoma gene and its products are blocked in large number of cancers.

Chromatin remodeling: Transcription factors are only able to act on the particular promoter sites and express specific gene when a portion of chromatin coil is opened up.

Box 5.8: Retinoblastoma protein.

- Rb is a recessive gene located in 13q14 chromosome
- Inactivated by mutation or deletion
- Functions
  - Cell cycle control:
    - pRB protein in its hypophosphorylated state binds with E2F transcription factor.
    - Phosphorylated Rb releases E2F that helps in cell cycle progression
  - *Chromatin remodeling*: pRB protein binds with histone deacetylases, histone methyltransferases, etc. to influence chromatin remodeling
  - *Genomic instability*: Functional inactivation of pRB may lead to aneuploidy, subchromosomal loss, endoreduplication, and consistently high rate of chromosomal missegregation
  - *DNA damage*: pRB protein controls the expression of various DNA damage repair factors

pRB protein binds with many factors (such as histone deacetylases, histone methyltransferases, etc.) and helps in chromatin remodeling.[46] Chromatin remodeling plays essential role in gene expression.

Genomic instability: The inactivation of pRB results in mitotic defects due to supernumerary centrosomes and centromeric defects. Various studies have demonstrated that the functional inactivation of pRB may lead to several types of genomic alterations such as aneuploidy, subchromosomal loss, endoreduplication, and consistently high rate of chromosomal missegregation.[47]

DNA damage: pRB protein controls the expression of various DNA damage repair factors and these factors also may affect DNA repair processes indirectly. Inactivation of pRB fails to check the damaged DNA to enter into the cell cycle and therefore renders cells more prone to DNA damage.

TUMOR MICROENVIRONMENT

Cancer is not the mere aggregation of malignant cells. Many other nonmalignant cells of the host also complexly and dynamically interact with the tumor cells to make the tumor microenvironment (TME). The components of TME include the cells of immune system (lymphocytes and NK cells), the tumor vasculature and lymphatics, adipocyte,

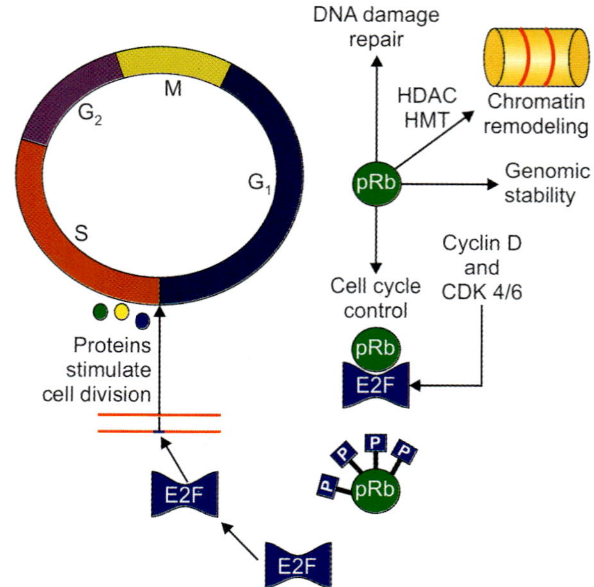

Fig. 5.16: The schematic diagram shows the various functions of pRB. pRB is related with cell cycle control, genomic stability, DNA repair and chromatin remodeling.

pericyte, cancer-associated fibroblasts, and extracellular matrix (ECM) around the cancer cells.[48]

T lymphocytes: Different types of T lymphocyte population infiltrate within the tumor—(1) CD4 positive T helper 2 (TH 2); (2) CD4 positive T helper 1 (TH1) cells; (3) CD8 T cells; (4) Regulatory T (Treg) cell.

B lymphocytes: B lymphocytes and Breg cells have tumor promoting activities.

Natural killer (NK) cells and natural killer T (NKT) cell: These cells also infiltrate in the tumor stroma and are linked with tumor killing activities.

Tumor-associated macrophages: These cells are present in large number in tumor and they have tumor promoting activities by helping in invasion, angiogenesis, and metastasis.

Cancer-associated fibroblasts[49]: Epigenetic changes in the fibroblasts transform the ordinary fibroblasts into cancer-associated fibroblasts. These cells help in the tumorigenesis by several ways: (1) angiogenesis by secreting stromal cell derived factor; (2) invasion by secreting several matrix metalloproteinases; (3) growth in metastatic sites by secreting various cytokines for cell survival; (4) survival of cancer cells by evading immune system; (5) altering cancer cell metabolism.

Adipocytes: Adipocytes secrets adipokines that helps in the recruitment of cancer cells. They also provide fatty acids, the fuel of cancer metabolism.

Vascular endothelial cells: Several growth factors such as vascular endothelial growth factor (VEGF), fibroblast growth factor (FGF), platelet derived growth factor (PDGF), etc. are released from the cancer cells, immune cells and cancer associated fibroblasts. These growth factors stimulate the endothelial cells and pericytes, and help in the angiogenesis of tumor.

The components of TME directly and indirectly help in carcinogenesis by supporting cell survival, invasion, metastasis, angiogenesis, metabolic alteration of tumor cells and evading immune system (Fig. 5.17).

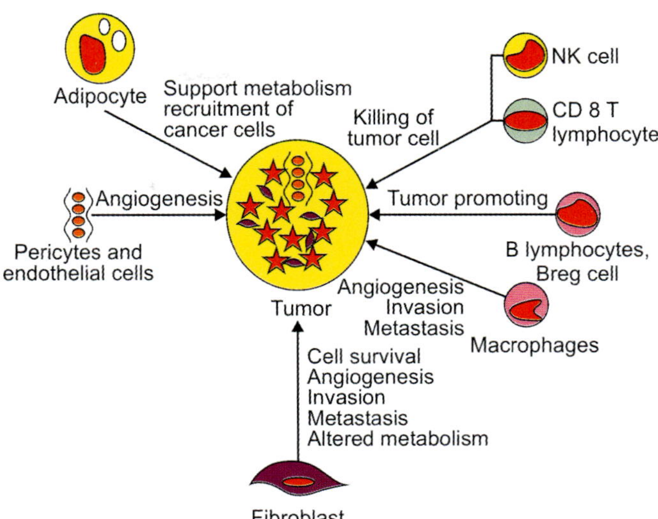

Fig. 5.17: The schematic diagram shows the various components of tumor microenvironment and their influence on tumor.

PRENEOPLASTIC LESIONS

Certain lesions of the epithelial origin are often restricted to the lining epithelium of the tissue and are related with cancer. They are called precancerous lesion. The various precursor lesions in the body include cervical intraepithelial lesions, atrophic gastritis of pernicious anemia, leukoplakia of vulva, penis or oral cavity, chronic ulcerative colitis and solar keratosis of skin. The terminology of "precancerous lesion" is not correct as many of such lesions may not develop malignancy in course of time. Precancerous lesion is often graded from I, II and III depending on the degree of nuclear atypia and relative involvement of the epithelial layer by the lesion. The essential characteristics of the precancerous lesions are:

- The cells are restricted to the epithelial layer only. There should not be any sign of invasion to the deeper tissue.
- The individual cells show mild to moderate nuclear enlargement and pleomorphism.
- Most of the time, these lesions are asymptomatic and a thorough search is needed to detect such lesions. Cytologists have a great role in detection of preneoplastic condition from scraping or smear so that the lesion could be excised to block the progression of the disease.
- The exact biological future of the precancerous lesion is unpredictable.

Most of the benign lesions of our body do not undergo malignant change. Therefore, there is no general rule that a cancer should always pass through a precancerous condition.

MORPHOLOGY OF CANCER CELL

It is very important for a cytologist to identify the cancer cell by light microscopy. Many of the morphological characteristics of benign and malignant cells are overlapping. Table 5.5 shows the differentiating morphological features of benign and malignant cell (Fig. 5.18).

Table 5.5: Benign versus malignant cell.

Features	*Benign cell*	*Malignant cell*
Nuclear size	Usually not enlarged	Nucleus enlarged and high nucleocytoplasmic ratio
Nuclear shape	Not variable	Variable shaped nucleus
Nuclear margin	Regular	Irregular
Nucleoli: Number Size	 Single Regular, small	 Single to multiple, Irregular, enlarged
Nuclear hyper-chromasia	Normochromatic	Hyperchromatic
Chromatin texture	Fine, nondescriptive	Coarse, irregular clumped
Micronuclei	Occasionally seen	Increased number of micronuclei
Mitotic rate	Low	High
Atypical Mitosis	Not present	Tripolar-star shaped atypical mitosis

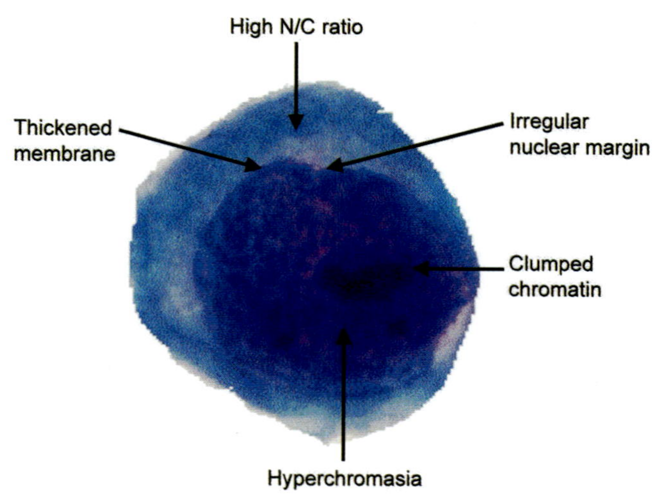

Fig. 5.18: The figure highlights the morphological features of the malignant cells.

Box 5.9: Characteristic morphological changes.

Background
- Tumor diathesis
- Blood
- Necrosis

Cell
- Enlarged cells
- Pleomorphic
- Loss of cell polarity

Nucleus
- Nuclear pleomorphism
- High nucleocytoplasmic (N/C) ratio
- Irregular and focally thickened nuclear margin
- Nuclear budding and fragmentation
- Nucleolar abnormalities: Enlarged, multiple, pleomorphic
- Nuclear hyperchromasia
- Alteration of chromatin pattern: Fine, reticular, irregular clumped
- *Mitosis:*
  - Increased in number
  - Qualitative abnormality: Tripolar and multipolar shaped mitotic figures
- *Other changes:*
  - Multinucleation
  - Intranuclear inclusions
  - Cell cannibalism
  - Excess Barr body
  - Excess micronuclei

Therefore, the combinations of cytomorphologic changes are important for identification of a cancer cell (Box 5.9).

Overall pattern: The overall pattern of the background of cancer has certain characteristic features. Cytology smear of cancer shows hemorrhagic and necrotic background. In addition tumor diathesis may also be present.

Cell and Cytoplasm

The cancer cell may show cytoplasmic changes. These changes may or may not be helpful in diagnosis because benign cells may also show similar features.

Size

Cancer cells are usually bigger than its normal counterpart. However, this may not be true all the times. Cytoplasm of the cancer cell may not always be more in amount relative to enlargement of nuclei. Therefore there may be gross alteration of the nucleocytoplasmic (N/C) ratio. Cancer cells may show variation of size among themselves known as anisocytosis.

Shape

The cancer cells usually show variable shapes and even grotesque shaped. Benign cells usually do not show much variation in shape. However, occasionally regenerative cells may show bizarre shapes. Shape is not a reliable criterion to identify malignant cells.

Cell Membrane and Cell to Cell Junction

Cell to cell junction is usually disrupted in cancer cell. The cell polarity is lost in epithelial malignancy. Therefore, the specific polar location of villi is not maintained. There may be variable sized microvilli over the entire surface of the cancer cell. In contrast, the benign cell maintains the polarity (epithelial) and the villi are located in one end.

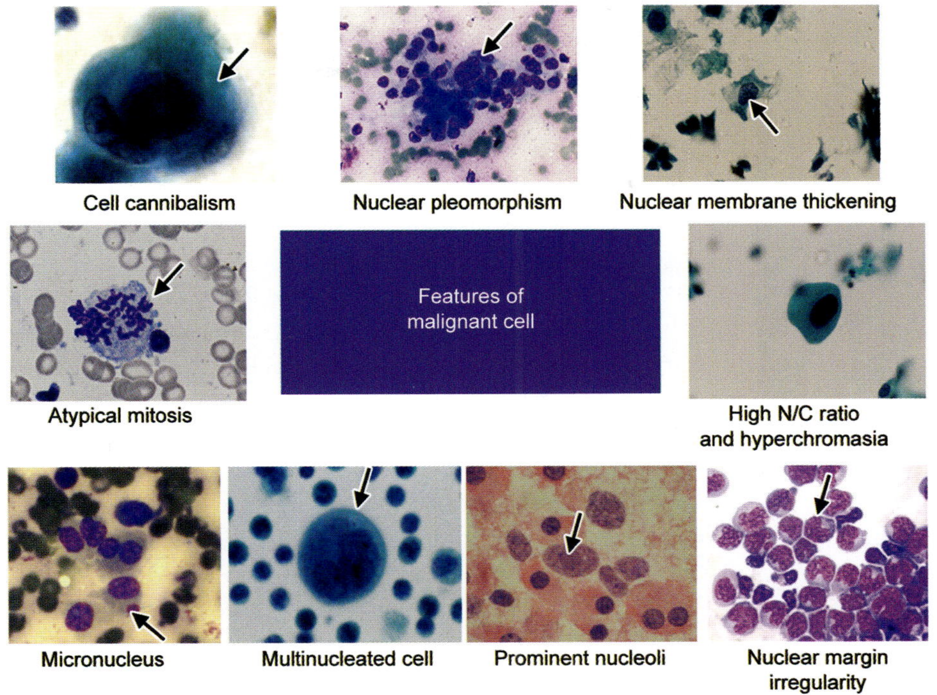

Fig. 5.19: Microphotograph highlights various nuclear features of malignant cells (*see* arrows).

The size of the villi is regular in benign cells. Malignant epithelial cells undergo a process of transition, known as epithelial mesenchymal transition, which is responsible for tumor progression and metastasis. This has been discussed previously.

Nucleus

The major changes of a malignant cell are seen in the nucleus (Fig. 5.19).

The characteristic light microscopic changes of cancer cells are:

- Nuclear enlargement and pleomorphism
- Nuclear margin irregularity
- Thickening of nuclear membrane
- Nuclear budding and fragmentation
- Nucleolar abnormalities
- Nuclear hyperchromasia and change of chromatin pattern
- Mitosis
- Other changes.

Nuclear Enlargement and Pleomorphism

Malignant cell shows nuclear enlargement. As the nucleus occupies the major part of cytoplasm so the N/C ratio is increased. The exact cause of nuclear enlargement is difficult to say. However the possible causes are:

- Increased DNA content and aneuploidy
- Increased amount of histone and nonhistone proteins in the nucleus.

In addition, the nuclei of the malignant cells often show variation of size (nuclear pleomorphism). Mutator phenotype theory tried to explain the etiology of nuclear pleomorphism.[50] It says that large number of genetic mutations occurs at the time of carcinogenesis. The cancer cells pick up the most appropriate mutational change for progression of carcinoma. So there may be mixed population of many subclones of cell with unique genetic mutation. These malignant cells have a set of biological changes along with variation of nuclear pleomorphism.

Nuclear Margin Irregularity

Nuclear contour irregularity is often noted in the malignant cell. There may be nuclear cleaving, convolution or molding. The abnormality of nuclear membrane may subtle in the form of nuclear protrusion or notch. These are difficult to detect and careful observation is needed for identification of membrane abnormalities. The factors responsible for change of nuclear contour are (Box 5.10):

Box 5.10: Nuclear margin irregularity.

- Nuclear cleaving, convolution or molding noted in cancer cell

Probable causes:
- *Quantitative or qualitative changes of lamin*: Lamin is altered in different cancers
- *Gene silencing by Rb protein*: pRB binds with inner nuclear membrane proteins and causes conformational changes of chromatin and silencing of gene
- *RET-PTC oncogenic changes*
- *Nuclear Matrix Protein*: Alteration of NMP in various cancers

- *Quantitative or qualitative changes of lamin*: Nuclear margin and shape may change due to qualitative or quantitative changes of nuclear lamin of nuclear envelope.[50] If the lamin protein is biochemically knocked out then the nuclei become small and fragile.[50]

Alteration of lamin is present in small cell carcinoma of lung with nuclear molding, colonic carcinoma, and gastric carcinomas.[51]

- *Gene silencing by Rb-protein*: pRB binds with inner nuclear membrane protein and other factors such as histone deacetylase, DNA methyltransferases, histone methyltransferases, and heterochromatin protein 1. This protein complex causes chromatin remodeling and silencing of gene leading to carcinogenesis. Therefore membrane abnormality is expected in cancer nuclei.[52]
- *RET-PTC oncogenic changes*: RET-PTC oncogenic transformation is present in papillary thyroid carcinoma with nuclear grooves. However, the exact cause and effect relationship of RET-PTC oncogenic transformation and nuclear groove is not known so far.[53]
- *Nuclear matrix, nuclear shape and tumor*: An alteration of nuclear shape may occur due to change in the composition of the nuclear matrix protein, the internal skeleton of the nucleus. NMP is tissue and cancer specific and its composition varies depending on nuclear activities.

Thickening of Nuclear Membrane

Thickening of nuclear membrane is often present in cancer nuclei, which is due to the heterochromatin formation on the nuclear membrane.

Nuclear Budding or Fragmentation

Nuclei of the malignant cells often show budding, fragmentation, ring-shape, and nuclear holes.

Nucleoli

Nucleoli of the malignant cell are often multiple, enlarged and pleomorphic. The nucleoli are easily detectable by light microscope. In hematoxylin and eosin stained histological section, the nucleoli are stained as deep eosinophilic round structures and in May-Grunwald Giemsa (MGG) stained cytology smears, the nucleoli are stained as light blue colored structures (*see* Fig. 5.19). Nucleoli are related with ribosome synthesis. The proliferating cells have increased demand for protein synthesis, and therefore need increased rate of ribosomal biogenesis. As the cancer cells have higher growth fraction and metabolic activity, so it is expected that the cancer cells show enlarged nucleoli. However, the cell proliferation rate may not be the sole factor of nucleolar change. Several tumor suppressor gene products particularly p53 and pRB asccumulate in nucleoli and lead to increased rRNA transcriptional activity. Alteration of the pathway of p53 and pRB in cancer cell may be directly related with nucleolar changes.

Nuclear Chromatin

Nuclei of the cancer cell are usually dark colored known as hyperchromatic. The dark color of the nucleus may be due to increased amount of DNA, increased histone and nonhistone proteins. Changes of chromatin pattern of nucleus are the hallmark of cancer cell. Cancer nuclei may show salt-and-pepper chromatin, opened up reticular chromatin, irregular coarse clumped chromatin, and vesicular chromatin (Figs. 5.20A to D). Fine chromatin pattern is seen in leukemia, adenocarcinoma and many lymphoma cases. Salt and pepper chromatin is noted in nuclei of neuroendocrine tumor and carcinoid. Nuclei of lymphoblastic lymphoma show reticular chromatin. Any high grade carcinoma shows irregular clumped chromatin.

The etiology of abnormal chromatin pattern is obscured. However, the probable causes are (Box 5.11):
- Chromatin relocation
- Chromatin remodeling
- DNA aneuploidy
- Change of nuclear matrix protein
- Change of nuclear pore.[54,55]

Chromatin relocation: Each chromosome is located in a specific position in the nucleus. The gene poor chromosomes are present in the peripheral part of the nucleus, whereas the gene rich chromosomes are present in the central part of the nucleus. The malignant cells often show increased gene expression and therefore the chromosomal location may be altered. This relocation of chromosome may be responsible for chromatin pattern alteration.

Chromatin remodeling: The activation or repression of genes by acetylation and deacetylation are related with

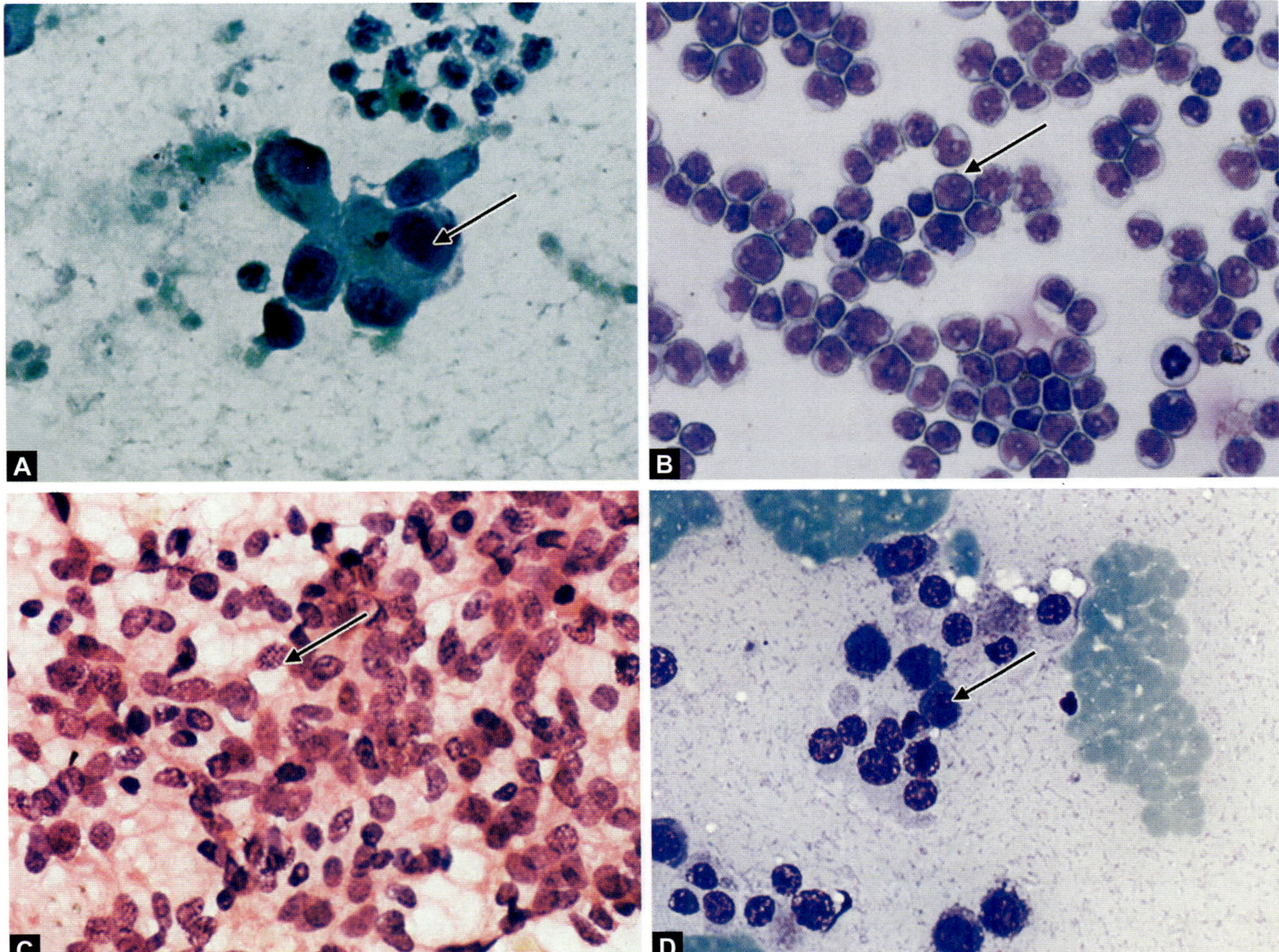

Figs. 5.20A to D: Microphotograph highlights different types of chromatin pattern. (A) Irregular clumped chromatin (arrow) in urothelial cell carcinoma (Papanicolaou's stain X HP); (B) Fine chromatin (arrow) in acute lymphatic leukemia (May-Grunwald Giemsa X HP); (C) Salt and pepper chromatin (arrow) in peripheral neuroectodermal tumor (Hematoxylin and eosin HP); (D) Cartwheel like chromatin (arrow) pattern in plasma cells tumor (May-Grunwald Giemsa X HP).

Box 5.11: Nuclear chromatin.

- Change of chromatin pattern is the identification mark of cancer cell
- *Different pattern:*
  - Salt-and-pepper: Neuroendocrine tumor and carcinoid
  - Fine chromatin pattern: Leukemia, adenocarcinoma, lymphoma cases
  - Reticular chromatin: Lymphoblastic lymphoma
  - Irregular clumped chromatin: Any high grade carcinoma
- *Etiology:*
  - Chromatin
    - » Reorientation
    - » Remodeling
  - DNA aneuploidy
  - Change of nuclear matrix protein
  - Change of nuclear pore

chromatin remodeling. In case of various malignancies the alteration of histone acetylation has been noted.[37] The altered histone acetylation may change the conformation of chromosome resulting in change of chromatin pattern.

DNA aneuploidy: Aneuploidy (abnormal DNA content) of the cancer cell may change the packaging of chromatin resulting in change of chromatin texture.

Nuclear pore: The abnormal diffusion of various materials through the nuclear pore may affect the nuclear chromatin pattern.

Mitosis

Abnormality in mitosis may be either quantitative or qualitative.

Quantitative abnormality: Cell proliferation is one of the important hallmarks of cancer. This is reflected as increased number of mitosis in the tumor tissue. Mitotic phenomenon is also noted in case of proliferating cells of regenerative tissue. However, the rate of mitosis is almost equal to death rate of the cells in proliferating tissue and the mitotic phenomenon is a temporary event.

Qualitative abnormality of Mitosis: Qualitative abnormality of the mitotic phenomenon is an important characteristic of cancer. Instead of bipolar mitotic figure, there may be tripolar, multipolar or incomplete multipolar mitotic figures. The various causes of mitotic abnormality and chromosomal instability have been described in detail in Chapter 4.

Other Nuclear Changes

Various other nuclear changes are often associated with malignancy such as:

- *Multinucleation*: Multinucleated cells may be seen in malignancy (Fig. 5.19). However, the multinucleated cells can also be seen in benign tumors and in chronic inflammation. So it is a nonspecific feature.
- *Intranuclear inclusion*: Intranuclear pseudoinclusions (INI) are the invagination of the cytoplasm into the nucleus. The INIs are readily appreciable in cytology smear than histopathology sections. It appears as round to oval pale structure within the nucleus. It looks like a pink colored round structure in MGG stained smears and a grayish to light-greenish appearance in Papanicolaou stained material.[55] Electron microscopic study clearly shows that the INI is of cytoplasmic origin and contains cytoplasmic structures such as mitochondria, premelanosomes, melanosomes, microfilaments, ribosomes, rough endoplasmic reticulum, and annulate lamellae. INIs are separated from the nuclear matrix by a double-layered membrane.[28] INIs are commonly seen in papillary thyroid carcinoma, malignant melanoma, papillary renal cell carcinoma, choroid plexus carcinoma and human ovarian surface epithelial cells.[55] However, benign lesions such as meningioma or lymphocytic thyroiditis may also show INIs. The exact pathogenesis of the INI is unknown. The probable causes of INIs are:
    - Altered ratio of nuclear surface to volume: Leduc and Wilson propose that INI formation is an attempt to preserve the normal nuclear surface:nuclear volume ratio.[28]
    - Swollen excess cytoplasm: Sobel et al. think that INI develops due to the swollen cytoplasm protruding into the nucleus.[29]
    - Nuclear grooves followed by inclusion: It may also be possible that the folding of nuclear membrane is the initial stage of the deep cytoplasmic protrusion that ultimately forms INIs.
- *Excess Barr bodies or sex chromatin*: The Barr body is the inactive X chromosome in a female somatic cell. It is present on the nuclear membrane as a planoconvex structure of 2–3 µm in diameter. Number of Barr body in a nucleus is less than one of the total numbers of X chromosome. This means female with two X chromosomes will have one Barr body. However, the malignant cell shows more than one Barr body. This is an interesting finding in cancer cell.
- *Cell cannibalism (Fig. 5.19)*: Cellular cannibalism is defined as "a large cell enclosing a slightly smaller one within its cytoplasm".[56] The cannibalistic cell contains a crescent-shaped nucleus and it engulfs another cell that has round faded nucleus. The cannibalistic cells have the unique property to engulf the fellow tumor cells. The cannibalized cell remains alive within the cannibalistic cell at a certain period of time. Cannibalism is different than phagocytosis, entosis, emperipolesis and autophagy.

Cell cannibalism is a helpful morphologic feature to identify the malignant lesion.

- *Excess micronuclei*: A micronucleus (MN) is a small nonretractile, round to oval shaped structure. It is present near the main nucleus and is visible by light microscope. The diameter of MN is 1/16 to 1/3 of the main nucleus. The shape, color, and texture of MN are like the main nucleus (*see* Fig. 5.19). MN can be demonstrated on simple MGG stain or Papanicolaou's stain. However, specific DNA stain such as Feulgen stain or Acridine orange stain can be used to demonstrate it. Micronucleus is the chromosomal segments that fail to be incorporated in main nuclei during cell division. The MN represents both chromosome breakage as well as chromosome loss.[57] Therefore, simple counting of MN may be used as a biomarker of chromosomal damage and cancer risk.

Characterization of Type of Cancer Cell

After the initial diagnosis of malignancy in cytology it is often necessary to characterize the type of malignancy. As described previously, the malignant cells usually try to simulate the tissue of origin. The cancer cells either morphologically mimic the cell of origin or they produce the substance derived from the parental tissue.

Table 5.6: Morphological resemblance and products of cancer cell.

Malignancy	*Morphological features*	*Products*
Squamous cell carcinoma	Polyhedral squamoid cells with eosinophilic cytoplasm, keratin pears	Keratin
Adenocarcinoma	Columnar looking cells with eccentric nuclei and vacuolated cytoplasm	Mucin
Malignant melanoma	Round to oval pleomorphic cell with intracytoplasmic melanin	Intra and extracellular melanin
Hepatocellular carcinoma	Polyhedral hepatocyte like cells	Cells may contain bile pigment
Osteosarcoma	Cells look like osteoblasts	Osteoid
Chondrosarcoma	Cells look like chondrocytes	Cartilaginous material

Table 5.7: Ancillary immunological tests for broad categorizations of cancer.

Malignancy	*Immunocytochemistry*
Carcinoma	Epithelial membrane antigen, cytokeratin
Lymphoma	CD45 (leukocyte common antigen)
Melanoma	HMB45, Melan-A
Hepatocellular carcinoma	Hep Per 1, Glypican-3
Sarcoma	Vimentin
Rhabdomyosarcoma	Desmin
Leiomyosarcoma	Smooth muscle actin
Nerve sheath tumor	S-100
Neuroendocrine tumor	Chromogranin, neuron specific enolase

Table 5.6 shows the various examples of morphological resemblance of malignant cells with the parental tissue. The duty of the cytologist is to find out these features for exact subtyping of the cancer. At times the products of the cancer cells are also important (Table 5.6) such as keratin in squamous cell carcinoma, mucin in adenocarcinoma, osteoid in osteosarcoma, cartilaginous material in chondrosarcoma, melanin in melanoma, etc.

Ancillary Tests

At times it is necessary to have further confirmation of subtype of cancer. In fact, in poorly differentiated malignancy, it is very difficult to categorize the tumor by morphology alone. In these circumstances ancillary tests are needed (Table 5.7). Immunocytochemistry may be very helpful for exact subtyping in most of the cases.

Box 5.12: Potential pitfalls in diagnosis of cancer.

False positive
- *Inflammation*: Inflammatory atypia in bacterial or viral infections
- *Chemotherapy and radiotherapy* induced changes
- *Reactive changes*: Reactive mesothelial hyperplasia, lithiasis, etc.
- *Benign neoplasm showing nuclear pleomorphism:* Paraganglioma, Schwannoma, pleomorphic lipoma, etc.
- *Metaplasia*: Endometriosis

False negative
- *Malignancy with monomorphic nuclei*: Lobular carcinoma of breast, low grade non-Hodgkin lymphoma, follicular carcinoma, etc.

Diagnostic Pitfalls of Malignancy

There are various mimickers of malignant cells (Box 5.12). The cytologist should carefully assess this condition. Enlarged nucleus, mild pleomorphism and prominent nucleoli are the main misleading features. Cytologist should give more importance on nuclear chromatin pattern, N/C ratio and overall cytological features. Clinical histories of the individual cases are also very important factor to avoid false positive cases.

REFERENCES

1. Willis RA. The Spread of Tumors in the Human Body. London: Butterworth & Co.; 1952.
2. Hanahan D, Weinberg RA. Hallmarks of cancer: the next generation. Cell. 2011;144(5):646-74.
3. Dyson N, Howley PM, Munger K, et al. The human papillomavirus-16 E7 oncoprotein is able to bind to the retinoblastoma gene product. Science. 1989;243:934-7.
4. Markowitz S, Wang J, Meyeroff L, et al. Inactivation of the type II TGF-b receptor in colon cancer cells with microsatellite instability. Science. 1995;268:1336-8.
5. Hueber AO, Zornig M, Lyon D, et al. Requirement for the CD95 receptor-ligand pathway in c-Myc-induced apoptosis. Science. 1997;278:1305-9.
6. Blasco MA. Telomeres and human disease: ageing, cancer and beyond. Nat Rev Genet. 2005;6:611-22.
7. Baeriswyl V, Christofori G. The angiogenic switch in carcinogenesis. Semin Cancer Biol. 2009;19:329-37.
8. Cavallaro U, Christofori G. Cell adhesion and signalling by cadherins and Ig-CAMs in cancer. Nat Rev Cancer. 2004;4:118-32.
9. Chambers AF, Matrisian LM. Changing views of the role of matrix metalloproteinases in metastasis. J Natl Cancer Inst. 1997;89:1260-70.
10. Negrini S, Gorgoulis VG, Halazonetis TD. Genomic instability—an evolving hallmark of cancer. Nat Rev Mol Cell Biol. 2010;11:220-8.
11. Loeb LA. Mutator phenotype may be required for multistage carcinogenesis. Cancer Res. 1991;51:3075-9.
12. Yang L, Pang Y, Moses HL. TGF-beta and immune cells: an important regulatory axis in the tumor microenvironment and progression. Trends Immunol. 2010;31:220-7.

13. Renan MJ. How many mutations are required for tumorigenesis? Implications from human cancer data. Mol Carcinogenesis. 1993;7:139-46.
14. Kinzler KW, Vogelstein B. Lessons from Hereditary Colorectal Cancer. Cell. 1996;87:159-70.
15. Nowell PC. The clonal evolution of tumor cell populations. Science.1976;194:23-8.
16. Merlo LM, Pepper JW, Reid BJ, et al. Cancer as an evolutionary and ecological process. Nature Rev. Cancer. 2006;6:924-35.
17. Press MF, Bernstein L, Thomas PA, et al. HER-2/neu gene amplification characterized by fluorescence in situ hybridization: poor prognosis in node-negative breast carcinomas. J Clin Oncol. 1997;15:2894-904.
18. Schwab M, Alitalo K, Klempnauer KH, et al. Amplified DNA with limited homology to myc cellular oncogene is shared by human neuroblastoma cell lines and a neuroblastoma tumour. Nature. 1983;305:245-8.
19. Rodenhuis S. RAS and human tumors. Semin Cancer Biol. 1992;3:241-7.
20. Davies H, Bignell GR, Cox C, et al. Mutations of the BRAF gene in human cancer. Nature. 2002;417:949-54.
21. Heldin CH, Westermark B. Mechanism of action and in vivo role of platelet derived growth factor. Physiol Rev. 1999;79:1283-316.
22. Kaziro Y, Itoh H, Kozasa T, et al. Structure and function of signal-transducing GTP-binding proteins. Annu Rev Biochem. 1991;60:349-400.
23. Jenuwein T, Allis CD. Translating the histone code. Science. 2001;293:1074-80.
24. Nakamura T, Mori T, Tada S, et al. ALL-1 is a histone methyltransferase that assembles a supercomplex of proteins involved in transcriptional regulation. Mol Cell. 2002;10: 1119-28.
25. Bartel DP. MicroRNAs: genomics, biogenesis, mechanism, and function. Cell. 2004;116(2):281-97.
26. Metias SM, Lianidou E, Yousef GM. MicroRNAs in clinical oncology: at the crossroads between promises and problems. J Clin Pathol. 2009;62(9):771-6.
27. Geigl JB, Obenauf AC, Schwarzbraun T, et al. Defining "chromosomal instability". Trends Genetics. 2007;24(2):64-9.
28. Leduc EH, Wilson JW. An electron microscopic study of intranuclear inclusions in mouse liver and hepatomas. J Biophys Biochem Cytol. 1959;6:427-30.
29. Sobel HJ, Schwartz R, Marquet MS, et al. Nonviral nuclear inclusions. Cytoplasmic invaginations. Arch Pathol. 1969; 87:179-92.
30. Li Y, Benezra R. Identification of a human mitotic checkpoint gene: hsMAD2. Science. 1996;274:246-8.
31. Cahill DP, Lengauer C, Yu J, et al. Mutations of mitotic checkpoint genes in human cancers. Nature. 1998;392:300-3.
32. Lentini L, Amato A, Schillaci T, et al. Simultaneous Aurora A/STK15 overexpression and centrosome amplification induce chromosomal instability in tumor cells with a MIN phenotype. BMC Cancer. 2007;7:212.
33. Maney T, Hunter AW, Wagenbach M, et al. Mitotic centromere-associated kinesin is important for anaphase chromosome segregation. J Cell Biol. 1998;142:787-801.
34. Thompson SL, Bakhoum SF, Compton DA. Mechanisms of chromosomal instability. Curr Biol. 2010;20(6):R285-95.
35. Arzimanoglou IA, Gilbert F, Barber HR. Microsatellite instability in human solid tumors. Cancer. 1998;82: 1808-20.
36. Wilson AS, Power BE, Molloy PL. DNA hypomethylation and human diseases. Biochim Biophys Acta. 2007;1775,138-62.
37. Dey P. Chromatin remodeling, cancer and chemotherapy. CMC. 2006;13(24);2909-19.
38. Sharma S, Kelly TK, Jones PA. Epigenetics in cancer. Carcinogenesis. 2010;31(1):27-36.
39. Kern SE, Pietenpol JA, Thiagalingam S, et al. Oncogenic forms of p53 inhibit p53-regulated gene expression. Science. 1992;256(5058):827-30.
40. Bosari S, Viale G. The clinical significance of p53 aberrations in human tumours. Virchows Arch. 1995;427:229-41.
41. Woods DB, Vousden KH. Regulation of p53 function. Exp Cell Res. 2001;264:56-66.
42. Harper JW, Adami GR, Wei N, et al. The p21 Cdk-interacting protein Cipl is a potent inhibitor of GI cyclin-dependent kinases. Cell. 1993;75:805-16.
43. Wu GS, Bums TF, McDonald ER, et al. KILLER/DR5 is a DNA damage-inducible p53-regulated death receptor gene. Nat Genet. 1997;17:141-3.
44. Lowe SW, Bodis S, McClatchey A, et al. p53 status and the efficacy of cancer therapy in vivo. Science. 1994;266: 807-10.
45. Weinberg RA. The retinoblastoma protein and cell cycle control. Cell. 1995;81:323-30.
46. Hernando E, Nahlé Z, Juan G, et al. Rb inactivation promotes genomic instability by uncoupling cell cycle progression from mitotic control. Nature. 2004;430:797-802.
47. Manning AL, Longworth MS, Dyson NJ. Loss of pRB causes centromere dysfunction and chromosomal instability. Genes Dev. 2010;24(13):1364-76.
48. Balkwill FR, Capasso M, Hagemann T. The tumor microenvironment at a glance. J Cell Sci. 2012;125(Pt 23):5591-6.
49. Kalluri R. The biology and function of fibroblasts in cancer. Nat Rev Cancer. 2016;16(9):582-98.
50. Dey P. Nuclear margin irregularity and cancer: a review. Anal Quant Cytol Histol. 2009;31(5):345-52.
51. Broers JL, Raymond Y, Rot MK, et al. Nuclear A-type lamins are differentially expressed in human lung cancer subtypes. Am J Pathol. 1993;143:211-20.
52. Luo RX, Postigo AA, Dean DC. Rb interacts with histone deacetylase to repress transcription. Cell. 1998;92:463-73.
53. Peculis BA. Ribosome biogenesis: ribosomal RNA synthesis as a package deal. Curr Biol. 2002;12:R623-4.
54. Dey P. Chromatin pattern alteration in malignant cells: an enigma. Diagn Cytopathol. 2005;32(1):25-30.
55. Arora SK, Dey P. Intranuclear peudoinclusions: morphology, pathogenesis, and significance. Diagn Cytopathol. 2012; 40(8):741-4.
56. Sharma N, Dey P. Cell cannibalism and cancer. Diagn Cytopathol. 2011;39(3):229-33.
57. Samanta S, Dey P. Micronucleus and its applications. Diagn Cytopathol. 2012;40(1):84-90.

Review Questions

1. **Which one is the definitive sign of malignancy?**
   a. Rapid growth
   b. Poor encapsulation
   c. High mitosis
   d. Distant metastasis
2. **The hallmark/s of cancer is/are:**
   a. Sustained proliferation without any growth signal
   b. Insensitivity to antigrowth signal
   c. Reprogramming cellular metabolism
   d. All of the above
3. **Characteristics of cancer stem cell:**
   a. Poorly regulated self-renewal
   b. Sensitive to apoptosis
   c. Differentiates to produce tumor
   d. Long life span
4. **The rate-limiting step that initiates the tumorigenesis of normal colonic epithelial cells:**
   a. Mutation of K-RAS gene
   b. Mutation of DCC gene
   c. Mutation of p53 genes
   d. Mutation of adenomatous polyposis coli (APC) gene
5. **RAS oncogene causes tumor as:**
   a. Growth factor receptors
   b. Signal transducers
   c. Transcription factors
   d. Chromatin remodelers
6. **Which one is *true* about miRNA?**
   a. Anneals to the complementary strand of messenger RNA
   b. Causes cellular differentiation
   c. Causes translational repression
   d. All of the above
7. **Alteration of the pattern of polymorphic short tandem repeat segments of DNA is seen in:**
   a. SiRNA
   b. miRNA
   c. Microsatellite instability
   d. RNA-induced silencing complex (RISC)
8. **Epigenetic changes are caused by all *except*:**
   a. Methylation of cytosine at the CpG islands of DNA
   b. Post-translation modification of linker histone
   c. Nucleosome remodeling by ATP dependent chromatin complexes
   d. miRNA modification
9. **Which tumor suppressor gene is working as CDK inhibitor?**
   a. p53
   b. BRCA1
   c. WT1
   d. p16(INK4A)
10. **Mode of activation of ERB-B2 oncogene is:**
    a. Point mutation
    b. Amplification
    c. Translocation
    d. None of the above
11. **The tumor suppressor gene that binds and degrades β catenin and causes inhibition of signal transduction:**
    a. APC
    b. p53
    c. Retinoblastoma
    d. WT 1

Answers

1. d. Distant metastasis
2. d. All of the above
3. b. Sensitive to apoptosis
4. d. Mutation of adenomatous polyposis coli (APC) gene
5. b. Signal transducers
6. d. All of the above
7. c. Microsatellite instability
8. b. Post-translation modification of linker histone
9. d. p16(INK4A)
10. b. Amplification
11. a. APC

CHAPTER 6

Tissue and Cell Organization

INTRODUCTION

There are approximately 200 distinct cell types in our body. These cells are arranged and organized to form tissues. Different types of tissues are organized to form a complete organ. The cytologist's prime duty is to identify the tissue, types of cells and then to assess the basic character of the cell (benign versus malignant).

The four basic tissue types are: (1) epithelial, (2) connective, (3) muscle, and (4) neural tissue.

Epithelial Tissue

Classification of epithelial tissues is based on: (1) The number of the constituent cell layer, such as single layer of epithelium is known as simple epithelium, whereas the multiple layer of epithelium is known as stratified epithelium; (2) individual cell morphology such as flattened cell, columnar cell, or cuboidal cell; and (3) the presence of surface specializations such as cilia or keratin.

Classification of Epithelial Tissue

- Simple
  - Squamous
  - Cuboidal
  - Columnar
- Pseudostratified
- Stratified
  - Squamous keratinized
  - Squamous nonkeratinized
  - Cuboidal
  - Columnar
  - Transitional.

Simple squamous epithelium: This is defined as the surface epithelium with single layer of squamous cells. This type of lining epithelial cells are present in pulmonary alveoli, loop of Henle, parietal layer of Bowman capsule, and the lining of the pleural, pericardial and peritoneal cavities (Fig. 6.1).

Simple cuboidal epithelium: It is composed of a single layer of cuboidal cells. When the epithelial cells are viewed in cut section or smears, the cells present a square profile with centrally placed round nuclei. The simple cuboidal epithelium forms the lining of many small ducts, kidney collecting tubules, and ovarian surface (Fig. 6.2).

Simple columnar epithelium: This is a single layer of tall columnar epithelial cells. In longitudinal view, the cells look like tall with basally placed nuclei. Simple columnar epithelium forms the lining of the intestine, gall bladder, and large ducts or glands (Fig. 6.3). The epithelial cells often show surface microvilli or cilia.

Pseudostratified columnar epithelium: As the name indicates, the cells appear as stratified but actually are present in single layer. All the cells are attached to the basal lamina but only some cells reach to the free surface of the

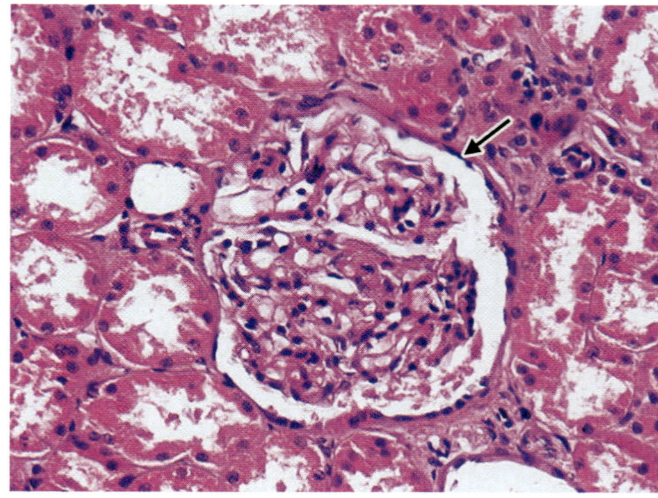

Fig. 6.1: Simple squamous epithelium: lining of parietal layer of Bowman's capsule is indicated by arrow (Hematoxylin and eosin stain X HP).

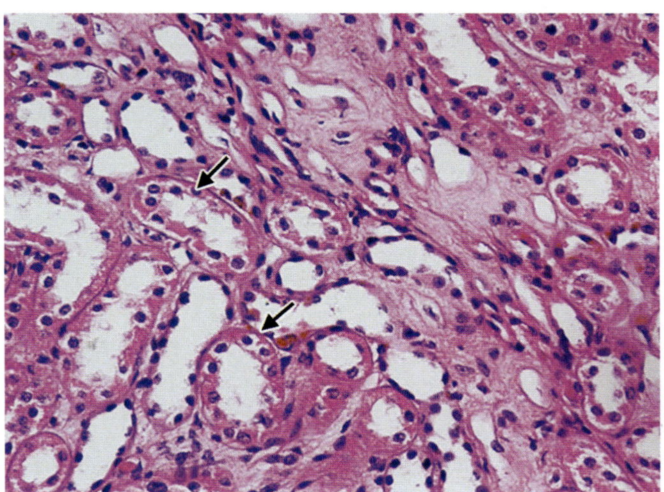

Fig. 6.2: Simple cuboidal epithelium: lining of collecting tubules of kidney. The arrows indicate the cuboidal cells (Hematoxylin and eosin stain X HP).

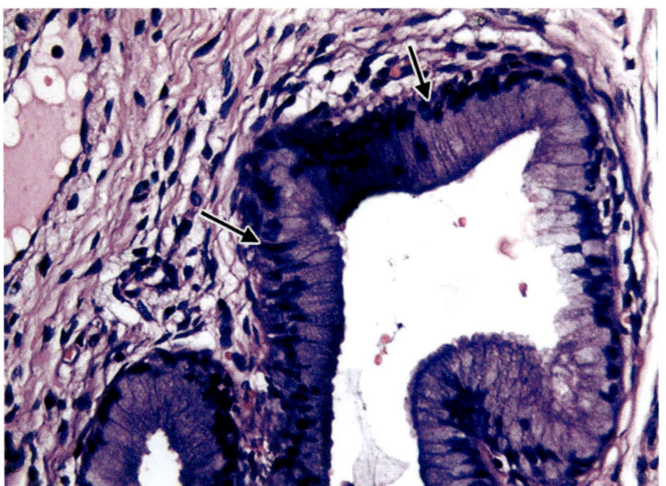

Fig. 6.3: Simple columnar epithelial cell on the lining of endocervical gland is pointed by the arrows (Hematoxylin and eosin stain X HP).

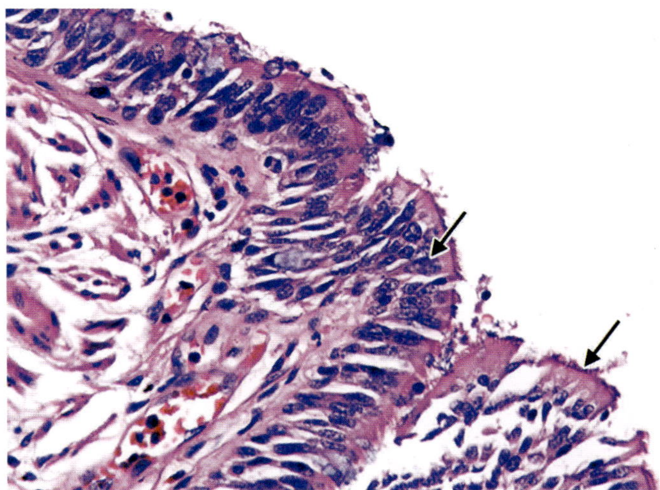

Fig. 6.4: Pseudostratified columnar epithelium of bronchial lining cells are pointed by the arrows (Hematoxylin and eosin stain X MP).

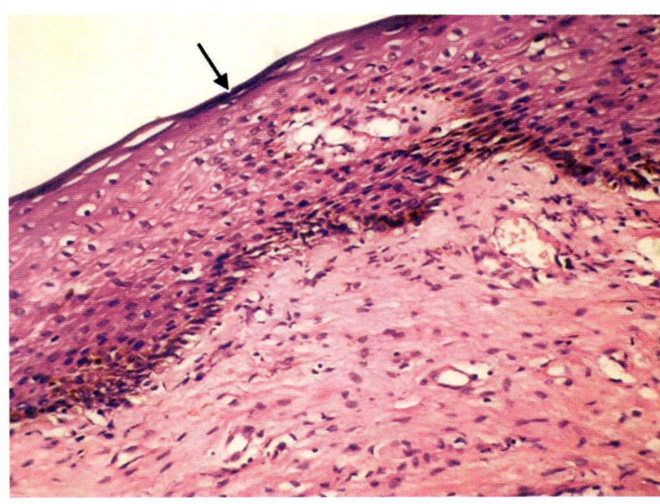

Fig. 6.5: Keratinized stratified squamous epithelium in skin. The arrow indicates the upper layer of the squamous cells (Hematoxylin and eosin stain X MP).

membrane. The cells are columnar-looking and many of them show cilia on their apical surface (Fig. 6.4). The lining of most of the trachea, primary bronchi, epididymis, ductus deferens, auditory tube, part of the tympanic cavity, the nasal cavity, lacrimal sac, and male urethra show pseudostratified ciliated columnar epithelium.

Stratified squamous epithelium: It is comprised of several layers of epithelial cells. Only the cells of basal layer are in contact with basement membrane. These basal cells are cuboidal in shape. The cells located in the intermediate portion are more polyhedral and the cells on the surface layer are flattened in shape. This is found in the lining of mouth, epiglottis, esophagus, vocal folds, and the cervix.

In case of keratinizing stratified squamous epithelium, the cells in the superficial layers are dead and replaced by keratin. This is found in the epidermal layer of skin (Fig. 6.5).

Stratified cuboidal epithelium: It is made of only two layers of cuboidal cells. It lines the large duct of sweat glands.

Stratified columnar epithelium: Stratified columnar epithelium contains more than one layer of cells. The cells adjacent to basal lamina are cuboidal and superficial layer

Table 6.1: Different types of epithelium.

Types of epithelium	*Description*	*Location*
Simple		
Squamoid	Single layer of flattened cells	Lining of pulmonary alveoli, loop of Henle, parietal layer of Bowman capsule and delicate lining of the pleural, pericardial and peritoneal cavities
Cuboidal	Single layer of cuboidal cells	Lining of many small ducts, kidney collecting tubules and ovarian surface
Columnar	Single layer of columnar cells	Lining of the intestine, gall bladder and large ducts or glands
Pseudostratified	Single layer of cells. All the cells are attached with the basal lamina but only some cells reach to the free surface of the membrane	Lining of most of the trachea, primary bronchi, epididymis, the auditory tube, part of the tympanic cavity, the nasal cavity, lacrimal sac, and male urethra
Stratified		
Non-keratinized squamous epithelium	Multiple layers of epithelial cells The basal cuboidal cells to intermediate polyhedral cells to superficial flattened cells	Lining of mouth, epiglottis, esophagus, vocal folds, vagina
Keratinized squamous epithelium	Same as above but the cells in the superficial layers are dead and replaced by keratin	Epidermis of skin
Cuboidal	Only two layers of cuboidal cells	Lining of the large duct of sweat glands
Columnar	Multiple layers of cells The cells adjacent to basal lamina are cuboidal and superficial layer of cells are columnar in appearance	Lining of conjunctiva of the eye and large excretory ducts
Transitional	Multiple layers of cells, basal superficial cells to polyhedral to dome-shaped superficial cells	Lining of renal pelvis, ureter, bladder, and urethra

of cells are columnar in appearance. The lining of the conjunctiva of the eye and large excretory ducts are composed of stratified columnar epithelium.

Transitional epithelium: Transitional epithelium is composed of multiple layers of cells. The basal cells are cuboidal or columnar, and the intermediate groups of cells are polyhedral in shape. The cells on the top are dome-shaped with bulge into the luminal side. The linings of almost all the parts of urinary system such as renal pelvis, ureter, bladder, and urethra are made up of transitional epithelium (Fig. 6.6).

The brief description and locations of different types of epithelial cells are listed in Table 6.1 and schematic cytomorphology of different types of epithelium has been highlighted in Figure 6.7.

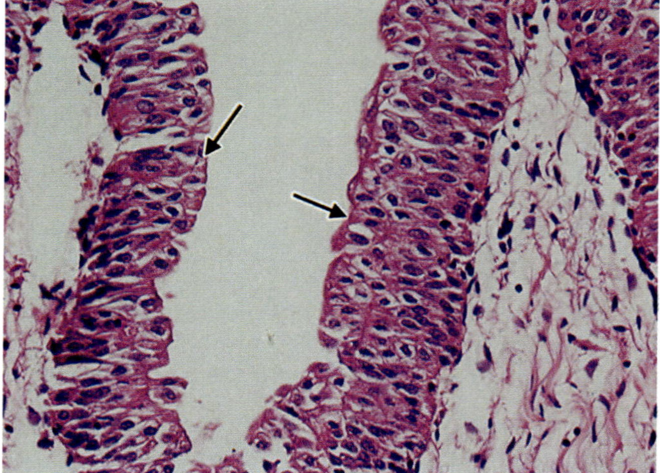

Fig. 6.6: Transitional lining epithelium of urinary bladder. The arrows indicate the lining transitional lining epithelial cells (Hematoxylin and eosin stain X HP).

Connective Tissue

Connective tissue connects different tissues in our body. Mature connective tissue is classified as:

- Connective tissue proper
  - Loose areolar tissue
  - Dense connective tissue
- Specialized connective tissue
  - Adipose tissue
  - Hematopoietic tissue
  - Bone
  - Cartilage

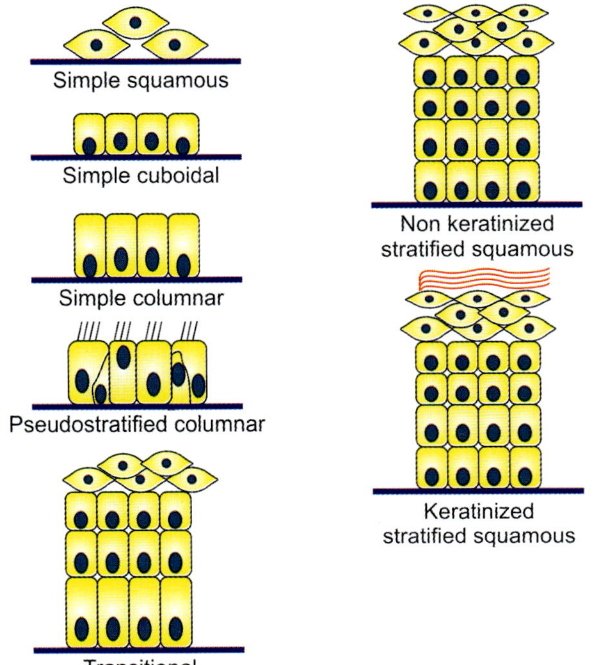

Fig. 6.7: Schematic diagram of different types of epithelial cells.

Major cells in the connective tissue are divided into:

Fixed cells:

- Fibroblasts
- Adipose cells
- Macrophages
- Pericytes
- Mast cells

Transient cells:

- Plasma cells
- Lymphocytes
- Neutrophils
- Monocytes
- Eosinophils
- Basophils

Fixed Cells

- *Fibroblast*: These cells may present in the active or inactive form as fibrocyte. Fibroblast is oval to elongated cells with ample amount of cytoplasm. Nuclei of the fibroblasts are oval to elongated with single prominent nucleoli. In contrast, inactive fibroblast or fibrocyte is smaller with eosinophilic cytoplasm and elongated nuclei.
  Markers: Vimentin, fibroblast specific protein 1, fibroblast surface antigen, HSP47 is a good marker of skin fibroblast.
  - Myofibroblasts are modified fibroblasts with properties of both fibroblast and smooth muscle.

  Markers: Vimentin, alpha smooth muscle actin
- *Adipose cells*: The fat cells or adipocytes are large cells with abundant vacuolated cytoplasm having eccentric nuclei. The cells often look like signet ring cells.
  Markers: Pref-1 is the marker of preadipocyte, vimentin
- *Macrophages*: Macrophages are the normal constituents of the connective tissue. The cells are large with abundant amount of vacuolated cytoplasm. The nucleus is central to eccentric, and ovoid to kidney bean in shape with condensed chromatin. The nucleolus is inconspicuous. The cytoplasm of the macrophages often contains phagocytosed debris.
  Markers: CD68, CD163, and Mac 2 (galectin-3).
- *Pericytes*: These cells are arranged around the endothelial cells of capillaries and small venules. Pericytes are pale-staining cells with moderate cytoplasm and oval to elongated nuclei.
  Markers: CD146, CD31, and PECAM 1.
- *Mast cells*: Mast cells are originated from the bone marrow stem cells. They are large cells with a centrally placed round to ovoid nuclei. The cytoplasm of the mast cell contains abundant metachromatic blotchy granules comprised of histamines, heparin, aryl sulfatase, and neutral proteases.
  Markers: The high-affinity IgE receptor, CD117
- *Transient Cells*
  - *Plasma cells*: Plasma cells are scattered throughout the connective tissue and they are often concentrated in chronic inflammation. These cells are round to oval cells with intensely basophilic cytoplasm and eccentric nuclei. Nucleus of the cell has peripheral clumped chromatin giving a cart-wheel appearance.

  Markers: CD138, CD38, CD78
  - *Lymphocytes*: Lymphocytes are originally present in blood. They accumulate in the connective tissue during chronic inflammation from blood. The lymphocytes are mixed population of cells with great difference in origin, lifespan, surface immunophenotyping, and function. Morphology of lymphocytes provides no clue to their immunophenotpying features.

Morphology: Lymphocytes are small round cells with 6–9 microns in diameter. They have scanty deeply basophilic rim of cytoplasm with round nuclei having condensed chromatin and inconspicuous nucleoli. Large granular lymphocytes are a bit larger in size and they possess azurophilic granules in the cytoplasm.

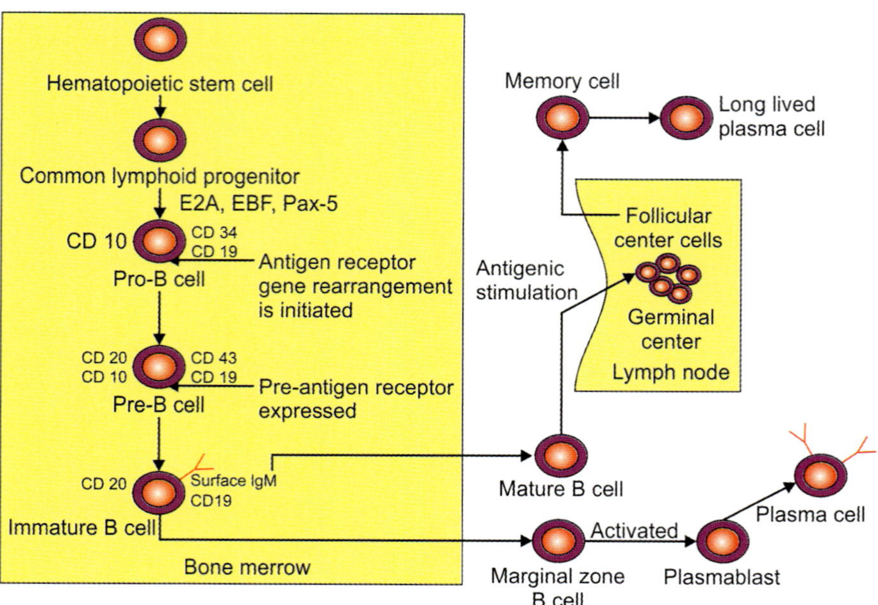

Fig. 6.8: Schematic diagram shows development of B lymphoid cells.

Lymphocytes are principally classified as B lymphocyte, T lymphocyte, and Null cell.

The hematopoietic stem cells (HSC) generate distinct progenitors of cells known as common lymphoid progenitors (CLP) from which both B and T lymphocytes develop (Fig. 6.8).

B lymphocyte: From the CLPs the successive development of Pro-B cell, pre-B cell and immature B cell occur. The CLPs are committed to the B lineage cells by the influence of early B cell factor (EBF) and E2A transcription factors and later on by Pax-5. Pro-B cells express CD34, CD10, and also CD19. Antigen receptor gene rearrangement is initiated in Pre-B cell. Subsequently, Pre-B lymphocytes develop that express the antigen receptors on the cell surface and both cytoplasmic and surface μ heavy chain are demonstrated in these cells. The cells are also positive for CD10, CD19, CD20, and CD43. Immature B cells develop from the Pre-B cells. Immature B cells show surface IgM. The cells are also positive for CD19, CD20, CD21, and CD22. From the immature B cells, mature B cell develops and comes to the circulation. These mature naïve B cells migrate to the primary follicles of lymph node. When they encounter with antigen, they migrate to the T cell zone of the lymph node and are converted into large B blast. The antigen-primed B cells further migrate into the primary follicles to form the germinal center. Each B lymphocyte is destined to generate only one specific antibody or immunoglobulin. Immunoglobulin has two major components: (1) heavy chains and (2) light chains. Heavy chains are of five types: alpha, beta, gamma, delta, and epsilon. Similarly, there are two types of light chains: kappa and lambda. Each immunoglobulin contains only one type of heavy chain and light chain. There are five isotypes of immunoglobulin IgM, IgA, IgG, IgD, and IgE. In the bone marrow B lymphoid cell undergoes gene rearrangement known as V, D, and J gene rearrangement. With the help of this VDJ gene rearrangement a unique immunoglobulin is formed. VDJ gene rearrangement is initiated from the pre- B cell. A subset of B cells develops as memory cells and long-lived plasma cells. The two subsets of B cells are present: B-1 and marginal zone (MZ) B cells. B-1 cells are unique population of B cells that are positive for CD5. MZ B cells are the sources of naive and memory B cells in spleen.

T lymphocytes: T lymphocytes are small round to oval cell with scanty light blue cytoplasm having round nuclei with condensed chromatin. Morphologically they are indistinguishable from B lymphocytes.

T lymphocytes at first develop in the bone marrow and then migrate to thymus to become immunocompetent. T lymphocytes contain surface receptor known as T cell receptor (TCR). The constant portion of TCR is attached with the membrane and the variable amino terminal region that binds with the antigen is extending away from the membrane. TCR makes a complex with other membrane proteins CD4, CD8, and CD3.

Box 6.1: Types of T cells.

- *Helper T cells*: CD4 protein on cell surface
- *Cytotoxic T cell*: CD8 protein on their surface
- *Memory T cell*: CD45RO, and either CD4 or CD8 positive
- *T regulatory cell*:
  - *Naturally occurring T_{reg} cells*: Contains intracellular FoxP3
  - *Adaptive T_{reg} cells*: Developed from naïve T cells
- *Natural killer T cells*: Recognize glycolipid antigen presented to them in conjunction with CD1d molecules.

T lymphocytes have several subtypes based on the surface molecules and functions (Box 6.1):

- *Helper T cells*: T helper (Th) cells show CD4 protein on their surface. They work in collaboration with antigen-presenting cells and help in the development of B cells into plasma cells and memory cells.
- *Cytotoxic T cell*: T cytotoxic (Tc) cells show CD8 protein on their surface and are responsible for killing virally infected cells, foreign cells, and tumor cells.
- *Memory T cell*: Memory T cells are responsible for long-term memory of the immune system. These cells rapidly proliferate to large number of effector cells when they are exposed to the antigen. These cells show cell surface protein CD45RO, and they are either CD4 or CD8 positive.
- *T regulatory cell*: T regulatory cells possess CD4 molecules on the surface and are related to immunosuppression, so they were previously known as T suppressor cells. There are two types of T regulatory cells:
  1. *Naturally occurring T_{reg} cells*: These cells develop in thymus and when they interact with antigen-presenting cell, they suppress the immune response in a nonantigen-specific manner. Naturally occurring T_{reg} cells show characteristic intracellular FoxP3.
  2. *Adaptive T_{reg} cells*: They are also known as Th3 cells. These cells develop from naïve T cells.
- *Natural killer T cells*: Natural killer T (NKT) cells are the effector T cells that resemble NK cells. NKT cells recognize glycolipid antigen presented to them in conjunction with CD1d molecules. Activated NKT cells can function as both Th and Tc cells.

Cluster of Differentiation

Cluster of differentiation (CD) commonly abbreviated as CD markers are special molecules present on the surface of the cells of our body.[1] These CD molecules are also expressed on the cell surface during various stages of differentiation of white blood cells. CD nomenclature was first proposed in the human leukocyte differentiation antigen (HLDA) workshops for the standardization and recognition of many such molecules with important functions. This system has standardized the various monoclonal antibodies that are developed against the epitopes of the surface molecules of white blood cells in many laboratories. Since the first workshop held in Paris in 1984, about 326 CD markers have been enlisted so far. Presently, CD markers have been used widely for cell type identification by immunocytochemistry or flow cytometric immunophenotyping. Table 6.2 highlights CD expression in different types of lymphoid cells.

Table 6.2: CD markers of lymphoid cells and macrophage.

Cell type	*CD markers*
T lymphocytes	
All T lymphocyte	CD45, CD3,
T helper	CD45, CD3, CD4
T cytotoxic	CD45, CD3, CD8
T regulator	CD45, CD3, CD25, CD4, FOXP3
T memory	CD45, CD3, CD44, CD4/CD8
B lymphocytes	
All B lymphocytes	CD45, CD19,CD20
Pro-B cell	CD34, CD10, CD19
Pre-B cell	CD10, CD19, CD20
Immature B cell	CD19, CD20, CD21, CD22
Plasma cell	CD138
Macrophages	CD14, CD68
Natural killer cell	CD16, CD56

Neutrophils: They are multilobated nucleated cells with moderate amount of cytoplasm. These cells accumulate in the tissue during acute inflammation.

Eosinophils: Eosinophils show multilobated nucleus with cytoplasmic eosinophilic granules. They accumulate in tissue during allergic reaction or parasitic infection.

Basophils: Basophils contain blotchy cytoplasmic metachromatic granules. They contain heparin in the cytoplasm.

Monocytes: The cells have been described in macrophages.

REFERENCE

1. Zola H, Swart B, Banham A, et al. CD molecules 2006—human cell differentiation molecules. J Immunol Methods. 2007;319(1-2):1-5.

Review Questions

1. **Simple squamous epithelium is seen in all except:**
   a. Lining of pulmonary alveoli
   b. Lining of the pleural and peritoneal cavities
   c. Parietal layer of Bowman capsule
   d. Lining of kidney collecting tubules
2. **Pseudostratified columnar epithelium is seen in:**
   a. Lining of the epididymis
   b. Lining of the epiglottis
   c. Lining of the conjunctiva of the eye
   d. Lining of the ureter
3. **Identify the lining epithelium of the histopathology section of Figure 6.9.**
4. **Match the cells in Figures 6.10A to F.**

a.	(1).	Plasma cell
b.	(2).	Mesothelial cell
c.	(3).	Salivary acinar cell
d.	(4).	Respiratory epithelial cells
e.	(5).	Endocervical cell
f.	(6).	Hepatocytes

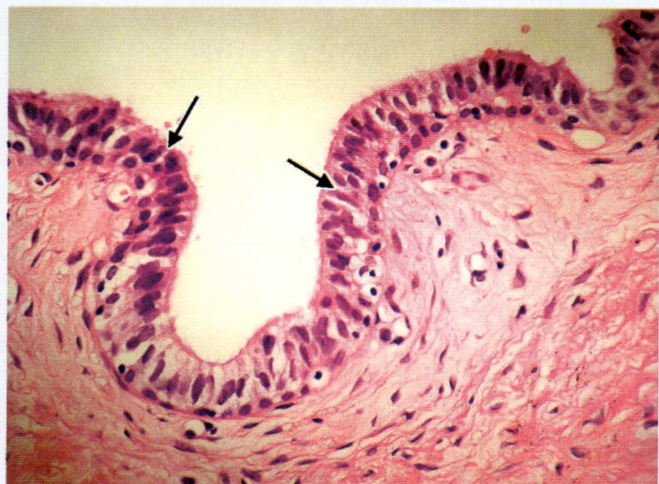

Fig. 6.9: The microphotograph shows the histopathology section of question 3.

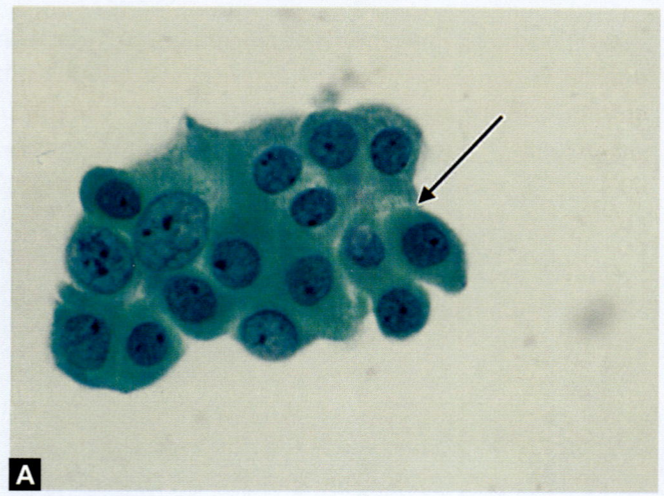

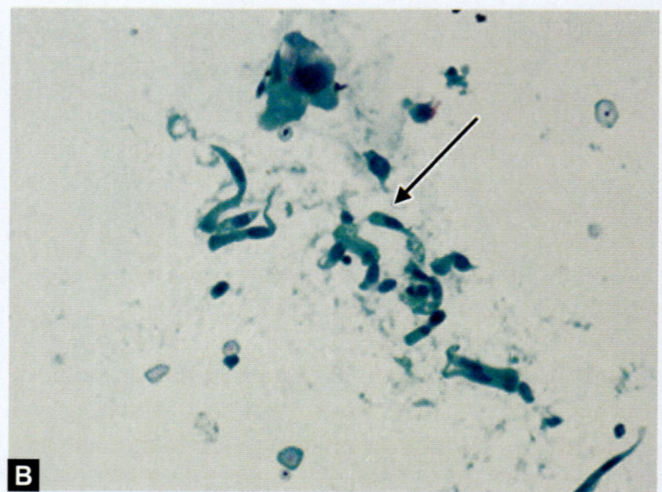

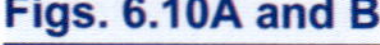

Figs. 6.10A and B

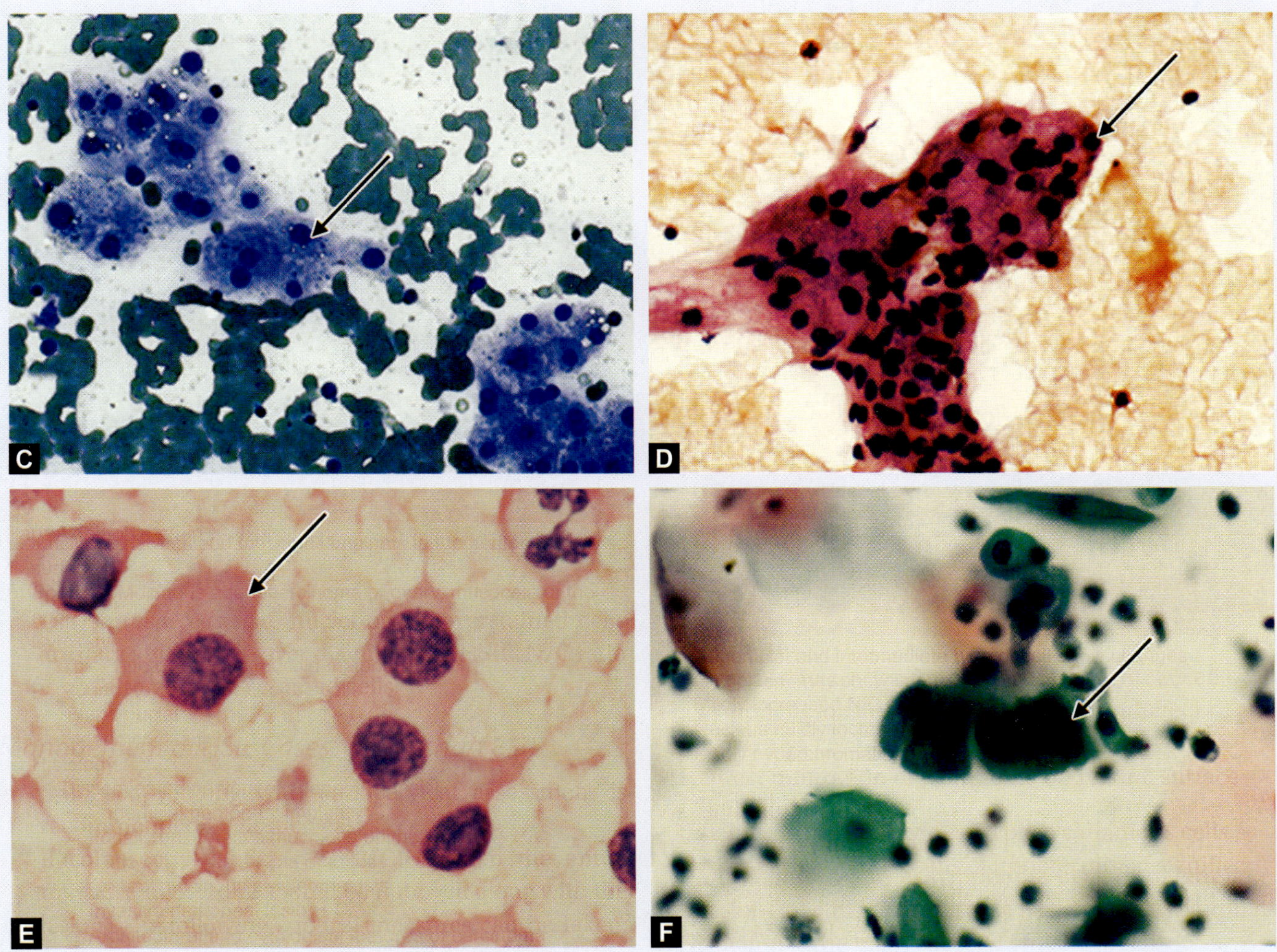

Figs. 6.10C to F: The microphotographs show the different cytology smears of question 4.

Answers

1. d. Lining of kidney collecting tubules
2. a. Lining of the epididymis
3. Transitional lining epithelial cells
4. a. (2) Mesothelial cell
   b. (4) Respiratory epithelial cells
   c. (6) Hepatocytes
   d. (3) Salivary acinar cell
   e. (1) Plasma cell
   f. (5) Endocervical cell

Section 2

Clinical Cytology (Exfoliative)

Chapter Outline

CHAPTER 7

Normal Anatomy, Histology and Cytology of Female Genital Tract

INTRODUCTION

Normal female genital tract is made of following components: vulva, vagina, uterus (with cervix), fallopian tubes and ovaries. Figure 7.1 shows the schematic diagram of the female genital tract.

VULVA

Vulva is the outermost part of the female genital tract that includes labia majora and labia minora. The labia majora are the two large soft folds of the outer part of vulva and labia minora are the two smaller inner folds. Clitoris, the rudimentary counterpart of penis, is the small erectile tissue situated within the anterior two folds of labia minora.

VAGINA

Vagina is 8–9 cm fibromuscular tubal structure that joins the uterus and the outer vulva. The opening of the vagina is caudal to the urethral opening in between the labia minora. The upper part of the vagina is continuous with the cervical canal. The free space between the upper part of vaginal pouch and cervix is known as posterior vaginal fornix. This is a potential space and cells are usually accumulated here. Urinary bladder is located anterior to vagina and rectum is located posterior to vagina.

Histology

Vaginal wall has three layers: (1) inner mucosal lining made of non-keratinizing stratified squamous epithelium; (2) muscular layer; and (3) outermost connective tissue layer. The epithelial cells of vaginal mucosa are stimulated by estrogen and contain large amount of glycogen. This glycogen serves as nutrients of the naturally occurring bacterial flora of the genital tract. Lactic acid is released as metabolic byproduct of utilization of glycogen that lowers the pH of that region. Low pH helps to protect from pathogenic invasion.

UTERUS

This is the pear-shaped thick muscular organ measuring 7 cm long, 4 cm wide and 2.5 cm thick. Uterus has three parts: (1) fundus, (2) body, and (3) cervix.

Fundus

This is the uppermost part of the uterus situated above the opening of the fallopian tubes.

Body

This is the central board portion where the two fallopian tubes open laterally.

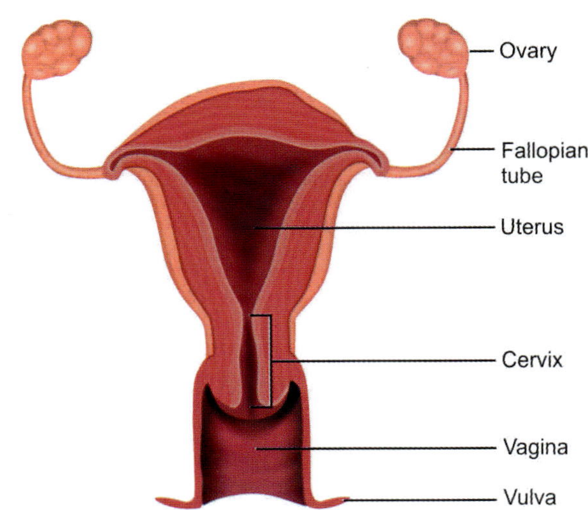

Fig. 7.1: The schematic diagram shows the different parts of the female genital tract.

Cervix

This is the lowermost circular portion of the uterus that opens into vagina. The cervix has two parts: (1) ectocervix and (2) endocervix. The portion of the cervix protruding within the vagina is known as "ectocervix". This is about 3 cm long. The rest of the cervix within the vaginal wall is labeled as "endocervix". The ectocervix opens into vagina through a circular orifice known as external os. The endocervical canal is the connective passage between the external os and uterine cavity. The opening of endocervical canal into the uterine cavity is known as internal os.

Histology

Body and fundus: The wall of the body and fundus of uterus has three layers: (1) inner endometrium, (2) myometrium, and (3) outer serosa.

Endometrium: Endometrium is the mucosal lining of the uterus and consists of two layers:

1. *Outer functionalis layer*: This layer is the superficial layer and is shedded regularly during menstruation.
2. *Inner basalis layer*: This is the deeper layer from which the glands and connective tissue elements proliferate after menstrual shedding.

The mucosal lining of the endometrium is made of secretory columnar cells. Lamina propria contains many tubular glands and arterioles.

Myometrium: It is composed of three layers of smooth muscles: (1) inner longitudinal, (2) middle circular and (3) outer longitudinal.

Serosa: The outer part of the uterus is lined by mesothelial cells.

Histology of Cervix

Ectocervix: It is lined by non-keratinizing stratified squamous epithelium (Fig. 7.2). The epithelium can be divided into three parts: (1) Lower zone (Basal/parabasal cell layer): This is the lowermost layer and contains basal and parabasal cells; (2) Mid zone (intermediate cell layer): This occupies the major part of the epithelium and is composed of intermediate cells; (3) Superficial zone (superficial cell layer): This is the most differentiated superficial part of the epithelium and is composed of flattened superficial cells.

Endocervix: Mucosal membrane of the endocervix is a single layer of mucus secreting columnar lining epithelium (Fig. 7.3). These cells are tall columnar with basally placed nuclei giving rise to picket fence-like appearance.

Cervical stroma is composed of predominantly fibrous, muscle and elastic tissue. There are many endocervical mucus-secreting glands in the endocervical submucosal tissue.

Transformation zone (Box 7.1): This is the junction between the stratified squamous epithelium and mucin-secreting columnar epithelium of the endocervix (Figs. 7.4A and B). This is also known as squamocolumnar junction. The transformation zone is not a fixed area and depending on the situation, it may shift toward ectocervix or endocervix. Original transformation zone at the time of birth is toward the upper part of cervix. At the time of childbearing age or pregnancy, the cervix enlarges and the transformation

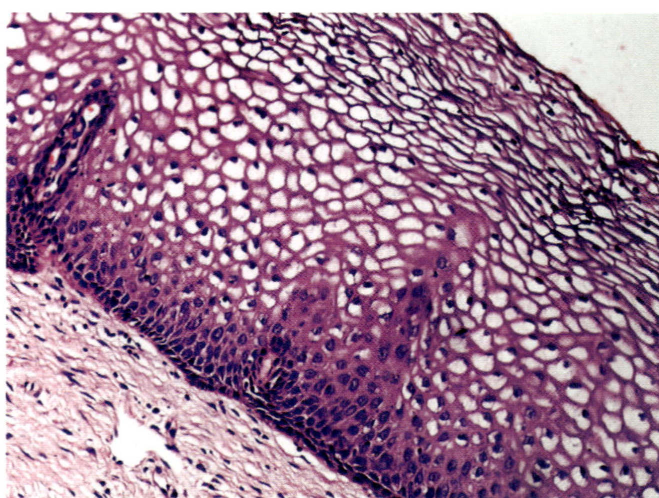

Fig. 7.2: Histology section of the normal ectocervical squamous epithelial lining (Hematoxylin and Eosin stain × HP).

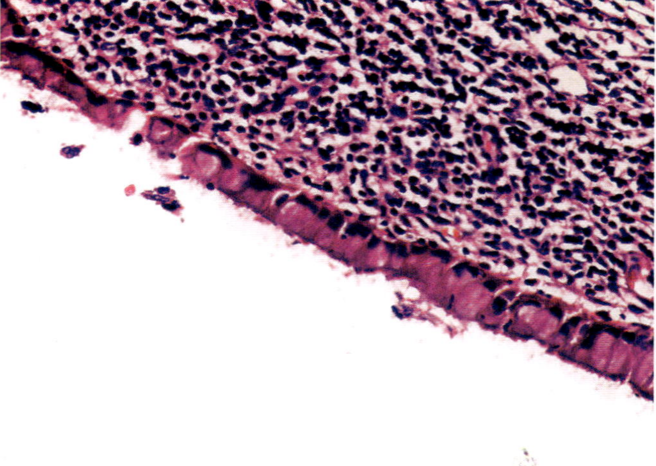

Fig. 7.3: Histology section of the normal endocervical lining epithelium (Hematoxylin and Eosin stain × HP).

zone moves toward the external os. As the age increases, the squamocolumnar junction moves toward the upper part of the endocervical canal. In case of physiologic transformation zone, the endocervical epithelium undergoes squamous metaplasia, and the new transformation zone is formed by metaplastic squamous epithelium and columnar epithelium.

The concept of the transformation zone is important because all the cervical squamous cell carcinoma originates from the new transformation zone, and also the cervical preneoplastic conditions develop from this area. Therefore, sampling from transformation zone is important during cervical cancer screening.

OVARIES

These are two ovoid-shaped 3–5 cm diameter structures situated lateral to fallopian tubes and uterus. Each ovary is attached to the uterus at its medial pole by utero-ovarian ligament. The ovary is divided into highly cellular outer cortex and less cellular richly vascular inner medulla.

Box 7.1: Transformation zone.

- Junction between the stratified squamous epithelium and columnar epithelium of the endocervix
- Sampling target

  Original transformation zone: The junction between the stratified squamous epithelium and mucin secreting columnar epithelium of the endocervix

  Physiologic transformation zone: The junction between the metaplastic squamous epithelium and columnar epithelium

  Significance of TZ: (1) It is vulnerable to HPV infection; (2) Squamous cell carcinoma of cervix arise from TZ; (3) Surveillance of this area is needed to detect early cases of dysplasia.

Surface Epithelium

The surface epithelium of the ovary is a single layer of modified mesothelial cells. The individual cells are cuboidal to columnar in appearance.

Stroma: Ovarian stroma shows spindle-shaped stromal cells along with multiple ovarian follicles in various stages of maturation.

FALLOPIAN TUBES

Fallopian tubes extend from the cornual ends of uterus laterally up to each ovary. It is of 9–11 cm in length. Fallopian tubes end directly to the peritoneal cavity in the ovarian end with 25 irregular fingers like extensions around the opening part.

Histology

The fallopian tube has three layers: (1) mucosal membrane, (2) muscular layer, and (3) outer serosal layer. Mucous membrane consists of three types of columnar cells: (1) ciliated, (2) nonciliated secretory and (3) intercalary. There is no lamina propria and the mucosa is directly in contact with muscle layer. The muscle layer is made of outer longitudinal and inner circular layer. The outermost serosa is lined by flattened mesothelial cells.

NORMAL CELLS IN CERVICAL SMEAR

The various normal cells are seen in routine cervical cytology smear on Papanicolaou's stained smear. It is necessary to identify these cells. Table 7.1 highlights the

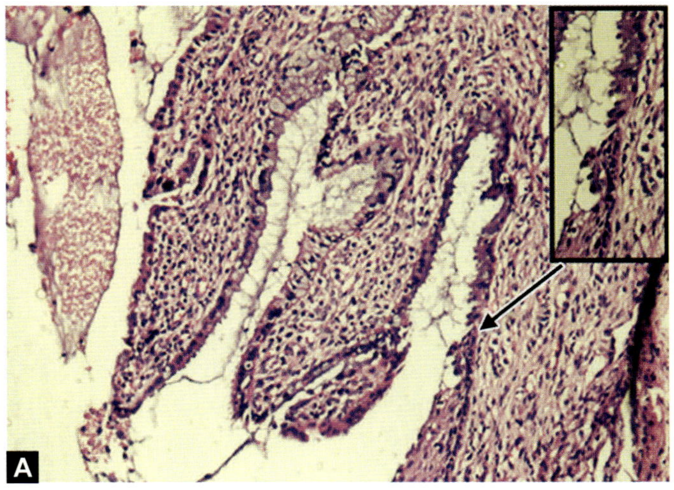

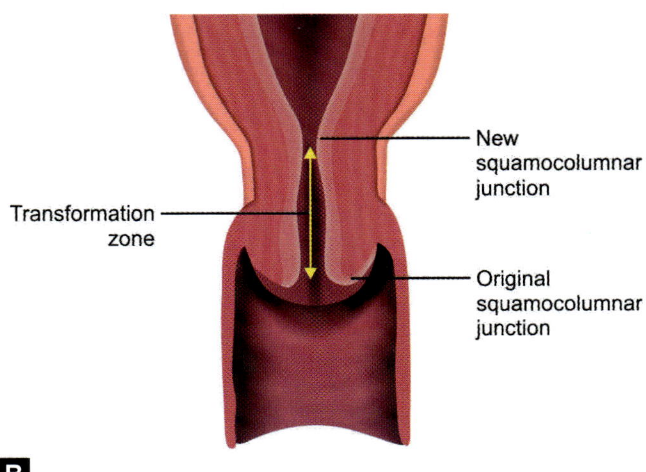

Figs. 7.4A and B: (A) Transformation zone or squamocolumnar junction of the cervix (Hematoxylin and Eosin stain X MP). (B) Schematic diagram of transformation zone of the cervix.

Table 7.1: Comparison of epithelial cells of cervical lining epithelium.

Features	*Superficial*	*Intermediate*	*Parabasal*	*Endocervical*
Cell arrangement	Discrete	Discrete	Discrete	Honeycomb shaped clusters
Cell size	Largest, 30–40 micron diameter	Larger: 30–40 micron diameter	Smaller: 25–30 micron diameter	Smallest: 20 micron diameter
Cell shape	Polyhedral	Polyhedral	Round	Round to columnar
Nucleus	Central pyknotic	Vesicular to fine granular chromatin	Round Occupies most of the cytoplasm chromatin is finely granular	Round, central to eccentric
Cytoplasm	Orangeophilic	Pink to greenish cytoplasm	Dense cytoplasm	Vacuolated cytoplasm

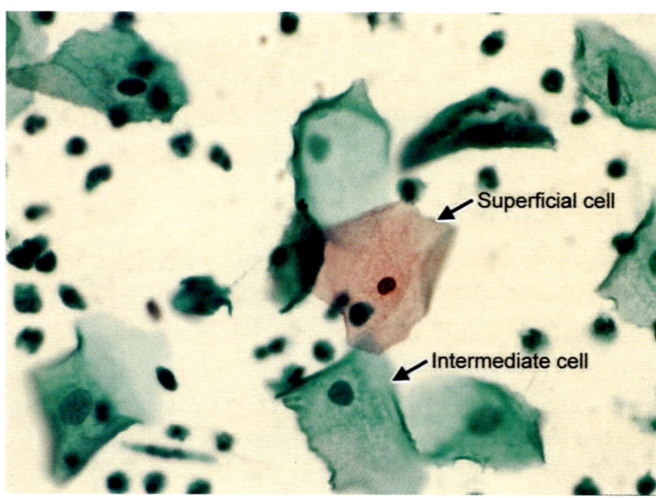

Fig. 7.5: Cytology smear showing superficial cell with abundant orangeophilic cytoplasm and central pyknotic nucleus. Smear also shows intermediate cell with abundant cytoplasm and vesicular nucleus (Papanicolaou's stain × HP).

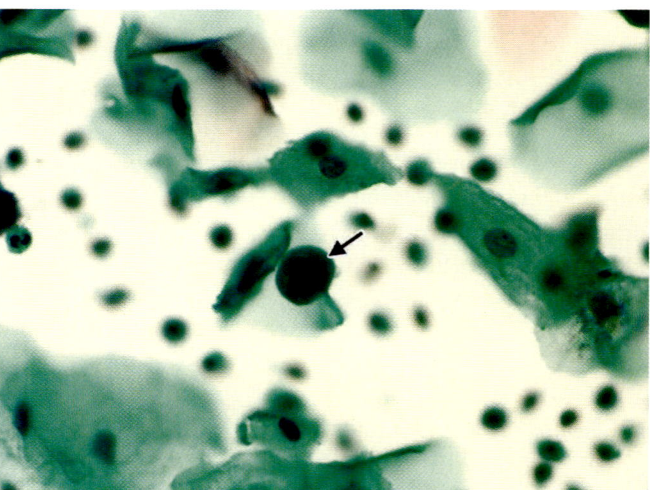

Fig. 7.6: Cytology smear showing parabasal cell with thick cytoplasm and centrally placed large nucleus (*see* arrow) (Papanicolaou's stain × HP).

differentiating features of various types of squamous cell on cervical cytology.

The lining of the ectocervix is non-keratinizing stratified squamous epithelium. The scraping of ectocervix therefore shows predominantly superficial squamous cells and intermediate cells. Occasionally parabasal cells are also noted on the smear.

Superficial Squamous Cells

These are large polyhedral cells with abundant thin pink to green cytoplasm and centrally placed small pyknotic nuclei. The diameter of the superficial cell is usually 30–45 μ and nucleus is about 5–7 μ (Fig. 7.5). The cells often show orangeophilic cytoplasm indicating intracellular keratin.

Intermediate Cells

These are large polyhedral cells with abundant pale green cytoplasm and centrally placed vesicular nucleus. The diameter of intermediate cell is usually 35–45 μ and nucleus is about 8–10 μ. Nucleus is the main differentiating point between superficial and intermediate cell (Fig. 7.5). The nucleus of the intermediate cell is vesicular with fine granular chromatin. Nuclear groove may be seen in intermediate cells as deep longitudinal fold. Intermediate cells with peripheral boat-like folding are known as navicular cells. This is due to progesterone effect on cervical epithelium. Navicular cells are seen in pregnant patients.

Parabasal and Basal Cells

These are small round to oval cells with dense cytoplasm and relatively large nucleus. Diameter of parabasal cell is 10–25 μ and nucleus is 6–8 μ, round with condensed chromatin (Fig. 7.6). Basal cells have almost same appearance except they are small in size. Parabasal cells are frequently seen in atrophic smear of postmenopausal patient.

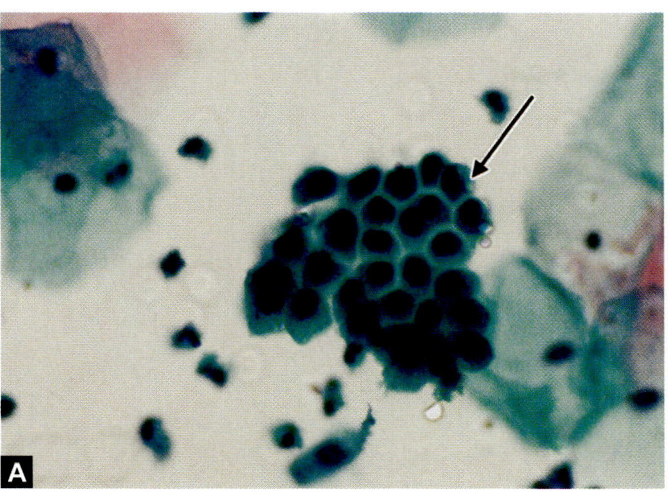

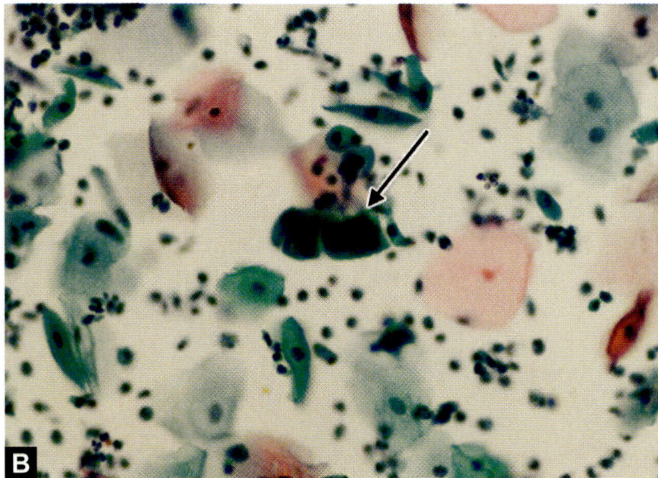

Figs. 7.7A and B: (A) Endocervical cells in flat sheet. Individual cells have moderate vacuolated cytoplasm and round monomorphic nuclei (*see* arrow) (Papanicolaou's stain × HP). (B) Tall columnar endocervical in row (*see* arrow) (Papanicolaou's stain × HP).

Box 7.2: Endocervical cells.

- Honeycomb-shaped clusters of cells
- On side view, picket fence appearance at times
- Columnar cells with basally placed nuclei
- Cytoplasm moderate
- Vesicular nucleus with fine chromatin
- Small nucleoli
- Endocervical cells with tuft of cilia from terminal plate in tubal metaplasia

Box 7.3: Squamous metaplasia.

- Single or sheets of cells
- Smaller parabasal type of cell
- Cytoplasm
  - Spider like cells with angulated projections
  - Cyanophilic
  - Dense
  - Sharp border
- Nucleus
  - Round to oval
  - Smooth outline
  - Fine chromatin
  - Small nucleoli
- High nucleocytoplasmic ratio

Fig. 7.8: Tubal metaplasia of the endocervical cells. Inset highlights endocervical cell with basal plate and cilia (*see* arrow) (Papanicolaou's stain × HP).

Endocervical Cells (Box 7.2)

The cells are small round to columnar shaped with vacuolated cytoplasm and basally placed nuclei. The diameter of endocervical cell is about 18–20 μ and nucleus is 8–10 μ. The nucleus is vesicular with finely granular chromatin having occasional small nucleoli (Figs. 7.7A and B). These cells are usually present in tight honeycomb shaped clusters. On side view, the cells may give the appearance of picket fence. Endocervical cells may undergo *tubal metaplasia* (Fig. 7.8). The individual cells are columnar shaped with cilia attached on terminal plate.

Metaplastic Squamous Cells (Box 7.3)

This is the most common change of endocervical cells. It usually occurs in transformation zone. The glandular surface of the endocervix is replaced by squamous cell. The metaplastic cells are composed of immature parabasal cell. The cells are arranged in interlocking manner and one cell fits within another (Fig. 7.9). This gives a mosaic-like pattern. The cells of squamous metaplasia are relatively

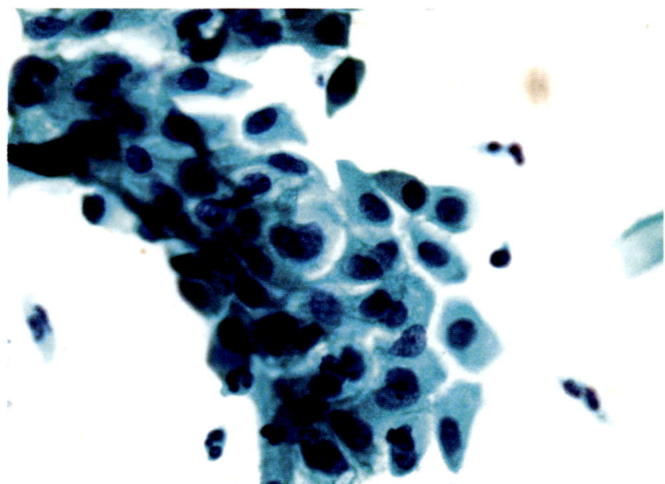

Fig. 7.9: Metaplastic endocervical cell in SurePath liquid-based cytology smear. Cells are arranged in interlocking manner and one cell fits within another (Papanicolaou's stain × HP).

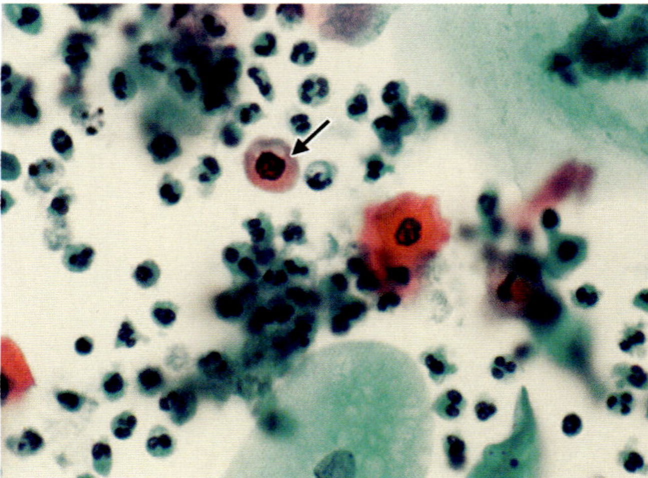

Fig. 7.10: Parakeratotic cells showing small squamous cell with pyknotic nucleus (*see* arrow) (Papanicolaou's stain × HP).

small with scanty cytoplasm. The nuclei are enlarged with slightly irregular contour and mildly hyperchromatic.

CHANGES OF SQUAMOUS EPITHELIUM

The following changes may occur in the squamous epithelium:

Hyperkeratosis

The term hyperkeratosis is characterized by the presence of thick keratin layer over the squamous lining of the cervix. In cervical cytology smear hyperkeratosis is represented by single or clusters of anucleated squamous cells. The nuclei of the cells may be only seen as clear central zone.[1] Hyperkeratosis is a nonspecific finding and may be seen in inflammation, postcryotherapy or uterine prolapse. However, hyperkeratosis may be an associated finding in HPV infection.[2]

Parakeratosis

The term parakeratosis means the presence of nucleated squamous cells in keratin layer of the hyperkeratosis. On cytology smear, the parakeratotic cell is characterized by superficial squamous cells with small, pyknotic or hyperchromatic nuclei[2] (Fig. 7.10). The presence of parakeratosis is also a nonspecific finding. Probably, the female with the presence of parakeratosis in the cervical smear has higher chance of HPV infection.

Box 7.4: Endometrial cells.

- Tight spherical clusters of cells
- Small round cells with scanty cytoplasm
- Cytoplasmic vacuolations
- Round dark nuclei with nuclear molding or angulated contour
- No nucleoli

Differential diagnosis: High-grade squamous intraepithelial lesion, small cell nonkeratinizing squamous cell carcinoma, endometrial adenocarcinoma.

Pseudoparakeratosis

The term "pseudoparakeratosis" indicates the glandular cells with deep orangeophilic cytoplasm simulating parakeratotic cells. These types of cells are seen in patients who receive oral contraceptive. The pseudoparakeratotic cells may also be seen as degenerated parabasal cells in atrophic background.

Dysplastic cells: Discussed later.

Endometrial Cells (Box 7.4)

Endometrial cells are spontaneously shed in first few days of the menstrual cycle and may be present in the cervical smear at that time. Both glandular and superficial stromal cells may be present. Spontaneously exfoliated normal looking endometrial cells are expected also after birth of baby, abortion, endometrial polyp, endometritis, and endometriosis. At times, clusters of endometrial cells may show dual population of cells with central small dark stromal cells and peripheral glandular cells with moderately vacuolated cytoplasm.

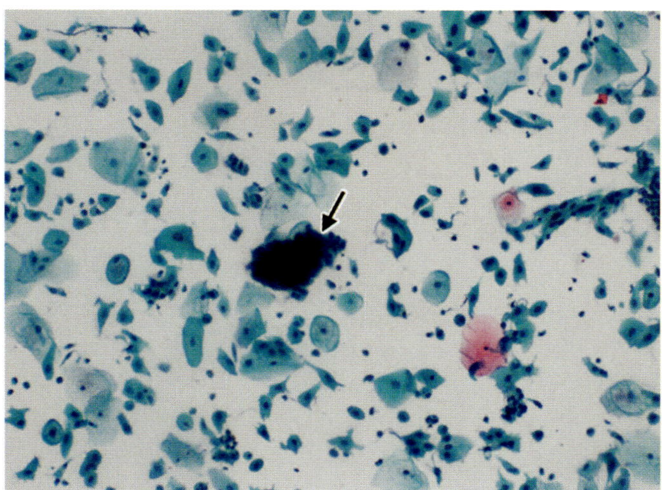

Fig. 7.11: Low-power magnification of endometrial cells in small tight clusters (*see* arrow) (Papanicolaou's stain X MP).

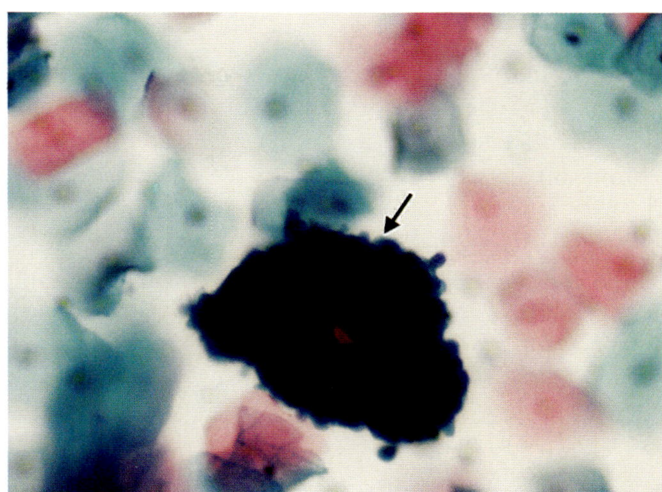

Fig. 7.12: High-power magnification of endometrial cells in tight clusters. Individual cells have scanty cytoplasm and small hyperchromatic nucleus (*see* arrow) (Papanicolaou's stain × HP).

Endometrial cells are commonly present in small tight spherical clusters (Figs. 7.11 and 7.12). Individual cells are small round shaped with round dark nuclei. The nuclei often show molding. Nucleoli are not seen in endometrial cells. Cytoplasm of the cells is scanty and occasionally may show vacuolations.

Exfoliated Endometrial Cells in Cervical Smear

In these following conditions, endometrial cells may be seen in cervical smear: (1) Menstruation, (2) Endometritis, (3) Endometriosis, (4) Endometrial polyp, (5) Submucosal leiomyoma, (6) Intrauterine instrumentation, (7) Tamoxifen therapy, (8) Endometrial adenocarcinoma.

During menstruation, the endometrial cells are normally exfoliated and are known as exodus. These cells are noted from 6th to 10th day of the menstrual cycle and their presence after 12th day of the menstrual cycle is unusual. The cytological features of exodus are: (1) tight cohesive clusters of cells with central dense stromal cells, and (2) peripheral larger endometrial cells.

The endometrial cells should always be distinguished from endocervical cells. The differentiating points are:

- Endometrial cells are present in 3-D (dimensional) cohesive clusters, whereas endocervical cells are present in 2-D sheet or discretely.
- Endometrial cells have scanty cytoplasm whereas endocervical cells have moderate cytoplasm
- Nuclear chromatin of the endometrial cells is dense compared to the fine chromatin of the endocervical cells.
- Absence of nucleoli in endometrial cells compared to single small nucleoli in endocervical cells.

Mimickers of Endometrial Cells

There are few mimickers of endometrial cells.

- *High-grade squamous intraepithelial lesion (HSIL)*: The cells of HSILs are usually bigger than endometrial cells. The nuclei are markedly hyperchromatic with irregular nuclear contour. Usually, these cells are arranged discretely or in loose clusters compared to tight spherical arrangement of endometrial cells.
- *Well-differentiated adenocarcinoma*: Occasionally, it is very difficult to distinguish well-differentiated adenocarcinoma of uterus from benign endometrial cells on cervical smears. In this condition, it is better to have complete investigations to exclude or confirm adenocarcinoma.
- *Lymphocytes*: Smaller size and condensed nuclei of lymphocytes may simulate endometrial cells.
- *Histiocytes*: Occasionally, histiocytes may simulate endometrial cells; however the histiocytes are usually discrete having bean-shaped nuclei with cytoplasmic debris.
- *Parabasal cells*: Parabasal cells are present in small two-dimensional flat sheet or discrete. The cells have relatively more amount of dense cytoplasm.

Inflammatory Cells

Various inflammatory cells such as polymorphonuclear leukocytes, lymphocytes, and histiocytes may be present in cervical smear.

Leukocytes

Polymorphonuclear leukocytes are often seen in cervical smears and their presence does not always indicate acute inflammation. Lymphocytes and plasma cells are noted in chronic inflammatory conditions.

Histiocyte (Macrophage)

These cells are often noted in cervical smears. The individual cells are large with centrally placed nuclei. The nuclear shape may be kidney shaped. Cytoplasm often shows phagocytosed material. The presence of histiocytes in the cervical smear is a nonspecific finding and is noted in many conditions such as pregnancy, foreign body reactions, endometrial cancer, etc. Occasionally, multinucleated histiocytes are seen in foreign body granuloma, chronic inflammation or in postmenopausal atrophic smear (Fig. 7.13).

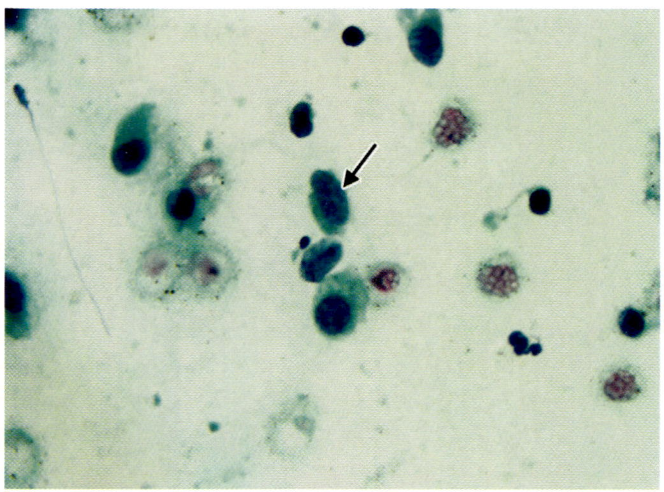

Fig. 7.13: Histiocytes in cervical smear (*see* arrow) (Papanicolaou's stain × HP).

Trophoblastic and Decidual Cells

Rarely, trophoblastic cells may be seen in cervical smear. The trophoblastic cell is large with abundant cytoplasm having multiple nuclei. Nuclei show mild irregular nuclear margin and fine granular chromatin (Fig. 7.14). Decidual cell is large mononuclear cell with abundant cytoplasm. The nuclei are large vesicular with prominent nucleoli. In lack of history, it is difficult to identify the decidual cells with certainty and the cell may be confused with malignant cell.

Others

Spermatozoa

At times, sperms may be seen in cervical smear if the smear is taken sometimes after sexual intercourse (Fig. 7.15).

Ova of Parasites

Occasionally, ovum of parasites may be seen in cervical smears.

Cells of Adjacent Organ

Urothelial cells: Rarely in case of uterovesical fistula, urothelial cells from urothelium of bladder may contaminate cervical smear. These cells may be difficult to identify.

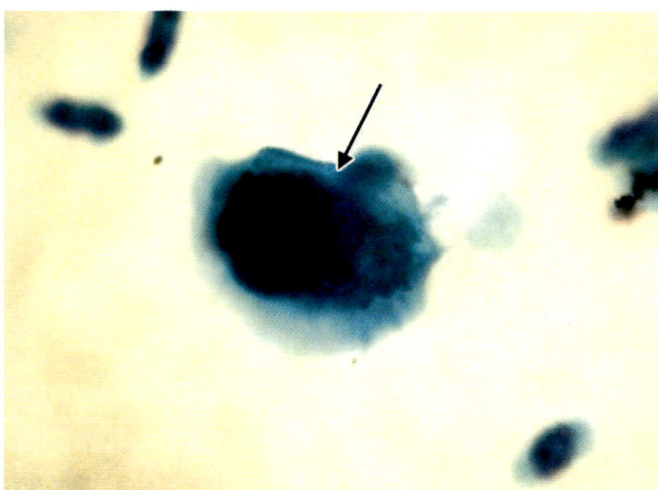

Fig. 7.14: Trophoblastic cell with large multiple nuclei (*see* arrow) (Papanicolaou's stain × HP).

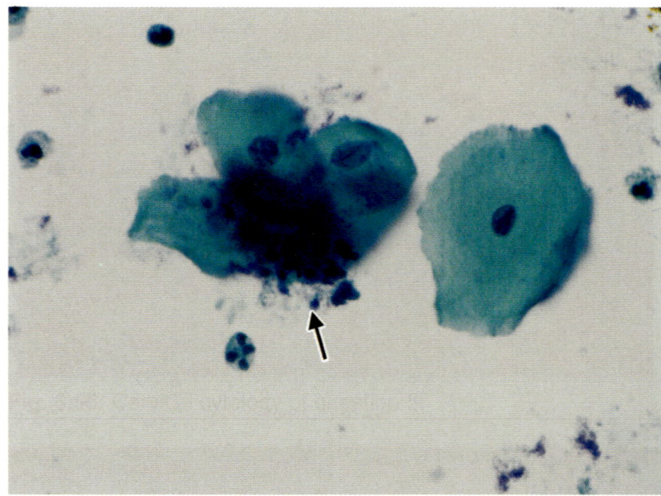

Fig. 7.15: Sperm heads in cervical smear (*see* arrow) (Papanicolaou's stain × HP).

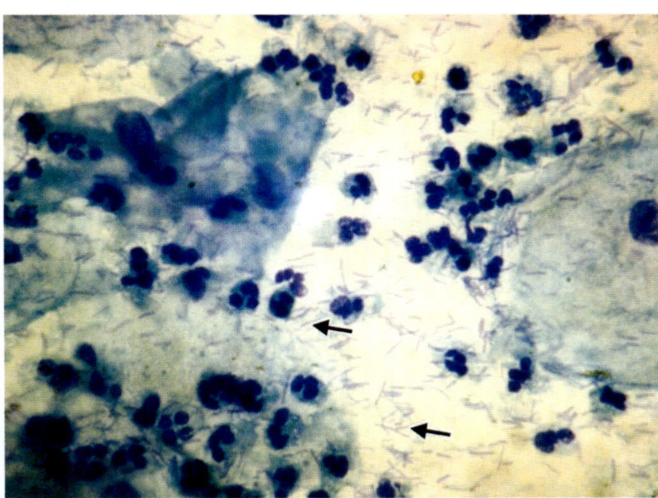

Fig. 7.16: Small scattered rod-shaped lactobacilli (*see* arrows) (Papanicolaou's stain × HP).

Colonic cells: These are sheets of columnar epithelial cells and can be identified as rows of columnar cells similar to that of endocervical cells.

Acellular Material

Contaminants: Cervical smears may often show contaminants by dust of surgical gloves, lubricant jellies, etc.

Lactobacilli

Lactobacilli are seen in cervical smear. These are Gram-positive rod-shaped bacilli normally present in the vaginal flora (Fig. 7.16). Lactobacilli metabolize the glycogen content of the exfoliated squamous cells and produce lactic acid. Lactic acid decreases pH of the vaginal tract and protects it from pathogenic invasion.

BETHESDA SYSTEM OF REPORTING

The Bethesda system (TBS) workshop was first held in 1988 followed by 1991 and 2001 at the National Institutes of Health in Bethesda, Maryland. In 1988 TBS, the fundamental principles and terminology of the Bethesda system of reporting cervical smear was formulated.[3] In this workshop, the two-tier system of reporting cervical squamous intraepithelial lesion was given on the basis of knowledge of HPV infection and progression. Specimen adequacy criteria were also provided.

The diagnostic terms of specimen adequacy were further provided in TBS 1991 along with TBS interpretive categories.[4] In the Bethesda system 2001, the following changes were done:[5]

1. Specimen adequacy criteria have been changed and "satisfactory but limited" terminology was withdrawn. Only two categories "satisfactory" and "unsatisfactory" have been kept.
2. The word "diagnosis" has been replaced by "interpretation/result".
3. The category Negative for Intraepithelial Lesion or Malignancy has been kept and the reporting non-neoplastic findings are kept as optional category (other than organism).
4. The modification was done in atypical squamous cells of undetermined significance (ASCUS). Only two terminologies were kept here: "atypical squamous cells of undetermined significance (ASC-US)" and "atypical squamous cells, cannot exclude HSIL" (ASC-H). There was no provision of ASCUS possibly reactive.
5. Atypical glandular cells: The classification in this category was extensively revised and the term "atypical glandular cells of undetermined significance" (AGCUS) was removed. The glandular cell abnormality was kept as Atypical Glandular Cells (AGC) and Atypical Glandular Cells possibly neoplastic. It was recommended to mention the possible origin of the glandular cells.
6. It was recommended to mention the name of the ancillary tests in cervical smear

In 2014, there was minor modification of Bethesda system:[6]

- The criteria of mentioning the presence of endometrial cells was raised from 40 years to 45 years.
- The details of TBS 2001 and 2014 have been discussed in Table 7.2.
- The Bethesda system 2001/2014 can be divided into three parts: (1) specimen adequacy, (2) general categorization, and (3) terminologies.

Specimen Adequacy

The Bethesda system 2001 maintains only "satisfactory for evaluation" and "unsatisfactory" categories and eliminates "satisfactory but limited" category as the "satisfactory but limited" category was confusing to many clinicians. So, the elimination of this category gives clear and reproducible indications about the adequacy of the sample. However, the option was kept about providing information on transformation zone to improve the quality of the sample collection.

Table 7.2: The Bethesda System 2014.[6]

Specimen type
• Conventional or liquid-based cytology • Specimen adequacy
Satisfactory for evaluation • Adequate number of squamous cells: - Conventional smear: 8,000–12,000 squamous cells - Liquid-based cytology: 5,000 squamous cells • Mention the presence or absence of endocervical cells or transformation zone components: at least 10 endocervical or metaplastic cells should be present, no need for cell clusters. • Any other quality elements such as drying artifact, obscured by blood or inflammation, etc. Partially obscured: 50–75% epithelial cells cannot be visualized; unsatisfactory: when more than 75% epithelial cells cannot be visualized
Unsatisfactory for evaluation
• Specimen rejected: Specimen rejected due to broken slide or mislabeled specimen • Fully evaluated unsatisfactory specimen: Specimen processed but unsatisfactory because: - Insufficient squamous cells - More than 75% of smear is obscured by blood or inflammatory cells
General categorization (optional)
Negative for intraepithelial lesion or malignancy Epithelial cell abnormality
Interpretation/Result
Negative for intraepithelial lesion or malignancy
Non-neoplastic findings (optional to report)
• Non-neoplastic cellular variations - Squamous metaplasia - Keratotic changes - Tubal metaplasia - Atrophy - Pregnancy-associated changes • Reactive cellular changes associated with: - Inflammation (includes typical repair) - Lymphocytic (follicular) cervicitis - Radiation - Intrauterine contraceptive device (IUD) • Glandular cells status post-hysterectomy
Organisms
• *Trichomonas vaginalis* • Fungal organisms morphologically consistent with *Candida* spp. • Shift in flora suggestive of bacterial vaginosis • Bacteria morphologically consistent with *Actinomyces* spp. • Cellular changes consistent with herpes simplex virus • Cellular changes consistent with cytomegalovirus
Other: Endometrial cells (in a woman aged more than 45 years) (Also specify if "negative for squamous intraepithelial lesion")
EPITHELIAL CELL ABNORMALITY
Squamous cell
Atypical squamous cell (ASC)
• Of undetermined significance (ASC-US) • Cannot exclude HSIL (ASC-H)
Low-grade squamous intraepithelial lesion (LSIL) High-grade squamous intraepithelial lesion (HSIL) Squamous cell carcinoma

Contd...

Contd...

Glandular cell
• Atypical - Endocervical in origin - Endometrial in origin - Glandular cell, not otherwise specified • Atypical - Endocervical, favor neoplastic - Glandular favor neoplastic, not otherwise specified • Endocervical adenocarcinoma in situ • Adenocarcinoma - Endocervical - Endometrial - Extra uterine - Not otherwise specified • Other malignant neoplasm
ADJUNCTIVE TESTING
Provide a brief description of the test method(s) and report the result so that it is easily understood by the clinician
COMPUTER-ASSISTED INTERPRETATION OF CERVICAL CYTOLOGY
If case examined by an automated device, specify the device and result
EDUCATIONAL NOTES AND COMMENTS APPENDED TO CYTOLOGY REPORTS (optional)
Suggestions should be concise and consistent with clinical follow-up guidelines published by professional organizations (references to relevant publications may be included)

Cellularity

The Bethesda system 2001 provided the quantitative numerical estimate for the adequacy of squamous cells.

Adequate Number of Cells

Conventional smear: 8000–12000 squamous cells
Liquid-based cytology: 5000 squamous cells

Only the well-visualized and well-preserved squamous cells should be taken into consideration for cellular adequacy. Endocervical cells, endometrial cells and inflammatory cells should not be considered for cellular adequacy. The approximate number of cells should be estimated only and the cytologists are not expected to count individual cells. TBS 2001 published the reference images in their website to help in the estimation of the number of cells on conventional smear and liquid based preparations.[7]

Endocervical Cells

In TBS 2001, mention of the presence of endocervical cell or transformation zone component is needed. At least 10 well-preserved endocervical cells or metaplastic cells should be present to represent the transformation zone; however, the clusters of cells are not required.

The absence of endocervical cell is not considered as unsatisfactory smears.

General Categorization

"General categorization" is kept as an optional component in TBS 2001/2014. The previous two categories "within normal limit" and "benign cellular changes" are combined together in a single category as "negative for intraepithelial lesion or malignancy" in TBS 2001.

Others

The presence of benign looking endometrial cells over 45 years of age should be labeled as "others" in 2014 TBS.

The above-mentioned categories in TBS are mutually exclusive. However, in case of multiple different findings in one smear, the smear may be labeled according to the most clinically significant lesion.

Interpretation and Result

In the 2001 TBS, the term "diagnosis" has been replaced by interpretation or result because the cervical smear report is primarily a screening test.

Negative for Intraepithelial Lesion or Malignancy

The specimen in absence of epithelial cell abnormality is reported as Negative for Intraepithelial Lesion or Malignancy (NILM). The term "infection" has been replaced by "organism" in TBS 2001 because the presence of some organisms may not indicate clinical infection.

There is optional choice to report other non-neoplastic findings such as changes due to reparative processes, radiation, atrophy, and intrauterine contraceptive devices. The cytological features of these lesions are important to recognize to avoid false positive cases because the cellular features of these cases may resemble intraepithelial lesions.

Epithelial Cell Abnormalities

Atypical Squamous Cells

In 2001 TBS, "atypical squamous cell" is qualified as "atypical squamous cells of undetermined significance (ASC-US)" and "atypical squamous cells, cannot exclude HSIL" (ASC-H). The category ASC-favors reactive atypia is eliminated and the cytologists have to take decision judiciously to put the cases either as NILM or in ASC. Atypical squamous cells, cannot exclude HSIL suggests that cytological features are close to HSIL but do not fully support the definitive interpretation of HSIL. According to TBS 2001, ASC-H includes HSIL and its mimics and will include 5–10% of ASC cases overall.

Squamous Intraepithelial Lesion

The Bethesda system 2001 workshop kept two-tiered low-grade squamous intraepithelial lesion (LSIL)/HSIL terminology as was suggested by previous TBS. The dichotomous division of SIL is kept because it was thought that LSIL and HSIL are clinically different. The supporting evidences of this two-tiered system are:

- Low-grade squamous intraepithelial lesion is a transient infection of HPV and rarely progress to higher grade, whereas HSIL is due to persistent infection and has higher risk of progression.[8]
- To separate minor low-risk LSIL from significant high-risk HSIL on the basis of morphology
- Low-grade squamous intraepithelial lesion versus HSIL is reproducible
- Subdividing HSIL into CIN2 and CIN3 may not be reproducible.

High-grade squamous intraepithelial lesion cannot exclude invasion: In certain situation, it may be difficult to distinguish HSIL from an invasive carcinoma on the basis of cytological features. In this situation, cytologists may apply this terminology to increase clinician's concern on that particular case.

Squamous Cell Carcinoma

It represents the invasive squamous cell carcinoma. Usually tumor diathesis is present in invasive squamous cell carcinoma. In TBS, there is no option to differentiate keratinizing from nonkeratinizing squamous cell carcinoma in cytology smear.

Atypical Glandular Lesion

The terminology of atypical glandular cells has been significantly changed in TBS 2001 and the term "atypical glandular cells of undetermined significance (AGUS)" has been eliminated to avoid confusion with ASC-US. The glandular cell abnormalities have been classified as:

- Atypical glandular cells: Endocervical, endometrial, or not otherwise specified
- Atypical glandular cells favor neoplastic: Endocervical, or not otherwise specified.

The pathologists are encouraged to identify the origin of the atypical glandular cells (whether endocervical or endometrial) and specify in report, if not possible, then they may just mention "atypical glandular cell".

Endocervical Adenocarcinoma in situ

Adenocarcinoma in situ (AIS) category has been kept as a separate entity. There may be some amount of overlapping between AIS with invasive carcinoma in one hand and AIS with atypical glandular cells favor neoplastic in other hand.

Automated Review and Ancillary Testing

If the slides are scanned in automated scanning system then in cytology report, there should be complete mention of the name of the instrumentation, and the results of the automated system. Similarly, if any other ancillary test is done such as screening of high-risk HPV test then the result should be mentioned concurrently or as an addendum with cytology report.

Educational Notes and Suggestions

The cytologists may write brief educational notes or suggestions in the report. The comments and suggestions should be according to guidelines of the professional societies. It is preferable not to communicate with the patient directly because as this may adversely affect the patient-clinician relationship.

Negative for Intraepithelial Lesion or Malignancy

Organisms and Infection

Bacterial vaginosis (BV): This is a fairly common infection and affects large number of patients worldwide. The patients have thin milky vaginal discharge with foul fishy smell. Many of them may be asymptomatic also. Previously it was believed that *Gardnerella vaginalis* is solely responsible for this infection. However now, it is evident that BV can be caused by infections with other bacteria in Clostridiales order. It is now suggested to report as "*shift in bacterial flora*" rather than to make the specific diagnosis of *G. vaginalis* infection. Bacterial vaginosis cases are positive for *Whiff's test*. In this test, 10% potassium hydroxide is added on the slide of vaginal fluid. The production of fishy smell indicates a positive test.

Cytology: Smear shows numerous small coccobacilli replacing the normal lactobacilli giving a filmy background (Box 7.5). There may be variable amount of acute inflammatory cells. Clue cells are the squamous cells filled with numerous small coccobacilli. These cells are one of the diagnostic features of BV (Fig. 7.17); however, they are not specific for BV.

Trichomonas: *Trichomonas vaginalis* is the most common infection in the female genital tract (Box 7.6). The patient usually complains of burning sensation, severe itching, and foul smelling vaginal discharge. In addition, the patient may have lower urinary tract infection. Considerable number of patients (up to 50%) may be asymptomatic.

Trichomonas vaginalis is well visualized in Papanicolaou's stained cervical smear as 15–30 μ long, round-to-oval "pear-shaped" organisms with an indistinct eccentric

Box 7.5: Bacterial vaginosis (shift in bacterial flora).

- The patient has thin milky vaginal discharge with foul fishy smell
- Caused by *Gardnerella vaginalis* and other bacteria
- Positive for Whiff's test: Adding 10% potassium hydroxide on vaginal fluid produces fishy smell

Cytology smear
- Filmy background
- Absence of lactobacilli
- Numerous small coccobacilli and curved bacilli
- *Clue cells*: Polygonal squamous cells filled with small coccobacilli.

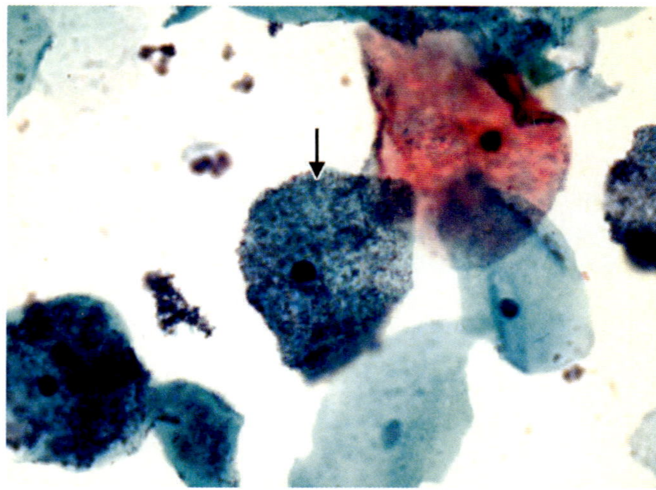

Fig. 7.17: Classical clue cells with multiple coccobacilli in the cytoplasm in bacterial vaginalis infection (*see* arrow) (Papanicolaou's stain × HP).

vesicular nucleus and red cytoplasmic granules (Fig. 7.18). Flagella may be seen in liquid-based cytology (LBC) preparation. In majority of the cases, TV is associated with long branching curved bacilli known as "Leptothrix". The background of smear is usually dirty and often shows aggregates of neutrophils around the surface of the squamous cells known as "cannon ball" or "pus ball". In addition, squamous cells show perinuclear halo and increased eosinophilia.

Candida (Box 7.7): *Candida albicans* and *Candida glabrata* are the two common Candidal species that infect lower female genital tract. The patient complains of burning, itching, and thick white discharge. However, a good number of patients may be asymptomatic.

Cytology: Candida may be in two forms: (1) conidia (yeast) form and (2) fungus (pseudohyphae) form. The yeast forms are pink colored, oval 3–7 micron diameter encapsulated regular structure. The fungus forms are long slender nonseptate structures which are known as pseudohyphae (Fig. 7.19).

The associated squamous cells show nuclear enlargement, perinuclear haloes, and increased eosinophilia. In addition, background shows many fragmented neutrophils. At times, the smears also show herringbone or fern-like arrangement of the epithelial cells which is also known as "sheish kabab" like arrangement (Fig. 7.20).

Differential Diagnosis

- Thin mucous strands may often be mistaken as Candidal pseudohyphae. However, they are pale blue in color.
- Perinuclear halo in the squamous cells may often be mistaken as koilocytosis.
- Nuclear atypia of the squamous cell may simulate atypical squamous cell.

Box 7.6: Trichomonas vaginalis (TV).

- Burning sensation, severe itching, and foul smelling vaginal discharge

Morphology of TV
- 15–30 micron long
- Round-to-oval "pear-shaped" organisms
- Indistinct vesicular nucleus: Important feature
- Red cytoplasmic granules

Background
- Dirty, fuzzy
- "Cannon ball" or "pus ball": Aggregates of neutrophils around the surface of the squamous cells
- Associated with Leptothrix (80% cases)

Differential diagnosis: Cytoplasmic fragments of epithelial cells

Box 7.7: Candida.

- Two common candidal infection: Candida albicans and Candida glabrata
- Complaints: Burning, itching and thick white discharge
- Conidia (yeast) form: Pink colored, oval 3–7 micron diameter encapsulated regular structure
- Fungus (pseudohyphae) form: Long slender nonseptate structure

Other changes
- Squamous cells: Nuclear enlargement, perinuclear haloes and increased eosinophilia
- Background: Many fragmented neutrophils

Comments
- Perinuclear halo in the squamous cells may often be mistaken as koilocyosis.
- Nuclear atypia of the squamous cell may simulate atypical squamous cell.

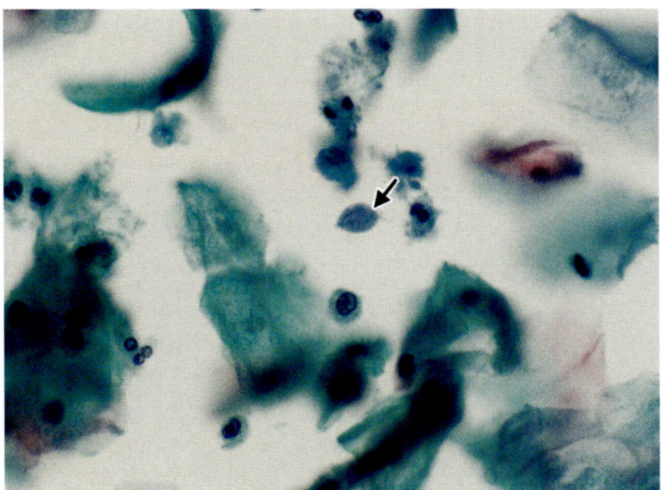

Fig. 7.18: Round-shaped *Trichomonas vaginalis* in cervical smear (*see* arrow) (Papanicolaou's stain × HP).

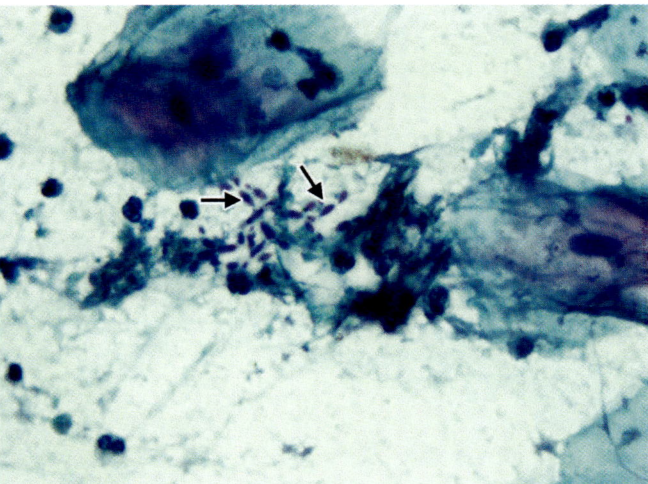

Fig. 7.19: Candidal spores in cervical smear (*see* arrows) (Papanicolaou's stain × HP).

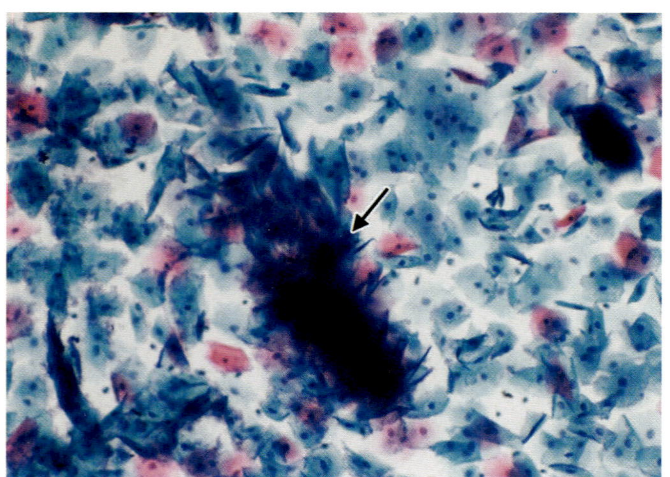

Fig. 7.20: Cervical smear shows "sheish kabab" like arrangement in candidal infection (*see* arrow) (Papanicolaou's stain X MP).

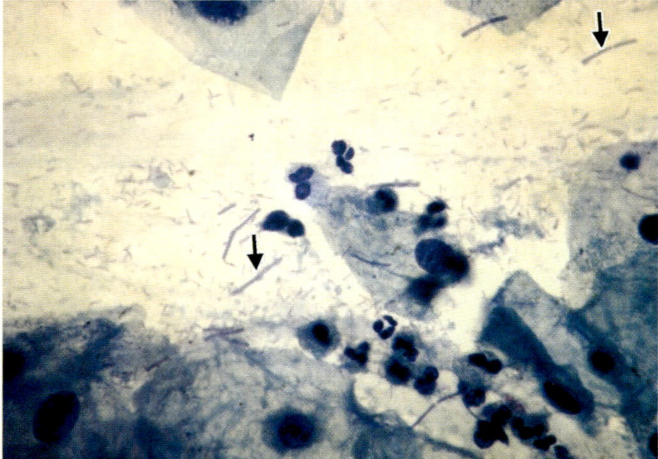

Fig. 7.21: Long slender leptothrix in cervical smear (*see* arrows) (Papanicolaou's stain × HP).

Box 7.8: Actinomycosis.

- Gram-positive aerobic organism
- Commonly associated with intrauterine contraceptive devices (IUCD)
- Asymptomatic or may show foul smelling vaginal discharge containing sulfur granules
- Clumped of grayish blue filamentous bacteria radiate from a dense center
- Cotton ball appearance
- Background: Numerous polymorphonuclear leukocytes, macrophages, and occasional multinucleated giant cells

Box 7.9: Herpes simplex.

- Sexually transmitted infection
- Infected cells are large
- Multinucleated with molding of the nucleus
- Ground glass appearance
- Large eosinophilic intranuclear inclusion
- Bizarre nucleus may be noted

Fig. 7.22: Actinomycosis of cervical smear. The filamentous bacteria radiate from a dense center (Papanicolaou's stain × HP).

Leptothrix: It is a type of lactobacillus and is a Gram-negative, nonspore-forming anaerobic organism. They are thin, segmented, long filamentous organism (Fig. 7.21). Leptothrix are commonly associated with Trichomonas infection.

Actinomycosis (Box 7.8): These are Gram-positive aerobic organism and commonly associated with intrauterine contraceptive devices (IUCD). The patients are asymptomatic or may show foul smelling vaginal discharge.

Cytology: The clumped of grayish blue filamentous bacteria radiate from a dense center. The organisms are thick and beaded in appearance. Overall, they give a cotton ball or "wooly body" appearance (Fig. 7.22). Background of the smear shows numerous polymorphonuclear leukocytes, macrophages, and occasional multinucleated giant cells.

Herpes Simplex (Box 7.9): Herpes simplex type II causes genital infection. This is a sexually transmitted infection. Clinically, there are multiple small vesicles filled with clear fluid. Pustules may appear. Within 10–15 days, the ulcerative lesions heal and re-epithelialization occurs.

Cytomorphology: Infected cell are large, multinucleated with molding of the nucleus. Homogenization of nuclear content gives rise to ground glass appearance. Large eosinophilic intranuclear inclusion with surrounding clear area is noted. Cytoplasm of the infected cell is dense and opaque (Fig. 7.23).

Chlamydia trachomatis (Box 7.10): *Chlamydia trachomatis* is the most common sexually transmitted infection. It is a

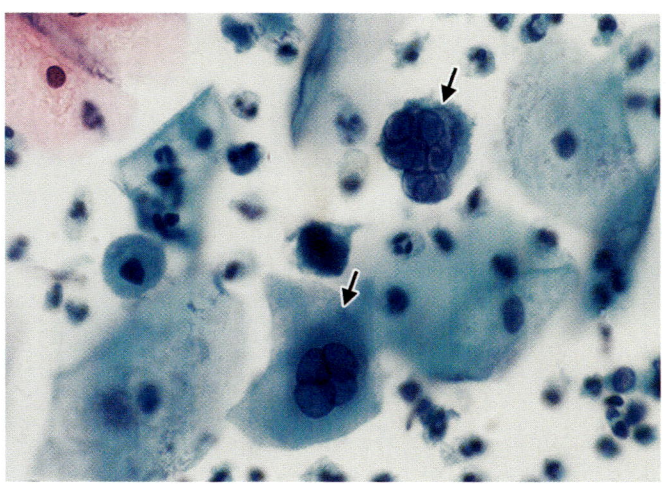

Fig. 7.23: Typical multinucleated cells with faceted nuclei and ground glass nuclear appearance (*see* arrows) (Papanicolaou's stain × HP).

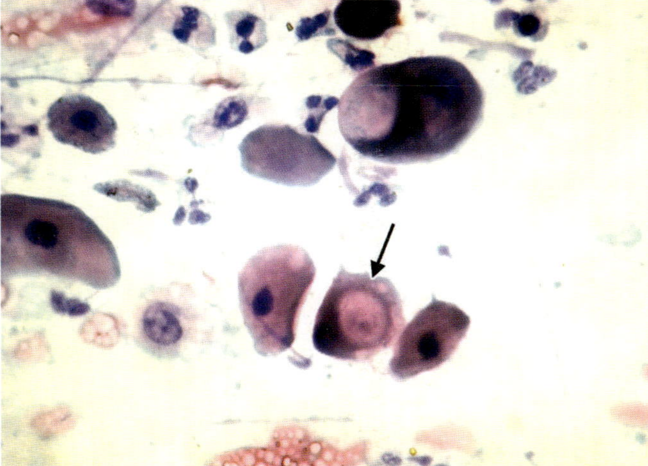

Fig. 7.24: Intracytoplasmic inclusion in case of Chlamydia trachomatis infection (*see* arrow) (Papanicolaou's stain × HP).

Box 7.10: Chlamydia trachomatis.

- The most common sexually transmitted infection
- Tiny coccoid bodies surrounded by narrow clear zones are noted in the cytoplasm of squamous and endocervical cells
- Moth-eaten appearance of the cytoplasm
- Central acidophilic or basophilic inclusion bodies in the cytoplasm
- Culture is mandatory for confirmation

Box 7.11: Inflammation.

- Polymorphonuclear leukocytes infiltration
- Necrotic debris
- Inflammatory cells stick to the epithelial cells
- Increased number of parabasal cells
- Eosinophilia of the cell cytoplasm
- Degenerative changes
  - Cytoplasm: Vacuoles
  - Nucleus: Pyknosis, karyorrhexis, karyolysis

Gram-negative organism. Most of the patients are asymptomatic. The symptomatic patient may have urethritis, vaginitis, cervicitis, and pelvic inflammatory disease.

Initially, tiny coccoid bodies surrounded by narrow clear zones are noted in the cytoplasm of squamous and endocervical cells. The infected cells in course of time may give the moth-eaten appearance of the cytoplasm. Later on clearly visible central acidophilic or basophilic inclusion appears in the cytoplasm (Fig. 7.24). *Chlamydia trachomatis* infection is associated with heavy infiltration by acute inflammatory cells. This may obscure the cytoplasmic detail. Therefore, it is difficult to distinguish degenerative changes due to other causes and infection by *Chlamydia trachomatis*. The diagnosis of *Chlamydia trachomatis* should always be confirmed by culture.

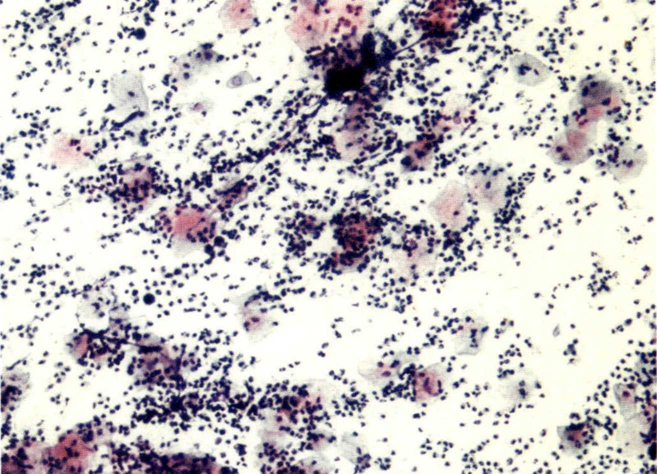

Fig. 7.25: Inflammatory cervical smear shows polymorphs adhered with epithelial cells (Papanicolaou's stain X MP).

Reactive Cellular Changes

Inflammatory Smear

Acute cervicitis: In case of acute inflammation, the smear shows heavy inflammatory exudates predominantly composed of polymorphonuclear leukocytes, necrotic debris, and inflammatory changes in the epithelium (Box 7.11). The inflammatory cells are usually adhered to the epithelial cells (Fig. 7.25). Usually, the parabasal cells are increased in number and the epithelial cells often show eosinophilia. The individual cells also show degenerative changes such as cytoplasmic perinuclear vacuoles, nuclear pyknosis, karyorrhexis, and karyolysis.

Chronic inflammation: Smears of chronic inflammation show abundant lymphocytes, histiocytes, and benign squamous cells. Occasionally, epithelioid cell granulomas may be seen in granulomatous inflammation.

Follicular cervicitis is a type of chronic inflammatory condition characterized by abundant reactive lymphoid cells, many tangible body macrophages, and polymorphs in a dirty necrotic background. The reactive lymphoid cell population may be falsely interpreted as lymphoma.

Intrauterine Contraceptive Device-related Changes (Box 7.12)

In intrauterine contraceptive devices, both endocervical and endometrial cells show abnormality. Tail and body of IUD cause irritation of adjacent endocervical epithelium and endometrium. As mentioned before, IUD is often associated with actinomycosis infection. Two distinct types of cells may be noted in IUD users.[9] One type of cell is glandular and arranged singly or in small clusters. Individual cells have vacuolated cytoplasm with enlarged nucleus having prominent nucleoli. These cells with large vacuolated cytoplasm are often referred as "bubble gum cell". The other cell type is small round to oval with high nucleocytoplasmic ratio and hyperchromatic nucleus. These cells are probably of endometrial in origin and are known as "IUD" cells (Fig. 7.26). Occasionally, psammoma bodies or calcification may be seen (Fig. 7.27).

Box 7.12: IUD-related changes.

- Associated with actinomycosis infection (25%)
- Two distinct types of cells:
  - "Bubble gum cell":
    - Cells with large vacuolated cytoplasm
    - Enlarged nucleus having prominent nucleoli
  - IUD cells
    - Small round to oval cell with high nucleocytoplasmic ratio
    - Hyperchromatic nucleus
- Background: Psammoma bodies or calcification may be seen

Mimicker: Adenocarcinoma: Features such as absence of tumor diathesis, degenerative changes, background inflammation are common in IUD smears

Differential Diagnosis

Adenocarcinoma: The large cells with vacuolated cytoplasm of the "bubble gum" cells may be misinterpreted as adenocarcinoma. The following features may be helpful in diagnosis: (1) clinical history of IUCD; (2) absence of "tumor diathesis"; (3) presence of degenerative changes in the nuclei; and (4) presence of inflammation.

Radiation-induced Changes

Radiation-induced changes in cervix may be acute or chronic. The effects of radiotherapy are on benign epithelial cells and on cancer cells (Box 7.13).

Changes in acute radiation effect: The cells are enlarged with marked nucleomegaly. The cytoplasm is abundant and vacuolated. The nuclear chromatin is smudged with single to multiple prominent nucleoli (Fig. 7.28). Nuclear

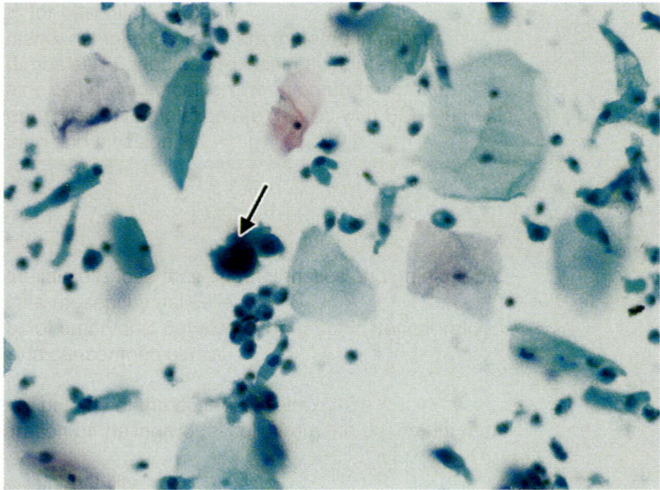

Fig. 7.26: IUD cell in smear used in intrauterine contraceptive device (*see* arrow) (Papanicolaou's stain × HP). (IUD: Intrauterine contraceptive device).

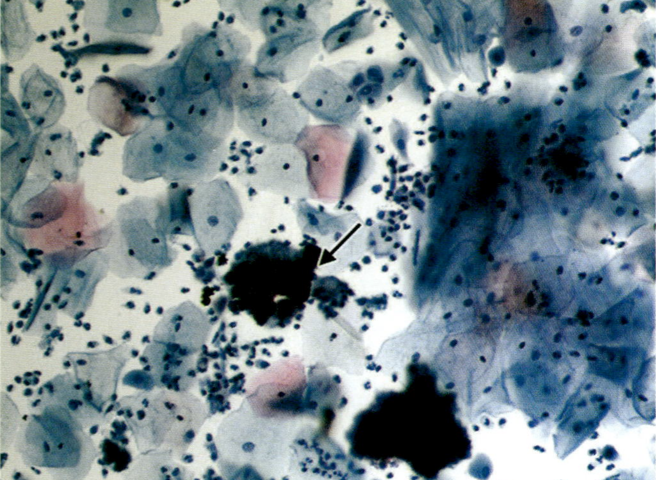

Fig. 7.27: Dense calcified material in case of IUCD use in LBC preparation (SurePath) (*see* arrow) (Papanicolaou's stain × HP). (IUCD: Intrauterine contraceptive device; LBC: Liquid-based cytology).

Box 7.13: Radiation effect.

Acute effect
- Cells: Markedly enlarged
- Cytoplasm: Abundant and vacuolated
- Multinucleation is frequent
- Nucleus: Enlarged mildly pleomorphic
- Nucleo-cytoplasmic ratio low
- Nuclear chromatin: Smudged
- Nucleoli: Single to multiple prominent

Chronic effect
- Cell: Mildly enlarged
- Sheets of squamous cell with spindle-shaped elongated nuclei resembling smooth muscle cell

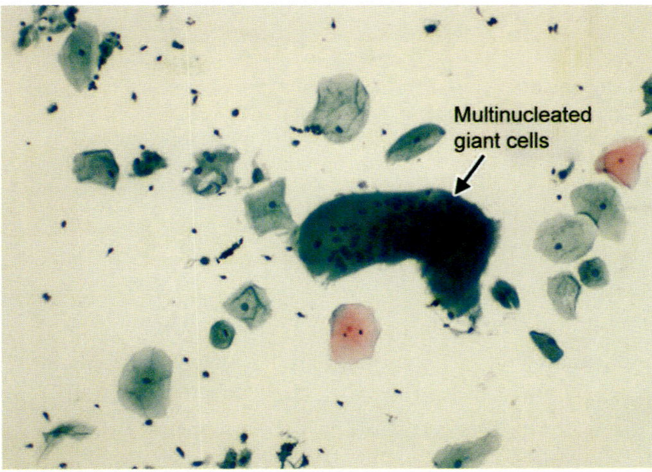

Fig. 7.28: Radiation changes in cervical smear in LBC preparation showing multinucleated giant cells (*see* arrow) (Papanicolaou's stain × HP). (LBC: Liquid-based cytology).

vacuolations may also be seen. The squamous cells may show multinucleation, bizarre form, and hyperchromasia. These cells may resemble malignant cells; however, the following features are helpful to differentiate them from malignant cells:

- No change of nucleo/cytoplasmic ratio
- Smudged nuclei and ill preserved nuclear morphology
- History of radiation.

These acute changes in the squamous epithelium regress in course of time.

Differential diagnosis

- *Recurrence of malignancy*: As mentioned before, the radiation-induced changes may simulate malignancy. However, the malignant cells show preserved nuclear morphology with coarsely granular chromatin and significant nuclear pleomorphism.
- *Herpes simplex infection*: Herpes simplex viral infection shows multinucleated giant cells and may simulate radiation-induced changes. However, clinical history and absence of viral inclusion are helpful in exclusion of herpex simplex infection.

Chronic radiation effect: The cells show mild nuclear enlargement. However, no cytoplasmic vacuolations and nuclear changes are seen. The number of multinucleated cells reduces. There may be sheets of squamous cell with spindle-shaped elongated nuclei resembling smooth muscle cell.

Glandular Cell Status Post-hysterectomy

This is an uncommon finding and is seen only in 2% cases of cervical smear after total hysterectomy. The cervical smear shows benign looking columnar endocervical cells. The cells are present in small groups. The cytoplasm shows pale mucinous material. In addition, inflammatory cells, atrophic pattern and occasional atypical cells may also be seen.[10]

Box 7.14: Repair.

- Occurs after injury or chronic irritation
- Two-dimensional flat cohesive sheets
- Individual cell are arranged in one direction: school of fish appearance
- Nucleus
  - Enlarged
  - Pleomorphic
  - Smooth nuclear border
  - Hyperchromatic
  - Single to multiple prominent nucleoli
- Cytoplasm: Abundant may be vacuolated
- Low N/C ratio
- Neutrophils are often seen
- Mitotic activity may be seen
- Mimics malignancy.

Cytological Features of Reparative and Regenerative Changes (Box 7.14)

In case of injury or chronic irritation, the reserve cells of the cervical lining epithelium proliferate and replenish the loss. Injury of the lining epithelium of the cervix may be due to various causes such as recent hysterectomy, severe cervicitis, history of conization of cervix, etc.

Cytology: The cells are often arranged as two-dimensional flat cohesive sheets. Individual cell are arranged in one direction giving the appearance of "school of fish". The cells are enlarged with well-defined cytoplasmic margin. Nuclei are enlarged and pleomorphic. Nuclear chromatin is fine with single to multiple prominent nucleoli. Mitotic activity may be seen. In addition, background may show inflammatory exudates and blood.

Box 7.15: Atrophic smear.

- Predominant parabasal and basal cell population
- Degenerated orangeophilic or eosinophilic parabasal cells and histiocytes in the smear
- "Blue blobs": Dark blue round-shaped amorphous material
- Cells with uniform nuclear enlargement
- Elongated spindle-shaped cells may be confused with malignancy
- *D/d:* HSIL, invasive carcinoma

Differential diagnosis

- *Carcinoma*: The cytological features of repair may simulate carcinoma and therefore one should be careful in interpretation of this type of smear. The cells in repair are almost always cohesive and single discrete pleomorphic cells are rarely seen.
- *Parakeratosis*: At times, the superficial layer of squamous cell of cervix may show small nucleated squamous cells. This is caused by chronic irritation. The cells are arranged in isolated or loose sheets. Individual cells are small polygonal with eosinophilic to orangeophilic cytoplasm. Nuclei are small, uniform, and pyknotic. The persistence presence of these cells in cervical smear needs close follow-up.
- *Tubal metaplasia*: Occasionally due to chronic irritation, the cervical lining epithelium undergoes tubal metaplasia. Cervical smear normally may show small number of ciliated columnar cells. However, in case of tubal metaplasia, the number of such cell is more. The cells are arranged in small groups or in pseudostratified strips. Individual cells are columnar in appearance with discrete vacuoles. One end of the cell has a terminal bar and cilia arise from the terminal bar. Nuclei of the cells are centrally located round to oval, with mildly enlarged and atypical. Occasionally tubal metaplasia may shed abnormal cells that may be mistaken for malignancy.

Atrophic Smears

In case of atrophic smear, the predominant cell population is parabasal and basal cells (Box 7.15). There are minimal number of superficial squamous cells and intermediate cells. The parabasal cells are often present in sheets with crowded appearance (Fig. 7.29). In liquid-based cytology (LBC) preparation, the parabasal cells may be discrete. There may be drying artifact and uniform nuclear enlargement. Atrophic epithelium is vulnerable to injury and inflammation. Therefore, the cells may show eosinophilic cytoplasm and nuclear changes of inflammation such as nuclear pyknosis and karyorrhexis. This should not be taken as significant. The smear may often show dark blue round-shaped amorphous material known as "blue blobs". This is most likely mucous globules or degenerated cells. In addition, the atrophic smear often contains elongated spindle shaped cells that are probably artifact. These cells may be confused with spindle cell type of squamous cell carcinoma. In addition, blue blobs and background granular material may resemble necrosis and tumor diathesis and thereby may mislead the cytologists.

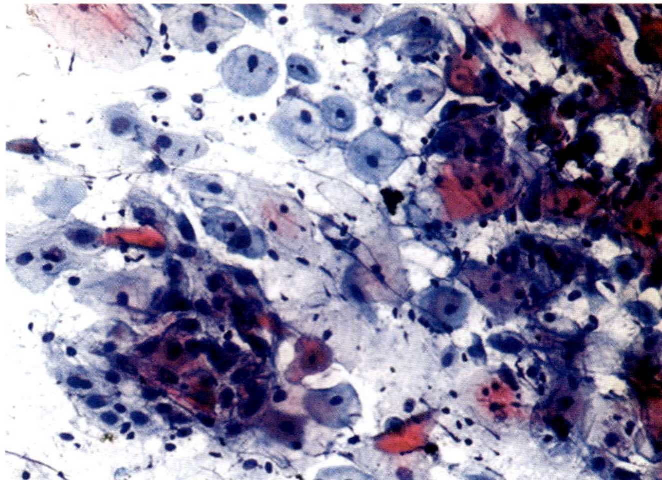

Fig. 7.29: Atrophic smear showing large number of parabasal cells (Papanicolaou's stain × HP).

Differential Diagnosis

- *High-grade squamous intraepithelial lesion*: The atrophic smear may be mistaken as HSIL due to the presence of small cells with high N/C ratio. However, the cells in atrophic smears lack nuclear hyperchromasia and nuclear margin irregularity as noted in SIL.
- *Invasive carcinoma*: Atrophic smear may simulate tumor diathesis of invasive carcinoma due to fine granular dirty background and blue blobs. The individual cells do not show any cytological features of malignancy.

REFERENCES

1. Izadi-Mood N, Sarmadi S, Alijani S, et al. The significance of hyperkeratosis in pap smears with squamous intraepithelial lesion. Acta Cytol. 2012;56(4):379-82.

2. Zahn CM, Askew AW, Hall KL, et al. The significance of hyperkeratosis/parakeratosis on otherwise normal Papanicolaou smears. Am J Obstet Gynecol. 2002;187:997-1001.
3. National Cancer Institute Workshop. The 1988 Bethesda System for reporting cervical/vaginal cytologic diagnoses. JAMA. 1989;262:931-4.
4. National Cancer Institute Workshop. The Bethesda System for reporting cervical/vaginal cytologic diagnoses. Acta Cytol. 1993;37:115-24.
5. Solomon D, Davey D, Kurman R, et al. The 2001 Bethesda System—terminology for reporting results of cervical cytology. JAMA. 2002;287:2114-9.
6. Nayar R, Wilbur DC. The Pap test and Bethesda 2014. Cancer Cytopathol. 2015;123(5):271-81.
7. Bethesda System Web Atlas. Online Available from the American Society of Cytopathology website: http://www.cytopathology.org.
8. Park TW, Richart RM, Sun XW, et al. Association between human papillomavirus type and clonal status of cervical squamous intraepithelial lesions. J Natl Cancer Inst. 1996;88(6):355-8.
9. Risse EK, Beerthuizen RJ, Vooijs GP. Cytologic and histologic findings in women using an IUD. Obstet Gynecol. 1981;58(5):569-73.
10. Tambouret R, Pitman MB, Bell DA. Benign glandular cells in posthysterectomy vaginal smears. Acta Cytol. 1998;42(6):1403-8.

Review Questions

1. **Identify the cell in the cervical smear (Fig. 7.30):**
   a. Endocervical cells
   b. Endometrial cell
   c. Parabasal cell
   d. Histiocytes collection
2. **Identify (Fig. 7.31):**
   a. Metaplastic cells
   b. Cytomegalovirus infection
   c. Clue cell
   d. Herpes infection
3. **Identify (Fig. 7.32):**
   a. Histiocytes
   b. Trichomonas vaginalis
   c. Parabasal cell
   d. Cytoplasmic fragment
4. **Identify (Fig. 7.33):**
   a. Actinomycosis
   b. Tubal metaplasia
   c. Bacterial vaginosis
   d. Acellular contaminant
5. **Identify (Fig. 7.34):**
   a. Candidal pseudohyphae
   b. Leptothrix
   c. Cotton thread
   d. Actinomycosis
6. **A 48-year-female was irradiated for squamous cell carcinoma of cervix 2 years back. Figures 7.35A to D show the follow-up cervical smear.**
   What is your interpretation?

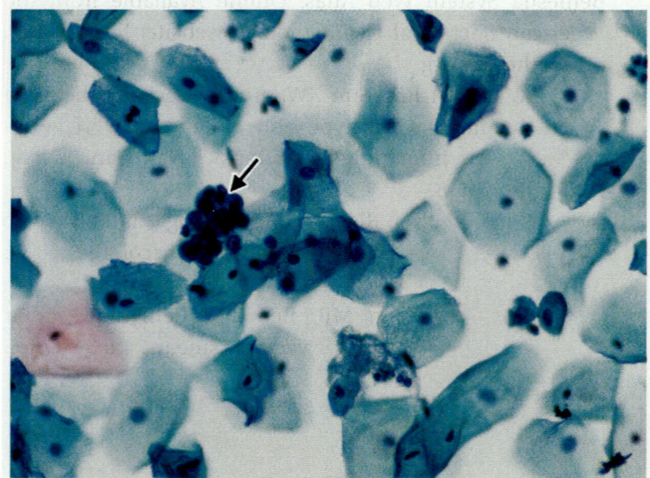

Fig. 7.30: Cervical smear of question 1.

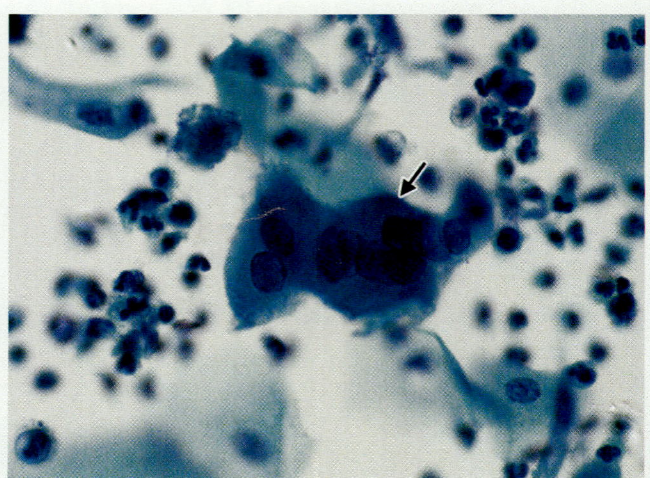

Fig. 7.31: Cervical smear of question 2.

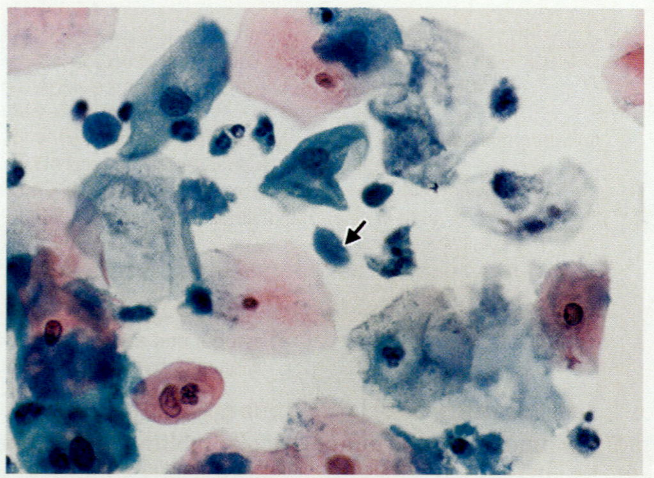

Fig. 7.32: Cervical smear of question 3.

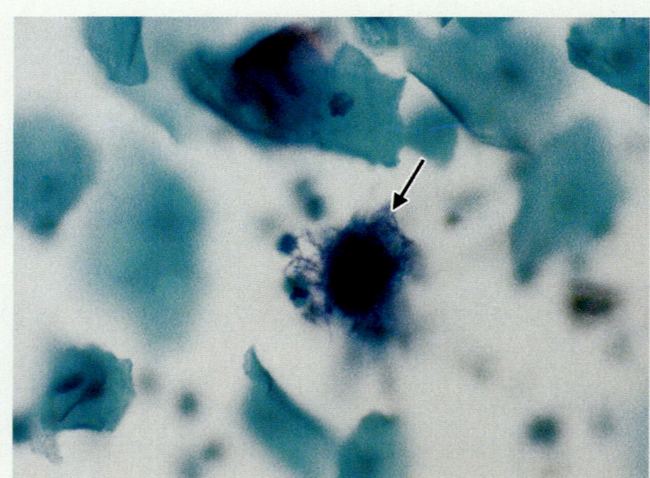

Fig. 7.33: Cervical smear of question 4.

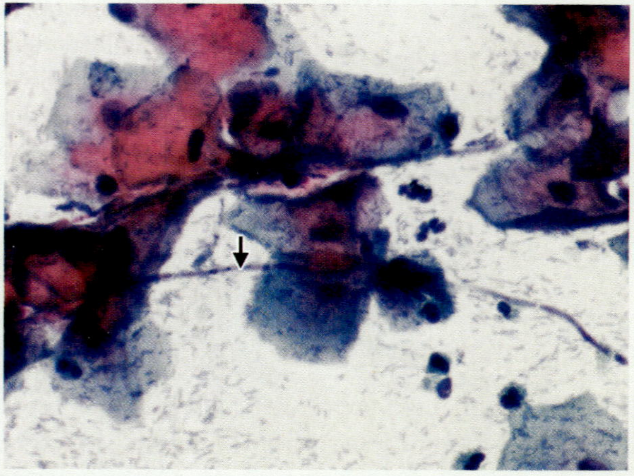

Fig. 7.34: Cervical smear of question 5.

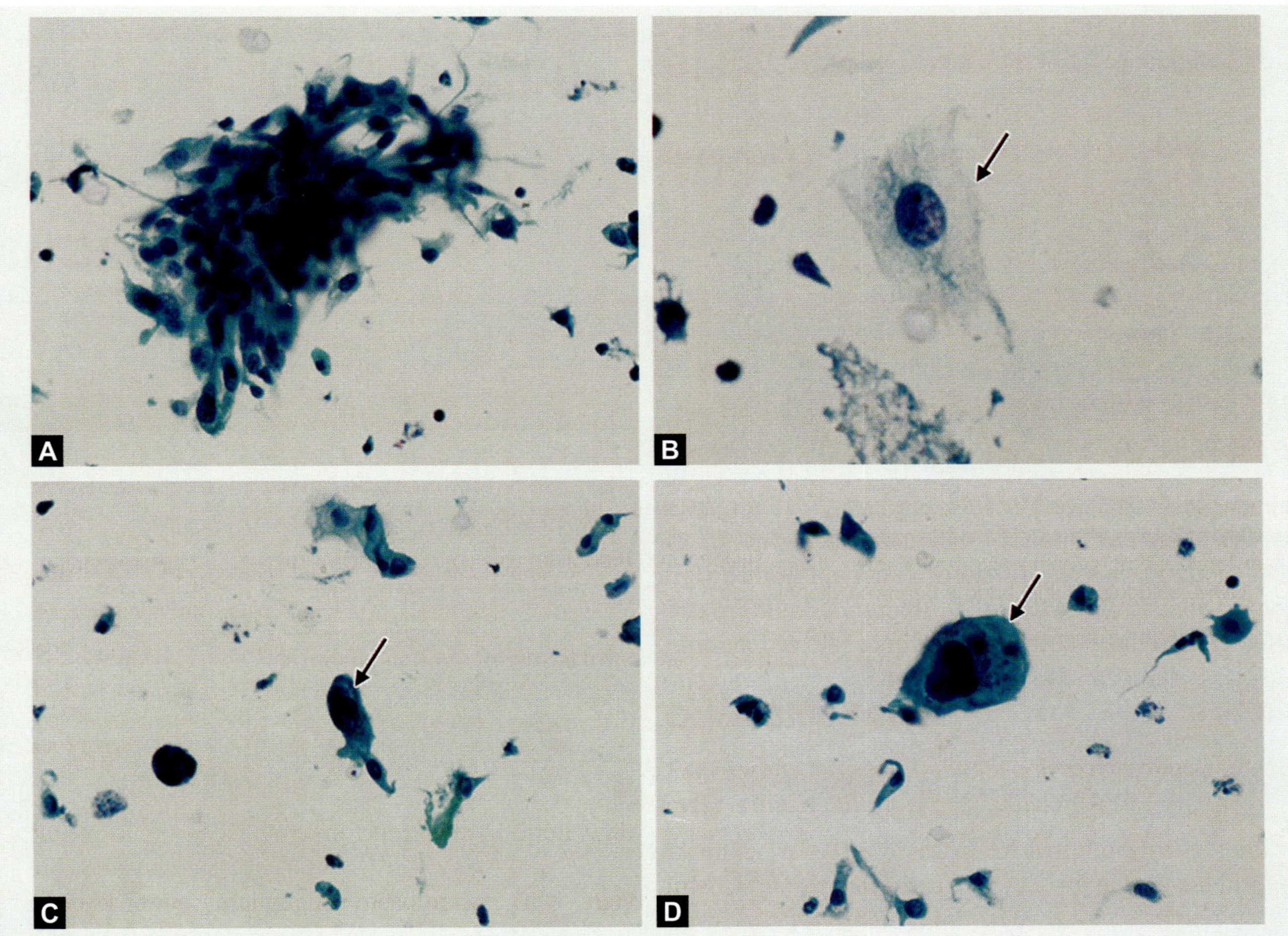

Figs. 7.35A to D: Microphotographs of the cervical smear of question 6.

Answers

1. b. Endometrial cell
   Note: The tight cluster of cells with scanty cytoplasm indicates endometrial cells.
2. d. Herpes infection
   Note: Typical multinucleated cells with ground glass nuclei is the characteristic of herpes virus infection.
3. b. Trichomonas vaginalis
   Note: The arrow points to green pear-shaped trichomonas vaginalis. Note the nucleus in the cell that helps it to distinguish from simple cytoplasmic fragments.
4. a. Actinomycosis
   Note: The cotton ball-like extension of the actinomycosis organisms from the central bluish aggregates.
5. a. Candidal pseudohyphae
   Note: Typical long thin candidal pseudohyphae along with spores are present.
6. Radiation induced changes
   Note: There are many large cells with unaltered nucleocytoplasmic ratio. Multinucleated giant cells are also present (Figs. 7.35C and D).

CHAPTER 8

Cervical Carcinogenesis, Preneoplastic and Neoplastic Conditions

HUMAN PAPILLOMAVIRUS AND CERVICAL CARCINOGENESIS

Human papillomavirus (HPV) infection is the main etiological factor of carcinoma of cervix cervical. It is a sexually transmitted infection occurring in both men and women. HPV infection is very common and most infected indivisduals eliminate HPV without any recognizable evidence of disease. Almost all the cases of cervical carcinoma are positive for HPV deoxyribonucleic acid (DNA).

Prevalence of Human Papillomavirus

It is estimated that HPV prevalence in world's woman population is about 2–44%.[1] This wide variation of range may be due to difference of sensitivity of DNA assay and age range of the population studied.

Different Subtypes of Human Papillomavirus

More than 100 different subtypes of HPV are known and only minorities of them are involved in cervical carcinogenesis. About 30 subtypes of HPV infect genital tract and only minority of them cause cervical cancer. Based on their oncogenic potential, HPV subtypes are divided into two groups: low risk and high risk. Low-risk HPV types are 6, 11, 42–44, 54, 61, 70, 72, and 81 and high-risk HPV types are 16, 18, 31, 33, 35, 39, 45, 51, 52, 56, 58, 59, 61, 66, 68, 73, and 82 (Table 8.1). Low-risk HPV subtypes usually cause condyloma warts and high-risk subtypes are related with squamous intraepithelial lesions (SIL) and are at higher risk for progression of malignancy.

Risk Factors of Cervical Cancer

In addition to HPV infection, other cofactors are also required for cervical carcinogenesis such as smoking, nutritional deficiency, high parity, absence of male circumcision, prolonged use of oral contraceptive pill (OCP), immune suppression and coinfection with human immunodeficiency virus, herpes simplex virus, and *Chlamydia trachomatis*.

Table 8.1: Types of human papillomavirus (HPV).

Risk classification	*HPV types*	*Lesions*
Low risk	6, 11, 42, 43, 44, 54, 61, 70, 72, 81	Condyloma, LSIL
High risk	16, 18, 31, 33, 35, 39, 45, 51, 52, 56, 58, 59, 61, 66, 68, 73, 82	LSIL, HSIL, carcinoma

(LSIL: Low-grade squamous intraepithelial lesion; HSIL: High-grade squamous intraepithelial lesion).

Natural Course of Infection

The majority of HPV infections happen after initiation of the sexual activity and the infections are transitory. Prevalence of HPV is highest at 18–25 years of age, and then declines as the age increases. The majority of women infected with a specific HPV type do not show the infection of same type about 1 year later. The initial HPV infection clears of rapidly within 12–18 months.[2] Infection by multiple types of HPV is common and there is higher chance of persistence of HPV infection in this situation.[2] Long back, it was postulated that there is a natural progression of cervical intraepithelial neoplasia 1 (CIN1) to CIN2 and CIN2 to CIN3 followed by invasive carcinoma.[3] However, it is now known that the large number of CIN1, regress without treatment, and a good proportion of high-grade lesions progress to invasive cancer.

More than 95% of squamous-cell carcinomas of cervix are caused by HPV 16, 18, 45, 31, 33, 52, 58, and 35. Out of these subtypes, HPV 16 is responsible for 52–56% cases followed by HPV 18 (13–22%) to develop invasive

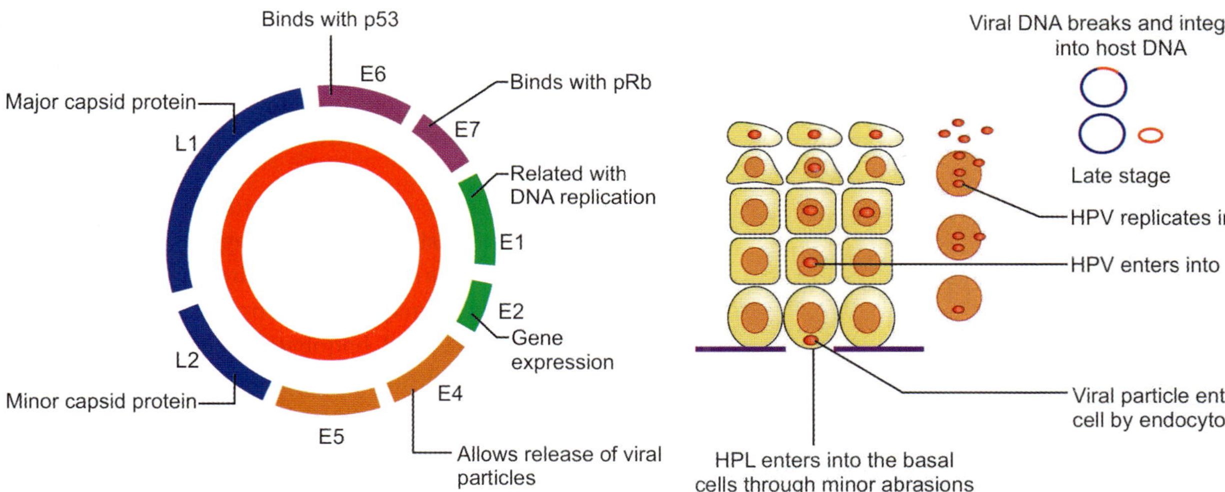

Fig. 8.1: Schematic diagram of human papillomavirus (HPV) structure shows an outer protein capsid and inner circular genome. The circular genome contains 8,000 nucleotides and encodes 8 viral proteins. Early region (E) encodes nonstructural proteins such as E1, E2, E4, E5, E6 and E7. Late region (L) encodes viral capsid proteins L1 and L2 that are expressed late in viral life.

Fig. 8.2: Schematic diagram shows the lifecycle of human papillomavirus (HPV) infection. In the early stage of viral infection, HPV virus remains within the nucleus as episome and proliferates within the nucleus. In late stage, the viral deoxyribonucleic acid (DNA) integrates within the host DNA. Viral E2 genomic portion is lost and that promotes overexpression of oncoproteins E6 and E7.

squamous cell carcinoma (SQC).[4] The patients with high-grade squamous intraepithelial lesion (HSIL) usually have persistent high-risk HPV (16 and 18) and uncommonly regress. Low-grade squamous intraepithelial lesion (LSIL) associated with HPV 16 and 18 are more frequently progress to higher grade of SIL.

Structure of Human Papillomavirus

Human papillomaviruses are the member of Papillomavirus family of DNA viruses. These are circular DNA viruses with 55 nm in diameter, and consist of an outer protein capsid and inner circular genome. The circular genome contains 8,000 nucleotides and encodes 8 viral proteins. HPV genome contains three regions (Fig. 8.1):

1. *An upstream regulatory region (URR) (also known as non-coding region)*: It contains the viral promoter that regulates transcription and replication of virus.
2. *An early (E) region*: E region contains open reading frames (ORF) and encodes nonstructural proteins such as E1, E2, E4, E5, E6, and E7. These proteins are involved in viral replication, transcription, and transformation. They also help in viral adaptation in changing environment. E1 protein is related with the viral replication and E2 protein controls viral transcription and replication. E2 also interacts with viral oncogenes E6 and E7 and helps in carcinogenesis.
3. *A late (L) region*: L region encodes viral capsid proteins L1 and L2. These proteins are produced in late viral life. The capsid proteins help in the formation of the structure of the virus and facilitate in DNA maturation and packaging.

Viral Lifecycle

During sexual intercourse, HPV enters into the female genital tract by small superficial abrasions. The virus particles are attached within the basement membrane. Within a few hours the virus particles enter within the basal layer of the epithelial cell by endocytosis (Fig. 8.2). In the epithelial cells, the envelope protein of the virus is dissolved and viral DNA enters in the host nucleus. In the nucleus of the epithelial cells, the viral particle remains as episome and the virus is not integrated within the host DNA. No cytological abnormality is noted in this stage. The viral episomes are maintained in the basal cells. One daughter basal cell retained the basal characteristics and other daughter cell differentiates with the viral episomes. The viral assembly takes place in the mature squamous epithelium and amplified viruses are released. The whole process takes usually 3 weeks that corresponds to the maturation time of basal cells to squamous cells. Uncommonly, HPV infection persists and viral DNA integrates within the host DNA. The circular E2 becomes

Flowchart 8.1: Major events in the human papillomavirus (HPV) infection.

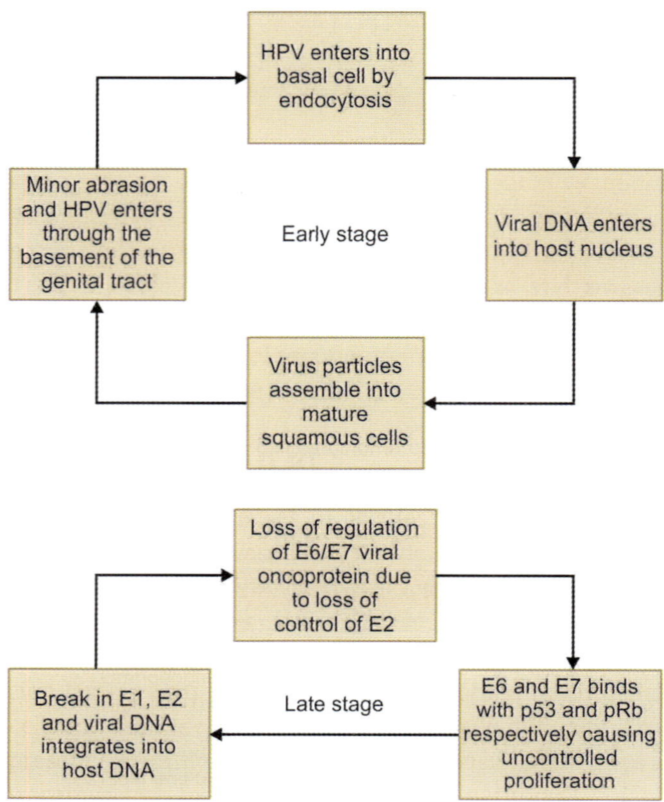

linear and is incorporated within host DNA. Loss of the function of E2 permits overexpression of oncoproteins E6 and E7 (Flowchart 8.1).

Viral Protein Interaction and Oncogenic Transformation

Human papillomavirus DNA is usually extrachromosomal or episomal in benign proliferative lesions of cervix. During persistent infection, HPV DNA integrates within the host DNA. There is breakage in E1/E2 region and loss of E1 and E2. Loss of E2 results in uncontrolled expression of E6 and E7 oncoproteins.

E6 Protein

E6 protein interacts with several host cell proteins (Box 8.1). E6 particularly binds with tumor suppressor protein p53 and inhibits the function of p53. E6 also binds with E6 associated protein, BAK, Paxillin, p16 (INK4A), etc. The overall effects of E6 are immortalization of cell, telomerase activation, chromosomal destabilization, and anti-apoptosis.[5]

Box 8.1: Viral early protein functions.

E2: Controls viral transcription and replication
E1: Helps in the viral replication protein
E4:
- Interacts with the cytoskeletal structure of host
- Interacts with the mitotic spindle formation and cytokinesis

E6: Binds with tumor suppressor protein p53 and inhibits the function of p53
E7: Binds with several host proteins particularly retinoblastoma protein and releases transcription factor E2F

E7 Protein

E7 protein also binds with several host proteins particularly retinoblastoma protein (pRb) and its related pocket proteins. Binding of E7 with pRb releases transcription factor E2F. Released E2F facilitates cell cycle progression.[6] E7 protein also binds with E2F cyclin A complex, histone H1 kinase, cyclin E and TATA box binding protein.

E4 Protein

E4 gene is a part of early region. This E4 protein is necessary for viral maturation. E4 protein interacts with the cytoskeletal structure of the host epithelial cells and permits HPV to leave the cell. E4 and cytoskeleton interaction is responsible for koilocytotic changes. E4 protein interacts with the mitotic spindle formation and cytokinesis and therefore causes multinucleation.[6]

E5 Protein

E5 protein facilitates the interaction of growth factor receptors and ligands of the cell and therefore enhances cellular growth.

CERVICAL PRENEOPLASTIC LESIONS

Dysplasia

Reagan et al. in the year 1953 introduced the term "dysplasia" to indicate disordered maturation of the squamous epithelium.[7] In 1975, World Health Organization (WHO) proposed unified terminology to describe precursor lesions of cervical carcinoma. Dysplasia was graded as mild, moderate, and severe form.[8] In this classification, carcinoma in situ was considered as distinct entity from severe dysplasia rather than a spectrum of a single disease process with variable severity.

Cervical Intraepithelial Neoplasia

Richart in 1981 mentioned the term "cervical intraepithelial neoplasia (CIN)" to avoid confusion between severe dysplasia and carcinoma in situ.[9] The CIN terminology graded the preneoplastic lesions into three categories, CIN1, CIN2, and CIN3, with carcinoma in situ being incorporated into the CIN3 category. Therefore, this new terminology of CIN replaced arbitrary difference between severe dysplasia and carcinoma in situ. CIN is graded depending on the amount of undifferentiated cells from basement membrane to the superficial squamous epithelium. Grade 1 is labeled when up to one-third of basal layer is involved. When more than one-third to two-thirds is involved the grade is labeled as 2, and when more than two-thirds is involved the grade is labeled as 3 (Figs. 8.3 to 8.6).

Bethesda System

Currently, the Bethesda system (TBS) reporting is the most popular and widely used. Bethesda system is a two-tiered system and classified the SIL as LSIL and HSIL.

1. *Low-grade squamous intraepithelial lesions*: LSIL includes both HPV-induced changes and cervical intraepithelial lesions grade 1.

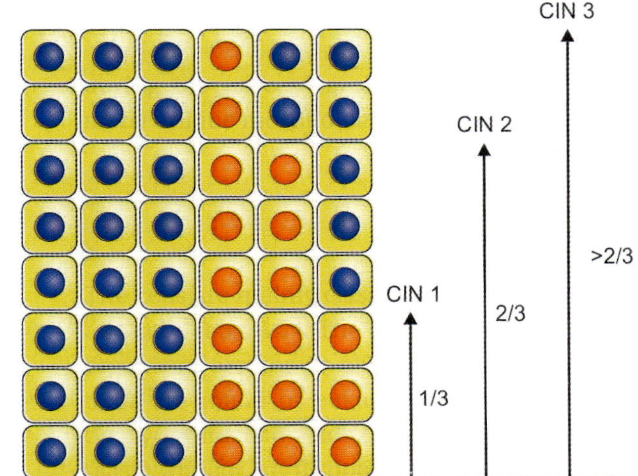

Fig. 8.3: Schematic diagram shows CIN1, CIN2 and CIN3. CIN1 involves up to one-third of the basal layer, CIN2 involves one-third to two-thirds of the epithelium, and CIN3 involves more than two-thirds of the epithelium.

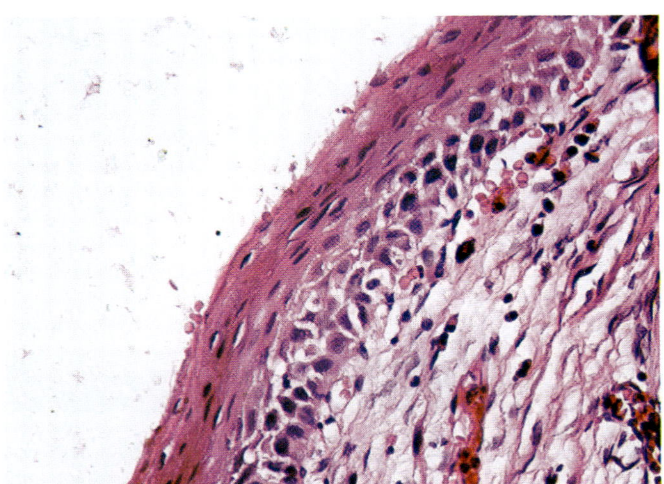

Fig. 8.4: Histology section of CIN1 involves less than one-third of the basal epithelium (H&E X MP).

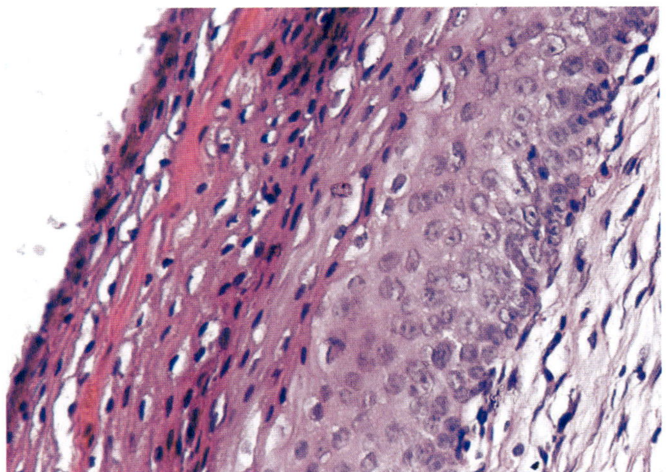

Fig. 8.5: Histology section of CIN2 involves less than two-thirds of the epithelium (H&E X MP).

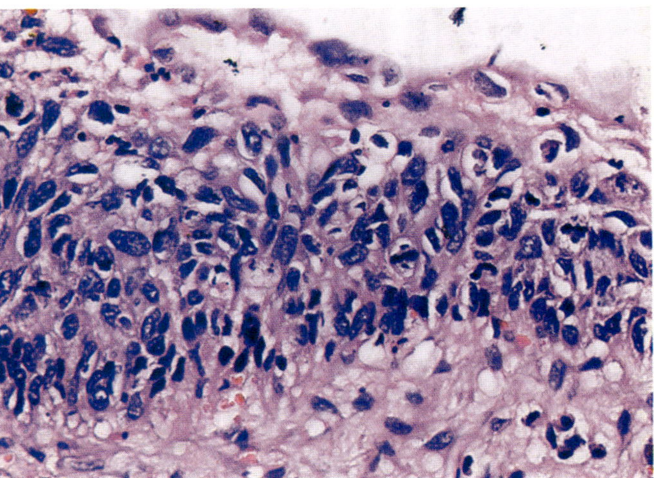

Fig. 8.6: Histology section of CIN3 involves full thickness of the epithelium (H&E X MP).

2. *High-grade squamous intraepithelial lesions*: HSIL includes cervical intraepithelial lesions grade 2, grade 3 and also carcinoma in situ.

Bethesda system closely reflects the biology of cervical preneoplastic lesions and unifies the cervical cytology and histology reporting. Table 8.2 shows the comparison of different classification of cervical preneoplastic lesions.

Natural History of Cervical Intraepithelial Neoplasia

Natural history of CIN is mentioned in Table 8.3.

Table 8.2: Nomenclature of cervical preneoplastic lesions.

Classification	*Grades*				
WHO	Mild dysplasia	Moderate dysplasia	Severe dysplasia	Carcinoma in situ	Carcinoma
CIN	CIN1	CIN2	CIN3	CIN3	Carcinoma
Bethesda	LSIL	HSIL	HSIL	HSIL	Carcinoma

(WHO: World Health Organization; CIN: Cervical intraepithelial neoplasia; LSIL: Low-grade squamous intraepithelial lesion; HSIL: High-grade squamous intraepithelial lesion).

Table 8.3: Natural history of cervical intraepithelial neoplasia (CIN) cases.

	Regression	*Persist*	*Progression CIN3*	*Progression to invasion*
CIN1	60%	30%	10%	1%
CIN2	40%	40%	20%	5%
CIN3	33%	56%	–	12%

Low-grade Squamous Intraepithelial Lesion (Box 8.2)

Low-grade SIL is caused by both low-risk and high-risk HPV. In fact, many LSIL regresses if not treated and approximately 21% LSIL progresses to HSIL. Only 1% of LSIL cases may progress to invasive cancer if left untreated.

Cytology (Figs. 8.7 to 8.12)

Smears show abnormality of superficial and intermediate squamous cells. The cells are usually present singly or in small sheets. There is mild nuclear enlargement and the nucleus occupies one-third of the cytoplasmic area (Fig. 8.7). The nucleocytoplasmic ratio is usually low. There is mild nuclear enlargement and hyperchromasia with irregular nuclear margin (Figs. 8.8 to 8.10). Chromatin is finely granular. Nucleoli are either inconspicuous or absent.

Box 8.2: Low-grade squamous intraepithelial lesion (LSIL).

- Single or sheets of superficial and intermediate cells
- Abundant cytoplasm
- Nucleus:
  - Enlarged nucleus: Nucleus occupy more than one-third of the cytoplasmic area (3–5 times of a normal intermediate cell nucleus)
  - Moderate pleomorphism
  - Mild hyperchromasia
  - Irregular margin
  - Evenly distributed fine granular chromatin
  - Nucleoli absent
- Low nucleocytoplasmic (N/C) ratio
- Koilocytosis: Distinct perinuclear cytoplasmic vacuoles with sharp condensed thick cytoplasmic margin. Nuclei are enlarged.

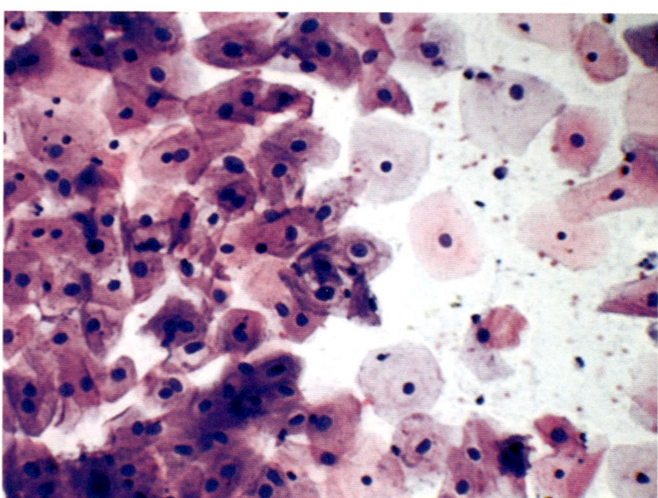

Fig. 8.7: Cervical smear of low-grade squamous intraepithelial lesion (LSIL) showing many koilocytes (Papanicolaou's stain X MP).

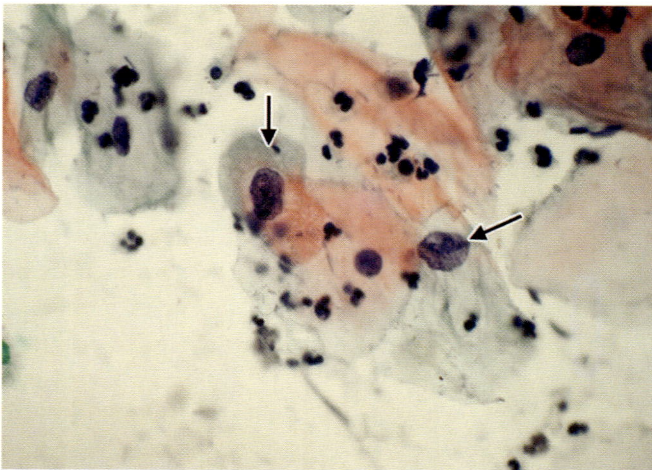

Fig. 8.8: Cervical smear of low-grade squamous intraepithelial lesion (LSIL) showing mild enlargement of the nucleus and altered nucleocytoplasmic ratio (*see* arrows) (Papanicolaou's stain X HP).

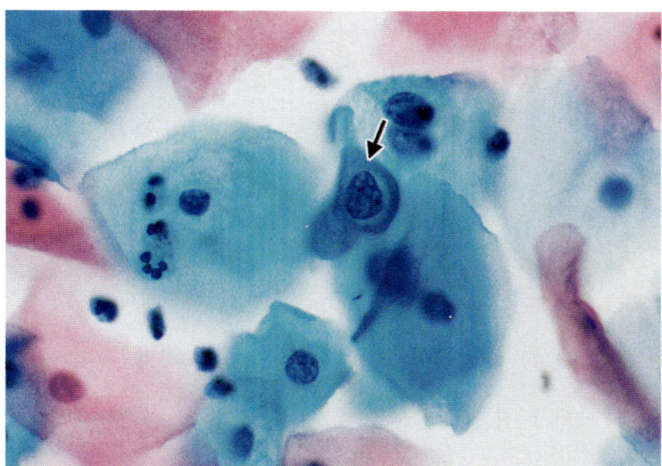

Fig. 8.9: Nucleus occupies more than one-third of the cytoplasmic area in a low-grade squamous intraepithelial lesion (LSIL) case (*see* arrow) (Papanicolaou's stain in SurePath X HP).

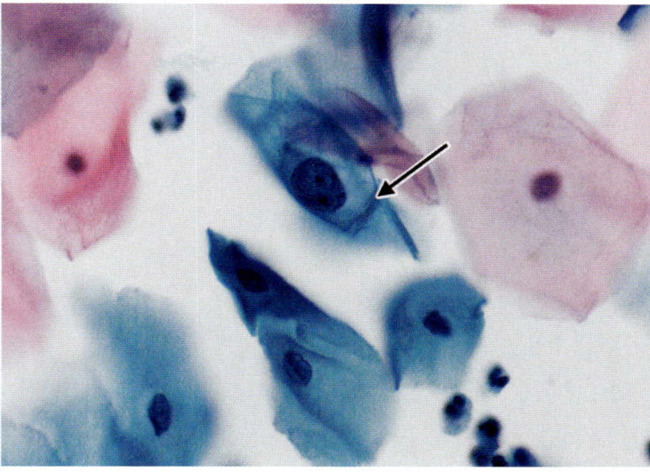

Fig. 8.10: Mildly hyperchromatic nuclei in low-grade squamous intraepithelial lesion (LSIL) (*see* arrow) (Papanicolaou's stain in SurePath X HP).

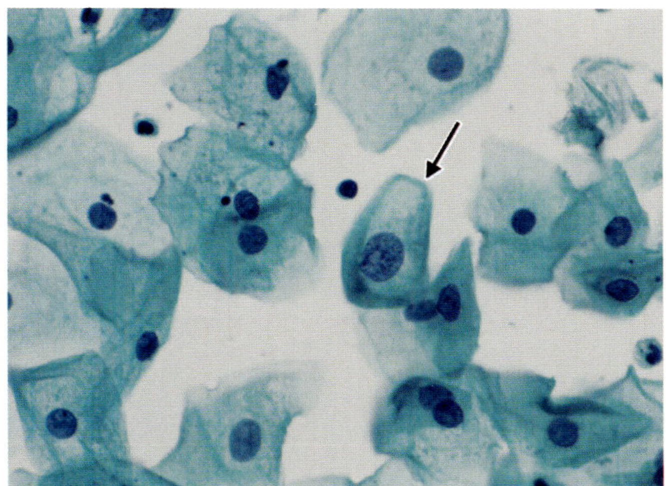

Fig. 8.11: Koilocytes in a case of low-grade squamous intraepithelial lesion (LSIL) showing large perinuclear halo wisth clear distinct thick cytoplasmic margin (*see* arrow) (Papanicolaou's stain in SurePath X HP).

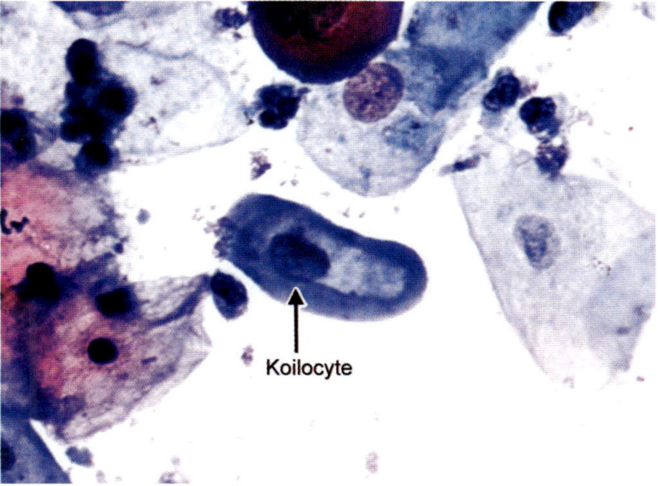

Fig. 8.12: Koilocytes in conventional smear in low-grade squamous intraepithelial lesion (LSIL) (*see* arrow) (Papanicolaou's stain X HP).

Koilocytosis is seen in LSIL cases (Figs. 8.11 and 8.12). It is characterized by cells with distinct perinuclear cytoplasmic vacuoles with sharp condensed thick cytoplasmic margin and enlarged nuclei (Box 8.3). The presence of koilocytosis is the characteristic feature of LSIL but it is not an essential feature to interpret LSIL.

Box 8.3: Koilocytosis.

Morphology:
- Distinct perinuclear cytoplasmic vacuoles
- Sharp condensed thick cytoplasmic margin
- Enlarged nuclei
- Irregular nuclear margin
- Hyperchromasia

Significance: Koilocytic cells indicate human papillomavirus (HPV) infection

Mechanism of formation: E4 of HPV reacts with cytoskeleton of the cells and damage it to produce halo around nucleus

Mimickers: *Trichomonas vaginalis* infection, artifact, enlarged endocervical cells

Differential Diagnosis of LSIL

Differential diagnosis of LSIL includes:

- *Reactive inflammatory changes in squamous epithelial cells*: Nuclear enlargement is often seen in squamous

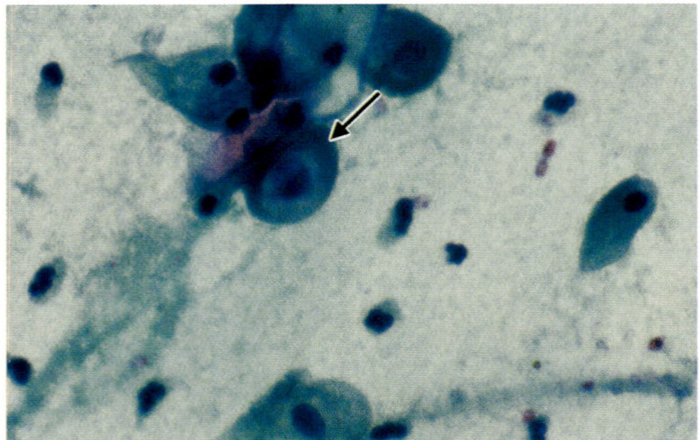

Fig. 8.13: Nonspecific perinuclear halo resembling koilocytosis (*see* arrow) (Papanicolaou's stain in SurePath X HP).

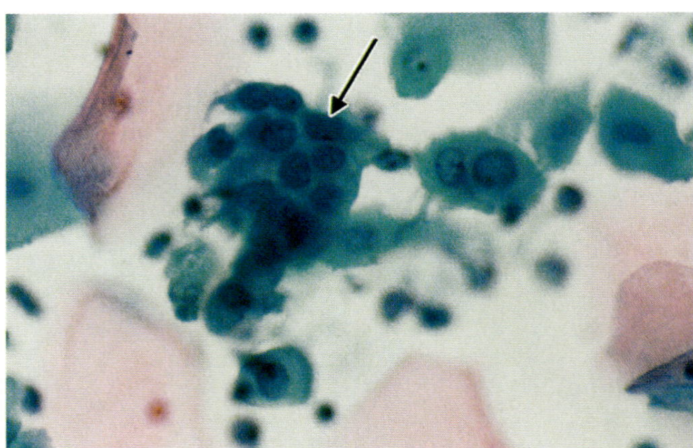

Fig. 8.14: Reactive endocervical cells showing nuclear enlargement (*see* arrow) (Papanicolaou's stain in SurePath X HP).

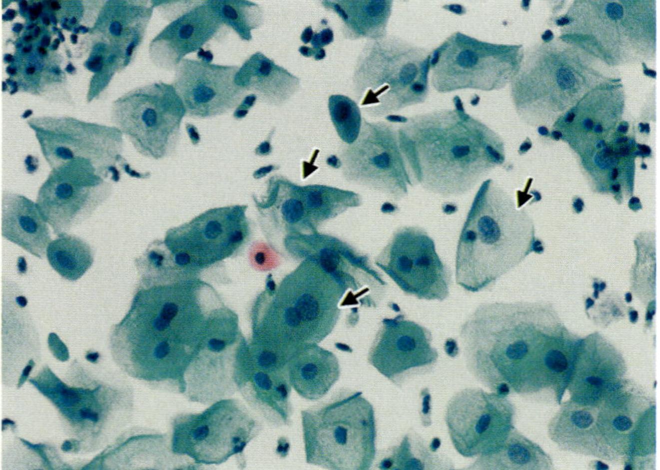

Fig. 8.15: Nuclear enlargement in all the squamous cells in folic acid deficiency (*see* arrows) (Papanicolaou's stain in SurePath X HP).

Flowchart 8.2: Outline of management of low-grade squamous intraepithelial lesion (LSIL) cases.

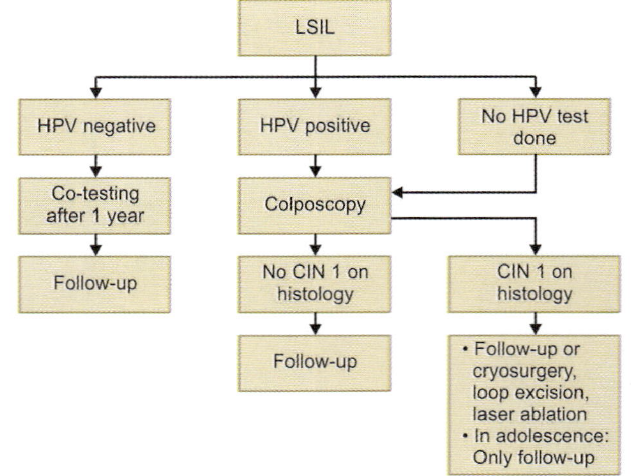

cells due to the effect of inflammation. However other nuclear abnormalities are not noted in these cells.

- *Air drying artifact*: Air drying may cause nuclear enlargement and may be mistaken as LSIL.
- *Nonspecific perinuclear halos*: It may be seen in inflammation or trichomonas infection. No nuclear atypia is seen in these conditions (Fig. 8.13).
- *Reactive changes in endocervical cells*: Reactive endocervical cells may have enlarged nucleus and polygonal shape. These cells may mimic LSIL. However, accompanying more recognizable endocervical cells may indicate their character (Fig. 8.14).
- *Atypical cells of undetermined significance (ASC-US)*: It is often difficult to distinguish ASC-US from LSIL cases.
- *Folic acid deficiency (Fig. 8.15)*: Folic acid deficiency shows uniform nuclear enlargement of the cells. Other than nuclear enlargement no other nuclear abnormalities are seen.
- *Radiation-induced nuclear enlargement*: Radiation injury shows both nuclear and cytoplasmic enlargement and the nucleocytoplasmic ratio of the cell is not altered.

Management of LSIL Cases (Flowchart 8.2)

Management of LSIL cases includes:

- Colposcopy and/or HPV testing should be done.
- If HPV test is negative then the patient is followed up and repeat cervical cytology and HPV test to do after 1 year.
- In case of positive HPV or abnormality in colposcopy then histopathology should be done.
- If there is CIN1 in histology then following should be done: (1) follow-up, (2) cryosurgery, loop excision,

laser ablation. In case of adolescence, no such treatment is required and follow-up is sufficient.
- If colposcopic-guided biopsy shows CIN2 or CIN3, then surgical ablation could be done.
- In case of no lesion in histopathology, follow-up is sufficient.

High-grade Squamous Intraepithelial Lesions

High-grade squamous intraepithelial lesion in TBS encompasses CIN2 and CIN3. Only 0.5% of all cervical smears show HSIL. High-risk HPV is found in 97% of HSIL cases.[10] HSIL usually develops in the endocervical epithelium either in the transformation zone or in the endocervical canal.

Cytology (Figs. 8.16 to 8.20 and Box 8.4)

Cells in HSIL are usually parabasal, basal or metaplastic type. They are arranged in small sheets, three-dimensional crowded groups or singly. Individual cells are round with scanty cytoplasm and high nucleus-to-cytoplasm (N/C) ratio. Cytoplasm is dense or lacy in character. In case of

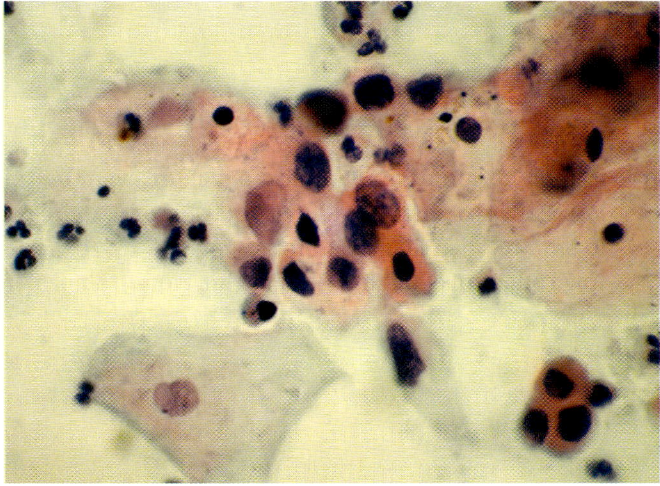

Fig. 8.16: Discrete dysplastic cells in high-grade squamous intraepithelial lesion (HSIL) case (Papanicolaou's stain X HP).

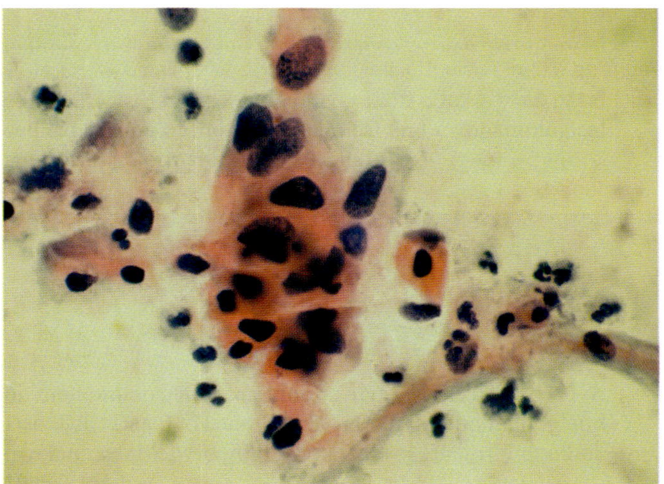

Fig. 8.17: Cervical smear of a high-grade squamous intraepithelial lesion (HSIL) case shows enlarged nuclei occupying more than two-thirds of the cytoplasmic area (Papanicolaou's stain X HP).

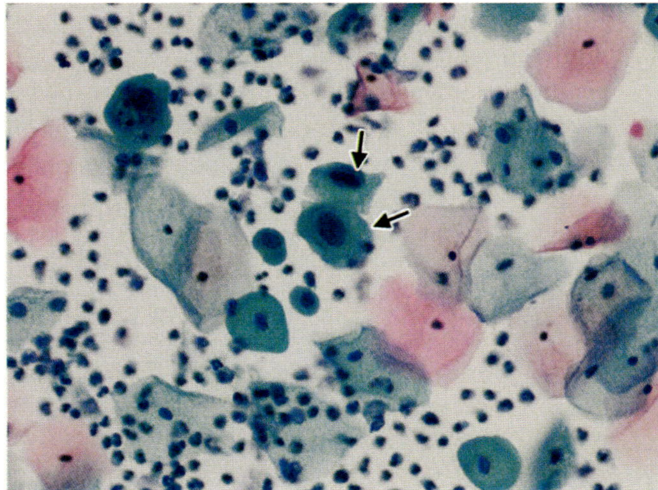

Fig. 8.18: Many discrete cells with moderate nuclear pleomorphism (*see* arrows) (Papanicolaou's stain in SurePath X HP).

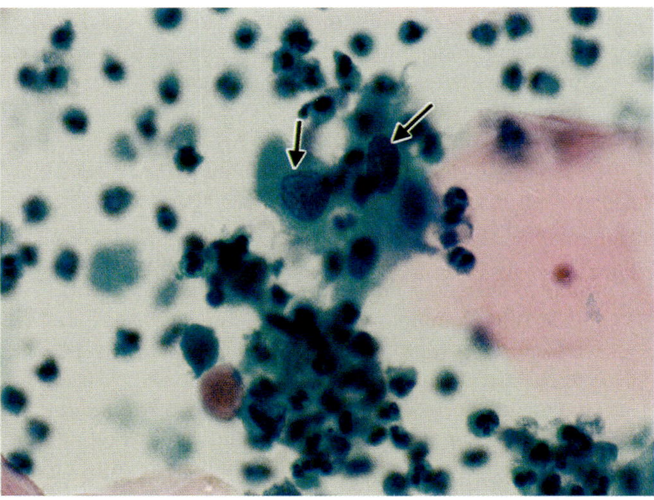

Fig. 8.19: Nuclei show hyperchromasia in high-grade squamous intraepithelial lesion (HSIL) (*see* arrows) (Papanicolaou's stain in SurePath X HP).

keratinizing variant, there may be orangeophilia in the cytoplasm. Nuclei of the cells are enlarged, moderately pleomorphic, hyperchromatic with coarse chromatin. Nuclear contour is markedly irregular. Nucleoli of HSIL are commonly absent.

Keratinizing HSIL is characterized by multiple clusters of dysplastic cells with orangeophilic cytoplasm and enlarged pleomorphic nuclei (Fig. 8.21). Many spindle-shaped cells and tadpole cells are seen that may simulate keratinized SQC (Fig. 8.22). However, the absence of tumor diathesis is helpful to eliminate the possibility of SQC.

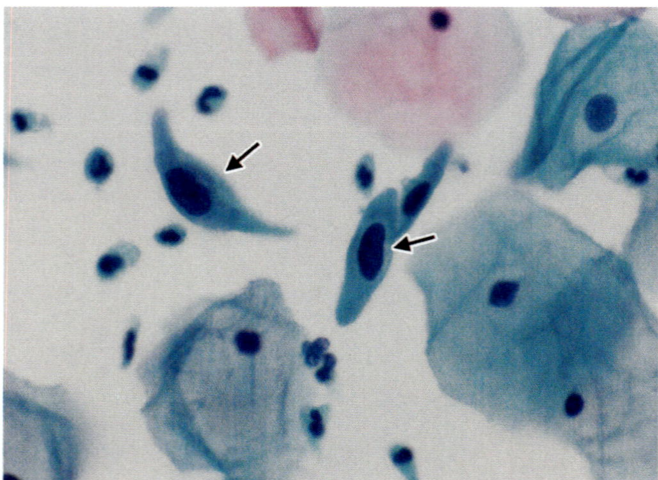

Fig. 8.20: Discrete cells with pleomorphic enlarged nuclei in high-grade squamous intraepithelial lesion (HSIL) (*see* arrows) (Papanicolaou's stain in SurePath X HP).

Potential Pitfalls in High-grade Squamous Intraepithelial Lesion Diagnosis

Pale cell dyskaryosis[11] *(Box 8.5)*: The presence of hyperchromasia in dysplastic cells is probably overemphasized and therefore the dysplastic cells with hypochromatic pale nuclei may be missed. *Pale cells* are usually seen in small groups or singly (Fig. 8.23). As the name indicates pale, the nuclei of the cells are pale hypochromatic with regular nuclear contour. Irregularly clumped chromatin producing a speckled appearance of chromatin pattern is characteristic of pale dyskaryotic cells. The pale cells are often present in addition to classical hyperchromatic dysplastic cells and therefore the identification of these cells is not very difficult. However, predominant population of pale cell in the cytology smear may pose diagnostic

Box 8.4: High-grade squamous intraepithelial lesion (HSIL).

- Single or sheets of cells
- Parabasal or basal type of cell
- Cells are relatively smaller than low-grade squamous intraepithelial lesion (LSIL)
- Cytoplasm is dense or lacy and orangeophilic in keratinized variant
- Nucleus:
  - Three times of the nucleus of intermediate cell
  - Moderately pleomorphic
  - Hyperchromatic
  - Marked irregular nuclear membrane
  - Coarse chromatin
  - Inconspicuous nucleoli
- Nucleocytoplasmic ratio is high

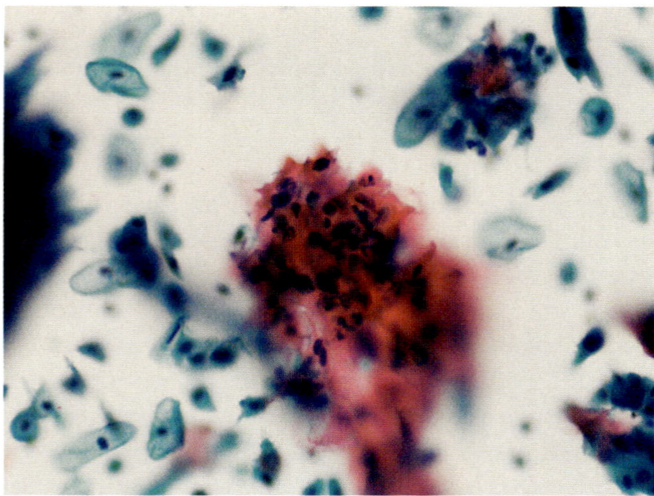

Fig. 8.21: Clusters of dysplastic cells with orangeophilic cytoplasm and enlarged pleomorphic nuclei in keratinizing high-grade squamous intraepithelial lesion (HSIL) (Papanicolaou's stain in SurePath X HP).

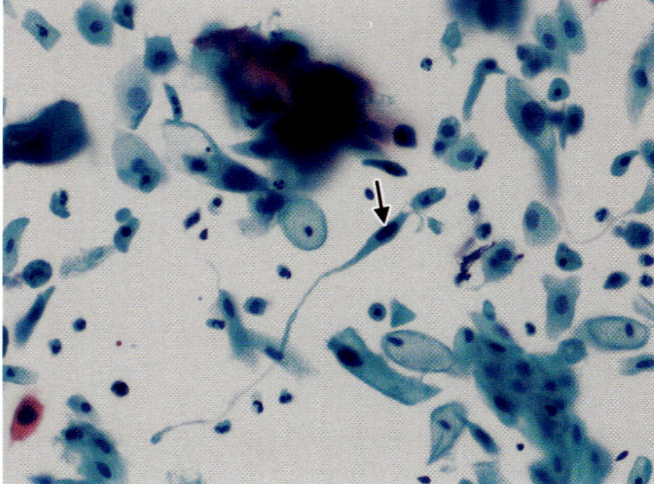

Fig. 8.22: Tadpole-like cells in keratinizing high-grade squamous intraepithelial lesion (HSIL) (*see* arrow) (Papanicolaou's stain in SurePath X HP).

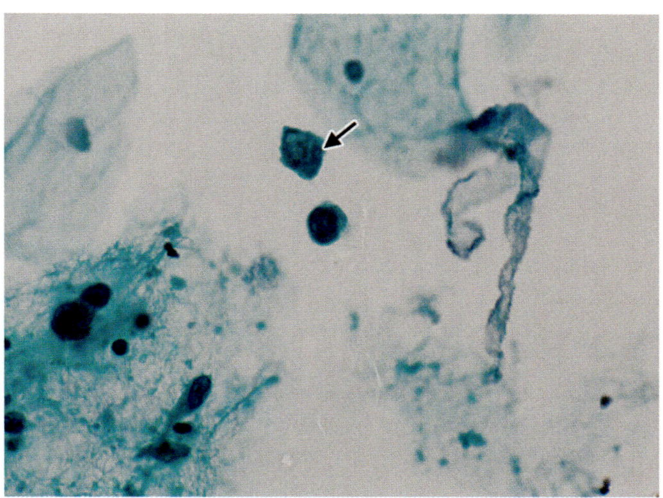

Fig. 8.23: Pale cells in pale cell dyskaryosis (*see* arrow) (Papanicolaou's stain in SurePath X HP).

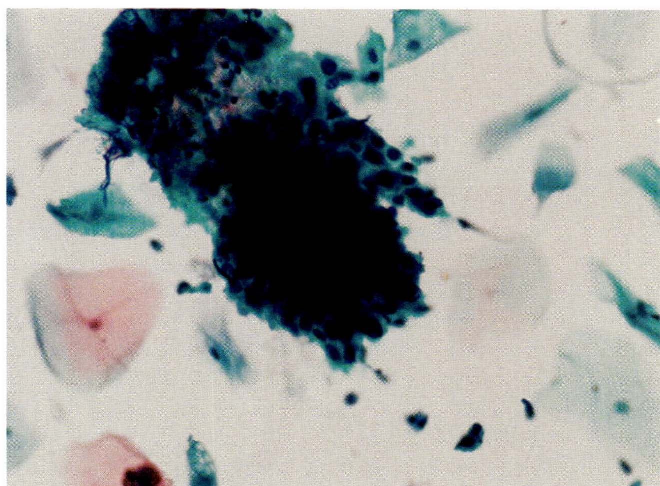

Fig. 8.24: Hyperchromatic crowded group of cells in high-grade squamous intraepithelial lesion (HSIL). Note the irregular ragged margin of the cluster (Papanicolaou's stain in SurePath X HP).

Box 8.5: Pale cell dyskaryosis.

- Small groups or discrete cells
- Pale nuclei
- Speckled chromatin
- Regular nuclear margin
- Minimal chromatin abnormality

Differential diagnosis: Inflammatory cells, endocervical cells and histiocytes, benign immature metaplastic cells and reserve cells

Box 8.6: Bland dyskaryosis.

- Disorganized group of cells
- Enlarged nuclei with high N/C ratio
- Hyperchromatic nuclei
- Regular nuclear contour
- Bland chromatin in low power view
- Speckled chromatin in higher magnification

Differential diagnosis: Immature metaplastic cells or endocervical cells

Box 8.7: Hyperchromatic crowded groups.

- Three-dimensional tight cluster of cells
- Hyperchromatic nuclei
- Noted in:
- Benign: Endometrial cells, endocervical cells, atrophic smear and in tubal metaplasia
- Neoplastic (or preneoplastic): HSIL, adenocarcinoma, SQC, and metastatic carcinoma
- Characteristic of neoplastic HCG:
- Chaotic architecture of the cells
- Irregular ragged peripheral margin
- Coarse chromatin
- Nuclear margin irregularity
- Occasional mitosis within the cluster

(HSIL: High-grade squamous intraepithelial lesion; SQC: Squamous cell carcinoma; HCG: Hyperchromatic crowded groups).

challenge as these cells may be overlooked. Pale cells are often mistaken as inflammatory cells, endocervical cells, and histiocytes.

Bland dyskaryosis: The bland dyskaryosis shows loose clusters of cells with hyperchromatic nuclei, having regular nuclear margin and bland chromatin pattern in low power examination (Box 8.6). However, in high power view the chromatin is speckled in appearance.

These cells are commonly mistaken as immature metaplastic cells or reactive endocervical cells.[12]

Hyperchromatic crowded groups (HCG) (Box 8.7): HCG of cells is three-dimensional clusters of cells with overlapping nuclei (Fig. 8.24). The nuclei of the cells are hyperchromatic.[13] HCG may be present both in non-neoplastic and neoplastic conditions. HCG in benign conditions is seen in endometrial cells, endocervical cells, atrophic smear and also in tubal metaplasia (Fig. 8.25). Whereas, HCG associated with neoplastic (or preneoplastic) lesions are HSIL, adenocarcinoma, SQC, and metastatic carcinoma. It is important to differentiate HCG from a benign and neoplastic lesion. The following features may be helpful to suggest neoplastic (or preneoplastic) HCG: (1) chaotic architecture of the cells that means loss of polarity of the nuclei, (2) irregular ragged margin of the periphery of HCG, (3) coarse chromatin, (4) nuclear margin irregularity, and (5) occasional mitosis within the cluster.

The HSIL with glandular involvement: HSIL may involve the endocervical glands and the smears of such cases may pose diagnostic problems. The cytology smears show

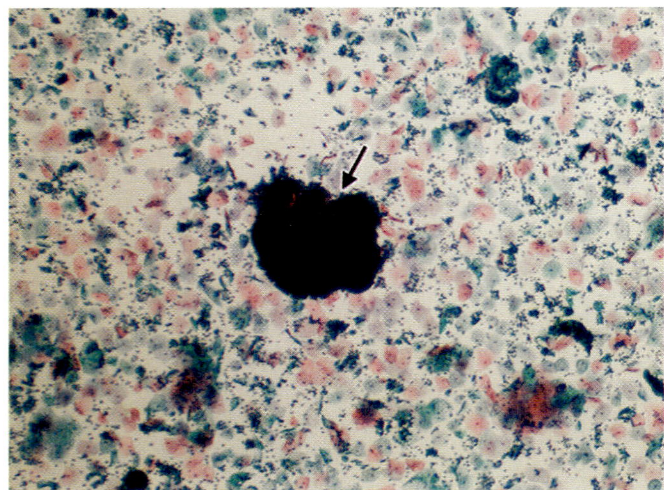

Fig. 8.25: Hyperchromatic crowded group of cells in benign condition (endocervical cell cluster) (Papanicolaou's stain in SurePath X HP).

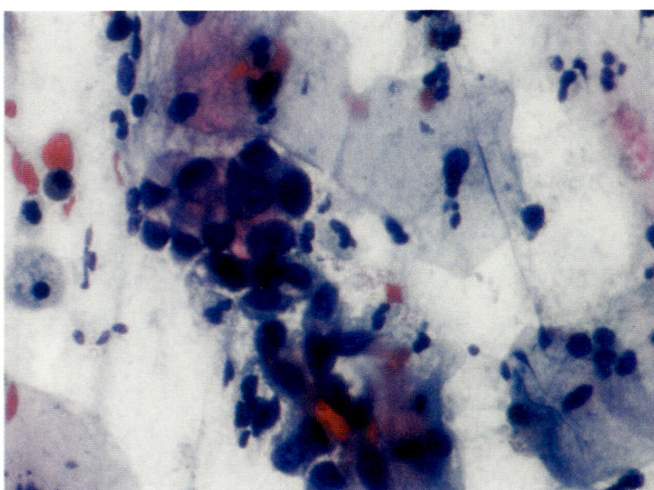

Fig. 8.26: High-grade squamous intraepithelial lesion (HSIL) with glandular involvement showing cluster of cells having vacuolated cytoplasm. Nucleolar prominence is also seen (Papanicolaou's stain in SurePath X HP).

Table 8.4: Comparison of LSIL and HSIL.

Cytological features	*LSIL*	*HSIL*
Cell arrangement	Singly and in clusters	Singly and in clusters
Cell type	Superficial and intermediate	Parabasal, basal and metaplastic
Koilocytes	Present	Usually absent
Cell cytoplasm	More	Less
N/C ratio	Low	High
Nucleus:		
• Size	Mild enlargement	Moderate enlargement
• Pleomorphism	Mild	Moderate
• Contour	Mildly irregular	Moderately irregular
• Hyperchromasia	Mild	Moderate
• Chromatin	Fine	Coarse
Mitosis	Rare	Frequent

(LSIL: Low-grade squamous intraepithelial lesion; HSIL: High-grade squamous intraepithelial lesion; N/C: Nucleus-to-cytoplasm).

HCG. The individual cells show pleomorphic nuclei, vacuolated cytoplasm, and prominent nucleoli (Fig. 8.26). It is necessary to have a close look to such cells for any evidence of squamous differentiation.

Differential diagnosis of high-grade squamous intraepithelial lesion:

- *Squamous cell carcinoma*: The cells of SQC and HSIL may simulate each other. The degree of nuclear abnormality is more in SQC; however, this may not be helpful due to overlapping cytological features of HSIL and SQC. The presence of tumor diathesis is the most important diagnostic feature of SQC. In addition, the other helpful features of SQC are the presence of fiber cells and tadpole cells.
- *LSIL*: HSIL should be distinguished from LSIL. Table 8.4 compares the cytological differentiating points between them. The degree of the cellular abnormality is less in LSIL than HSIL. The following features are helpful for the diagnosis of HSIL such as: (1) high N/C ratio, (2) significant nuclear margin irregularity, (3) moderate to marked hyperchromasia, and (4) coarse irregular chromatin.
- *Atrophic smear*: Small parabasal cells with enlarged nuclei in atrophic smear may simulate HSIL at times. However, careful observation of nuclear character such as absence of coarse chromatin and irregular nuclear margin may be helpful in differentiating atrophic smear from HSIL (Fig. 8.27).
- *Squamous metaplastic cells*: Relatively enlarged nucleus and dense chromatin of squamous metaplastic cells may simulate as HSIL.
- *Histiocytes*: Mononuclear histiocytes with enlarged nucleus may also simulate HSIL. However, nuclei of histiocytes have fine chromatin texture.
- *ASC-H*: The cells with enlarged and pleomorphic nuclei in ASC-H closely simulate HSIL.
- *Intrauterine device (IUD) effect*: Small cells in IUD are often difficult to distinguish from HSIL.
- *Endometrial cells*: At times, endometrial cells may be difficult to distinguish from HSIL. However, HSIL clusters are less well circumscribed and individual cells are larger than endometrial cells.

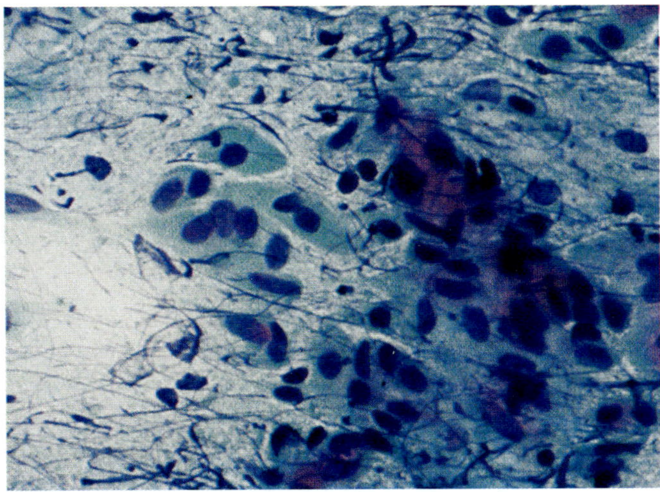

Fig. 8.27: Atrophic smear showing moderate nuclear enlargement and simulate high-grade squamous intraepithelial lesion (HSIL) (Papanicolaou's stain X HP).

- *Overstained cells*: The nuclei of the overstained cells are dark and may be over diagnosed as HSIL. N/C ratio is not altered in overstained cells.

Management of HSIL Cases[14] (Flowchart 8.3)

- Colposcopy along with endocervical assessment is recommended in all such cases.
- If colposcopy confirms CIN2/CIN3, then the entire transformation zone should be removed along with the lesion. The following surgical measures can be taken: (1) cryotherapy, (2) loop electrosurgical excision procedure (LEEP)/large loop excision of the transformation zone (LLETZ), and (3) cold knife conization (CKC).
- In case of negative colposcopy: (1) A diagnostic excisional biopsy, (2) repeat cervical smear 6 monthly twice, and (3) repeat colposcopy.
- In case of HSIL in repeat cervical cytology: The diagnostic excisional procedure should be taken.
- Two successive negative cytology smears at 6 monthly interval, negative colposcopy, and endocervical sampling: The patient should be in routine cervical cytology program.

Atypical Squamous Cells

The term "ASC-US" is used when cytology smear is suggestive of SIL but there are not enough evidences to have a definitive interpretation of SIL. ASC-US terminology has evoked lot of confusion because of low reproducibility, heterogeneous mixture of diagnoses and variable outcomes.

Flowchart 8.3: Outline of high-grade squamous intraepithelial lesion (HSIL) management.

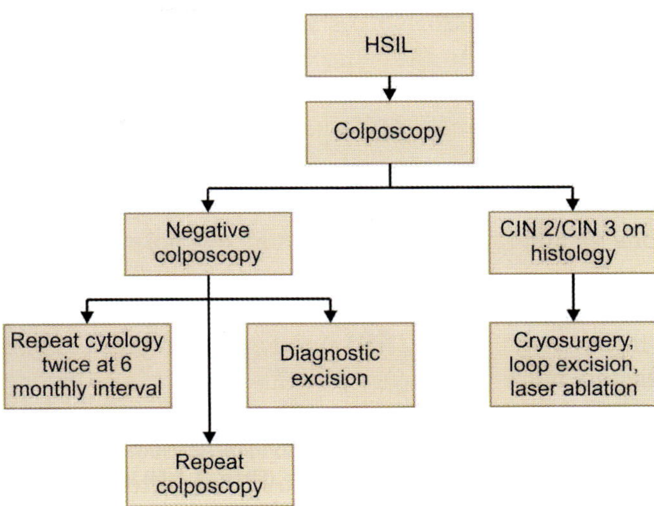

Box 8.8: Atypical cells of undetermined significance (ASC-US).

Cytology:
- Superficial and intermediate type of cell show changes
- Cytoplasm may show vague perinuclear halos
- Mildly increased N/C ratio
- Nucleus mildly increased in size
- Mildly hyperchromatic nucleus

Bethesda system divides atypical squamous cells as:
- Atypical squamous cells of undetermined significance
- Atypical squamous cells cannot exclude high-grade SIL (ASC-H).

The ASC-US is a diagnosis of exclusion. The interpretation of ASC-US is subjective and depends on pathologist's diagnostic threshold. ASC-US should be reported as minimum as possible. There is no correct rate of ASC-US and the prevalence of ASC-US is indirectly proportional with the reporting of LSIL. It is suggested that the rate of ASC-US diagnosis should be less than 5% of total cervical smear. The reporting rate of ASC-US in cervical smear should not exceed 2–3 times of the SIL.

Cytology (Box 8.8)

Cytology smear of ASC-US shows predominantly atypia in superficial and intermediate group of cells. Cytoplasm of the cell is dense orangeophilic. The atypical cells show mildly increased nucleocytoplasmic ratio and the nuclear enlargement of the atypical squamous cell is 2.5–3.0 times enlarged than the nucleus of the normal intermediate cell. The cells show regular nuclear margin with mild nuclear hyperchromasia with fine granular chromatin (Figs. 8.28 and 8.29).

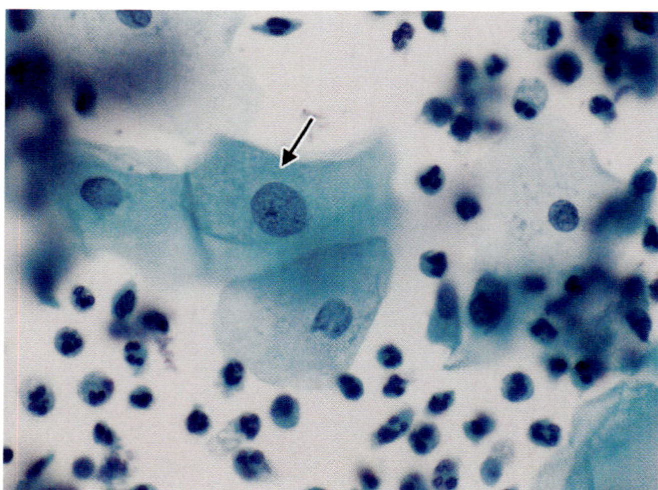

Fig. 8.28: Atypical squamous cells of undetermined significance (ASC-US): Atypical squamous cell with mature intermediate type cytoplasm (*see* arrow) (Papanicolaou's stain in SurePath X HP).

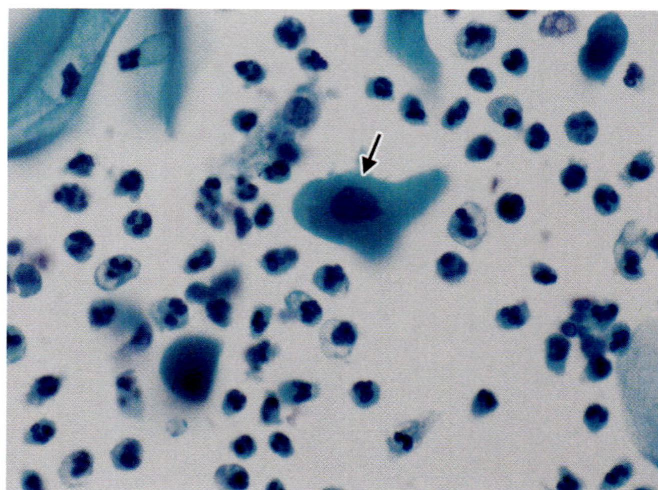

Fig. 8.29: Atypical squamous cells of undetermined significance (ASC-US): The cells show only mild nuclear enlargement. Nucleus occupies half of the cytoplasmic area (*see* arrow) (Papanicolaou's stain in SurePath X HP).

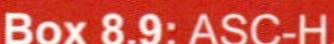

Box 8.9: ASC-H.

- Single and loose cohesive group of cells
- Immature small squamous cells
- Nucleus: Mild-to-moderate enlargement, hyperchromasia, and pleomorphism
- Increased nucleocytoplasmic ratio

Reproducibility of ASC-US

Reproducibility of ASC-US is poor due to its high interobserver and intraobserver variabilities. Even after adequate experience or review of criteria by TBS atlas, the reproducibility of ASC-US is poor. Complete consensus of ASC-US cases can be reached only in 30% cases.[15]

Differential Diagnosis

Differential diagnosis includes:

- *Inflammatory atypia*: Inflammation-induced atypia in the cervical smear may simulate ASC-US.
- *LSIL*: Nuclear atypia in LSIL may overlap with ASC-US. However, nuclear changes are qualitatively more in LSIL than in ASC-US.
- *Artifact-producing changes*: Occasionally staining artifact may show nuclear enlargement and may simulate ASC-US.
- *Radiation- and chemotherapy-induced atypia*: In case of radiation- and chemotherapy-induced atypia, the nuclear chromatin is smudgy and overall nuclear preservation is poor. Moreover, both the cytoplasmic and nuclear areas are increased and N/C ratio is not altered in such cases.
- *Folic acid deficiency*: In case of folic acid deficiency, the smear shows nuclear enlargement in most of the cells and the nuclei are normochromatic.

Atypical Squamous Cell-High-grade Squamous Intraepithelial Lesion

Atypical squamous cell-high-grade squamous intraepithelial lesion cannot be excluded. The ASC-H cases are close to HSIL but a definitive interpretation of HSIL is difficult or impossible in such cases. ASC-H cases are less common and represent only 5–10% of all ASC cases.[16] Subsequent HSIL is seen in 30–40% of cases of ASC-H.

Cytology (Box 8.9)

The cytology smears of ASC-H cases show immature small squamous cells (Figs. 8.30 to 8.32). Nuclei are moderately enlarged and nuclear size is 1.5–2.5 times more than normal metaplastic cells. The nuclei are hyperchromatic and pleomorphic with absent to inconspicuous nucleoli. There may be overlapping tight cohesive group of cells known as "hyperchromatic crowded group of cells".

Differential Diagnosis of ASC-H

Differential diagnosis of ASC-H includes:

- *Endometrial cells*: Endometrial cells in tight clusters may simulate ASC-H. The nuclei of the endometrial cells are homogeneously dark with regular nuclear margin.
- *Histiocytes*: The discrete and pale histiocytes are easily distinguishable from ASC-H cells.

- *Atypical glandular cells (AGCs)*: AGCs in clusters may mimic ASC-H. However, these cells have vacuolated cytoplasm with vesicular nuclear chromatin.
- HSIL involving the endocervical glands may mimic ASC-H.
- *Atypia in radiation*: Atypical cells in radiation may mimic ASC-H.

Management of ASC-US Cases (Flowchart 8.4)

Three approaches are recommended in these cases:[17]

1. Repeat cervical cytology at 6 monthly intervals
2. High-risk HPV testing
3. One time colposcopic examination.

According to guideline[18] high-risk HPV DNA testing (HPV 16 and 18) is recommended in such cases.

- If HPV DNA test is negative: Repeat cervical cytology and HPV test after 1 year.
- If HPV DNA test is positive: Colposcopy should be done:
  - If two successive Pap test are negative then the patient may undergo routine screening scheme.
  - If any of the two Pap test shows ASC-US or greater then colposcopy is recommended.

Management of ASC-H

Management of ASC-H includes:

- Colposcopy is always recommended in all ASC-H patients.
- If colposcopic examination is negative for CIN2 or CIN3 then high-risk HPV DNA test can be done.
- Alternately cytology smear examination can be done at 6-month and 12-month intervals.
- If HPV DNA test is positive or any of the cytology tests shows ASC or above then repeat colposcopy should be done.

Squamous Cell Carcinoma

Squamous cell carcinoma is the most common carcinoma of the cervix. It occurs between 40 years and 55 years of age. Early invasive carcinoma is asymptomatic, however, as the progression of carcinoma the patient presents with vaginal bleeding and postcoital or intermenstrual bleeding.

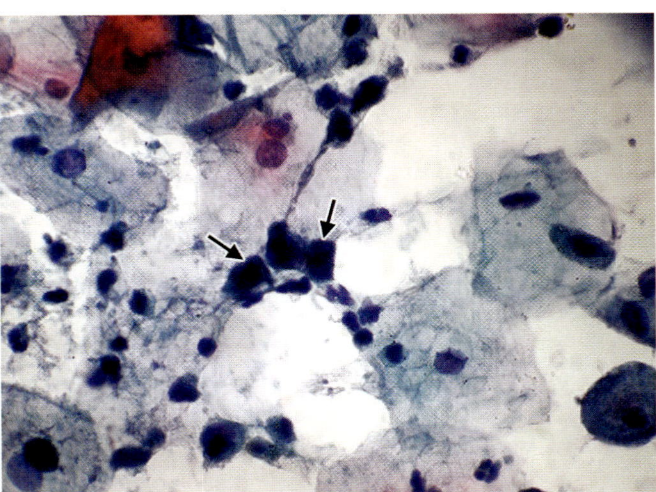

Fig. 8.30: Small cluster of cells with enlarged hyperchromatic nuclei in ASC-H case (*see* arrows) (Papanicolaou's stain in SurePath X MP).

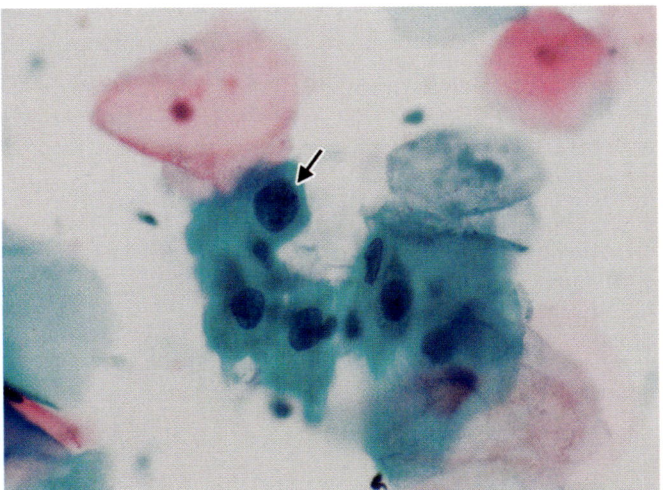

Fig. 8.31: ASC-H: Loose cluster of cells with high nucleocytoplasmic ratio. Nuclei occupying more than two-thirds of the cytoplasm (*see* arrow) (Papanicolaou's stain in SurePath X HP).

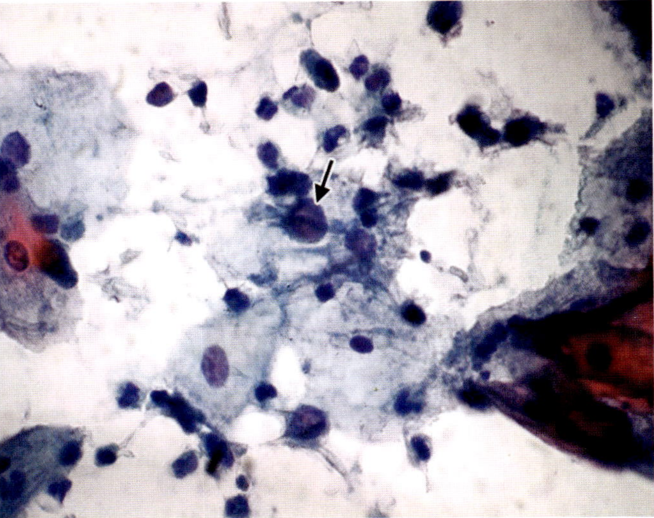

Fig. 8.32: Discrete dysplastic cells with enlarged nuclei in ASC-H case (*see* arrow) (Papanicolaou's stain X HP).

Flowchart 8.4: Outline of management in atypical cells of undetermined significance (ASC-US) and ASC-H cases.

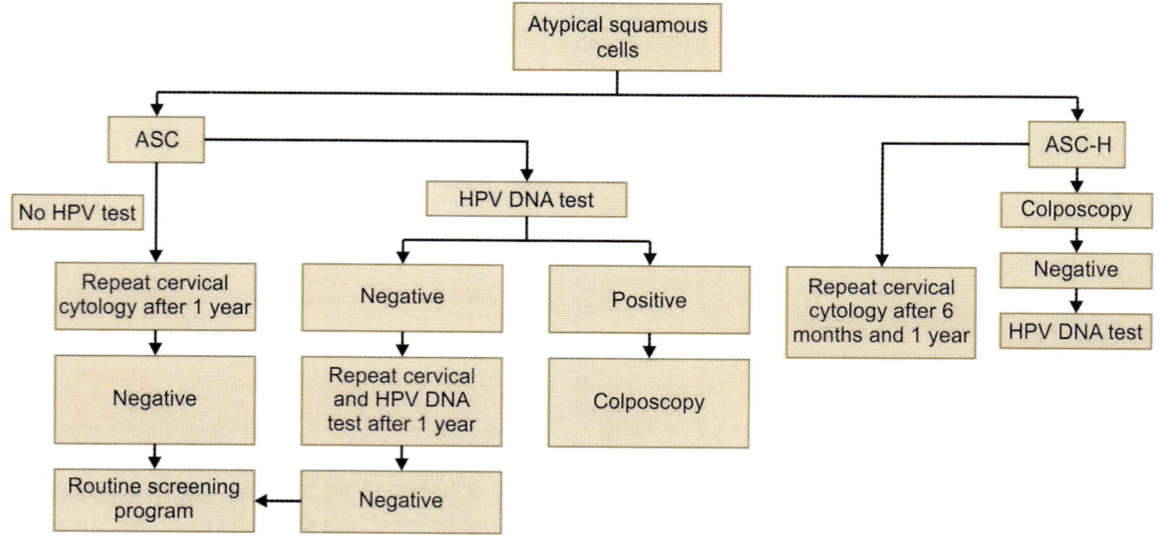

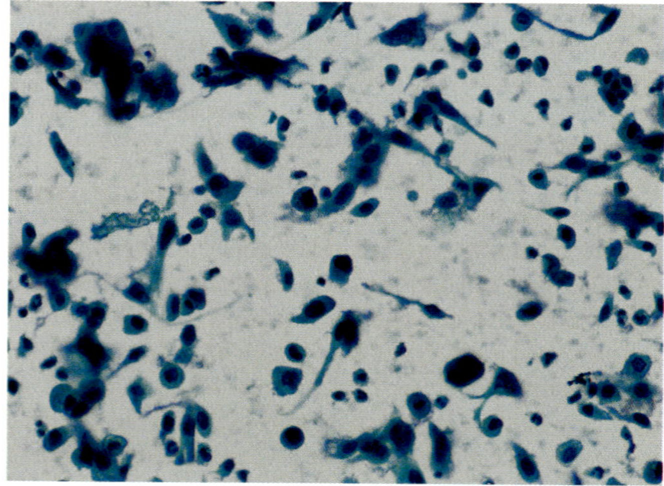

Fig. 8.33: Squamous cell carcinoma (SQC): Abundant discrete cells with moderate to marked nuclear pleomorphism (Papanicolaou's stain in SurePath X LP).

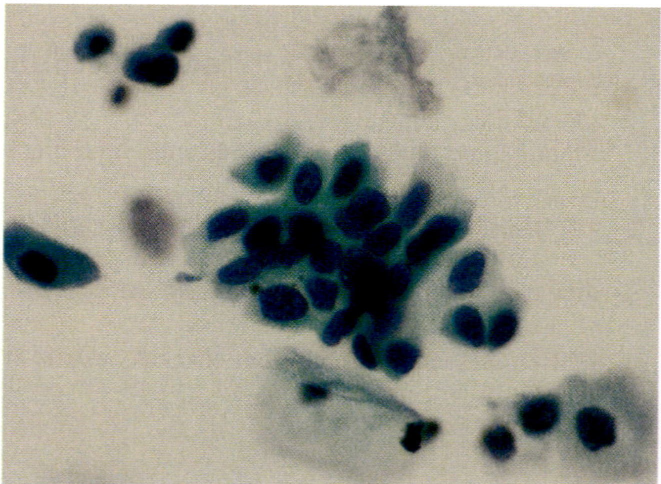

Fig. 8.34: Squamous cell carcinoma (SQC): Loose cluster of cells with hyperchromatic nuclei (Papanicolaou's stain in SurePath X HP).

In late-invasive cases, the patient may show features of infiltration into the surrounding tissue such as back pain, hematuria, rectal bleeding, and obstructive uropathy.

World Health Organization recommends two-tiered system of classification of SQC of cervix:

1. Keratinizing SQC
2. Nonkeratinizing SQC.

Cytology (Figs. 8.33 to 8.39 and Box 8.10)

Smear shows discrete and small groups of malignant cells. Individual cells show moderately pleomorphic, hyperchromatic nuclei with irregular clumped chromatin. Cytoplasm of the cell is orangeophilic with well-defined border. The characteristic of tadpole cells and fiber cells are noted. Tadpole cells are elongated in shape with large abnormal nuclei in one corner. Fiber cells are spindle-shaped with elongated hyperchromatic nucleus (Figs. 8.36 and 8.37).

Background tumor diathesis is an important feature of invasive carcinoma. Smear shows nuclear debris, red blood cells (RBCs) and small necrotic tissue fragments (Fig. 8.38). Atrophic smear and heavy menstrual blood may simulate similar pattern. In liquid-based cytology (LBC), the smear may show more clean background;

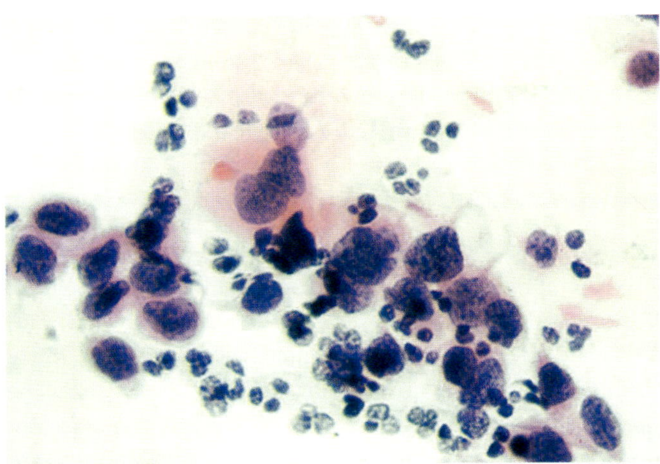

Fig. 8.35: Squamous cell carcinoma (SQC): Coarse and clumped chromatin (Papanicolaou's stain X HP).

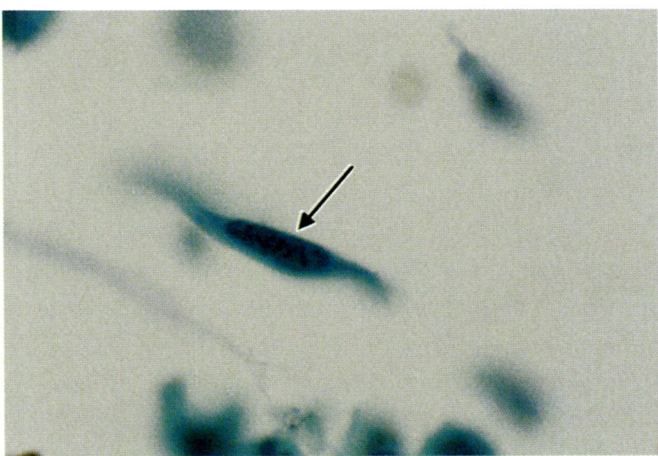

Fig. 8.36: Squamous cell carcinoma (SQC): Fiber cell (*see* arrow) (Papanicolaou's stain in SurePath X HP).

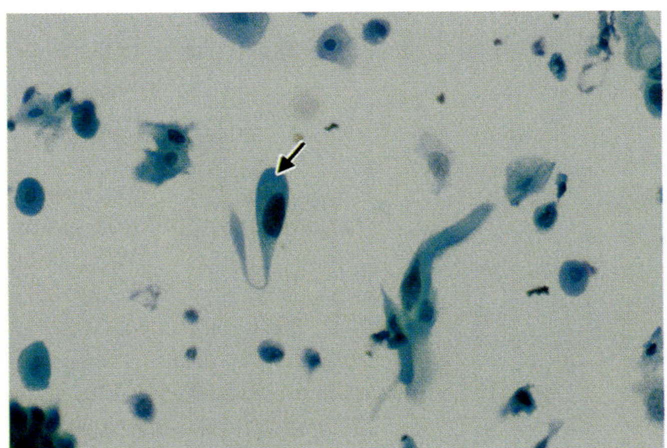

Fig. 8.37: Squamous cell carcinoma (SQC): Tadpole cell (*see* arrow) (Papanicolaou's stain in SurePath X HP).

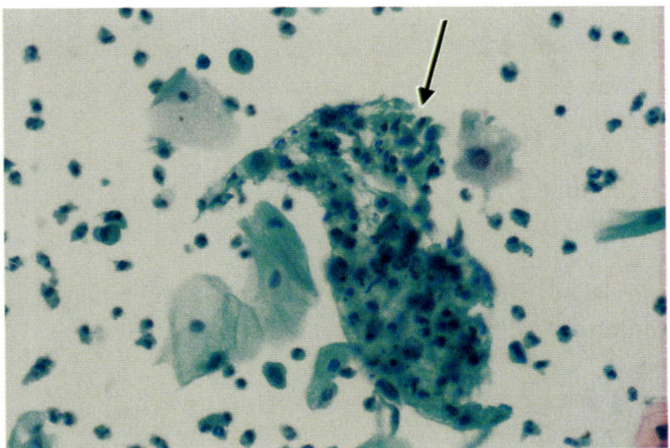

Fig. 8.38: Squamous cell carcinoma (SQC): Tumor diathesis (*see* arrow) (Papanicolaou's stain in SurePath X MP).

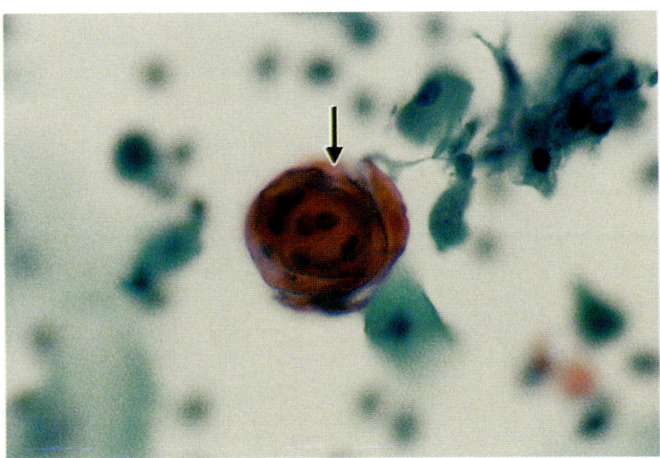

Fig. 8.39: Squamous cell carcinoma (SQC): Squamous pearl (*see* arrow) (Papanicolaou's stain in SurePath X MP).

Box 8.10: Squamous cell carcinoma.

Keratinizing:

- Scattered and small clusters of tumor cells
- Moderately pleomorphic cell with high N/C ratio
- Nuclei:
  - Pleomorphic
  - Hyperchromatic
  - Irregular coarse chromatin
  - Nucleoli present
- *Cytoplasm*: Dense orangeophilic
- *Tadpole cells*: Elongated cell with large abnormal nuclei in one corner
- *Fiber cell*: Spindle shaped hyperchromatic nuclei
- *Tumor diathesis*: Dirty background with necrotic tissue fragments and red blood cells (RBCs)

Nonkeratinizing:

- Cells are smaller
- Cytoplasm: Basophilic
- Prominent nucleoli

however, the typical malignant cells are easily recognized. Careful observation may reveal tumor diathesis and other salient features of SQC.

Differential Diagnosis

- *High-grade squamous intraepithelial lesion*: It is the closest differential diagnosis of SQC. Tumor diathesis is the most important differentiating feature between HSIL and invasive carcinoma. However, in the absence of tumor diathesis it may be difficult to distinguish invasive carcinoma from HSIL.
- *Atypia of repair*: Marked reparative changes may mimic invasive carcinoma. Cells may show moderate nuclear enlargement and pleomorphism with large prominent nucleoli in reparative changes. However, nuclear chromatin is fine and granular in reparative cells in comparison to coarse irregular clumped chromatin in carcinoma.
- *Atrophic smear*: Dirty background along with cells having orangeophilic cytoplasm and moderately enlarged dark nuclei of atrophic smear may often mimic invasive cancer. However, chromatin pattern of these cells is usually smudgy and help in differentiating from carcinoma.
- *Endometrial cells*: Small spherical clusters of endometrial cells in a menstrual background may simulate small cell nonkeratinizing SQC. A careful history of growth in cervix may be helpful in this condition.

Box 8.11: Adenocarcinoma in situ (AIS).

- Hyperchromatic crowded groups, rosettes, strips of cells
- Feathering effect
- Columnar cells
- Nuclei more than twice the size of normal endocervical cells
- Hyperchromatic
- Small nucleoli
- No tumor diathesis

Endocervical Adenocarcinoma in situ

Adenocarcinoma in situ (AIS) represents only 1% of all in situ carcinoma of cervix. This entity is difficult to recognize in cytology smear. The cytology smear of AIS shows HCG, strips and rosette-like arrangement of cells (Box 8.11). Unlike adenocarcinoma, the tumor diathesis is absent in AIS. The tumor cells are columnar in shape having enlarged nuclei that are twice the size of normal endocervical cells. The nuclei are pleomorphic with prominent nucleoli and coarse chromatin. The smear may show feathering effect characterized by peripheral protrusion of nuclei and cytoplasmic fragment.

Endocervical Adenocarcinoma

Endocervical adenocarcinoma comprises of 15% of all cervical carcinomas.[19] The incidence of adenocarcinoma of cervix has increased about 5–20% during the last few decades. In contrast to SQCs, which are associated with HPV 16, adenocarcinomas of cervix are more frequently related with HPV 18.[20] Mean age of the patient is 55 years. Majority of the patients are asymptomatic. However, some patients may present with vaginal bleeding, discharge, and pain.

Cytology (Figs. 8.40 to 8.45 and Box 8.12)

Cytology smear of the endocervical adenocarcinoma usually shows abundant malignant cells. The cells are present

Fig. 8.40: Adenocarcinoma: Abundant discrete and clusters of cells with columnar appearance (Papanicolaou's stain in SurePath X MP).

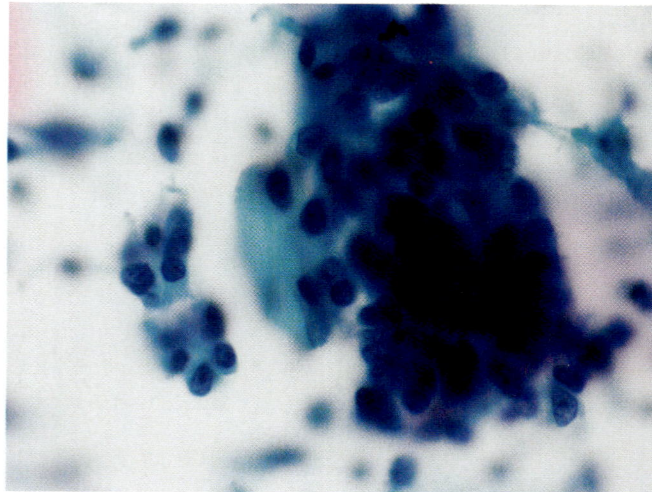

Fig. 8.41: Adenocarcinoma: Cells with overlapping nuclei (Papanicolaou's stain in SurePath X HP).

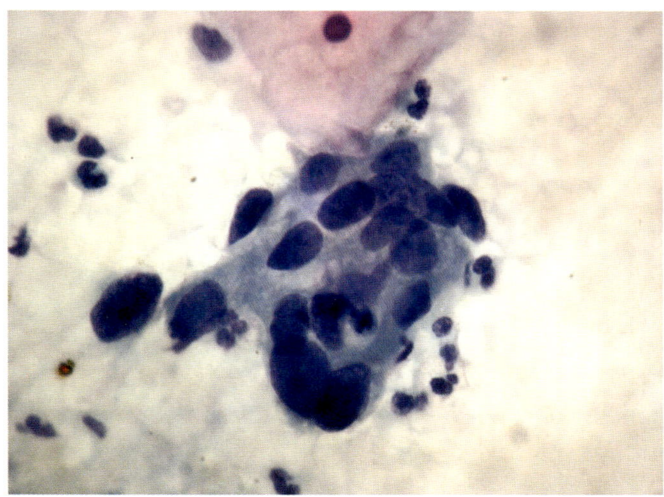

Fig. 8.42: Adenocarcinoma: Cells with enlarged nuclei and moderate amount of vacuolated cytoplasm in adenocarcinoma of cervix (Papanicolaou's stain X HP).

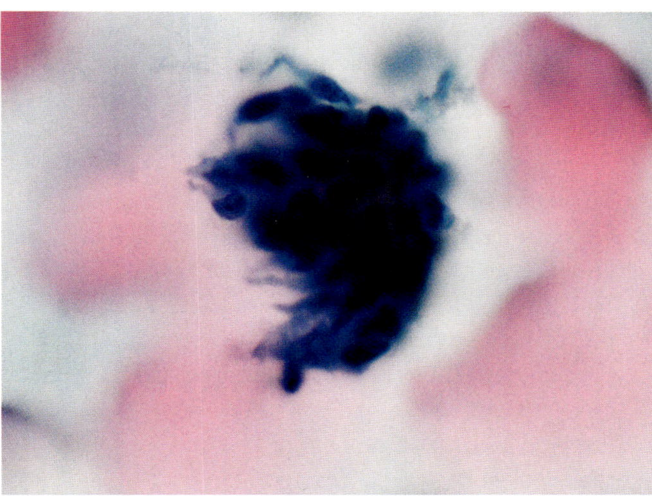

Fig. 8.43: Adenocarcinoma: Feathering of cells (Papanicolaou's stain in SurePath X HP).

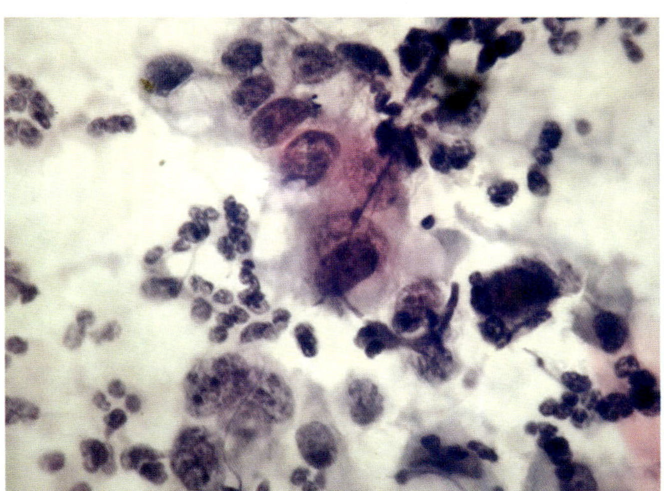

Fig. 8.44: Adenocarcinoma: Many discrete cells with moderate nuclear pleomorphism, coarse chromatin and large prominent nucleoli (Papanicolaou's stain X HP).

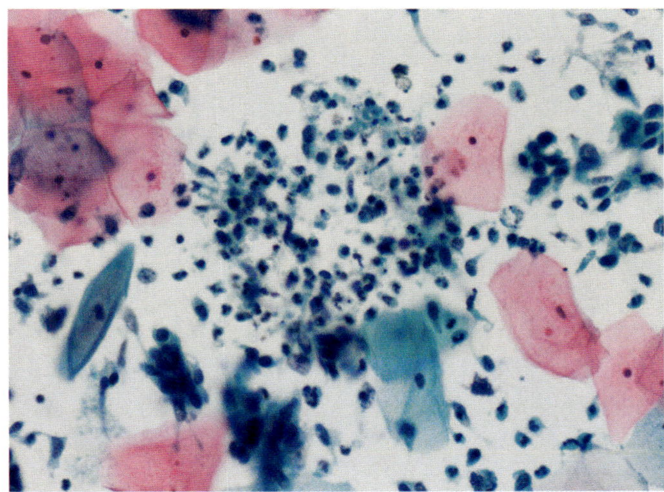

Fig. 8.45: Adenocarcinoma: Thin tumor diathesis (Papanicolaou's stain in SurePath X MP).

Box 8.12: Adenocarcinoma.

- High cellularity
- Single and loose clusters of cells
- Well-defined scalloped borders of the cluster
- Columnar to cuboidal cells
- Nucleus:
  - Large and round
  - Nuclear overlapping
  - Prominent nucleoli
  - Macronucleoli may be present
  - Coarse chromatin
- Cytoplasm: Abundant and vacuolated
- Tumor diathesis present

discretely or in small loose clusters (Fig. 8.40). The margin of the cluster shows scalloped border. There is overcrowding of the nuclei in the cluster. Individual cells show round to oval nucleus with moderate amount of vacuolated cytoplasm (Fig. 8.42). Nuclei show moderate pleomorphism with coarse chromatin and large prominent nucleoli. In addition, smears show tumor diathesis (Fig. 8.45).

Differential Diagnosis

Differential diagnoses of adenocarcinoma are discussed under different leadings.

- *Reactive endocervical cells*: Reactive endocervical cells with nuclear pleomorphism may simulate as endocervical adenocarcinoma. However, cells are in monolayer sheets and other nuclear features of adenocarcinoma are absent.
- *Microglandular hyperplasia*: Reactive endocervical cells in microglandular hyperplasia may often mimic as endocervical adenocarcinoma. Nuclear enlargement, pleomorphism, and cytoplasmic vacuoles may mislead the cytologist. A careful history (such as history of pregnancy or the presence of endocervical polyp) may be needed in such case.
- *Endometrial adenocarcinoma*: The differentiating features of endocervical and endometrial adenocarcinoma are highlighted in Table 8.5.

Table 8.5: Differentiating features of endocervical and endometrial adenocarcinoma.

Features	*Endocervical adenocarcinoma*	*Endometrial adenocarcinoma*
Age	Premenopausal younger patient	Postmenopausal, older patient
Cellularity	Abundant	Relatively scanty
Cell arrangement	Discrete and sheets	Discrete and spherical clusters
Cell appearance	Columnar	Round to oval
Nucleus	Moderate enlargement	Relatively smaller
Nucleus-to-cytoplasm (N/C) ratio	Low	High
Histiocytes	Absent	Present

Endometrial Adenocarcinoma

Most of the endometrial adenocarcinoma patients are postmenopausal and majority of the patients present with postmenopausal bleeding. Cervical smear is not a screening test of endometrial adenocarcinoma.

Cytology (Figs. 8.46 to 8.49 and Box 8.13)

Cytology smear of endometrial cells shows tight clusters and discrete tumor cells. The nuclei in the clusters show loss of polarity. There may be numerous histiocytes in the smear and less number of malignant cells. Individual cells show nuclear enlargement, hyperchromasia, and pleomorphism.

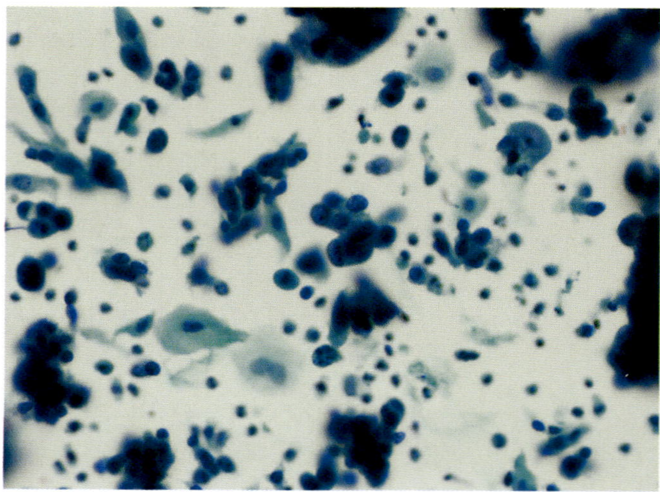

Fig. 8.46: Endometrial adenocarcinoma: Cervical smear showing loose clusters and discrete tumor cells (Papanicolaou's stain X HP).

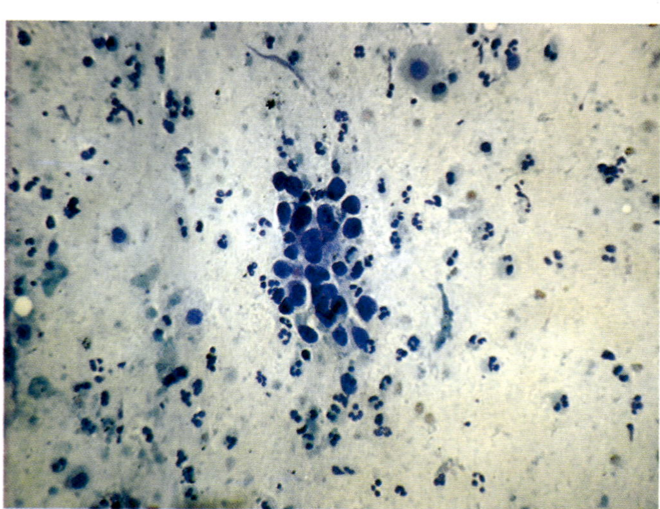

Fig. 8.47: Endometrial adenocarcinoma: Loose cluster of tumor cells (Papanicolaou's stain X HP).

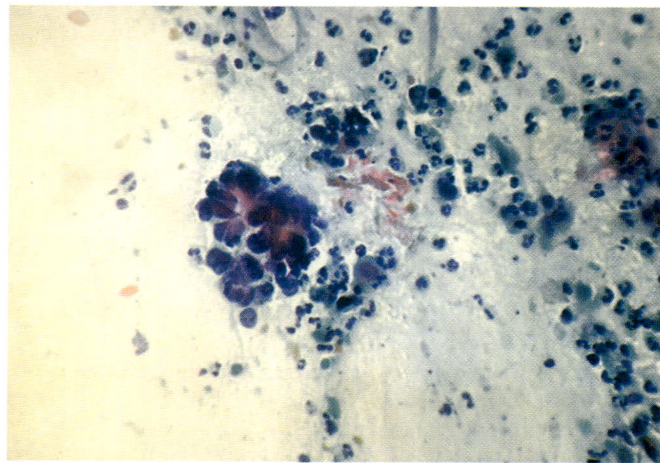

Fig. 8.48: Cluster of cells with overlapping nuclei in endometrial adenocarcinoma. The nuclei are dark and occupy whole of the cytoplasm (Papanicolaou's stain X HP).

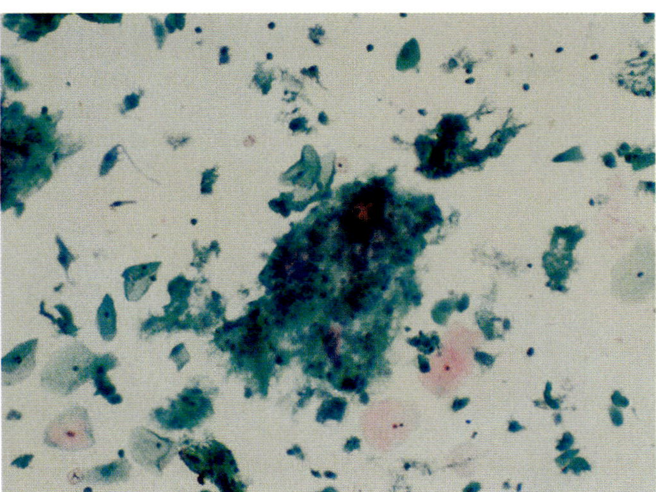

Fig. 8.49: Endometrial adenocarcinoma: Thin tumor diathesis (Papanicolaou's stain in SurePath X MP).

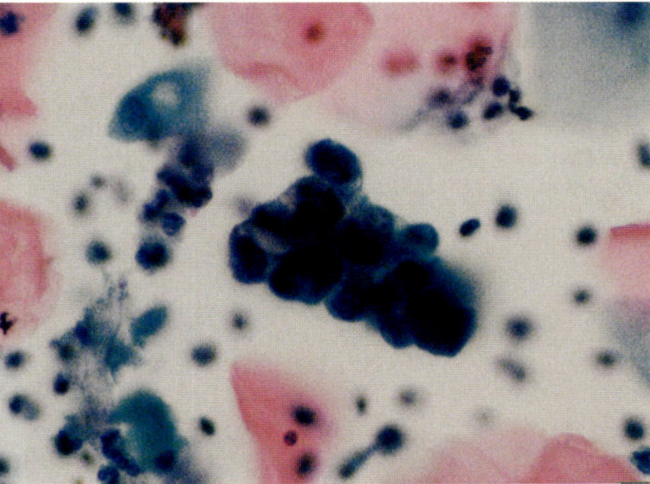

Fig. 8.50: Atypical glandular cell (AGC) possibly endocervical origin: Cells in tight cluster with moderate amount of vacuolated cytoplasm diathesis (Papanicolaou's stain in SurePath X MP).

Box 8.13: Endometrial adenocarcinoma.

- Highly cellular smear
- Cells are present predominantly in tight clusters
- Nuclei show: Loss of polarity, enlargement, hyperchromasia, pleomorphism, multiple nucleoli
- Cytoplasm: Scanty, vacuolated and often contains many polymorphs giving "bag of poly" appearance
- Finely granular watery tumor diathesis

Box 8.14: Atypical glandular cell (AGC), endocervical.

- Cells are in sheets or small overcrowded groups
- Cytoplasm: Abundant, vacuolated with distinct cell border
- Nucleus:
  - Mild enlargement: Three times than normal endocervical nuclei
  - Mildly pleomorphic
  - Hyperchromatic
  - Small nucleoli
- Rare mitotic figures

Nucleoli are prominent. Cytoplasm of the cells often shows vacuoles. Cytoplasm of the cells is scanty and vacuolated. The cytoplasm contains many polymorphs giving "bag of poly" appearance. The background of the smear shows characteristic finely granular watery tumor diathesis. In fact, the cytological features of endometrial carcinoma depend predominantly on the grade of endometrial adenocarcinoma. Relative abundance of cells increases from lower to higher grade of tumor. Similarly nuclear enlargement and pleomorphism increase in severity depending on the grade of the endometrial carcinoma.

Atypical Glandular Cell

Atypical glandular cell is defined as atypical cell with nuclear atypia more than reactive or reparative changes, however, fall short of unequivocal diagnosis of adenocarcinoma. AGC is less common than ASC-US and comprises of less than 1% of all abnormal cervical smear.[21] According to TBS 2001, AGC should always be specified as:

- Atypical:
  - Endocervical in origin
  - Endometrial in origin
  - Glandular cell, not otherwise specified
- Atypical favors neoplasm:
  - Endocervical cells favor neoplastic
  - Glandular cell favors neoplastic, not otherwise specified.

Atypical Glandular Cell, Endocervical in Origin (Fig. 8.50 and Box 8.14)

Smear shows discrete and small clusters cells with crowded nuclei. Cytoplasm of the cell is abundant and vacuolated with distinct cell border. The nuclei of the cells are 3–5 times larger than the normal endocervical nuclei and are mildly pleomorphic and hyperchromatic.

Atypical Glandular Cell, Endocervical in Origin, Favors Neoplasia

Cytology (Box 8.15): Cervical smear shows sheets and tight clusters of cells and HCG. The margin of the cluster often shows nuclear palisading and feathering effect (Fig. 8.51). Individual cells show moderate nuclear enlargement,

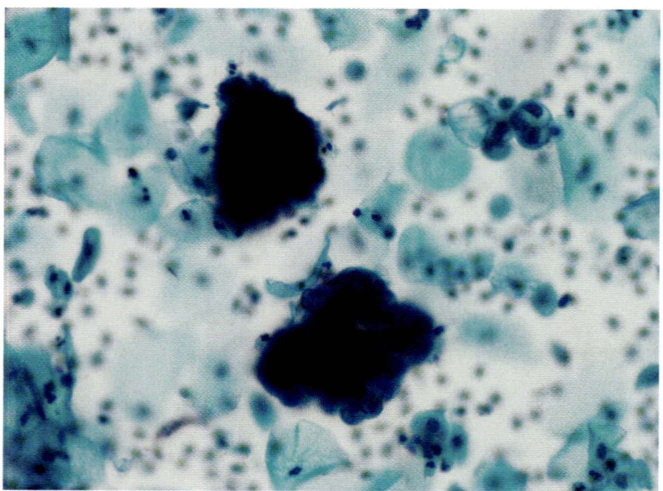

Fig. 8.51: Atypical glandular cell (AGC) favors neoplasia: Clusters of cells with moderate nuclear pleomorphism (Papanicolaou's stain in SurePath X MP).

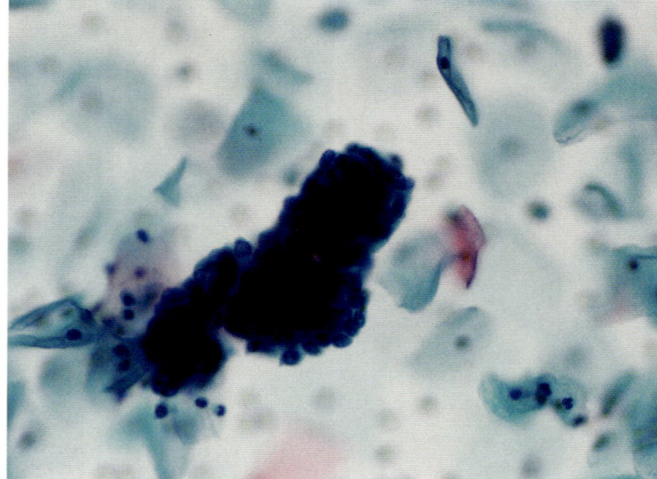

Fig. 8.52: Atypical glandular cell (AGC) possibly endometrial in origin: Tight cohesive cluster with scanty cytoplasm (Papanicolaou's stain in SurePath X MP).

Box 8.15: Atypical glandular cell (AGC), endocervical origin, favors neoplasia.

- Sheets and hyperchromatic crowded groups of cell
- Feathering effect
- Nucleus: enlarged, hyperchromatic, pleomorphic with irregular margin
- N/C ratio increased
- Mitosis increased

Box 8.16: Atypical endometrial cells.

- Small groups of cells
- Nucleus:
  - Mildly enlarged than normal endometrial cell
  - Mildly hyperchromatic
  - Small nucleoli
- Cytoplasm: Vacuolated

pleomorphism, and hyperchromasia. The nuclear abnormality of the cells falls short of AIS or adenocarcinoma. Mitotic figures may be seen frequently.

Atypical Endometrial Cells

Cytology (Fig. 8.52 and Box 8.16)

Smear shows small tight spherical cluster of cells. Individual cells have mildly enlarged hyperchromatic nuclei with small nucleoli and vacuolated cytoplasm.

Differential Diagnosis of Atypical Glandular Cell

These include:

- *Reactive endocervical cells*: The cells are present in flat sheet with minimal pleomorphism and bland chromatin.
- *Tubal metaplasia*: The presence of terminal plate and cilia of the cells indicate tubal metaplasia.
- *Intrauterine contraceptive device (IUCD)*: The clinical history of using IUCD, cytoplasmic vacuoles giving bubblegum appearance, degenerative changes in the cells, presence of psammoma bodies, and frequent presence of actinomycosis help in the distinguishing IUCD from AGC.
- *Radiation-induced changes*: Unaltered N/C ratio and degenerative changes of the cells are seen in radiation effect.
- *Endocervical polyp*: The presence of necrosis, inflammatory background, hyperchromatic crowded groups of cells, and reactive endocervical cells are diagnostic helpful features of endocervical polyp.

Management of AGC-US

They include:

- Colposcopy with endocervical sampling.
- Woman with atypical endometrial cells should have endometrial sampling.
- If no abnormality is identified then repeat PAP smears at 4–6 months interval should be done until four consecutive samples are negative.

Extrauterine Carcinoma

Uncommonly cervical smear may show malignant cells from ovary, Fallopian tube, colon, and breast. The malignant

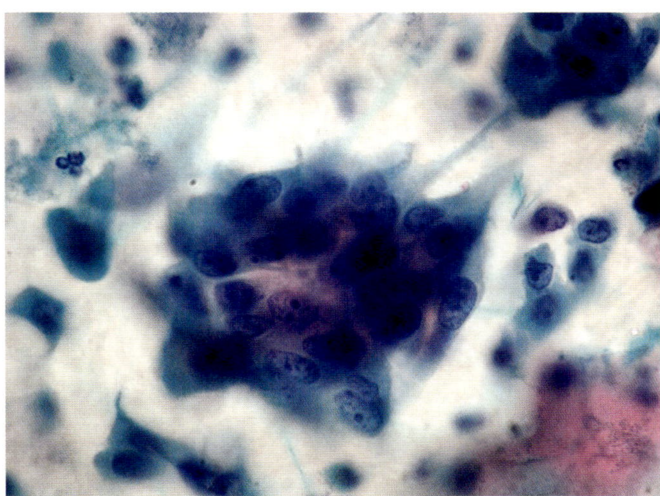

Fig. 8.53: Liquid-based cytology (LBC) smear (SurePath) of a case of adenocarcinoma of the ovary showing clusters and discrete malignant cells (Papanicolaou's stain X HP).

cells may either come to the cervix through the transtubal and uterine passage or they may be present due to the metastasis of the tumor in cervix. The cytomorphology of the malignant cells depends on the histological features of the primary malignancy. The thorough clinical history is helpful for the exact diagnosis of metastatic carcinoma. Adenocarcinoma of the ovary usually shows clusters and discrete malignant cells in cervical smear (Fig. 8.53). Individual cells show moderately pleomorphic nuclei with single to multiple prominent nucleoli. Unlike uterine or cervical adenocarcinoma, tumor diathesis is not seen in such cases.

REFERENCES

1. Bosch FX, de Sanjose S. Chapter 1: Human papillomavirus and cervical cancer—burden and assessment of causality. J Natl Cancer Inst Monogr. 2003;31:3-13.
2. Ho GY, Bierman R, Beardsley L, et al. Natural history of cervicovaginal papillomavirus infection in young women. N Engl J Med. 1998;338(7):423-8.
3. Richart RM, Barron BA. A follow up study of patients with cervical dysplasia. Am J Obstet Gynecol. 1969;105:386-93.
4. Ostor AG. Natural history of cervical intraepithelial neoplasia: a critical review. Int J Gynecol Pathol. 1993;12:186-92.
5. Burk RD, Chen Z, Van Doorslaer K. Human papillomaviruses: genetic basis of carcinogenicity. Public Health Genomics. 2009;12:281-90.
6. Motoyama S, Ladines-llave CA, Villanueva SL, et al. The role of human papilloma virus in the molecular biology of cervical carcinogenesis. Kobe J Med Sci. 2004;50(1):9-19.
7. Reagan JW, Seidemann IL, Patten SF. Developmental stages of in situ carcinoma in uterine cervix: an analytical study of cells. Acta Cytol. 1953;6:538-46.
8. Poulsen ME, Taylor CW, Sobin LM. Histological Typing of Female Genital Tract Tumours. Geneva: World Health Organization; 1975;15-18, 55-62.
9. Richart RM, Barron BA. Screening strategies for cervical cancer and cervical intraepithelial neoplasia. Cancer. 1981;47:1176-81.
10. Solomon D, Schiffman M, Tarone R. Comparison of three management strategies for patients with atypical squamous cells of undetermined significance: baseline results from a randomized trial. J Natl Cancer Inst. 2001;93: 293-9.
11. Smith PA, Turnbull LS. Small cell and pale dyskaryosis. Cytopathology. 1997;8:3-8.
12. Denton K, Rana DN, Lynch MA, et al. Bland dyskaryosis: a new pitfall in liquid-based cytology. Cytopathology. 2008;19(3):162-6.
13. Demay RM. Hyperchromatic crowded groups: pitfalls in pap smear diagnosis. Am J Clin Pathol. 2000;114(Suppl): S36-43.
14. Wright TC Jr, Cox JT, Massad LS, et al. 2001 Consensus Guidelines for the management of women with cervical cytological abnormalities. JAMA. 2002;287(16):2120-9.
15. Smith AE, Sherman ME, Scott DR, et al. Review of the Bethesda System atlas does not improve reproducibility or accuracy in the classification of atypical squamous cells of undetermined significance smears. Cancer. 2000;90: 201-6.
16. Davey DD, Neal MH, Wilbur DC, et al. Bethesda 2001implementation and reporting rates: 2003 practices of participants in the College of American Pathologists Interlaboratory Comparison Program in Cervicovaginal Cytology. Arch Pathol Lab Med. 2004;128(11):1224-9.
17. Wright TC Jr, Massad LS, Dunton CJ, et al. 2006 consensus guidelines for the management of women with abnormal cervical cancer screening tests. Am J Obstet Gynecol. 2007;197(4):346-55.
18. Massad LS, Einstein MH, Huh WK, et al. 2012 updated consensus guidelines for the management of abnormal cervical cancer screening tests and cancer precursors. Obstet Gynecol. 2013;121(4):829-46.
19. Wang SS, Sherman ME, Hildesheim A, et al. Cervical adenocarcinoma and squamous cell carcinoma incidence trends among white women and black women in the United States for 1976-2000. Cancer. 2004;100(5): 1035-44.
20. Castellsague X, Diaz M, de Sanjose S, et al. Worldwide human papillomavirus etiology of cervical adenocarcinoma and its cofactors: implications for screening and prevention. J Natl Cancer Inst. 2006;98(5):303-15.
21. Schnatz PF, Guile M, O'Sullivan DM, et al. Clinical significance of atypical glandular cells on cervical cytology. Obstet Gynecol. 2006;107(3):701-8.

Review Questions

1. **What is associated with this condition in the cervical smear (Fig. 8.54)?**
   a. HSV
   b. HPV 16
   c. *Trichomonas vaginalis*
   d. Nonspecific inflammation
2. **High-risk HPV type is/are:**
   a. HPV 6
   b. HPV 11
   c. HPV 16
   d. All of the above
3. **The function of p53 is inhibited by HPV protein:**
   a. E4
   b. E6
   c. E7
   d. E2
4. **Progression of CIN1 to CIN3 occurs in:**
   a. 60% cases
   b. 50% cases
   c. 30% cases
   d. 10% cases
5. **The probable management of this patient with cervical smear (Fig. 8.55) should be:**
   a. HPV test
   b. Repeat cervical smear after 6 months
   c. Colposcopy and biopsy
   d. Routine test after 3-year interval
6. **The most probable diagnosis of this routine cervical smear (Figs. 8.56A to D) is:**
   a. HSIL
   b. LSIL
   c. ASCUS
   d. Squamous cell carcinoma
7. **A 39-year-old female is presented with adnexal mass. Routine cervical smear is shown in Figures 8.57A to D. What is your diagnosis?**
   a. Adenocarcinoma
   b. Endometrial cells
   c. HSIL
   d. Benign endocervical cells

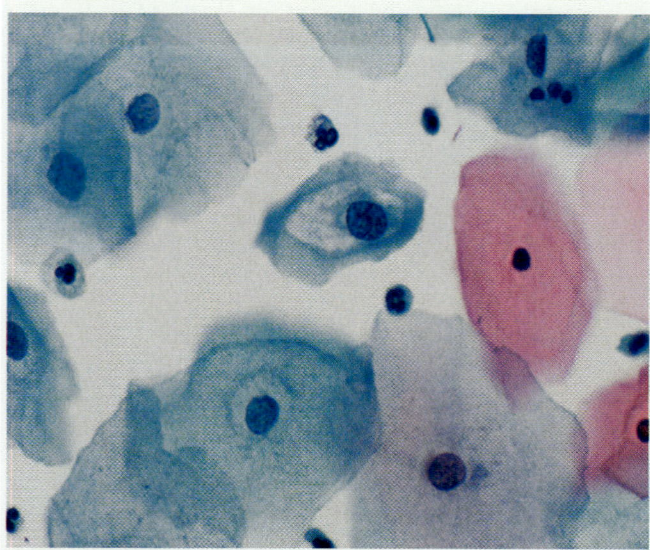

Fig. 8.54: Cervical cytology of question 1.

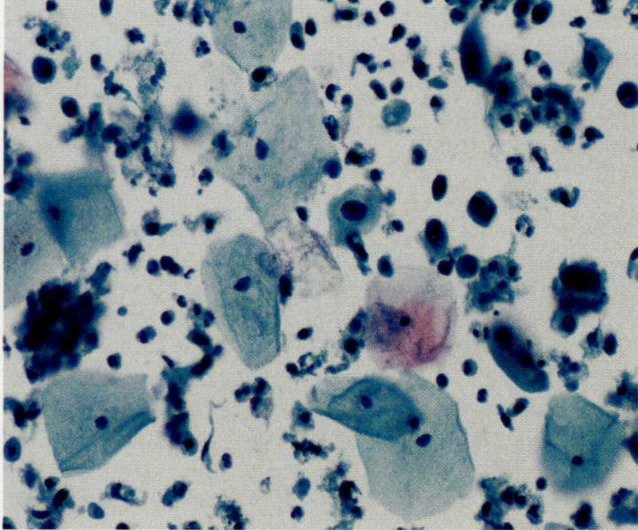

Fig. 8.55: Cervical cytology of question 5.

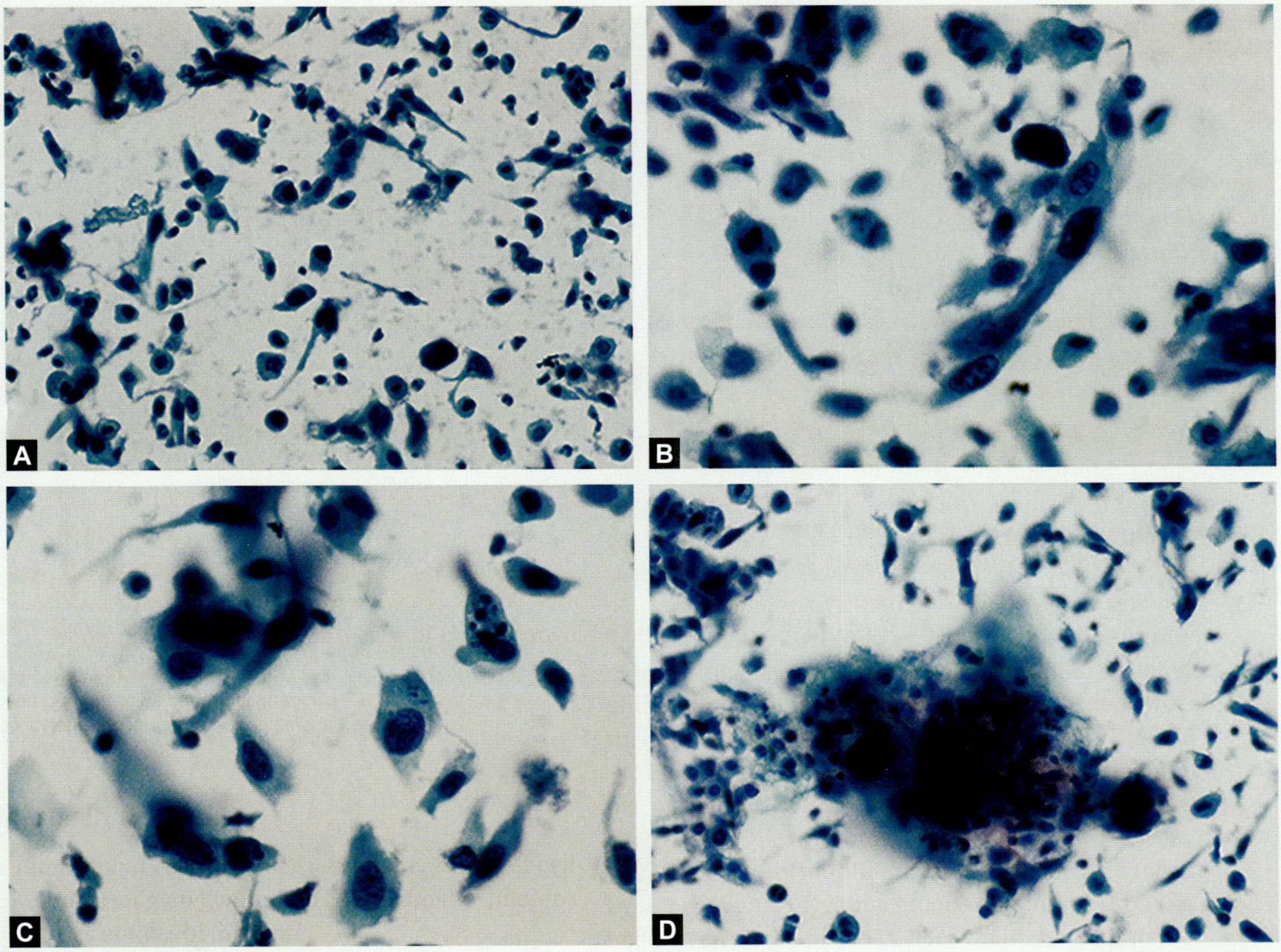

Figs. 8.56A to D: Cervical cytologyof question 6.

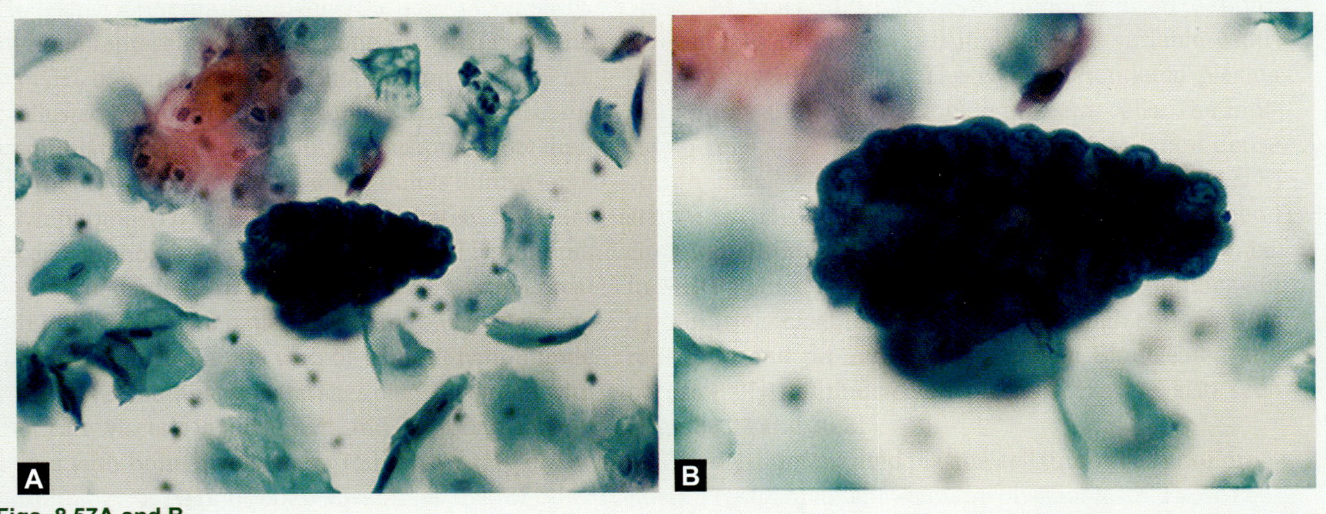

Figs. 8.57A and B

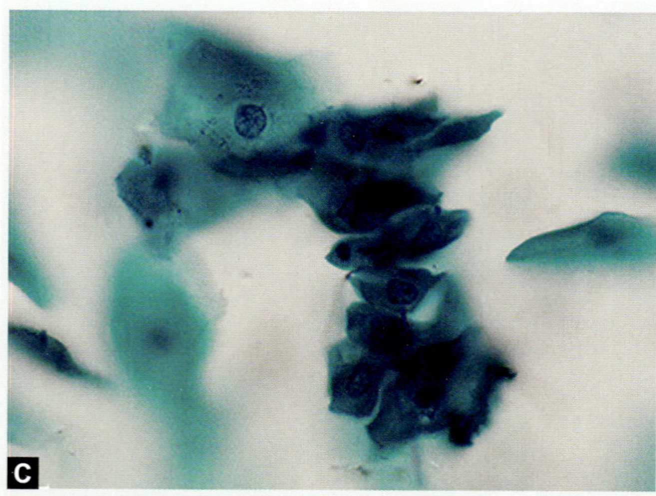

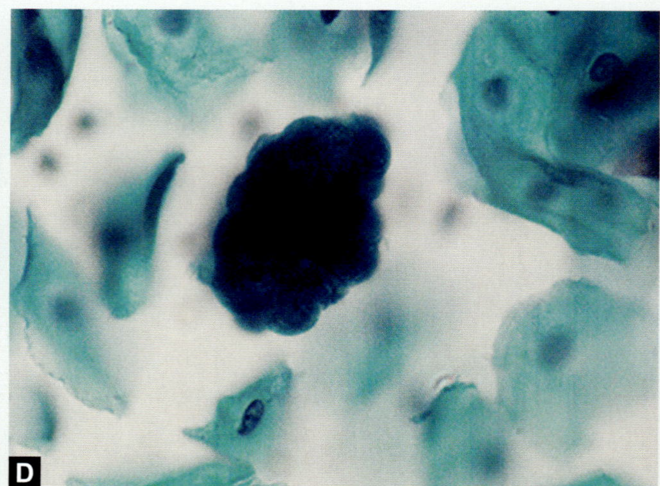

Figs. 8.57A to D: Cervical cytology of question 7.

Answers

1. b. HPV 16
   Note: This is typical koilocytotic cells and HPV 16 causes koilocytoctic changes.
2. c. HPV 16
3. b. E6
4. d. 10% cases
5. c. Colposcopy and biopsy
   Note: The smear shows HSIL and a possibility of squamous cell carcinoma cannot be ruled out in this smear. Colposcopy and biopsy is preferable in this case.
6. d. Squamous cell carcinoma
   Note: The smears show moderately pleomorphic cells with hyperchromatic nuclei. Many tadpole cells and also tumor diathesis (Fig. 8.56D) are present that indicate invasive carcinoma.
7. a. Adenocarcinoma
   Note: The tight cohesive tumor cells with round nuclei and high N:C ratio and prominent nucleoli indicate adenocarcinoma.

CHAPTER 9

Cervical Cancer Screening Program

INTRODUCTION

Cervical cancer is the second most common cancer in women in the world and the most common cancer in developing countries.[1] It is considered as a leading public health problem. Detection of cervical cancer on cervical cytology helped a lot to decrease the incidence of cervical cancer in developed countries.

PARAMETERS TO MEASURE THE VALIDITY OF SCREENING TESTS

There are several parameters to measure the efficacy of a screening test.

- *Sensitivity*: Sensitivity refers to the ability of the test to detect the disease that means it detects the proportion of positive result among the total number of disease positive cases.

$$\text{Sensitivity} = \frac{\text{True positive}}{\text{True positive} + \text{false negative}} \times 100\%$$

- *Specificity*: This term means ability to exclude the presence of disease that means it indicates the percentage of negative cases reported among the total number of negative cases.

$$\text{Specificity} = \frac{\text{True negative}}{\text{True negative} + \text{false positive}} \times 100\%$$

  True positive means a genuine indication of the presence of disease and true negative means genuine absence of the disease. Similarly, false positive means the test reported as positive but in reality the person is free of disease. False negative indicates that the test reported as negative, but in reality, the case is positive of the disease.

- *Positive predictive value*: Positive predictive value (PPV) measures the reliability of positive tests in predicting the presence of disease. So, PPV measures the proportion of real positives among all positive results reported by the test.

  Positive predictive value

$$= \frac{\text{True positive}}{\text{True positive} + \text{false positive}} \times 100\%$$

- *Negative predictive value*:

$$= \frac{\text{True negative cases}}{\text{True negative cases} + \text{false negative cases}}$$

The sensitivity and specificity of conventional Papanicolaou (PAP) test varies widely ranging from 30 to 80% and 86 to 100%, respectively.[2] The mean sensitivity of cervical smear is 47% and the mean specificity is 95%.

SCREENING GUIDELINES

Start Age of the Target Population

World Health Organization (WHO): It recommends 30 years[3] as start age because most of the females with human papillomavirus (HPV) infection spontaneously improve.

American Society for Colposcopy and Cervical Pathology (ASCCP): It recommends 21 years as start age.

Stop of Age

Majority of the program considers 65 years as stop age provided the female has previous normal cervical cytology report.

Frequency

ASCCP: 3 years interval.
WHO: Every 3–5 years.

Mode of Screening

ASCCP: *21–30 years*: The women should be primarily screened by cervical cytology alone.[4]

31–65 years: (1) The screening of women between 31 to 65 years should be done either by cervical cytology 3 yearly with HPV testing as a triage of atypical squamous cells of undetermined significance (ASCUS) patients, (2) Alternatively cervical cytology with HPV cotesting at 5-year interval.

WHO: Either by cervical cytology or HPV high-risk testing or visual inspection of cervix with acetic acid (VIA) depending on resource.

TYPES OF MODALITIES FOR CERVICAL CANCER SCREENING

There are different modalities for cervical cancer screening. These are:

- Conventional cervical PAP test
- Liquid-based cytology
- HPV testing
- Colposcopy
- VIA
- Automated cervical screening techniques.

Table 9.1 has compared different modalities of cervical cancer screening.

Conventional PAP Smear

Conventional PAP smear is still considered as gold standard in cervical cytology screening. It is moderately sensitivity but highly specific. Effective PAP smear screening needs well-organized program, dedicated trained personnel and good laboratory support.

Liquid-based Cytology

The sample is collected in liquid media instead of directly spreading on the glass slide. Later on, the collected sample in liquid media is processed accordingly. Liquid-based cytology helps in avoiding in air-drying artifact and increased adequacy of the samples. The monolayered cellular smear is easy to screen. Moreover, the residual sample in the vial can be used for further ancillary investigations such as HPV DNA testing. The overall adequacy rate of liquid-based cytology (LBC) is higher than the conventional PAP smear. However, the sensitivity and specificity of LBC is not remarkably high compared to conventional PAP test. The current evidence is not adequate enough to recommend replacing conventional PAP smear testing by LBC.[8] The cost-effectiveness of LBC needs to be assessed very carefully in developing countries.

Human Papillomavirus DNA Test

Human papillomavirus DNA testing for high-risk HPV such as HPV 16, 18, 31, 33, 35, 39, 45, 51, 52, 56, 59, and 68 is a potentially useful screening test. There is a recent trend to use high-risk HPV testing as a primary screening technique because all cervical cancer is primarily related with HPV infection. Studies have shown that HPV-based screening provides 70% greater protection against carcinoma of cervix compared to cytology-based screening.[9]

Advantages of Human Papillomavirus Test

- Highly sensitive 95–100%
- Sample is easy to collect

Limitations

- High cost of the test
- *Low-specificity*: 75–84%.

There are three ways to use HPV testing:

1. *ASCUS triage*: Selected HPV testing only in ASCUS cases to reduce colposcopic burden.

Table 9.1: Comparison of different modalities of cervical cancer screening.

Methods	*Sensitivity*	*Specificity*	*Advantages*	*Disadvantages*
Conventional PAP test	30–80%	86–100%	Easy, cheap, effective	Needs organized approach, laboratory-based, stringent quality control needed
Liquid-based cytology[5]	61–66%	82–91%	No air drying effect, adequate, clean background, multiple smears and HPV DNA test possible from residual material	Costly, trained personnel for interpretation
VIA[6]	67–79%	49–86%	Low cost, easy to do, high sensitivity	Low specificity and high false positivity. Stringent quality control is needed
Colposcopy	44–77%	85–90%	High specificity	Expensive, slow, not possible to cover large population and in low resource area
HPV test[7]	88–100%	61–96%	Highly sensitive, objective, reproducible, robust	Costly

(PAP: Papanicolaou; HPV: Human papillomavirus; VIA: Visual inspection of cervix with acetic acid).

2. *Cotesting of cytology and HPV testing*: Both cervical cytology and HPV testing at the same time to increase the sensitivity of the screening. High sensitivity of HPV testing and high specificity of cervical cytology provide the balance. Therefore, screening interval can be raised if contesting is used.
3. *Primary HPV testing*: HPV testing is done as primary screening test and cytology to do only in positive HPV cases. HPV as primary screening test is recommended only in women after 30 years of age.

Types of Human Papillomavirus Testing

A large number of commercially available HPV tests are present in the market. However, only a few HPV tests are the Food and Drug Administration (FDA) approved.

Primary Screening over 30-year of Age and ASCUS Triage over 21-year

Hybrid capture 2 (HC 2), Cervista HPV HR, Cobas 4800 System, and Aptima mRNA.

Hybrid Capture 2

It is a quantitative test for HPV. In this test, patient's DNA is hybridized with a specific RNA cocktail probe of HPV virus. The RNA-DNA hybrid is captured on the surface of microplate well that is coated with anti-RNA-DNA antibody and is demonstrated by antibody against DNA-RNA hybrid conjugated with alkaline phosphatase and chemiluminescent substrate. HC 2 has high analytical sensitivity and can detect 1,000–5,000 copies/reaction.

Cervista Human Papillomavirus High Risk

Cervista HPV HR identifies 14 high-risk HPV subtypes including HPV 16 and 18. It is a qualitative in vitro diagnostic test that uses nucleic acid signal amplification method to detect specific nucleic acid sequence of the HPV. Its analytical sensitivity is 1,250–2,500 copies/reaction.

Cobas 4800 System

This is polymerase chain reaction (PCR)-based highly sensitive method. Its analytical sensitivity is 150 copies/mL.

Aptima mRNA

It is a qualitative nucleic acid amplification test that detects E6/E7 mRNA of high-risk HPV. Its analytical sensitivity is 24–488 copies/reaction.

Visual Inspection of Cervix with Acetic Acid

This is a relatively simple technique with high sensitivity and low specificity.

Method

Dilute acetic acid (3–5%) is applied to cervix using a cotton swab or a spray and then the cervix is inspected after 2 minutes. Detection of well-defined acetowhite area near transformation zone is regarded as positive for VIA. Acetowhite area in cervical intraepithelial neoplasia (CIN) is well demarcated, intensely opaque, and localized to the squamocolumnar junction. Acetowhite area is possibly due to a reversible coagulation of intracellular proteins following acetic acid application.

Advantages

- Easy to do and so can be done in remote area by health care personnel
- Low cost
- Immediate result.

Limitations

High false positivity as acetowhite area can also be seen in squamous metaplasia, inflammation and repair.

Colposcopy

It is one of the important modes of cervical cancer screening. Colposcopy helps to find out the source of abnormal cells in cytology smear. It is a binocular stereotactic microscope that produces magnified image of the cervical mucosa. The colposcopic appearance of the cervical mucosa depends mainly on the architecture of the surface epithelium, connecting tissue stroma and vasculature of the tissue. The normal cervical epithelium is translucent and gives pink color, whereas the dysplastic epithelium is thickened with altered vascular pattern and therefore produces the white opaque appearance (Fig. 9.1). This is further accentuated by prior application of 3% acetic acid over the cervical mucosa. Colposcopic examination needs to consider the following points:

- *Surface alteration*: Any growth over the surface.
- *Color*: Alteration of normal pink color to white opaque area. This is due to thick surface epithelium and epithelial cells with increased nucleocytoplasmic ratio.

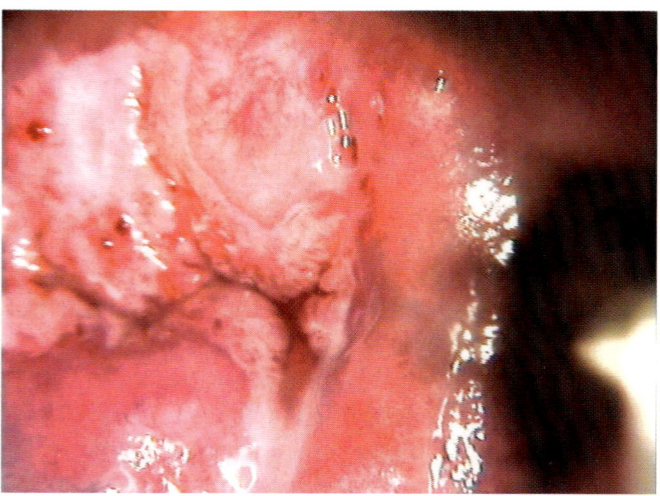

Fig. 9.1: Opaque white area on colposcopy in a case of cervical intraepithelial neoplasia.
Source: Courtesy by Dr Subhash Chandra Saha, Additional Professor, Department of Gynecology and Obstetrics, PGIMER, Chandigarh, India.

- *Vascular pattern*: There may be significant variation of vascular pattern in dysplastic epithelium. The following changes of vascular pattern are seen:
  - *Mosaicism*: Capillaries are arranged in such a way that the tissue looks like honeycomb.
  - *Punctuation*: End of the capillaries shows a red dot-like appearance.
  - *Atypical vessels*: Vessels show variable thickness and complex branching pattern.

Colposcopy cannot be used in routine screening because it is a time-consuming procedure, expensive, and needs a lot of experience.

Automated Cervical Screening Techniques

Described in Chapter 21.

Essential Elements for Successful Cervical Cancer Screening

World Health Organization recommended certain essential elements of a successful cervical screening program.[1] Cervical screening program should be:

- The part of a national screening program and ministry of health should provide the budget.
- Adequate healthcare system is mandatory for the implementation of a successful cervical screening program.
- Target population to be screened should be well-defined.
- Target population should be properly educated.
- Adequate means to identify and invite the target population.
- Training of the healthcare personnel is needed.
- There should be well-defined referral center and further management of the patient whenever needed.
- Proper guideline or protocol of the management.
- There should be proper means to identify the failure of the program.

Problems of Screening in Developing Countries

In developing and underdeveloped countries, cervical cancer screening program faces several hurdles. These hurdles are related with political motivation, financial strictures, proper education, etc. Important obstacles against successful cervical screening in these countries are:

- Poor healthcare budget on cervical screening
- Poor financial and healthcare resources
- Poorly organized healthcare system
- Ill-educated target population
- Poor laboratory and other pathology facilities.[10]

False-negative Cytology

This is one of the important indicators of successful cervical cytology screening. It can be simply said that a report is a false negative when the patient has actually the disease process. Van der Graff reported false-negative cytology as "cervical epithelial abnormality is diagnosed in a woman who had previously been negative but the former negative smear did not contain the abnormality or when an existing abnormality, present at that time of initial investigation, was not recognized through interpretative error or sampling error",[11] whereas Davey described false-negative cytology as an originally negative test report that is found to have sufficient number of dysplastic or carcinoma cells on review.[12] These abnormal cells should always be verified by more than one experienced cytologists.

The false-negative fraction is defined as:[13]

False negative fraction

$$= \frac{\text{Estimated false negative results}}{(\text{True positive results} + \text{estimated false negative results})} \times 100\%$$

The exact incidence of false-negative cytology is difficult to assess due to differences in the definition of this entity. However, false-negative cytology varies from 1.6 to 2.7%.[14]

The etiological causes of false-negative cytology are:

- *Sampling error*: Abnormal cells are not present in the smear due to faulty sampling technique or faulty smear preparation.
- *Interpretation error*:
  - *Abnormal cells are not detected at all*: This may be due to too little cells or cells are obscured by blood or mucus.
  - Abnormal cells are wrongly interpreted as normal.

Various studies have shown that sampling error is the main source of false-negative cytology.[15] The quality of the smear may be hampered by air-drying effect, blood, mucus, or necrotic material. Moreover, in conventional cytology the major amount of cells is not transferred to the slide. Failure to obtain samples from transformation zone and lack of endocervical may be another possible cause of false-negative cytology.[16]

Screening error may be another important cause of false-negative cytology. The abnormal cells may be missed due to loss of concentration, fatigue, or inadequate training.

Remedies to Avoid False-negative Cytology

Sampling error: This can be avoided by

- Adequate training for healthcare personnel for better sampling
- Liquid-based cytology to obtain more representative cells in clean background.

Interpretation error: This can be avoided by

- Adequate training of the screener and cytologist.
- *Rescreening*: Negative cytology cases may be rescreened in various ways such as
  - *100% rapid review*: To screen all negative cases rapidly within 30 seconds.
  - *Rescreening of 10% smear*: To screen only 10% of the negative cases randomly.
  - *Selective rescreening*: To screen only high-risk individuals such as previous history of atypical cytology, prostitutes, patients with postmenopausal bleeding, etc.
  - *Automated rescreening*: To take the help of machine for the detection of abnormal cells and then further confirmation by a cytologist.

REFERENCES

1. Castellsagué X, Sanjosé SD, Aguado T, et al. HPV and Cervical Cancer in the World. 2007 Report. WHO/ICO Information Centre on HPV and Cervical Cancer (HPV Information Centre). Available from www.who.int/hpvcentre.
2. Nanda K, McCrory DC, Myers ER, et al. Accuracy of the Papanicolaou test in screening for and follow-up of cervical cytologic abnormalities: a systemic review. Ann Intern Med. 2000;132:810-9.
3. WHO. (2013). Guidelines for screening and treatment of precancerous lesion for cervical cancer prevention. [online] Available from www.who.int/reproductivehealth/publications/cancers/screening_and_treatment_of_precancerous_lesions/en/ [Accessed March 2017].
4. Saslow D, Solomon D, Lawson HW, et al. American Cancer Society, American Society for Colposcopy and Cervical Pathology, and American Society for Clinical Pathology Screening Guidelines for the Prevention and Early Detection of Cervical Cancer. CA Cancer J Clin. 2012;62: 147-72.
5. Coste J, Cochand-Priollet B, de Cremoux P, et al. Cross sectional study of conventional cervical smear, monolayer cytology, and human papillomavirus DNA testing for cervical cancer screening. BMJ. 2003;326(7392):733.
6. Sankaranarayanan R, Gaffikin L, Jacob M, et al. A critical assessment of screening methods for cervical neoplasia. Int J Gynaecol Obstet. 2005;89(Suppl 2):S4-12.
7. Kulasingam SL, Hughes JP, Kiviat NB, et al. Evaluation of human papillomavirus testing in primary screening for cervical abnormalities comparison of sensitivity, specificity, and frequency of referral. JAMA. 2002;288(14):1749-57.
8. Hartmann EK, Nanda K, Hall S, et al. Technological advances for cervical cancer screening-Is newer better? Obstet Gynecol Surv. 2001;56:765-74.
9. Valentine K, Vanden Broeck D, Benoy I, et al. Cytology at the time of HPV: Some things to think about when discussing HPV. Acta Cytol. 2016;60(6):527-33.
10. Denny L, Quinn M, Sankaranarayanan R. Screening for cervical cancer in developing countries. Vaccine. 2006;24 (Suppl 3):S3/71-7.
11. van der Graaff Y, Vooijs GP, Gaillard HL, et al. Screening errors in cervical cytologic screening. Acta Cytol. 1987;31 (4):434-8.
12. Davey DD. Quality and liability issues with the Papanicolaou's smear. Arch Pathol Lab Med. 1997;121:261-9.
13. Dolinar J, Ollayos CW, Tellado M, et al. The false-negative fraction: a statistical method to measure the efficacy of cervical smear screening laboratories. Mil Med. 1999;164(6):410-1.
14. Naryshkin S. The false-negative fraction for Papanicolaou smears: how often are "abnormal" smears not detected by a "standard" screening cytologist? Arch Pathol Lab Med. 1997;121(3):270-2.
15. Sodhani P, Singh V, Das DK, et al. Cytohistological correlation as a measure of quality assurance of cytology screening. Cytopathology. 1997;8(2):103-7.
16. Mitchell H, Medley G. Cellular differences between true negative and false negative Papanicolaou smears. Cytopathology. 1993;4(5):285-90.

Review Questions

1. **World Health Organization (WHO) recommends that start age of the cervical screening program should be:**
   a. 21 years
   b. 30 years
   c. Just after the sexual activity
   d. 35 years
2. **Polymerase chain reaction (PCR)-based highly sensitive method for human papillomavirus (HPV) DNA detection is:**
   a. Hybrid capture 2
   b. Cervista HPV HR
   c. Cobas 4800 System
   d. Aptima mRNA
3. **The percentage of negative cases reported among the total number of negative cases is known as:**
   a. Sensitivity
   b. Specificity
   c. Positive predictive value
   d. Negative predictive value
4. **Which is not true for human papillomavirus (HPV) test in cervical screening:**
   a. Highly sensitive compared to cytology
   b. Highly specific compared to cytology
   c. Primary HPV testing is recommended only after 30 years of age
   d. Same sample can be processed for cytology and HPV test both.

Answers

1. b. 30 years
2. c. Cobas 4800 System
3. b. Specificity
4. b. Highly specific compared to cytology

CHAPTER 10

Effusion Cytology

ANATOMY AND HISTOLOGY OF BODY CAVITIES

There are three body cavities: (1) pleural, (2) pericardial, and (3) peritoneal (Fig. 10.1). These cavities and visceral organs are lined by a thin layer of mesothelial cells. In normal healthy person these cavities are collapsed and retain only a potential space with thin lubricating fluid. The mesothelial layer that covers the visceral organ is called as visceral layer and the outer layer is known as parietal layer. Each lung in the thoracic cavity is lined by visceral pleura and the potential space is known as the pleural cavity. The pleural that is attached to the chest wall is known as parietal pleura. There is no anatomical connection between the two pleural spaces. Similarly, the heart is within the pericardial sac and most of the abdominal organs are within the peritoneal cavity. The peritoneal cavity is the largest serosal sac in our body and it is derived from the coelomic cavity of the embryo. It contains about scanty fluid that has lubricant and anti-inflammatory effect.

The visceral layer of pleura consists of a single layer of small cuboidal mesothelial cells (Fig. 10.2). These cells rest on fibrovascular connective tissue, blood vessels, and nerves.

Fig. 10.1: Schematic diagram of body cavities: pericardial, pleural, and peritoneal.

EFFUSION

Under normal physiologic condition, fluid is produced by the parietal pleura and is absorbed by capillaries and lymphatic of visceral pleura. Accumulation of excess fluid in the body cavity is labeled as "effusion". Effusion is always a pathologic process. Clinically effusion can be divided as: transudative and exudative.

Transudative Effusion

Transudative fluid is caused by the disturbance of hydrostatic pressure and/or osmotic pressure, and it represents the ultrafiltrate of plasma. The wall of the blood vessels in transudative effusion is intact. The common causes of

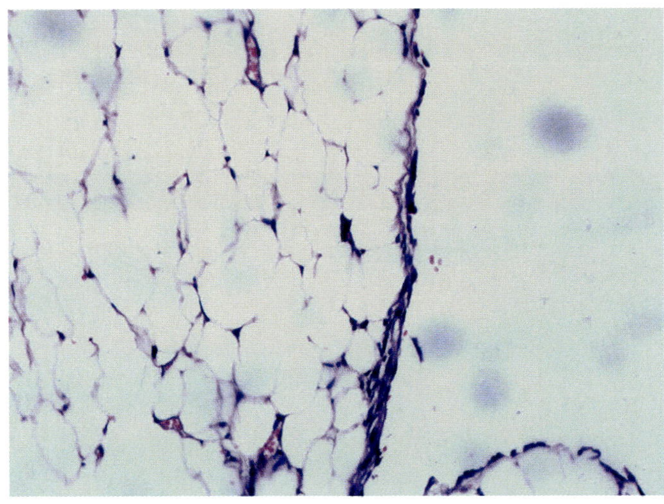

Fig. 10.2: A single layer of flat to small cuboidal mesothelial cells as lining of peritoneal surface (hematoxylin and eosin × MP).

transudate are congestive cardiac failure, cirrhosis of liver, and renal failure. Transudate has a low specific gravity (less than 1.015), low protein content, and scanty cellularity. The cells in transudate are usually mesothelial cells and occasional lymphocytes or polymorphs.

Exudative Effusion

Exudate is caused by the damage to the wall of the blood capillaries of the mesothelial lining. This damage of the capillaries may be due to inflammation or by direct damage by malignant cells. The common causes of transudative effusions are infection, collagen vascular disease, and malignancy. Comparison of transudative and exudative effusion is shown in Table 10.1. Exudative effusion has a higher specific gravity (more than 1.015), high protein content (more than 3 g/100 mL), high lactate dehydrogenase content, high in fibrin, and rich in cells.

Malignancy usually causes exudative effusion by damaging the wall of the blood vessels. However, the tumor may block the lymphatic channels by pressure effect and may cause transudative effusion.

Appearance of Effusion Sample

The following thing should be noted carefully in all effusion fluid.

Volume

Exact amount of fluid should be recorded.

Color

Color of the fluid is important. Transudative fluid is usually light straw color. Blood-tinged fluid is reddish in color. The gross presence of blood may be due to direct trauma of vessels during collection of fluid, or it may indicate malignancy. Chylous fluid is milky in color that is usually noted in lymphatic obstruction. Dark brown fluid may be due to old hemorrhage. Chocolate brown fluid is noted in malignant melanoma.

Table 10.1: Difference between transudate and exudate.

Features	*Transudate*	*Exudate*
Appearance	Clear	Turbid
Specific gravity	Less than 1.015	More than 1.015
Protein content	Less than 3 g/100 mL	Above 3 g/100 mL
Fibrin	Low, does not coagulate	High, coagulates if kept
Lactate dehydrogenase	Low	High
Cells	Scanty cells	Rich in cells
Significance	Rarely contains malignant cells	Often contains malignant cells

Consistency

Viscosity of the fluid may give important information. Fluid in mesothelioma is rich in hyaluronic acid and may have increased consistency like honey. Thick gelatinous consistency of fluid is seen particularly in pseudomyxoma peritonei.

Smell

Any unusual smell of the fluid should be noted.

SPECIMEN COLLECTION AND PROCESSING

A collection of effusion fluid from the body cavity is a relatively easy process. This is done under local anesthesia by inserting a wide bore needle into the body cavity affected by effusion. Thus, the collection of effusion fluid from the thoracic cavity, pericardial cavity, and peritoneal cavity is known as thoracocentesis, pericardiocentesis, and paracentesis, respectively. At a time one should not draw more than 1.5 L of fluid from the pleural cavity as this may cause rebound phenomenon and development of pneumothorax. The effusion fluid should be collected in a clean container. We prefer to collect fluid in anticoagulant solution (9:1, fluid:ammonium oxalate). However, many laboratories prefer fresh sample without any anticoagulant. If necessary, effusion fluid can be kept in refrigerator at 4°C for a few days. Under any circumstances fluid should not be frozen.

Processing (Box 10.1)

Centrifugation

The specimen of fluid should be shaken before the processing so that the cells are well dispersed. Approximate 50 mL fluid is centrifuged and the supernatant is discarded. Three to four smears are made from the sediment.

Box 10.1: Processing of effusion sample.

- *Centrifugation*: Specimen centrifuged and supernatant is discarded. Multiples smears for Papanicolaou's stain and May-Grünwald Giemsa stain.
- *Cell block*: Centrifuged sample treated with plasma followed by thrombin. Clot fixed by 10% formalin and then processed in tissue processor.
- Liquid-based preparation
- Ancillary technique:
  - Sample for flow cytometry
  - Other techniques.

We usually make one air-dried smear for May-Grünwald Giemsa (MGG) stain and three alcohol fixed (95% ethanol) smears for Papanicolaou's stain. Extra smears are kept for further special stains, if required.

Liquid-based Preparation

As cells in effusion fluid is in liquid media so it is not necessary to keep sample for liquid-based cytology. However, liquid-based cytology preparation may yield good cellularity and the cells are spread in a small area.

Cell Block

It is always advisable to make a cell block from the residual sample. The residual sediment is mixed with plasma and then drops of thrombin. The sample is clotted. The clot is fixed with 10% buffered formalin for 30 minutes. The fixed clot is then wrapped in filter paper and is processed for paraffin embedding.

Advantages of Cell Block

- Cell block sample allows to perform special stains, immunocytochemistry (ICC), etc. because multiple slides can be made from the block.
- Tissue can be kept as archival material for future use.
- Morphologic comparison with histopathology section is possible.
- As cell blocks enmesh all cells in clots so chances of detection of malignancy is high in the cell block.

ANCILLARY TESTS

Immunocytochemistry: From cell block.

Flow cytometry: The residual fluid after routine processing can be used for DNA flow cytometry and dual color flow cytometry.

BENIGN CELL POPULATION IN EFFUSION

The benign effusion fluid consists of mesothelial cells, macrophages, lymphocytes, polymorphs, etc.

Mesothelial Cells (Box 10.2)

These are the most common cells noted in effusion. Effusion, due to irrespective of the causes, contains mesothelial cells. These cells are shaded from the visceral or parietal lining and freely proliferate in the effusion fluid. Therefore, mesothelial cells may often show reactive changes and simulate malignant cells.

The mesothelial cells in smear are usually present discretely or as small monolayer clusters (Figs. 10.3 and 10.4). The individual cells are round in shape with moderate

Box 10.2: Mesothelial cells.

- Single and small clusters
- Uniform cell population
- Window-like pattern in between two adjacent cells
- Round cells with round nuclei
- Central to eccentric nuclei
- Prominent nucleoli
- Well-defined cytoplasmic border
- Cells appear to be surrounded by adjacent cell
- Cytoplasmic outpouchings or blebs
- Aggregates of cell may be arranged around a central lumen
- Cytochemistry:
  - Alcian blue positive
  - Periodic acid-Schiff's positive
- Immunocytochemistry
  - Positive for calretinin.

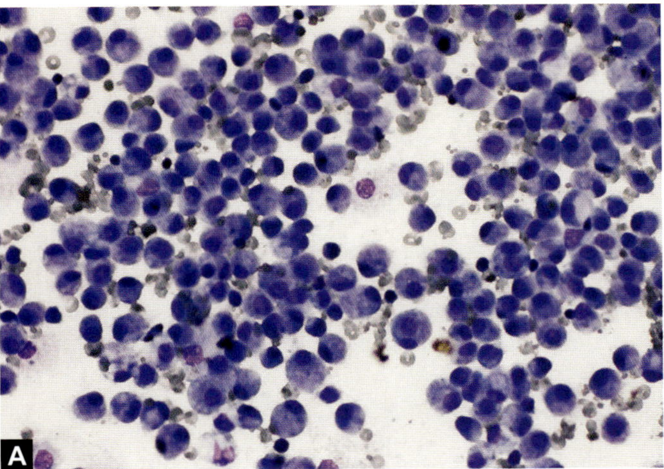

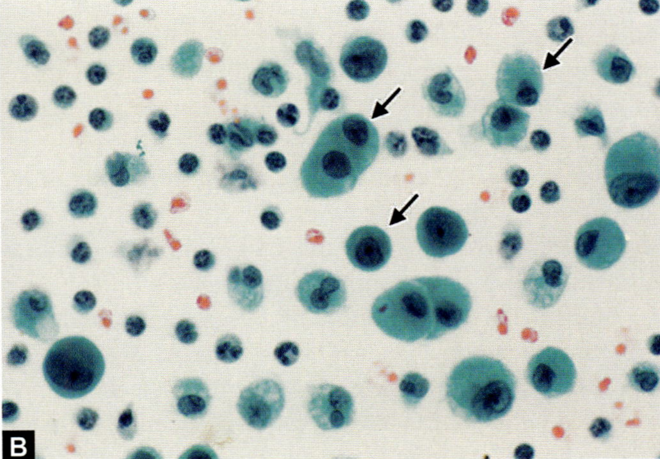

Figs. 10.3A and B: (A) Clusters and discrete mesothelial cells in peritoneal effusion (May-Grünwald Giemsa × MP) and (B) Discrete mesothelial cells in a benign effusion (*see* arrows) (Papanicolaou's stain × MP).

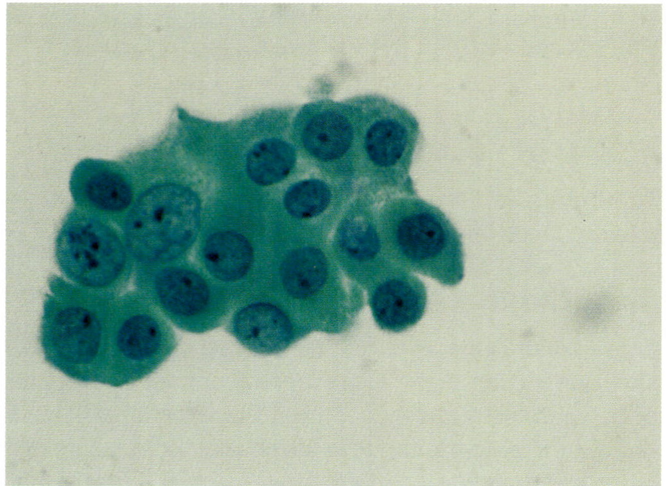

Fig. 10.4: Flat sheet of mesothelial cells with window-like gaps in between the cells (Papanicolaou's stain × HP).

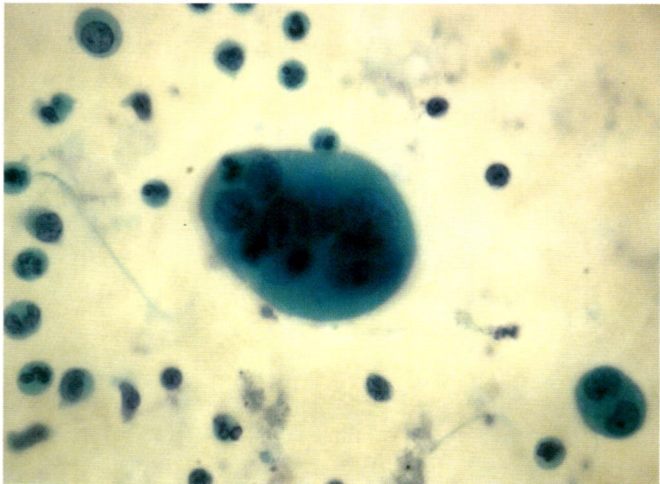

Fig. 10.5: Multinucleated giant cells in a benign effusion (Papanicolaou's stain × MP).

Box 10.3: Interpretation of mesothelial cells.

- **Do not over interpret** nuclear atypia of mesothelial cells
- Appropriate **importance** should be given to
  - Clinical details
  - Background cellular details such as intense inflammation
- Do not interpret a compromised smear
- Two cell population usually indicates malignancy
- Intense mesothelial cell hyperplasia is seen in
  - Cirrhosis
  - Uremia
  - Pulmonary infarct
- "Atypical mesothelial cell" terminology should be avoided.

amount of cytoplasm and central to eccentric nucleus. The nuclei show mild nuclear pleomorphism, smooth contour with uniformly granular chromatin and readily visible nucleoli. Mesothelial cells often show bi-nucleation, multinucleation (Fig. 10.5), nuclear pleomorphism, and multiple prominent nucleoli. However, the nuclei of the cells do not show marked atypia and these cells often attach to the other mesothelial cells that give indication of their mesothelial origin.

The groups of mesothelial cells often show a window-like space in between the cells. Which is due to the long slender microvilli of the cells that have been demonstrated ultrastructurally by scanning electron microscopy.

Mesothelial cells often show binucleation, multinucleation, and marked nuclear pleomorphism. This nuclear atypia depends upon the duration and intensity of inflammation. Therefore, the interpretation of effusion cytology smear should be carefully done and overall cellular background and clinical history should be given importance (Box 10.3).

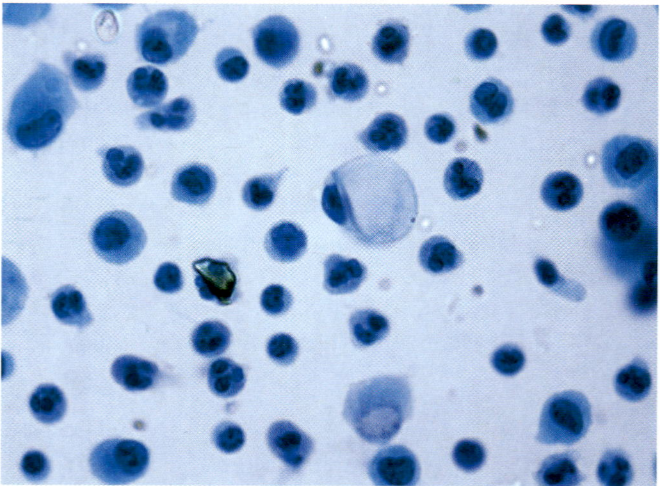

Fig. 10.6: Signet ring-like cells in a benign effusion in liquid based cytology preparation (Papanicolaou's stain × MP).

Longstanding effusion may cause small to large vacuoles within the cytoplasm of the mesothelial cells. Occasionally the large vacuoles may push the nucleus to the periphery and the cells may look signet ring (Fig. 10.6). Benign mesothelial cells with signet ring appearance should be distinguished from the malignant cells with signet ring cell. Nuclear morphology is the most important distinguishing feature to differentiate these two entities (Box 10.4).

Differential Diagnosis

- *Macrophages*: Mesothelial cells are difficult to distinguish from the macrophages (Table 10.2). Macrophages often contain phagocytosed material in their cytoplasm.

Box 10.4: Signet ring-like cells in effusion.

- Longstanding effusion may show such cells
- Round cells with abundant vacuolated cytoplasm and peripherally pushed nuclei
- Nuclear morphology is helpful in distinguishing the character of such cells
- Other conditions where such cells may be seen:
  - Signet ring carcinoma of stomach
  - Breast carcinoma
  - Ovarian adenocarcinoma
  - Therapy-related changes.

Table 10.3: Comparison of reactive mesothelial cells and mesothelioma.

Features	*Reactive mesothelial cells*	*Mesothelioma*
Cell cluster	Small loosely adhesive	Large clusters of cells, more than 10–12 cells
Cell size	Small	Relatively large
Nuclear pleomorphism	Mild	Moderate
Nucleoli	Small	Large
EMA	Weak positive	Strong positive
Glucose-transport protein 1 (GLUT-1)	Negative	Positive

Nuclei of macrophages are central in position with indistinct nucleoli.

- *Mesothelioma*: Malignant mesothelial cells may simulate reactive mesothelial cells (Table 10.3). The mesothelioma cells are in large groups, with moderate nuclear pleomorphism and often show macronuclei. Clinical history of asbestos exposure, rapidly developing effusion, mass lesion near mesothelial surface, etc. may be helpful in difficult situations.

Histiocytes (Macrophages)

Histiocytes are almost invariably present in all sorts of effusion fluid. The number of histiocytes in effusion fluid varies. In case of chronic infection, the number of macrophages or histiocytes may be increased. These cells originate in the bone marrow and come to the effusion fluid by circulation.

Histiocytes are usually present as dispersed population of cells (Table 10.2). However, occasionally they may form loose aggregates. In contrast to mesothelial cells they do not form any window pattern. Individual cells are round to oval with moderate amount of vacuolated cytoplasm that often contains phagocytosed particles. The cytoplasmic margin of the histiocytes is ill defined and blends with the background. Cytoplasm may contain single large vacuole or multiple small vacuoles. Nucleus of the cell is in a central position and reniform in shape with small nucleoli and fine granular chromatin. The nucleus is usually single in number but they may be bi or multiple in number.

Table 10.2: Comparison of mesothelial cells and macrophages.

	Mesothelial cells	*Macrophages*
Cell arrangement	Cluster of cells showing window pattern	No such window pattern
Cytoplasm	Vacuolated cytoplasm	Phagocytosed material
Cytoplasmic margin	Sharp distinguishable from background	Ill-defined and blends with the background
Nuclear position	Eccentric	Central
Nuclear shape	Round	Kidney shaped, indented
Nucleoli	Small conspicuous	Indistinct

Other Blood Cells

Polymorphs: Scanty number of polymorphonuclear leukocytes is invariably present in effusion fluid.

Lymphocytes: The presence of lymphocytes is common in effusion. Reactive lymphocytes are polyclonal in origin however most of the lymphocytes are T cell type.

Eosinophils: Occasional eosinophils may be seen in effusion. The term eosinophilic effusion is labeled when the predominant population of cells (more than 50%) in effusion is eosinophils.

Mast cells: The presence of mast cell is not rare in effusion fluid. These are mononuclear cells with blotchy purple colored metachromatic granules in the cytoplasm in MGG stain. These cells are not recognizable in Papanicolaou's stain.

Other Cellular and Noncellular Substances

Various other cellular and noncellular substances may be present in the effusion fluid that may be helpful in diagnosis.

Psammoma bodies: Concentric laminated dark blue calcified material known as psammoma body may be seen in effusion fluid. Psammoma body is usually related with metastatic papillary adenocarcinoma of ovary (Fig. 10.7). However,

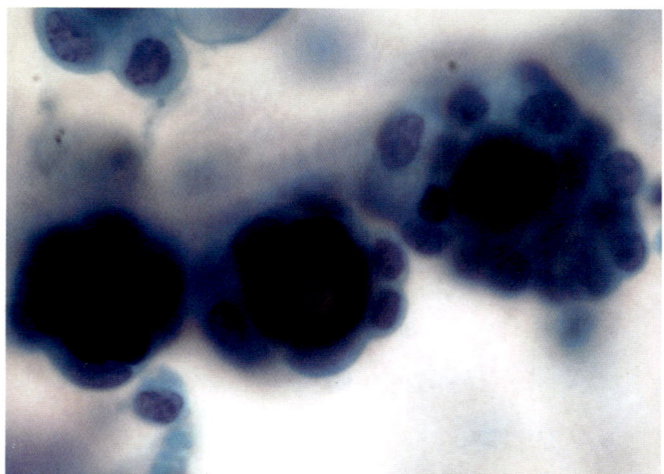

Fig. 10.7: Concentric calcified psammoma bodies in effusion smear (Papanicolaou's stain × HP).

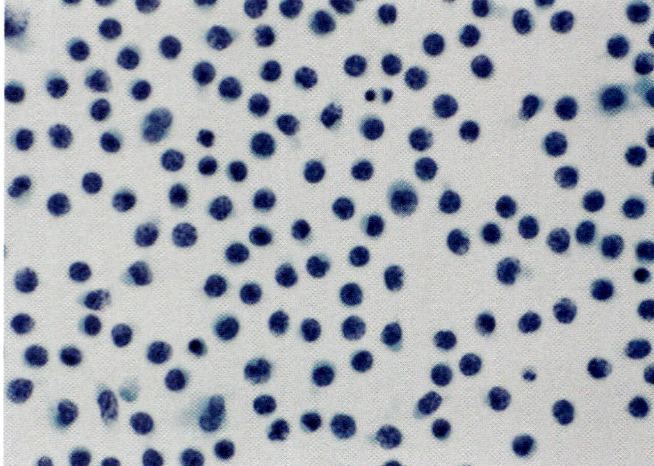

Fig. 10.8: Effusion fluid shows predominantly lymphocytes in a case of tuberculous effusion in liquid based cytology (SurePath) preparation (Papanicolaou's stain × MP).

Box 10.5: Tuberculosis.

- Indirect involvement of pleura:
  - Predominantly lymphocytes
  - Occasional plasma cells, polymorphs and mesothelial cells
- Direct involvement of pleura:
  - Large number of mesothelial cells.

the presence of psammoma body does not always indicate malignancy. It may be noted in benign effusion also.

Melanin-containing cells: Cells with dark brown melanin-containing pigment may be noted in effusion with malignant melanoma.

Hemosiderin laden crystal: Golden brown hemosiderin laden macrophages may be seen in chronic hemorrhagic effusion.

Crystals: Various types of crystal such as oxalate crystal, cholesterol crystal, Charcot-Leyden crystal, etc. may be noted in effusion.

EFFUSION DUE TO NON-NEOPLASTIC CAUSES

Effusion may be caused by a large number of diseases. However, the cytological features of effusion are nonspecific and do not indicate the exact cause.

Tuberculous Effusion (Box 10.5)

In tuberculosis, two things may happen:

- *Indirect involvement of pleura*: This may occur due to a hypersensitivity reaction. In this condition effusion fluid shows predominantly lymphocytes (Fig. 10.8). Occasional plasma cells, polymorphs, and mesothelial cells are also noted.
- *Direct involvement of pleura*: In case of direct involvement of pleural surface, effusion fluid shows a large number of mesothelial cells. Multinucleated giant cells or epithelioid cell granulomas are rarely noted (Fig. 10.9).

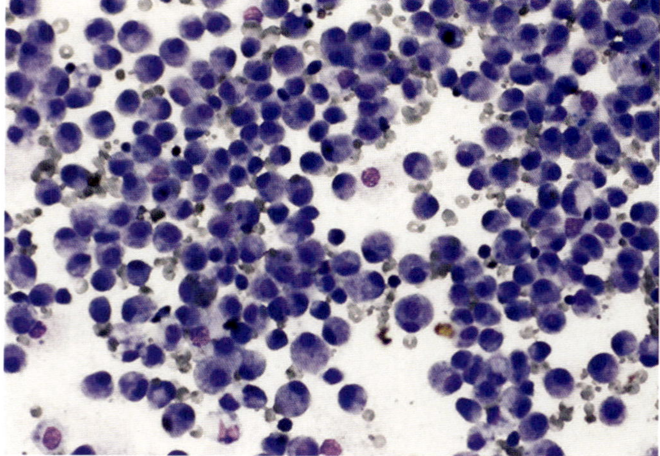

Fig. 10.9: Effusion fluid shows predominantly mesothelial cells in a case of tuberculous effusion (Papanicolaou's stain × MP).

In tuberculous effusion predominantly T lymphocytes are seen and out of which majority are $CD4^+$ subpopulation. Diagnosis of tuberculous effusion is not possible on the basis of cytological examination of effusion fluid. However, the presence of tuberculosis can be confirmed by demonstration of bacterial genome with the help of polymerase chain reaction (PCR).[1]

Rheumatoid Arthritis

Only a small population of rheumatoid arthritis patients develops pleural effusion (less than 5%). The pleural manifestation of rheumatoid arthritis generally precedes joint manifestation.

Cytological features of effusion fluid in rheumatoid arthritis are pathognomonic and diagnostic (Box 10.6). Smears show greenish, pink, or orange color granular debris on the background in Papanicolaou's stain. This granular material is developed from the breakdown of macrophages. The material is amorphous, soft, and fluffy looking. The majority of the cells are macrophage. Individual cells are round to spindle shaped. Occasionally spindle-shaped elongated histiocytes with single to multiple nuclei are also present. The nuclei of each cell may be 10–20 in number. The cells have moderate cytoplasm with elongated ends. In addition, there may be polymorphs and lymphocytes with a striking absence of mesothelial cells.

Effusion Associated with Pneumonia

Pneumonia is the inflammation of lung parenchyma. If this inflammation extends to the pleural surface then effusion develops. The nature of the inflammatory cells in effusion depends on the nature of inflammation in the lung parenchyma. In bacterial pneumonia the effusion cytology shows predominantly polymorphs in the early stage of pneumonia (Fig. 10.10). However, in course of time the effusion fluid shows lymphocytes as are seen in the lung parenchyma. In viral pneumonia the predominant cell population is lymphocytes.

Box 10.6: Rheumatoid arthritis.

- Granular necrotic debris
- Oval to elongated macrophages
- Multinucleated histiocytes
- Absent mesothelial cells.

Systemic Lupus Erythematosus

Systemic lupus erythematosus (SLE) patients may also present (one-third cases) with pleural, pericardial, and peritoneal effusion. The characteristic cell in SLE is lupus erythematous cell (LE). It is probably an in vitro phenomenon. LE cell is the neutrophil or less often macrophage with an eccentric nucleus and glassy homogenous ingested cytoplasmic particle known as hematoxylin body (Box 10.7). The color of hematoxylin body is purple or blue in Papanicolaou's stain and magenta in MGG stain. Nucleus of the LE cell is crescent shaped and pushed to the periphery of the cell (Fig. 10.11). *The tart cell* may also be seen in the effusion of SLE cases. These cells are neutrophils with an ingested bare

Box 10.7: Systemic lupus erythematosus.

- Lupus erythematosus cell is the characteristic cell:
  - Neutrophil or macrophages
  - Crescent shaped nucleus pushed to periphery
  - *Hematoxylin body*: Homogenous, glassy, cytoplasmic material filling whole of the cell.
- *Tart cell*: Neutrophils with ingested bare nucleus of another cell
- Scanty polymorphs and mesothelial cells.

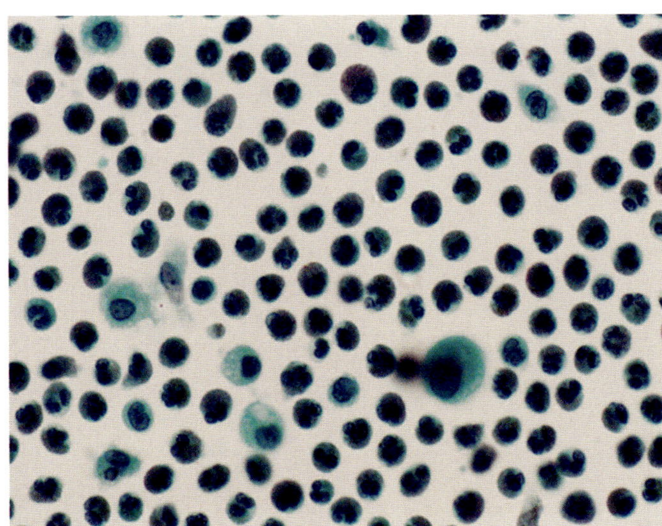

Fig. 10.10: Large number of polymorphs in early stage of pneumonia (Papanicolaou's stain × MP).

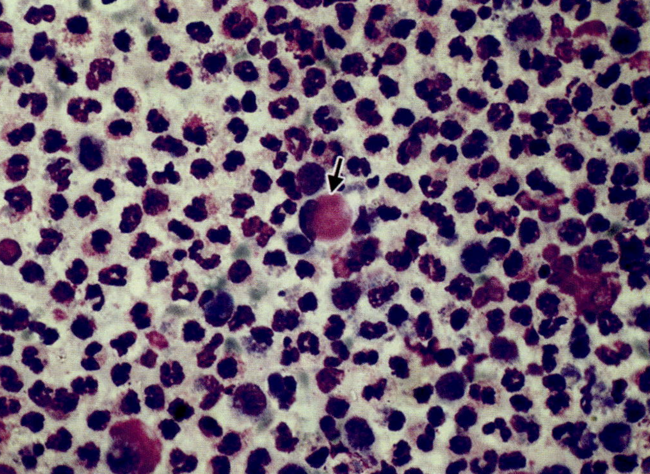

Fig. 10.11: Lupus erythematous (LE) cell in effusion fluid. Nucleus of the LE cell is crescent shaped and pushed to the periphery of the cell (*see* arrow) (May-Grünwald Giemsa × HP).

nucleus of another cell. The chromatin of the dead degenerated nuclei may be noted. In addition to LE cell, the smears may also show polymorphs and occasional mesothelial cells.

Congestive Heart Failure

Effusion in congestive heart failure is due to high hydrostatic pressure and the fluid is usually transudative unless secondarily infected. As the cause of effusion is very obvious, so practically there is no need of cytological examination.

Cytological feature is quite nonspecific and smears usually show scanty mesothelial cells, lymphocytes and polymorphs. In case of secondary infection large number of polymorphs may be noted.

Cirrhosis (Box 10.8)

The predominant causes of ascities in hepatic cirrhosis are decreased intravascular osmotic pressure because of hypoalbumenimia and increased hydrostatic pressure due to portal hypertension. Smears usually show scanty mesothelial cells. However in case of longstanding effusion large number of reactive hypertrophied mesothelial cells may be seen and may pose diagnostic difficulty. The presence of numerous polymorphs in effusion fluid gives a warning signal of spontaneous bacterial peritonitis.

Box 10.8: Cirrhosis.

- Scanty reactive mesothelial cells and lymphocytes
- *Longstanding effusion*: Abundant reactive mesothelial cells and large fragments of mesothelial cells
- Numerous polymorphs indicate spontaneous bacterial peritonitis.

Box 10.9: Etiologies of eosinophilic effusion.

- Pleural effusion
  - Pneumothorax
  - Cancer
  - Postsurgical
  - Traumatic
  - Pulmonary embolus
  - Parasitic
  - Pancreatitis
  - Pneumonic
  - Tuberculosis
  - Allergic
  - Idiopathic
- Pericardial
  - Pulmonary eosinophilia
  - Hypersensitivity reaction
- Peritoneal
  - Allergic
  - Peritoneal dialysis
  - Parasitic.

Eosinophilic Effusion

Eosinophilic pleural effusions contain at least 10% eosinophils. Common etiologic factors are listed in Box 10.9.

Out of these causes hemothorax and pneumothorax are the most common causes of eosinophilic effusion. Repeated thoracocentesis may also cause eosinophilic effusion because the procedure may introduce a small amount of air into the pleural cavity that may generate eosinophilic reaction. About one-third of cases no exact etiologic cause may be identified. Most of the eosinophilic effusions are self limiting and resolve spontaneously.

Cytology smear shows a large number of eosinophils that can be easily identified both in MGG and Papanicolaou's stain (Fig. 10.12). In addition, there may be polymorphs and mesothelial cells. The amount of mesothelial cells varies greatly from scanty to abundant. In case of secondary infection the smear may contain large numbers of polymorphs.

MALIGNANT EFFUSION

Malignant tumors often metastasize in the body cavity producing effusion. The relative frequency of pleural and peritoneal effusion in man and woman is different (Table 10.4).

In malignant pleural effusion, lung and breast are the most common sites in male and female patient, respectively. Similarly, in case of malignant peritoneal effusion lung and gynecologic tumors are the most common primary sites in male and female patients.

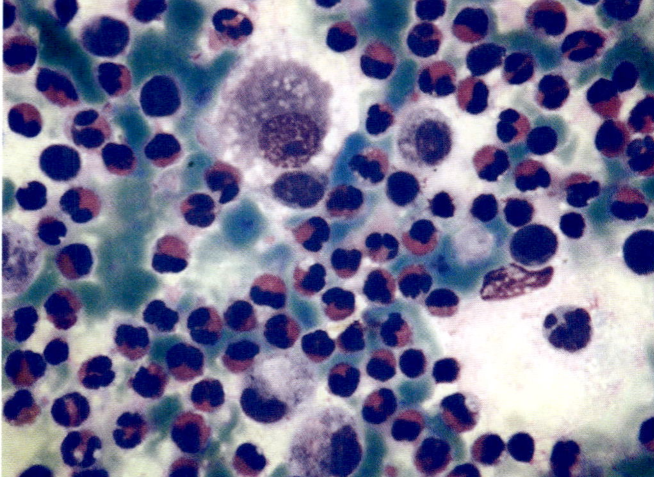

Fig. 10.12: Large number of eosinophils in a case of eosinophilic effusion (May-Grünwald Giemsa × HP).

Table 10.4: Common primary sites of malignancy in malignant effusion.

	Male	*Female*
Pleural	• Lung	• Breast
	• Hematologic	• Lung
	• Gastrointestinal tract	• Gynecologic
		• Gastrointestinal tract
Peritoneal	• Gastrointestinal tract	• Gynecologic
	• Miscellaneous	• Breast
	• Lung	• Lung

Box 10.11: Cannonball in effusions.

- Ovarian carcinoma
- Breast carcinoma
- Lung carcinoma
- Mesothelioma.

Box 10.12: Single row of cells in effusion.

- Gastric carcinoma
- Lobular carcinoma of breast
- Small cell carcinoma of lung.

In children non-Hodgkin's lymphomas and hematological malignancies are the most common malignant tumors in effusion sample.

In most of the cases during cytological examination of fluid the primary malignancy is known. However in certain cases the malignant effusion may be associated with occult primary neoplasm. Lung cancer is the most common occult malignancy in malignant pleural effusion whereas ovarian and pancreatic carcinomas are the most common occult malignancy in peritoneal effusion.

The recognition of malignant cells in effusion fluid is necessary for appropriate management of the patient. The primary duties of the cytologist are: (1) recognizing malignant cell, and (2) exact type and origin of malignant cell.

The *main challenges* of the cytologist are:

- To differentiate malignant cells from the mesothelial cells
- To differentiate adenocarcinoma from mesothelioma
- To differentiate mesothelial cells from the mesothelioma.

Identification of Malignant Cell

The identification of malignant cells in effusion depends on the constellation of features rather than one or two cytological features. It is important to note the overall smear pattern, background cell, and cytological features of individual cells for diagnosis of malignancy in effusion fluid. In majority of the cases morphologically recognizable malignant cells are seen in the effusion smears. Recognition of foreign or alien cells in the smear is an important step in the diagnosis of malignancy. Ancillary techniques such as cytochemistry or ICC are rarely helpful in the diagnosis of malignancy in effusion cytology and these techniques mainly help in diagnosis of specific subtypes of malignancy. Cytologists, therefore, have to rely mainly on the morphological characteristic of the cell (Box 10.10).

Box 10.10: Cytological features of malignant cells in effusion.

- Cell arrangement
  - Cannon ball-like tight three-dimensional cell clusters
  - Papillary cluster
  - Single dissociated cells in small cell carcinoma of lung
  - Small rows of cells in lobular carcinoma of breast
- Cytoplasm
  - Single to multiple vacuoles in cytoplasm
  - *Keratin*: In squamous cell carcinoma
  - *Mucus*: Adenocarcinoma
  - *Melanin*: Melanoma
- Nucleus
  - High nucleocytoplasmic ratio
  - Large nucleus
  - *Pleomorphism*: Mild to moderate
  - Irregular nuclear margin
  - Single to multiple prominent nucleoli
  - Coarse chromatin
- Mitosis
  - Atypical tripolar mitosis
- Other features:
  - Cell cannibalism
  - Psammoma bodies.

Box 10.13: Discrete cells in effusion.

- Non-Hodgkin lymphoma
- Gastric carcinoma
- Breast carcinoma
- Malignant round cell tumors.

Cytology

Cell Arrangement

Malignant cells are arranged in different patterns that include:

- *Cannonball-like cell clusters (Box 10.11)*: The cohesive three-dimensional (3D) clusters of cells are characteristics of many carcinomas in effusion.
- *Single row of cells (Box 10.12)*: At times the malignant cells in effusions are present in a single row.
- *Discrete cells (Box 10.13)*: Discrete cells in the effusion are difficult to identify. A careful observation of the individual cells may help in this situation.

Cell Shape

The malignant cells in the metastatic effusion fluid are recognizable on light microscopy. In fact, identification of the distinct different population of cell other than mesothelial cell is very helpful (Fig. 10.13A). Individual malignant cells are usually round to oval. Multinucleated cells are also present in malignant effusion (Box 10.14). Occasionally the cells are spindle shaped particularly in case of sarcoma.

Cytoplasm

Cytoplasm of the cells in case of adenocarcinoma often shows large single to multiple vacuoles. The vacuoles often displace the nucleus toward the periphery giving rise to the signet ring appearance. Signet ring types of cells are present in both benign and malignant conditions (Box 10.15). Therefore, these cells must be distinguished from the signet ring type of macrophages. Nuclei of the macrophages are small, reniform with inconspicuous nucleoli. At times it is difficult to determine the exact character of the signet ring cell.

Cytoplasmic Product

Mucin: Mucin in the cytoplasm produces clear vacuoles and special stain such as mucicarmine is needed to demonstrate mucin. As benign cells rarely produce mucin so the demonstration of mucin by mucicarmine indicates malignancy.

Melanin: The presence of dark brown melanin granules in the cytoplasm of cells in malignant melanoma is characteristics. This can be confirmed by HMB45 immunostain in smear or cell block.

Keratin: The presence of keratin within the cytoplasm is indicated by orange color in Papanicolaou's stain.

Nucleus

Nucleocytoplasmic ratio: In malignant cell the nucleocytoplasmic (N/C) ratio is almost always high (Fig. 10.13B).

Nuclear chromatin: Nucleus usually shows vesicular chromatin. Cells also show irregular clumped chromatin.

Nuclear margin irregularity: The margin of the malignant cells shows an irregular outline. It is often thickened focally (Fig. 10.13C).

Nucleoli: The presence of multiple nucleoli of variable shape and size (nucleolar pleomorphism) is one of the important characteristics of malignant cells in effusion (Fig. 10.13D).

Mitosis: Qualitative abnormality of mitosis is more important rather than simply increased mitotic figures in the smear. The abnormal mitotic figures show tripolar or multipolar mitotic figures.

Cell Cannibalism: We have noted that the increased number of cell cannibalism is one of the reliable features of malignant cell in effusion cytology smear.

Psammoma Bodies

Concentric calcified bodies are often seen in malignant effusion due to metastatic serous adenocarcinoma of ovary, papillary thyroid carcinoma, and carcinomatous mesothelioma.

Sites of Origin to Predict from the Cytomorphology in Effusion Fluid

Careful observation of cytomorphology may help to indicate the primary sites of origin of malignancy.

- *Knobby-like clusters*: Mesothelioma
- *Single file arrangement*: Lobular carcinoma, gastric carcinoma
- *Psammoma body*: Usually noted in papillary serous ovarian carcinoma
- *Signet ring cells*: Gastric carcinoma
- *Intranuclear pseudoinclusions*: Papillary carcinoma
- *Melanin*: Melanoma
- *Keratin or squamous pearls*: Squamous cell carcinoma.

METASTATIC TUMORS

Adenocarcinomas

This is the most common malignancies in the effusion fluid and the common primary sites are ovary, gastrointestinal tract, lung, and breast. In case of malignant effusion with adenocarcinoma the morphologically distinct foreign cell populations along with mesothelial cells are seen. Depending on the primary location of the tumor there may be some amount of variation in morphology of the cells; however, the basic characteristics of the malignant cells are almost same. The cells are usually in a tight spherical ball-like clusters (Fig. 10.14). The nuclei of the cells show overlapping and crowding. There may be hollow sphere of cells. On smear preparation, the empty space is seen in the central part of the cluster and two different layers of the cells are also identified (Fig. 10.15). In cell block section, the hollow sphere is seen as a central clear space with

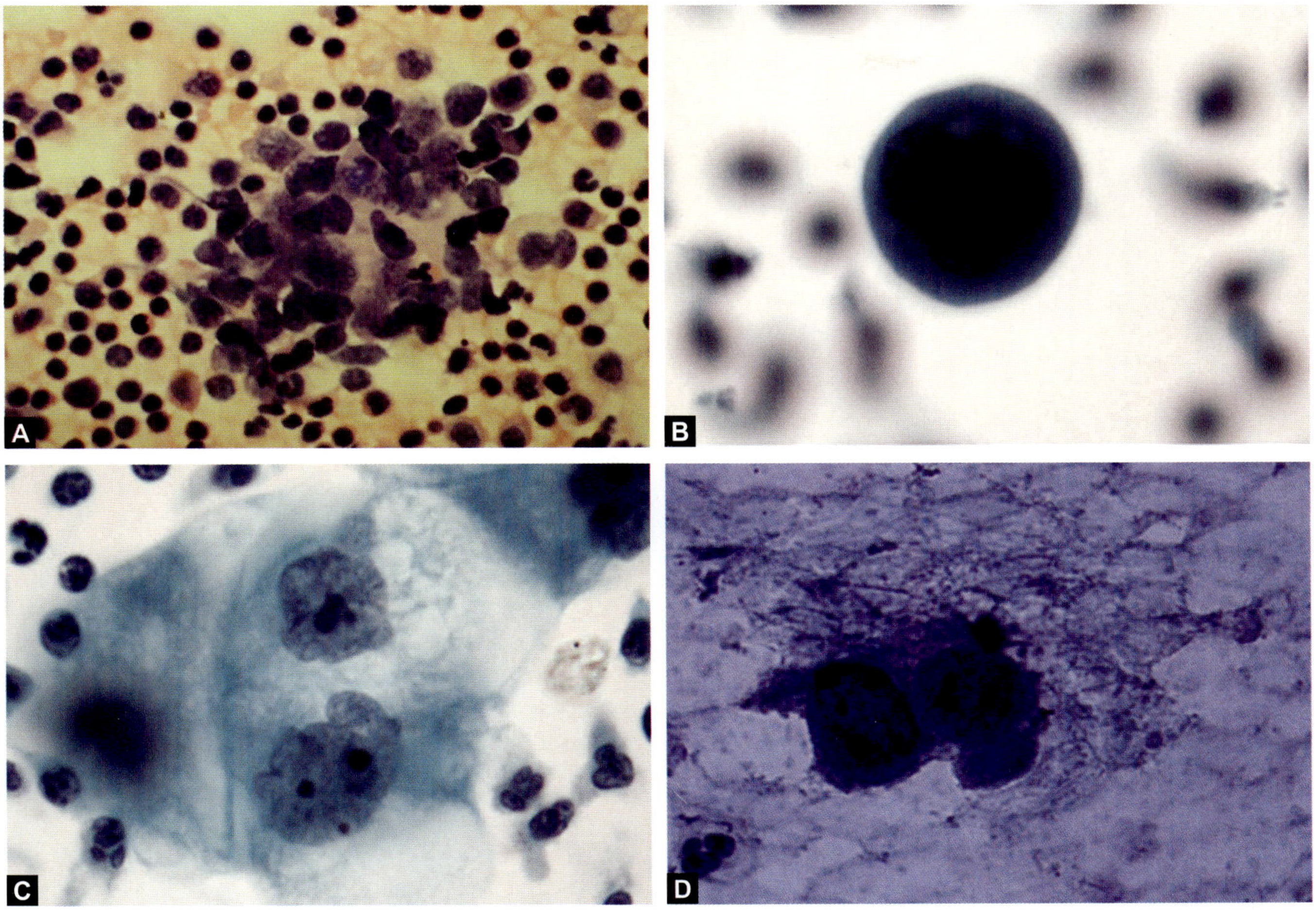

Figs. 10.13A to D: (A) Distinct two cell population is evident in metastatic carcinoma in effusion (Papanicolaou's stain × MP). (B) Malignant cell with high nucleocytoplasmic ratio (Papanicolaou's stain × OI). (C) The margin of the malignant cells show irregular outline in LBC preparation (SurePath) (Papanicolaou's stain × OI). (D) Multiple nucleoli of variable shape and size in malignant cells in effusion in LBC preparation (SurePath) (Papanicolaou's stain × OI).

Box 10.14: Multinucleated cells in effusion.

- Sarcoma
- Malignant melanoma
- Hepatocellular carcinoma
- Large cell anaplastic carcinoma of lung
- Reactive mesothelial cells.

Box 10.15: Signet ring cells.

- Gastric adenocarcinoma
- Breast carcinoma
- Any mucinous adenocarcinoma
- Mesothelial cells.

surrounding cells resembling glandular appearance. The cells may be present in single layers admixed with many mesothelial cells. Discrete recognizable malignant cells

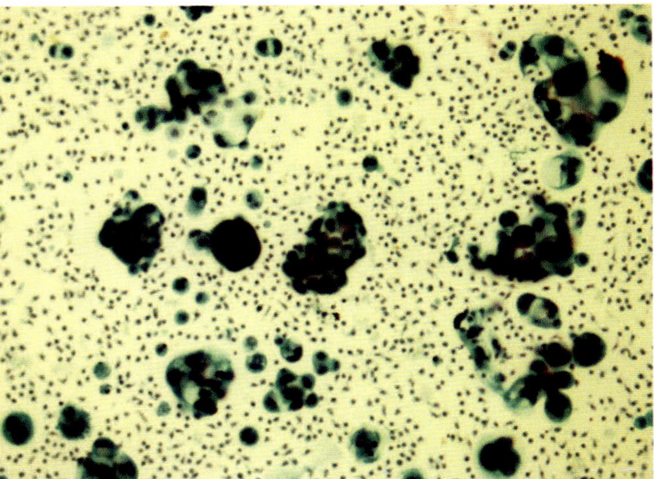

Fig. 10.14: Tight spherical ball-like clusters of malignant cells in effusion (Papanicolaou's stain × HP).

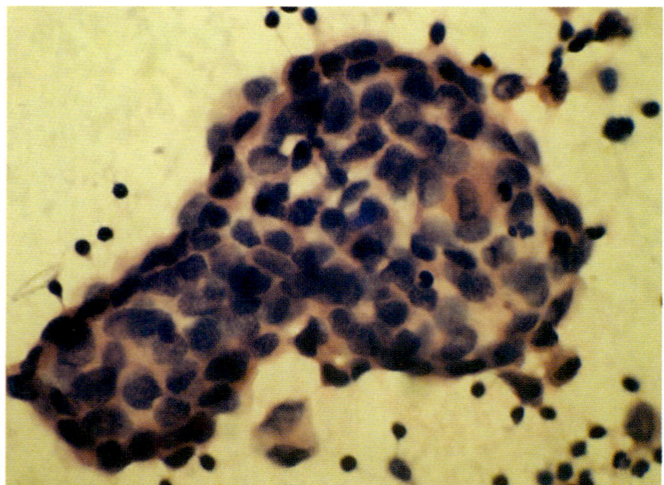

Fig. 10.15: The cells with overlapping nuclei in the cluster of cells in metastatic carcinoma in effusion (Papanicolaou's stain × HP).

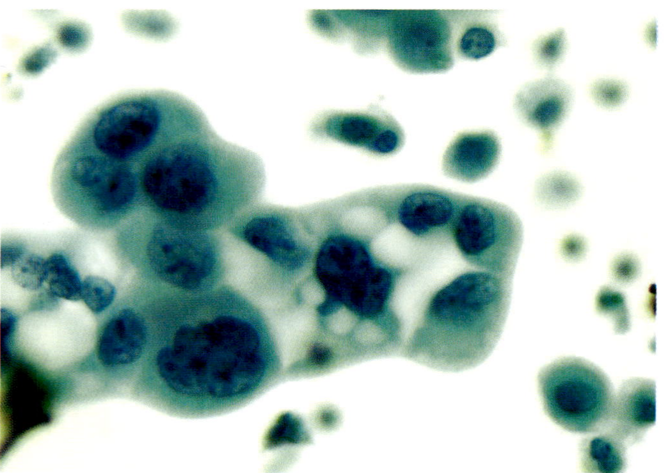

Fig. 10.16: Discrete moderately pleomorphic malignant cells in metastatic carcinoma in effusion (Papanicolaou's stain × HP).

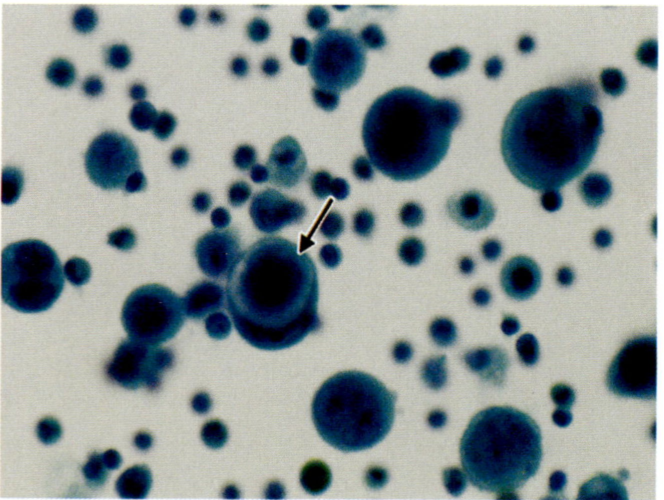

Fig. 10.17: Cell cannibalism in malignant effusion (*see* arrow) (Papanicolaou's stain × HP).

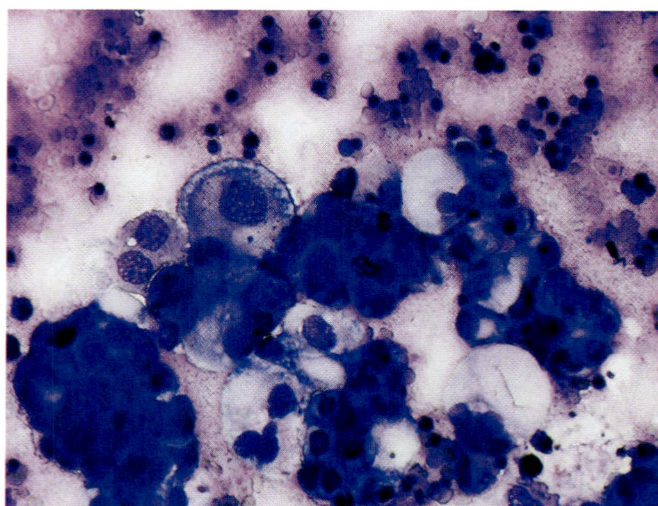

Fig. 10.18: Discrete malignant cells with vacuolated cytoplasm and large prominent nucleoli (Papanicolaou's stain × HP).

are also seen (Fig. 10.16). Cell cannibalism is frequently noted in malignant effusion (Fig. 10.17). There may be frequent bi- and multinucleation. The individual cells are relatively large with moderately pleomorphic nuclei and prominent nucleoli (Fig. 10.18). The cytoplasm of the cells shows single to multiple large vacuoles. Vacuoles may not contain mucin. However, they often contain glycogen and are Periodic acid-Schiff's (PAS) positive.

There may be predominant discrete cells in gastric and breast carcinoma. The individual cells are round to oval with eccentric nuclei containing large vacuoles giving a signet ring-like appearance.

Differential Diagnosis

- *Reactive mesothelial cells versus adenocarcinoma*: It is a great challenge to the cytopathologist to differentiate reactive mesothelial cells from adenocarcinoma. At times the morphology of reactive mesothelial cells may simulate the cells of adenocarcinoma (Table 10.5). The important distinguishing points between reactive mesothelial cells and adenocarcinoma are mentioned in Box 10.16.

  In case of doubt a panel of ICC or other ancillary techniques should be applied.

Table 10.5: Differentiating points between reactive mesothelial cells and adenocarcinoma.

Cytological features	*Reactive mesothelial cells*	*Adenocarcinoma*
Ball-like spherical clusters	Absent	Present
Two cell population	Absent	Present
Cell with high nucleocytoplasmic ratio	Absent	Present
Large pleomorphic nucleoli	Absent	Present
Irregular nuclear margin	Absent	Present
Sharply demarcated cytoplasmic margin	Absent	Present
Cytochemistry		
• Mucicarmine	• Negative	• Positive
• Periodic acid-Schiff	• Positive	• Positive
Immunocytochemistry		
• CEA (carcinoembryonic antigen)	• Negative	• Positive
• Ber-Ep4	• Negative	• Positive
• Leu-M1	• Negative	• Positive
• B72.3	• Negative	• Positive

Box 10.16: The most important features to distinguish reactive mesothelial cells from adenocarcinoma.

- Ball-like three-dimensional clusters of cells
- High nucleocytoplasmic ratio
- Large pleomorphic nucleoli
- Cells with irregular nuclear margin.

- *Adenocarcinoma versus mesothelioma*: Another challenge to the cytologist is to differentiate adenocarcinoma from mesothelioma. Cells from both mesothelioma and adenocarcinoma may show almost similar morphology. In this situation the cytologist should depend on (1) clinical history, (2) radiological features, and (3) ancillary tests such as ICC.

Characteristic Features of Different Metastatic Carcinoma

Breast (Box 10.17): Metastatic breast carcinoma is the most common tumor in pleural effusion of a female patient. The cytology features suggestive of breast carcinoma are multiple cannonballs-like hollow spheres, acini, chain-like arrangement of the cells, and intracytoplasmic lumina. The nuclei are often rectangular in shape without any molding. The cells of infiltrating duct carcinoma are usually larger and show nuclear enlargement and pleomorphism. These cells are easily recognizable. However, the cells of lobular carcinoma are smaller cells with minimal nuclear pleomorphism. These cells are often arranged as small rows simulating Indian file-like arrangement (Fig. 10.19). Therefore, these cells are difficult to identify in effusion.

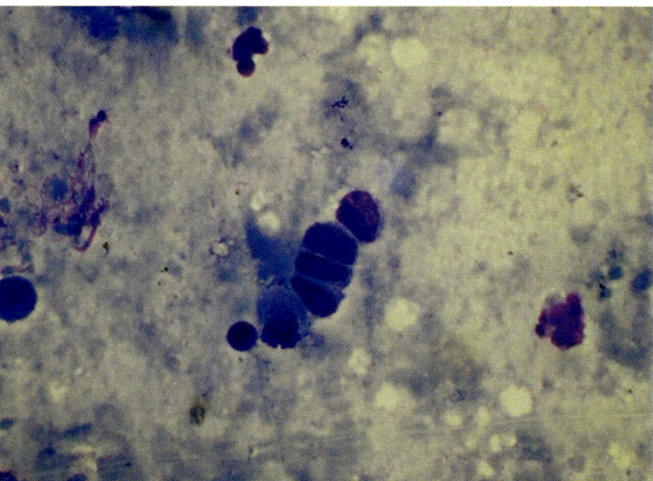

Fig. 10.19: Small rows of cells simulating Indian file-like arrangement in a case of lobular carcinoma (May-Grünwald Giemsa × HP).

Box 10.17: Breast carcinoma.

- Hollow spheres (cannonballs)
- Small chains or Indian file-like arrangement
- Rectangular-shaped nuclei
- Intracytoplasmic lumina
- *Immunocytochemistry*: Estrogen and progesterone receptor positive, gross cystic disease fluid protein.

Colonic carcinoma: Cells of colorectal carcinoma may show acini-like arrangement. Individual cells are elongated columnar like with hyperchromatic nuclei and prominent nucleoli. The cells are positive for cytokeratin 20 immunostain.

Gastric carcinoma: Cytomorphology of metastatic gastric carcinoma depends on whether the primary tumor is intestinal or gastric type. In gastric type of cancer the effusion smears show dispersed cells. Individual cells are large with peripherally pushed eccentric nuclei and large vacuolated cytoplasm (Figs. 10.20A and B). Vacuoles contain mucin and this is demonstrable by mucicarmine stain. In intestinal type, the effusion smear shows large pleomorphic cells with hyperchromatic nuclei.

Ovarian carcinoma: Metastatic ovarian cancer usually presents with ascities. Isolated pleural effusion is not seen in ovarian carcinoma. The cells are usually present as large 3D ball-like clusters (Fig. 10.21). Individual cells show large vacuoles that displaced the nucleus toward periphery of the

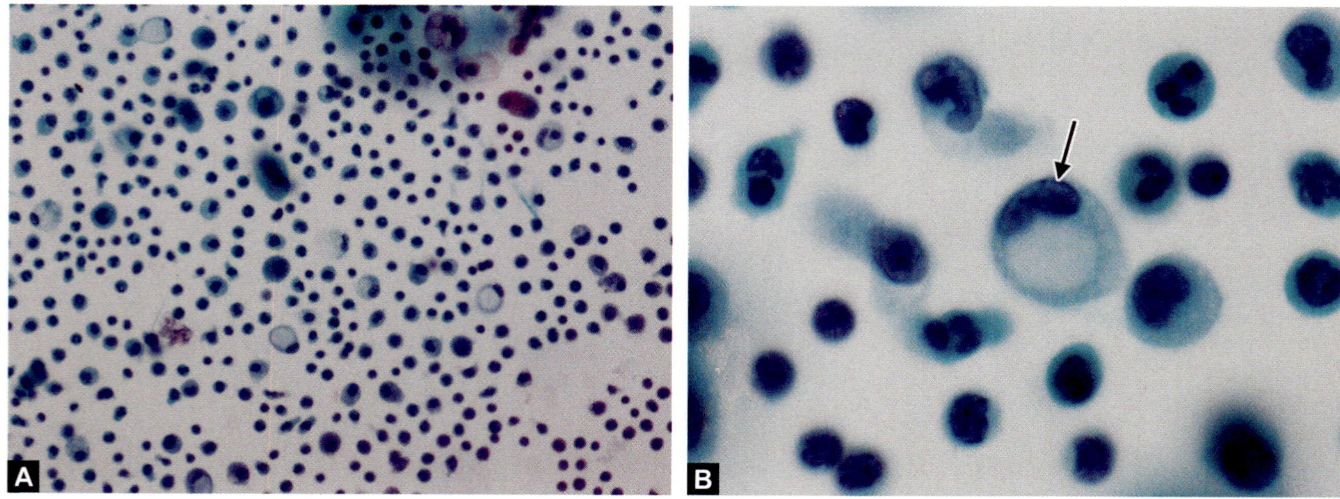

Figs. 10.20A and B: (A) Discrete cells with signet ring appearance in a signet ring carcinoma (Papanicolaou's stain × LP) and (B) Cells with abundant cytoplasm and peripherally pushed nuclei (*see* arrow) (Papanicolaou's stain × HP).

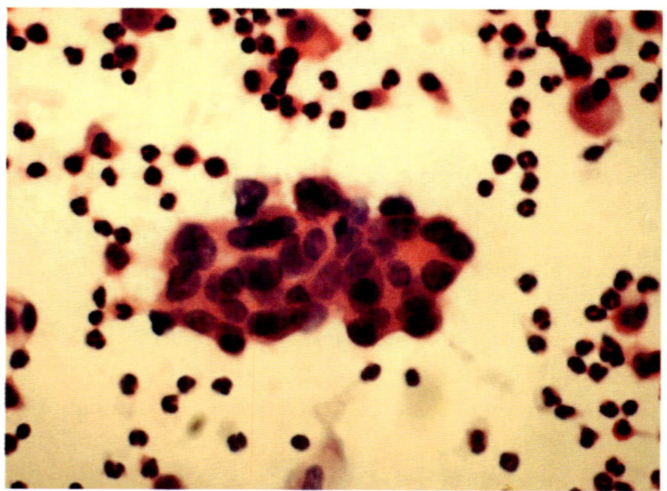

Fig. 10.21: Large three-dimensional ball-like cluster in an ovarian carcinoma (Papanicolaou's stain × HP).

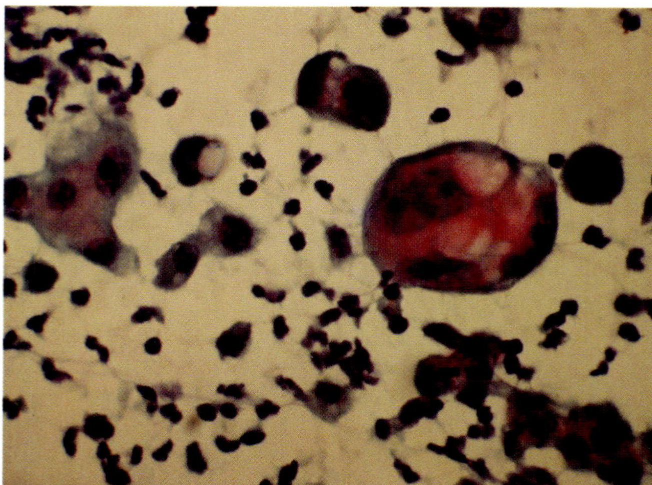

Fig. 10.22: Cells with abundant vacuolated cytoplasm with peripherally pushed nuclei (Papanicolaou's stain × HP).

cell. The nuclei show large prominent nucleoli (Fig. 10.22). Psammoma bodies may be present in serous ovarian carcinomas. The cells are positive for cytokeratin 7 immunostain.

Lung carcinoma: Lung carcinoma is commonly noted metastatic carcinoma in pleural effusion fluid. The cytomorphology of metastatic lung carcinoma depends mainly on tumor type. In case of moderately differentiated bronchogenic adenocarcinoma the cells are usually arranged in tight 3D clusters. Individual cells show moderately pleomorphic nuclei with prominent nucleoli. Therefore, the cells do not show any distinguishing cytological features. In bronchioloalveolar carcinoma the smears show uniform population of monomorphic cells with vacuolated cytoplasm. Small cell carcinoma of lung often shows characteristic small rows of cells in effusion (Fig. 10.23).

Renal cell carcinoma: Metastatic renal cell carcinoma usually shows tight papillary clusters or acinar arrangement of cells. The individual cells are large with granular or clear cytoplasm with hyperchromatic nucleus and prominent nucleoli. The vacuoles in the cytoplasm contain glycogen or lipid (Fig. 10.24).

Squamous cell carcinoma (Box 10.18): Squamous cell carcinoma uncommonly metastasizes in the serous

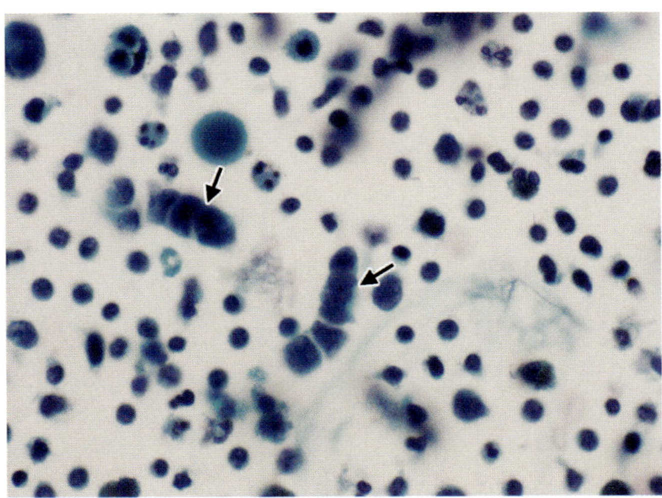

Fig. 10.23: Single row of cells in a metastatic small cell carcinoma of lung in pleural effusion (*see* arrows) (Papanicolaou's stain × MP).

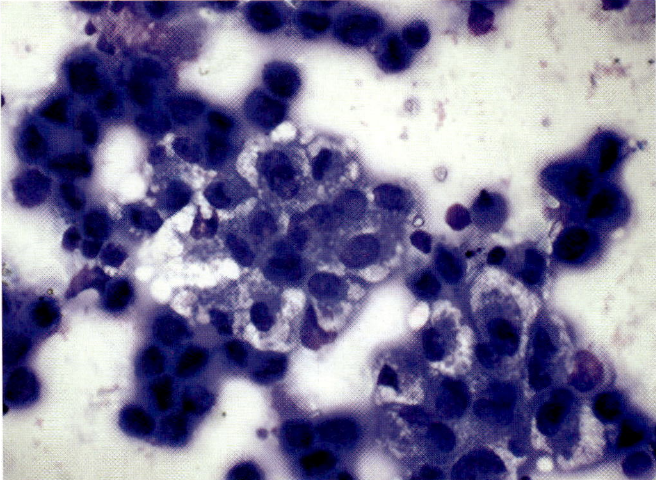

Fig. 10.24: Malignant cells with vacuolated cytoplasm in a case of metastatic renal cell carcinoma (May-Grünwald Giemsa × HP).

Box 10.18: Squamous cell carcinoma.

- Rarely metastasize in effusion fluid
- Small clusters or discrete cell population
- Oval cells in nonkeratinizing squamous cell carcinoma
- Polyhedral and occasional spindle cells in keratinizing squamous cell carcinoma
- Dense and orangeophilic cytoplasm
- Hyperchromatic nucleus with inconspicuous nucleoli
- Cytoplasmic vacuole usually indicates degenerative changes.

Box 10.19: Small cell carcinoma.

- Cells in small clusters, discrete and small chain
- Small cells twice the diameter of the lymphocyte
- Scanty cytoplasm
- Nuclear molding or angulations
- Granular chromatin and inconspicuous nucleoli.

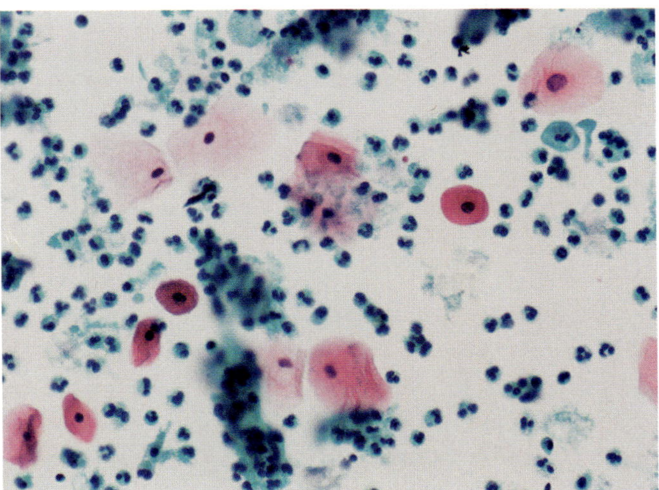

Fig. 10.25: Metastatic squamous cell carcinoma in effusion fluid. Note mature looking squamous cells in the smear (Papanicolaou's stain × MP).

cavities and the primary diagnosis is known in most of the effusion positive cases. The common primary sites are lung, larynx, and cervix.

Cytology (Fig. 10.25): The cells are usually arranged as isolated discrete or small clusters. Individual cells are oval to polyhedral and occasionally spindle shaped. Cytoplasm is orangeophilic and dense. The nucleus is hyperchromatic with inconspicuous nucleoli. Occasionally anucleated squames may also be noted. The presence of cytoplasmic vacuoles should not be misinterpreted as glandular differentiation.

Small cell carcinoma (Box 10.19): Metastatic small cell carcinoma is commonly derived from the lung.

Cytology: The cells are usually arranged discretely or in small chain. The individual cells are small and just two to three times larger than the lymphocytes. The cells show scanty cytoplasm and small hyperchromatic nuclei with granular chromatin and inconspicuous nucleoli. The nucleus may be fitted with each other giving angulated appearance (Fig. 10.23).

Melanoma (Box 10.20)

Metastatic malignant melanoma is uncommon. It is usually associated with cutaneous or ocular melanoma. Effusion may be present without a known primary tumor or many years after the complete therapy of the primary malignancy (Figs. 10.26A and B).

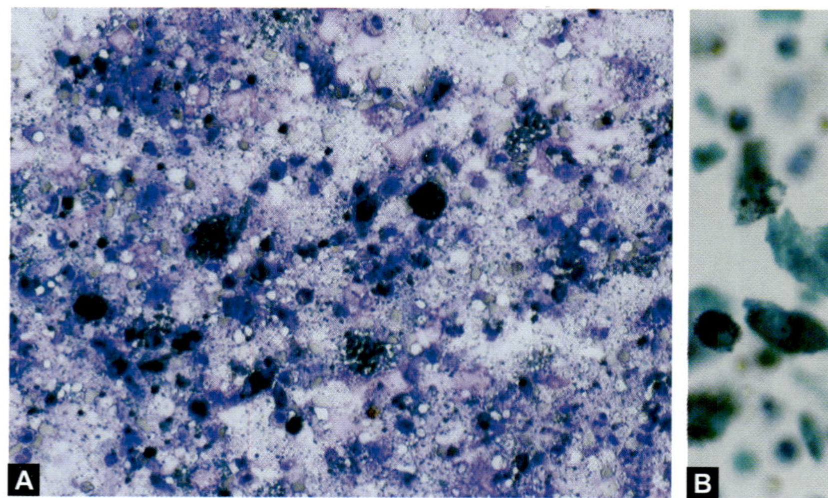
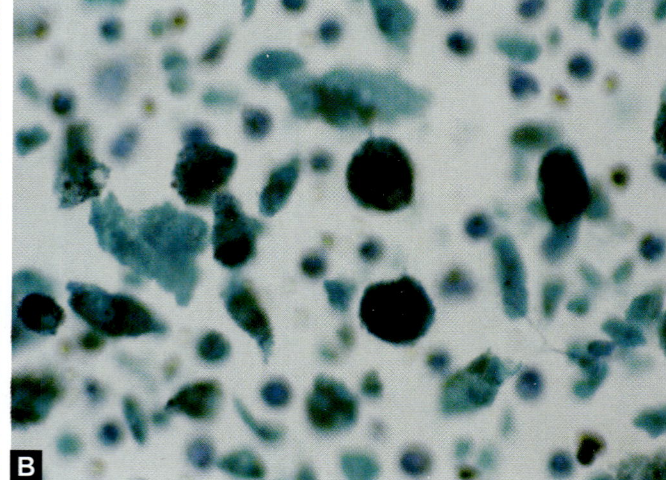

Figs. 10.26A and B: (A) Discrete tumor cells containing melanin pigment in a metastatic melanoma (May-Grünwald Giemsa × MP) and (B) Metastatic melanoma in effusion (Papanicolaou's stain × MP).

Box 10.20: Malignant melanoma.

- Uncommon, may present without any history of primary melanoma
- Discrete cells
- Variable sized cytoplasmic vacuoles
- Cytoplasmic brown melanin pigmentation
- Large prominent nucleoli
- Intracytoplasmic intranuclear cytoplasmic inclusions
- *Immunocytochemistry*: Positive for HMB 45, S-100, melan A.

The cells are usually discrete and admixed with reactive mesothelial cells. Individual cells are round to oval with moderate to severe pleomorphism. The cytoplasm of the cell shows single to multiple vacuoles of variable sizes. Brownish melanin pigmentation may be noted in the cytoplasm. Nuclei of the cells are central to eccentric in position with prominent large nucleoli. Intranuclear cytoplasmic inclusions are often noted.

Diagnostic difficulties: Cells of amelnotic malignant melanoma may not show pigmentation. In addition, the absence of significant nuclear enlargement or pleomorphism may simulate melanoma cells as reactive mesothelial cells. ICC particularly HMB-45 and S-100 protein positivity helps in the diagnosis of malignant melanoma.

Sarcomas

Metastatic sarcoma to the serosal cavity is uncommon. However, a range of sarcomas consisting of osteogenic sarcoma, malignant fibrous histiocytoma, leiomyosarcoma, liposarcoma, synovial sarcoma, and chondrosarcoma have been reported in effusion cytology.[2] Smears usually show scanty discrete malignant cells. The cytomorphology depends mostly on the exact diagnosis of the primary sarcoma. However, the cells are usually large with indistinct cell border. Cells frequently show multinucleation with bizarre nuclei (Fig. 10.27). Spindle-shaped, fusiform- or oval-shaped cells have also been described.

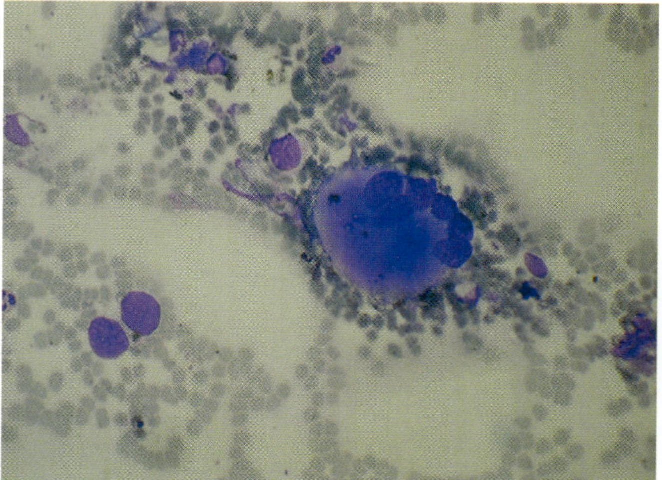

Fig. 10.27: Multinucleated bizarre cells in a sarcoma in effusion (May-Grünwald Giemsa × HP).

Pseudomyxoma Peritonei (Box 10.21)

Pseudomyxoma peritonei (PMP) is a poorly understood low-grade neoplastic condition. It shows mucinous ascities and diffuse mucinous implants in the peritoneal surfaces.[3] The most common sources of the primary tumor are mucinous adenocarcinoma of ovary, mucocele of the appendix, and gastric carcinoma.

The peritoneal fluid in such cases is thick and gelatinous and difficult to spread on the slide. On MGG stain, the material looks like purple and Papanicolaou's staining shows orange to red color. The cells are scanty and are usually discrete or in small clusters. The tumor cells are round to columnar in shape with bland nuclei and clear cytoplasm (Figs. 10.28 and 10.29). Ronnett et al.[3] classified PMP as disseminated peritoneal adenomucinosis (DPAM) and peritoneal mucinous carcinomatosis (PMCA). DPAM is characterized by superficial peritoneal implants composed of abundant extracellular mucin containing scanty simple to focally proliferative mucinous epithelium with little cytological atypia or mitotic activity. DPAM has a benign and indolent clinical course. PMCA shows invasive peritoneal lesions with more abundant mucinous epithelium. The cells show the architectural and cytological features of carcinoma. The prognosis of PMCA is worse than that of DPAM. This above classification is histological and has not been applied to cytology till now.

Box 10.21: Pseudomyxoma peritonei.

- Mucinous ascities and mucinous implants in the peritoneal surfaces.
- *Sources*: Mucinous adenocarcinoma of ovary, mucocele of the appendix
- Cytology:
  - Thick and gelatinous mucoid materials
  - Round- to columnar-shaped cells
  - Bland nuclei
  - Clear cytoplasm
- Histology
  - Disseminated peritoneal adenomucinosis:
    - Superficial peritoneal implants
    - Focally proliferative mucinous epithelium
    - Little cytological atypia or mitotic activity
  - Peritoneal mucinous carcinomatosis
    - Invasive peritoneal lesions
    - Architectural and cytological features of carcinoma.

Hematological Malignancies

Serous effusion is commonly seen in lymphomas and usually the patient presents with a known history of lymphoma. About 10–20% of malignant effusion is caused by non-Hodgkin's lymphoma (NHL) and Hodgkin's lymphoma (HL).[4] Serous effusion caused by lymphoma has distinct sex and age variation. Male has higher frequencies of involvement by lymphomas than female. In case of children more than 50% of malignant effusion is caused by lymphoma and leukemia.[5] Altogether involvement by the NHL in serous effusion is much more common than HL. T-cell NHLs are more frequently associated with effusion than B-NHL.[4]

Pleural effusion by lymphomas is mainly caused by:

- Lymphatic obstruction due to pressure effect of thoracic duct
- Direct infiltration of lymphoma on pleural surface
- Radiation effect
- Pulmonary infraction.

Direct infiltration of lymphoma cells in pleura is the main cause of effusion in cases of NHL, whereas lymphatic obstruction is the main cause of effusion in HL.

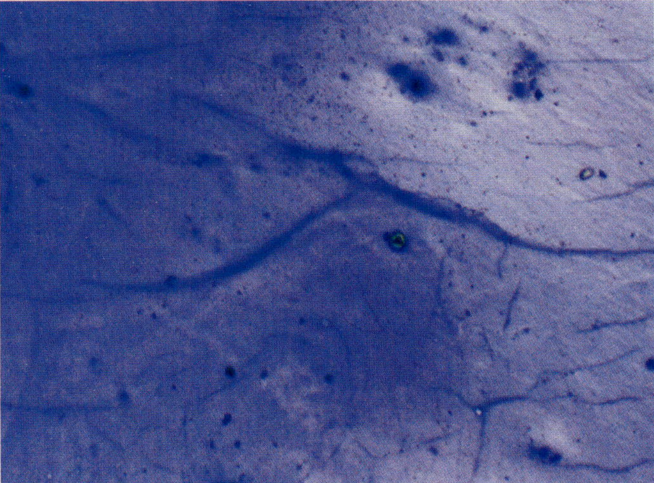

Fig. 10.28: Occasional round to oval cells in a background of thick mucinous material in pseudomyxoma peritonei (May-Grünwald Giemsa × HP).

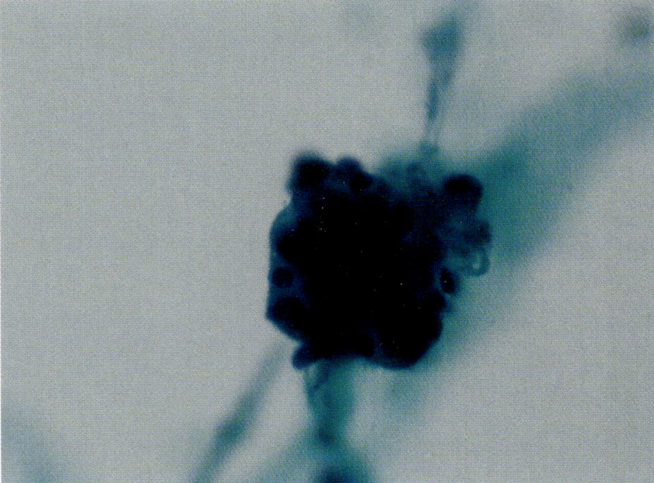

Fig. 10.29: Small loose cluster of cells in pseudomyxoma peritonei (Papanicolaou's stain × HP).

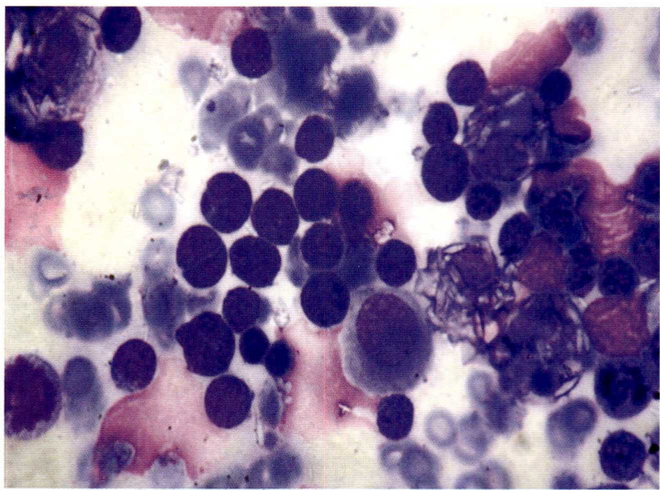

Fig. 10.30: Medium-sized cells with scanty cytoplasm and reticular nuclear chromatin in a case of lymphoblastic lymphoma (May-Grünwald Giemsa × HP).

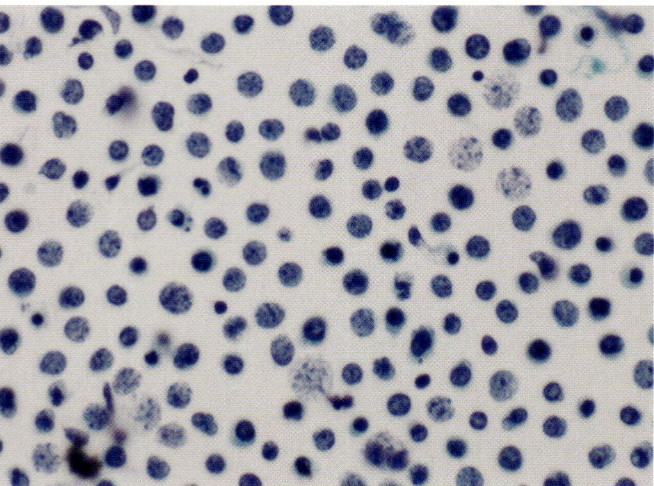

Fig. 10.31: Mixed population of small and large cells with nuclear cleaving in follicular center cell lymphomas (Papanicolaou's stain × HP).

Cytomorphology

Non-Hodgkin's lymphoma: Almost all types of NHL have been reported in effusion fluid. Cytomorphological features mainly depend on the primary type of NHL. The cells are always arranged discretely and they may frequently exhibit necrosis. Lymphoblastic lymphoma in effusion shows medium-sized cells with nuclear convolution and fine nuclear chromatin (Fig. 10.30). Burkitt's lymphoma shows cells with noncleaved nuclei and prominent multiple nucleoli. The cytoplasm of the cell is deeply basophilic and vacuolated. The follicular center cell lymphomas show a mixed population of small and large cells with nuclear cleaving (Fig. 10.31). Anaplastic large cell lymphoma shows many large lymphoid cells with nuclear cleaving and large mononuclear and multinuclear cells. Doughnut cells with wreath-like arrangement are also present. In case of small lymphocytic lymphoma or mantle cell lymphoma the effusion cytology smear shows small cells with irregular clumped chromatin. Without any known history of lymphoma it may be difficult to diagnose such cases as the cells may often be mistaken with reactive lymphoid cells. Monoclonal origin of the lymphoma cells can be demonstrated by flow cytometry.

Hodgkin's lymphoma: Hodgkin's lymphoma usually shows a polymorphic population of cells consisting of lymphocytes, plasma cells, and eosinophils. The typical Reed-Sternberg cell may be difficult to find out. A careful search of several smears may be needed to find out classical Reed-Sternberg cells. However, large mononuclear type of Hodgkin's cell and multinuclear cells may be noted in smear. In most of the cases of HL, the diagnosis is already known and therefore it may not be difficult to diagnose such cases.

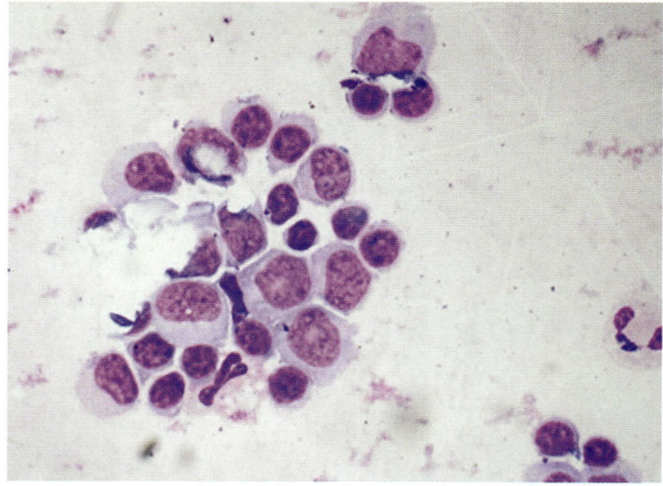

Fig. 10.32: Leukemic blasts in a case of leukemic infiltration (May-Grünwald Giemsa × HP).

Leukemia: In case of leukemic infiltration it is very important to distinguish leukemic infiltration from admixture with peripheral blood in effusion fluid (Fig. 10.32). A differential count of peripheral blood and in effusion cytology smear may be helpful in this instance. The detailed cytological features of the leukemic cells are best demonstrable in the MGG-stained smear.

Box 10.22: Primary effusion lymphoma.

- Serous effusion without any solid tumor mass
- Noted in advanced AIDS and cases with Kaposi sarcoma
- Possibly a rare subtype of diffuse large B-cell lymphoma
- Associated with human herpes virus 8 (HHV-8)
- Cytomorphology
  - Plasmablastic or immunoblastic differentiation
    - » Large lymphoid cells with abundant basophilic cytoplasm
    - » Round nuclei with prominent nucleoli
  - Anaplastic differentiation
    - » Moderately pleomorphic nuclei
    - » Large, irregular multilobated nuclei
- Immunocytochemistry
  - *Positive for*: CD45, CD19, CD20, CD23, CD38
  - HHV-8 positive
- Differential diagnosis
  - Anaplastic large cell lymphoma
  - Diffuse large B cell lymphoma
  - Carcinoma.

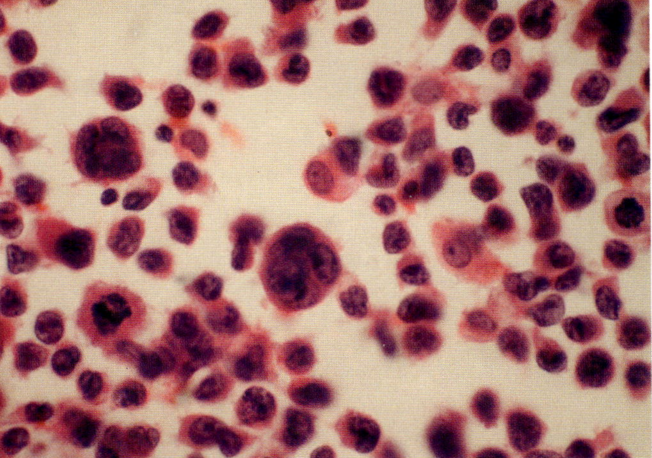

Fig. 10.33: Moderately pleomorphic, large, irregular multilobated nuclei in primary effusion lymphoma (Papanicolaou's stain × HP).

Primary Effusion Lymphoma

Primary effusion lymphoma (PEL) or body cavity lymphoma is a distinct clinicopathological entity which shows only serous effusion and no solid tumor mass (Box 10.22).[6,7] The PEL is a rare subtype of diffuse large B-cell lymphoma. It is associated with human herpes virus 8 (HHV-8). It is predominantly found in advanced AIDS and cases with Kaposi sarcoma. The exact histogenesis and pathogenesis of this entity is still unclear. It has been suggested that vascular endothelial growth factor (VEGF) or vascular permeability factor (VPF) liberated by PEL cells may cause vascular leakage.[8]

Cytomorphology: The smears show large lymphoid cells with abundant basophilic cytoplasm and round nuclei with prominent nucleoli having a plasmablastic or immunoblastic differentiation. The cells may also have moderately pleomorphic, large, irregular multilobated nuclei indicating anaplastic differentiation (Fig. 10.33). Smears may show frequent mitosis and apoptosis. Rare cases of PEL with Burkitt's-like lymphoma have also been described.[9] It is suggested that PEL is a unique subgroup of B-NHL. PEL cells usually express CD45 and also positive for the following CD markers: CD19, CD20, CD23, CD38.[10] With the available history of immunodeficiency along with cytomorphology of the lymphoid cells, a possibility of PEL in effusion fluid should be suspected. Detailed ICC and demonstration of HHV-8 are necessary for the final diagnosis.[11]

Differential Diagnosis

- *Anaplastic large cell lymphoma (ALCL)*: Large lymphoid cells with marked nuclear atypia may simulate ALCL. However, typical history of immunodeficiency and HHV-8 positivity may help in diagnosis of PEL.
- *Diffuse large B cell lymphoma (DLBCL)*: The cells of DLBCL may simulate PEL. However, the presence of lymph nodal mass or any solid tumor mass and negative HHV-8 may exclude DLBCL.
- *Carcinoma*: The presence of large pleomorphic cells may simulate carcinoma in effusion. However, discrete cell population along with ICC (CD45 positive) helps in exclusion of carcinoma.

PRIMARY SEROSAL TUMOR

Primary serosal tumors are uncommon. Mesothelioma and PEL are two malignant neoplasms that may arise from the serosal surface.

Mesothelioma

Mesothelioma can be diffuse and localized variety. Diffuse mesotheliomas are always malignant in nature. Localized mesothelioma may be either benign or malignant in nature. Only malignant mesothelioma (MM) causes effusion. Only the epithelial variants of diffuse MM have characteristic diagnostic features in effusion fluid.

Diffuse Malignant Mesothelioma

Diffuse MM is often associated with asbestos exposure. It develops in the pleura, peritoneum, pericardium, and tunica vaginalis. Pleural surface is the most common site

Box 10.23: Malignant mesothelioma.

- Pattern:
  - Two cell populations absent
  - Spherical clusters with knobby edges and papillae-like clusters
  - Dissociated cells
  - Cell in cell (cell cannibalism)
- Mesothelial cell morphology
- Window-like gaps in between the cells
- Enlarged cells
- Low nucleocytoplasmic ratio
- Frequent binucleation and multinucleation
- Centrally placed nucleus with large prominent nucleoli (macronucleoli)
- Condensed cytoplasm with ring-like peripheral clear zone.

of development of MM. It usually occurs in sixth or seventh decade of life. Initially diffuse MM shows multiple tiny seed-like nodules that may not be detected in X-ray. Later on, the small nodules coalesce and large plaque-like nodule appears on the pleural or peritoneal surface. This is mostly seen in the basal or posterior surface of the lung. Later on this may encase the whole lung. On histological examination, MM can be classified as epithelial, sarcomatoid, or biphasic types.

The patient usually presents with chest pain, shortness of breath, and unilateral pleural effusion.

Cytology (Box 10.23): Cells in MM are arranged in 3D spherical clusters with knob-like projections and papillae. Many discrete cells are also noted. Cells often show "cell in cell pattern" or cell cannibalism. For the cytological diagnosis of MM, primary duties of the cytologists are (1) to identify the cells as mesothelial in nature, and (2) to decide the neoplastic nature of the mesothelial cells. The individual cells are round to oval with a window-like gap in between two cells (Fig. 10.34). Surface projections may also be seen. Cells usually show abundant dense cytoplasm with peripheral clear halo. Cells are enlarged with deceptively low nucleocytoplasmic ratio. Nuclei are usually central in position with frequent binucleation. Occasionally multinucleated cells are seen. Nuclei show mild pleomorphism with large prominent macronucleoli.

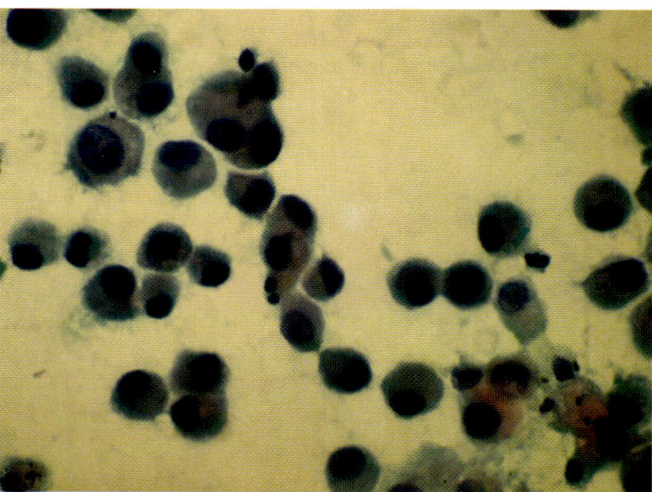

Fig. 10.34: Abundant malignant cells resembling mesothelial cells in a case of malignant mesothelioma (Papanicolaou's stain × HP).

Table 10.6: Distinguishing features between malignant mesothelioma and metastatic adenocarcinoma.

Distinguishing points	*Malignant mesothelioma*	*Metastatic adenocarcinoma*
Two cell population	Absent	Present
Cell clusters	Spherical clusters with knobby edges	Hollow clusters
Cell in cell (cell cannibalism)	Frequent	Less common
Window-like gaps	Present	Absent
Cytoplasmic peripheral halo	Present	Absent
Nucleocytoplasmic ratio	Low	High
Nuclear pleomorphism	Mild	Moderate
Nuclear position	Central	Central to eccentric
Multinucleated giant cells	More frequent	Less frequent
Cytochemistry		
• Mucin stain (mucicarmine)	• Negative	• Positive
• Alcian blue	• Positive and diastase sensitive	• Positive and diastase resistant
Electron microscopy		
• Intermediate filaments	• Abundant	• Scanty
• Microvilli	• Long	• Short
Immunocytochemistry		
• Calretinin	• Positive	• Negative
• WT1	• Positive	• Negative
• CEA	• Negative	• Positive
• BER-EP4	• Negative	• Positive
• Leu-M1	• Negative	• Positive
• B72.3	• Negative	• Positive
• Vimentin	• Positive	• Negative

Differential Diagnosis

- *Metastatic adenocarcinoma*: MM may often simulate as metastatic adenocarcinoma and vice versa. In MM, there is a striking absence of two cell populations and individual cells resemble like mesothelial cells with a window-like pattern, dense cytoplasm, and peripheral haloes. Table 10.6 shows detailed distinguishing features between MM and metastatic adenocarcinoma.
- *Reactive mesothelial cells*: To distinguish between reactive mesothelial cells and MM is a great diagnostic challenge to the cytopathologist. The cells of MM look like mesothelial cells. Reactive mesothelial cells often show mild nuclear enlargement and pleomorphism. Moreover, the cells of MM may not show much

nuclear enlargement. In this condition clinical history of asbestos exposure, radiological evidences of nodular mass on the serosal surface along with other cytomorphological features such as a spherical cell cluster with a knobby appearance may be helpful. The cells of MM often show cytogenetic abnormalities such as deletion of 1p, 3p, 6q, 9p, and 22q.[12]

Ancillary Techniques

The routine cytomorphological examinations are very helpful in the diagnosis of malignancy in most of the cases. Different studies have shown that the conventional cytology has near about 57% sensitivity and 89% specificity.[13] The positive and negative predictive values for detection of malignancies in effusion cytology are 89.3% and 69.4%, respectively.[13] However, in gray zone lesions the cytologists often face difficulties in diagnosis and subtyping of malignancies. In this condition, ancillary investigative techniques are helpful.

Cytochemistry

Simple cytochemistry is also helpful in diagnosis of metastatic adenocarcinoma. The cells of adenocarcinoma are often positive for mucicarmine stain. This stain may be helpful in diagnosis of gastric carcinoma in ascitic fluid. The cells of adenocarcinoma are often positive for alcian blue and sensitive to hyaluronidase. Whereas mesothelial cells are positive for alcian blue and resistant to hyaluronidase.

Box 10.24: Basic approach to immunocytochemistry.

- Any relevant history of primary
- Sex and age
- Location of the effusion
- Cytomorphology of the cells
- Working diagnosis
- Differential diagnosis
- Antibody selection
  - In a limited differential diagnosis only 2/3 markers sufficient
  - Alternatively a panel of markers may be used
- Final diagnosis: Based on immunocytochemistry, cytology, and clinical history.

Box 10.25: Basic panel of markers in effusion.

- *CEA*: Strongly positive in adenocarcinoma
- EMA:
  - *Cytoplasmic positivity*: Adenocarcinoma
  - *Membranous positivity*: Malignant mesothelioma
- *Leu-M1*: Adenocarcinoma
- *BER-EP4*: Adenocarcinoma.
- *Calretinin*: All mesothelial cells
- *Desmin*: Reactive mesothelial cells

Immunocytochemistry

Immunocytochemistry is the most important ancillary technique in diagnosis, classification, and detecting the source of primary site in malignant effusion. Judicious selection of antibody solves majority of the problems in effusion cytology (Box 10.24).

The most commonly used antibodies in effusion sample are (Box 10.25): EMA, CEA (carcinoembryonic antigen), Leu-M1, BER-EP4, calretinin, and desmin. EMA is one of the most helpful markers in effusion containing atypical cells. Adenocarcinoma shows cytoplasmic positivity whereas MM shows membranous positivity of EMA. Reactive mesothelial cells are negative for EMA.

In case of evaluation of effusion fluid, the cytologist has to face three primary challenges:

1. Are the cells mesothelial or nonmesothelial in origin?
2. Are the mesothelial cells malignant or benign?
3. What is the type of nonmesothelial cells?

1. *Mesothelial versus nonmesothelial*: There are several markers which help in distinguishing mesothelial versus nonmesothelial cells. Table 10.7 shows the different immunocytochemical markers or antibody to differentiate mesothelial cells from epithelial cells.

   Epithelial cells are positive for CEA, BER-EP4, Leu-M1 and B72.3, and MOC-31, whereas mesothelial cells are positive for calretinin, WT1, OV-CAR3, thrombomodulin, HBME-1, and N-cadherin.[13]
2. *Malignant versus benign reactive mesothelial cells*: Truly speaking, there is no immunohistochemical stain that firmly separates benign from malignant mesothelial proliferations. It has been suggested that a panel of ICC consisting of EMA, desmin, glucose-transport protein 1

Table 10.7: Markers of mesothelial cells and epithelial cells.

Antibody	*Mesothelial cells*	*Epithelial cells*
CEA	Negative	Positive
BER-EP4	Negative	Positive
Leu-M1	Negative	Positive
B72.3	Negative	Positive
MOC-31	Negative	Positive
Calretinin	Positive	Negative
WT1	Positive	Negative
Low and high molecular weight cytokeratin	Both positive	Positive for low molecular weight keratin
N-cadherin	Positive	Negative
CD44	Positive	Negative
Thrombomodulin	Positive	Negative

(GLUT-1), Ki67, and p53 may be helpful to distinguish reactive mesothelial cells and MM[14] (Box 10.26). The combination of positive EMA and negative desmin strongly favors MM; conversely, negative EMA and positive desmin usually indicates a reactive process. In addition, strong membranous positivity for GLUT-1 and/or strong p53 positivity favors a diagnosis of mesothelioma. High Ki67 proliferative index has probably no value in the diagnosis of malignancy.

3. *Type of primary tumor and possible source of primary site*: Immunocytochemistry greatly helps in categorization of the nonmesothelial cells and therefore the source of origin of the primary tumor. For the determination of primary source and type of tumor in effusion following data are necessary:

Clinical History of the Patient

Age: Older age group patients usually show carcinomas. The common tumors in the young age are lymphomas and leukemia.

Sex: Breast and ovarian carcinomas are more frequent in female patients whereas lung carcinomas are more frequent in male.

Location: As mentioned previously, location of effusion is very important. Certain tumors are more frequent in pleural than peritoneal effusion.

History of previous diagnosis of malignancy: This is the most important clue to primary tumor's type.

Cytomorphology: As mentioned before, cytomorphological features are very helpful to decide the possible type of tumors.

Therefore, depending on the history one can apply the panel of ICC to identify the source or type of primary tumor. In case of pleural effusion with possible lung origin TTF-1, CK7, and p63 can be done (Figs. 10.35A to D). Tables 10.8 and 10.9 highlight the relevant ICC for detection of primary source of the tumor.

Other Ancillary Techniques for the Detection of Malignancy

DNA flow cytometry: Flow cytometric (FCM) analysis of DNA content to detect aneuploid malignant cells in effusion sample may help in detection of malignancy. DNA flow cytometry has 55–100% sensitivity and 86–100% specificity.[15] Many malignant tumors are diploid and may not be detected by DNA FCM.

Flow cytometric immunophenotyping: Flow cytometry immunophenotyping (FCI) helps in the diagnosis of hematological malignancies (Box 10.27). In comparison to ICC, FCI is rapid, reproducible, sensitive, and reliable. Multicolor FCI can be used by a panel of antibody consisting of BER-EP4, EMA, CD15 (epithelial markers), CD45 (leukocyte), and N-cadherin (mesothelial cell marker).

A combination of CD56 and cytokeratin is also helpful to detect neuroendocrine tumors in effusion fluid. A panel of antibodies consisting of cytokeratin, desmin, vimentin, neuron-specific enolase (NSE), and CD99/MIC2 on FCM detects most of the cases of small round cell tumors in effusion.[16]

Electron microscopy: Transmission electron microscopy is helpful in differentiating MM from metastatic adenocarcinoma. Ultrastructurally the mesothelioma cells show abundant long branching microvilli with absence of any glycocalyceal bodies. Whereas in adenocarcinoma the villi are short and stubby.[17] In addition, the mesothelial cell shows abundant perinuclear tonofilaments, glycogen, and apical tight junctions with well-developed desmosomes. Unfortunately, there may be overlapping features with poorly differentiated malignancies and a specific diagnosis may be difficult.

Argyrophilic nucleolar organizer region (AgNOR): The argyrophilic nucleolar organizer region (AgNOR) technique detects specialized nucleolar protein by applying the silver impregnation method. The number and size of NORs indicate cellular metabolic and indirectly proliferation activity. Rapidly proliferating malignant cells show an increased number of large irregular NORs in comparison to less number of smaller NOR dots in reactive mesothelial cells.[18]

Fluorescence in situ hybridization: Numerical chromosomal abnormalities are frequently present in the chromosomes of malignant cells and this can be demonstrated by fluorescence in situ hybridization (FISH) technique. Various centromeric probes have been used to demonstrate numerical chromosomal abnormalities for the detection of malignant cells. Fiegl et al. by using centromeric probes representing chromosomes 7, 8, 11, 12, 17, and 18 detected significantly more malignancy in effusions than conventional cytology alone.[19] FISH can also detect hyperdiploid malignant cells and is particularly helpful when the malignant cells cannot be distinguished from reactive atypical cells.

Telomerase activity: Telomeres are specialized repetitive DNA sequence at the ends of the chromosomes in eukaryotic cells. The telomerase enzyme prevents telomeric loss. High telomerase activity is present in neoplastic condition.

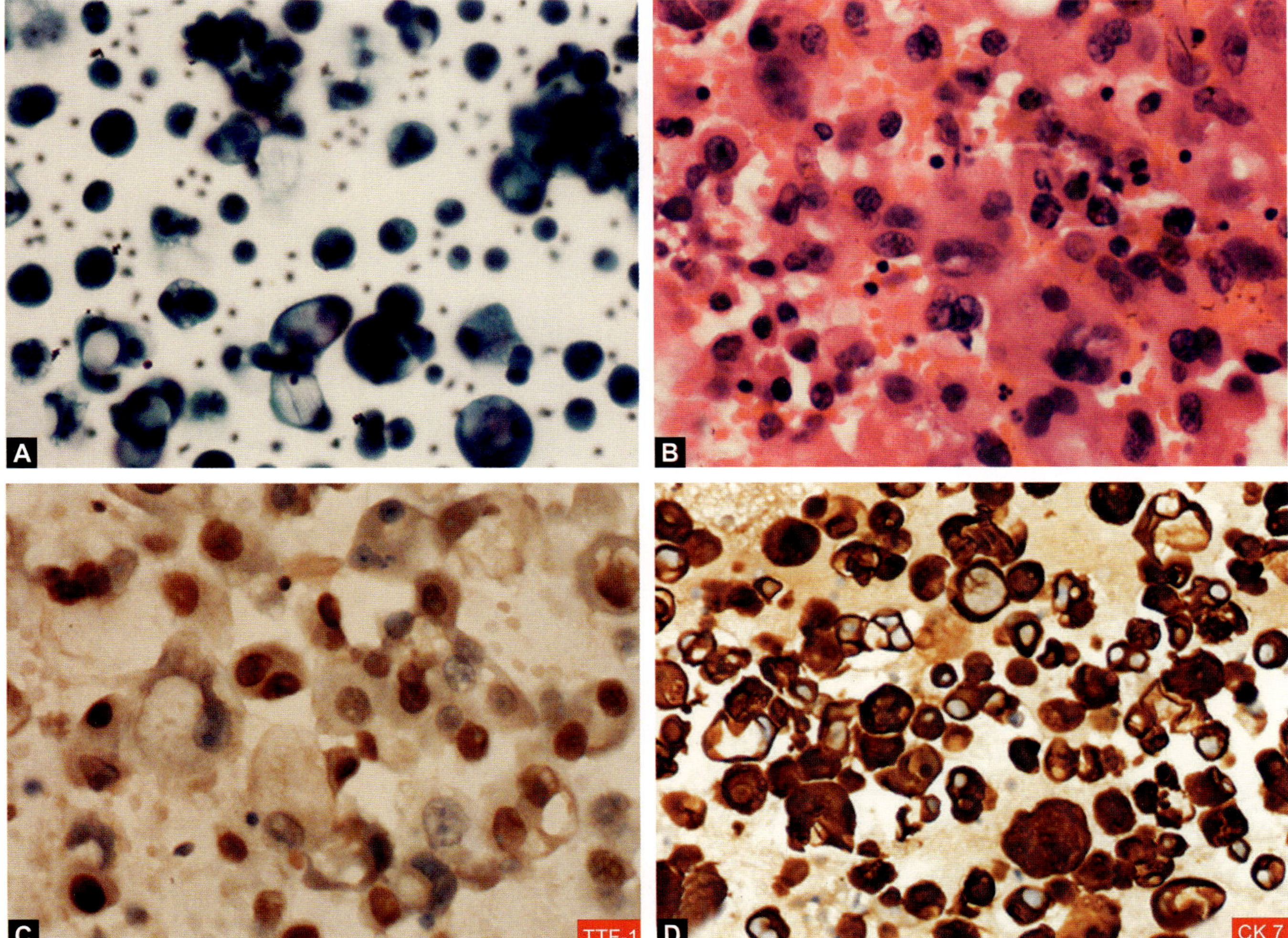

Figs. 10.35A to D: (A) Cytology smear of pleural effusion in a 54-year-old male (Papanicolaou's stain × HP); (B) Cell block of the effusion fluid (hematoxylin and eosin stain × HP); (C) Strong TTF-1 positivity of the cells indicating lung adenocarcinoma; and (D) Strong CK7 positivity of the cells again confirms adenocarcinoma.

Table 10.8: Immunocytochemistry for primary neoplasm detection.

Primary	*Antibody panel*
Colonic adenocarcinoma	CK20, CDX2, CEA
Ovary: adenocarcinoma	CK7, CA125
Prostate	PSA
Breast	Estrogen and progesterone receptor, GCDP
Melanoma	HMB-45
Thyroid	TTF, thyroglobulin
Neuroendocrine	Synaptophysin, neuron-specific enolase, chromogranin
Liver	Alpha-fetoprotein, alpha 1 antitrypsin
Lung adenocarcinoma	CK7, TTF-1
Lung: Squamous cell carcinoma	CK5/6, P63

Box 10.26: Immunostain of malignant mesothelial cells.

- Strong EMA positivity and negative desmin
- Strong membranous positivity for GLUT-1
- Strong nuclear staining for p53.

Table 10.9: Immunocytochemistry in different lesions.

	TTF-1	*CK7*	*CK20*	*ER/PR*	*PSA*	*CEA*	*Calretinin*
Lung	+	+	–	–	–	–	–
Breast	–	+	+	+	–	–	–
Colon	–	–	+	–	–	+	–
Ovary	–	+	–	–	–	+	–
Prostate	–	+	+	–	+	–	–
Mesothelioma	–	–	–	–	–	–	+

Flowchart 10.1: Schematic diagram of overall approach of effusion cytology.

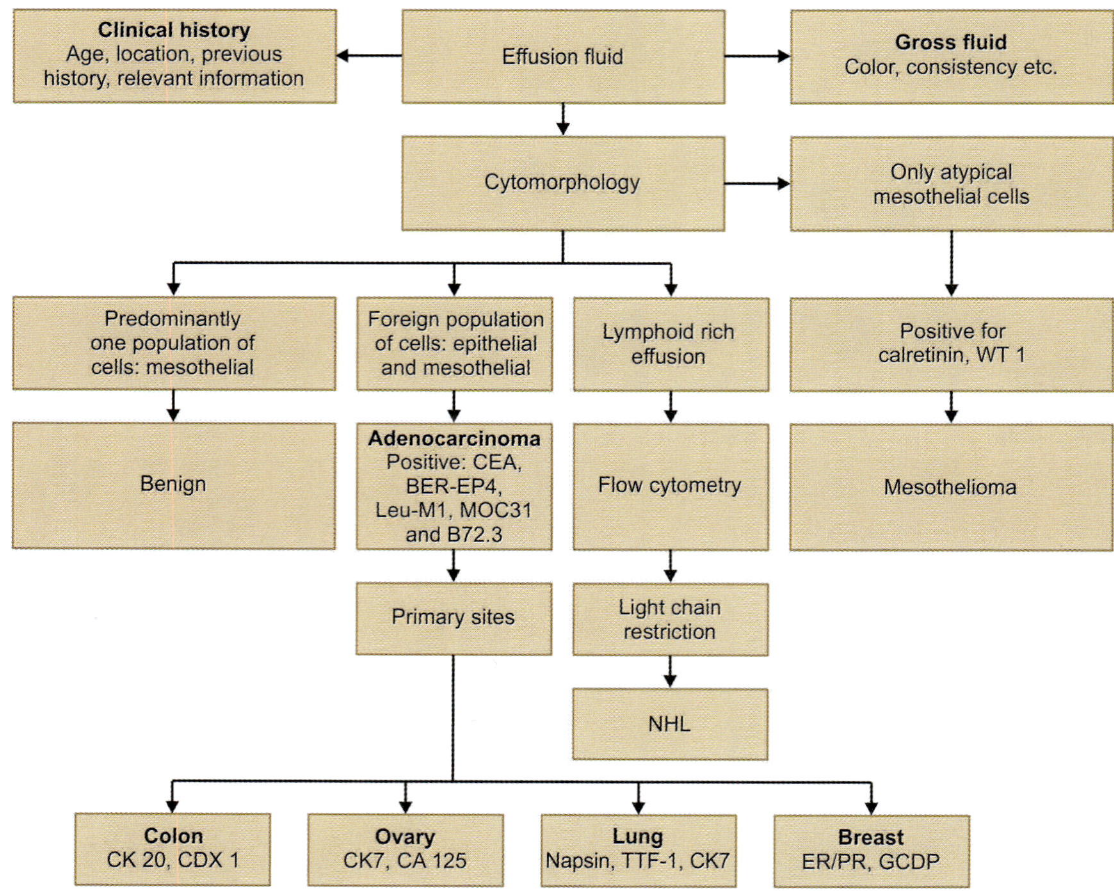

Box 10.27: Flow cytometric immunophenotyping.

- Rapid
- Reproducible
- Sensitive
- Reliable
- Markers:
  - *Epithelial*: BER-EP4, EMA, CD15
  - *Mesothelial*: N-cadherin
  - *Lymphoid*: CD45
- *Monoclonality*:
  - *B-cell*: Light chain restriction (kappa or lambda)
  - *T-cell*: Aberrant expression of T cell markers.

A PCR-based method is applied to detect telomerase activity, i.e. telomeric repeat amplification protocol (TRAP).[20] Various studies have shown increased telomerase activity in 52–91% of pleural effusions, diagnosed as malignant in routine cytology.[21,22] It can be suggested that telomerase activity demonstrated by TRAP can be a valuable complementary technique in the assessment of malignancy in pleural effusions.

Image morphometry: Image morphometry alone has questionable role in the diagnosis of malignancy in effusion.

Overall approach in a case of effusion fluid is described in Flowchart 10.1.

REFERENCES

1. Reechaipichitkul W, Lulitanond V, Sungkeeree S, et al. Rapid diagnosis of tuberculous pleural effusion using polymerase chain reaction. Southeast Asian J Trop Med Public Health. 2000;31(3):509-14.
2. Abadi MA, Zakowski MF. Cytologic features of sarcomas in fluids. Cancer. 1998;84(2):71-6.
3. Ronnett BM, Zahn CM, Kurman RJ, et al. Disseminated peritoneal adenomucinosis and peritoneal mucinous carcinomatosis. A clinicopathologic analysis of 109 cases with emphasis on distinguishing pathologic features, site of origin, prognosis, and relationship to "pseudomyxoma peritonei". Am J Surg Pathol. 1995;19(12):1390-408.
4. Das DK. Serous effusions in malignant lymphomas: a review. Diagn Cytopathol. 2006;34:335-47.

5. Wong JW, Pitlik D, Abdul-Karim FW. Cytology of pleural, peritoneal and pericardial fluids in children. A 40-year summary. Acta Cytol. 1997;47:467-73.
6. Huang Q, Chang KL, Gaal K, et al. Primary effusion lymphoma with subsequent development of a small bowel mass in an HIV-seropositive patient: a case report and literature review. Am J Surg Pathol. 2002;26:1363-7.
7. Carbone A, Cilia AM, Gloghini A, et al. Establishment of HHV-8 positive and HHV-8-negative lymphoma cell lines from primary lymphomatous effusions. Int J Cancer. 1997; 73:561-9.
8. Aoki Y, Tosato G. Vascular endothelial growth factor/vascular permeability factor in the pathogenesis of primary effusion lymphomas. Leuk Lymphoma. 2001;41:229-37.
9. Shimazaki M, Fujita M, Tsukamoto K, et al. An unusual case of primary effusion lymphoma in a HIV-negative patient not pathogenetically associated with HHV8. Eur J Haematol. 2003;71:62-7.
10. Perez CL, Rudoy S. Anti-CD20 monoclonal antibody treatment of human herpesvirus associated body cavity-based lymphoma with an unusual phenotype in human immunodeficiency virus-negative patient. Clin Diagn Lab Immunol. 2001;8:993-6.
11. Wakely PE Jr, Menezes G, Nuovo GJ. Primary effusion lymphoma: cytopathologic diagnosis using in situ molecular genetic analysis for human herpesvirus 8. Mod Pathol. 2002;15(9):944-50.
12. Granados R, Cibas ES, Fletcher JA. Cytogenetic analysis of effusions for malignant mesothelioma: a diagnostic adjunct to cytology. Acta Cytol. 1994;38:711-7.
13. Mohanty SK, Dey P. Serous effusions: diagnosis of malignancy beyond cytomorphology. An analytic review. Postgrad Med J. 2003;79(936):569-74.
14. Hasteh F, Lin GY, Weidner N, et al. The use of immunohistochemistry to distinguish reactive mesothelial cells from malignant mesothelioma in cytologic effusions. Cancer Cytopathol. 2010;118(2):90-6.
15. Evans D, Thornthwaite J, Ng ABP, et al. DNA flow cytometry of pleural effusions: comparison with pathology for the diagnosis of malignancy. Anal Quant Cytol Histol. 1982;5:19-27.
16. Gautam U, Srinivasan R, Rajwanshi A, et al. Comparative evaluation of flow-cytometric immunophenotyping and immunocytochemistry in the categorization of malignant small round cell tumors in fine-needle aspiration cytologic specimens. 2008;114(6):494-503.
17. Leong AS-Y, Stevens MW, Mukherjee TM. Malignant mesothelioma: cytologic diagnosis with histologic, immunohistochemical, and ultrastructural correlation. Semin Diagn Pathol. 1992;9:141-50.
18. Mohanty SK, Dey P, Rana P. Manual and automated AgNOR count in differentiating reactive mesothelial from metastatic malignant cells in serous effusion. Anal Quant Cytol Histol. 2003;25(5):273-6.
19. Fiegl M, Kaufmann H, Zojer N, et al. Malignant cell detection by fluorescence in situ hybridization (FISH) in effusions from patients with carcinoma. Hum Pathol. 2000; 31:448-55.
20. Kim NW, Piatyszek MA, Prowse KR, et al. Specific association of human telomerase activity with immortal cells and cancer. Science. 1994;226:2011-5.
21. Cunningham VJ, Markham N, Shroyer AL, et al. Detection of telomerase expression in fine-needle aspirations and fluids. Diagn Cytopathol. 1998;18:431-6.
22. Mu XC, Brien TP, Ross JS, et al. Telomerase activity in benign and malignant cytologic fluids. Cancer. 1999;25(87):93-9.

Review Questions

1. **These cells in the effusion (Fig. 10.36) are positive for:**
   a. CEA (carcinoembryonic antigen)
   b. Leu-M1
   c. MOC-31
   d. Calretinin
2. **Ascitic fluid (Fig. 10.37) in a case of chronic renal failure:**
   a. Candida
   b. Bacterial infection
   c. Positive for malignancy
   d. None of the above
3. **Pleural effusion (Fig. 10.38) in a 59-year-old female. Possible primary may be:**
   a. Colonic adenocarcinoma
   b. Small cell carcinoma of lung
   c. Ovarian adenocarcinoma
   d. Gastric carcinoma.
4. **Pleural effusion in a 55-year-old male (Fig. 10.39):**
   a. Chronic myeloid leukemia
   b. Non-Hodgkin's lymphoma (NHL)
   c. Reactive mesothelial cell
   d. Carcinoma of stomach
5. **Peritoneal effusion (Fig. 10.40) in a 65-year-old male with massive loss of weight. What cytochemistry will be helpful in diagnosis?**
   a. Mucicarmine positivity
   b. Periodic acid-Schiff positivity
   c. Alcian blue positive and hyaluronidase resistant
   d. Congo red positive

6. Pleural effusion in a 49-year-old female (Figs. 10.41A to D). What is the diagnosis?
   a. Metastatic carcinoma from stomach
   b. Metastatic carcinoma from lung
   c. Metastatic carcinoma from breast
   d. Metastatic carcinoma from colon

7. The characteristics of transudate effusion is:
   a. Rich in cells
   b. Specific gravity more than 1.015
   c. High fibrin content and coagulates if kept
   d. Usually turbid

8. A 57-year-old male presented with ascites. The patient had nephrectomy 1 year back for renal cell carcinoma. Now, he has 3 cm space occupying lesion in right upper lobe of lung. Figures 10.42A to F represent the cytology, cell block, and immunocytochemistry (CD10, CK7, vimentin, and napsin). What is your diagnosis?
   a. Adenocarcinoma of lung
   b. Metastatic renal cell carcinoma
   c. Reactive mesothelial cells
   d. Malignant mesothelioma

9. Which one is the epithelial marker?
   a. Thrombomodulin
   b. WT1
   c. N-cadherin
   d. MOC-31

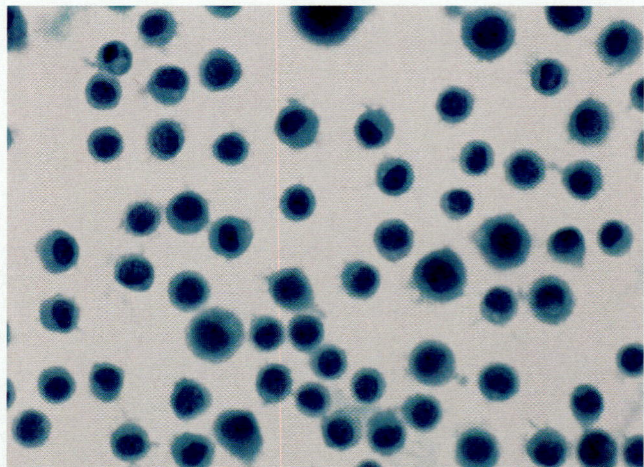

Fig. 10.36: Cytology smear of effusion fluid of question 1.

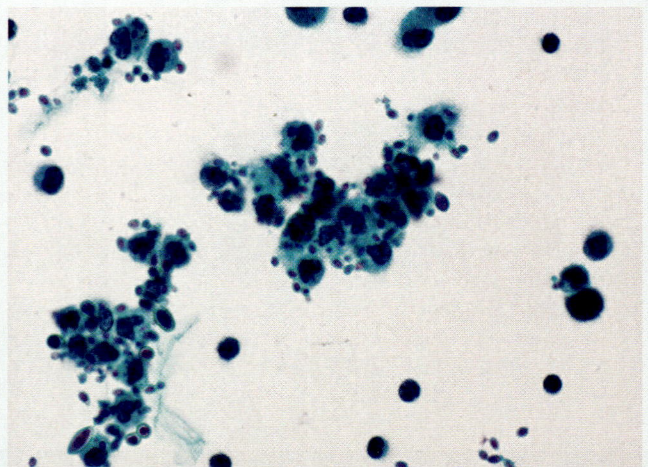

Fig. 10.37: Cytology smear of effusion fluid of question 2.

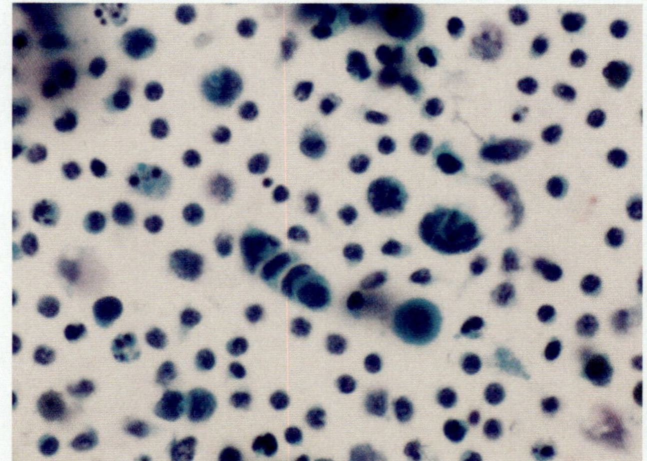

Fig. 10.38: Cytology smear of effusion fluid of question 3.

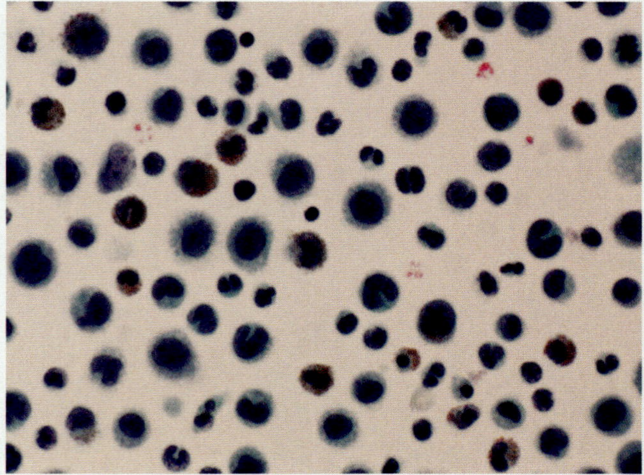

Fig. 10.39: Cytology smear of effusion fluid of question 4.

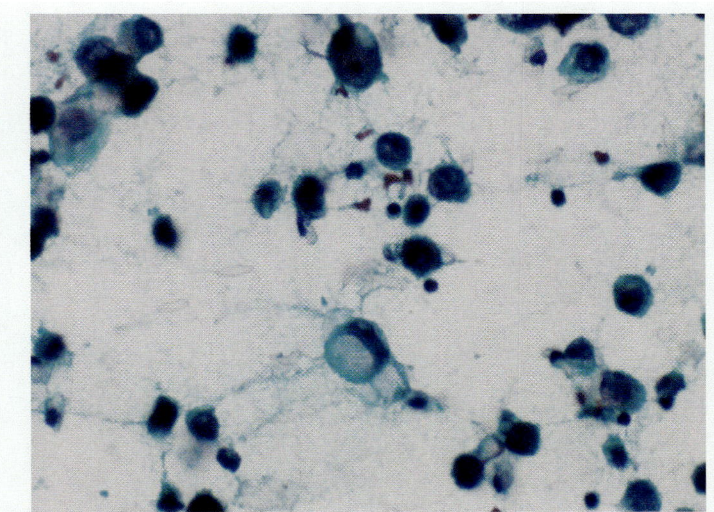

Fig. 10.40: Cytology smear of effusion fluid of question 5.

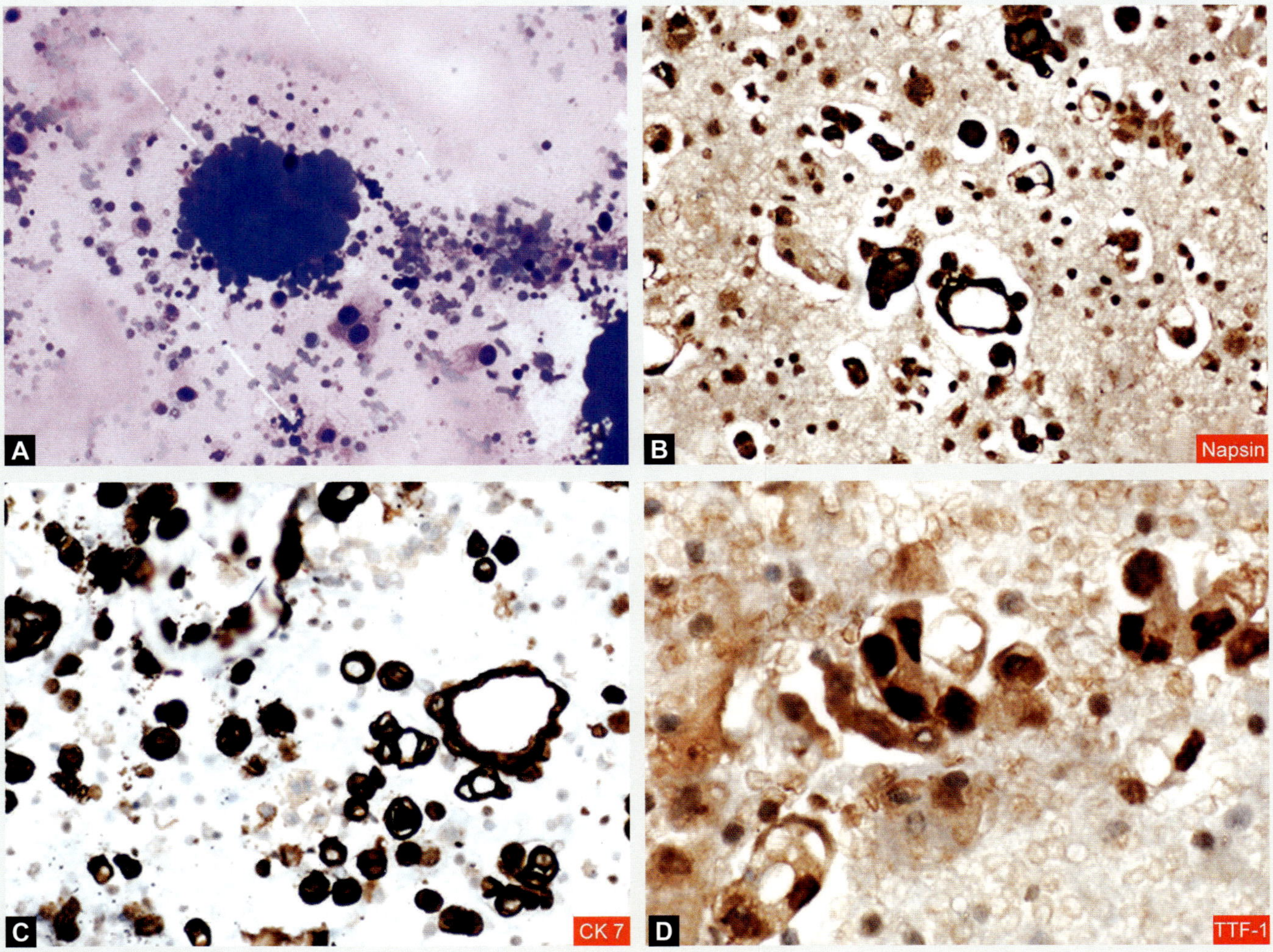

Figs. 10.41A to D: Cytology smear of effusion fluid of question 6.

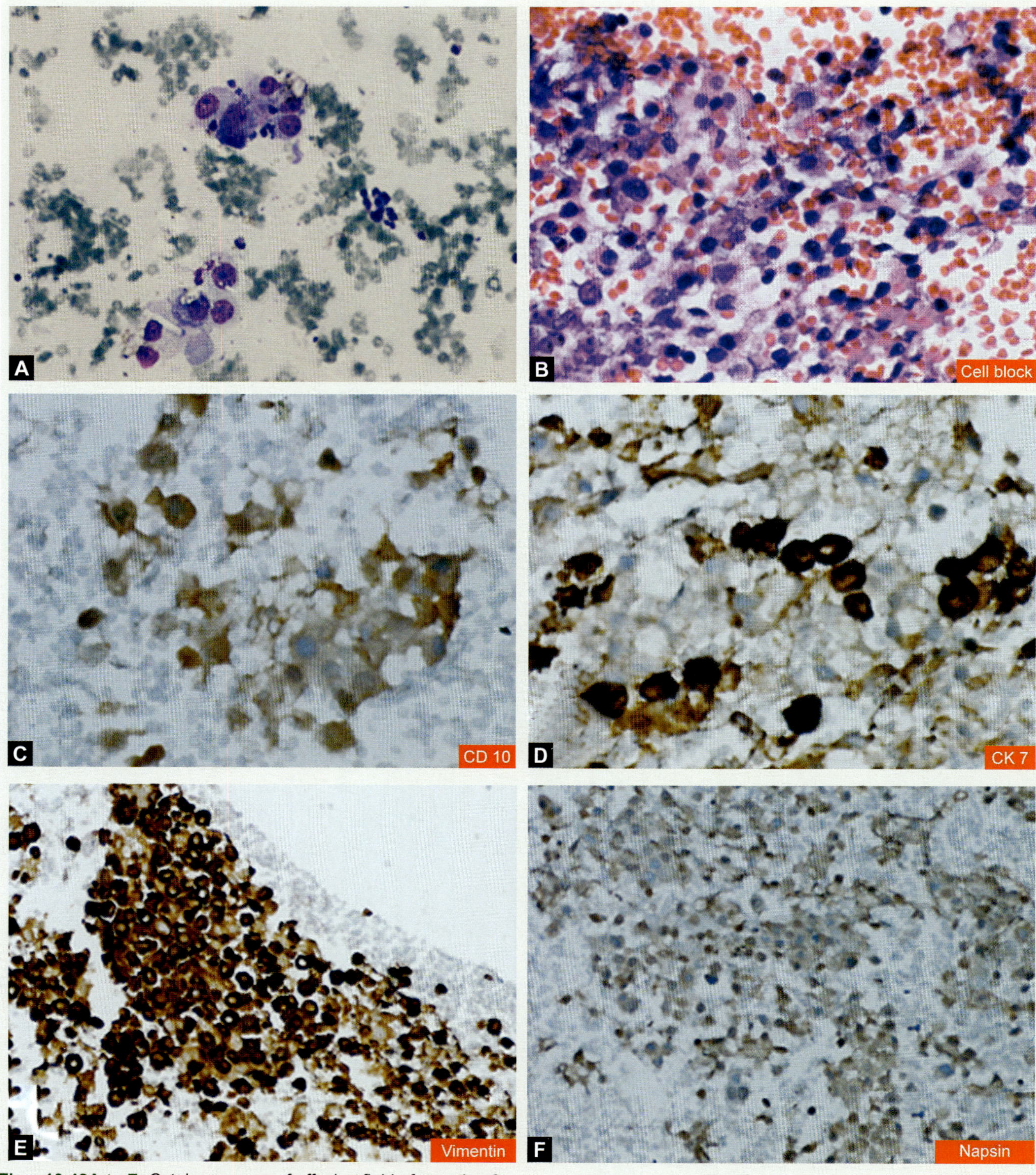

Figs. 10.42A to F: Cytology smear of effusion fluid of question 8.

Answers

1. d. Calretinin
   Note: The cells are mesothelial cells and they are positive for calretinin and WT1.
2. a. Candida
   Note: There are abundant candidal spore. The renal failure patients may have candidal infection in the effusion fluid.
3. b. Small cell carcinoma of lung
   Note: This typical vertebroid appearance of malignant cells is a feature of small cell carcinoma. Lobular carcinoma of breast may also show rows of cells in effusion.
4. a. Chronic myeloid leukemia
   Note: Many myeloid and metamyeloid cells are present in the smear. This is a case of chronic myeloid leukemia
5. a. Mucicarmine positivity
   Note: The signet ring cells and many discrete atypical cells indicate signet ring type of carcinoma possibly gastric carcinoma. The tumor cells are mucicarmine positive.
6. b. Metastatic carcinoma from lung
   Note: The tumor cells in this case are positive for napsin, CK7 and TTF-1. The immunocytochemistry result indicate a primary lung origin of the tumor.
7. a. Rich in cells
8. b. Metastatic renal cell carcinoma
   Note: The tumor cells are positive for both CK and vimentin. The cells are also positive for CD10. The above features indicate possible renal origin of tumor in this case.
9. d. MOC-31

CHAPTER

11 Urine Cytology

INTRODUCTION

George Papanicolaou and Marshal[1] first time introduced urinary cytology for detection of malignancy. Later on it was considered as a well-established technique for the detection of malignancy in the urinary tract. Despite its low sensitivity, urinary cytological examination is still considered as a useful adjunct to the cystoscopy. It is an inexpensive, rapid, and highly reliable technique for screening of bladder cancer. The major advantage of urine cytology is to detect the malignant lesions that are either not visible by cystoscopy or difficult to see on cystoscopy. The major disadvantages of urinary cytology are its low detection rate and failure to ascertain the exact anatomical localization of the lesion.

The *major indications* of urinary cytology are:

- To investigate the cause of hematuria
- Screening of recurrence of bladder cancer
- To screen asymptomatic high-risk cases for bladder cancer.

The most common presentation of bladder carcinoma is hematuria. A simple examination of urine sample can readily detect malignant cells. These cases should be further confirmed by cystoscopy and cystoscopy-guided biopsy (Box 11.1).

Box 11.1: Urine cytology examination.

Indications
- Investigation for hematuria cases
- Screening test for follow-up of bladder cancer
- Screening test for asymptomatic high-risk cases for bladder cancer

Advantages
- Simple
- Inexpensive
- Wide area of mucosal lesion is covered
- Especially helpful in lesions that are not visualized by cystoscopy
- High specificity

Disadvantages
- Low sensitivity particularly in low-grade urothelial tumors
- Exact anatomical location of tumor not possible.

Urine examination is particularly helpful in follow-up of patients with bladder cancer. High-grade urothelial carcinoma (UC) is prone to recur. Cystoscopy may be helpful in the detection of the recurrent cases. However, urine examination is particularly helpful in case of tumors that are not visualized by cystoscopy. It is a simple and inexpensive test of bladder cancer in asymptomatic people. Urine examination can be done to the high-risk asymptomatic people such as persons who are exposed to aniline dyes or cyclophosphamide therapy.

ANATOMY

The lower urinary tract acts as a passage to transmit and store urine. It consists of renal pelvis, ureters, urinary bladder, and urethra (Fig. 11.1).

Renal Pelvis

The renal pelvis is the funnel-like dilated portion of the proximal end of the ureters within the kidney. It receives the final product of urine from the renal calyces.

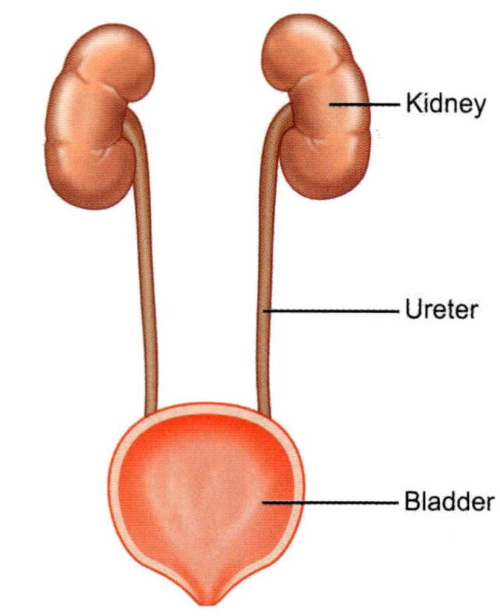

Fig. 11.1: Schematic diagram of the urinary tract.

Ureter

The ureter is a muscular tube-like long slender structure which transmits urine from the kidney to the bladder. Each ureter is 25–30 cm long and 3–4 mm in diameter. The ureter is a retroperitoneal structure and passes through the abdominal cavity and then opens in the back of the urinary bladder.

Urinary Bladder

The urinary bladder is the muscular bag that receives urine from the two ureters and temporarily stores urine. It is superior to the prostate. In the male the urinary bladder is situated in between the rectum posteriorly and pubic bone anteriorly. In females the bladder is situated in between posteriorly vagina and anteriorly pubic bone. Urine exits from bladder via the urethra.

Urethra

Urethra connects the urinary bladder to the external part of the body. In females it is used for urination and in male urethra serves as a conduit of semen and also urine. Male urethra starts from the internal urethral orifice of the bladder to the external urethral orifice of the penis. It is about 17–20 cm long. The female urethra is a membranous tube of 4–5 cm long and extends from the internal urethral orifice of the urinary bladder to the external genitalia in between the clitoris and vagina.

HISTOLOGY

Ureter

Ureter has three layers:

1. *Inner mucosal layer*: Mucosa of the ureter is lined by 3–5 layers of transitional epithelium and is rested on dense fibroconnective tissue, known as lamina propria.
2. *Muscular layer*: Muscle layer consists of inner longitudinal, middle circular, and outer longitudinal layer.
3. Outer fibroconnective tissue coat.

Urinary Bladder

Urinary bladder has three layers: (1) inner mucosal layer, (2) submucosal layer, and (3) muscular layer.

1. *Mucosal layer*: Mucosa of the urinary bladder is lined by transitional epithelial cells (Fig. 11.2). There are three different zones of cells: (1) basal cell layer, (2) intermediate cell layer, and (3) surface cell layer. Basal layer is composed of only one cell layer and the cells are compact and cuboidal in shape. The intermediate cell layers are made of 4–5 layers of columnar cells. The superficial layer is composed of only one layer of cell. These cells are also known as umbrella cells or dome cells and have the unique characteristics that allow them to maintain impermeability to urine to mucosal layer. The cells are large and oval in shape having abundant eosinophilic cytoplasm and round centrally placed nuclei. The surface outline of the cell is fuzzy and indistinct. Many cells are binucleated and a few are multinucleated. The superficial transitional epithelial cells have certain unique ultrastructural features that help them to expand greatly and rapidly when the bladder is distended with urine and the epithelium is at full stretch. The plasma membrane of the umbrella cell has specialized, rigid, thickened regions, known as plaques (also called as asymmetrical unit membrane). These plaques are interspersed with narrow zones of normal interplaque regions. The plaques probably play an important role in maintaining urine-blood barrier and intervening interplaque parts take part in the expansion of the bladder wall during the stretch.

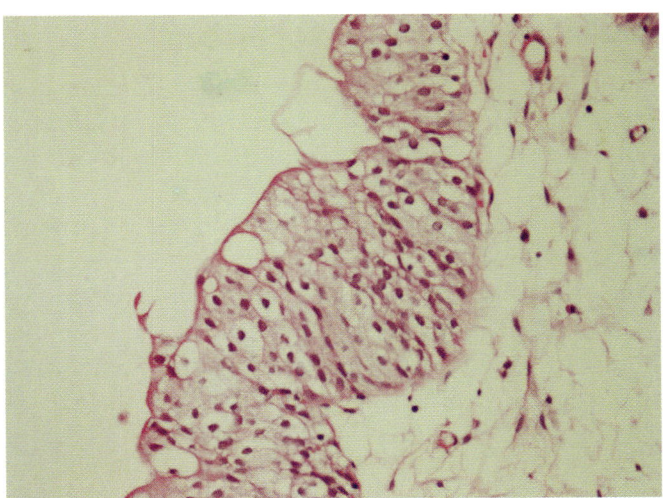

Fig. 11.2: Histology section shows transitional epithelial layer of bladder mucosa (hematoxylin and eosin × MP).

2. *Submucosal layer*: Mucosal membrane of the bladder rests on the submucosal layer. It consists of connective tissue and dense capillary plexus. This capillary plexus serves not only as vascular supply but it also acts as a urinary blood barrier.
3. *Muscular layer*: The muscle layer consists of innermost longitudinal, middle circular, and outermost longitudinal layers that are often difficult to distinguish.

Urethra

The female urethra is lined by transitional epithelium near the bladder and the rest of the part is lined by nonkeratinized stratified squamous epithelium with intervening pseudostratified columnar epithelium.

The prostatic part of the male urethra has transitional epithelial cell lining. The cavernous urethra is lined by stratified columnar epithelium interspersed with portions of the pseudostratified columnar epithelium. The penile urethra has stratified and pseudostratified columnar epithelial lining, except near the meatus that is lined by stratified nonkeratinized squamous epithelium.

NORMAL CYTOLOGY

The normal voided urine sample shows scanty cells. The predominant cell population is transitional cells. However, the other cells may also be noted (Box 11.2).

Transitional Cells

The cells are usually present in discrete or in small loose clusters.

Voided urine sample usually shows discrete superficial cells whereas the catheterized specimen shows clusters or papillary groups of cells containing intermediate and parabasal cells.

Box 11.2: Normal cells in urine.

- Urothelial cells
  - Superficial umbrella cells
  - Intermediate cell
  - Basal cells
- Reactive transitional cells
- Columnar cells
- Squamous cells
- Others
  - Renal tubular cells
  - Seminal vesicle cells
  - Prostatic cells
  - *Blood cells*: polymorphs, lymphocytes, histiocytes, giant cells, etc.

Box 11.3: Superficial umbrella cells.

- Large cell
- Abundant cytoplasm
- Well-defined cytoplasmic margin
- Centrally placed nucleus
- Very low nucleocytoplasmic ratio
- Finely granular nuclear chromatin
- Frequent bi- and multinucleation.

Superficial Cells (Umbrella Cells) (Box 11.3)

Superficial cells are the largest epithelial cells in our body. They are also known as umbrella cells as they protect the underneath cells from the toxic urine of bladder. These cells are about 100 micron in diameter. The cells are round to oval in shape with abundant eosinophilic finely granular cytoplasm. The cytoplasmic margin of the cell is well defined. The nucleus is round and central in position with very low nucleocytoplasmic (N/C) ratio (Fig. 11.3A). The chromatin is granular with inconspicuous nucleoli. The umbrella cells are often bi- or multinucleated and may show even 10–20 nuclei. At times, the superficial cells may show mild nuclear hyperchromasia and pleomorphism. However, the cells maintain low N/C ratio and usually easily recognizable from a neoplastic cells. Degenerated urothelial cells often contain large round eosinophilic cytoplasmic inclusions that are known as Melamed-Wolinska bodies. These structures are seen more frequently in catheterized urine sample than voided urine sample.

Intermediate Cells

The basal/parabasal cells are small round to oval cells with well-defined cell margin and scanty cytoplasm that often shows diffuse fine vacuoles. The nuclei are relatively larger with fine granular chromatin (Box 11.4). The intermediate cells are a bit larger compared to basal cells. The cells show basophilic cytoplasm with central round nuclei and prominent nucleoli (Fig. 11.3B). Bi- and multinucleated cells are infrequent compared to superficial cells.

Reactive Transitional Cells (Box 11.5)

Reactive transitional cells are commonly seen in bladder stone, viral or bacterial cystitis, catheterization or other

Box 11.4: Intermediate and parabasal cells.

- Smaller cells
- Round to oval
- Diffuse fine vacuoles in the cytoplasm
- Central to eccentric round nuclei
- One to two nucleoli
- Bland chromatin.

Box 11.5: Reactive transitional cells.

- Round to oval cells
- Enlarged nucleus with increased nucleocytoplasmic (N/C) ratio
- Mild nuclear pleomorphism
- Mild hyperchromasia
- Prominent nucleoli
- Vacuolated cytoplasm.

Commonly seen: Stone, cystitis, instrumentation, radiation, drugs.

instrumentation, and radiation or drugs. The superficial transitional cells show nuclear enlargement, mild nuclear pleomorphism, hyperchromasia, and even coarse chromatin (Fig. 11.3C). Nuclear membrane may be thickened focally. There may be prominent nucleoli. Low-grade transitional cell carcinoma usually does not show prominent nucleoli.

Squamous Cells

Squamous cells are often present in urine (Box 11.6). Both superficial and intermediate types of squamous cells may be noted. The squamous cells are commonly exfoliated from squamous metaplasia of trigone of the bladder (Fig. 11.3D). This is more frequent in female than male. In addition, the squamous cells may come from the terminal part of urethra as this is lined by squamous epithelium. The other sources of squamous cells are lithiasis, infections, and inflammation.

Columnar Cells (Box 11.7)

The presence of columnar cells in voided urine is uncommon; however, these cells are frequently present in the catheterized urine sample. They are also present due to response to chronic irritation of the bladder. The other sources of columnar cells are cystitis cystica, the lacunae of Morgagni and the glands of Littre of the urethra, seminal vesicles, prostatic epithelium, renal tubules, and rarely from endometrium in endometriosis.

The cells are elongated, columnar in shape with moderate amount of cytoplasm and basally placed nuclei. The cytoplasm of the cells may have small vacuoles (Fig. 11.3E).

Box 11.6: Squamous cells.

- Commonly seen in urine
- Both superficial and intermediate squamous cells
- Common sources are trigone of the bladder, meatus of penis, and vaginal contamination
- Other sources: Stone, infection such as schistosomiasis, exogenous hormone treatment.

Box 11.7: Columnar cells.

- Commonly present in
  - Instrumentation
  - Cystitis cystic
  - Renal tubules
  - Intestinal metaplasia
  - Periurethral glands
  - Prostate
  - Endometriosis
  - Adenocarcinoma
- Morphology
  - Columnar in shape
  - Moderate amount of cytoplasm
  - Small vacuoles
  - Basally placed nuclei.

Pseudopapillary Clusters of Urothelial Cells (Box 11.8)

Clusters of urothelial cells forming papillae-like structures are frequently seen in catheterized urine samples, bladder washing, lithiasis, and cystitis. The pseudopapillary arrangement of the cells may often pose diagnostic difficulty with urothelial cell carcinoma (UCC). However, the pseudopapillary cluster in reactive condition is ball shaped, cohesive with smooth margins. The cytomorphology of the discrete cells is also very important to differentiate the reactive condition form UCC.

Other Cells

There may be sparse polymorphs in the normal urine. Histiocytes, lymphocytes, and plasma cells are present in inflammatory condition. Sperms are seen in urinary sample after a prostatic massage or retrograde ejaculation (Fig. 11.3F).

Seminal vesical cells, epididymal cells, prostatic epithelial cells, and cells from ileal loops may also be present at times.

SPECIMEN COLLECTION

There are five types of specimen collection techniques of urine:

1. Voided urines specimen
2. Catheterized specimen
3. Bladder wash and brush cytology
4. Ureteric sample or from renal pelvis
5. Ileal conduits sample.

Box 11.8: Papillary clusters.

Causes
- Instrumentation
- Infections
- Bladder catheterization
- Stone
- Low-grade urothelial carcinoma

Distinguishing points in favor of benign lesions
- Margin of the papillae is smooth and regular
- Discrete cells have monomorphic and normochromatic nuclei.

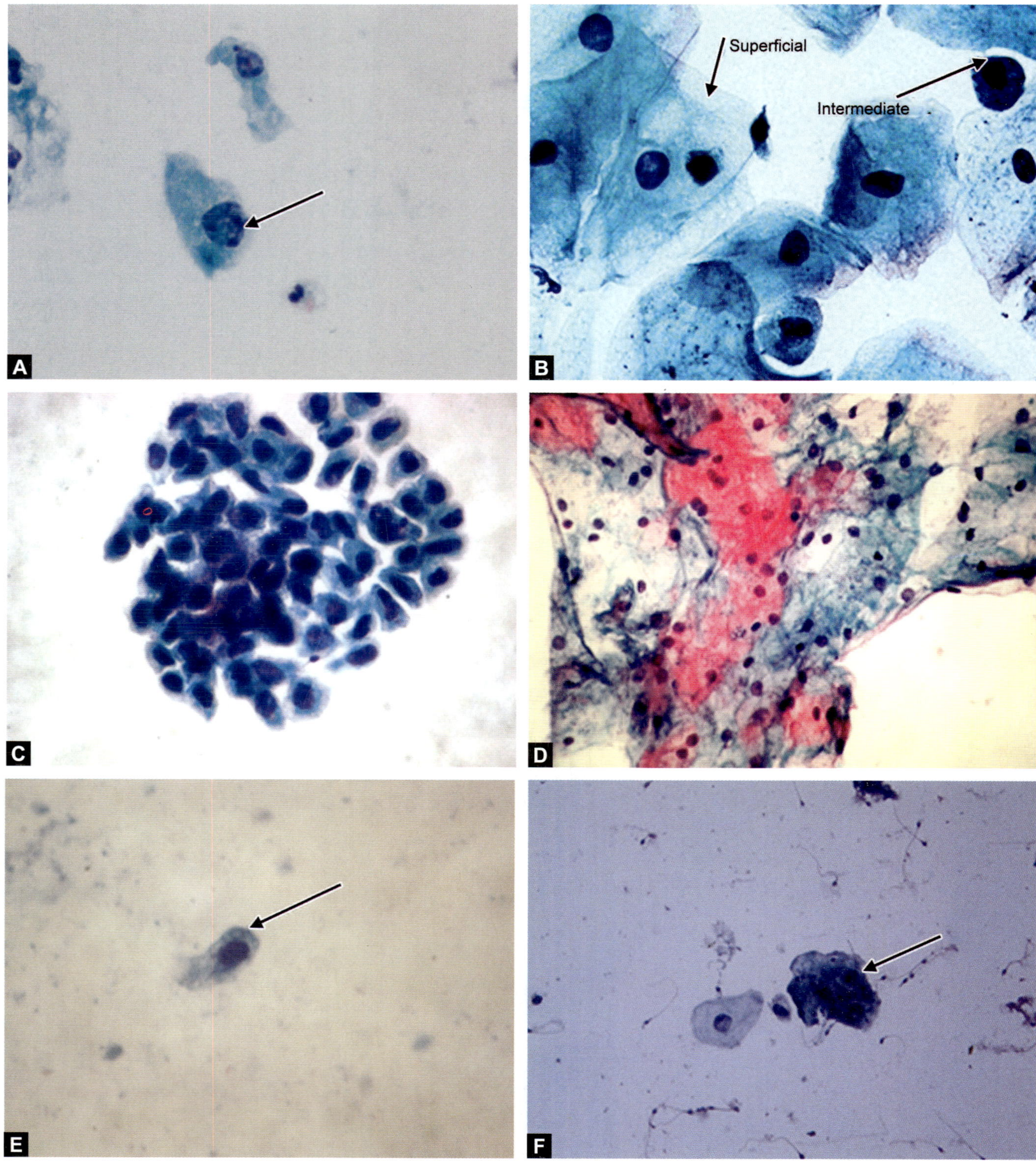

Figs. 11.3A to F: (A) Umbrella cell on urine cytology smear is indicated by arrow (Papanicolaou's stain × HP). (B) Superficial and intermediate cell in urine cytology smear (indicated by arrows) (Papanicolaou's stain × HP). (C) Reactive atypia of transitional cells in urine cytology smear showing nuclear enlargement and pleomorphism (Papanicolaou's stain × HP). (D) Benign squamous epithelial cells in urine cytology smear (Papanicolaou's stain × MP). (E) Columnar cell in urine cytology smear is indicated by arrow (Papanicolaou's stain × HP). (F) Many spermatozoa and seminal vesicle cell in urine cytology smear (*see* arrow) (Papanicolaou's stain × HP).

Box 11.9: Voided sample.

- Choice of sampling in screening of symptomatic patient

Collection
- Three to four hours after last urination with adequate hydration
- Fresh urine in clean container
- At least 50 mL urine
- No preservative

Advantages
- Easy technique
- No artifact due to instrumentation
- Noninvasive technique

Disadvantages
- Degenerative changes
- Contamination of vaginal cells in female.

Voided Urine (Box 11.9)

The specimen of choice for screening of bladder cancer is voided urine sample. The urine sample should be collected 3–4 hours after last micturation. First morning voided urine should better be avoided as it shows considerable amount of degeneration because of prolonged stagnation. Fresh randomly voided urine specimen should be collected in a clean container and should be sent to a laboratory for immediate processing to avoid degenerative changes. About 50 mL of urine is sufficient for cytological examination.

Voided urine is easy to collect; however, the urine sample shows sparse cellularity and considerable degenerative changes. In addition, in female patients there may be high chances of contamination from vaginal cells.

Catheterized Urine

A catheterized urine sample is used in cases of follow-up of a patient of known neoplastic lesion of the lower urinary tract (Box 11.10). Catheterized urine sample yields better cellularity and shows less degenerative changes. However, it may cause breaking up of large tissue fragments that may simulate malignancy. Another important disadvantage of this technique is introduction of urinary tract infection by the tip of the catheter.

Bladder Wash and Brush

Bladder wash and brush are indicated in cases of suspected urothelial neoplasm or follow-up of a case of known neoplastic lesion (Box 11.11). The bladder wash specimen is obtained by rinsing the bladder with 50 mL of sterile normal saline for 3–4 times. The collected fluid is processed. Bladder brushing is done by direct supervision under cystoscopy. The *main advantages* of these techniques are: (1) good cellularity and (2) better preservation of the cells. The major *disadvantages* are: (1) instrumental artifact, (2) invasive technique, and (3) uncomfortable to the patient.

Box 11.10: Catheterized urine.

- Indication
  - Follow-up of a patient of known neoplastic lesion of the lower urinary tract
- Advantages
  - Good cellularity
  - Better preservation than voided urine sample
- Disadvantages
  - Instrumental artifact: Large papillary clusters of cells
  - Urinary tract infection
  - Invasive.

Box 11.11: Bladder wash.

- Indications
  - Suspected urothelial neoplasm
  - Follow-up of a case of known neoplastic lesion
- Advantages
  - Good cellularity,
  - Better preservation of the cells.
- Disadvantages
  - Instrumental artifact,
  - Invasive technique
  - Uncomfortable to the patient.

Other Sampling Techniques

Ureteric Sample

Urine may also be collected by introducing a catheter to the ureter. Urine can be collected separately from each ureter to localize the specific pathology in the ureter or kidney. Smear from each side can be compared for subtle cytological abnormalities.

Ileal Conduits

In case of total cystectomy surgeon makes a duplicate bladder with the help of ileum to provide a conduit of urine. Urine samples are often taken to examine the recurrence of bladder cancer. The sample from ileal conduit usually contains lots of intestinal epithelial cells.

PROCESSING OF URINARY SAMPLE

The urine sample should be processed immediately after receiving the specimen. The exact technique of processing of urine depends on the amount, appearance, and laboratory facility:

- *Simple centrifugation*: Approximately 50 mL urine is centrifuged for 10 minutes with 1,200 rounds per minute. Multiple smears are prepared from the sediment and alcohol fixed smears are kept for staining.
- *Millipore technique*: Large amount (more than 200 mL) of clear urine is processed by this technique.
- *Cytocentrifugation*: Small amount of clear urine particularly ureteric urine sample is processed by cytocentrifugation.
- *Liquid-based preparation*: Liquid-based preparation may be used in urine specimen preparation.[2] This technique provides better morphology and cell preservation along with better cellularity. However, it may not be a cost-effective technique.
- *Cell block*: If fleshy tissue is visible in urine specimen, then cell block could be done.

CRYSTALS AND CASTS IN URINE

The following crystals may be seen in urinary examination (Fig. 11.4).

Normal crystals in urine: Uric acid, calcium phosphate, calcium oxalate, calcium carbonate, and triple phosphate.

Abnormal crystals in urine: Cholesterol, bilirubin, tyrosine, cysteine, etc.

The presence of crystals may be related with renal calculi or crystal nephropathy. However, crystals may be formed after urination outside in the body due to prolonged storage in refrigerators or change of pH.

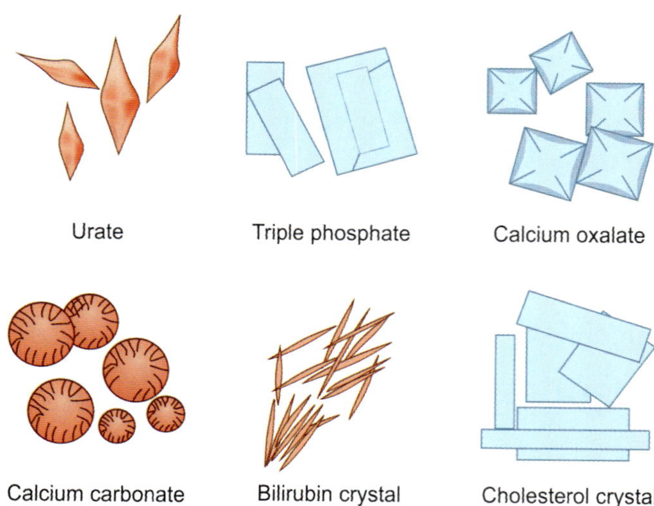

Fig. 11.4: Line diagram of various crystals in urine.

Common Crystals

Uric Acid Crystals

These are amber-colored rhomboid, needle-shaped or polygonal crystals of variable size. Urate crystals may be seen in normal person. However, these crystals are more common in urate nephropathy and urate nephrolithiasis.

Triple Phosphate Crystals

These are rectangular-shaped crystals and typically described as "coffin-lid". Triple phosphate crystals are present in alkaline pH of urine. Urinary tract infections by urea-splitting organism usually produce such crystals.

Calcium Oxalate Crystals

These are colorless envelope-shaped crystals of variable size. They are noted in normal person with high ingestion of oxalate containing food and in nephrolithiasis.

Hippuric Acid Crystals

These are colorless prism-shaped crystals.

Calcium Carbonate Crystals

These are variable sized spheroid- or dumbbell-shaped crystals with radial striations.

Amorphous Crystals

These are finely granular crystals without any specific shape and are seen in acidic urine.

Bilirubin Crystals

These are needle-shaped yellowish crystals due to high conjugated bilirubin and are related with hepatic disorders.

Cholesterol Crystals

These are rectangular-shaped colorless crystals and are often associated with nephrotic syndrome.

NON-NEOPLASTIC LESIONS IN THE URINARY TRACT

Lithiasis (Box 11.12)

The patient of urinary lithiasis may present with hematuria and pain. However, many patients may be totally

Box 11.12: Urinary calculi.

- Symptoms: Pain and hematuria or asymptomatic
- Cytology
- Papillary clusters
- Smooth border of papillae
- Cells with centrally placed nuclei
- Predominantly normal nuclear size and shape but mild nuclear enlargement may be present
- Regular nuclear membrane
- Nuclear hyperchromasia
- Prominent nucleoli
- Squamous metaplasia
- Stone fragments
- Acute inflammatory cells
- *Differential diagnosis*: Urothelial cell carcinoma.

Box 11.13: Similarity and dissimilarity of lithiasis and urothelial cell carcinoma (UCC).

Simulating features
- Both lithiasis and UCC show papillary clusters.
- Nuclear atypia
- Nuclear hyperchromasia and coarse chromatin
- Necrosis, blood, and polymorphs simulate tumor diathesis

Distinguishing points

In lithiasais
- Papillae are usually smooth bordered
- Prominent nucleoli
- Stone fragments
- Nuclear atypia is not so severe
- Clinical history of stone such as pain or radiological features.

asymptomatic. Radiolgically there may be filling defect in the bladder. The cytology smear of urinary lithiasis may simulate malignancy and is the common source of false positive diagnosis.[3] The smears are hypercellular with large fragments of urinary epithelial cells. The cells are often sloughed as papillary clusters. The papillae have usually smooth borders unlike ragged margin of the papillae of UCC (Box 11.13). The individual cells show mild nuclear enlargement and pleomorphism (Fig. 11.5). The nuclear chromatin is coarsely clumped and dark. Nucleoli are prominent. Metaplastic squamous cells may also be present. In addition, background shows acute inflammatory cells, blood, and necrosis. This may simulate tumor diathesis. Fragments of stone may also be noted as calcified and laminated structures.

Infections: Cystitis

Bacterial Infection

Most cases of bacterial cystitis are due to Gram-negative organisms particularly *Escherichia coli*, *Proteus*, *Klebsiella*, and *Pseudomonas aeruginosa*. Gram-positive infections

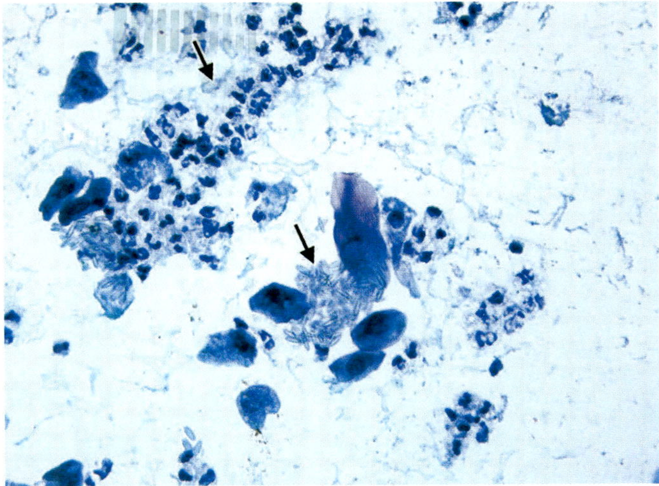

Fig. 11.5: Atypical cells in urinary lithiasis along with crystals (*see* arrows) (Papanicolaou's stain × HP).

rarely cause cystitis. The patient usually presents with dysuria, increased frequency of micturation, and suprapubic tenderness.

Cytology: The smears show abundant polymorphs, RBCs, and necrotic debris. The urothelial cells may be obscured by the inflammatory cells. The transitional cells often show reactive atypia with mild nuclear enlargement, pleomorphism, hyperchromasia, and prominent nucleoli.

Differential diagnosis
- *Urothelial cell carcinoma*: Reactive atypia in urothelial cells should always be distinguished from that of UCC. The presence of abundant polymorphs, mild nuclear atypia, and degenerative changes in nucleus usually indicate reactive changes. In the presence of chromatin smudging or poor preservation of nucleus one should always be careful in the diagnosis of UCC.

Fungal Infections

Fungal infections are commonly seen in diabetic patients and other immunocompromised patients. Candida is the most common fungal infection and other fungal infections are aspergillus, histoplasma, and cryptococcus. Cytological features of fungal infections are similar to that of bacterial infections. The presence of candidal spores in the absence of inflammatory reaction usually indicates contamination in urine.

Viral Infections

Human polyomavirus (Box 11.14): Human polyomavirus is also known as BK virus. It is a DNA virus. BK virus is

Box 11.14: Human polyomavirus.

BK virus
- DNA virus, papova family group
- Present in renal transplant patient, cancer patient, steroid therapy.

Cytology
- Enlarged cells with eccentric nuclei (comet cell)
- Enlarged nucleus
- Hyperchromatic nuclei
- Evenly dispersed chromatin
- Regular nuclear membrane
- Large basophilic intranuclear inclusion body
- Smudgy degenerated nucleus

Differential diagnosis: UCC.

the member of papova virus family. It commonly infects the lower urinary tract with apparently no clinical significance. They commonly affect the patients with renal transplant, steroid therapy, cancer, and AIDS. However, BK virus infection may produce cytological changes in the urinary tract that may simulate UCC.[4] The cells are usually enlarged with eccentric nuclei giving a comet-like appearance (comet cell). Individual cells show mild nuclear enlargement, high N/C ratio, hyperchromatic nuclei, and irregular nuclear contour. The nucleus may have a large basophilic inclusion body that completely replaces the nuclei and only a peripheral rim of the nucleus may remain intact (Fig. 11.6). The nuclei look smudgy. As the infected urothelial cells simulate high-grade UCC so they are also known as "decoy cells".

Distinguishing features between "decoy cells" and urothelial cell carcinoma.

The cells of UCC have following features:
- Larger in size
- Homogenous chromatin
- Irregular nuclear membrane
- Present in clusters.

Human papillomavirus: These are DNA viruses and commonly infect urothelial lining of bladder and squamous lining of cervix. The patient commonly presents as condylomatous lesion of bladder. Cells with koilocytic changes are diagnostic. In voided urine of female patients the possibility of contaminated cells from the lower genital tract should always be excluded.

Cytomegalovirus: It commonly infects the renal convoluted tubular cells. The infected cells are rarely seen in urine specimen. The cells are enlarged with large nuclei having a large intranuclear inclusion and perinuclear clearing.

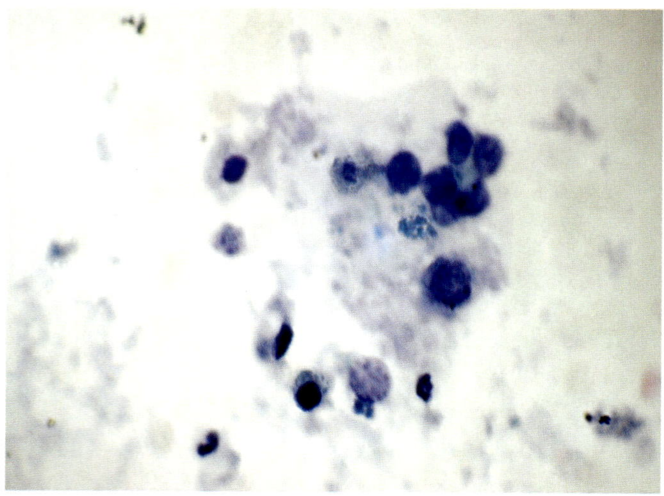

Fig. 11.6: Decoy cell in urine (Papanicolaou's stain × HP).

Chemotherapeutic Effect

Chemotherapeutic drugs like cyclophosphamide, busulfan, thiotepa, and mitomycin may show significant changes of the urothelial cells that simulate malignancy.

Some drugs like cyclophosphamide and busulfan are introduced systemically and are concentrated in the bladder. Other drugs like mitomycin C, thiotepa, adriamycin, etc. are used locally.

Cyclophosphamide: The active metabolite of cyclophosphamide is concentrated in the urine and produces hemorrhagic cystitis. There is necrosis and sloughing out of the bladder mucosal lining resulting profuse hematuria.

Cytology: On cytological examination, the urothelial cells show:
- Cellular smear
- Necrosis
- High N/C ratio (Fig. 11.7)
- Mild nuclear pleomorphism
- Irregular nuclear outline
- Coarse chromatin
- Large prominent nucleoli.

These atypical cells closely mimic high-grade UCC. The cells often show considerable nuclear degenerative changes.

Differential Diagnosis

High-grade UCC: Significant nuclear atypia of the cells may mislead to the diagnosis of UCC. Without proper clinical history it may be impossible to diagnose cells with cyclophosphamide effect.

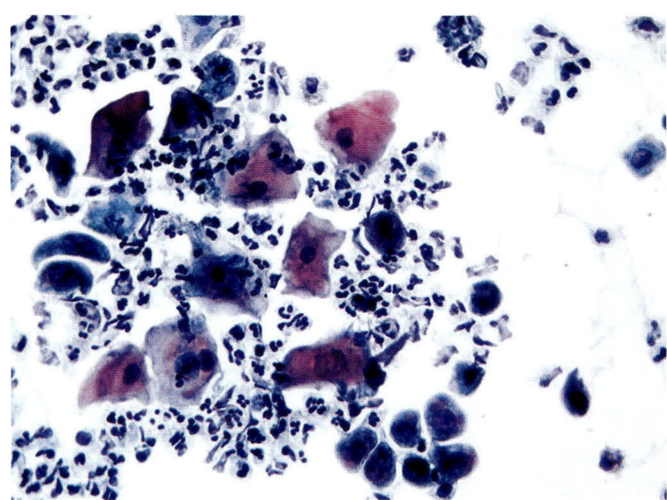

Fig. 11.7: Chemotherapy-induced changes in urine. Nucleus is enlarged with smudgy outline (Papanicolaou's stain × HP).

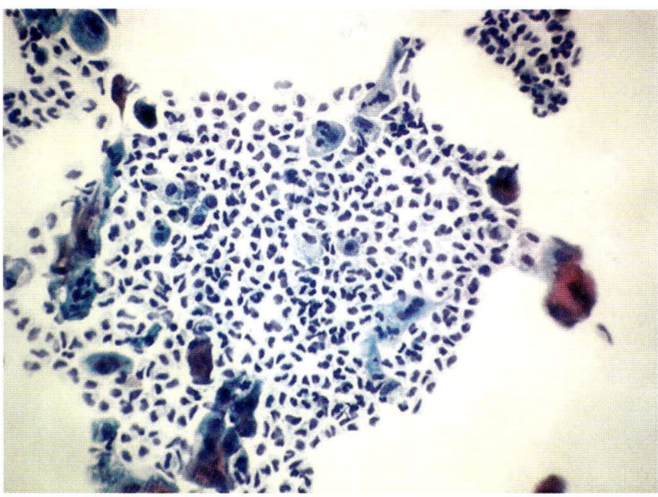

Fig. 11.8: Loose collection of histiocytes and ill-formed epithelioid cell granulomas in BCG-induced changes in urine (Papanicolaou's stain × MP).

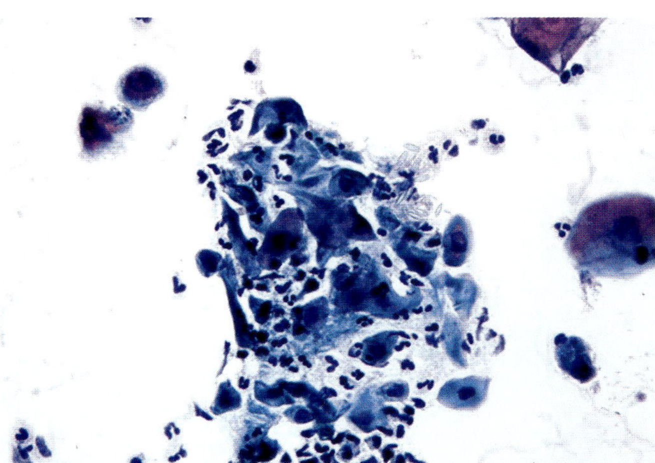

Fig. 11.9: Mild nuclear atypia in BCG-induced changes in urine (Papanicolaou's stain × HP).

Viral infection: Enlarged atypical nucleus may often simulate polyomavirus infection.

Busulfan

Busulfan therapy usually affects lung and occasionally it may cause hemorrhagic cystitis. The cells show nuclear enlargement, pleomorphism, and hyperchromasia. These cells simulate high-grade UCC.

Mitomycin C and Thiotepa

These drugs are locally used intravesically. They also cause sloughing and degeneration of both normal and neoplastic urothelial cells. Urothelial cells show nuclear enlargement and pleomorphism; however, the N/C ratio is not altered. Nuclei often show multiple small nucleoli. Cytoplasm shows polychromasia and vacuolations.

Box 11.15: BCG therapy.

- Attenuated Mycobacterium bovis strain used for carcinoma in situ of bladder
- Initial: polymorphs, degenerated urothelial cells
- Later stage: Lymphocytes, histiocytes
- Epithelioid cell granulomas
- Multinucleated giant cells
- Atypical transitional cells: Nuclear enlargement, hyperchromasia
- No change in nucleocytoplasmic ratio.

BCG Vaccine (Box 11.15)

Immunotherapy with the attenuated *Mycobacterium bovis* strain, Bacillus Calmette-Guérin (BCG) is also used as chemotherapeutic agents for bladder cancer particularly carcinoma in situ. Cytological examination of urine of the patients initially shows neutrophilic reaction along with degenerated urothelial cells. Later on lymphocytes and histiocytes appear. The smear often shows a loose collection of histiocytes and ill-formed epithelioid cell granulomas[5] (Figs. 11.8 and 11.9). Individual cells may show mild nuclear enlargement and hyperchromasia. The N/C ratio of these cells is usually maintained.

Radiation Effect (Box 11.16)

Pelvic irradiation is commonly used in cervical cancer, bladder cancer, and other pelvic malignancies. Radiation

Box 11.16: Radiation changes.

- Marked cytomegaly (macrocytes)
- Nuclear enlargement
- No alteration of nucleocytoplasmic ratio
- Cytoplasmic eosinophilia and vacuoles
- Nuclear vacuoles
- Prominent and multiple nucleoli (macronucleoli)
- Nuclear hyperchromasia
- Multinucleated cells.

causes mucosal edema, congestion, and ulceration. The urothelial cells show degenerative changes.

Cytology

The smear shows markedly enlarged cells known as macrocytes.

Both cytoplasm and nucleus are enlarged and therefore there is no change of N/C ratio. Cytoplasm shows polychromasia or eosinophilia and contains multiple degenerative vacuoles. Nuclei also show vacuoles, mild hyperchromasia, and multiple prominent nucleoli. Nuclear membrane is usually regular. Nuclear chromatin may be smudgy and featureless. Chronic radiation change may show multinucleated giant cells and similar type of cells as seen in acute radiation effect (Fig. 11.10).

Differential diagnosis: Malignant cells: Radiation changes may simulate malignant cells because of markedly enlarged cells and nuclear hyperchromasia. However, the cells in radiation effect do not show any alteration of N/C ratio. Both cytoplasm and nuclei of these cells show degenerative vacuoles. Nuclei show smudged featureless chromatin.

NEOPLASTIC LESIONS

Urothelial carcinoma of the bladder represents more than 90% of all malignant bladder neoplasms.[6] UC is three times more common in male than female and is more common over 50 years of age; however, it may occur in young adults and children. The common environmental factors related to UCC are exposure to aromatic amines used in rubber, plastic and dye, cigarette smoking, Schistosoma hematobium infection, long-term use of analgesics particularly phenacetin, cyclophosphamide, and lithiasis.

The common presenting symptoms of the patient are hematuria, dysuria, and increased urinary frequency. The urothelial neoplasms are fundamentally classified as two types: (1) Flat lesions and (2) papillary lesions. Currently World Health Organization (WHO) has classified bladder tumors as mentioned in Box 11.17.[7]

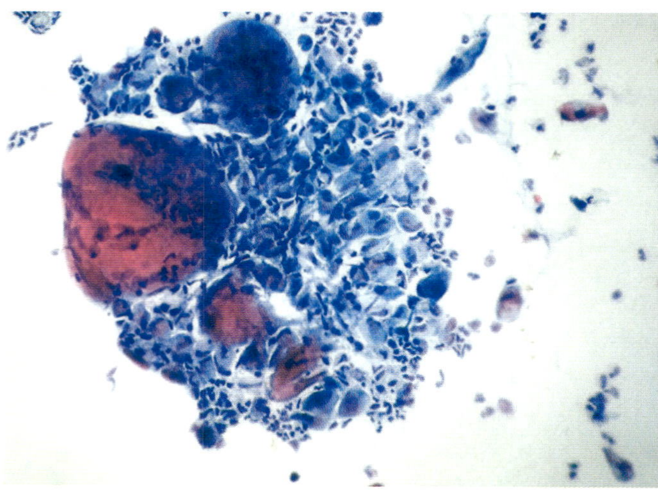

Fig. 11.10: Multinucleated cells along with polymorphs and lymphocytes in urine cytology smear (Papanicolaou's stain × MP).

Box 11.17: WHO classification of urothelial tumors (2016).

- Infiltrating urothelial carcinoma
  - Microcystic, micropapillary, nested, signet ring type, sarcomatoid, giant cell type
- Noninvasive urothelial neoplasms
  - Urothelial carcinoma in situ
  - Noninvasive papillary urothelial carcinoma, low grade
  - Noninvasive papillary urothelial carcinoma, high grade
  - Papillary urothelial neoplasm of low malignant potential
  - Urothelial papilloma
  - Inverted urothelial papilloma
  - Urothelial proliferation of uncertain malignant potential
  - Urothelial dysplasia
- Squamous cell neoplasm
  - Squamous cell carcinoma
  - Verrucous carcinoma
- Glandular neoplasm
  - Adenocarcinoma
  - Villous adenoma

Urachal carcinoma

- Tumors of Müllerian type
  - Clear cell carcinoma
- Neuroendocrine tumor
  - Small cell neuroendocrine carcinoma
  - Large cell neuroendocrine carcinoma
  - Well-differentiated neuroendocrine carcinoma
- Mesenchymal tumor
- Melanocytic tumor
- Hematopoietic and lymphoid tumor
- Miscellaneous.

Basically the urothelial neoplasm can be divided into flat and papillary neoplasm. The flat lesions are classified as dysplasia and carcinoma in situ. The papillary neoplasm is divided into four groups: (1) papilloma, (2) papillary urothelial neoplasm of low malignant potential (PUNLMP), (3) low-grade papillary carcinoma, and (4) high-grade papillary carcinoma.

PARIS SYSTEM OF CLASSIFICATION

The urinary sample is usually of low cellularity, having degenerated cells and there is an unrealistic expectation to diagnose low-grade UC. There was no standardized reporting format of urinary cytology. To combat these challenges a panel of cytopathologists and urologists met in Paris in May of 2013 at the 18th International Congress of Cytology. The consensus approach to the reporting of urinary cytology is reached. Box 11.18 highlights the Paris system of reporting urinary cytology.[8] The main goal of the system is to detect more number of high-grade UCC.

Nondiagnostic/Unsatisfactory or Criteria of Adequacy

Any urine cytology smear that shows abnormal cells is adequate. It was suggested in a meta-analytic study that the "presence of 2,600 cells or 2 well-visualized urothelial cells per high-power field in 10 consecutive high-power fields" in ThinPrep method is an adequate urine sample.[9]

Box 11.18: Paris system of reporting urinary cytology.[8]

1. Non-diagnostic/unsatisfactory
2. Negative for high grade urothelial cell carcinoma (NHGUC)
3. Atypical urothelial cells (AUC)
4. Suspicious for high grade urothelial cell carcinoma (SHGUC)
5. High grade urothelial cell carcinoma (HGUC)
6. Low grade urothelial cell carcinoma (LGUC)
7. Others: Primary and secondary malignancies and various other lesions

If the urine cytology smear is completely obscured by inflammatory cells or lubricant material then it should be considered unsatisfactory.

Negative for High-grade Urothelial Cell Carcinoma

Negative for high-grade urothelial cell carcinoma (NHGUC) includes those cases where the cells do not show any abnormality. The urine cytology smear with definite cause of atypia will be included in this group.

Atypical Urothelial Cells (Figs. 11.11A and B)

This is the challenging area and the diagnosis is difficult. The main diagnostic criteria are:

Mandatory Feature

1. *N/C ratio*: The N/C ratio of the urothelial cells more than 0.5 and less than 07. These cells should be nonsuperficial and nondegenerated urothelial cells.
   Minor Features
   Any one of these three should be present along with the high N/C ratio:
2. Hyperchromasia
3. Irregular clumped chromatin
4. Irregular nuclear membrane
   Note: One major feature along with any one minor feature.

Suspicious for High-grade Urothelial Cell Carcinoma (Figs. 11.12A and B)

Only few cells (less than five cells) show:

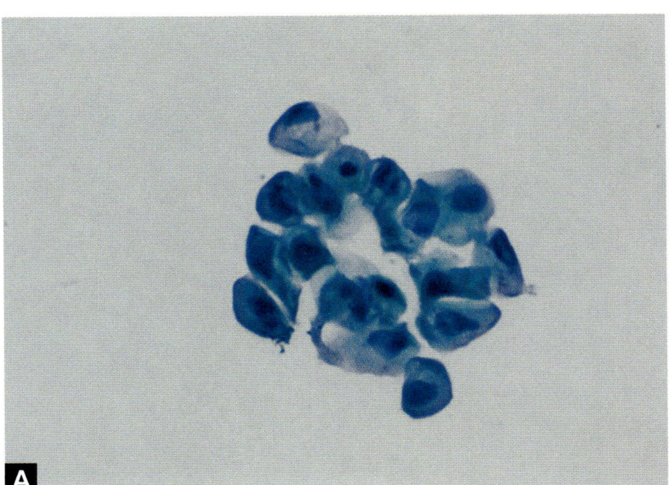

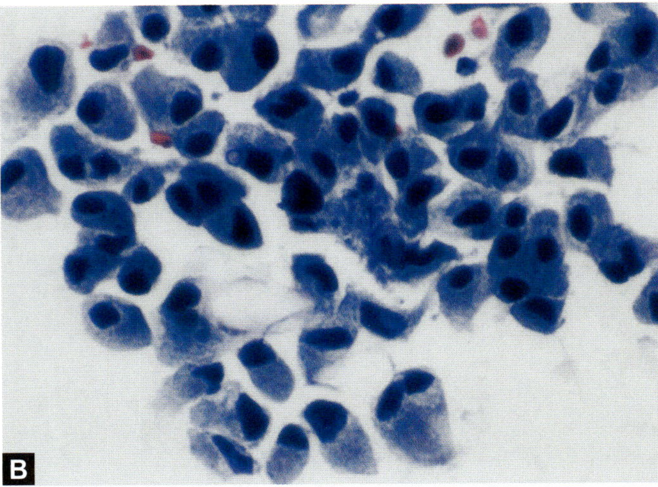

Figs. 11.11A and B: (A) Urine cytology smear shows enlarged nuclei (N/C ratio more than 0.5 but less than 0.7) with nuclear hyperchromasia (Papanicolaou's stain × MP). (B) Higher magnification of the atypical cells shows better morphology (Papanicolaou's stain × HP).

Mandatory features

1. *Nucleocytoplasmic ratio*: The N/C ratio of the urothelial cells should be more than 07.
2. Hyperchromasia.

Minor features

Any one of the two features should be present:

1. Irregular clumped chromatin.
2. Irregular nuclear membrane.

High-grade Urothelial Cell Carcinoma (Figs. 11.13 to 11.16)

At least 5–10 cells should have the following features:

Mandatory Features

1. *Nucleocytoplasmic ratio*: The N/C ratio of the urothelial cells should be more than 07.
2. Hyperchromasia.

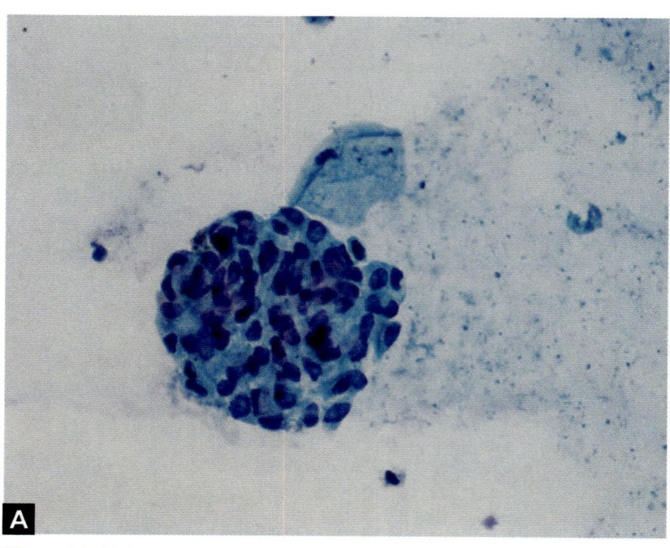

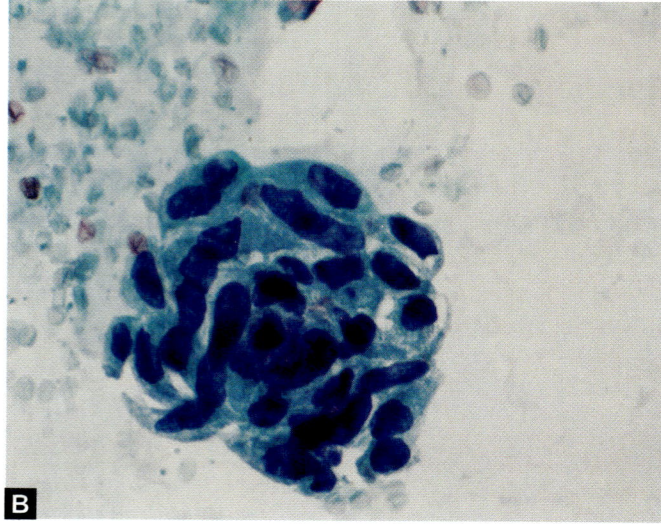

Figs. 11.12A and B: (A) Smear of atypia, suspicious for high-grade urothelial cell carcinoma. Note the nuclear enlargement, hyperchromasia, and irregular nuclear margin (Papanicolaou's stain × MP). (B) Smear of atypia, suspicious for high-grade urothelial cell carcinoma. Higher magnification of the cells (Papanicolaou's stain × HP).

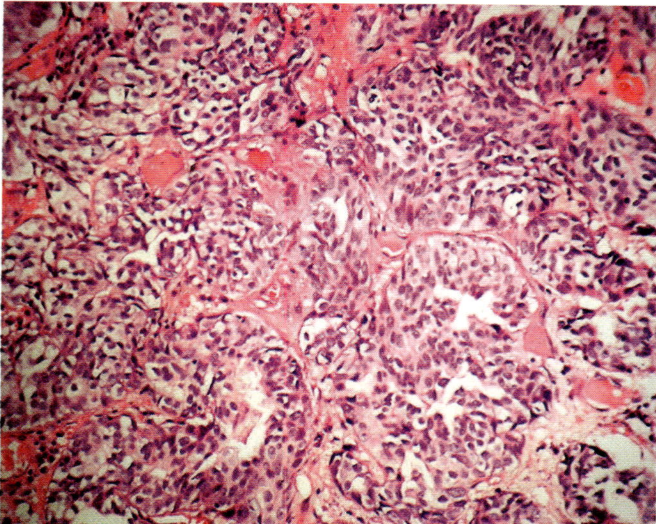

Fig. 11.13: Histology section of high-grade transitional cell carcinoma of bladder (hematoxylin and eosin × MP).

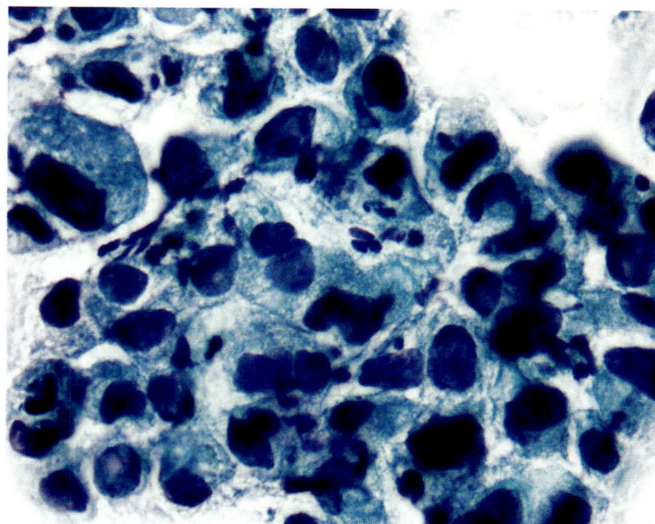

Fig. 11.14: Cytology smear of the high-grade transitional cell carcinoma of bladder showing moderate nuclear enlargement and pleomorphism (Papanicolaou's stain × HP).

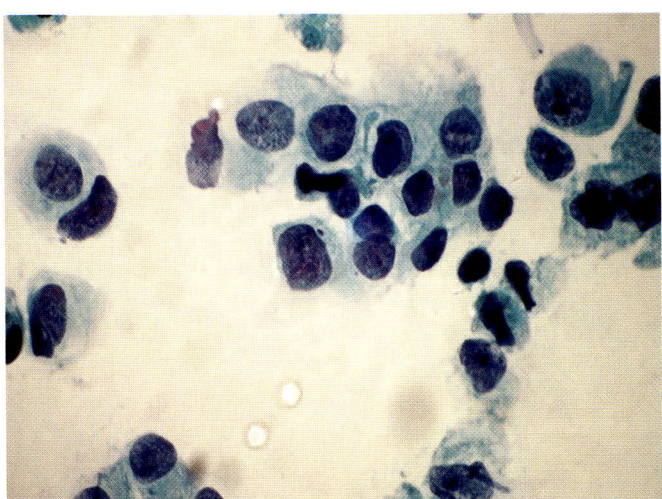

Fig. 11.15: Cytology smear of the high-grade transitional cell carcinoma of bladder showing discrete malignant cells with moderate nuclear enlargement, pleomorphism, and prominent nucleoli (Papanicolaou's stain × HP).

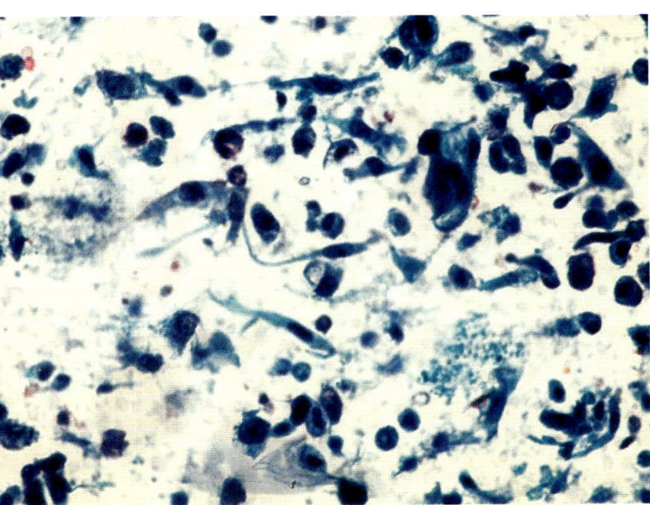

Fig. 11.16: Cercariform cells in high-grade transitional cell carcinoma of bladder (Papanicolaou's stain × HP).

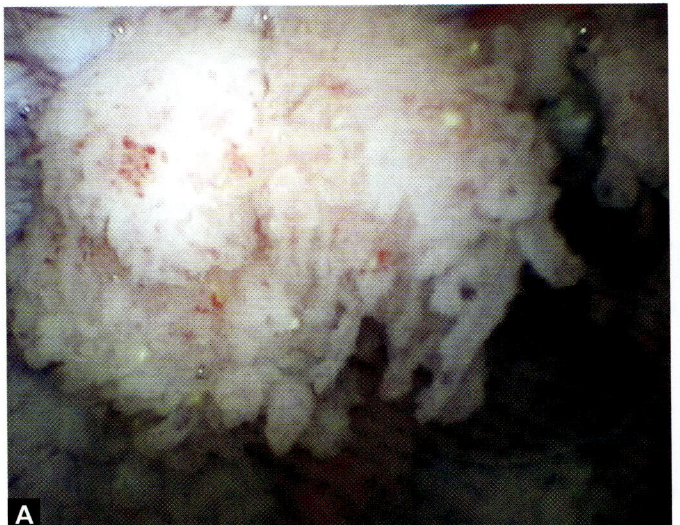

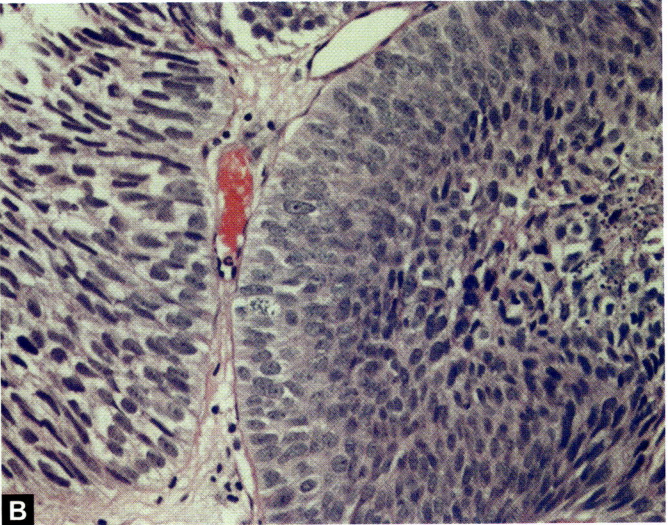

Figs. 11.17A and B: (A) Cystoscopic picture of a low-grade papillary urothelial carcinoma of urinary bladder and (B) Histology section of low-grade transitional cell carcinoma of bladder (hematoxylin and eosin × MP).
Courtesy: Dr Uttam Mete, Additional Professor, Department of Urology, PGIMER, Chandigarh, India (for Fig. 11.17A).

Minor Features

Any one of the two features should be present:

1. Irregular clumped chromatin
2. Irregular nuclear membrane.

In addition, the smear usually shows high cellularity, dissociated and loose clusters, moderately pleomorphic nuclei, large prominent nucleoli, and atypical mitosis.

Low-grade Urothelial Cell Carcinoma (Figs. 11.17 to 11.19)

Low grade urothelial cell carcinoma (LGUC): LGUC is difficult to diagnose in urine cytology smear. The presence of three-dimensional papillary clusters with fibrovascular core and tight clusters of cells with nuclear overlapping suggest LGUC. In addition, high N/C ratio and nuclear margin irregularity may be rarely present.

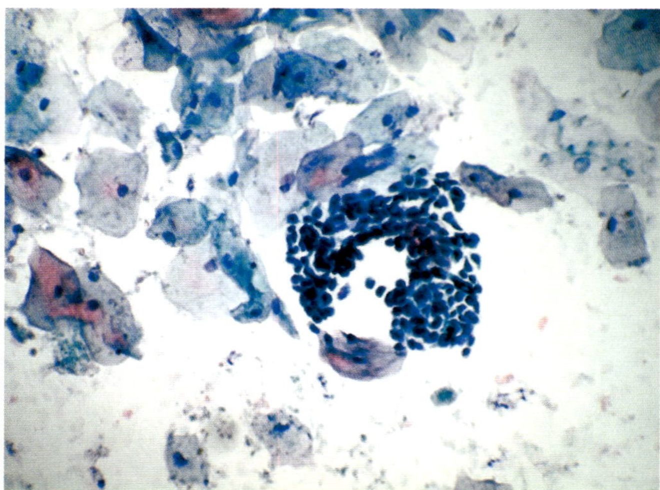

Fig. 11.18: Cytology smear of low-grade transitional cell carcinoma of bladder. The cells show scanty cytoplasm and mild nuclear enlargement (Papanicolaou's stain × MP).

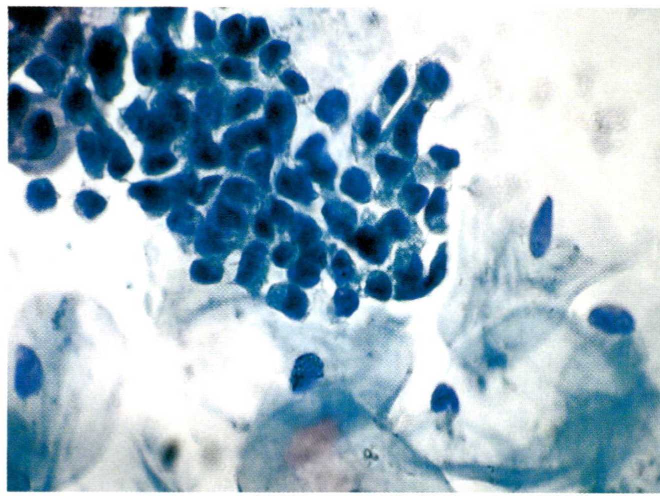

Fig. 11.19: High powered view of the same showing scanty cytoplasm and mild nuclear enlargement (Papanicolaou's stain × HP).

Others: Primary and Secondary Malignancies and Various Other Lesions

Miscellaneous other primary and secondary malignancies along with various benign lesions are included in this category.

Relative Risk of Malignancy in the Different Category

Unsatisfactory: Less than 5–10%
NHGUC: 0–10%
AUN: 8–35%
SHGUC: 50–90%
HGUC: More than 90%
LGUC: More than 90%.

Management

Repeat cytology should be done in unsatisfactory urine sample. Clinical follow-up is advised in both NHGUC and AUC categories. Intense follow-up and cystoscopy or biopsy are advised in SHGUC and HGUS categories. Whereas cystoscopy and biopsy are advised in LGUC.

CYTOLOGY OF MALIGNANCY IN URINE

Low-grade Papillary Carcinoma (Figs. 11.18 and 11.19)

Cytology smears of low-grade papillary UC show clusters of cells with irregular outline and multiple papillae-like structures with fibrovascular core and capillaries (Box 11.19).

Box 11.19: Low-grade papillary carcinoma.

- Papillary fragments of cells
- High cellularity
- Cells with enlarged nuclei
- High nucleocytoplasmic ratio
- Monomorphic to mild pleomorphic nucleoli
- Irregular nuclear membrane
- Small inconspicuous nucleoli.

Box 11.20: High-grade papillary carcinoma.

- High cellularity
- Dissociated and loose clusters
- Moderate pleomorphic nuclei
- Moderate to marked nuclear hyperchromasia
- High nucleocytoplasmic ratio
- Irregular nuclear membrane
- Coarse granular chromatin
- Large prominent nucleoli
- Atypical mitosis.

The cells show mild nuclear enlargement and pleomorphism. N/C ratio is mildly raised. Nucleoli are small and inconspicuous.

High-grade Urothelial Carcinoma and Carcinoma in situ Lesions (Box 11.20)

Cytological features of high-grade UC are similar to that of both high grade-papillary carcinoma and carcinoma in situ of flat lesions. The smears show high cellularity. The cells are predominantly discrete or in loose clusters (*see* Figs. 11.13 to 11.16). The individual cells show moderate to marked nuclear enlargement and pleomorphism with high N/C ratio. Nuclei are hyperchromatic with coarsely granular chromatin and prominent nucleoli. Nuclear membrane shows an irregular margin. Occasional cells show elongated nuclei and cytoplasmic extension resembling cercariform cells. The background may show RBCs, degenerated cells, and necrotic tissue fragments. The diagnosis of HGUC in voided sample is usually straight forward. However, if a diagnosis of HGUC is made but no lesion is seen in cystoscopy, then a possibility of carcinoma in situ or UC in the higher part of the urinary tract should be suggested.

Dysplasia

The term dysplasia is used in WHO classification of urothelial neoplastic lesions. In the voided urinary cytology specimen this entity is difficult to diagnose with confidence. Moreover, the clinical significance of the diagnosis of dysplasia in the urine sample is limited as it is mostly associated with high-grade UC. It is better to avoid the diagnosis of dysplasia in urine cytology.

Other Malignancies

Squamous Cell Carcinoma

Pure squamous cell carcinoma of urinary bladder is uncommon. It is usually related to Schistosoma hematobium infection which is more frequent near Nile river. The malignant cells are polyhedral in shape with hyperchromatic moderately pleomorphic nuclei. The cytoplasm of the cells shows orangeophilia indicating intracellular keratinization (Fig. 11.20).

Adenocarcinoma

The adenocarcinoma is rare in the urinary tract. The tumor resembles mucin secreting gastrointestinal carcinoma. The cells are columnar in appearance with moderately pleomorphic nuclei having prominent nucleoli. Occasionally the glandular arrangement is present. Abundant mucin may also be present in the background.

Small Cell Carcinoma

Small cell carcinoma of urinary bladder is a rare aggressive tumor. Cytomorphology is same as that of small cell carcinoma of other parts of the body. The cells are small round shaped with scanty cytoplasm (Figs. 11.21 and 11.22). Nuclei show salt and pepper like chromatin.

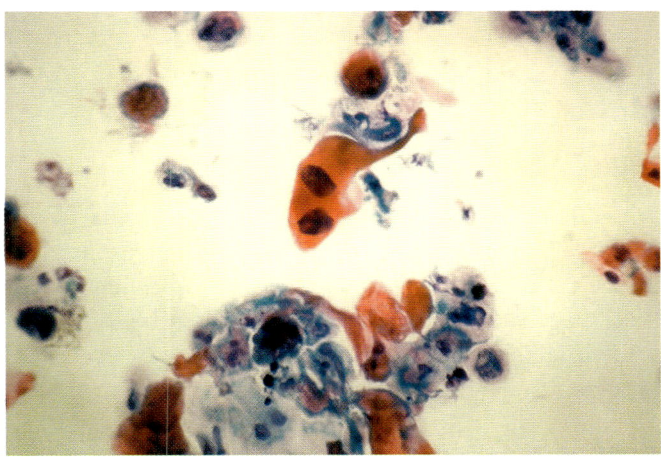

Fig. 11.20: Malignant cells with orangeophilic cytoplasm in a case of squamous cell carcinoma of bladder (Papanicolaou's stain × MP).

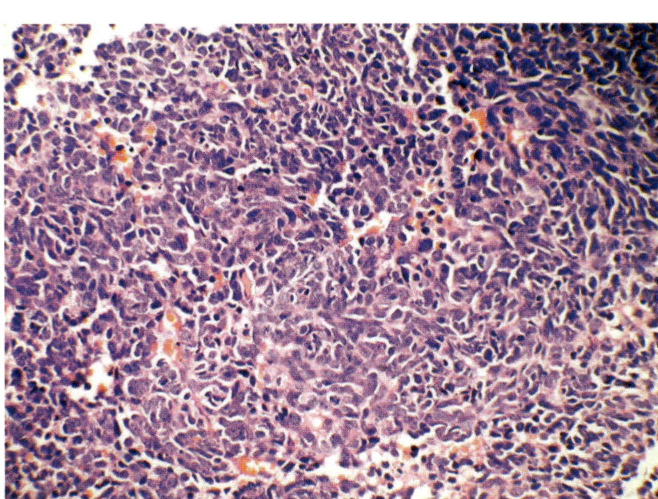

Fig. 11.21: Histology section of a small cell carcinoma of bladder (hematoxylin and eosin × MP).

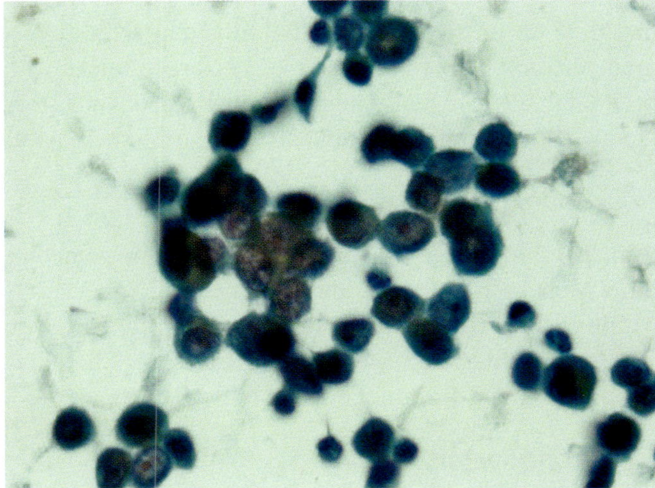

Fig. 11.22: Cluster of small cells with scanty cytoplasm in small cell carcinoma of bladder (Papanicolaou's stain × HP).

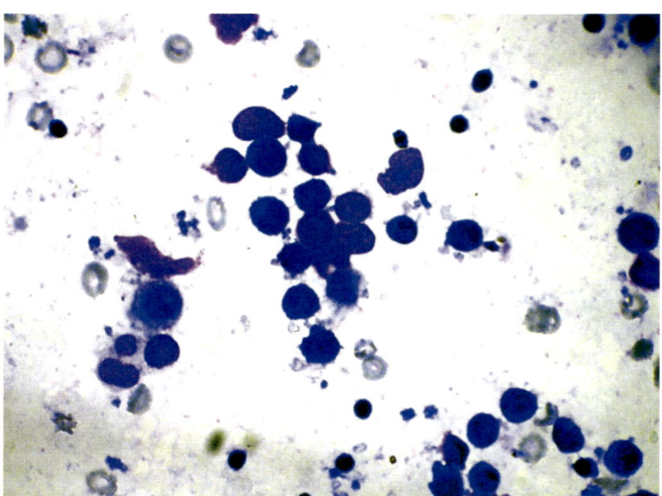

Fig. 11.23: High powered view of the immature lymphoid cells in non-Hodgkin's lymphoma (May-Grünwald Giemsa stain × MP).

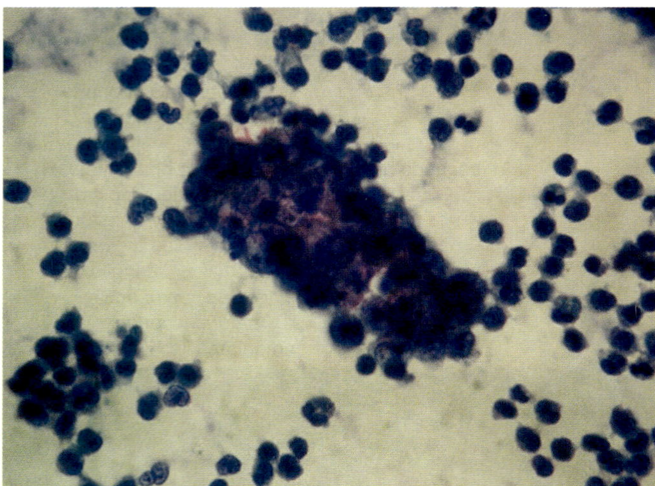

Fig. 11.24: Malignant cells with moderate nuclear enlargement and prominent nucleoli in urine in a case of rectal adenocarcinoma infiltrating into bladder (Papanicolaou's stain × HP).

Metastatic Carcinoma

Renal Cell Carcinoma

When renal cell carcinoma (RCC) invades the renal pelvis, urine cytology may show cells of renal cell carcinoma. The individual cells show abundant clear cytoplasm and centrally placed enlarged nuclei. Urine cytology has not much value in detecting such cells as most of the cases of RCC are diagnosed by other modalities such as CT scan or MRI.

Prostatic Carcinoma

Urine cytology often shows the presence of prostate carcinoma. In most of the cases the prior diagnosis of prostate carcinoma is known. Rarely, the primary diagnosis is made first time on urine cytology. The individual cells show a moderate amount of cytoplasm and enlarged nuclei with prominent nucleoli. Without prior knowledge of the history of prostatic carcinoma, it is difficult to diagnose such cases.

Non-Hodgkin's Lymphoma

Primary lymphoma of the urinary bladder is very uncommon. Most of the time bladder is secondarily involved by lymphoma. Occasionally urine shows discrete round to oval cells with scanty cytoplasm. Nuclei show fine chromatin and single prominent nucleoli (Fig. 11.23).

Metastatic Rectal Carcinoma

Occasionally the urinary bladder is infiltrated by rectal adenocarcinoma. Urine cytology examination may show malignant cells. The cells are usually round to oval with moderately pleomorphic nuclei and prominent nucleoli (Fig. 11.24).

ANCILLARY TECHNIQUES

Urine cytology is a specific but less sensitive technique particularly in low-grade UC. Cystoscopy is helpful for the detection of visible papillary growth; however, it is costly and invasive technique and may prove as inconclusive in cases of cystitis. Therefore, there is a need of simple, non-invasive, and reliable test to detect urothelial malignancy.

Food and Drug Administration-approved tests for the detection of urothelial carcinoma:

- Bladder tumor antigen test
- NMP22 (nuclear matrix protein 22)
- ImmunoCyt
- Urovysion.

The *point of care tests:*

- Bladder tumor antigen test
- NMP22.

Nuclear Matrix Protein (Box 11.21)

Nuclear matrix proteins (NMP) are the nonchromatic structure of the nucleus. They help to maintain the nuclear shape and also play significant role in DNA replication, transcription, and gene expression.[10] NMP22 is the fragmented nuclear mitotic apparatus protein present at a very low level in the interphase nuclear matrix. The level of NMP22 is 25-folds higher in urine of urothelial cancer.[10]

Box 11.21: Nuclear matrix protein 22.

Nuclear matrix protein 22 (NMP22) is nonchromatin structure related with nuclear shape, organizes DNA, and takes important role in cell division

- NMP22 concentration is very high in bladder cancer
- It is an enzyme-linked Immunoassay test
- It uses two monoclonal antibodies that are specific for NMP22
- FDA-approved test
- Point of care test
- *Advantages*
  - Simple test
  - No sample preparation needed
  - No intact cell needed
  - Result needs just 30 minutes.
- *False positive*
  - Cystitis
  - Bladder or renal stone
  - Prostate cancer.

The NMP22 test is a quantitative enzyme-linked immunoassay test. The sensitivity and specificity of NMP22 test varies from 68.5% to 88.5% and 65.2% to 91.3%, respectively.[11] NMP22 is an office-based test and is approved by the Food and Drug Administration (FDA) in the USA.

Advantages

- Simple test
- No sample preparation needed
- No intact cell needed
- Result needs just 30 minutes.

False Positive Test

Cystitis, bladder or renal stone, prostate cancer, and ileal conduit.

Bladder Tumor Antigen Test

This is FDA approved and a point of care test. The bladder tumor antigen (BTA) is made of basement membrane complexes derived from the urine of bladder cancer patients. The original BTA test is a latex agglutination assay that lacks adequate specificity particularly in patients with cystitis.[12] The two other tests, BTA stat and BTA TRAK assays measure human complement related H factor released from the basement membrane of bladder cancer. The sensitivity and specificity of BTA stat varies from 57% to 83% and 68% to 72%, respectively, whereas, the sensitivity and specificity of BTA TRAK are 62–77% and 50–75%, respectively.[11] False positivity of these tests may occur in cases of urinary tract inflammation, hematuria, and urinary stone.

Advantages

- A simple noninvasive assay
- No sample preparation.

False Positive

Urinary tract inflammation and bladder stone.

Fluorescent in situ Hybridization Technique (Urovysion Test)

This is a FDA-approved test. Cytogenetic abnormalities in UCC are seen in chromosome 1, 3, 4, 7, 8, 9, 11, and 17. These chromosomal abnormalities can be demonstrated by fluorescent in situ hybridization (FISH) technique using fluorescent-labeled DNA probes. Currently commercially available probes are against chromosome 3, 7, 17 and homozygous loss of 9p21. Each DNA probe is tagged with different fluorochrome to increase the sensitivity of the test.

Criteria of Positivity

- Five or more cells with gain of two or more chromosomes
- Ten or more cells with gain of one chromosome.

Sensitivity and specificity of urovysion test are 81% and 98%, respectively.[11]

Advantages

- *Anticipatory positive reading*: Detects the chromosomal change before the phenotypic expression of malignancy
- Not affected by inflammation, hematuria, stone effect
- Suitable for BCG-induced response.

UCyt/ImmunoCyt

It is a FDA-approved test. ImmunoCyt test is an immunofluorescence assay that detects cell markers specific for urothelial cancer. Two antibodies are used for CEA and mucin of urothelial cell:

- Antibody 19A21 labeled with Texas red against CEA
- Antibodies M344 and LDQ10 labeled with fluorescein against mucin.

Result

Positive tumor cells show both red and green dots.

The ImmunoCyt test is relatively sensitive test (86%) with moderate specificity (80%).[11]

Advantages

Relatively easy test and only 30 minutes incubation is needed.

Disadvantages

- Difficult to interpret for cytologist
- Fluorescence microscope needed
- Benign colonic cells may show positivity due to presence of CEA.

Flow Cytometry

The detection of an aneuploid population or demonstration of high synthetic (S) phase are indicators of malignancy in flow cytometry (FCM). The sensitivity and specificity of DNA FCM is variable and ranges from 45% to 95% and 83% to 100%, respectively.[13] The sensitivity of FCM can be enhanced further by using monoclonal antibodies cytokeratin 18 along with DNA FCM.[11]

Fibrin Degradation Product

Fibrin degradation product (FDP) is increased significantly in urine of bladder cancer patients.[11] Accu-Dx immunoassay device can qualitatively detect FDP. It has 68% sensitivity and 86.2% specificity.[11]

Hyaluronic Acid and Hyaluronidase

Hyaluronic acid (HA), a nonsulphated glucosaminoglycan, is elevated in urothelial cancer.[14] The overall sensitivity and specificity of HA tests are 83% and 90%, respectively.[11]

Telomerase

Telomerase is a specific ribonucleoprotein. Increased telomerase activity is present in urothelial cancer.[15] and is detected by specific telomerase repeat amplification protocol (TRAP). The sensitivity and specificity of telomerase activity are 70–86% and 60–90%, respectively.[11] The contaminated urine sample may produce false negative results. The false positive result may be noted in inflammation.

Quanticyt

Quanticyt system applies the image morphometric analysis and DNA content of the cell to detect urothelial cancer.[16] This technique requires bladder wash for optimal cellularity and technical expertise. Quanticyt system has 60% sensitivity and 70% specificity.[11]

Cytokeratin

Cytokeratin-20 (CK-20) is expressed mainly in malignant urothelial cells. The measurement of CK level in urine may be helpful to screen UC.[17] Sensitivity and specificity of CK-20 in urine sample are 91% and 67–100%, respectively.[11]

Table 11.1 shows sensitivity and specificity of different ancillary techniques used in urine specimen to detect malignancy.

In a cytology confirmed HGUC case, no ancillary test is recommended. Cytology along with Urovysion test increases the sensitivity of LGUC up to 75%. But in LGUC case cystoscopy clearly demonstrates the mass and ancillary test has little value. Probably ancillary tests are helpful in atypical urothelial cells.

Table 11.1: Comparison of different ancillary tests in urine sample.

Test	*Specific marker*	*Basic test type*	*Sensitivity (%)*	*Specificity (%)*
Flow cytometry	Aneuploid cell and high S-phase	Flow cytometry	45–95	83–100
NMP22	*Nuclear matrix protein*: Nuclear mitotic apparatus	Enzyme linked immunoassay	68–88	65–91
Bladder tumor antigen test	H factor of complement	Immunoassay	62–77	68–72
Accu-Dx	Fibrinogen degradation product	Immunoassay	68	86
Hyaluronic acid and hyaluronidase	Hyaluronic acid Hyaluronidase	Immunoassay	83	90
Telomerase	RNA polymerase	Telomeric repeat action protocol	70–86	90
Quanticyt	Nuclear morphometry and DNA	Image morphometry	59–69	70
Immunocyt	CEA and mucin	Immunofluorescence	86	79
Fluorescent in situ hybridization technique	Chromosomal aberration	In situ hybridization	81	98

Box 11.22: Causes of false positive urinary cytology.

- Viral cystitis
- Lithiasis
- *Instrumentation*: Catheterization, etc.
- *Chemotherapeutic drugs*: Cyclophosphamide, busulfan, BCG vaccine, etc.
- Radiation therapy
- Ileal conduit specimen
- Ill-preserved degenerated cell
- Inflammation causing atypia.

Diagnostic Accuracy of Urine Cytology

Sensitivity and specificity of urine cytological examination are 40–62% and 94–100%, respectively.[18] Diagnostic sensitivity and specificity of the urine cytological examination depends on several factors such as:

- *Specimen type*: Whether voided urine or bladder wash/brush: Bladder wash/brush usually yields better cellularity and diagnostic material.
- *Diagnostic category used*: Diagnostic criteria used in urinary cytology report influences the accuracy of the urinary cytological examination.
- *Grade of urothelial carcinoma*: Low-grade UC has low sensitivity and specificity. These cases are difficult to diagnosis in urinary cytology as the cytological features are subtle and difficult to find out, whereas high-grade UC has high sensitivity and specificity.
- *Screening or symptomatic patient*: Whether urinary examination is done as screening or in symptomatic patient. Sensitivity of urine cytology is much higher if the test is used in screening of symptomatic patients.

The false positive rate in urine cytology varies from 1% to 15%. The predominant causes of false positive urinary cytology are lithiasis, infection, and instrumentation (Box 11.22).

REFERENCES

1. Papanicolaou GN, Marshall VF. Urine sediment smears as a diagnostic procedure in cancers of the urine tract. Science. 1945;101:519-20.
2. Luthra UK, Dey P, George J, et al. Comparison of ThinPrep and conventional preparations: urine cytology evaluation. Diagn Cytopathol. 1999:21(5);364-6.
3. Highman W, Wilson E. Urine cytology in patients with calculi. J Clin Pathol. 1982;35:350-6.
4. Minassian H, Schinella R, Reilly JC. Polyomavirus in the urine: follow-up study. Diagn Cytopathol. 1994;10: 209-11.
5. Cohen J-M, Szporn AH, Unger P, et al. Noncaseating granulomata of the bladder following intravesical administration of Bacille Calmette-Guérin. Acta Cytol. 1991;35:600.
6. Harnden P, Parkinson MC. Transitional cell carcinoma of the bladder: diagnosis and prognosis. Curr Diagn Pathol. 1996;3:109-21.
7. Humphrey PA, Moch H, Cubilla AL, et al. The 2016 WHO classification of tumours of the urinary system and male genital organs-part B: prostate and bladder tumours. Eur Urol. 2016;70(1):106-19.
8. Barkan GA, Wojcik EM, Nayar R, et al. The Paris system for reporting urinary cytology: the quest to develop a standardized terminology. Acta Cytol. 2016;60(3):185-97.
9. Prather J, Arville B, Chatt G, et al. Evidence-based adequacy criteria for urinary bladder barbotage cytology. J Am Soc Cytopathol. 2014;4:57-62.
10. Manyak MJ, Becht E. A comparison of urinary nuclear matrix protein-22 and bladder tumor antigen tests with voided urinary cytology in detecting and following bladder cancer: the prognostic value of false-positive results. BJU Int. 2001;88:692-701.
11. Dey P. Urinary markers of bladder carcinoma. Clin Chim Acta. 2004;340(1-2):57-65.
12. Ianari A, Sernberg CN, Rossetti A, et al. Results of Bard BTA in monitoring patients with a history of transitional cell cancer of the bladder. Urology. 1997;49:786-9.
13. Kumar UN, Dey P, Mondal AK, et al. DNA flow cytometry and bladder irrigation cytology in detection of bladder carcinoma. Diagn Cytopathol. 2001;24:153-6.
14. Pham HT, Block NL, Lokeshwar VB. Tumor-derived hyaluronidase: a diagnostic urine marker for high-grade bladder cancer. Cancer Res. 1997;57:778-83.
15. Yoshida K, Sugino T, Tahara H, et al. Telomerase activity in bladder carcinoma and its implication for noninvasive diagnosis by detection of exfoliated cancer cells in urine. Cancer. 1997;79:362-9.
16. Van der Poel HG, Witjes JA, van Stratum P, et al. Quanticyt Karyometric analysis of bladder washing for patients with superficial bladder cancer. Urology. 1996;48:357-64.
17. Moll R, Lowe A, Laufer J, et al. Cytokeratin 20 in human carcinomas. A new histodiagnostic marker detected by monoclonal antibodies. Am J Pathol. 1992;140:427.
18. Landman J, Chang Y, Kavaler E, et al. Sensitivity and specificity of NMP-22, telomerase, and BTA in the detection of human bladder cancer. Urology. 1998;52:398-402.

Review Questions

1. **All are true about urine cytology *except*:**
   a. Wide area of mucosal lesion is covered
   b. Especially helpful in lesions that are not visualized by cystoscopy
   c. High specificity
   d. Highly sensitive
2. **More than 300 mL of clear urine sample is best processed by:**
   a. Simple centrifugation
   b. Millipore technique
   c. Cytocentrifugation
   d. Liquid-based preparation
3. **The cytology smear of urine in a 56-year-old male (Fig. 11.25). How will you label it according to Paris classification?**
   a. Atypia
   b. Atypia, suspicious for high-grade urothelial carcinoma
   c. High-grade urothelial cell carcinoma
   d. No abnormality
4. **The cytology smear of urine in a 67-year-old male (Fig. 11.26). How will you label it according to Paris classification?**
   a. Atypia
   b. Atypia, suspicious for high-grade urothelial carcinoma
   c. High-grade urothelial cell carcinoma
   d. No abnormality
5. **Which one is FDA approved and point of care test to detect malignancy in urine:**
   a. NMP22
   b. ImmunoCyt
   c. Quanticyt
   d. Fluorescent in situ hybridization technique (Urovysion test)
6. **"Decoy cells" in the urine are present in:**
   a. Urothelial cell carcinoma
   b. Lithiasis
   c. Human polyoma virus infection
   d. Human papilloma virus infection
7. **In this test the chromosomal abnormalities are detected using fluorescent labeled DNA probes:**
   a. NMP22
   b. Urovysion test
   c. ImmunoCyt test
   d. Quanticyt
8. **The urine cytology smear shows the multiple clusters (10–12 such clusters in high power field) of urothelial cells with: nucleocytoplasmic ratio more than 07, hyperchromatic nuclei and irregular nuclear membrane. What will be your diagnosis according to Paris classification?**
   a. Atypical urothelial cells
   b. Suspicious for high-grade urothelial cell carcinoma
   c. High-grade urothelial cell carcinoma
   d. Low-grade urothelial cell carcinoma

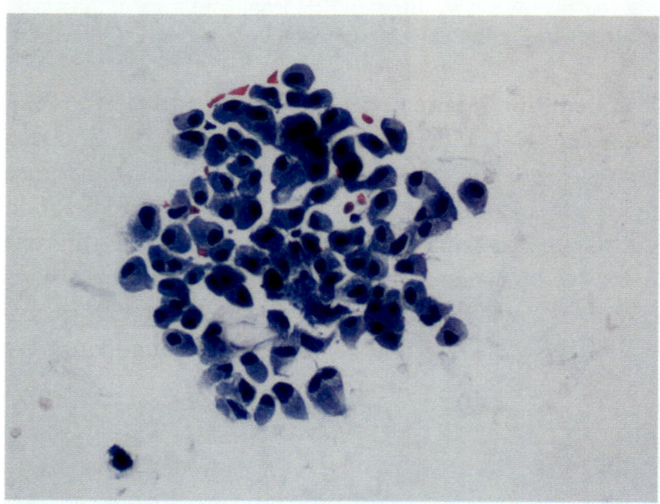

Fig. 11.25: Urine cytology smear of question 3.

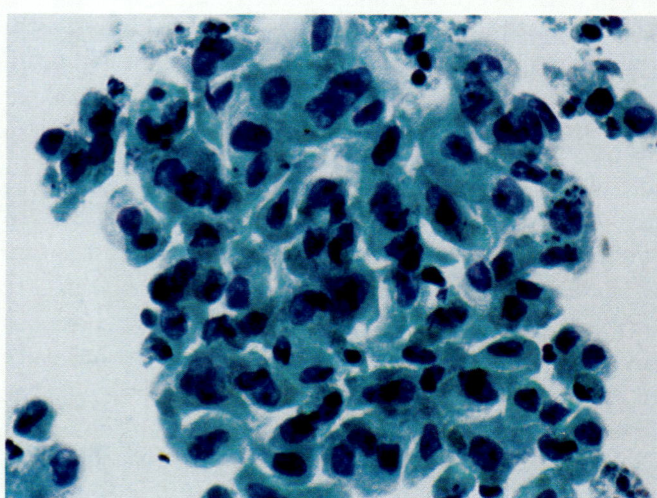

Fig. 11.26: Urine cytology smear of question 4.

Answers

1. d. Highly sensitive
2. b. Millipore technique
3. a. Atypia
   Note: The cells show N:C ratio between 0.05 to 0.07 and hyperchromasia. So the smear should be labelled as "atypia".
4. c. High grade urothelial cell carcinoma
   Note: Here the cells show more than 0.07 N:C ratio, hyperchromasia and irregular nuclear margin. Therefore this is a case of high grade urothelial cell carcinoma.
5. a. NMP 22
6. c. Human polyoma virus infection
7. b. Urovysion test
8. c. High-grade urothelial cell carcinoma
   Note: Multiple clusters of urothelial cells showing these abnormalities indicate high-grade urothelial cell carcinoma. In case of suspicious for high-grade urothelial cell carcinoma only a few cells show abnormality.

CHAPTER

12 Respiratory Cytology

NORMAL ANATOMY AND HISTOLOGY

The respiratory system is broadly divided into the upper respiratory tract, lower respiratory tract, and lungs (Fig. 12.1).

Upper Respiratory Tract

It extends from nose to larynx and comprises nose, paranasal sinuses, pharynx, and larynx.

Histology

The upper respiratory tract is lined by stratified squamous epithelium and ciliated columnar epithelial cells.

Lower Respiratory Tract

It extends from the trachea to the lungs and comprises trachea, bronchi, and bronchioles.

Lungs

It is made of respiratory bronchioles, alveolar ducts, alveolar sacs, and alveoli.

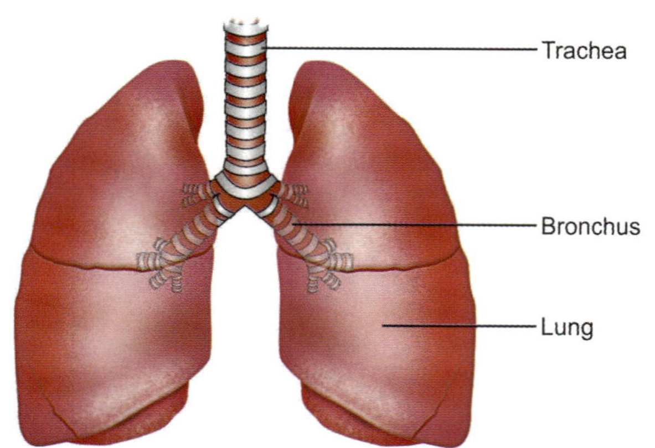

Fig. 12.1: Schematic diagram shows anatomy of respiratory tract.

Histology

Table 12.1 shows mucosal lining of the epithelium from the nose to the alveoli. Most of the portion of the respiratory tract from the nose to the bronchi is lined by ciliated columnar epithelium except vestibules of the nose, vocal cords and superior surfaces of the epiglottis are lined by nonkeratinizing stratified squamous epithelium.

Figure 12.2 shows histology of the lung alveoli. The alveolar epithelium of the lung is lined by type I and type II pneumocytes. Type I pneumocytes cover more than 95% of the alveolar surface. The cells are long, thin, and flattened. Type II pneumocytes cover less than 5% of the alveolar surface. The cells are round with vacuolated cytoplasm and centrally placed nuclei having prominent nucleoli. Electron microscopy of the type II pneumocytes shows membrane-bound lamellar bodies that contain pulmonary surfactant. Alveolar macrophages are large cells with abundant vacuolated cytoplasm that contain phagocytosed material. Nuclei are central in position and round monomorphic in shape.

Table 12.1: Lining of respiratory tract.

Parts	*Mucosal lining*
Nasal vestibules	Stratified squamous epithelium
Nasal sinuses	Ciliated columnar epithelium
Nasopharynx	Ciliated columnar epithelium
Larynx	• *Mostly*: Ciliated columnar epithelium • *Vocal cords and superior surfaces of the epiglottis*: Stratified squamous epithelium
Trachea and bronchi	Ciliated columnar epithelium, goblet cells, neuroendocrine cells
Terminal bronchioles	Simple columnar to cuboidal epithelium
Alveoli	Type I and II pneumocytes and alveolar macrophages

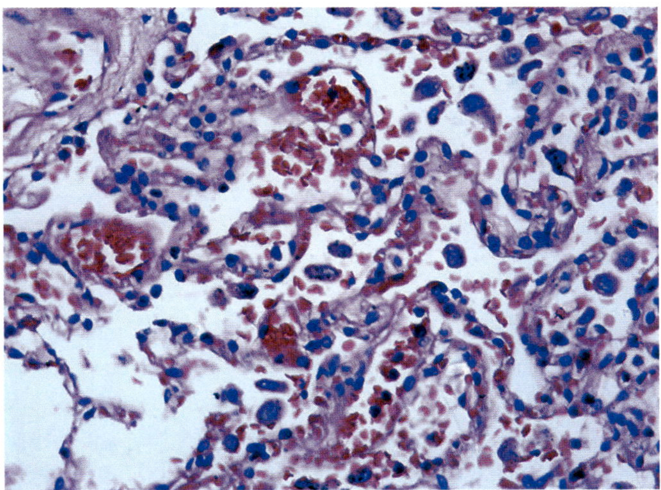

Fig. 12.2: Histology section of lung showing normal alveoli (hematoxylin and eosin × MP).

SAMPLING TECHNIQUES

Detailed knowledge of the sampling and preparation of respiratory specimen is very essential because the diagnostic accuracy depends vastly on sampling method. The commonly used sampling techniques are: sputum, bronchial wash and brush, bronchoalveolar lavage (BAL), transbronchial needle aspiration (TBNA) cytology, and USG-guided fine needle aspiration cytology (FNAC).

Sputum (Box 12.1)

It is the most commonly examined respiratory samples. Sputum is easy to collect and easy to examine. Early morning deep coughed sputum should be collected in a clean container. If the patient is unable to produce sputum then expectoration can be induced by inhalation of stream from saline water. Consecutive three morning sputum samples are recommended for better yield of cells and to increase diagnostic sensitivity. Examination of fresh sputum sample is recommended. However, if this is not possible then the sputum sample can be collected in 70% ethyl alcohol solution for fixation.

Sputum sample should be kept in a Petri dish on white background. Any tissue fragment or blood mixed material is taken and multiple smears are made. Both alcohol-fixed and air-dried smears should be kept for staining.

Box 12.1: Sputum.

- Early morning deep coughed sputum
- Fresh sample in clean wide bore container.

Advantages

- Easy to collect
- Wide area of respiratory tract is covered
- Simple and noninvasive
- Good sensitivity for central tumor
- Best for screening malignancy.

Disadvantages

- Exact localization of the tumor not possible
- Considerable degeneration of the cells
- Not good for peripheral tumors.

Bronchial Aspirate and Wash

Introduction of flexible fiberoptic bronchoscope enables the clinician to procure samples from the peripheral part of the lower respiratory tract. With the help of bronchoscope the bronchial secretion is aspirated directly. In case of bronchial washing technique, 3–5 mL of balanced salt solution or normal saline is introduced through the bronchoscope and the fluid is re-aspirated. The direct smear or multiple smears from the centrifuged fluid sample is made for staining.

Bronchial Brush

The lesion is directly visualized by the fiberoptic bronchoscope. The brush is applied to the lesion through the instrument. Multiple smears are made and fixed in 95% ethanol or the brush is rinsed in a collection solution and sent to the laboratory. The main advantage of the brush is that direct visualization of the lesion is possible and therefore diagnostic cellular yield is excellent.

Bronchoalveolar Lavage (Box 12.2)

Bronchoalveolar lavage is a powerful investigative technique in the field of pulmonary medicine.

Procedure

Bronchoalveolar lavage should be done before performing any other techniques such as bronchial wash/brush or biopsy. Under local anesthesia fiberoptic bronchoscope is wedged in a desired subsegmental bronchus at the desired location. At first 20 mL of normal saline is flushed through bronchoscope in the desired segment of the lung and gentle suction is done to collect the lavage specimen. The whole procedure is done for five times to get 40–50 mL solution. BAL specimen should be processed as early as possible.

Indications

The predominant clinical indications of BAL are:

- Any case of nonresolving pneumonia
- Interstitial lung disease

Box 12.2: Bronchoalveolar lavage.

Procedure
- Repeatedly (five times) 20 mL of normal saline is flushed through bronchoscope in the desired segment of the lung.
- Gentle suction is done to collect the lavage specimen.

Indications
- Nonresolving pneumonia
- Interstitial lung disease
- To diagnose opportunistic infection in an immunocompromised host
- Suspected case of peripheral lung carcinoma

Contraindications
- Severe coughing
- Dyspnea
- Cardiac arrhythmias

Adequacy of the sample
- Cell count more than 2×10^6
- More than 10 macrophages per high power field

Unsatisfactory sample
- Excessive blood
- Cellular degeneration
- Predominant squamous cells
- Artifacts changes.

- To diagnose opportunistic infection in an immunocompromised host
- Suspected case of peripheral lung carcinoma.

Bronchoalveolar lavage is particularly used for the diagnosis of *Pneumocystis carinii* infection. Other than diagnosis, BAL is also useful for therapy of alveolar proteinosis, cystic fibrosis, and pulmonary alveolar microlithiasis.[1]

Contraindications

Bronchoalveolar lavage is contraindicated in:
- Severe coughing
- Dyspnea
- Cardiac arrhythmias.

Ideally, BAL should be avoided in severe respiratory failure.

Adequacy of Bronchoalveolar Lavage Sample

There are no absolute indicators of adequacy of the BAL sample. However, it is considered that cell counts more than 2×10^6, or more than 10 macrophages per high power field are the markers of the adequacy of the sample.[2] The BAL sample is labeled unsatisfactory when it shows excessive blood, degeneration, and squamous cells.

Transbronchial Needle Aspiration

Transbronchial needle aspiration is done in those cases where the lesion is located in the sub-bronchial region. TBNA is done through the fiberoptic bronchoscope and multiple air-dried and alcohol-fixed smears are made. TBNA avoids other surgical procedures such as mediastinoscopy or surgical biopsy. Sensitivity of TBNA alone is near about 56% and specificity is 74%.

Transesophageal Fine Needle Aspiration

Fine needle aspiration cytology can be done by esophageal endoscopy and passing the needle through the esophagus. Ultrasound guidance in addition to the esophagoscope may improve the diagnostic accuracy of the technique. Transesophageal fine needle aspiration is particularly helpful in sampling of mediastinal lymph node.

Percutaneous Fine Needle Aspiration Cytology

Percutaneous fine needle aspiration cytology is an effective technique for rapid diagnosis of pulmonary mass lesions. It is usually done under USG or CT scan guidance with the help of 22 gauge needle. The sensitivity and specificity of percutaneous FNAC are 89% and 96%, respectively.[3]

Table 12.2 compares the different sampling techniques in the respiratory system.

NORMAL CYTOLOGY

The normal cellular components of the respiratory tract are squamous epithelial cells, ciliated columnar cells, alveolar macrophages, and goblet cells (Box 12.3).

Squamous Epithelial Cells

The squamous cells come from the oral cavity as contaminants and predominantly seen in sputum samples. The cells are superficial squamous cells and many of them are anucleated.

Columnar Cells (Box 12.4)

The ciliated columnar cells are the predominant lining cells of the lower respiratory tract. These cells are usually not seen in the sputum samples. They are mainly noted in bronchial washing/brushing and BAL specimens. The cells are columnar in appearance with moderate cytoplasm. Nuclei are located on one side of the cell. Cilia come out from the terminal plate of the columnar cells (Fig. 12.3).

Table 12.2: Comparison of different sampling techniques of respiratory system.

Techniques	*Procedure*	*Advantages*	*Disadvantages*
Sputum	Early morning sputum is collected in a container	• Easy to collect • The wider area of the respiratory tract is covered • Simple and noninvasive • Good sensitivity for central tumor • Best for screening malignancy	• Exact localization of the tumor not possible • Degeneration of the cells • Not good for peripheral tumors
Bronchial wash	Balanced salt solution or normal saline is introduced through the bronchoscope and the fluid is re-aspirated	• Cellularity more than sputum • Morphology is better preserved	• Better for central lesion • Lesion is not well visualized
Bronchial Brush	The brush is applied on the lesion through the bronchoscope and multiple smears are made	• Direct visualization of the lesion is possible • Morphology is well preserved • Much more sensitive than sputum or wash	• Sophisticated technique • Suitable only for central localized lesion
Bronchoalveolar lavage	Normal saline is flushed through bronchoscope in the desired segment of the lung and gentle suction is done to collect the lavage specimen	• Useful to diagnose peripheral lung lesions such as infection, alveolar diseases • High sensitivity in diagnosing bronchoalveolar carcinoma	• Technical skill is needed
Transbronchial needle aspiration	It is done through the fiberoptic bronchoscope	• Good for sub-bronchial lesion • Better morphology	• Swelling is needed • Sophisticated technique

Box 12.3: Normal constituents of lung samples.

Lining cells
- Squamous epithelial cells
- Ciliated columnar cells
- Alveolar macrophages
- Goblet cells

Associated cells
- Polymorphs
- Lymphocytes
- Histiocytes

Acellular material
- Curschmann's Spirals
- Ferruginous (asbestos) bodies
- Charcot-Leyden crystals
- Carbon particles
- Hemosiderin

Contaminants
- Pollen grains
- Vegetable materials
- Contaminants from food particles.

Fig. 12.3: Ciliated columnar cell of normal lining cells and alveolar macrophages in bronchoalveolar lavage. Cilia arise from the terminal plate of the cell (Papanicolaou's stain × HP).

Box 12.4: Ciliated columnar cell.

- Present singly and also in honeycomb-like clusters
- Columnar shaped
- Terminal bar with cilia in one end
- Nuclei present basally
- Round, regular monomorphic nuclei
- Inconspicuous nucleoli
- Nuclear chromatin fine.

Goblet Cells (Box 12.5)

These cells are present mainly in bronchial washing/brushing or BAL samples and are rarely seen in sputum. The individual cells have a moderate amount of vacuolated cytoplasm filled with mucin. The nuclei are round and monomorphic. Goblet cells are seen in abundant numbers in chronic tracheobronchial irritation and asthma.

Alveolar Macrophages (Box 12.6)

These are the *key cells* that indicate adequacy of sputum sample and in the absence of them the sputum sample has not much diagnostic value. The alveolar macrophages show moderate to abundant cytoplasm filled with

Box 12.5: Goblet cells.

- Present in small clusters
- Cells with moderate amount of vacuolated cytoplasm
- Round, monomorphic nuclei
- Abundant goblet cells seen in bronchial asthma, chronic bronchitis.

Box 12.6: Alveolar macrophages.

- Indicate adequacy of sputum sample
- Always present singly
- Round cells with abundant cytoplasm
- Cytoplasm filled with brownish to blackish dust particles
- Centrally placed kidney-shaped nuclei
- Bi- and multinucleation present
- Fine chromatin.

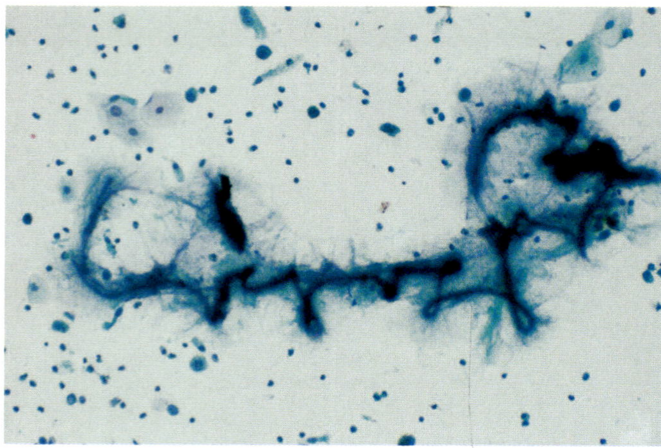

Fig. 12.4: Curschmann's spirals: corkscrew-shaped long inspissated mucus cast (Papanicolaou's stain × HP).

Table 12.3: Noncellular components in respiratory sample: Morphology and significance.

Material	*Morphology*	*Significance*
Curschmann's spirals	Corkscrew-shaped long inspissated mucus cast	Present in chronic bronchitis, asthma, and in smokers
Ferruginous (asbestos) bodies	Long rod-shaped golden brown structures with two terminal bulbous tips	Present in asbestos exposure
Charcot-Leyden crystals	Bipyramidal needle-shaped crystal with two pointed ends	Present in asthma patients, eosinophilic pneumonia, and allergic bronchopulmonary aspergillosis
Mucus	Acellular homogenous substances	Bronchial obstruction and bronchioloalveolar carcinoma
Psammoma body	Darkly stained concentric lamellated structures	Present in bronchioloalveolar carcinoma

phagocytosed brownish to blackish dust particles (Fig. 12.3). The nuclei are centrally in place with convoluted kidney shaped. Binucleation and multinucleation are common in alveolar macrophages.

Other Cells

Polymorphs and lymphocytes: In the absence of inflammation scattered occasional polymorphs and lymphocytes are also seen in respiratory sample.

Noncellular Components (Table 12.3)

Mucus

These are acellular homogenous substances. The largest amount of mucus is usually present in bronchial obstruction and bronchioloalveolar carcinoma.

Curschmann's Spirals (Fig. 12.4)

Curschmann's spirals are corkscrew-shaped long inspissated mucus cast produced in the small bronchioles due to excessive mucus production. These are commonly seen in condition with excessive mucus production such as chronic bronchitis, asthma, and in smokers.

Ferruginous (Asbestos) Bodies

The ferruginous bodies are approximately 50–200 micron long rod-shaped golden brown structures with two terminal bulbous tips. These are usually asbestos fibers coated with protein and iron. The presence of ferruginous bodies in the sputum or BAL usually indicates asbestos exposure.

Charcot-Leyden Crystals

These are bipyramidal needle-shaped crystal with two pointed ends. These crystals are composed of granules of eosinophils. Charcot-Leyden crystals are seen frequently in asthma patients, eosinophilic pneumonia, and allergic bronchopulmonary aspergillosis.

Psammoma Body

These are darkly stained concentric lamellated structures made up of calcium. Psammoma bodies are usually seen in bronchioloalveolar carcinoma.

Others: In addition, respiratory specimen may contain pollen grains, vegetable materials, or contaminants from food particles (Fig. 12.5).

BENIGN CELLULAR ABNORMALITIES

Various nonneoplastic lesions may affect the different components of the respiratory epithelial cells such as:

- Squamous cells
- Bronchial epithelium
- Reserve cell hyperplasia
- Hyperplasia of type II pneumocytes.

Abnormalities of Squamous Cells

Inflammatory Changes

The inflammatory changes of the squamous epithelial cells are very common. Nuclear atypia is seen in infection and trauma of lung. The cells show a mild nuclear enlargement, coarse chromatin, and hyperchomasia. Nuclei of these cells often show degenerative changes. These cells should not be misinterpreted as cancer. In contrast to malignant cells, the cells show regular nuclear membrane and monomorphic nuclei.

PAP Cells

PAP cells are small squamous cells with round hyperchromatic nuclei. The cells are related to inflammation of lower respiratory tract. These atypical cells should not be mistaken for cancer cells because of hyperchromasia and enlarged nuclei. Unlike cancer cells, they have regular monomorphic nuclei with regular nuclear margin. George Papanicolaou noted these atypical cells in his sputum after respiratory tract infection and the cells are named after his name.[4]

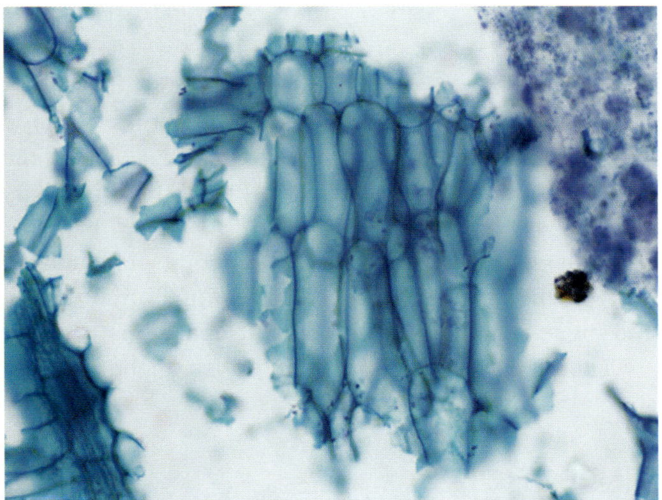

Fig. 12.5: Vegetable material in the sputum (Papanicolaou's stain × HP).

Abnormalities of Bronchial Epithelial Cells

Ciliocytophthoria

There is a very important point about cilia in respiratory epithelial cells. The cells in the presence of cilia degenerate and the cell may show only terminal plate. Infection particularly viral infection of the bronchial lining epithelial cells may cause detachment of cilia from the cell. This condition is known as ciliocytophthoria. The cytology smear shows detached fragment of cilia or cells with cytoplasm and nucleus without any cilia. There is no association of malignancy with ciliocytophthoria.

Hyperplastic Bronchial Epithelium

The chronic irritation or infection such as chronic bronchitis, tuberculosis, bronchial asthma, etc may cause hyperplasia of the bronchial epithelial cells (Box 12.7). The bronchial cells show the variable degree of nuclear enlargement and pleomorphism (Fig. 12.6). The cells may show prominent nucleoli and clumped chromatin. Bi- and multinucleated cells may also be seen. The hyperplastic bronchial epithelial cells show large three-dimensional (3D) papillary clusters of the bronchial cells with smooth peripheral outline (Fig. 12.7). The outer layer of the cell is often arranged as palisade manner. The cells on the surface of the clusters often show cilia. The cells are

Box 12.7: Bronchial cell hyperplasia (creola body).

Commonly seen
- Chronic bronchitis
- Tuberculosis, bronchial
- Asthma

Morphology
- Large three-dimensional papillary clusters of the bronchial cells
- Smooth peripheral outline
- Focal areas of the surface cells show cilia
- Outer cells in palisade arrangement
- Cells are small with monomorphic nuclei
- Fine nuclear chromatin
- Occasional prominent nucleoli

Differential diagnosis: Adenocarcinoma.

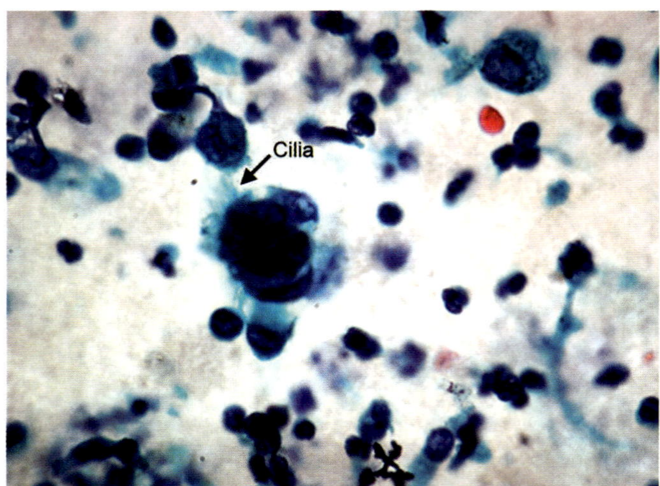

Fig. 12.6: Nuclear enlargement and pleomorphism in the reactive bronchial hyperplasia (Papanicolaou's stain × HP).

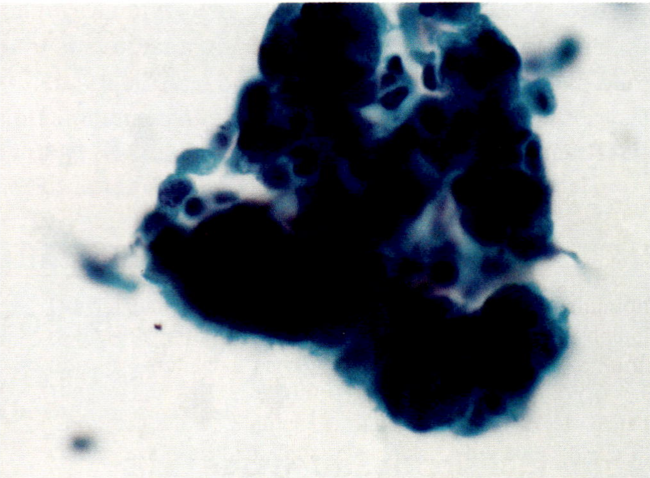

Fig. 12.7: Large three-dimensional papillary clusters of the bronchial cells with smooth peripheral outline in hyperplastic bronchial epithelial cells (Papanicolaou's stain × HP).

Box 12.8: Reserve cell hyperplasia.

Causes: Infection, injury

Morphology
- Tight cohesive small clusters
- Small cells
- High nucleocytoplasmic ratio
- Scanty cytoplasm
- Hyperchromatic nuclei
- Nuclear molding

Differential diagnosis: Small cell carcinoma.

Box 12.9: Hyperplastic type II pneumocytes.

Causes: Tuberculosis, pulmonary infraction, radiation injury, chemotherapeutic drugs, pneumonia, interstitial lung disease.

Morphology
- Tight papillary clusters
- Abundant vacuolated cytoplasm
- Enlarged nuclei
- Fine chromatin
- Prominent nucleoli

Differential diagnosis: Adenocarcinoma.

small with monomorphic nuclei, fine nuclear chromatin, and occasional prominent nucleoli. This cluster of cells is also called as Creola body. The name was kept by the name of the patient in whom it was first recognized. The Creola body may be mistaken for adenocarcinoma (ADC) due to the papillary arrangement of the cells. However, individual cells of the cluster do not show any evidence of malignancy.

Bronchial Reserve Cell Hyperplasia (Box 12.8)

During lung injury of infection, the superficial bronchial epithelial cells may be damaged and the basal layer of cells may proliferate. The hyperplastic basal cells are usually arranged in small tight clusters. The cells are small with scanty cytoplasm and round mildly hyperchromatic nuclei. Nucleoli are usually absent but may show prominent nucleoli. Nuclear molding is also noted at times. The cells may often resemble small cell carcinoma (SCC) because of small size, hyperchromatic nuclei, and nuclear molding. However, the basal cells are arranged most of the time in tight clusters and the nuclei have prominent nucleoli.

Hyperplasia of type II pneumocytes (Box 12.9): Hyperplasia of type II pneumocytes are seen in various conditions such as tuberculosis, pulmonary infarction, radiation injury, chemotherapeutic drugs, pneumonia, interstitial lung disease, etc. The cells are present in tight papillary clusters.

Individual cells show a moderate amount of vacuolated cytoplasm. Nuclei are mildly enlarged with fine chromatin and single to multiple prominent nucleoli.

The hyperplastic type II pneumocytes are the common source of false positive diagnosis as ADC.[5]

INFECTIONS

Cytological examination of the respiratory samples play good role in the diagnosis of various infective processes.

Bacterial Infections

Large varieties of Gram-positive and Gram-negative organisms cause bacterial pneumonia. The common organisms causing bacterial pneumonia are *Staphylococcus aureus, Pneumococci, Streptococcus, Klebsiella pneumonia, Pseudomonas, Haemophilus influenza*, etc. These organisms are identified by Gram stain and corresponding mycobacterial culture. The sputum or other respiratory specimen shows abundant polymorphs, necrotic debris, and degenerated bronchial epithelial cells. Cytologic examination is usually not performed in clinically diagnosed cases of bacterial pneumonia.

Tuberculosis (Box 12.10)

Mycobacterium tubercle infection of the lung provokes granulomatous inflammation. The cytology smear shows multinucleated giant cells, epithelioid cell granulomas, lymphocytes, and necrosis (Figs. 12.8 and 12.9). In sputum sample, the combination of multinucleated giant cells and epithelioid cell granulomas are pathognomonic for tuberculosis and can be seen in 60% tuberculosis cases.[6] However, these features are not specific for tuberculosis and may be noted in other granulomatous inflammations such as fungal infections, sarcoidosis, etc. Ziehl-Neelsen stain for acid fast bacilli or culture is necessary for confirmation.

Box 12.10: Mycobacterial infection.

- Fine needle aspiration cytology of lung lesion is mostly done in suspicion of malignancy
- Cytology
  - Multiple epithelioid cell granulomas
  - Multinucleated Langhans type giant cells
  - Necrosis

Confirmation

- Ziehl-Neelsen stain shows acid fast bacilli
- Atypical mycobacteria may stain weakly. Fite stain is better
- Culture
- PCR confirmation

Actinomycosis

Actinomyces species are commonly present in tonsilar crypts and gingival crevices. The organisms are usually noted as a contaminant in the sputum.

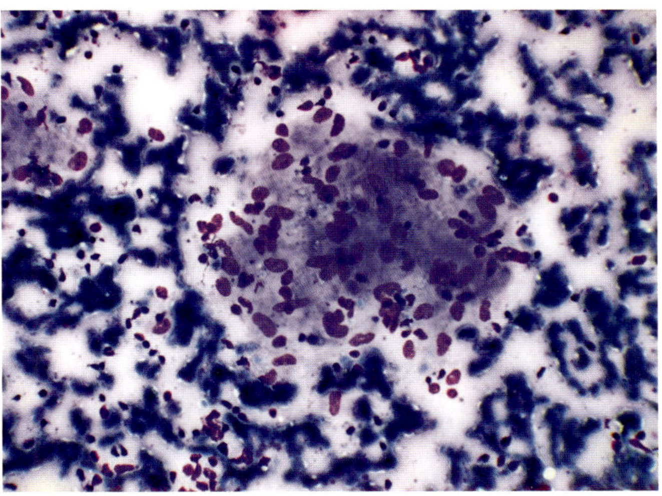

Fig. 12.8: Well-formed epithelioid cell granuloma in a case of tuberculosis of lung (May-Grünwald Giemsa stain × MP).

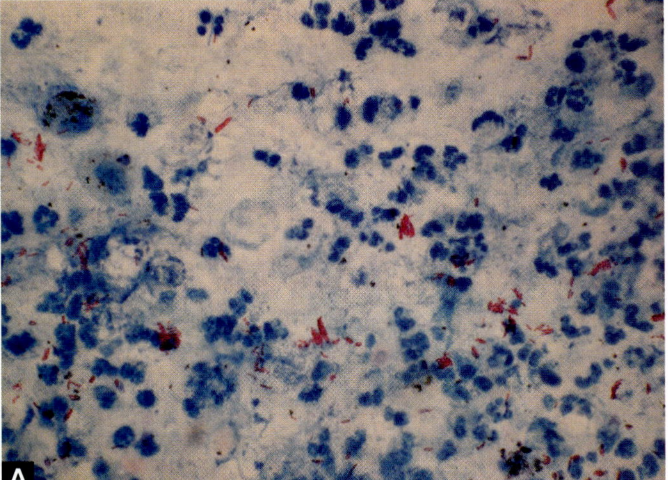

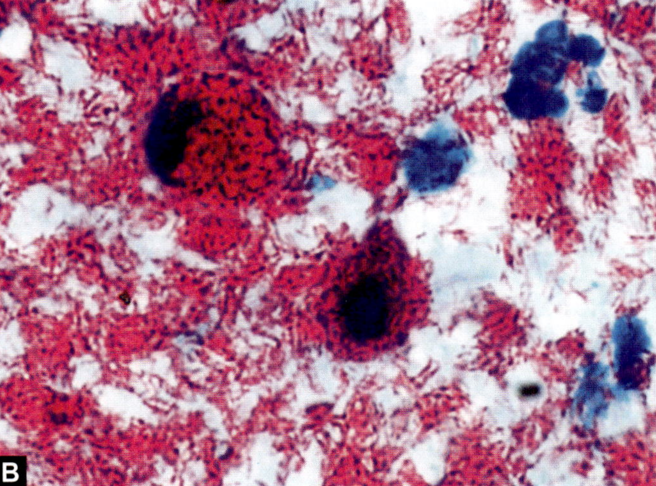

Figs. 12.9A and B: Strong positivity of acid fast bacilli in case of tuberculosis of lung (Ziehl-Neelsen stain × OI). (B) Atypical mycobacteria: Bunch of acid fast bacilli within the macrophages and in the background (Ziehl-Neelsen stain × OI).

They infect lung in anaerobic condition such as lung injury or infarct. The organisms are cotton ball-like floppy hematoxylin-stained tangled filamentous material with associated squamous cells. Background of the smear often shows polymorphonuclear leukocyte reaction. The presence of actinomycosis organisms in the BAL or fine needle aspiration cytology material usually indicates infection.

Nocardia

Nocardia is the aerobic filamentous organisms and commonly is the inhabitant of soil. They infect lung in the immunocompromised patient. Nocardia is slender, filamentous, branching organisms. They are Gram positive and weak acid fast positive organism (Fig. 12.10). They are usually diagnosed by BAL specimen.

Fungal Infections

Fungal infections are readily diagnosed in respiratory specimen because of the typical morphology of the fungi and most of the fungi are detectable in May-Grünwald Giemsa (MGG) stain; however, special stains and fungal culture may be needed for the final confirmation. On cytology smear different substances can be misinterpreted as fungus such as pollen grains, anthracotic pigment, talc, and red blood cells (Table 12.4).

The smears usually show multinucleated giant cells, epithelioid cell granulomas, polymorphs, and eosinophils along with necrotic material. Morphological characteristics of different fungi are mentioned in Box 12.11.

Aspergillus (Fig. 12.11)

Aspergillus infection of the lung may cause extrinsic allergic alveolitis, allergic bronchopulmonary aspergillosis, infection in the already existing lung cavity, tracheobronchitis, and diffuse parenchymal infection of the lung or

Table 12.4: Substances that simulate fungus.

Materials	*Comments*
RBCs: Variable depigmentation during Papanicolaou stain and may simulate fungal spore.	• RBCs are present as clusters.
Nuclear lobes of polymorphs	• They are of variable sized • Smaller sized • Block like nuclear chromatin
Talc	• Central hole or defect • Present in polarized light
Hemosiderin	• Variable sized particle • Absence of internal structure of fungus

Box 12.11: Common fungal infections.

- *Aspergillus*: Septate, uniform acute angle branching 30 μ width hyphae, septate
- *Special stain*: PAS, Mucicarmine, Methenamine silver.
- *Zygomycetes*: Broad, nonseptate, wide angel branching

Special stain: PAS, Mucicarmine.

- *Cryptococcus*: 5–10 μ diameter round, thick outer capsule. Narrow-based budding

Special stain: India ink.

- *Histoplasma*: Small round (2–5 μ), narrow budding, usually inside the macrophages.

Special stain: PAS, Z-N stain.

- *Candida*: Thin slender peseudohyphae with budding yeast Special stain: PAS.

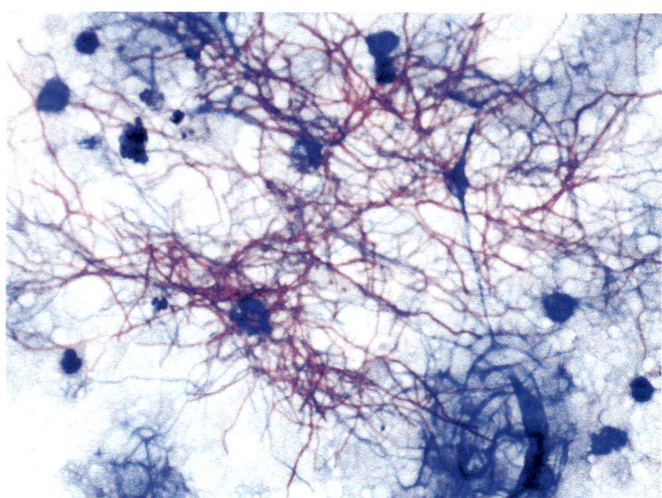

Fig. 12.10: Long filamentous Nocardia (Modified acid fast stain).

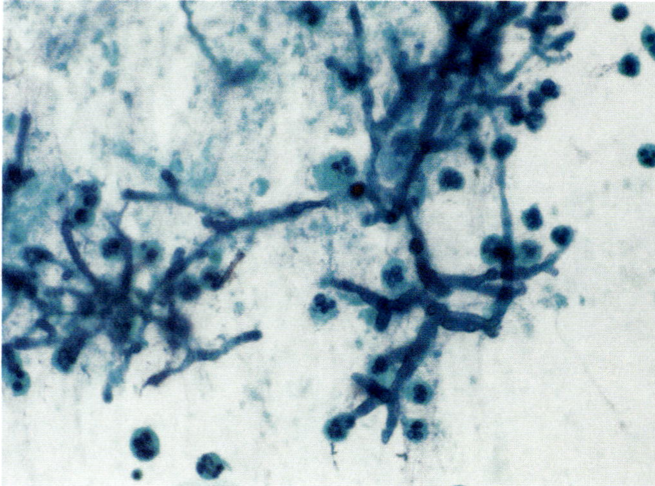

Fig. 12.11: Aspergilous in bronchoalveolar lavage showing acute angle branching and septae (Papanicolaou's stain × HP).

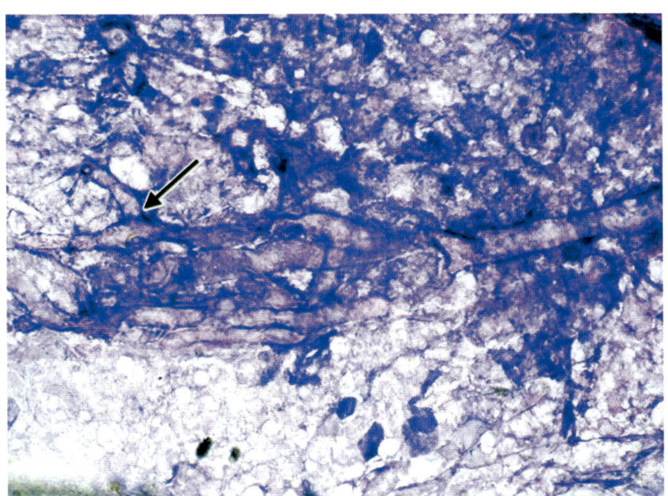

Fig. 12.12: Broad, nonseptate, wide angel branching hyphae of mucormycosis of lung infection (May-Grünwald Giemsa stain × HP).

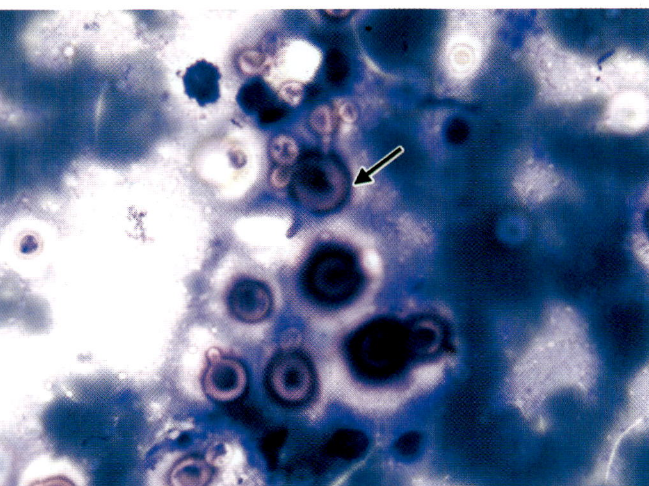

Fig. 12.13: Round capsulated *Cryptococcus* in lung infection (May-Grünwald Giemsa stain × OI).

solitary cavitary lesion. The Aspergillus infection usually occurs in severely immunocompromised patients particularly AIDS patient. The organism is usually invasive and enters the blood stream by invasion into the blood vessel. The organism is long septate, uniform, and acute angle branching. Intracavitary aspergillosis may show ball-like aggregation of Aspergillus, calcium oxalate crystal, and squamous cell atypia. The atypical squamous cells may simulate malignant cell because of nuclear enlargement, pleomorphism, and hyperchromasia.

Pulmonary Zygomycosis

These include Mucor, Absidia, Cunninghamella, and Rhizopus. The infection usually occurs in debilitated patients, diabetes mellitus, renal failure, and immunocompromised patient. Zygomycosis group of fungi overall show broad, nonseptate, wide angle branching hyphae (Fig. 12.12).

Pulmonary Cryptococcosis

Pulmonary cryptococcosis is caused by *Cryptococcus neoformans. C. neoformans* is found in soil contaminated by bird droppings. It causes systemic infection, and lung is also involved. The organism is 5–10 μ diameter round with thick outer capsule (Fig. 12.13). Narrow-based budding is often noted. Special stains such as Periodic acid-Schiff, mucicarmine, or alcian blue are needed for better visualization of the fungi.

Histoplasma

Histoplasma is the inhabitant of soil. Histoplasmosis is caused by inhalation of spore of *Histoplasma capsulatum.* Infection occurs particularly in immunocompromised patient and debilitated person. The organism is intracellular and remains within the macrophages. The organism is small round 2–5 μ in diameter and therefore difficult to recognize in Papnicolaou's stained smear; however, they are well visualized in MGG staining (Fig. 12.14). Special stains such as methenamine silver is needed to demonstrate the organism.

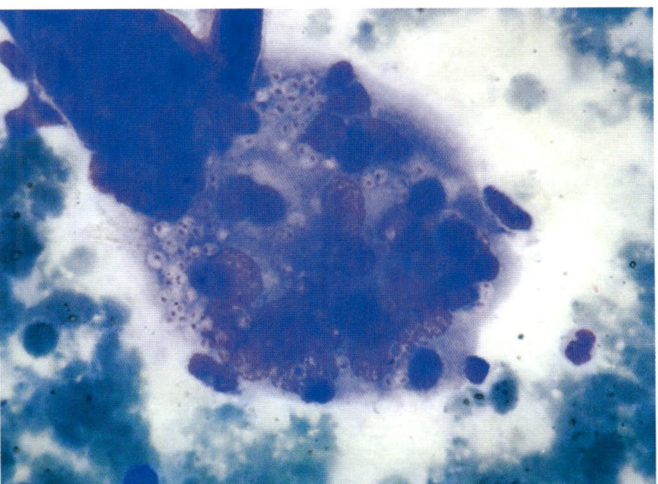

Fig. 12.14: Small round intracellular *Histoplasma* within the histiocyte (May-Grünwald Giemsa stain × OI).

Pulmonary Candidiasis

Candidiasis is caused by mainly *Candida albicans.* Candidiasis is an opportunistic infection and occurs in immunocompromised patient. Candida appears as small, oval,

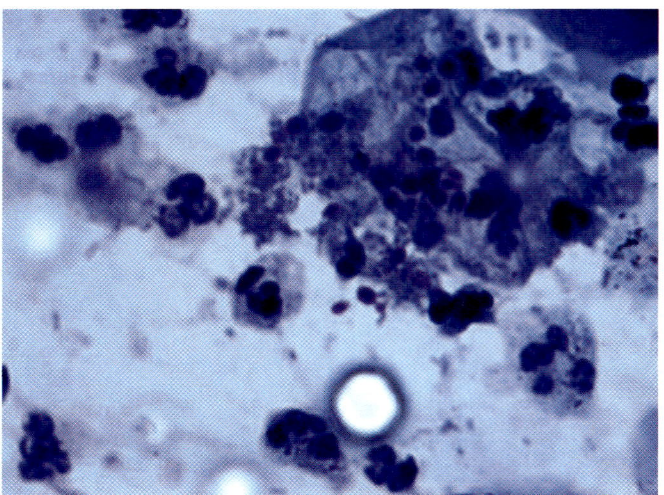

Fig. 12.15: Candidal spores and inflammatory cells in bronchoalveolar lavage sample (Papanicolaou's stain × OI).

Box 12.12: *Pneumocystis carinii* infection.

- Associated with immunocompromised patient particularly in AIDS
- *Best sampling method*: Bronchioloalveolar lavage
- Tissue response
  - Alveoli filled with frothy eosinophilic material
  - Granulomatous inflammation
  - Giant cell reaction
  - No tissue response

Cytology
- Frothy appearance
- Extracellular aggregate
- Not stained by Papanicolaou's staining
- Cup-shaped structure of 6–8 µm diameter
- One surface flat and a central dark zone

Special stain
- Methenamine silver

Mimickers
- Lubricant
- RBCs in aggregates
- Mucus.

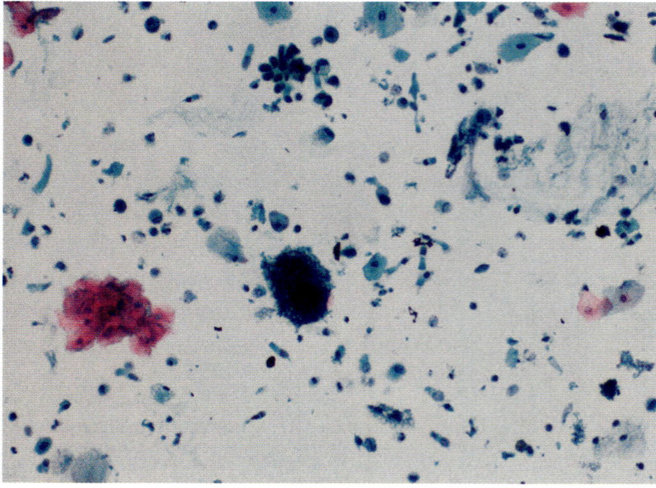

Fig. 12.16: *Pneumocystis carinii* in bronchoalveolar lavage showing amorphous foamy proteinaceous material (Papanicolaou's stain × HP).

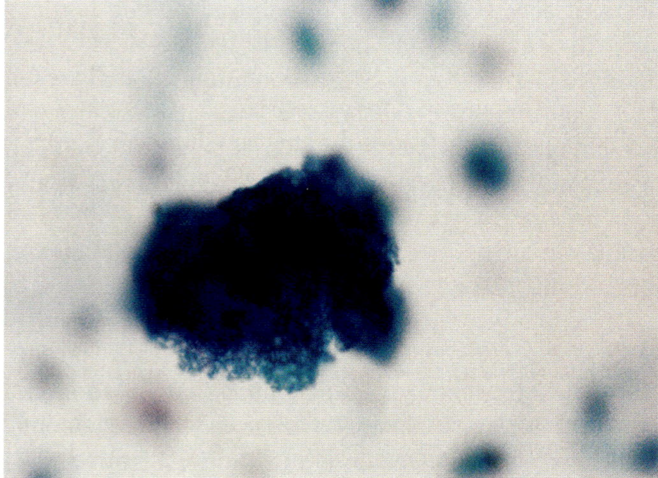

Fig. 12.17: *Pneumocystis carinii*: Organisms are embedded in eosinophilic material (Papanicolaou's stain × OI).

2–4-µm budding yeasts, or elongated pseudohyphae forms (Fig. 12.15). In the healthy person *Candida* is the commensal organism of the oral cavity and upper respiratory tract. Therefore, the simple presence of candidal spore may not indicate infection. However, the presence of candidal hyphae in the FNAC of lung indicates candidiasis.

Pneumocystis Carinii Infection (Box 12.12)

Pneumocystis carinii infection is seen in immunocompromised patient particularly in AIDS. BAL is the best way to diagnose *P. carinii* infection (Figs. 12.16 and 12.17). The cytology smear may show granulomatous inflammation and giant cell reaction. The organisms are not visualized in the Papanicolaou-stained smear. However, masses of organisms are embedded in eosinophilic amorphous foamy proteinaceous alveolar cast. In a proper clinical setting, this finding should be taken as suspicious. Special stains like methenamine silver should be done to demonstrate the organism. *P. carinii* is a cup-shaped structure of 6–8 µm diameter with one surface flat and a central dark zone. With the help of MGG stain intracystic trophozoites may be seen within the cyst.[7]

Viral Infection

Herpes Virus Infection

Herpes simplex virus (HSV) is a DNA virus and causes tracheobronchitis, pharyngitis, and lung infection in immunocompromised, diabetic, and debilitated patient. The cytological examination of sputum in HSV infection shows many multinucleated giant cells. The individual cells show multiple enlarged basophilic nuclei with ground-glass appearance, slaty gray homogenized chromatin, and large intranuclear eosinophilic inclusions. Nuclei of the giant cells are molded.

Cytomegalovirus

It is a DNA virus and affects immunocompromised and debilitated patient. The patient presents with fever, dyspnea, and cough. Cytology smears show markedly enlarged cells with enlarged nuclei. Large amphophilic intranuclear inclusion with a peripheral clear halo and margination of chromatin on the inner nuclear membrane are seen in the bronchial cells, macrophages, and endothelial cells. Small satellite basophilic cytoplasmic inclusions are seen. Occasional multinucleated cells are also noted along with the mononuclear cells.

Adenovirus

Adenovirus usually causes mild fever. The cytology smears show ciliocytophthoria of the respiratory epithelial cells. The virus affected cells show two types of inclusions. The first type shows small reddish well circumscribed inclusion surrounded by clear halo and other type shows large basophilic homogenous inclusion that completely fills the entire nucleus.

Measles Virus

This is an RNA virus and commonly infects children. It is a self limited infection and rarely becomes fatal except in immunocompromised patient. Cytology smear shows enormous multinucleated giant cells (Warthin-Finkelday cells) with more than 100 nuclei containing eosinophilic intracytoplasmic and intranuclear inclusions.

Parasitic Infection

Strongyloidiasis

Strongyloid stercoralis infection is caused by penetration of larva through the skin. The larva penetrates the blood vascular wall, comes to the circulation, and resides in the intestine. It comes to the lung through hematogenous migration from the intestine or skin. The larvae are long, 400 μ in length with a characteristic V-shaped notch in the tail.

LUNG CARCINOMAS

Carcinoma of the lung is the most frequent cancer in the world. It is the most common cause of death in male due to cancer.[8] Male to female ratio of lung cancer is 2.7:1. The peak age of lung cancer is 60–70 years. Lung cancer usually occurs after 40 years of age. Large amount of evidences suggest that the major etiological factor of lung cancer is cigarette smoking.[9] The smoke of cigarette and other tobacco products contain a large number of carcinogens and toxic products. Inhalation of smoke causes inflammation of the respiratory epithelium. Cigarette smoking increases the risk of all lung cancer but it is particularly associated with squamous cell carcinoma (SQC) followed by SCC and ADC.

The common complaints of the patient are progressive shortness of breath, chest pain, cough, dyspnea, and hemoptysis. Infections of lung due to bacterial, viral, or fungal agents may also produce space occupying lesions and may yield hyperplastic atypical bronchial cells. Reactive atypical cells are usually in cohesive clusters, scanty in number and have bland nuclear chromatin. The cells often preserve cilia. Table 12.5 highlights the differentiating points between reactive atypical bronchial cells from malignant cells.

Table 12.5: Differentiating points between reactive atypical bronchial cells from malignant cells.

Features	*Reactive atypical bronchial cells*	*Malignant cells*
Cell arrangement	Predominantly tight papillary clusters	Dissociated cells
Margin of the cluster	Smooth	Irregular
Nuclear crowding	No significant nuclear overlapping	Nuclear overlapping
Atypical cells	Scanty	Many
Cilia	Usually present	*Loss of cilia*: Ciliocytophoria
Nuclear margin	Regular	Irregular
Nuclear chromatin	Fine	Irregular coarsely clumped

CLASSIFICATION OF LUNG CANCER

In 2015, World Health Organization (WHO) classified lung carcinoma[10] as mentioned in Box 12.13. The box shows a mild modification of this classification.

Previously in cytology specimen we used to classify the lung carcinoma as two primary types:

1. Nonsmall cell carcinoma (NSCC)
2. Small cell carcinoma (SCC)

Previously, this major diagnostic identification on cytology sample was sufficient for cliniciains because there was no significant difference in therapy of SQC and ADC. However, following major advances of therapeutic advances have changed the scenario:

- *EGFR mutation of ADC*: Treated by EGFR (epidermal growth factor receptor) tyrosine kinase inhibitors
- *Positive for ALK fusion*: Treated with ALK inhibitor crizotinib
- Many other drugs are in clinical trial for targeted therapy.

Therefore, it is strongly recommended to omit the terminology of "nonsmall cell carcinoma" on cytology and to classify the nonsmall cell carcinoma (NSCC) as ADC, SQC, and NSCC—not otherwise specified.

The *new cytology and small biopsy terminology by WHO 2015*[11] is mentioned in Box 12.14.

To maintain uniformity and good practices in cytology and small biopsies WHO also provided important guidelines[11] (Box 12.15).

In all cases, if possible, cytology material should be also be collected in:

- *10% formalin for cell block*: For further immunocytochemistry (IC), PCR (polymerase chain reaction) or FISH (fluorescent in situ hybridization)
- *Phosphate buffer solution (PBS)*: For gene sequencing, PCR.

The essential ancillary techniques for diagnosis and classification of lung carcinomas include IC and molecular techniques (PCR or FISH, gene sequencing).

Immunocytochemistry

Immunocytochemistry is often required for the diagnosis of SQC, ADC, SCC, and carcinoid. In almost 50–70% of cases cytology smear alone can diagnose SQC and ADC. IC is very helpful in the diagnosis of SQC or ADC, and it

Box 12.13: WHO classification of lung tumors (2015).

- Epithelial tumors
  - Adenocarcinoma
    - » Lepidic adenocarcinoma
    - » Acinar adenocarcinoma
    - » Papillary adenocarcinoma
    - » Solid adenocarcinoma
    - » Invasive mucinous adenocarcinoma
    - » Minimally invasive adenocarcinoma
    - » Colloid adenocarcinoma
  - Squamous cell carcinoma
    - » Keratinizing squamous cell carcinoma
    - » Nonkeratinizing squamous cell carcinoma
    - » Basaloid squamous cell carcinoma
  - Neuroendocrine tumors
    - » Small cell carcinoma
    - » Large cell neuroendocrine carcinoma
    - » Carcinoid tumors
      - Typical carcinoid
      - Atypical carcinoid
  - Large cell carcinoma
  - Adenosquamous carcinoma
  - Pleomorphic carcinoma
  - Giant cell carcinoma
  - Carcinosarcoma
  - Pulmonary blastoma
  - Salivary gland type tumor
- Mesenchymal tumor
- Lymphohistiocytic tumor
- Tumors of ectopic origin
  - Metastatic tumors

Box 12.14: Cytology and small biopsy terminology by WHO, 2015.

- Squamous cell carcinoma
- Adenocarcinoma
- Adenocarcinoma with lepidic pattern
- Invasive mucinous carcinoma
- Nonsmall cell carcinoma favors adenocarcinoma
- Nonsmall cell carcinoma favors squamous cell carcinoma (poorly differentiated squamous or adenoca part is sampled)
- Nonsmall cell carcinoma, not otherwise specified (large cell carcinoma, solid component of adenocarcinoma, squamous cell carcinoma that does not express immunocytochemical markers).

Box 12.15: Important guidelines for the interpretation of cytology sample.

- *In all cytology specimen*: Avoid the terminology nonsmall cell carcinoma (NSCC) and mention the specific subtypes squamous cell carcinoma (SQC) or adenocarcinoma (ADC).
- *Mention whether the diagnosis is supported by other adjunctive studies*: Immunocytochemistry
- Both cytology and small biopsies should be interpreted together, if paired samples are available
- The markers of neuroendocrine carcinoma should be used only in suspected cases of neuroendocrine morphology.
- The term large cell carcinoma should not be used in cytology or small biopsy specimen as through sampling is necessary to avoid any differentiated component.
- Smears with sarcomatioid features should be classified as NSCC with suggestion of ADC or SQC or not otherwise specified. The presence of giant cells and spindle cells should be mentioned in the report.

Table 12.6: Immunocytochemistry of lung carcinomas.

Markers	*Squamous cell carcinoma*	*Adenocarcinoma*	*Small cell carcinoma*
CK7	Negative	Positive	Negative
CK 5/6	Positive	Negative	Negative
TTF-1	Negative	Positive	Positive
p63	Positive	Negative	Negative
p40	Positive	Negative	Negative
Napsin	Negative	Positive	Negative
CD56	Negative	Negative	Positive
Chromogranin	Negative	Negative	Positive

may avoid to put them in NSCC group. The accepted markers of ADC are TTF-1, napsin A, CK7; whereas accepted markers of SQC are p63, p40, and CK 5/6. Positivity of p63 is not entirely specific for SQC and almost 30% cases of ADC may also show p63 staining. In this respect p40 is a more reliable marker of SQC. If a tumor shows TTF-1 and p63 coexpression it should be taken as ADC. WHO recommends that only TTF-1 and p40 markers are sufficient to discriminate SQC and ADC. SCCs are positive for CD56 and chromogranin (Table 12.6). Algorithmic approach of IC has been given in Flowchart 12.1.

Molecular Study

Lung carcinoma shows certain genetic abnormalities that promote tumor growth and survival and these abnormalities include:

- Mutation of oncogene: EGFR, KRAS, BRAF, etc.
- *Translocation*: ALK, RET, and
- *Amplification*: MET.

Molecular Changes in Adenocarcinoma

Mutation: Predominant mutation of ADC includes EGFR (10–45%) and KRAS (35%). The mutation of EGFR occurs in kinase domain of the tyrosine kinase. In 90% cases of ADC mutation of EGFR affects

- Point mutation of codon 858 (L858R)
- In-frame deletions in exon 19.

Epidermal growth factor receptor (EGFR) mutation is highly specific for ADC and patients of this mutation are treated with tyrosine kinase inhibitor therapy. However, EGFR mutation of exon 20, in-frame insertion is associated with resistant to tyrosine kinase inhibitor therapy (Box 12.16). EGFR mutation can be demonstrated by PCR technique.

Gene rearrangement: ALK gene fused with EML4 (5%). ALK rearrangement (EML4-ALK) is specific for lung carcinoma

Flowchart 12.1: Algorithmic approach of TTF-1 positivity in lung carcinoma.

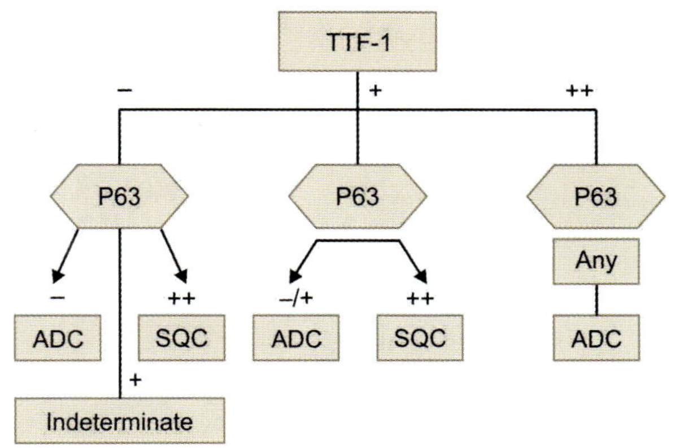

Box 12.16: Epidermal growth factor receptor mutation in adenocarcinoma of lung.

- Epidermal growth factor receptors (EGFR) mutation is commonly seen in female and nonsmokers.
- Mutation occurs in kinase domain of the tyrosine kinase.
- Frequency of mutation 15–45%. High in Asians.
- Point mutation of codon 858 (L858R) and in-frame deletions in exon 19.
- Highly specific for adenocarcinoma.
- EGFR mutation of exon 20, in-frame insertion is associated with resistant to tyrosine kinase inhibitor therapy.
- Tyrosine kinase inhibitor is given in EGFR mutation cases.

and mainly associated with ADC. The ALK arrangement needs to have ALK inhibitor therapy; however, the ALK arrangement is not related with prognosis of ADC.

Molecular changes in squamous cell carcinoma

- *Mutation*: Rb and p53 (>90%)
- *Amplification*: MYC (20–30%).

Significance: It is essential to know the specific mutational change of EGFR and activating fusion of ALK because specific targeted therapy of ADC of lung is available.

- *EGFR tyrosine kinase inhibitor*: Gefitnib, erlotinb
- *ALK inhibiting agent*: Crizotinib.

Flowchart 12.2 shows algorithmic approach of classification of lung carcinoma.

INDIVIDUAL TUMORS

Squamous Cell Carcinoma

This is one of the most common lung cancers. It is strongly associated with cigarette smoking and more than 90% of SQCs of lung occur in cigarette smoker. The majority of SQCs arises centrally from major bronchi or segmental bronchi and only 10% occur in the periphery. The salient cytological features are highlighted in Box 12.17.

Flowchart 12.2: Algorithmic approach of lung carcinoma on the basis of immunocytochemistry and molecular biology.

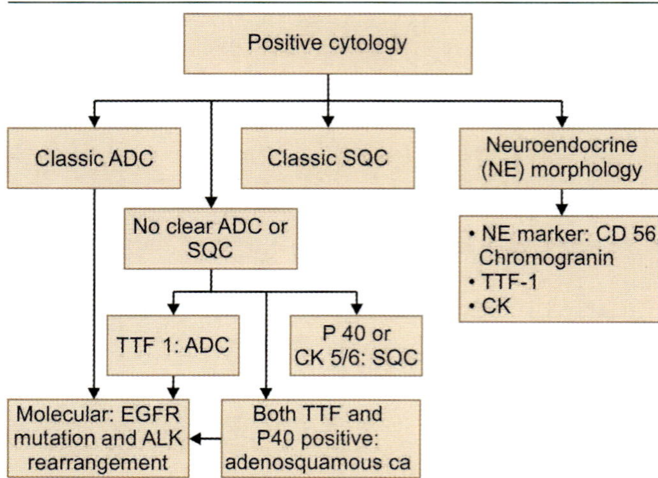

Cytology (Figs. 12.18 to 12.22)

Cytological examination of sputum provides a quick diagnosis of squamous cell cancer. Cytology smear shows clusters and discrete malignant cells in the background of

Box 12.17: Squamous cell carcinoma.

- Polyhedral cells
- Eosinophilic cytoplasm
- Intracellular keratin (orangeophilic cell)
- Round nucleus with moderate nuclear pleomorphism
- Hyperchromatic nucleus, inconspicuous nucleoli
- Fiber cells and tadpole cells
- Ghost of squamous cells
- Background necrosis and granular debris
- Keratin pearls

Immunocytochemistry: Positive for CK 5/6, CEA. Usually negative for TTF.

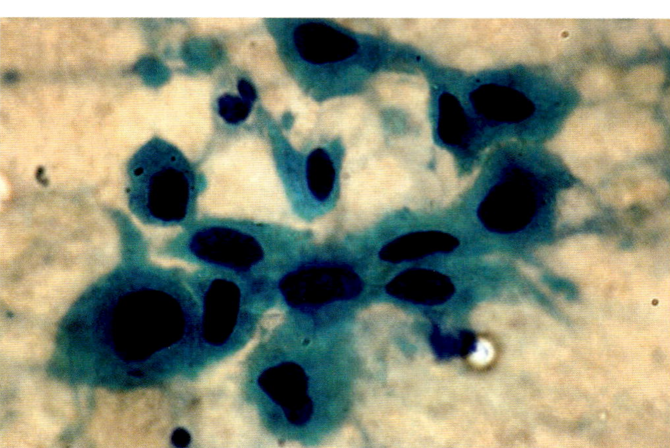

Fig. 12.18: Oval to polyhedral cells with moderately pleomorphic nuclei in squamous cell carcinoma of lung (Papanicolaou's stain × HP).

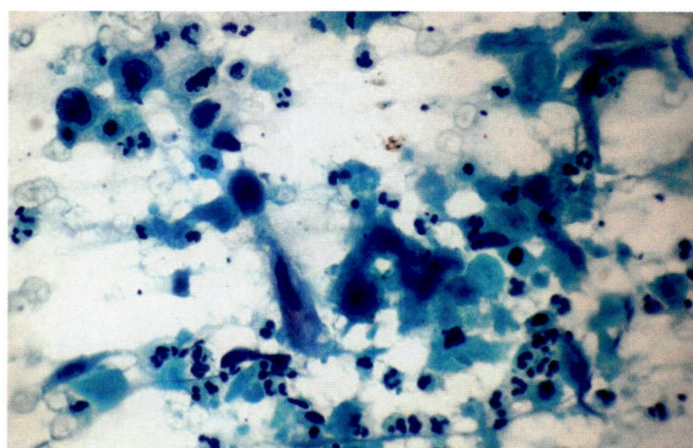

Fig. 12.19: Fiber-like cell with elongated nuclei in squamous cell carcinoma of lung (Papanicolaou's stain × HP).

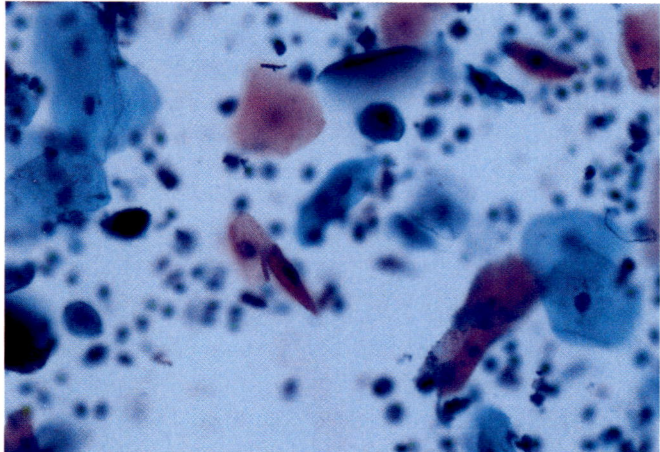

Fig. 12.20: Squamous cell carcinoma in sputum: Fiber-like cell with elongated nuclei (Papanicolaou's stain × HP).

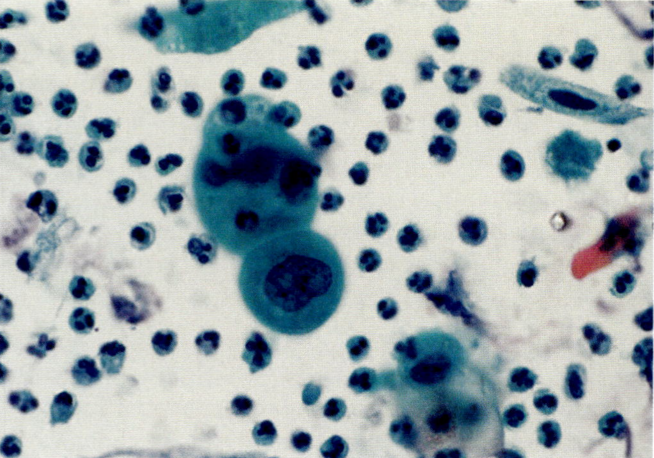

Fig. 12.21: Squamous cell carcinoma in bronchoalveolar lavage: Occasional discrete large atypical cells (Papanicolaou's stain × HP).

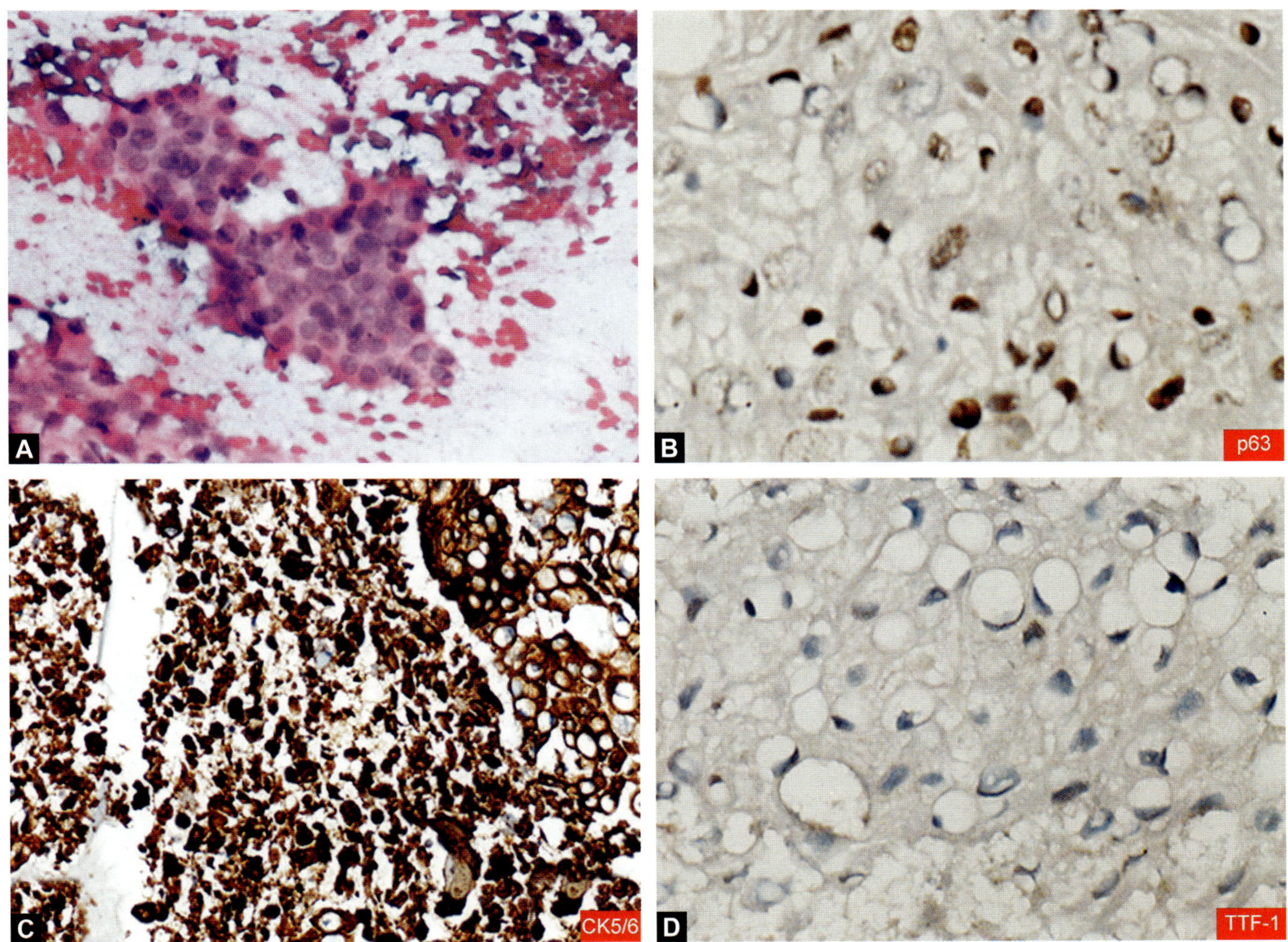

Figs. 12.22A to D: Squamous cell carcinoma of lung in a 55-year-old male: Cytology along with (a) p63, (b) CK 5/6, and (c) TTF-1. The cells are positive for p63 and CK 5/6. Tumor cells are negative for TTF-1.

necrosis and granular debris. The individual malignant cells are oval to polyhedral with centrally placed nuclei). The cytoplasm is moderate to abundant and shows orange color in Papanicolaou's stain. The dense orangeophilic cytoplasm of the cell is particularly noted in keratinizing SQC (Table 12.7). Keratinized cells are more evident in sputum than in bronchial washing or brushing specimen.

Nuclei show moderate to marked pleomorphism and marked hyperchromasia. Nuclear chromatin is irregular and coarse. Pyknotic dense ink dot like nuclear chromatin is more frequent in sputum samples. Nucleoli are usually not visible. In addition, many tadpole cells and fiber-like cells may be noted (Fig. 12.18). Occasionally keratin pearls are seen. The ghost of squamous cells along with necrosis in a clinically suspicious patient may suggest the possibility of malignancy.

Table 12.7: Differentiating features between keratinizing squamous cell carcinoma and nonkeratinizing squamous cell carcinoma.

Cytology features	*Keratinizing squamous cell carcinoma*	*Nonkeratinizing squamous cell carcinoma*
Cell clusters	Less, more discrete cells	More clusters
Cytoplasm	Orangeophilic	Basophilic
Nucleocytoplasmic ratio	Low	High
Nucleoli	Absent	Prominent
Chromatin	Coarse	Fine
Pyknotic nuclei	Frequent	Absent
Fiber and tadpole cells	More frequent	Less frequent

In moderately and poorly differentiated SQCs, the individual cells may not show features of keratinization and the cytoplasm is less eosinophilic and scanty in amount. The nuclear size is relatively large with more open chromatin and prominent nucleoli. Pyknotic nuclei are less frequent in nonkeratinizing SQC.

Immunocytochemistry

Positive for CK 5/6, p-63, p40 and usually negative for TTF. p40 is considered as most specific and sensitive marker of SQC.

Diagnostic Difficulties

Cytological features of SQC are characteristic however at times different conditions mimic this entity (Box 12.18).

- *Squamous metaplasia*: Squamous metaplasia occurs due to chronic bronchial irritation. These cells are smaller in size with relatively high nucleocytoplasmic (N/C) ratio. Metaplastic squamous cells may simulate SQC; however, these cells have monomorphic small round nuclei, smooth nuclear margin with homogenous chromatin.
- *Reactive squamous atypia*: Reactive squamous atypia are noted in cavitary Aspergillus lesions, radiation therapy, chemotherapeutic drugs, and infection of the lung. The nuclei of these atypical cells are monomorphic with regular nuclear margin.
- *Vegetable bodies*: Thick-walled plant cells with dark nuclei may rarely be mistaken as SQC of the lung. However the plant cells are very regular and their cellulose wall is thick.
- *Small cell carcinoma*: Small cell nonkeratinizing SQC may simulate SCC because of relatively smaller size and lack of typical squamous differentiation. Coarse chromatin, prominent nucleoli, absence of crushing artifact and nuclear molding are the characteristic differentiating points between SCC and SQC.
- *Adenocarcinoma*: At times poorly differentiated ADC is difficult to differentiate from poorly differentiated SQC. ADC cells often show cytoplasmic vacuoles that are positive for mucin. Nuclei of the cells show fine chromatin and prominent nucleoli.
- *Metastatic squamous cell carcinoma*: Without a proper history of another SQC, it is almost impossible to differentiate a primary form a metastatic SQC on cytological basis.

Box 12.18: Differential diagnosis of squamous cell carcinoma.

- *Squamous metaplasia*: Monomorphic small round nuclei with homogenous chromatin
- *Reactive squamous atypia*: Monomorphic with regular nuclear margin
- *Vegetable bodies*: Regular cell with thick cellulose wall
- *Small cell carcinoma*: Hyperchromatic nuclei, absence of nucleoli, crushing artifact, molding
- *Adenocarcinoma*: Cytoplasmic vacuoles, fine nuclear chromatin, prominent nucleoli
- *Metastatic squamous cell carcinoma*: Clinical history.

Adenocarcinoma

Adenocarcinomas of the lung are the most common subtype in females. These are commonly located in the peripheral part of the lung and may be detected in an asymptomatic patient.

The salient cytological features of ADC are mentioned in Box 12.19.

Cytology (Figs. 12.23 to 12.26)

The cytology smears of ADC show single and small clusters of cells. The cells are occasionally arranged as acini or honeycomb-like sheets. The gland may not be well-formed and often are absent. There may be 3D cell balls of malignant cells with nuclear overcrowding. The

Box 12.19: Adenocarcinoma of lung.

- Discrete, cluster, and glandular pattern.
- Sheets of cells with honeycomb pattern
- Round cells with moderate vacuolated cytoplasm
- Central to eccentric nucleus
- Fine chromatin
- Prominent nucleoli.

Immunocytochemistry: Positive for TTF-1, napsin A, CK7

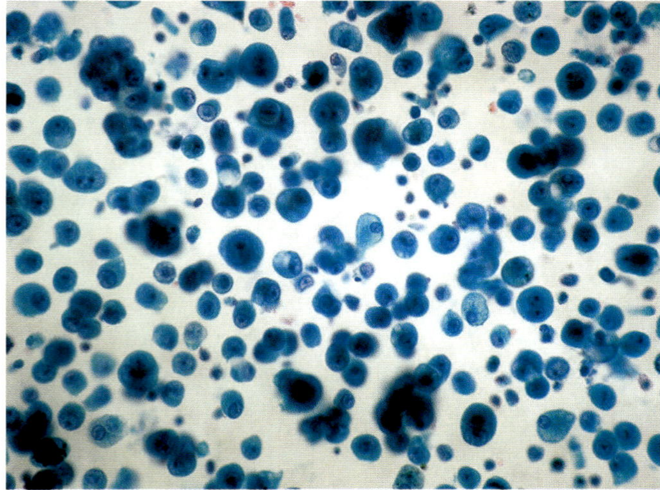

Fig. 12.23: Bronchoalveolar lavage sample shows discrete and loose clusters of malignant cells in adenocarcinoma of lung (Papanicolaou's stain × MP).

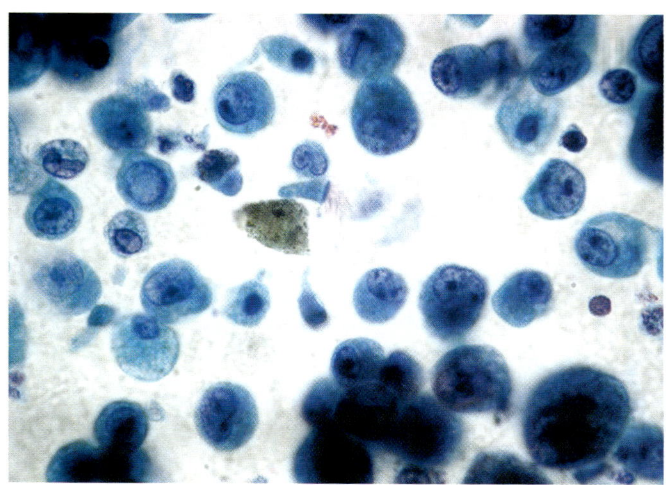

Fig. 12.24: Bronchoalveolar lavage sample shows malignant cells with moderate amount of cytoplasm and enlarged nuclei with prominent nucleoli in adenocarcinoma of lung (Papanicolaou's stain × HP).

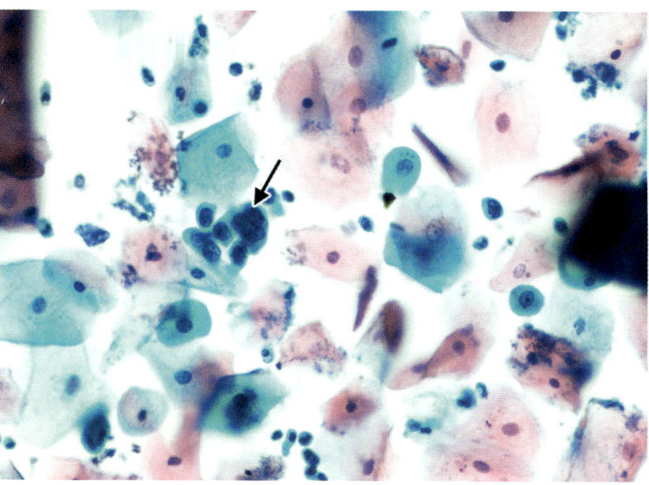

Fig. 12.25: Sputum smear shows discrete malignant cells entangled in adenocarcinoma of lung (*see* arrow) (Papanicolaou's stain × MP).

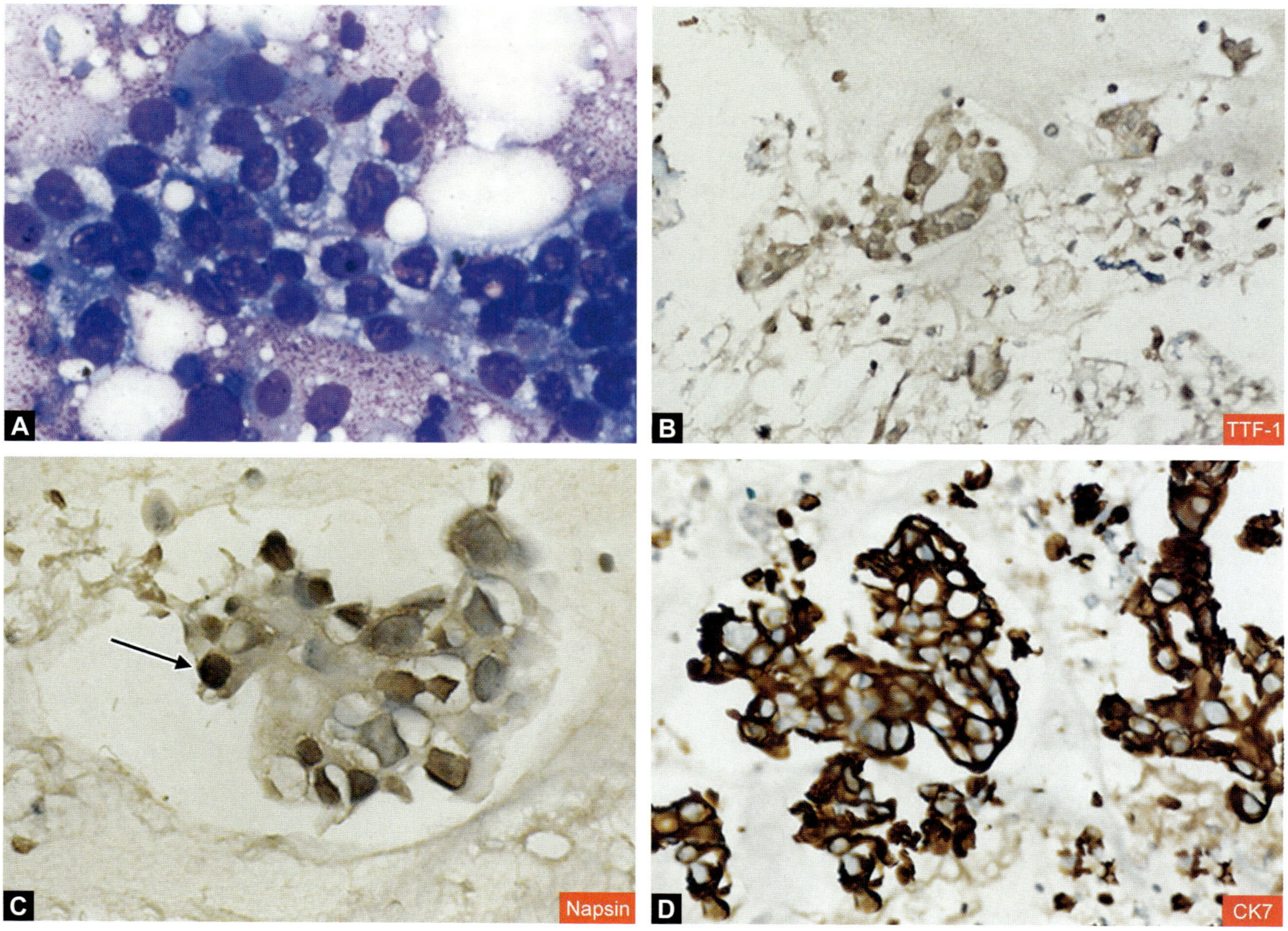

A B TTF-1 C Napsin D CK7

Figs. 12.26A to D: Cytology smear (A), and immunocytochemistry (B, C, and D) in a lung fine needle aspiration biopsy. Tumor cells are positive for TTF-1, napsin (*see* arrow), and CK7.

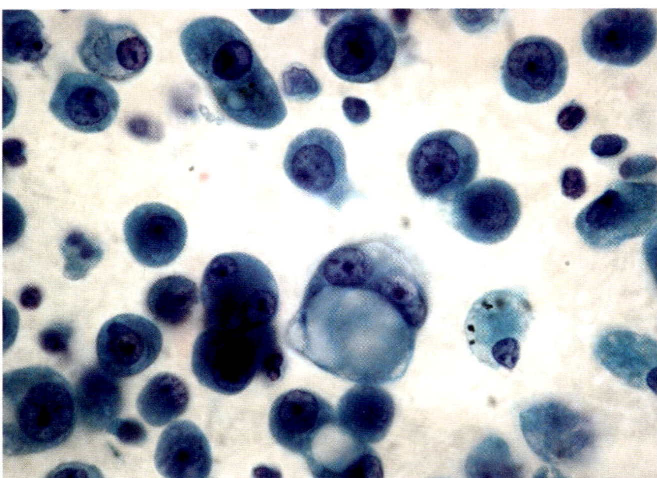

Fig. 12.27: Bronchoalveolar lavage sample shows small clusters and discrete cells with abundant vacuolated cytoplasm and enlarged nuclei with prominent nucleoli in a case of bronchioloalveolar carcinoma (Papanicolaou's stain × HP).

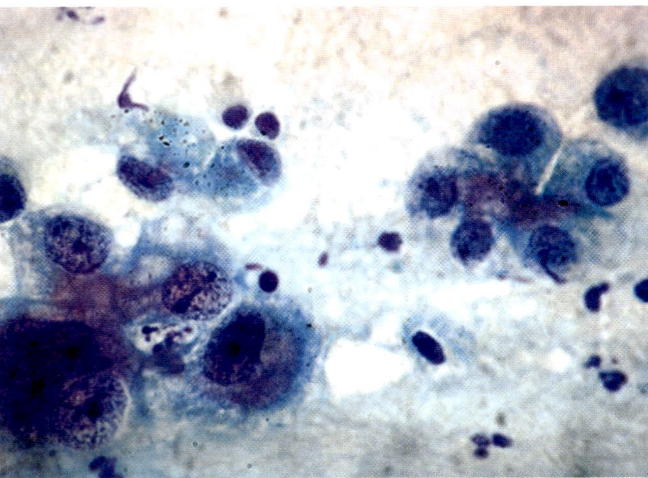

Fig. 12.28: Smear shows malignant cells with abundant vacuolated cytoplasm in a case of bronchioloalveolar carcinoma. Nuclei are mildly pleomorphic with single to multiple prominent nucleoli (Papanicolaou's stain × HP).

cytoplasm of the cell is moderate to abundant and often contains large vacuoles filled with mucin. Large vacuoles may push the nucleus to the periphery of the cell causing indented margin of the nucleus. The background mucinous material may also be noted in a small number of cases (less than 25%). The nuclei are central to eccentric in position with smooth margin having moderate pleomorphism. Nuclear chromatin is fine and evenly distributed. In poorly differentiated ADC, nuclear chromatin is coarse and hyperchromatic. Nucleoli are usually prominent and characteristically large and regular. One important feature of ADC is the presence of nucleocytoplasmic polarity. The nuclei of the cells are almost always in basal position.

Immunocytochemistry

Adenocarcinoma of lung is positive for TTF-1, napsin A, CK7.

Lepidic Adenocarcinoma (Bronchioloalveolar Carcinoma)

This tumor typically occurs in the peripheral part of the lung as a single nodule, multiple nodules, or diffuse lesions. The key cytological features are mentioned in Box 12.20.

Cytology

Lepidic ADC may be mucinous and nonmucinous types with overlapping cytomorphology. The cells are often arranged in monolayered sheets, ball-like tight clusters and papillae without any fibrovascular core. Cells of the mucinous type of BAL show abundant vacuolated cytoplasm with monomorphic nuclei having prominent nucleoli. In comparison, the cells of nonmucinous type of lepidic ADC shows smaller cells with relatively pleomorphic nuclei (Figs. 12.27 and 12.28). Intranuclear cytoplasmic inclusions are one of the diagnostic features of lepidic ADC. Psammoma bodies are present in occasional cases.

Box 12.20: Lepidic adenocarcinoma.

- Monolayer sheet, ball-like clusters.
- Papillary fragments of cells.
- Round to oval cells with mild to moderate vacuolated cytoplasm.
- Mild to moderate nuclear atypia.
- Finely granular nuclear chromatin.
- Inconspicuous nucleoli.
- Intranuclear inclusions.

Differential Diagnosis

Various differential diagnosis of ADC is highlighted in Box 12.21.

- *Poorly differentiated squamous cell carcinoma*: At times poorly differentiated ADC is difficult to distinguish from nonkeratinizing SQC. The problem has been discussed in the previous section.
- *Metastatic adenocarcinoma*: It is not possible to differentiate primary from a metastatic ADC on the basis of cytology alone. A clinical history may be helpful in this aspect.

Box 12.21: Differential diagnosis of adenocarcinoma and lepidic adenocarcinoma.

- *Poorly differentiated squamous cell carcinoma*: Cytoplasmic vacuoles, fine nuclear chromatin, prominent nucleoli
- *Metastatic adenocarcinoma*: Impossible without clinical history
- *Reactive bronchial cell hyperplasia*: Clusters have regular outline. Individual cells show presence of cilia. Nuclei monomorphic with regular margin.
- *Goblet cell hyperplasia*: Monomorphic nuclei
- *Reactive mesothelial cells*: Honeycomb sheet, window pattern, and regular nuclear margin.
- *Vegetable cell*: Thick cell wall
- *Hamartoma*: Presence of myxofibroid tissue, cartilaginous fragments, and cells with preserved cilia helps in the diagnosis of hamartoma.
- *Viral inclusions*: Halo around inclusion and beaded chromatin are helpful differentiating features.

- *Reactive bronchial cell hyperplasia*: This has been highlighted previously in the Table 12.5. The clusters of reactive atypical cells have a more regular outline. There is no significant nuclear overlapping. In addition, the individual cells show cilia. The nuclei of the cells are also monomorphic with regular margin.
- *Goblet cell hyperplasia*: Goblet cells with large vacuolated cytoplasm may mimic ADC. However, these cells have monomorphic benign looking nuclei that help in diagnosis.
- *Reactive mesothelial cells*: The mesothelial cells often show nuclear enlargement and pleomorphism with prominent nucleoli. Mesothelial cells are usually arranged in monolayerd sheets unlike 3D clusters in ADC. The individual cells show a typical window-like pattern. Differential diagnosis of ADC and reactive mesothelial cells have been discussed in detail in the next section.
- *Vegetable cells*: Vegetable cells are recognized by their thick cell wall.
- *Hyperplasia of pneumocytes*: At times there may be hyperplasia of pneumocytes type II that may resemble lepidic ADC.
- *Hamartoma*: This may be a source of false positive diagnosis as hamartoma contains good amount of glandular material. The presence of myxofibroid tissue, cartilaginous fragments, and cells with preserved cilia helps in the diagnosis of hamartoma.
- *Viral inclusions*: At times large viral inclusions may mimic prominent nucleoli and may be mistaken as ADC. However other features such as halo around inclusion and beaded chromatin are helpful differentiating features.

Box 12.22: Small cell carcinoma.

- Dissociated cells
- Small cells, resembling lymphocytes
- Scanty cytoplasm
- Hyperchromatic nucleus with inconspicuous nucleoli
- Nuclear molding
- Paranuclear blue bodies
- Crushing artifact and nuclear threading.

Small Cell Carcinoma

Small cell carcinoma accounts for 20% of lung cancer and 90% of these tumors are centrally located. It is strongly associated with cigarette smoking. Male to female ratio of this tumor is 2:1. The WHO has classified SCC as (1) pure SCC, and (2) combined SCC with other carcinomas. This is a highly aggressive malignancy and metastasizes quickly. The surgical resection is ineffective in this malignancy. This tumor is sensitive to chemotherapy. The key cytological features are mentioned in Box 12.22.

Cytology (Figs. 12.29 to 12.32)

The cytology smears of the SCC shows a predominant discrete population of the small round cells about one and half times larger than mature lymphocytes. In sputum smears, the cells are entangled in the mucus and arranged in small rows like Indian file arrangement. The tumor cells show nuclear threading and crushing artifact due to the fragile nature of the cells. The individual cells are round with scanty cytoplasm. Occasional spindle cells are also seen. The nuclei are relatively monomorphic with finely granular "salt and pepper" like chromatin. Nucleoli are absent. Nuclear molding is characteristic of SCC. Cytoplasm may contain round light blue to dark homogenous bodies known as paranuclear blue bodies. In the sputum sample the detailed morphology of the cells may not be seen as they are enmeshed in mucus. However, the presence of small round cells with hyperchromatic nuclei and scanty cytoplasm indicate the diagnosis of SCC. In comparison, bronchial washing or brushing specimen show better nuclear morphology. The nuclei show cell to cell compression and characteristic nuclear molding.

Immunocytochemistry

The SCC is positive for CD56, chromogranin, synaptophysin, and cytokeratin.

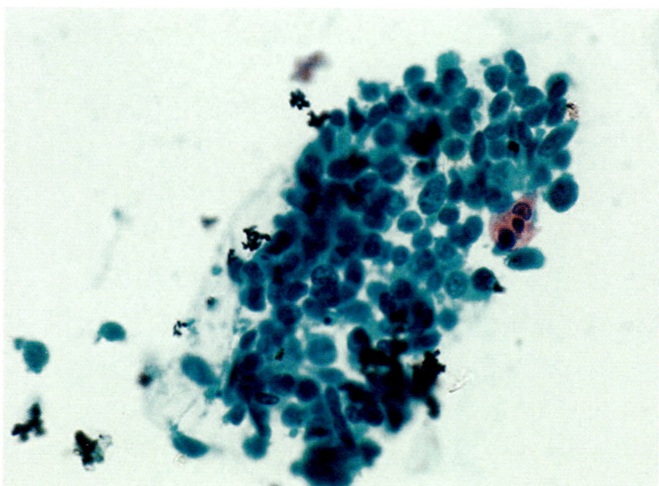

Fig. 12.29: Small cell carcinoma of lung in sputum: Loose cluster malignant cells with scanty cytoplasm (Papanicolaou's stain × HP).

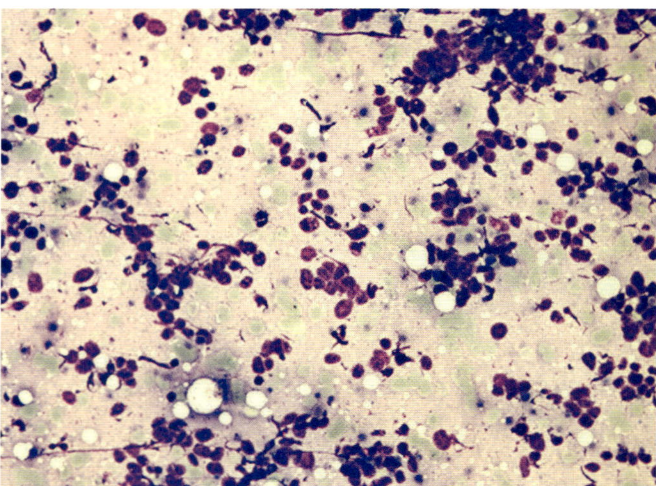

Fig. 12.30: Abundant small cells with scanty cytoplasm and hyperchromatic nuclei in small cell carcinoma of lung (Papanicolaou's stain × MP).

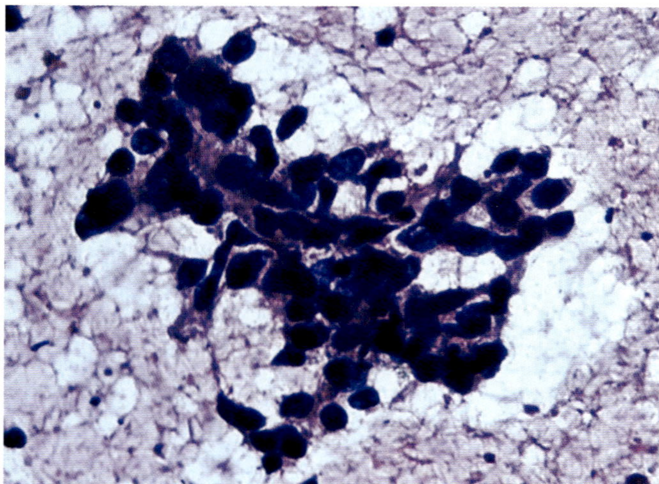

Fig. 12.31: Malignant cells are often compressed with each other in small cell carcinoma of lung (Papanicolaou's stain × HP).

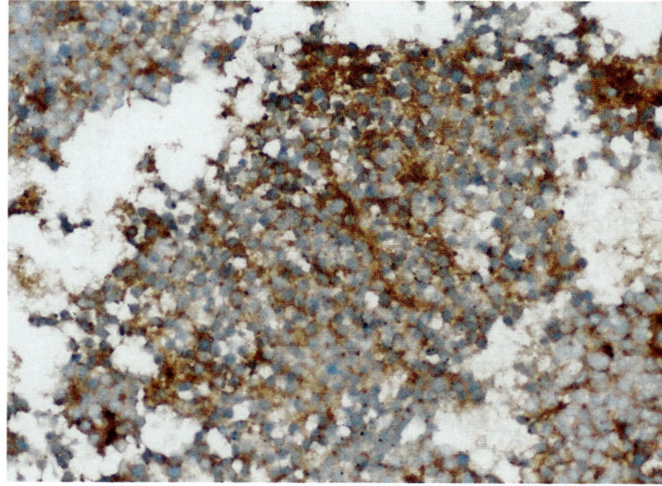

Fig. 12.32: Malignant cells are positive for chromogranin in small cell carcinoma of lung.

Differential Diagnosis

- *Reserve cell hyperplasia*: Reserve cells show much smaller cells with smudged nuclei and featureless chromatin.
- *Lymphocytes*: Lymphocytes in chronic inflammation may be mistaken as SCC. Lymphocytes are usually dissociated and smaller than the cells of SCC.
- *Poorly differentiated carcinoma*: Poorly differentiated SQC and ADC with small round cells may be confused with SCC. Cellular dissociation, scanty cytoplasm, and nuclear molding favor the diagnosis of SCC.
- *Carcinoid tumor*: Discrete cells with relatively monomorphic nuclei may pose a diagnostic dilemma with carcinoid tumor. However, the presence of abundant granular cytoplasm, salt and pepper chromatin, and prominent nucleoli favor the diagnosis of carcinoid.
- *Lymphomas*: Small round dissociated cells with scanty cytoplasm may simulate non-Hodgkin lymphoma (NHL). The presence of lymphoglandular bodies is characteristic of NHL.
- *Nonkeratinizing squamous cell carcinoma*: Small cells of nonkeratinizing SQC may be difficult to distinguish from SCC. However, nuclear morphology is helpful in diagnosis of SCC.

Table 12.8 shows differential diagnosis of SCC of the lung.

Table 12.8: Differential diagnosis of small cell carcinoma of lung.

	Small cell carcinoma	*Squamous cell carcinoma*	*Carcinoid*	*Lymphoma*
Cell clusters	Discrete	Present	Discrete	Discrete
Indian file arrangement	Present	Absent	Absent	Absent
Nuclear threading	Present	Absent	Absent	Absent
Lymphoglandular bodies	Absent	Absent	Absent	Present
Cell cytoplasm amount	Scanty to nil	Moderate	Moderate, reddish granular	Scanty
Cytoplasm character	Thin rim of basophilic	Orangeophilic dense cytoplasm	Reddish granular	Deep blue in Giemsa stain
Nuclear molding	Present	Absent	Absent	Absent
Nucleus	Small, one to two times larger than lymphocyte	Relatively low nucleocytoplasmic ratio, small nucleus	Larger	Twice the size of mature lymphocyte
Chromatin	Granular and Salt and pepper	Irregular coarse	Salt and pepper	Fine
Immunochemistry • Chromogranin • Synaptophysin • TTF • LCA	 • Positive • Positive • Positive • Negative	 • Negative • Positive • Mostly negative • Negative	 • Positive • Positive • Variable positivity • Negative	 • Negative • Negative • Negative • Positive
Electron microscopy	Neuroendocrine granules	Desmosomal junction	Neuroendocrine granules	Non-specific

Box 12.23: Undifferentiated large cell carcinoma.

- Large cell with marked nuclear pleomorphism
- Moderate to abundant cytoplasm
- Ill-defined cytoplasm
- Severely pleomorphic bizarre nuclei
- Multiple prominent nucleoli
- Large tumor giant cell
- Polymorphs sticking to the cells.

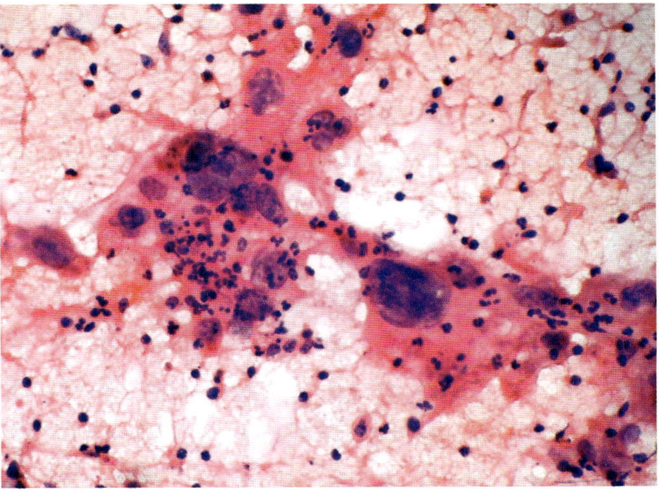

Fig. 12.33: Discrete malignant cells with enlarged markedly pleomorphic nuclei along with many ploymorphs (Papanicolaou's stain × HP).

Undifferentiated Large Cell Carcinoma

Large cell carcinoma (LCC) accounts for 10% of all lung carcinomas. These are undifferentiated LCCs without any particular evidence of differentiation toward squamous or ADC. Majority of LCCs are located in the peripheral part of lung. WHO discourages in the diagnosis of LCC on cytology smear, and it recommends to put this entity as NSCC. Overall the key cytological features of LCC are mentioned in Box 12.23.

Cytology (Fig. 12.33)

The cells are usually arranged in syncytial clusters and also discretely. No acinar or glandular differentiation is seen. The individual cells show moderate to abundant dense cytoplasm with ill-defined margins. Nuclei show marked pleomorphism, nuclear margin irregularity, irregular coarse chromatin, and multiple enlarged prominent nucleoli. Many large mono/multinuclear giant cells are also noted. The characteristic feature of LCC is sticking of polymorphs with the malignant. The malignant cells also engulf the polymorphs. Giant cell carcinoma is one of the varieties of the undifferentiated LCC. Here, the smear shows many large multinuclear and mononuclear tumor giant cells along with heavy polymorphonuclear leucocytes infiltration. The large cell neuroendocrine tumor shows a rosette-like structures and nuclear molding.

Differential Diagnosis (Box 12.24)

- *Sarcomas*: Large bizarre cells may give rise to the possibilities of sarcomas. However, sarcoma of the lung is rare. Immunostaining such as vimentin is helpful for confirmation of sarcoma.
- *Amelanotic melanoma*: Large cells with large prominent nucleoli may simulate amelanotic melanomas. Malignant melanoma cells are positive for HMB45.
- *Reactive changes*: Different types of lung injury may produce large bizarre reactive bronchial cells and pneumocytes. Nuclear margin irregularity and chromatin pattern help in diagnosis of LCC.
- *Squamous cell carcinoma*: Poorly differentiated nonkeratinizing SQC may often show moderate nuclear enlargement and pleomorphism. SQC often shows orangeophilic cells, fiber cells, and tadpole cells.
- *Adenocarcinoma*: Gland-like arrangement and background mucin may help in diagnosis of ADC.

Carcinoid

Carcinoid tumor comprises of a small proportion of primary lung tumors. WHO classified carcinoid as typical carcinoid and atypical carcinoid tumor. The key cytological features are mentioned in Box 12.25.

Box 12.24: Differential diagnosis of large cell carcinoma.

- *Sarcomas*: Rare, immunostain: Vimentin for sarcoma, CK for large cell carcinoma
- *Amelanotic melanoma*: HMB45 immunostaing.
- *Reactive changes*: Regular nuclear margin and no significant chromatin abnormality
- *Squamous cell carcinoma*: Orangeophilic cells, fiber cells, and tadpole cells
- *Adenocarcinoma*: Gland-like arrangement and background mucin.

Cytology (Figs. 12.34 to 12.36)

Sputum sample of carcinoid tumor is usually paucicellular because the tumor cells rarely shed in the sputum as the overlying mucosa of the tumor remains preserved.

Box 12.25: Carcinoid.

- Dissociated cells
- Rosettes
- Monomorphic cells
- Moderate to abundant cytoplasm with red granularity
- Round monomorphic nuclei with salt and pepper chromatin
- Mitosis is uncommon.

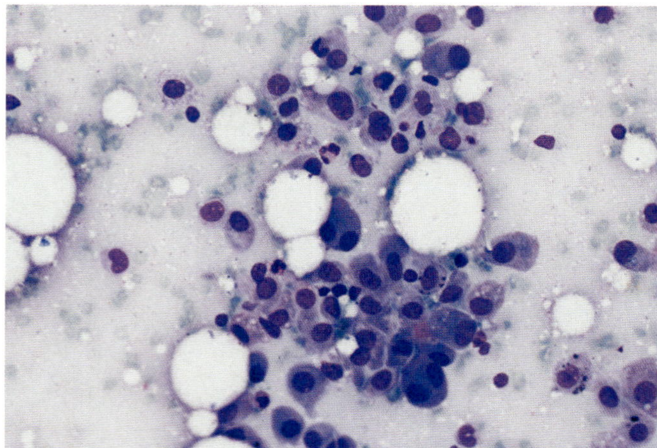

Fig. 12.34: Carcinoid of lung: Smears show discrete small round monomorphic cells (May-Grünwald Giemsa stain × MP).

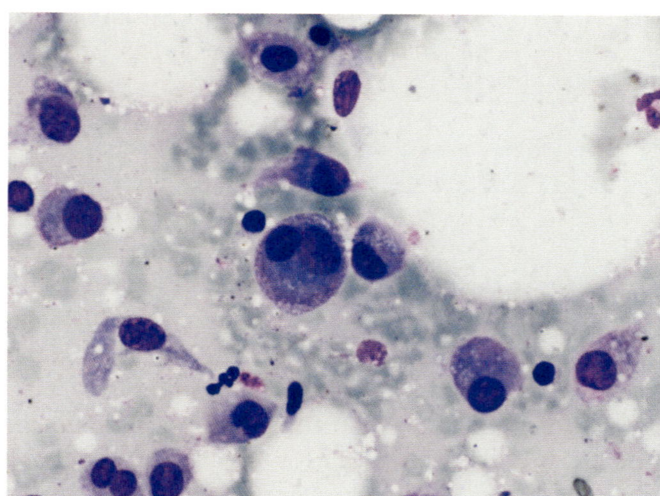

Fig. 12.35: Carcinoid of lung: Individual cells show abundant cytoplasm with reddish granularity (May-Grünwald Giemsa stain × HP).

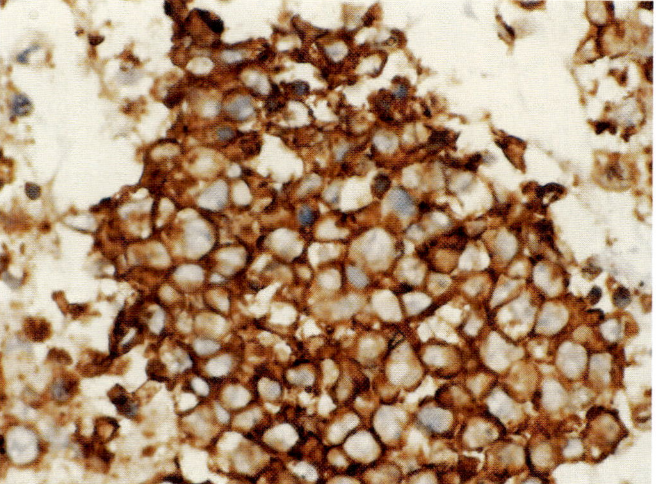

Fig. 12.36: Carcinoid of lung: Strong synaptophysin positivity of the tumor cells.

The cells are usually seen in bronchial brushing. Cytology smears of the carcinoid tumor usually show dissociated cells. Occasional rosette-like structures may be seen. Individual cells are small to moderate amount of cytoplasm having fine reddish granules. The nuclei are central in location and relatively monomorphic. Chromatin is finely stippled and gives the characteristic salt and pepper appearance. Nucleoli are usually small and inconspicuous.

Cells of atypical carcinoid show large nuclei with moderate pleomorphism. The individual cells have moderate to abundant reddish granular cytoplasm.

Differential Diagnosis

- *Small cell carcinoma*: See in SCC.
- *Other lung carcinomas*: Cells of bronchioloalveolar carcinoma (BAC) with monomorphic nuclei may create diagnostic confusion with carcinoid. However, cytological features such as monolayered sheets, frequent aggregation of cells, cells with vacuolated cytoplasm favor BAC.

Lymphomas

Primary NHL and HL (Hodgkin lymphoma) are uncommon in the lung. In fact less than 10% of extranodal lymphomas occur in the lung. Primary pulmonary HLs are exceedingly rare. The common primary NHLs of the lung are marginal zone lymphoma and diffuse B cell lymphoma.

Metastatic Malignancies

The lung is the most common sites of metastasis and the large varieties of malignancies metastases in the lung. However, metastatic carcinomas are uncommonly seen in sputum or bronchial washing or brushing specimen. The most common primary sites of metastatic lung carcinomas are breast, colon, stomach, pancreas, kidney, prostate, liver, male genitalia, and female genital tract. This happens because lung is the sole organ that receives the entire blood and lymphatic flow. A thorough clinical history with the detailed knowledge of previous histological diagnosis is needed for the exact diagnosis. TTF and napsin A positivity on immunostaining usually confirm the primary origin of ADC of lung.

REFERENCES

1. Daniele RP, Elias JA, Epstein PE, et al. Bronchoalveolar lavage: role in the pathogenesis, diagnosis and management of interstitial lung disease. Ann Intern Med. 1985;102:93-9.
2. Rankin JA, Naegel GP, Reynolds HY. Use of a central laboratory for analysis of bronchoalveolar lavage fluid. Am Rev Respir Dis. 1986;133:186-90.
3. Zarbo RJ, Fenoglio-Preiser CM. Interinstitutional database for comparison of performance in lung fine-needle aspiration cytology: a College of American Pathologists Q-probe study of 5264 cases with histologic correlation. Arch Pathol Lab Med. 1992;116:463-70.
4. Koss LG, Richardson HL. Some pitfalls of cytological diagnosis of lung cancer. Cancer. 1955;8:937-47.
5. Kitamura H, Kameda Y, Ito T, et al. Atypical adenomatous hyperplasia of the lung. Implications for the pathogenesis of peripheral lung adenocarcinoma. Am J Clin Pathol. 1999;111:610-22.
6. Nasiell M, Roger V, Nasiell K, et al. Cytologic findings indicating pulmonary tuberculosis: I. The diagnostic significance of epithelioid cells and Langhans' giant cells found in sputum or bronchial secretions. Acta Cytol. 1972;16:146-51.
7. Jacobs JA, Dieleman MM, Cornelissen EI, et al. Bronchoalveolar lavage fluid cytology in patients with *Pneumocystis carinii* pneumonia. Acta Cytol. 2001;45: 317-26.
8. Wynder EL, Graham EA. Tobacco smoking as a possible etiologic factor in bronchogenic carcinoma: a study of 684 proven cases. JAMA. 1950;143:329-36.
9. Frank AL. The epidemiology and etiology of lung cancer. Clin Chest Med. 1982;3:219-28.
10. Travis WD, Brambilla E, Nicholson AG, et al. The 2015 World Health Organization Classification of Lung Tumors: Impact of Genetic, Clinical and Radiologic Advances Since the 2004 Classification. J Thorac Oncol. 2015;10(9):1243-60.
11. Travis WD, Brambilla E, Müller-Hermelink HK, et al. (Eds). World Health Organization Classification of Tumors: Pathology and Genetics of Tumors of the Lung, Pleura, Thymus and Heart. Lyon: IARC Press; 2015.

Review Questions

1. **Bronchoalveolar lavage (Fig. 12.37) in a 38-year-old male with fever and lung opacity in radiograph. The most likely diagnosis is:**
   a. Candida
   b. Histoplasma
   c. Cryptococci
   d. Artifact
2. **Bronchoalveolar lavage (Fig. 12.38) in a 28-year-old male with history of longstanding steroid intake for autoimmune disease:**
   a. Pneumocystis infection
   b. Alveolar cast
   c. Talc
   d. RBC in clump
3. **The lung carcinoma that is positive for p40, p63, and CK7 band negative for TTF-1 is most likely:**
   a. Adenocarcinoma
   b. Carcinoid
   c. Small cell carcinoma
   d. Squamous cell carcinoma
4. **The most common site of EGFR mutation of adenocarcinoma of lung is:**
   a. Exon 20
   b. In-frame deletions in exon 19
   c. Exon 18
   d. Exon 21
5. **ALK rearrangement (EML4-ALK) is specific for:**
   a. Adenocarcinoma
   b. Carcinoid
   c. Small cell carcinoma
   d. Squamous cell carcinoma
6. **A 71-year-old male presented with a 3 cm diameter space occupying lesion in the upper lobe of right lung. The most likely diagnosis of this cytology smear (Figs. 12.39A and B) and immunocytochemistry (synaptophysisn, chromogranin, TTF-1, and CK7, Figs. 12.39C to F) of this lung tumor is:**
   a. Adenocarcinoma
   b. Anaplastic large cell carcinoma
   c. Small cell carcinoma
   d. Squamous cell carcinoma
7. **Cytology (Fig. 12.40A) and immunocytochemistry of TTF-1 (Fig. 12.40B), napsin (Fig. 12.40C), and CK (Fig. 12.40D) have been shown. The most likely diagnosis is:**
   a. Adenocarcinoma
   b. Carcinoid
   c. Small cell carcinoma
   d. Squamous cell carcinoma

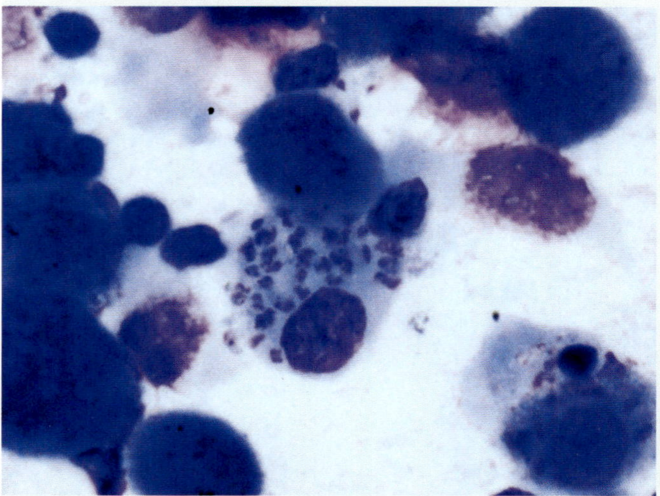

Fig. 12.37: Smear of bronchoalveolar lavage of question 1.

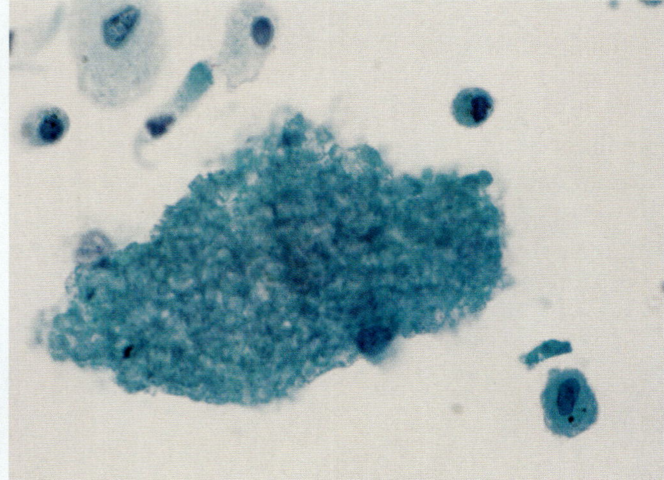

Fig. 12.38: Smear of bronchoalveolar lavage of question 2.

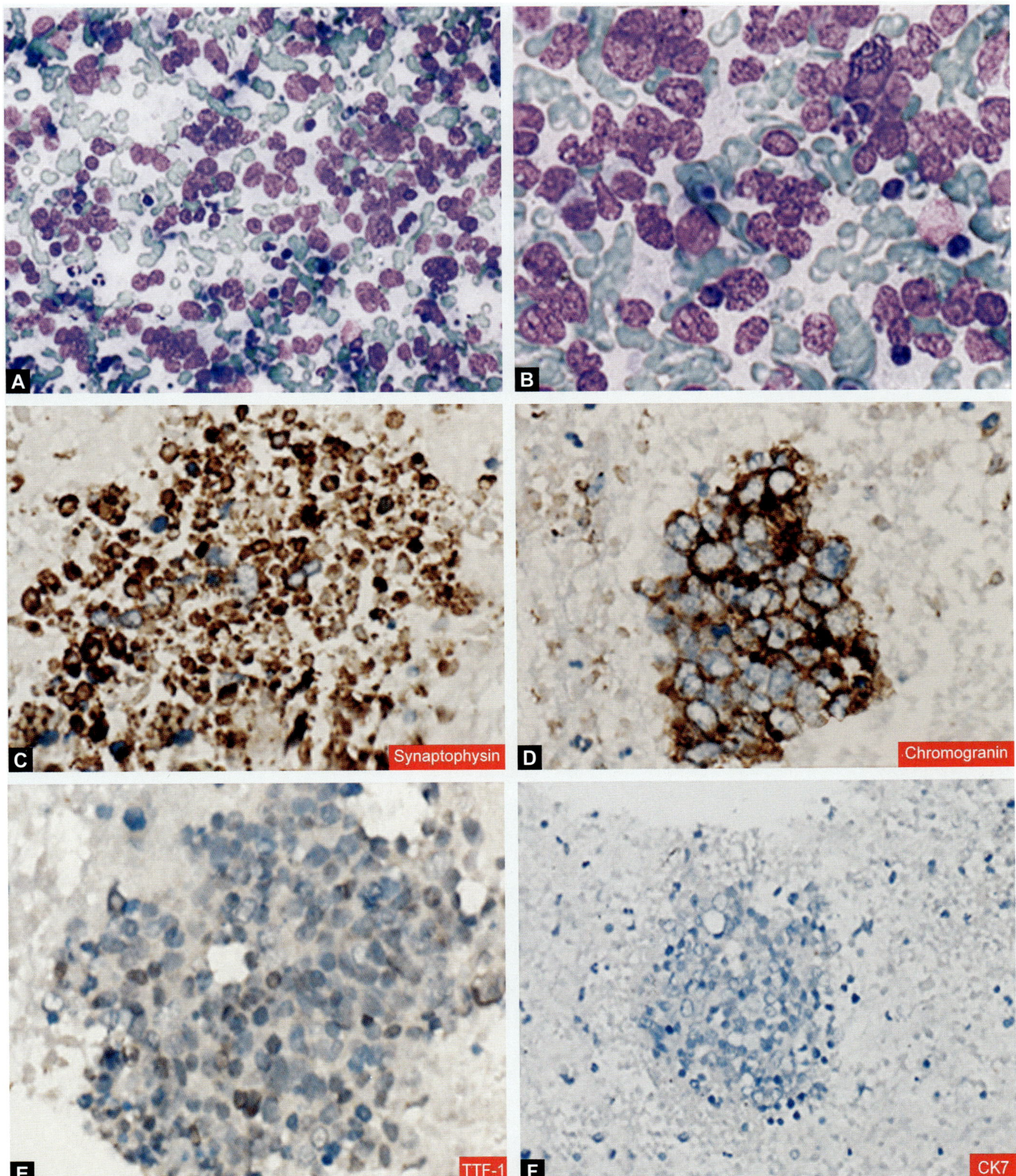

Figs. 12.39A to F: Cytology smear and immunocytochemistry of question 6.

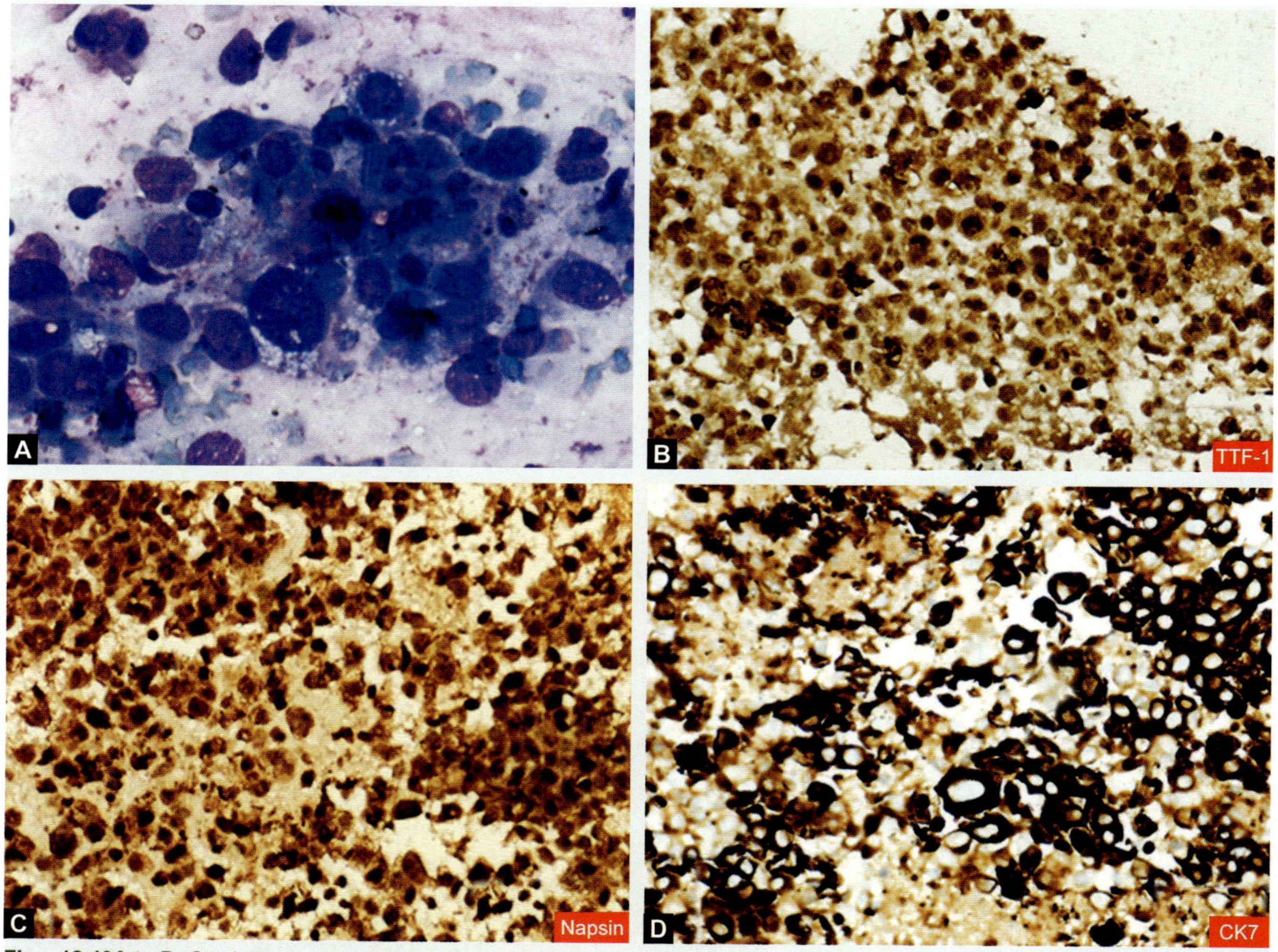

Figs. 12.40A to D: Cytology smear and immunocytochemistry of question 7.

8. Aspiration cytology smear (Fig. 12.41) from a 3 cm diameter lung lesion (right upper lobe) for 2 months. The tumor is likely to be strongly positive for:

a. CK 5/6
b. Chromogranin
c. p63
4. TTF-1

9. Aspiration cytology smear (Figs. 12.42A to D) from a 5 cm diameter lung lesion (left lower lobe) for 15 days. Cytology smear (Fig. 12.42A) along with immunocytochemistry of pancytokeratin (Fig. 12.42B), desmin (Fig. 12.42C), and p63 (Fig. 12.42D) have been provided. The most likely diagnosis is:

a. Adenocarcinoma
b. Carcinosarcoma
c. Adenosaquamous carcinoma
d. Squamous cell carcinoma

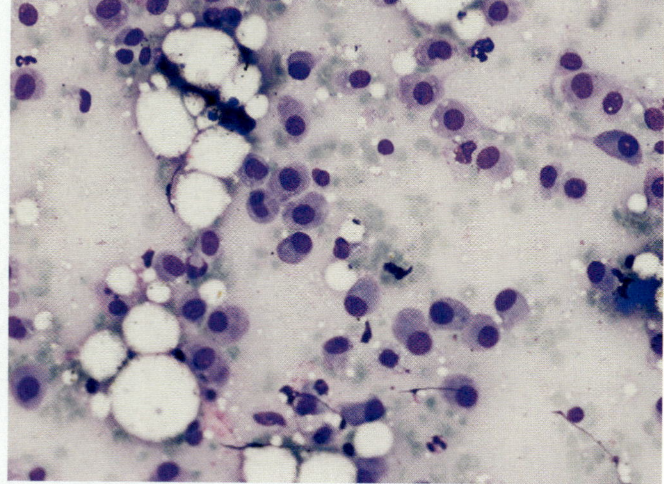

Fig. 12.41: Cytology smear of question 8.

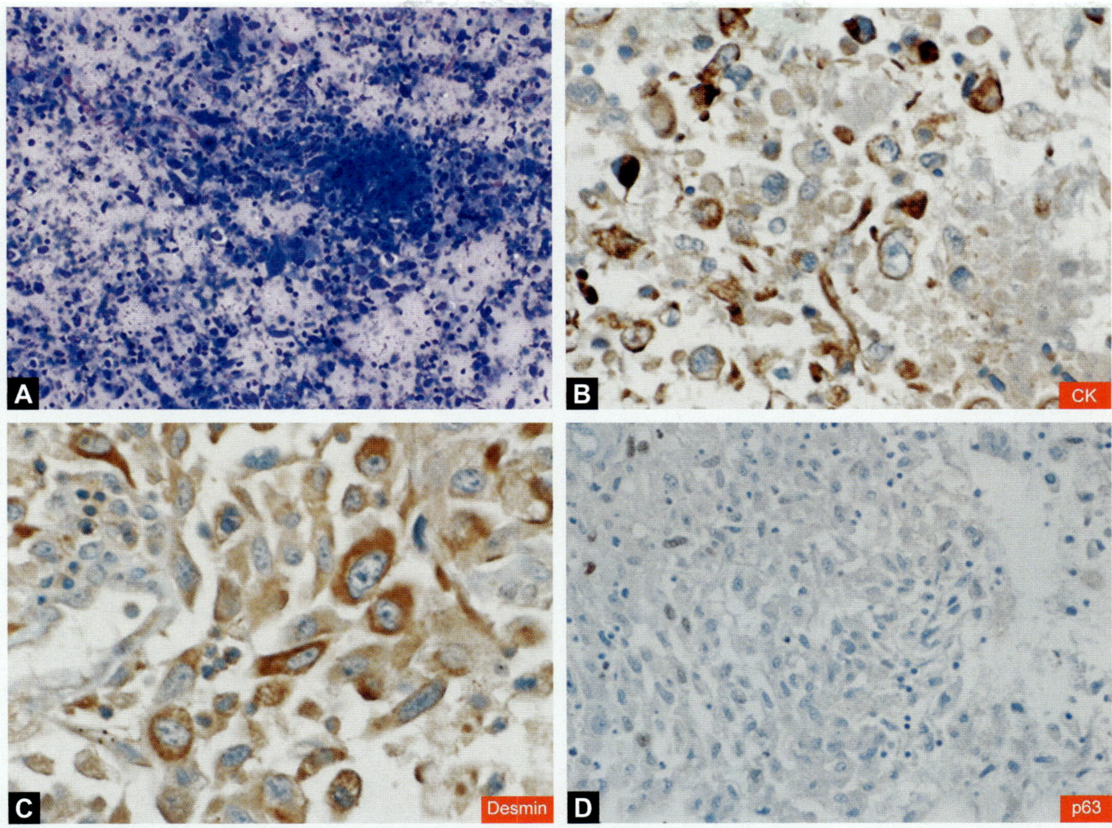

Figs. 12.42A to D: Cytology smear and immunocytochemistry of question 9.

Answers

1. b. Histoplasma
   Note: The organisms show characteristic features of histoplasma. They are small, ring shaped, intracellular and 2 to 3 micron in size. On or more chromatid substances are present in the periphery of the parasite.
2. a. Pneumocystis infection
   Note: This typical frothy alveolar cast is highly suggestive of pneumocystis infection. Careful observation shows cup shaped organism. The fungi are well visualized by Methenamine silver stain.
3. d. Squamous cell carcinoma
4. b. In-frame deletions in exon 19
5. a. Adenocarcinoma
6. c. Small cell carcinoma
   Note: The cells show stippled chromatin. In addition, the tumor cells are positive for synaptophysin and chromogranin and are negative for TTF-1 and CK7. All these features indicate a small cell carcinoma of lung.
7. a. Adenocarcinoma
   Note: The tumor cells are strongly positive for TTF-1, napsin and CK7, The immunocytochemistry findings confirm the diagnosis of adenocarcinoma of lung.
8. b. Chromogranin
   Note: The discrete cells with moderate amount of cytoplasm having central to eccentric monomorphic nuclei indicate the possibility of a neuroendocrine tumor. Therefore the cells are expected to be chromogranin positive.
9. b. Carcinosarcoma
   Note: The tumor shows oval to spindle cells that are positive for both CK and desmin. The features are in favour of carcinosarcoma.

CHAPTER

13 Gastrointestinal Tract

INTRODUCTION

Cytology plays an important role in the diagnosis of various lesions of gastrointestinal tract (GIT) particularly due to rapid improvement of technology of the sampling method and visualization techniques. It is now proved as an efficient technique for the diagnosis of various lesions in GIT. There are several added advantages of exfoliative and endoscopic aspiration cytology in GIT. These are:

- Wide area of the mucosal surface can be covered
- Quick turn over time
- Less invasive technology
- Deeper and stenotic part of the canal can be reached.

SAMPLING TECHNIQUES (BOX 13.1)

Endoscopic Brush Cytology

Procurement of the sample under direct visualization of the abnormal mucosa with the help of flexible fiberoptic endoscopy is a major advance in detection of lesions of GIT.[1] This is one of the most common techniques to obtain samples from upper GIT under direct visualization.

Procedure

To obtain the brush sample, a flexible fiberoptic endoscopy is introduced in the GIT. The flexible nature of the tube allows it to pass through the tortuous food canal. The endoscope contains specific channels for biopsy forceps and brush. The brush is made of nylon and is covered by a Teflon® sheath to prevent the loss of cytology material. When the mucosal lesion is visualized, the brush is taken out from the outer Teflon® sheath and gently rubbed on the lesion to get the material. Finally the brush is retracted into the Teflon® sheath and is withdrawn from the endoscope. Multiple smears are made by rubbing the brush on the glass slide.

Box 13.1: Sampling techniques in gastrointestinal tract (GIT).

- Endoscopic brush cytology
- Salvage cytology
- Endoscopic FNAC
- Endoscopic ultrasound-guided (EUS) FNAC
- Balloon technique
- Fine needle aspiration cytology by endoscopic retrograde cholangiopancreatography.

(FNAC: Fine needle aspiration cytology).

Major Advantages

Major advantages are: (1) It can procure samples from the large surface area of the mucosa under visual surveillance. As brush cytology it covers a large surface area so it is the most suitable technique for detection of infections (Box 13.2). (2) Brush cytology can be done from the deepest part of a stenotic canal when the usual tissue biopsy forceps cannot enter through the narrowed canal. (3) Brush cytology is comparatively less expensive, cost effective and less invasive technique than other sampling modalities. Brush cytology is complementary to biopsy. Combined use of biopsy and brush cytology increases the sensitivity of detection of malignancy near about 100%.[2]

Box 13.2: Brush cytology.

Procedure: With the help of flexible fiberoptic endoscopy, the lesion is visualized and endoscopic brush is taken through the channel of endoscope.

Advantages:

- Large surface area of the mucosa is covered
- Deeper part of a stenotic canal can be sampled
- Comparatively cost effective and less invasive.

Disadvantages:

- Difficult to differentiate severe dysplasia from invasive carcinoma
- Low sensitivity to detect Barrett's esophagus.

Comments: Combined use of biopsy and brush cytology has 100% sensitivity.

Major Problems

Major problems are: (1) It is difficult to differentiate severe dysplasia from invasive carcinoma on cytology and therefore the clinicians may prefer biopsy rather than brush cytology; (2) It is difficult to detect goblet cell metaplasia in esophageal brush and therefore the sensitivity of brush cytology to detect Barrett's esophagus is low.[3]

Salvage Cytology

This is rarely used for diagnosis. However it is a relatively rapid and easy technique.

Procedure

After obtaining the biopsy, the endoscopic channel is flushed through normal saline and the fluid is collected and processed for smear preparation. The idea of the lavage cytology is to retrieve the material from the endoscopic tube that is dislodged from the external surface of the forceps during withdrawal of the forceps after biopsy.

Endoscopic Fine Needle Aspiration Cytology

The endoscopic fine needle aspiration cytology (FNAC) helps in obtaining samples from the lesions located deep in the mucosa.

Procedure

The FNAC needle is introduced through the channel of the fiberoptic endoscope. After localizing the lesion the needle is introduced and moved to and fro in the lesion maintaining negative suction. Finally, the needle is withdrawn and the aspirated material is spread on the glass slide.

Endoscopic FNAC is particularly helpful in submucosal tumors and is complementary to biopsy. The combined use of biopsy, brush cytology and endoscopic FNAC gives 100% sensitivity.[4]

Endoscopic ultrasound-guided (EUS) FNAC is a very useful sampling technique in the diagnosis of the submucosal lesion such as carcinoid tumor, infiltrative tumor, lymphomas and stromal tumor. EUS helps in localizing along with an assessment of the size and extent of the lesion that is situated underneath the mucosa. EUS guidance helps in better placement of the needle in the submucosal lesion and therefore sensitivity of this technique is high.

Balloon Technique

It is predominantly used in some of the areas of China where the incidence of esophageal malignancy is very high.[5] It is an inexpensive and minimally invasive technique. This technique does not need any endoscope. The abrasive balloon technique is used for population screening of the high risk area of esophageal cancer.

A deflated balloon is swallowed by the patient. Within the stomach the balloon is inflated and dragged through the esophageal wall. Ultimately the balloon is deflated at the level of cricoids cartilage and the whole thing is withdrawn and rubbed on a glass slide to make the smear.

Endoscopic Retrograde Cholangiopancreatography

Endoscopic retrograde cholangiopancreatography (ERCP): It is a complex technique by which the endoscope is passed through the second part of the duodenum and a plastic catheter is introduced into the ampulla of vater. Radiographic dye is injected through the catheter to the bile duct and pancreatic ducts and the photographs are taken. The stenotic portion of the bile or pancreatic duct is brushed with the help of a brush introduced through the endoscope.

ESOPHAGUS

Normal Histology and Cytology (Fig. 13.1)

Figure 13.1 shows a schematic diagram of anatomy of GIT. The esophagus is a muscular tube of 25 cm long. It has four layers: (1) mucosal, (2) submucosal, (3) muscular and (4) adventitial. Almost the entire esophagus is lined with non-keratinizing stratified squamous epithelium. The distal 1–2 cm part of the esophagus is lined by simple columnar epithelium.

Immediately under the mucosal lining is the lamina propria which contains loose connective tissue and multiple esophageal cardiac glands. The submucosal of the esophagus contains dense fibroconnective tissue and esophageal glands.

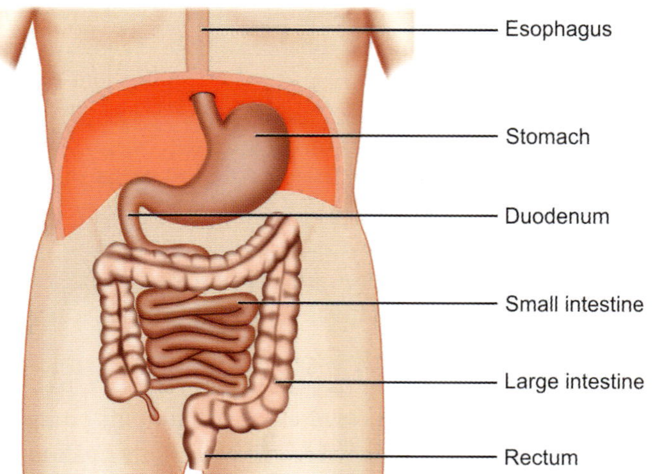

Fig. 13.1: Schematic diagram of gastrointestinal tract.

Box 13.4: Candidal esophagitis.

- Candidal pseudohyphae and budding yeast
- Squamous cells with mild atypia
- Acute inflammatory cells.

Cytology

Cytological specimen of the esophagus contains squamous epithelial cells. The cells are large, polygonal with abundant eosinophilic cytoplasm and centrally placed nuclei. Nuclear chromatin is fine with inconspicuous nucleoli.

Benign Diseases of Esophagus (Box 13.3)

Box 13.3: Diseases of esophagus.

- Infection
  - Fungal: Candida
  - Viral: Herpes, cytomegalovirus
- Esophagitis
- Radiation and chemotherapy induced changes
- Barrett's esophagitis
- Neoplasm
  - Benign: Leiomyoma
  - Malignant
    - Squamous cell carcinoma
    - Adenocarcinoma
    - Small cell carcinoma.

Infection

Brush cytology is commonly used for detection of various infections of the esophagus. Candida, herpes virus and cytomegalovirus are common infections in the esophagus that are diagnosed by brush cytology. These infections are commonly seen in immunocompromised patients.

Candida (Box 13.4)

Candidal esophagitis is the most common fungal infection of the esophagus. It usually occurs in the immunocompromised patient. Whitish pseudomembrane is seen in esophageal mucosa under endoscopic examination (Fig. 13.2A). Cytological diagnosis is relatively straightforward (Box 13.4). Smear shows many candidal pseudohyphae and yeast form along with squamous cells and polymorphs. Delicate thin elongated and constricted pseudohyphae can be readily evident in the Papanicolaou (PAP) stained smear. Small round spore is also noted by careful examination (Fig. 13.2B). The squamous cells may show reactive nuclear atypia. Candidal contamination from oral area is usually not a problem as the endoscopic brush is covered by a sheath.

Herpes simplex viral esophagitis: Herpes simplex virus infection is the most common cause of viral esophagitis. It usually occurs in immunocompromised patient, diabetic patient, carcinoma cases and patients who receive radiation and chemotherapy. Endoscopic examination classically shows multiple small reddish shallow ulcers with sharp margin in the distal part of the esophagus (Fig. 13.3A). Cytological features of herpetic esophagitis are similar as seen in other parts of the body (Box 13.5).

The cytology smear shows many multinucleated giant cells. Nuclei are closely spaced and often show characteristic nuclear molding (Fig. 13.3B). Individual cells show large intranuclear inclusions with a clear halo at the periphery and thick nuclear membrane. In many cells nuclear chromatin looks like refractile ground-glass. In addition, the squamous cells often show nuclear atypia. The atypical squamous cells may be mistaken as malignant cell. However, the nucleus-cytoplasm (N/C) ratio of the cell is not increased and nuclear margin is regular (Table 13.1).

Cytomegalovirus infection: Cytomegalovirus (CMV) infection in the esophagus is uncommon and it usually occurs in immunocompromised patient (Box 13.6). The endoscopic and clinical features are nonspecific. CMV mainly infects the endothelial cells and fibroblasts and glandular elements. Squamous cells in the mucosa are not involved by CMV. Therefore, endoscopic biopsy rather than brush is the choice of diagnostic modality.

Cytology smears of the esophageal brush rarely show the characteristic CMV infected cell. The infected cell shows

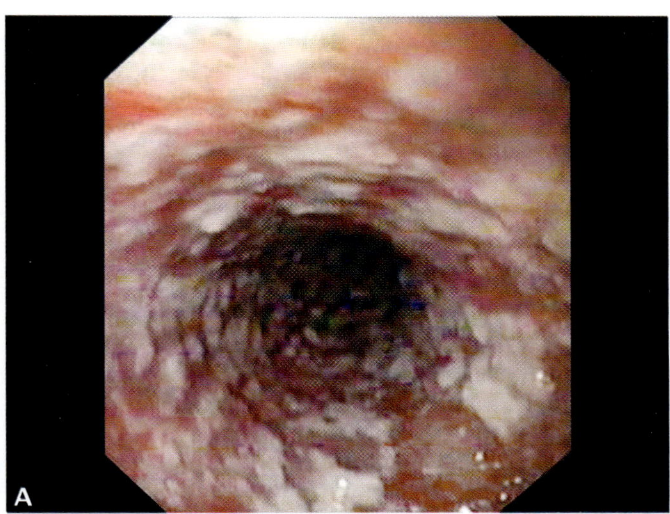

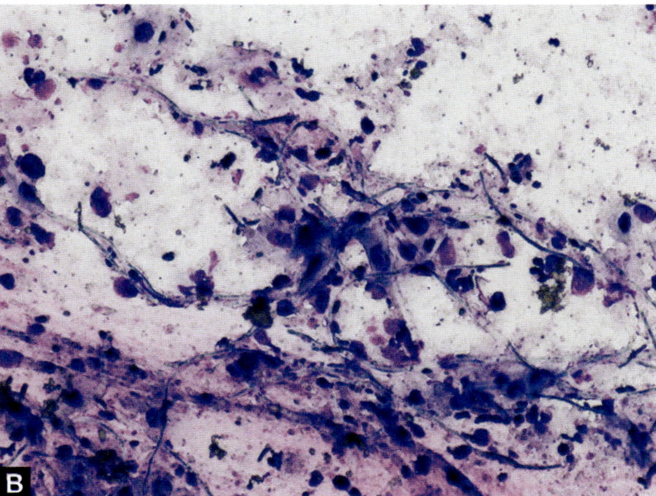

Figs. 13.2A and B: (A) Endoscopic examination shows whitish patches in candida infection of esophagus. (B) Candidal spores and pseudohyphae in a case of candidal esophagitis (May-Grünwald Giemsa stain X HP).
Courtesy: (A) Dr S Sinha, Professor of Gastroenterology, PGIMER, Chandigarh, India.

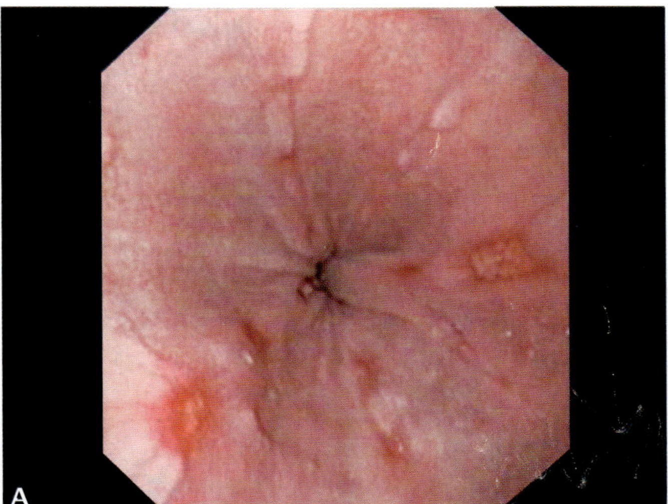

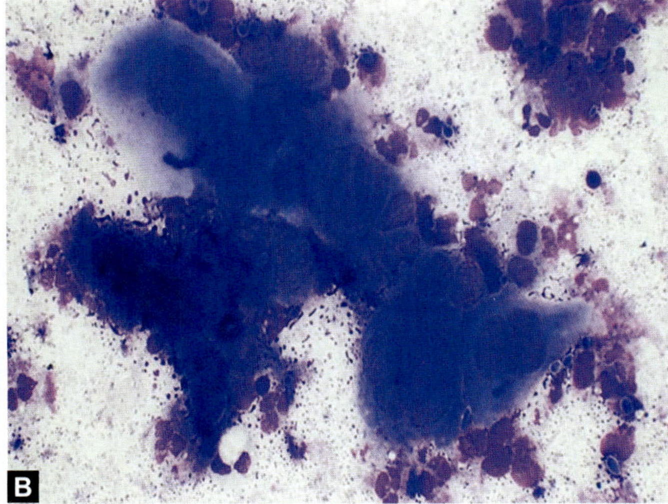

Figs. 13.3A and B: Endoscopic examination shows multiple small reddish shallow ulcers with sharp margin in herpetic esophagitis. (B) Multinucleated cells with nuclear molding in a case of herpetic esophagitis (May-Grünwald Giemsa stain X HP).
Courtesy: (A) Dr S Sinha, Professor of Gastroenterology, PGIMER, Chandigarh, India.

Box 13.5: Herpetic esophagitis.

- *Risk factors:* Immunocompromised patient, cancer, radiation and chemotherapy
- *Endoscopic features:* Multiple small reddish shallow ulcers with sharp margin
- *Cytology:*
  - Multinucleated giant cells
  - Molded nuclei
  - Large intranuclear inclusions
  - Clear halo around the inclusion with thick margin
  - Homogenized ground-glass chromatin
  - Reactive atypia in squamous cells.

Table 13.1: Differentiating features between HSV and squamous cell carcinoma.

Features	*HSV*	*Squamous cell carcinoma*
Multinucleation	Present	Occasionally present
N/C ratio	Increased	Moderately increased
Chromatin	Smudgy	Hyperchromatic, coarse granular
Intranuclear inclusion	Present	Absent

(HSV: Herpes simplex virus; N/C ratio: Nucleus-cytoplasm ratio).

Box 13.6: Cytomegalovirus esophagitis.

- *Endoscopic feature:* Nonspecific
- Infects the endothelial cells and fibroblasts and glandular elements
- The choice of diagnostic modality: endoscopic biopsy
- Immunocompromised patient is affected
- *Cytology*
  - Enlarged cell
  - Both cell and nuclei are enlarged
  - Large amphophilic intranuclear inclusion
  - Peripheral clear halo and margination of chromatin
  - Small satellite basophilic cytoplasmic inclusions.

Box 13.8: Distinguishing features between repair and malignancy.

Favorable points for malignancy:
- Many discrete cells
- Overcrowded cells and loss of polarity
- Enlarged nuclei
- High N/C ratio
- Irregular and thickened nuclear margin
- Irregular shaped multiple nucleoli
- Hyperchromatic coarse nuclei
- Abnormal mitotic figures
- Tumor diathesis

cytomegaly with preserved N/C ratio. Nuclei show large intranuclear inclusion with a peripheral clear halo and margination of chromatin on the inner nuclear membrane. Small satellite basophilic cytoplasmic inclusions are also noted.

Esophagitis: Esophagitis may be noted in various conditions such as reflux esophagitis, corrosive ingestion, alcohol, drugs, etc. (Box 13.7). Endoscopy shows erosion and ulceration.

Cytology smear from the brush sample shows cohesive clusters of cells with flowing or streaming pattern of cells giving "school of fish" appearance. The individual squamous cells show nuclear enlargement and prominent nucleoli. However, N/C ratio is well preserved and nuclear margin is regular. Nuclear chromatin is fine. In addition background of the smear shows inflammatory cells, increased mitosis and atypical stromal cells.

Differential diagnosis: The atypical squamous cells may be mistaken as malignant cells. The distinguishing cytological features are preserved N/C ratio, regular nuclear margin and fine nuclear chromatin (Box 13.8).

Radiation and Chemotherapy-induced Changes

Both radiation and chemotherapeutic drugs show similar changes (Box 13.9). Endoscopy shows reddish, friable and hemorrhagic areas.

Box 13.7: Esophagitis/Repair changes.

- *Causes:* Reflux esophagitis, corrosive ingestion, alcohol, drug ingestion
- *Endoscopy:* Hyperemia, erosion, ulceration
- *Cytology*
  - Reactive squamous cells with "school of fish" appearance, i.e. streaming pattern of cells.
  - Enlarged nuclei
  - Preserved N/C ratio
  - Regular nuclear margin
  - Evenly distributed chromatin
  - Prominent nucleoli
  - Mitosis
  - Inflammatory cells and atypical stromal cells

Differential diagnosis: Carcinoma.

(N/C ratio: Nucleus-cytoplasm ratio).

Box 13.9: Radiation and chemotherapy effects.

- *Endoscopy:* Reddish, friable and hemorrhagic areas
- *Cytology*
  - Enlarged cells
  - Frayed cytoplasmic border
  - Vacuolated cytoplasm
  - Nuclear enlargement
  - Preserved N/C ratio
  - Smudged chromatin
  - Multinucleation.

The cytology smear of brushing sample shows discrete atypical cells with enlarged nuclei. The N/C ratio of the cell is well preserved. Individual cells have frayed cytoplasmic border with intracytoplasmic vacuoles. Nuclei show smudgy chromatin with irregular outline. Occasional multinucleated cells are also seen.

Barrett's Esophagus

Barrett's esophagus (BE) is an acquired condition where the lower part of the squamous epithelial lining is replaced by columnar epithelial cells with intestinal metaplasia containing goblet cells (Box 13.10). It is thought as a protective mechanism to save the lower distal part of the esophagus from the recurrent gastric reflux. It is considered as a preneoplastic condition and the majority of the esophageal adenocarcinoma develops from the Barrett's esophagitis.

Clinical symptoms of the patients are heartburn and dysphagia. Endoscopic examination shows characteristic salmon-pink color with an admixture of intestine-like epithelium.

Cytology smear of BE show cohesive sheets of epithelial cells with monomorphic nuclei. The outline of the clusters is regular. The nuclear polarity of the cell is well maintained. Identification of goblet cell is essential for the diagnosis of BE. The cells have abundant vacuolated cytoplasm. The size of the vacuole is three times more than the nucleus. Cytological diagnosis of BE has low sensitivity and specificity. This may be due to sampling error.[6]

Dysplasia in Barrett's esophagus (Box 13.11): Almost all esophageal adenocarcinoma develop from Barrett's esophagus.[7] A series of dysplastic changes in the mucosal epithelium occurs before the development of adenocarcinoma. Therefore, the diagnosis of the degree of dysplasia is important in a setting of BE.

Cytology features of dysplasia in BE depend on the degree of dysplastic changes. The smears of high-grade dysplasia show loose cohesive groups of cells with irregular border. There is significant nuclear crowding, overlapping and loss of polarity. The individual cells are columnar in appearance with enlarged hyperchromatic nuclei. The nuclear margin is irregular and thickened. Nucleoli are large. The atypical cells are sparse in number compared to adenocarcinoma (Figs. 13.4A and B). The background of the smear is clean and no tumor diathesis is seen.

Box 13.10: Barrett's esophagus.

Definition: Lower part of the squamous epithelial lining is replaced by columnar epithelial cells with intestinal metaplasia.
- Premalignant condition
- *Clinical features:* Heart burn and dysphagia
- *Endoscopy:* Characteristic salmon-pink color with admixture of intestine-like epithelium.
- *Cytology*
  - Cohesive sheets of epithelial cells
  - Regular border of the cluster
  - No nuclear overlapping
  - "Goblet cells"
    - Cells with large cytoplasmic vacuoles three times the size of nucleus.

Squamous Cell Carcinoma

Squamous cell carcinoma (SQC) is the most common malignancies of the esophagus and includes more than 85% of esophageal malignancies. The patients are usually in 6th decade. The usual clinical symptoms are dysphagia and loss of weight. The common risk factors of SQC of the esophagus are cigarette smoking, alcohol abuse and vitamins A, C, E and riboflavin deficiency.

The cytological features (Box 13.12) of SQC are similar to that of other organs. Smears show small clusters and discrete cells. In case of keratinizing SQC the individual cells are polyhedral with well-defined cytoplasmic border (Fig. 13.5). The cytoplasm shows orangeophilic appearance. Nuclei are hyperchromatic, moderately pleomorphic nuclei with inconspicuous nucleoli. Occasional

Box 13.11: Dysplasia in Barrett's esophagus.

- Small clusters of cells with irregular outline
- Nuclear overlapping and loss of polarity
- Columnar cells
- Nuclear enlargement, pleomorphism, thickened nuclear membrane
- Hyperchromasia with prominent nucleoli
- Clean background.

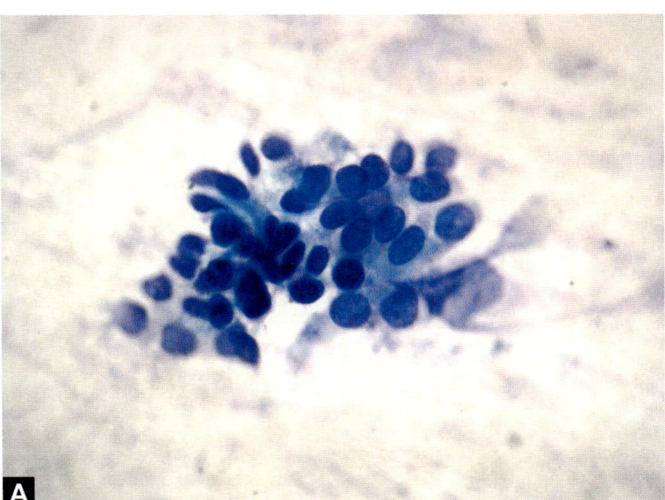

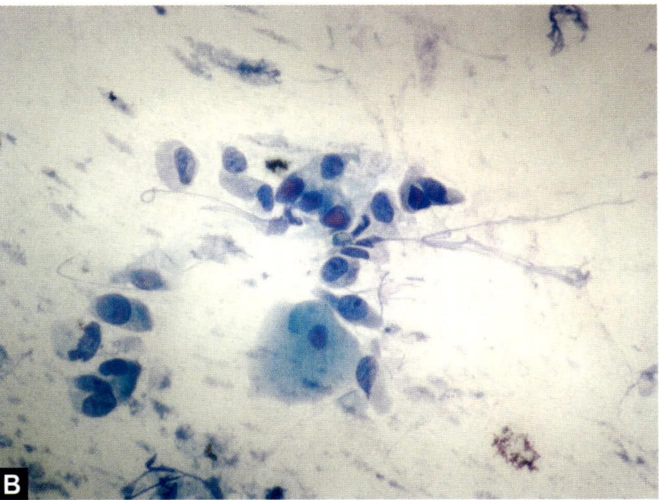

Figs. 13.4A and B: Dysplasia in esophagus: Smear shows cohesive cluster of cells with mild nuclear atypia (Papanicolaou's stain X MP). (B) Dysplasia in esophagus: Smear shows dissociated cells moderate amount of cytoplasm and mild nuclear atypia (Papanicolaou's stain X MP).

Box 13.12: Squamous cell carcinoma.

- Discrete and loose cluster of cells
- Polyhedral shaped
- Orangeophilic cytoplasm
- Hyperchromatic nuclei
- Moderate nuclear pleomorphism
- Inconspicuous nucleoli
- Irregular clumped chromatin
- Keratin pearls
- Background necrosis.

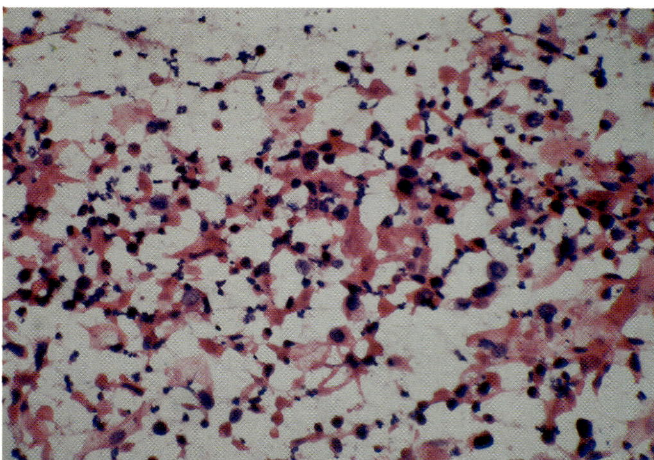

Fig. 13.5: Many discrete oval to polyhedral malignant cells with centrally placed nuclei having moderate nuclear pleomorphism in squamous cell carcinoma (Papanicolaou's stain X MP).

keratin pearls are also noted. In nonkeratinizing SQC smear shows round to oval cells with relatively scanty cytoplasm. Nucleus shows moderate pleomorphism, hyperchromasia and clumped irregular chromatin. Poorly differentiated carcinoma may show prominent nucleoli.

Adenocarcinoma (Box 13.13)

Adenocarcinoma of the esophagus arises from the lower part of the esophagus. EUS-guided FNAC is a preferable sampling modality than brush cytology for the detection of adenocarcinoma of the esophagus. Smears show the glandular arrangement of cells, loose clusters and discrete cells. Individual cells show a moderate amount of vacuolated cytoplasm. Nuclei are moderately pleomorphic with prominent nucleoli (Figs. 13.6A and B).

Small Cell Carcinoma (Box 13.14)

Small cell carcinoma (SCC) is an uncommon tumor of the esophagus. SCC accounts for less than 5% of esophageal carcinoma. It is a highly aggressive tumor.

Box 13.13: Adenocarcinoma of esophagus.

- Occurs in lower part of esophagus
- Rich cellularity
- *Background:* Tumor diathesis
- *Arrangement*
  - Multiple gland like arrangement of cells, clusters of cells
  - Overlapping or crowded arrangement of cells
  - Peripheral feathering of cell
- *Nuclei*
  - Enlarged
  - Pleomorphic
  - Irregular margin
  - Prominent nucleoli
- *Cytoplasm:* Moderately vacuolated.

Smears show predominantly discrete cells with scanty cytoplasm. Nuclei are small hyperchromatic. Chromatin is finely granular and gives a salt and pepper appearance. Nuclear molding is also noted.

STOMACH

Anatomy and Histology

The stomach has four regions: (1) cardiac, (2) fundus, (3) body and (4) pyloric region.

Cardiac: It is the narrow region at the gastroesophageal junction and frequently filled with gas.

Fundus: This is the small dome-shaped part situated left of the esophagus.

Body: This is the main part of the stomach.

Pylorus: This is the narrow-constricted part in between the body and duodenum.

The whole stomach has multiple longitudinal folds of mucosa and submucosal known as "rugae". Rugae permit distension of the stomach when food is ingested and in distended stomach the rugae disappear. The epithelial lining of the stomach invaginates within the mucosa forming gastric pits. Gastric glands open in the gastric pits.

Histology

The gastric mucosa is lined by simple columnar epithelium. The surface and neck of the glands are lined by mucous secreting columnar cells. The mucosal glands produce thick mucin that protects the stomach from the irritant substances and acid digestion. In addition, the glands in the fundus and body of the stomach also contain parietal and chief cells. The parietal cells manufacture hydrochloric acid and intrinsic factors. The parietal cells are round in shape with eosinophilic cytoplasm and basally placed

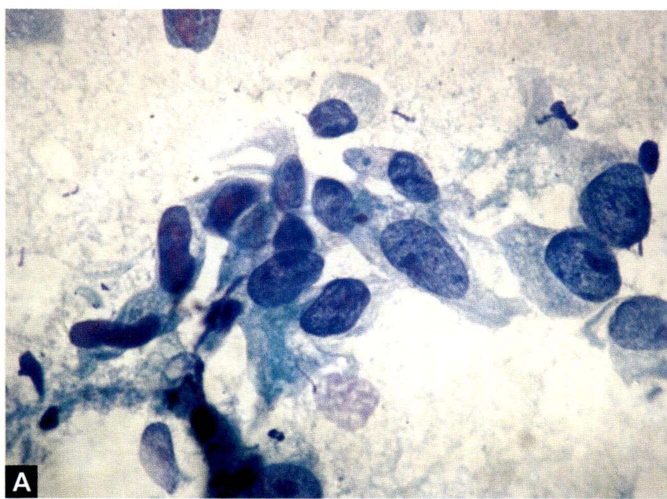
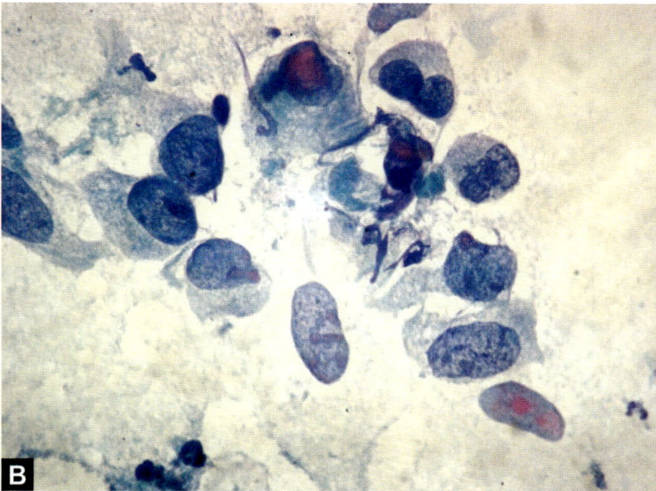

Figs. 13.6A and B: Moderately pleomorphic nuclei with prominent nucleoli in a case of adenocarcinoma in esophageal brush cytology (Papanicolaou's stain X HP). (B) Malignant cells with moderate amount of cytoplasm and moderately pleomorphic nuclei with prominent nucleoli in a case of adenocarcinoma in esophageal brush cytology (Papanicolaou's stain X HP).

Box 13.14: Small cell carcinoma.

- Discrete cells
- Small cells slightly larger than lymphocytes
- Scanty cytoplasm
- Nuclear molding present
- Hyperchromatic nuclei
- Salt and pepper chromatin
- Absent nucleoli

nuclei. The chief cells produce various enzymes such as pepsinogen, renin, and gastric lipase. These are columnar looking cells with basophilic cytoplasm and basally placed nuclei. In addition of these cells, scattered endocrine cells are also present.

Cytology

Mucous secreting cells: The mucous cells are usually present in small clusters and in flat sheets. The cells are usually in monolayer and polarity of the cells is well maintained. Dispersed single cells are infrequent in brush cytology. The individual cells are tall, columnar in appearance with abundant vacuolated cytoplasm (Fig. 13.7). The nuclei are central in position, round, and monomorphic with fine nuclear chromatin and inconspicuous nucleoli. Occasionally nuclear protrusion may be noted.

Chief cells: These are cuboidal cells with numerous coarse basophilic cytoplasmic granules. Nuclei are central in position and round in shape.

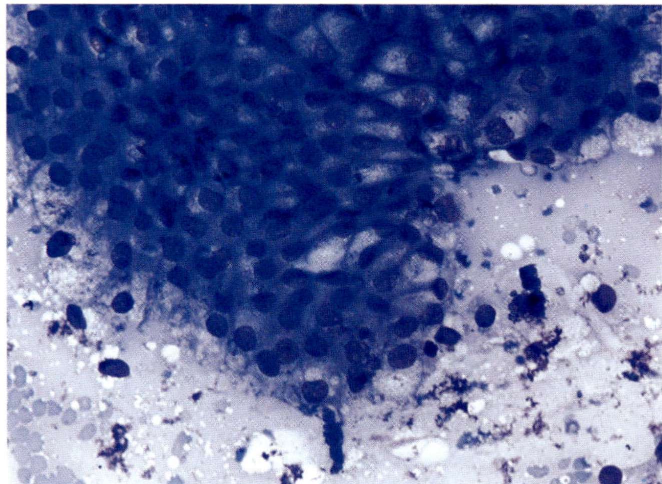

Fig. 13.7: Normal columnar epithelium of gastric mucosa (May-Grünwald Giemsa stain X HP).

Parietal cells: These are round cells with marked vacuolization of the cytoplasm. Cytoplasmic eosinophilic granules are seen. Nuclei are centrally placed having coarse chromatin.

Benign Diseases of Stomach

Acute Gastritis (Box 13.15)

Acute gastritis is caused by various factors such as aspirin ingestion, alcohol ingestion, heavy smoking, chemotherapy, burn, trauma, etc. Cytology is not done for diagnosis of acute gastritis. The cytology smear of acute gastritis

Box 13.15: Acute gastritis.

- *Etiological causes:* Aspirin ingestion, alcohol, heavy smoking, chemotherapy, burn or trauma, etc.
- *Cytology*
  - Polymorphs
  - Degenerated cells
  - Cohesive sheets of glandular cells
  - Reactive changes of the epithelial cells.

Box 13.17: Gastric adenocarcinoma.

Intestinal type
- Single cells, loose cohesive clusters of cells
- Columnar or cuboidal cells
- Marked nuclear pleomorphism
- Enlarged nuclei with high N/C ratio
- Hyperchromatic nuclei
- Irregular nuclear margin
- Prominent nucleoli

Diffuse or gastric type
- Predominantly single cells and occasional loose clusters
- Round cells with abundant vacuolated cytoplasm
- Crescent-shaped nucleus pushed to the periphery
- Hyperchromatic nucleus
- Prominent large nucleoli
- Pool of mucin.

shows cohesive sheets of glandular cells (Box 13.15). The cells may show reactive atypia. Nuclei of the cells may be enlarged; however, N/C ratio is well preserved. In addition the background of the smear shows abundant polymorphs.

Chronic Gastritis

Cytology smears of chronic gastritis show multiple cohesive sheets of glandular cells with reactive atypia. Nuclei may show a mild increase of the N/C ratio with relatively enlarged nuclei, nuclear pleomorphism and hyperchromasia. Nucleoli may be prominent. In case of gastric ulcer, there may be necrotic debris and inflammatory cells. Marked nuclear atypia of the gastric epithelial cells may mimic malignancy. At times it is very difficult to distinguish reactive atypia and carcinoma. The absence of significant nuclear pleomorphism and regular nuclear margin are in favor of reactive atypia.

Helicobacter Pylori

Helicobacter pylori is usually associated with chronic gastritis and peptic ulcer disease (Box 13.16). It can be easily detected by gastric crush smear, brush cytology or imprint smear. Brush cytology is preferable to demonstrate this organism as it covers the wide surface area of the mucosal membrane. The organisms are best demonstrated in the May-Grünwald Giemsa (MGG) staining. The organisms are mainly seen in the thin mucus as 2–3 μ long, curved, or spiral-shaped structure. In addition, the cytology smears also show sheets of epithelial cells with mild reactive atypia.

Box 13.16: Helicobacter pylori.

- Associated with chronic gastritis and peptic ulcer disease
- May-Grünwald Giemsa staining is the best
- 2–3 μ long, curved, or spiral-shaped structure
- Risk factor for gastric carcinoma and NHL of stomach.

Benign Tumors

Gastric polyp

Most of the gastric polyps are hyperplastic polyp with no risk factor for development of carcinoma. These polyps are small and may be single or multiple. Cytology smears show multiple clusters of epithelial cells with mild reactive atypia.

Gastric Adenocarcinoma

Adenocarcinoma is the most common malignant tumor of the stomach. A steady decline in the incidence of gastric carcinoma has been noted worldwide in the last few decades. Several strong associations of gastric carcinoma are known such as *Helicobacter pylori* infection, smoking, intake of large amount of smoked fish, pickled vegetables, and low socioeconomic setting. Early gastric carcinoma may not produce any symptoms and some of the patients may have only dyspeptic symptoms. Absence of any symptoms is responsible for detection of gastric carcinoma in advanced stage. In advanced stages it may cause pain, vomiting, hematemesis and melena. Patients may also have severe anemia.

There are two types of gastric adenocarcinoma, intestinal and diffuse (gastric) type.

Cytology (Box 13.17)

Intestinal carcinoma: The cytology smear shows loose clusters and discrete cells. The cells are in three-dimensional clusters. Individual cells show marked nuclear enlargement and high N/C ratio. Nuclei are moderately pleomorphic and hyperchromatic with irregular nuclear margin (Fig. 13.8). Prominent nucleoli and frequent mitosis are also noted.

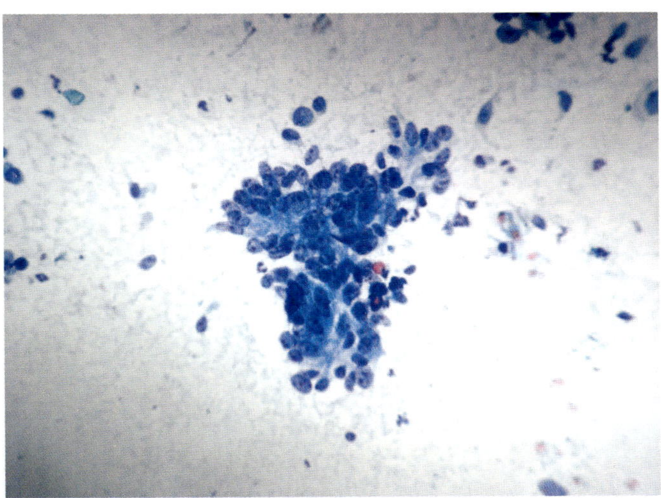

Fig. 13.8: Cluster of malignant cells with moderate nuclear enlargement and pleomorphism in a case of intestinal type adenocarcinoma of stomach (Papanicolaou's stain X MP).

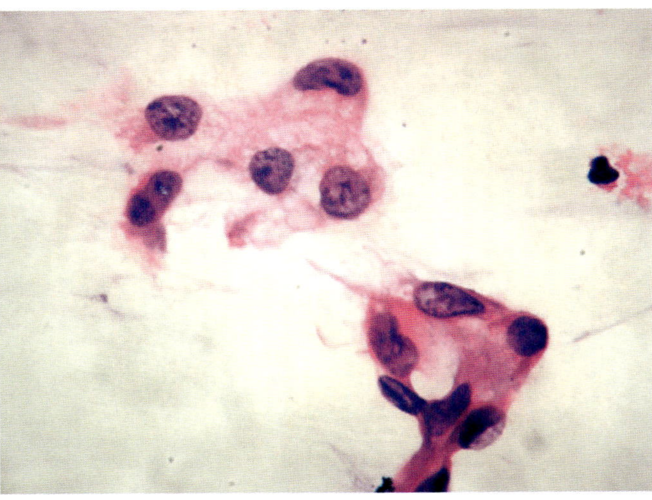

Fig. 13.9: Signet ring type adenocarcinoma of stomach showing malignant cells with abundant vacuolated cytoplasm and nuclei are pushed to the periphery (Hematoxylin and Eosin stain X HP).

Diffuse or gastric type: The diffuse type of gastric cancer is mainly made of the signet ring type of cells. The cells are mainly discrete with occasional loose small clusters. Individual cells are round to oval with the abundant vacuolated cytoplasm. Nuclei are eccentric in position and crescent in shape. Nuclear margin is irregular. Nucleoli are usually prominent (Fig. 13.9).

Differential diagnosis: Signet ring cells are often difficult to distinguish from macrophages. The signet ring cells are positive for pancytokeratin and epithelial membrane antigen (EMA) and negative for CD61.

Gastrointestinal Stromal Tumor

Gastrointestinal stromal tumor (GIST) comprises less than 1% tumors of the GIT. It commonly affects the older individual. GIST is most commonly seen in the stomach (60%) followed by the small intestine (30%) and rectum. The origin of the tumor is interstitial cell of Cajal or primitive stem cells. This cell is also known as "gastrointestinal pace maker cell".

Diagnosis of Gastrointestinal Stromal Tumor

The lesion is usually noted in endoscopy as submucosal mass protruding toward lumen. Endoscopy-guided FNAC is the best approach to get sample from the lesion. Cytomorphology along with immunocytochemistry and molecular markers (optional) are needed for the diagnosis of GIST. The tumor is positive for CD117 (c-KIT), CD34, and DOG1. It also shows mutation of KIT (80%) and platelet-derived growth factor receptor (PDGFRA) (10%).[8]

Steps of Diagnosis

- *Step 1*: Cytomorphology along with CD117 positivity by immunocytochemistry are sufficient to diagnose GIST. Approximately 95% cases of GIST are positive for CD117 (c-KIT). The other spindle cell tumors in GIT are not positive for c-KIT. The other c-KIT positive tumors in the body are seminoma, mesothelioma, melanoma, fibromatosis, chromophobe renal cell carcinoma and various sarcomas such as angiosarcoma, Ewing sarcoma, synovial sarcoma, and malignant fibrous histiocytoma.
- *Step 2*: CD34 or DOG1 immunostaining in CD117 negative cases confirm the diagnosis of GIST. CD34 is positive in 70–80% cases of GIST. DOG1, a newly developed marker, is positive in 95% cases of GIST.
- *Step 3*: In case of negative markers KIT/PDGFRA mutational analysis can confirm GIST.

  KIT mutation and GIST: CD117 (KIT) is a type III transmembrane receptor tyrosine kinase. The receptor KIT binds with its ligand on the cell surface and then activates a series of downstream pathway that ultimately causes cell survival and cell proliferation. Mutational change in KIT causes continuous activation of kinase pathway without binding the receptor with corresponding ligand. Near about 10% of GIST may not show any mutational change in KIT. These tumors usually show PDGFRA mutation.

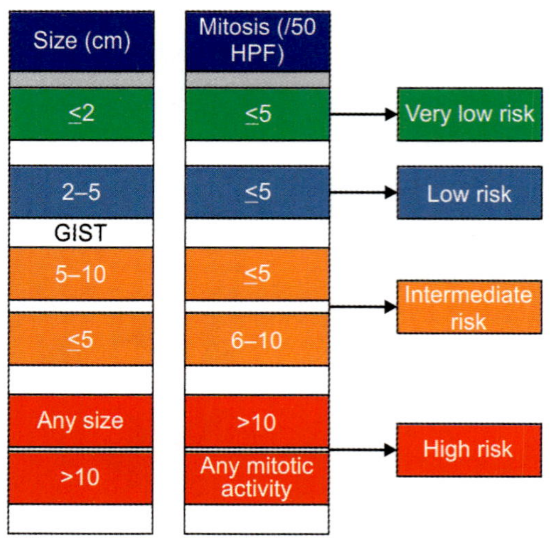

Fig. 13.10: Schematic diagram of the behavior of gastrointestinal stromal tumor (GIST).

Box 13.18: Gastrointestinal stromal tumor.

Cytology

- Clusters, fascicles and also dissociated cells
- Spindle cells with scanty to moderate cytoplasm
- Spindle-shaped nuclei with mild pleomorphism
- Coarse granular chromatin, indistinct nucleoli.

Immunocytochemistry: Positive for CD117 (c-KIT) and CD34.

Histological grade:

- High-grade tumor: Tumor with more than 10 mitosis per 10 high power field.
- Low-grade tumor: Tumor with 1–5 mitosis per 10 high power field.

Cytogenetics:

Malignant GIST usually shows:

- Losses in chromosomes 14 and 22.
- Gains and amplification of 3q, 8q, 5p and Xp region.
- Mutations of the c-KIT gene.

(GIST: Gastrointestinal stromal tumor).

Behavior

The behavior of the tumor depends on its size and mitotic activity (counted in 50 high power field). Figure 13.10 highlights the classification of GIST in relation to size and mitosis.

The patient presents with hematemesis and pain abdomen. Brush cytology of the stomach is not helpful for diagnosis of this tumor unless the tumor ulcerates the mucosa. Endoscopic ultrasound-guided FNA (EUS-FNA) is the best way to diagnose the submucosal GIST of the stomach. Percutaneous FNAC may also be helpful in relatively larger tumor under USG guidance.

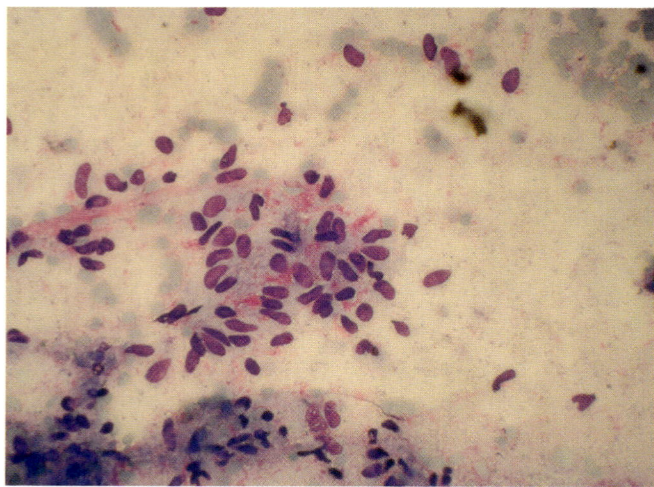

Fig. 13.11: Oval to elongated spindle cells with mild nuclear pleomorphism in gastrointestinal stromal tumor (May-Grünwald Giemsa stain X HP).

Cytology

Cytology smear shows loose cohesive clusters, small fascicles and dissociated spindle-shaped cells (Box 13.18). The individual cells show scanty to moderate cytoplasm and oval to elongated spindle-shaped nuclei (Fig. 13.11). Nuclei show mild-to-moderate pleomorphism, coarse granular chromatin and inconspicuous to absent nucleoli. CD117 (c-KIT) positivity is essential for diagnosis of GIST. In addition, the cells are also positive for CD34 (membranous pattern of positivity) and focally positive for smooth muscle actin.

Diagnostic Difficulties

Other spindle cell soft tissue tumor: Gastrointestinal stromal tumor always has a differential diagnosis of other spindle cell mesenchymal tumor such as leiomyoma, schwannoma and their malignant counterpart. At times it is difficult to differentiate GIST form these tumors on cytology alone. A panel of immunostaining may be helpful in this context (Table 13.2).

Carcinoid Tumors (Neuroendocrine Tumor)

The term "neuroendocrine tumor" is presently replaced by carcinoid tumor. These are potentially malignant tumors and often associated with hormone production with recognizable clinical syndromes. The appendix is the most common site of origin of carcinoid in GIT followed by the rectum, small intestine and stomach.[9] In stomach,

Table 13.2: Immunostaining of different spindle cell tumor.

Lesion	*C-Kit (CD117)*	*CD34*	*Desmin*	*S-100*	*SMA*	*CK*
GIST	+	+ (60%)	–	+ (occasional)	+ (30 – 40%)	–
Smooth muscle tumor	–	+	+	–	+	–
Schwannoma	–	–	–	+	–	–
Spindle cell carcinoma						+

(GIST: Gastrointestinal stromal tumor; SMA: Smooth muscle actin; CK: Cytokeratin).

Box 13.19: Carcinoid tumors.

- All carcinoid tumors are low-grade malignant tumor
- *Frequencies:* Appendix, rectum, small intestine (ileum, jejunum, duodenum), stomach
- Gastric carcinoid rare (less than 1%)
- *Clinical symptoms:* Classical symptoms rare
- *Stomach:* Hematemesis, pain
- *Carcinoid symptoms in intestine:* Diarrhea, flushing, bronchospasm

Cytology
- Singly and in loose aggregates
- Monomorphic round cells with scanty to moderate reddish granular cytoplasm
- Eccentric round nuclei, minimal pleomorphism
- Salt and pepper chromatin
- Small inconspicuous nucleoli.

Immunocytochemistry: Positive for chromogranin, synaptophysin.

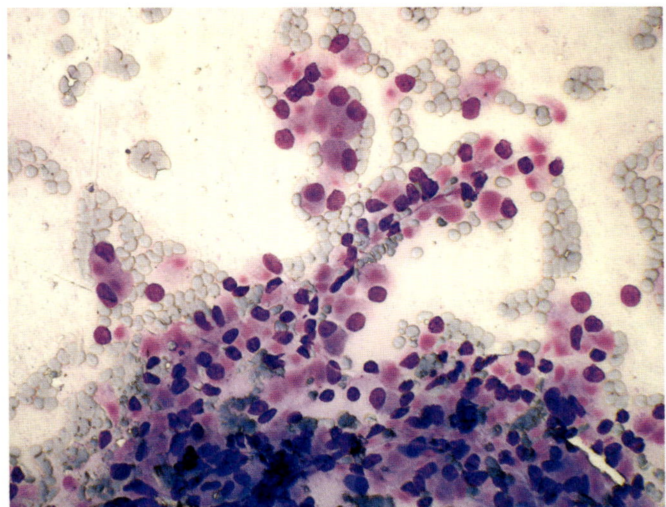

Fig. 13.12: Discrete tumor cells with monomorphic nuclei and moderate amount of pinkish granular cytoplasm in carcinoid of the stomach (May-Grünwald Giemsa stain X HP).

it is most frequently associated with atrophic gastritis. In nonatrophic gastritis it may occur from Zollinger-Ellison syndrome. Gastric carcinoid is infrequent and account for less than 1% of all gastric malignancies.[10]

Cytology (Box 13.19)

The cytology smear shows predominantly discrete, loose cohesive clusters, trabecular and rosette like arrangement of cells. The individual cells are monomorphic round cells with scanty to moderate reddish granular cytoplasm (Fig. 13.12). Many spindle-shaped cells may be seen. The nuclei are round monomorphic, with salt-and-pepper chromatin and inconspicuous nucleoli.

Diagnostic Difficulties

- *Adenocarcinoma*: Carcinoid tumor with acinar like arrangement of cells may simulate adenocarcinoma. The individual cell morphology of carcinoid such as reddish granular cytoplasm and monomorphic nuclei with salt and pepper chromatin are helpful in differentiating from adenocarcinoma. Immunocytochemistry may be helpful in certain situations. Carcinoid cells are positive for chromogranin and synaptophysin.
- *Small cell carcinoma*: Predominant discrete small cells in carcinoid tumor may often pose diagnostic difficulty with SCC. Nuclear threading, nuclear molding and condensed hyperchromatic nuclei favor a diagnosis of SCC.

Non-Hodgkin Lymphoma

Primary gastric lymphoma arises from the stomach and contiguous group of lymph nodes. It is considered as primary lymphoma of the stomach if the main tumor bulk is located in the stomach only. The majority of the gastric lymphomas are high-grade B cell lymphoma and some of these lymphomas have evolved from a mucosa associated lymphoma (MALT, B cell type). GIT is the most common extranodal site of the NHL. Lymphoma accounts about 10% of all gastric malignancies. There is a high association of *Helicobacter pylori* and low-grade MALT.[11]

Cytology smears show discrete cells with round nuclei. The nuclei are relatively monomorphic with scanty cytoplasm. Nuclear chromatin is condensed with inconspicuous nucleoli. Background shows lymphoglandular bodies (Fig. 13.13).

Brush cytology is helpful in the diagnosis of diffuse large B cell lymphoma. The cells are discrete with a relatively larger nucleus showing mild-to-moderate pleomorphism. Nuclei show coarse clumped chromatin, irregular nuclear membrane and prominent nucleoli.

Differential Diagnosis

- *Small cell carcinoma*: Small cell carcinoma often comes in the differential diagnosis of low-grade MALT (Table 13.3). Nuclear threading and molding are two important differentiating cytological features of SCC. In addition, the background lymphoglandular bodies are absent in SCC.
- *Poorly differentiated carcinoma*: Poorly differentiated carcinoma often poses diagnostic difficulty with diffuse large cell NHL. The cytology smears show loose clusters of cells, moderate cytoplasm, nuclear pleomorphism and absence of lymphoglandular bodies.
- *Carcinoid*: Cytology smears of carcinoid show cells with moderate reddish granular cytoplasm and absence of lymphoglandular bodies.
- *Lymphoid hyperplasia*: Benign lymphoid hyperplasia may pose diagnostic difficulty. The cytology smears of lymphoid hyperplasia show polymorphic population of cells with many tangible body macrophages. The lymphoid cells have regular nuclear contour.

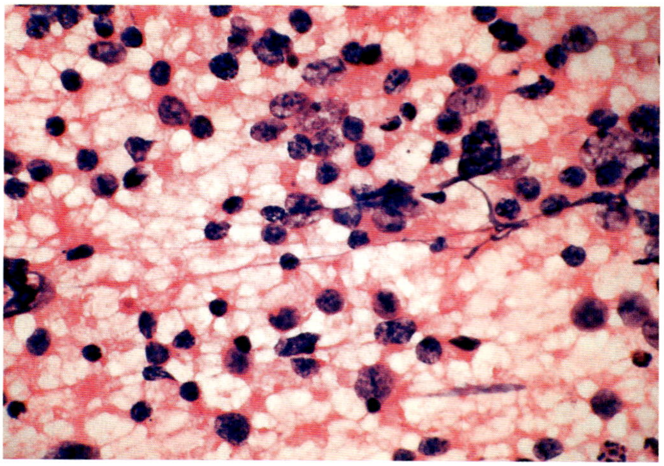

Fig. 13.13: Discrete immature lymphoid cells with fine nuclear chromatin in a case of non-Hodgkin lymphoma of stomach (Papanicolaou's stain X HP).

SMALL AND LARGE INTESTINE

Anatomy, Histology and Cytology

The small intestine is 7 m long tube. The surface area of the intestine is formed by transverse folds, multiple villi, microvilli, and crypts of Lieberkühn. The intestinal mucosa is composed of simple columnar epithelium, the lamina propria, and the muscularis mucosa. The surface mucosal lining of the intestine is made of surface absorptive cells, goblet cells, and diffuse neuroendocrine system (DNES) cells.

Surface Absorptive Cells

These are tall columnar cells with a basally placed round to oval nuclei. The cells have a low N/C ratio. The apical surface of the cell is covered by brush border.

Table 13.3: Differential diagnosis of MALToma.

Features	*Lymphoma*	*Small cell carcinoma*	*Carcinoid*	*Poorly differentiated carcinoma*
Cell dissociation	Predominantly discrete cells	Discrete and small clusters	Discrete and small clusters	Small clusters
Lymphoglandular bodies	Present	Absent	Absent	Absent
Cytoplasm	Scanty	Scanty	Scanty to moderate	Moderate
Cytoplasmic granularity	Absent	Absent	Present	Absent
Nuclear molding	Absent	Present	Absent	Absent
Nuclear threading	Absent	Present	Absent	Absent
Nucleoli	Absent	Absent	Absent	Present
Immunocytochemistry				
LCA	Positive	Negative	Negative	Negative
CK	Negative	Negative	Positive	Positive
Chromogranin	Negative	Positive	Positive	Negative

(MALToma: Mucosa-associated lymphoid tissue lymphomas; LCA: Leukocyte common antigen; CK: Cytokeratin).

Goblet Cells

Goblet cells are intermingled with surface absorptive cells. They are mucus producing cells and contain large vacuoles in the cytoplasm. Duodenum has the smallest number of goblet cells. The number of goblet cells increases from duodenum to ileum.

Neuroendocrine Cells

The mucosal surface of the small intestine also shows variable number of neuroendocrine cells that secrete various endocrine substances.

Cytology

Cytology smear shows flat monolayer sheets of cells. The cells are often arranged as honeycomb manner. The individual cells are tall columnar in appearance with round nuclei having a low N/C ratio. Nuclei are monomorphic with fine chromatin and small nucleoli. The goblet cells have large vacuolated cytoplasm and round small nuclei.

Infections

Giardia Lambia

Giardia lambia is a common parasite in the duodenum. The organism is noted either by endoscopic biopsy or by FNAC. Giardia lambia is usually located over the crypts of the mucosal surface of the duodenum. This is a 12–15 μ diameter, pear-shaped binucleated organism with four pairs of flagella.

Cryptosporidium

Cryptosporidium is usually seen in immunocompromised patients. The majority of the patients presents with watery diarrhea and fever. The protozoa are present on the luminal surface or within the glandular cells and are best seen in MGG stained smear. They are 2–3 μ sized round basophilic organism.

Tuberculosis

Tuberculosis is commonly noted in the small intestine. Percutaneous FNAC is the usual sampling technique in mass lesion of the abdomen. Cytology smears show multiple epithelioid cell granulomas, giant cells and necrosis. Ziehl-Neelsen stain shows acid fast bacilli.[12]

Adenocarcinoma

Adenocarcinoma of duodenum occurs more frequently than other malignancies. Cytology smears of adenocarcinoma show clusters and discrete cells with occasional glandular arrangement. The individual cells are columnar in appearance with moderate amount of vacuolated cytoplasm. Nuclei are moderately pleomorphic with prominent nucleoli.

Lymphoma

Non-Hodgkin's lymphomas are more frequent in small intestine than carcinomas. The patient usually presents with pain abdomen and weakness. MALT is a type of low-grade NHL. However, there may be transformation of low-grade NHL to high-grade NHL. Most of these MALTomas are B cell type. The cells are small to medium sized with scanty cytoplasm. Nuclei are round with fine chromatin. Plasma cell differentiation is common in intestinal MALTomas. There may be a good number of transformed centroblats or immunoblasts in MALtomas (Fig. 13.14).

LARGE INTESTINE

Large intestine includes cecum, colon, rectum and anal canal. Colon has no villi. Rectal and colonic mucosa are lined by a single or double layer of columnar cell and abundant goblet cells.

Cytology smear shows multiple small clusters and single columnar cells. The cells are columnar in shape

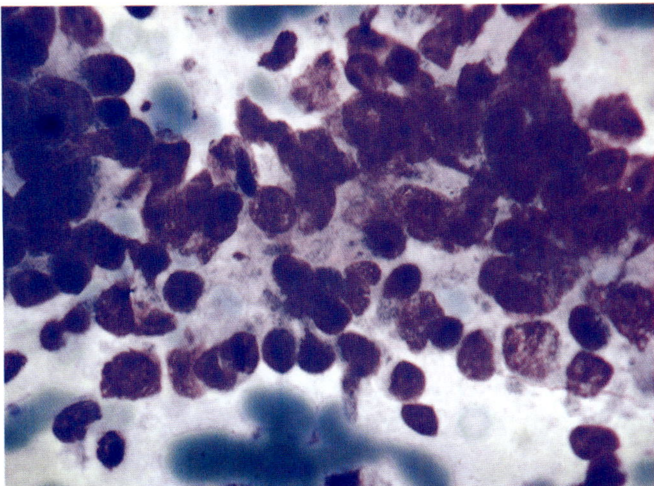

Fig. 13.14: USG-guided FNAC smear showing discrete immature lymphoid cells in a small intestinal lymphoma (May-Grünwald Giemsa stain X HP).

with distinct cell margin and round monomorphic nuclei. Many goblet cells are also seen.

Acute and Chronic Inflammation

Large intestine is affected by a wide variety of infections causing acute or chronic inflammation. Cytological sampling is rarely done for diagnosis of acute or chronic colitis. Colonoscopic examination can be performed easily along with colonic biopsy. Biopsy is more informative regarding dysplasia and presence of foci of infection.

Colorectal adenocarcinoma usually occurs in the 6th decade of life. The patient presents with sudden alteration of bowel habits, rectal bleeding and anemia. Brush cytology is helpful in diagnosis of adenocarcinoma. The cytomorphology of adenocarcinoma is similar to that of adenocarcinoma of duodenum. A cytology smear of well and moderately differentiated adenocarcinoma shows multiple clusters of columnar cells with gland like arrangement at places. The cells are columnar with moderately pleomorphic nuclei and prominent nucleoli.

ANAL CYTOLOGY

Cytology

Major portion of the anal canal is lined by stratified squamous epithelium except the proximal part of the anal canal adjacent to the rectum is lined by cuboidal to columnar epithelium.

Human papillomavirus infection of the anal canal and subsequent development of dysplastic lesions followed by SQC has promoted the screening of the anal canal region to detect dysplastic lesions. The incidence of SQC in the anal canal is about 35 per 100,000 population in homosexual man. This is a quite high incidence rate and is comparable to the incidence of cervical cancer in woman before the era of PAP screening. Both SQC of cervix of woman and anal canal in man has the same etiological link of infection of high risk HPV infection.[13] Screening of anal canal PAP test in high risk population for HPV related changes and dysplasia may have some effect in early diagnosis of dysplastic lesions.[14]

The anal PAP test is done by introducing a moistened swab blindly into the anal canal and then rotating firmly on the wall of the anal canal. Finally the smear is made by pressing the swab directly on the slide.

The cytologic reporting criteria of the anal PAP test are similar to that of Bethesda system classification of cervical cytology. However, the sensitivity of the anal PAP test is relatively lower than cervical cytology.

REFERENCES

1. Dowlatshahi K, Skinner DB, DeMeester TR, et al. Evaluation of brush cytology as an independent technique for detection of esophageal carcinoma. J Thorac Cardiovasc Surg. 1985;89:848-51.
2. Geramizadeh B, Shafiee A, Saberfirruzi M, et al. Brush cytology of gastric malignancies. Acta Cytol. 2002;46:693-6.
3. Wang HH, Sovie S, Zeroogian JM, et al. Value of cytology in detecting intestinal metaplasia and associated dysplasia at the gastroesophageal junction. Hum Pathol. 1997;28:465-71.
4. Kochhar R, Rajwanshi A, Malik AK, et al. Endoscopic fine needle aspiration biopsy of gastroesophageal malignancies. Gastrointest Endosc.1988;34:321-3.
5. Yang H, Berner A, Mei Q, et al. Cytologic screening for esophageal cancer in a high-risk population in Anyang County, China. Acta Cytol. 2002;46:445-52.
6. Wang HH, Sovie S, Zeroogian JM, et al. Value of cytology in detecting intestinal metaplasia and associated dysplasia at the gastroesophageal junction. Hum Pathol. 1997;28(4):465-71.
7. Haggitt RC. Barrett's esophagus, dysplasia, and adenocarcinoma. Hum Pathol. 1994;25(10):982-93.
8. Koo DH, Ryu MH, Kim KM, et al. Asian Consensus Guidelines for the Diagnosis and Management of Gastrointestinal Stromal Tumor. Cancer Res Treat. 2016;48(4):1155-66.
9. Modlin IM, Lye KD, Kidd M. A 5-decade analysis of 13,715 carcinoid tumors. Cancer. 2003;97(4):934-59.
10. Modlin IM, Sandor A. An analysis of 8305 cases of carcinoid tumors. Cancer. 1997;79(4):813-29.
11. Eidt S, Stolte M, Fischer R. Helicobacter pylori gastritis and primary gastric non-Hodgkin's lymphomas. J Clin Pathol. 1994;47:436-9.
12. Radhika S, Rajwanshi A, Kochhar R, et al. Abdominal tuberculosis: diagnosed by fine needle aspiration cytology. Acta Cytol. 1993;37:673-8.
13. Durante AJ, Williams AB, Da Costa M, et al. Incidence of anal cytological abnormalities in a cohort of human immunodeficiency virus-infected women. Cancer Epidemiol Biomarkers Prev. 2003;12:638-42.
14. Chiao EY, Giordano TP, Palefsky JM, et al. Screening HIV infected individuals for anal cancer precursor lesions: A systematic review. Clin Infect Dis. 2006;43(2):223-33.

Review Questions

1. **All are true about endoscopic brush cytology except:**
   a. Large surface area of the mucosa is covered
   b. Deeper part of a stenotic canal can be sampled
   c. Comparatively cost effective and less invasive
   d. Highly sensitive to detect Barrett's esophagus
2. **Which is true for *Helicobacter pylori*?**
   a. Easily detected by gastric crush smear
   b. The organisms are best demonstrated in May-Grünwald Giemsa staining
   c. Risk factor for gastric carcinoma and NHL of stomach
   d. All are true
3. **All are true for gastrointestinal stromal tumor except:**
   a. Most commonly seen in the intestine
   b. Approximately 95% cases of GIST are positive for CD117
   c. In case of negative markers KIT/PDGFRA mutational analysis can confirm GIST
   d. DOG1 marker is helpful in diagnosis of CD117 negative cases
4. **A 2-cm diameter gastrointestinal stromal tumor with 15 mitosis per 50 high power field will be:**
   a. Very low risk
   b. Low risk
   c. Intermediate risk
   d. High risk
5. **CD117 marker is positive in:**
   a. Gastrointestinal stromal tumor
   b. Seminoma
   c. Melanoma
   d. All of the above

Answers

1. d. Highly sensitive to detect Barrett's esophagus
2. d. All are true
3. a. Most commonly seen in the intestine
4. d. High risk
5. d. All of the above

CHAPTER

14 Cerebrospinal Fluid

INTRODUCTION

Cerebrospinal fluid (CSF) is normally found in the subarachnoid space. It helps in the nourishment and protection of the brain and spinal cord. CSF is formed in the ventricles by choroid plexus and bathes the brain and spinal cord. It circulates through the subarachnoid space of the spinal meninges. Unlike effusion fluid, CSF is normally produced in the ventricles and normal lining cells of the subarachnoid and pial meninges do not shed into CSF. Examination of CSF provides valuable information for diagnosis of various infective conditions, leukemic infiltration, metastatic tumor and some primary central nervous system (CNS) tumor. Indications of cytological examination of CSF are highlighted in Box 14.1.

ANATOMY

Choroid plexus is the complex folded membrane of the ependymal lining of the ventricles that generate CSF. CSF is continuously produced by the choroid plexus and circulates through the ventricles to subarachnoid space after passing through the ventricles via the midline foramen of Magendie (Fig. 14.1). Finally, it comes to the central canal of the spinal cord. CSF is absorbed in the arachnoid granulations and comes into the venous system.

Box 14.1: Indications of cerebrospinal fluid examination.

- Infections
  - Bacterial meningitis
  - Fungal meningitis
- Metastatic tumors
- Leukemia and lymphoma infiltration
- Primary central nervous system tumor rarely
- Ventricular disease
  - Trauma
  - Infarction
- Demyelinating diseases
  - Guillain-Barre syndrome
  - Multiple sclerosis

CYTOLOGY

Cerebrospinal fluid is a clear fluid and contains mainly water (90%), glucose, protein, and occasional lymphocytes. The lining cells of meninges such as pia and arachnoid very rarely shed into the CSF.

SAMPLING OF CEREBROSPINAL FLUID

Cerebrospinal fluid is collected by lumbar puncture technique and about 4–5 mL CSF is withdrawn during spinal tap. The portion of CSF should be collected in a clean plastic tube for cytological examination and should be sent immediately to the laboratory. No preservative is recommended for CSF collection. We recommend immediate processing of CSF.

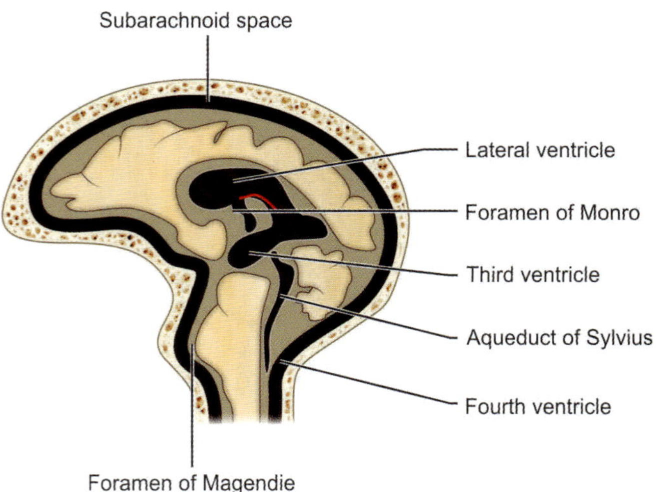

Fig. 14.1: Schematic view of circulation of cerebrospinal fluid in the central nervous system.

Flowchart 14.1: Laboratory evaluation of cerebrospinal fluid.

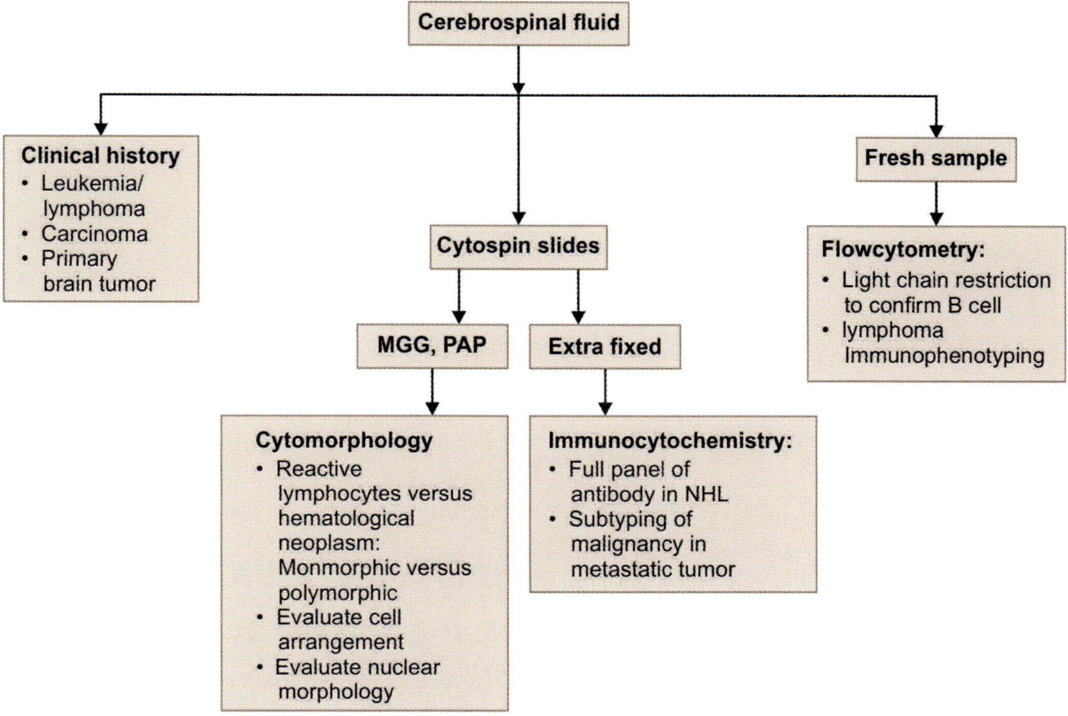

(MGG: May-Grünwald Giemsa; NHL: Non-Hodgkin's lymphoma; PAP: Papanicolaou).

Laboratory Techniques

Cerebrospinal fluid is processed by cytocentrifugation technique. At least two smears are made: one for Papanicolaou stain and the other for May-Grünwald Giemsa (MGG) stain. If necessary, multiple smears can be made for special stain. One portion of CSF can be kept for flow cytometry (Flowchart 14.1).

Normal Cells

Cerebrospinal fluid usually contains very scanty cellularity. It contains only a few lymphocytes. Mature lymphocytes have small round nuclei with condensed chromatin and scanty cytoplasm. Reactive lymphocytes have relatively more cytoplasm and enlarged nuclei having small nucleoli. There may be sparse monocytes. The monocytes have relatively more cytoplasm and kidney-shaped nuclei.

Neutrophils may also be present in CSF sample. Neutrophil count increases due to infection, particularly bacterial infection. Red blood cells (RBCs) are generally not seen in CSF sample. However, during the surgical procedure, RBCs may come to CSF. The presence of excess RBCs in CSF indicates trauma or hemorrhage. Rarely ependymal cells are seen in CSF sample. These cells have moderate cytoplasm with round to oval centrally placed nuclei.

Cerebrospinal fluid may occasionally be contaminated by starch granules from the gloves of the surgeon.

Box 14.2: Acute meningitis.

- Abundant polymorphs
- Bacteria: May or may not be present

INFECTIVE CONDITIONS

Acute Meningitis

Acute bacterial meningitis is caused by many gram-positive and gram-negative organisms. Smears show large numbers of polymorphonuclear leukocytes and occasional lymphocytes (Box 14.2). The overall cell count in CSF may be as high as 30–40 thousand per cubic mL. In addition, bacterial organisms can be demonstrated by Gram stain. Microbiological culture is the diagnostic test for exact identification of bacterial organisms.

Viral Meningitis

Viral meningitis is caused by mumps, herpes, enteroviruses and cytomegaloviruses. Most of the time, the course of infection is benign and self-recovery occurs except viral encephalomyelitis which has fatal course. Cytology smears show increased cell count (1,000–3,000 per cubic mL). The majority of the cells are lymphocytes (Box 14.3). In addition, transformed atypical lymphocytes are also (Fig. 14.2). The cells have relatively more cytoplasm and nuclei with opened up chromatin and single prominent nucleoli.

Tuberculous Meningitis

Tuberculosis of the meninges produces nonspecific changes. Cell count in CSF increases and predominant cell population are lymphocytes along with occasional plasma cells and histiocytes. The presence of multinucleated giant cell is a nonspecific finding.

AIDS Meningitis

- Acquired immune deficiency syndrome (AIDS) encephalopathy occurs directly or indirectly from infection of cells within the brain or spinal cord by the AIDS virus. In this condition, we get nonspecific chronic inflammatory infiltrate.

Box 14.3: Viral meningitis.
- Lymphocytes
- Atypical lymphocytes

- Opportunistic infections are most frequently produced by *Cryptococcus neoformans, Toxoplasma gondii*, mycobacteria, *Candida*, and viruses such as Cytomegalovirus (CMV).
- CNS lymphoma may be seen in AIDS patients.

Fungal Meningitis

Cryptococcal Meningitis

Cryptococcus neoformans is the most frequent fungal infection of CSF. It may occur both in healthy and also in immunocompromised patient (Box 14.4). The smear shows polymorphonuclear leukocytes and a yeast form of fungus. The yeast is round shaped 5–10 μm diameter structure that often shows narrow-based budding (Fig. 14.3). Cryptococci has a mucopolysaccharide capsule that stains with alcian blue and mucicarmine.

DEMYELINATING DISEASES

Multiple Sclerosis

It produces the normal cell count in CSF. T cell population increases. T helper/suppressor ratio decreases.[1]

In case of Guillain-Barre syndrome, the cytology smear of CSF is acellular. Occasionally, CSF may show lymphocytic response.

Box 14.4: Cryptococcal meningitis.
- Immunocompromised patient
- Polymorphonuclear leukocytes
- Yeast form of fungus: Round shaped 5–10 μ diameter structure that often shows narrow-based budding.
- Capsule of the fungus stains with alcian blue and mucicarmine

Fig. 14.2: Lymphocytes and activated lymphocytes in cerebrospinal fluid in a viral meningitis case (May-Grünwald Giemsa stain XMP).

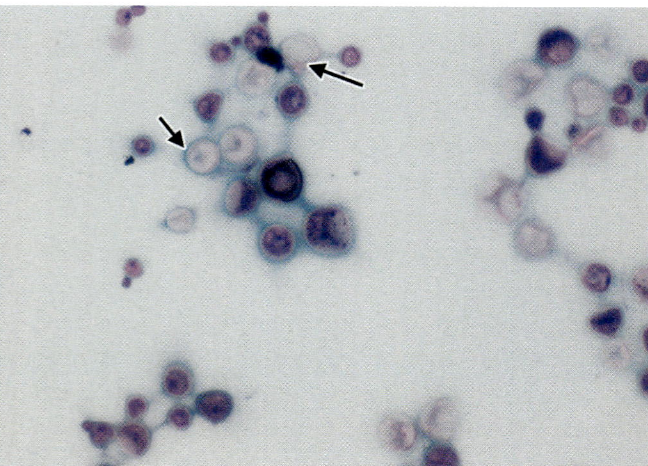

Fig. 14.3: Many round-shaped cryptococci in cerebrospinal fluid (Papanicolaou's stain XOI). Arrows show the cryptococci.

NEOPLASM

Metastatic Solid Tumor

Any malignancy may metastasize in the leptomeninges and may be detected in CSF. However, leukemia, lymphoma and carcinomas are more frequently seen in CSF. Majority of metastatic carcinomas in CSF are adenocarcinoma from lung, breast and gastrointestinal tract (GIT). Most of the time, meningeal carcinoma is associated with parenchymal involvement of brain.[2,3] Malignant cells come to CSF by direct extension from the parenchyma of the brain or by the extension of the tumor from bone to subdural space or by following the tracks of cranial or spinal nerve.

Proper clinical history of primary tumor and histological type of primary tumor are very important. Occult cases of breast or GIT tumor are very uncommon. However, occasionally pulmonary tumor may be small and asymptomatic. Cytological examination of CSF is very important to document the leptomeningeal involvement of the tumor.

Lung Carcinoma

Metastatic adenocarcinoma of the lung is more common than small cell carcinoma and squamous cell carcinoma. Cytology smears of CSF shows clusters and occasional dissociated cells with moderate to abundant cytoplasm. Nuclei are round with moderately pleomorphic having prominent nucleoli.

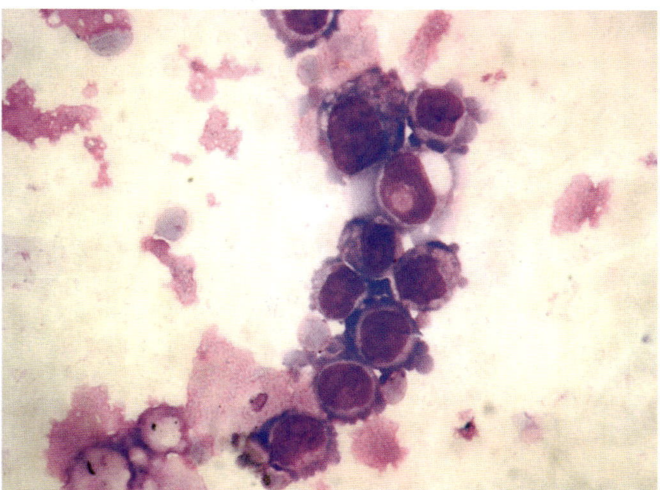

Fig. 14.4: Cells of infiltrating duct carcinoma of breast in cerebrospinal fluid. Smear shows enlarged cells with pleomorphic nuclei (May-Grünwald Giemsa stain XHP).

Small carcinoma of lung shows discrete cells. Cells may show linear arrangement with nuclear molding. The cytoplasm of the cells is scanty. Nuclei show small hyperchromatic nuclei.

Breast Carcinoma

Carcinoma of breast uncommonly metastasizes to CSF. Smears show discrete round cells with moderate cytoplasm. Nuclei are round with moderately pleomorphic nuclei and prominent nucleoli (Fig. 14.4).

Cytology smears of lobular carcinoma show discrete cells with occasional rows of cells. Cells are smaller in size with scanty cytoplasm and round relatively monomorphic nuclei. Signet ring type of cell is also seen.

Melanoma

Melanoma may metastasize from the skin or other organs. The cells are large with moderately pleomorphic nuclei having prominent macronucleoli. The cells may also contain melanin pigment in the cytoplasm.

LEUKEMIA

Leukemic infiltration of leptomeninges may be noted without any involvement of brain parenchyma. Many patients with leukemic infiltration are asymptomatic. Therefore, the routine CSF examination is very useful for diagnosis of leukemic infiltration.

Acute Lymphoblastic Leukemia

Acute lymphoblastic leukemia (ALL) is the most common leukemia in childhood. CNS relapse of ALL occurs in more than 50% cases. Periodic examination of CSF is required for detection of ALL infiltration in CSF. CSF of ALL infiltration usually shows excess lymphoid cells (Box 14.5). The cells are round with scanty deep blue cytoplasm and round nuclei with fine nuclear chromatin (Fig. 14.5). Nucleoli are large and prominent. In addition, nuclei often show large nipple like protrusion.

Box 14.5: Acute lymphoblastic leukemia.

- The most common childhood leukemia
- Excess lymphoid cells
- Round cells with scanty cytoplasm
- Nuclear chromatin (fine)
- Nipple like nuclear protrusion
- Large prominent nucleoli

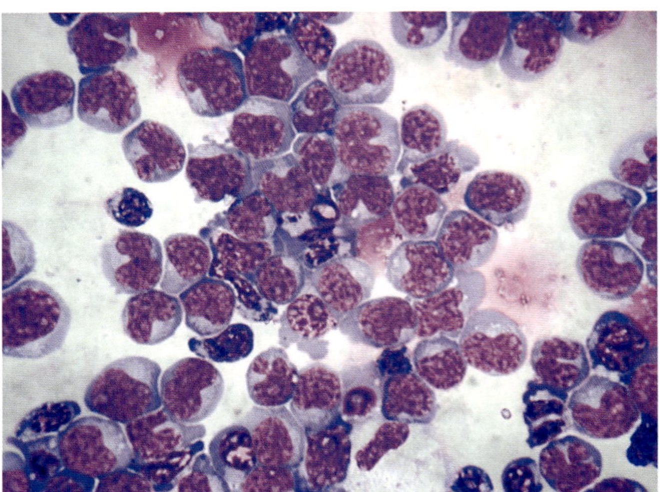

Fig. 14.5: Cerebrospinal fluid smear of acute lymphoblastic leukemia showing round cells with scanty deep blue cytoplasm and round nuclei with fine nuclear chromatin (May-Grünwald Giemsa stain XOI).

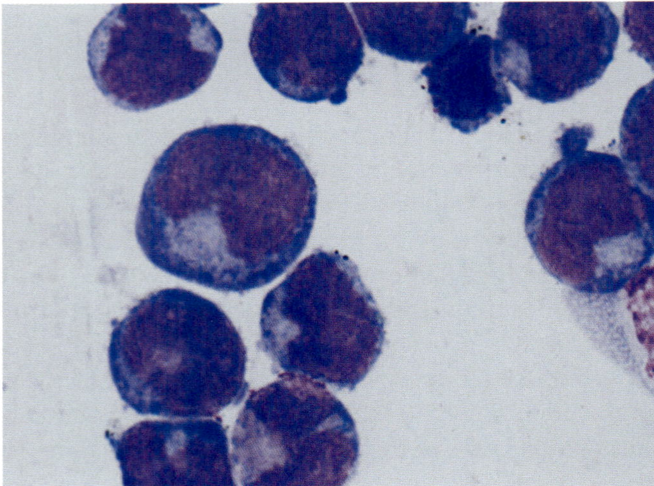

Fig. 14.6: Cerebrospinal fluid smear of acute myeloid leukemia: Large cells with scanty cytoplasm, convoluted nuclei having prominent nucleoli (May-Grünwald Giemsa stain XOI).

Box 14.6: Acute myeloblastic leukemia.

- Common in adults
- CSF involvement is less than ALL
- Blasts
  - Relatively large cells
  - Irregular nuclear margin
  - Fine chromatin
  - Multiple prominent nucleoli
  - Auer rods may be seen

(ALL: Acute lymphoblastic leukemia; CSF: Cerebrospinal fluid).

Interpretation Problems

- *Contamination with blood*: Cytology smear of CSF may be contaminated by blasts from the peripheral blood. Therefore, adequate precaution should be taken before the interpretation of such smear.
- *Too few cells*: At times, CSF may show scanty cells with occasional blasts. It is difficult to decide whether this patient should be treated as CNS relapse or not. If CSF contains more than 10 cells per cubic mL then these cases should be treated as CNS relapse.[4]

Acute Myeloblastic Leukemia

Acute myeloblastic leukemia (AML) commonly occurs in adulthood. The incidence of CNS infiltration in AML is much lower than ALL. It may be probably due to the lower survival period of AML. All subtypes of AML infiltrates in the leptomeninges and this may occur at the time of initial presentation or at relapse. The morphology of blasts is similar to that of blood (Box 14.6). The cells are large and round with irregular nuclear margin (Fig. 14.6). Nuclear chromatin is fine. Multiple prominent nucleoli are seen. In addition, the cytoplasm of the cells shows azurophilic granules. Auer rods are the linear slender structure in the cytoplasm formed by condensation of azurophilic granules. The presence of characteristic auer rods is pathognomonic of myeloblast.

Chronic Lymphocytic Leukemia

Leptomeningeal involvement of chronic lymphocytic leukemia (CLL) is very much uncommon. It is usually very difficult to differentiate small mature lymphocytes from the cells of CLL. Immunocytochemistry may be helpful in selected cases.

Chronic Myeloid Leukemia

Infiltration by chronic myeloid leukemia (CML) is also extremely uncommon. CSF smears in CML infiltration shows polymorphous population of cells consisting of myelocytes, metamyelocytes, promyelocytes and polymorphs. It is essential to eliminate the possibility of contamination by blood in such cases.

LYMPHOMAS

Leptomeningeal involvement of lymphoma is similar to that of leukemia. Lymphoma predominantly involves leptomeninges without any parenchymal involvement. About one-tenth of non-Hodgkin's lymphoma (NHL) involves CNS at the time of presentation or during the course of the disease. Some specific types of lymphoma such as diffuse large B cell lymphoma, Burkitt's and lymphoblastic lymphomas commonly affect leptomeninges (Fig. 14.7).[5] Most of the lymphomas in CSF are B cell NHL.

Adequate clinical information particularly the history of NHL and type of NHL are very helpful in diagnosis. In difficult cases immunocytochemistry or flow cytometry may be helpful. It has been noted that flow cytometry along with cytological examination, increases the sensitivity of diagnosis of NHL in CSF.[6]

Primary Central Nervous System Lymphoma

Primary CNS lymphoma accounts for 10–15% of all primary CNS tumors. Diffuse large B cell NHL is the most common type of primary CNS lymphoma.[7] In most of the cases, brain parenchyma is involved without leptomeningeal involvement. The diagnosis of primary CNS lymphoma is difficult in CSF examination. Flow cytometric immunophenotyping may be helpful to demonstrate monoclonality of the cells.

Box 14.7: Medulloblastoma.

- Small clusters and discrete cells
- Round cells with scanty cytoplasm
- Hyperchromatic round nuclei
- Nuclear molding
- Prominent nucleoli

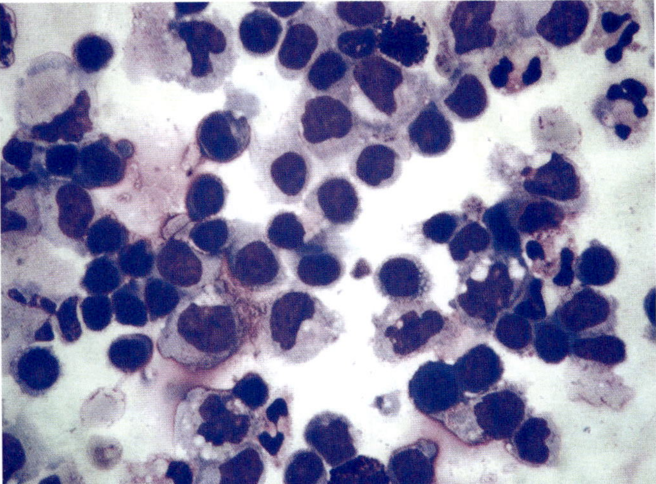

Fig. 14.7: Cerebrospinal fluid smear shows infiltration by a known case of non-Hodgkin's lymphoma (May-Grünwald Giemsa stain XOI).

Other Primary Central Nervous System Tumor

Primary neoplasm of the CNS is rarely noted in CSF except medulloblastoma. CSF is not examined for the investigation in primary CNS tumor.

Medulloblastoma

It is a childhood tumor and may invade the CSF through ventricles.[8] Cytology smears show small clusters and dissociated cells (Box 14.7). The individual cells have scanty cytoplasm and round to oval hyperchromatic nuclei having prominent nucleoli. Nuclear molding may be seen. The cells are positive for synaptophysin and negative for glial fibrillary acidic protein (GFAP).

Other Brain Tumor

Among the other primary neoplasms of the brain, germinoma and ependymoma may rarely shed into the CSF (Figs. 14.8A to D). The cells of ependymoma are usually arranged in small clusters, perivascularly and discretely. Individual cells are small, round with scanty cytoplasm and relatively monomorphic nuclei.

DIAGNOSTIC ACCURACY

Sensitivity of CSF examination for detection of malignancy is 54–60%.[2,9,10] However, the detection rate of malignancy in CSF increases if multiple samples are examined, the volume of CSF is more, and the extent of leptomeningeal involvement is diffuse and extensive. The major problems in CSF examination are relatively low cellularity in CSF, rapid degeneration of cells due to low sugar, low volume of samples examined, difficult to confirm histologically and difficult to obtain an additional sample (Box 14.8).

Box 14.8: Diagnostic problems.

Major problems

- Low cellularity in cerebrospinal fluid (CSF)
- Rapid degeneration of cells due to low sugar
- Lower volume of sample
- Malignancy in CSF are difficult to confirm histologically
- Difficult to obtain additional sample

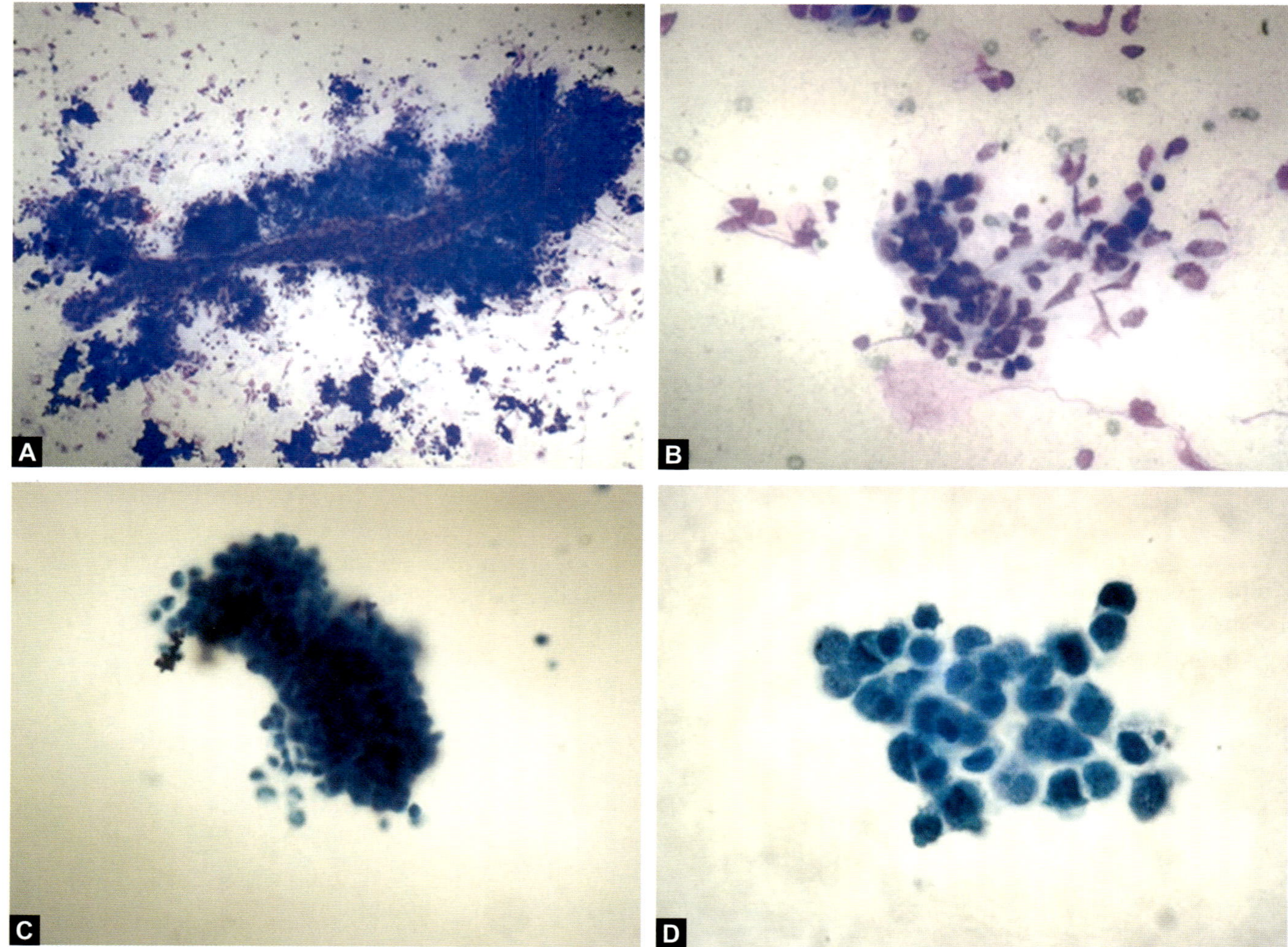

Figs. 14.8A to D: (A) Perivascular arrangement of cells in ependymoma of cerebrospinal fluid (May-Grünwald Giemsa stain XLP); (B) Round to oval cells with mildly pleomorphic nuclei having scanty cytoplasm in ependymoma (May-Grünwald Giemsa stain XMP); (C) Tight cluster of small cells in ependymoma (Papanicolaou's stain XMP); (D) Cells with mildly pleomorphic nuclei in ependymoma (Papanicolaou's stain XHP).

REFERENCES

1. Noronha A, Richman DP, Arnason GW. Multiple sclerosis: Activated cells in cerebrospinal fluid in acute exacerbations. Ann Neurol. 1985;18:722-5.
2. Glass JP, Melamed M, Chernik NL, et al. Malignant cells in cerebrospinal fluid (CSF): The meaning of a positive CSF cytology. Neurology. 1979;29:1369-75.
3. Gonzalez-Vitale JC, Garcia-Bunuel R. Meningeal carcinomatosis. Cancer. 1976;37:2906-11.
4. McIntosh S, Ritchey AK. Diagnostic problems in cerebrospinal fluid of children with lymphoid malignancies. Am J Pediatr Hematol Oncol. 1987;8:28-31.
5. Nolan CP, Abrey LE. Leptomeningeal metastases from leukemias and lymphomas. Cancer Treat Res. 2005;125:53-69.
6. French CA, Dorfman DM, Shaheen G, et al. Diagnosing lymphoproliferative disorders involving the cerebrospinal fluid: Increased sensitivity using flow cytometric analysis. Diagn Cytopathol. 2000;23:369-74.
7. Nuckols JD, Liu K, Burchette J, et al. Primary central nervous system lymphomas: A 30 year experience at a single institution. Mod Pathol. 1999;12:1167-73.
8. Jereb B, Reid A, Ahuja RK. Patterns of failure in patients with medulloblastoma. Cancer. 1982;50:2941-47.
9. Gondos B, King EB. Cerebrospinal fluid cytology: Diagnostic accuracy and comparison of different techniques. Acta Cytol. 1976;20:542-7.
10. Wasserstrom WR, Glass JP, Posner JB. Diagnosis and treatment of leptomeningeal metastases from solid tumors: Experience with 90 patients. Cancer. 1982;49:759-72.

Review Questions

1. **A 25-year-male had fever and headache for 5 days. Cerebrospinal fluid microphotograph (Fig. 14.9) indicates:**
   a. Lymphocytosis
   b. Normal
   c. Cryptococcus
   d. Leukemic infiltration
2. **A 17-year-boy had fever and headache. Cerebrospinal fluid microphotograph (Fig. 14.10) indicates:**
   a. Leukemic infiltration
   b. Reactive lymphocytosis
   c. Metastatic carcinoma
   d. Acute inflammation
3. **A 75-year-male was previously diagnosed as multiple myeloma and was treated accordingly. Now the patient presented with headache. Figures 11A and B show the cerebrospinal fluid cytology. What is your diagnosis?**

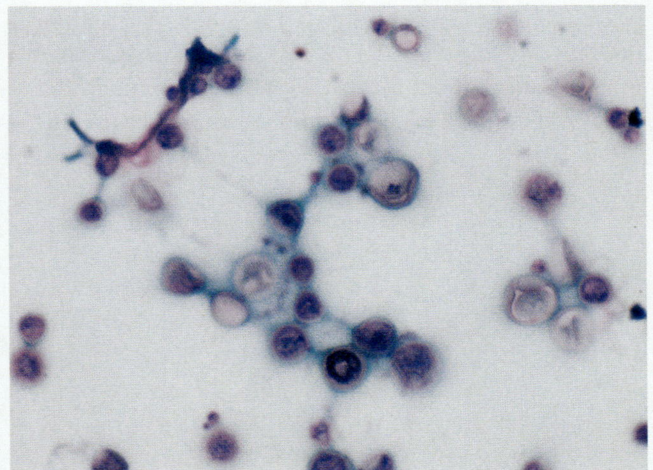

Fig. 14.9: CSF Smear in question 1.

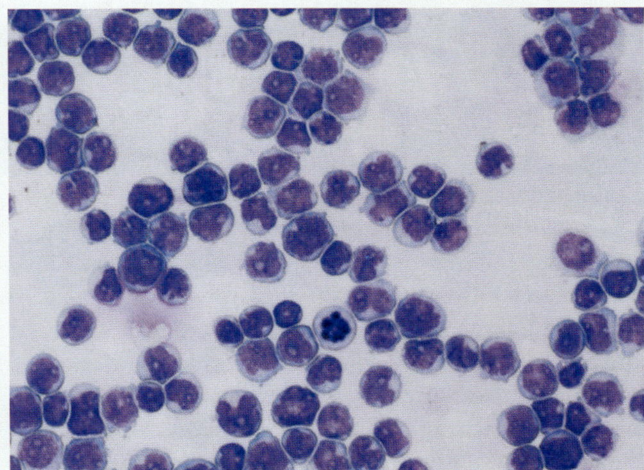

Fig. 14.10: CSF Smear in question 2.

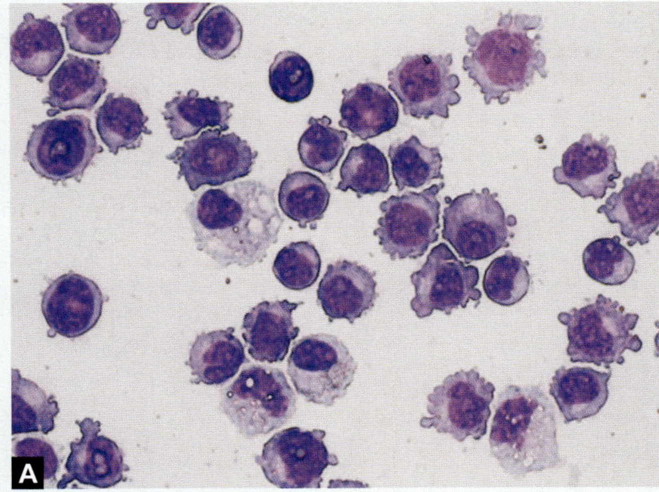

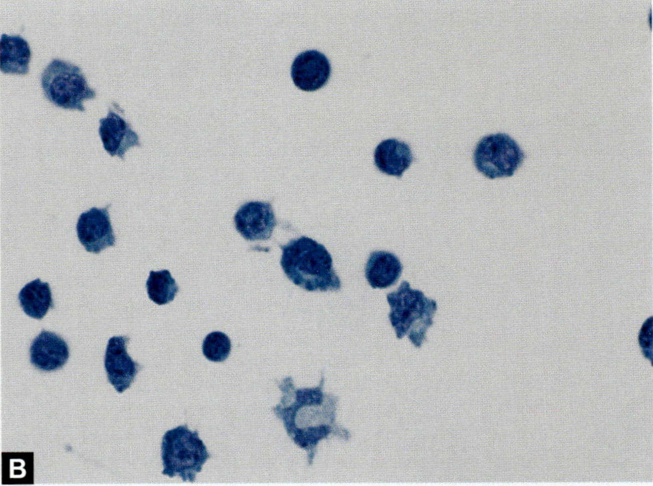

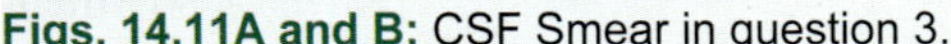

Figs. 14.11A and B: CSF Smear in question 3.

Answers

1. c. Cryptococcus

   Note: There are large number of cryptococci in the smear. The round unstained structures larger than the lymphocytes are the cryptococci. India ink rapidly stain the capsule of the organisms.
2. a. Leukemic infiltration

   Note: The CSF shows many cells with round nuclei having irregular margin and fine chromatin. The nuclei have single to multiple prominent nucleoli. The morphology of the cells are that of leukemic blasts.
3. Infiltration by plasma cell tumor (plasma blasts)

   Note: There are large number of immature cells (plasmablasts). Occasional typical plasma cells are also present.

Section 3

Laboratory Techniques

Chapter Outline

CHAPTER

15 Basic Technique and Approach to Fine Needle Aspiration Cytology

INTRODUCTION

Fine needle aspiration cytology (FNAC) is now an essential and integral part of cytology. It is also known as a fine needle aspiration biopsy (FNAB). In fact, FNAC procedure can be done in any organ of the body or any tissue or swelling.

ADVANTAGES

Fine needle aspiration cytology has several advantages over tissue biopsy (Box 15.1).[1] This procedure can be done anywhere in the laboratory, in outpatient department or in the hospital. No special precaution is needed for FNAC of a superficial mass. A patient can be called in the FNAC clinic or outpatient department and within just 1 hour the report can be delivered. This is a cost effective and rapid technique with high sensitivity and specificity. FNAC is comparable or even better than the frozen section in certain situations such as thyroid or breast lesions. This technique provides significant economical relief in developing countries where health-care cost is important. FNAC report provides a great psychological relief to the patient. It can convince the patient that the lesion is benign or infectious in origin. In case of malignancy, it can convince the patient to have an urgent treatment. Now-a-days with the help of ancillary technique on FNAC material, exact diagnosis is possible in most of the lesions. Therefore FNAC can avoid tissue biopsy in many situations.

Box 15.1: Advantages of fine needle aspiration cytology (FNAC).

- Simple technique
- Office procedure
- Rapid
- Economical
- Wide area of sampling
- High sensitivity and specificity
- Avoids further tissue biopsy in case of inoperable malignancy or infective conditions
- All most all the ancillary techniques are possible from FNAC material

LIMITATIONS OF FNAC (BOX 15.2)

Fine needle aspiration cytology has certain limitations over tissue biopsy such as loss of tissue architecture of tissue and inability to interpret capsular or vascular invasion. In many conditions, complex tissue architecture is helpful in diagnosis such as soft-tissue tumors or skin adnexal lesions. The exact classification of such lesions is difficult in FNAC. Follicular pattern of lymphoma is important in diagnosis of follicular lymphoma. It is difficult to diagnose follicular lymphoma on FNAC material alone. Another challenge in FNAC is to predict capsular or lymphovascular invasion. Similarly the diagnosis of "in situ" or invasive carcinoma is not always possible in FNAC material. Moreover, interpretation of FNAC sample is a bit different than tissue biopsy and considerable skill is needed to interpret FNAC material.[2]

In fact, FNAC interpretation is also different than exfoliative cytology. Unlike exfoliative cytology, interpretation of FNAC needs more importance on the overall cellular pattern (Table 15.1).

COMPLICATIONS (BOX 15.3)

Fine needle aspiration cytology of superficial masses are almost free of any complication. Minor hematoma may

Box 15.2: Limitations of fine needle aspiration cytology (FNAC) over tissue biopsy.

- Loss of tissue architecture
- Capsular invasion and lymphovascular invasions not possible to predict
- Not possible to comment on in situ versus invasive carcinoma
- Training is needed for accurate interpretation

Table 15.1: Exfoliative cytology versus fine needle aspiration cytology (FNAC).

Features	*FNAC*	*Exfoliative*
Cellular pattern	Important to examine	Not so important
Cellularity	High cellularity	Diagnostic cells are usually low
Nuclear morphology	Well preserved	Less well preserved
Nuclear detail	Less important	Very important

Box 15.3: Complications of fine needle aspiration cytology (FNAC).

- Minor hematoma
- Surgical emphysema
- Accidental rupture of aneurysmal vessel or spleen
- Anaphylaxis in hydatid cyst
- Biliary peritonitis and bowel perforation
- Infraction of lymph node and thyroid
- Needle tract seedling of cancer cells (if thick bore needle is used)

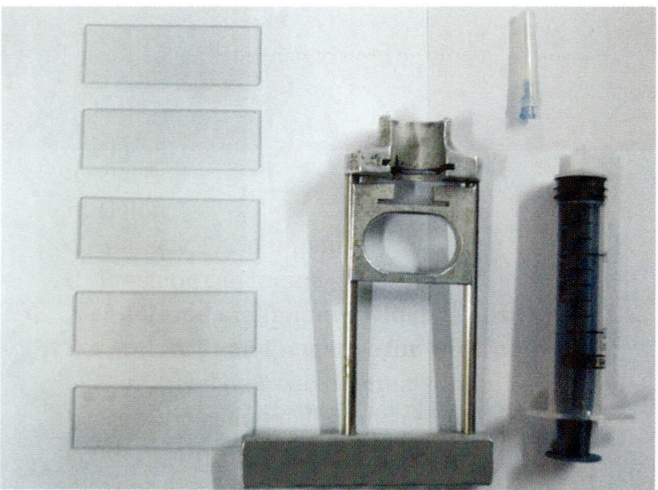

Fig. 15.1: Equipments needed for fine needle aspiration cytology (FNAC) is highlighted here: glass slides, pistol handle, needle, and syringe.

develop, if the area is not compressed after FNAC procedure. Anaphylactic reaction may occur due to accidental rupture of hydatid cyst during FNAC procedure. However even after FNAC of hydatid cyst this complication is rare unless there is spillage of the cyst fluid in the adjacent tissue.

Complications, if any, of the FNAC procedure mainly occurs in the deeper mass lesion or if the thick bore needle is used. In fact, incidence of complication is indirectly proportional to the diameter of the aspiration needle.[3,4] Surgical emphysema may occur in lung FNAC. However, in our experience most of such conditions can be managed conservatively. The spillage of tumor through the needle tract is not true if fine bore needle is used.[5] Truly speaking, FNAC can safely be used even in ovarian cyst if a thin needle is used and proper precautions are taken. Rarely FNAC needle may cause rupture of an aneurismal vessel or spleen. This can be avoided, if proper precautions are taken. In case of the spleen, gentle suction should be done and too much movement in different directions should be avoided. Occasionally biliary peritonitis and intestinal perforations have been reported[6] and this can be avoided if thin needle is used for FNAC.

CONTRAINDICATIONS (BOX 15.4)

There are no absolute contraindications of FNAC. However, one should be careful to do FNAC in coagulation disorders, particularly hemophilia. FNAC should better be avoided in such conditions. In case of severe thrombocytopenia, FNAC may cause hematoma and it should better be avoided in vascular organ in such disorders. In deep-seated lesion, a team approach with radiologist, surgeons, physician, and cytologists is needed.

Box 15.4: Contraindications of fine needle aspiration cytology (FNAC).

- Hemophilia or gross coagulation disorders
- Aneurysmal dilatation of blood vessels
- Hydatid cyst

EQUIPMENT

Following equipments are needed for the FNAC procedure to do:

- *Pistol handle to hold the syringe (Fig. 15.1)*: The pistol handle is made up of metal and is fit to hold the syringe properly. It also helps to give suction during the FNAC procedure. Its main advantage is that the other hand of the operator remains free to hold the swelling.
- *Syringe*: Depending on the size of the pistol handle 10 cc or 20 cc disposable plastic syringe is used.
- *Needles*: Ordinary disposable hypodermic needle of 22–27 Gauge is used for FNAC. The size of the needle depends on the situation. Large bore needle is especially helpful for hard and fibrotic lesion or cyst with viscous material. On the other hand, thin bore needle is used for small lymph node or vascular organ like thyroid.
- *Clean glass slides*: Frosted glass slides are preferable because they are easy to be labeled.

- *Spirit swabs*: Clean sterile swabs soaked with spirit are needed to clean the area of aspiration.
- *95% ethanol for fixation of slide*: This is needed to fix the slides for Papanicolaou's (Pap) stain.
- Few capped vials containing 10% formalin solution for cell blocks. Cell block is needed to do immunocytochemistry on FNAC sample.
- Few capped vials containing balanced salt solution for transport of the material in case flow cytometry is needed.

FINE NEEDLE ASPIRATION TECHNIQUE (BOX 15.5)

Clinical History

Before performing FNAC procedure a good clinical history is mandatory. It gives the idea of the provisional diagnosis so that the operator manages to take samples for ancillary tests. Clinical history is very important for interpretation of FNAC smears.

Preparation of the Patient

Many times the patient is apprehensive and therefore a good talk with the patient makes him/her relax. I have noted that the patient often feels that the biopsy is a cumbersome process so they themselves keep them overnight fast. These patients are vulnerable to collapse or faint. It is the duty of the cytologist to take special care of such patient. All the patients should be explained about the whole procedure. Explanation of the technique makes them more understandable and cooperative. Depending on the situation and country's law one should take proper consent from the patient for the FNAC procedure. This is particularly true for FNAC of deep-seated lesions and orbit. The area of the site of FNAC should be properly cleaned with a spirit swab.

Aspiration

It is generally recommended that the cytopathologist himself/herself should perform FNAC.[7,8] The plastic syringe with attached needle is properly fitted to the pistol handle (Figs. 15.2 to 15.8). The swelling is held in between the two fingers to make it immobilized. The needle is

Box 15.5: Fine needle aspiration procedure.

- *Clinical history*: Always take clinical details before fine needle aspiration cytology (FNAC)
- *Preparation of the patient*:
  - Explain the technique
  - Take proper consent
- *Aspiration*:
  - Clean the area by spirit swab
  - The swelling is hold in between the two fingers to make it immobilized
  - Needle is inserted within the mass
  - To and fro movement of the needle
  - Intermittent negative suction
  - Suction stopped
  - Needle is withdrawn
  - Needle is detached from the syringe
  - Syringe is filled with air
  - Material pushed on glass slide
  - Multiple smear made
  - Pressure by cotton swab is applied to the site of FNAC

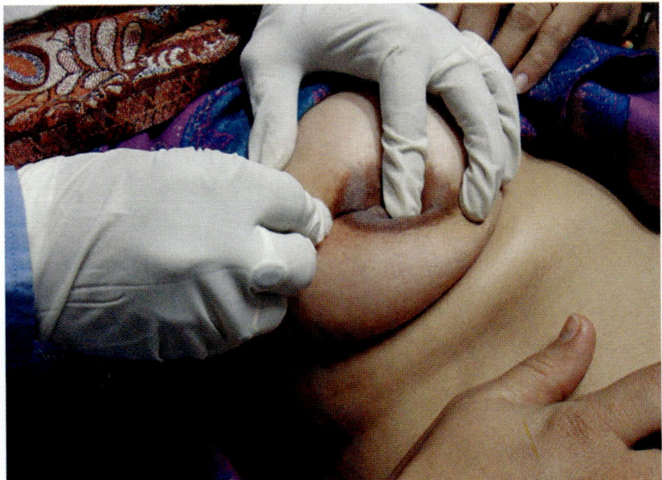

Fig. 15.2: Site of fine needle aspiration cytology (FNAC) is cleaned by a clean spirit swab.

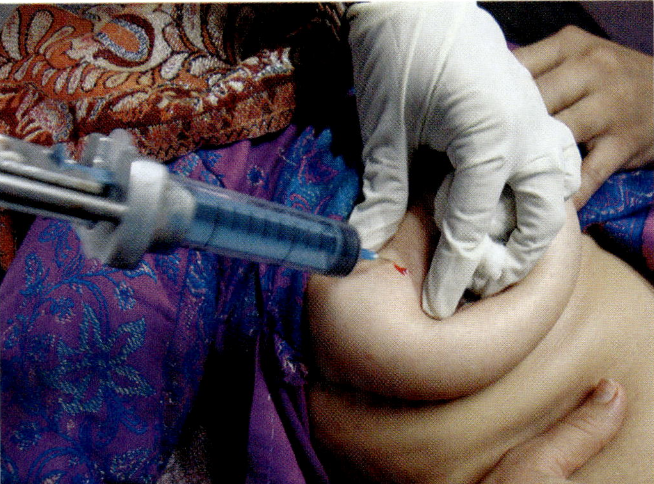

Fig. 15.3: The needle attached with the syringe is introduced into the swelling.

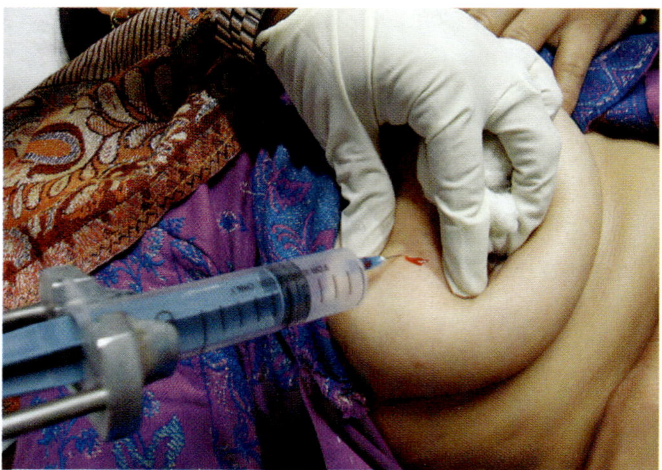

Fig. 15.4: The syringe and needle are moved to and fro and simultaneously negative suction is given.

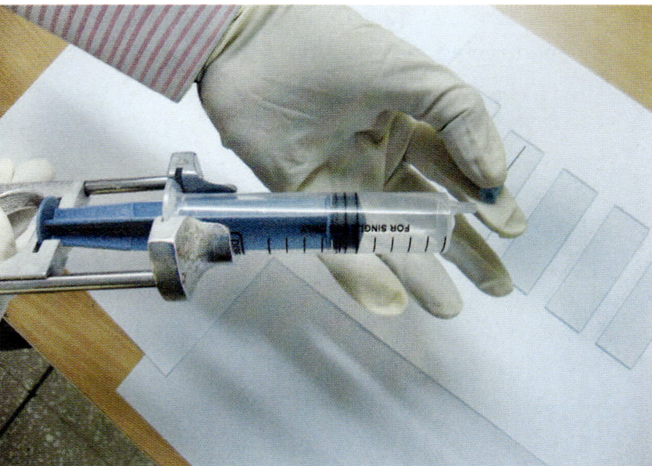

Fig. 15.5: The needle with the syringe is withdrawn from the swelling and the needle is detached from the syringe.

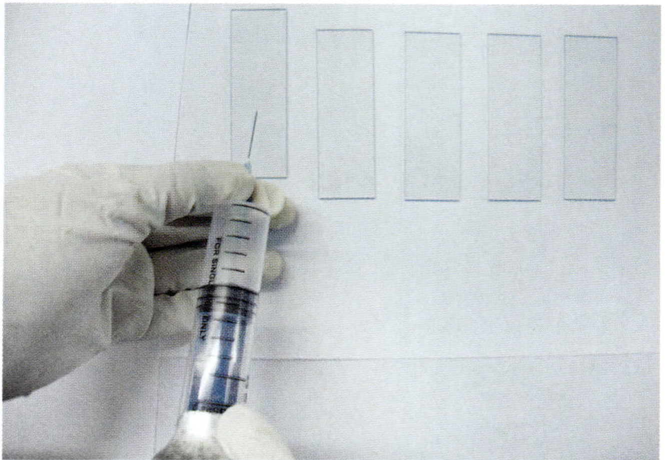

Fig. 15.6: Air is filled in the syringe and the material is expelled from the syringe and needle hub to the glass slide.

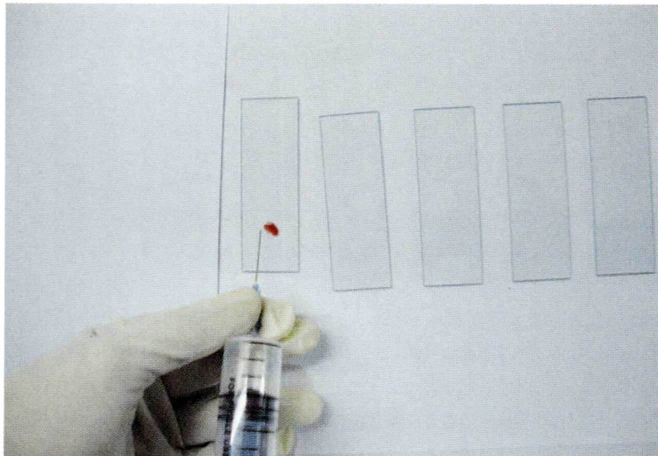

Fig. 15.7: Material is expelled on the glass slide.

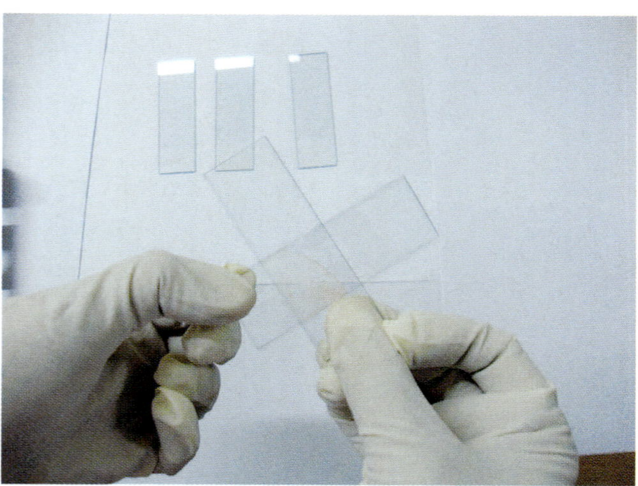

Fig. 15.8: Smear is made by putting another slide on the material and gently pushing the two slides apart.

gently and swiftly introduced within the mass. The needle should be directed perpendicular of the swelling and should penetrate adequately. There should be to and fro movement of the needle within the mass. In between gentle negative suction should be given. The needle may be withdrawn a little within the mass and the direction of the needle should be changed slightly. Major change of direction of the needle is not advisable as this may cut the tissue significantly. At the end of the FNAC the needle is withdrawn sharply along with the release of the plunger to stop the suction. The majority of times the material remains in the needle hub. Therefore, releasing the negative pressure before withdrawing the needle is a vital step to get adequate material. The needle is then rapidly detached from the syringe and the plunger is retracted to get enough air within the syringe. The needle is reattached and the air is pushed to eject the material on the glass slide. Firm pressure should be applied on the site of FNAC to prevent any hematoma formation.

Smear Preparation

The material is pushed on the clean glass slide a little away from the corner. The direction of the needle should be along the long-axis of the slide to avoid spillage of the material sideways. Now the smear is made by gently pressing a clean glass slide over it and moving the upper slide over the lower one to spread the material. Multiple smears are made and both air dried and alcohol fixed smears should be kept for staining. The residual material should be rinsed in balanced salt solution and can be processed for ancillary techniques. If needed a repeat FNAC should be undertaken to get more material for the ancillary techniques.

FINE NEEDLE SAMPLING (FIGS. 15.9 TO 15.11)

Fine needle sampling (FNS) is an alternative technique of FNAC and is helpful in certain situations like thyroid swelling, breast lesions, and small lymph nodes in a child.[9] In FNS procedure, no syringe or pistol handle is required during the procurement of the sample. The swelling should be pressed in between the two fingers and a thin bore needle is gently introduced. The needle is moved to and fro in the same direction and also in small inclination

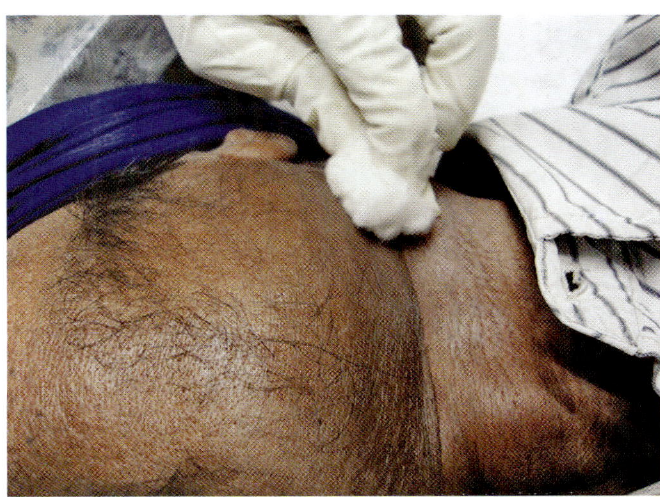

Fig. 15.9: Site of fine needle sampling (FNS) is cleaned.

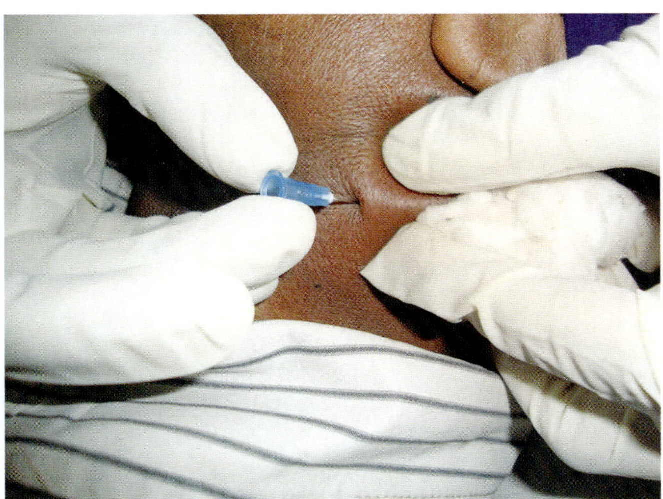

Fig. 15.10: The swelling is compressed in between the two fingers and the needle is introduced to the swelling gently.

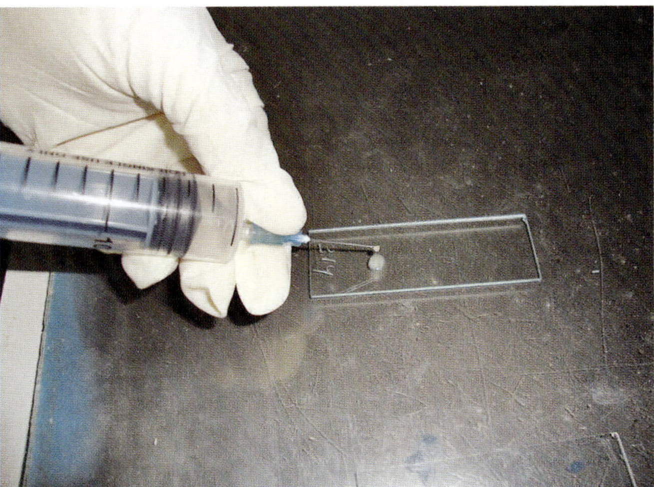

Fig. 15.11: The needle is withdrawn and the material is expelled on the glass slide.

in different directions. The material comes to the hub of the needle by capillary pressure. The needle is gently withdrawn and the syringe filled with air is attached to the needle hub. The aspirated material is expelled gently on the slide with the help of the syringe.

The major advantage of FNS is to get material without any admixture of blood (Box 15.6). Therefore FNS is particularly important in vascular organ like thyroid. The needle also can be easily manipulated as it is free of any attached syringe. However, the material is usually less in volume and cannot be divided into many slides. Moreover, FNS is not suitable for cystic lesion as the fluid is spilled over in this technique. In hard and fibrotic lesion this technique is unsuitable.

STAINING OF THE SMEAR

Fixation

Fixation includes:

- Air dried smears are used for MGG (May-Grünwald Giemsa) staining.
- For routine Papanicolaou's staining 95% ethanol, methanol, or isopropyl alcohol is used for fixation. The smears should be fixed at least 30 minutes. Commercially available spray fixatives can also be used as an alternate to wet fixation.

Staining

Air dried smear: MGG or Romanowsky stain, or Diff-Quik stain is done on the air dried smear. This is also a good stain for mucin and extracellular matrix.

Wet fixed smear: Papanicolaou's stain or hematoxylin and eosin stain is used. One great advantage of Pap stain is to demonstrate intracellular keratin and thereby identification of squamous cells.

Rapid staining: Commercially available Diff-Quick stain can be used for rapid staining within 2 minutes. Rapid Pap stain can also be done within 3 minutes.[10]

Box 15.6: Fine needle sampling technique.

Indications:
- Vascular tissue such as thyroid
- Small mobile lymph node
- Soft and mobile lesions in breast

Advantages:
- Least painful
- Easy to fix the lesion by needle
- Completely devoid of blood
- Good material

Limitations:
- Not good for cystic lesion due to spillage of fluid
- Material cannot be divided into many slides

ANCILLARY TECHNIQUES

All the ancillary techniques used in tissue section can also be done in FNAC sample.[11] Depending on the resource and the situation these tests should be done accordingly. However most of the laboratories routinely do a cell block for immunocytochemistry.

FNAC OF DEEP-SEATED LESIONS

Technique of FNAC of the deep-seated lesions in the body is almost similar to that of superficial lesion.[12] Radiological guidance is needed to perform FNAC of deeply seated lesion of the body. Certain information is required before performing FNAC of radiological-guided lesions (Box 15.7).

The deep-seated lesion can be aspirated under the guidance of ultrasonography (USG), computerized tomography (CT) or fluoroscopy (Figs. 15.12 to 15.15). Depending on individual situations radiologist decides the mode of guidance for FNAC of deeper lesions.

Box 15.7: Prior information needed for guided fine needle aspiration cytology (FNAC).

- Clinical history
- Location of the lesion
- Size of the lesion
- Consistency of the lesion
- Routine blood test
- Coagulation parameters

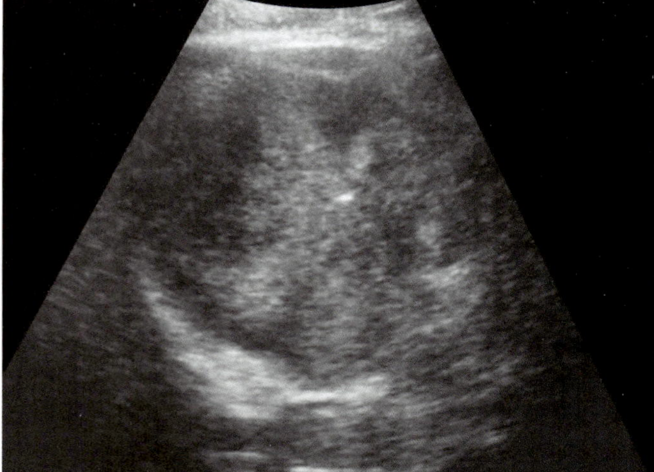

Fig. 15.12: Ultrasound-guided fine needle aspiration cytology (FNAC) of the space occupying lesion of the liver.
Courtesy: Dr Anupam Lal, Additional Professor, PGIMER, Chandigarh, India.

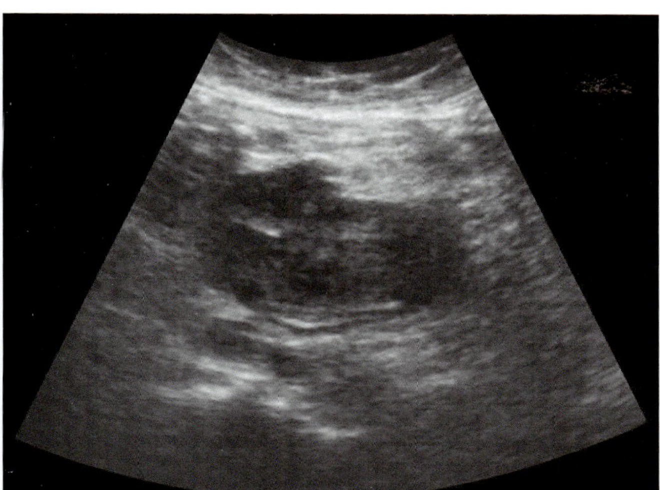

Fig. 15.13: Ultrasound-guided fine needle aspiration cytology (FNAC) of mass in the pancreatic head.
Courtesy: Dr Anupam Lal, Additional Professor, PGIMER, Chandigarh, India.

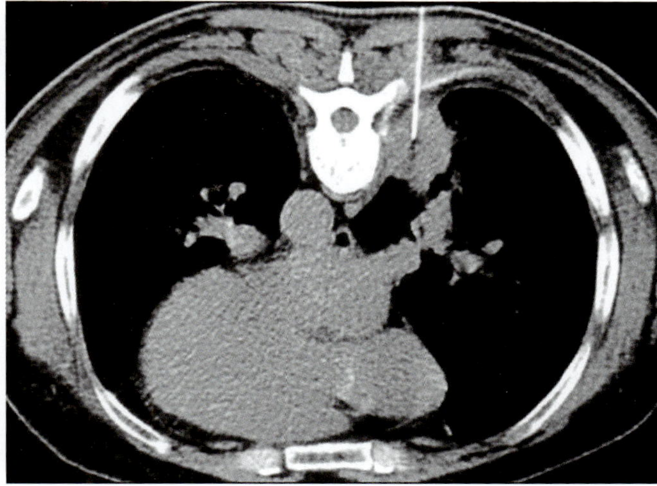

Fig. 15.14: Computerized tomography (CT)-guided fine needle aspiration cytology (FNAC) of a peripheral lung mass.
Courtesy: Dr Anupam Lal, Additional Professor, PGIMER, Chandigarh, India.

Box 15.8: Ultrasonography (USG)-guided fine needle aspiration cytology (FNAC).

- Easy to do
- Cheap
- Rapid
- Position of the patient can be changed
- Real time
- No radiation exposure
- Significant obscuration due to air or bone

Box 15.9: Computerized tomography (CT)-guided fine needle aspiration cytology (FNAC).

- High resolution
- Exact localization of the needle
- Image of the traversing needle visible
- Costly
- Time taken procedure
- Radiation exposure

Fig. 15.15: Computerized tomography (CT)-guided fine needle aspiration cytology (FNAC) of lung mass abutting the aorta.
Courtesy: Dr Anupam Lal, Additional Professor, PGIMER, Chandigarh, India.

Ultrasonography-guided FNAC

Ultrasonography guidance of FNAC is the most popular as it is easy to perform, less expensive and rapid technique (Box 15.8). There is no radiation hazard in USG-guided FNAC. At first radiologist identify the lesion and then introduce the needle with stylet. The pathway of the needle is assessed by real-time USG. After hitting the target, the stylet is withdrawn and suction is given with the help of syringe. The aspirated material is spreaded over the slide.

CT-guided FNAC

Computerized tomography-guided FNAC is more appropriate for small lesion which needs precise localization (Box 15.9). Thoracic lesion near the great vessels or deep-seated intra-abdominal lesions are the best targets for CT scan guided FNAC. However this is a time consuming and expensive procedure with good amount of radiation exposure. Moreover, no real-time guidance is possible in CT-guided FNAC.

Endoscopic Ultrasound-guided FNAC

In this technique, FNAC is done through endoscope under USG guidance. The needle with stylet is introduced through the endoscope and simultaneously the mass is localized by USG. Endoscopic ultrasound-guided FNAC (EUS-FNAC) technique is very much popular for mediastinal, lung, esophageal, and pancreatic lesion.

Others

In addition mammographic-guided FNAC is used for breast lesion. In fact, mammographic-guided core needle biopsy is more popular now-a-days. Fluoroscopic-guided FNAC can also be done. However, radiation exposure is significantly more in this type of guided FNAC.

Transrectal FNAC of the Prostate

Fine needle aspiration cytology is widely used for transrectal FNAC of the prostate. This procedure is easy to perform and multiple sampling can be done from the different areas of the prostate.

Franzen's guide and needle are needed for doing transrectal FNAC of the prostate. Franzen's guide is the long guide with a central hole inside (Fig. 15.16). Franzen's needle is introduced within the guide hole for FNAC of the prostate (Fig. 15.17). At first, the patient should lie down in his left lateral position with the lower leg extended and upper leg folded to chest firmly. The prostate should be palpated to assess initially. Franzen's guide should be fixed with the left index finger of the aspirator with the help of finger stall. Now the Franzen's guide is introduced gently through the rectum to the area of the prostate to be aspirated (Fig. 15.18). FNAC is now done with the help of Franzen's needle within the guide and syringe (Fig. 15.19).

SUBOPTIMAL MATERIAL IN FNAC (BOX 15.10)

The FNAC material may be suboptimal for various reasons. The excessive blood in the smear may be present due to too much suction in a vascular lesion. This can be avoided by intermittent suction when applying negative

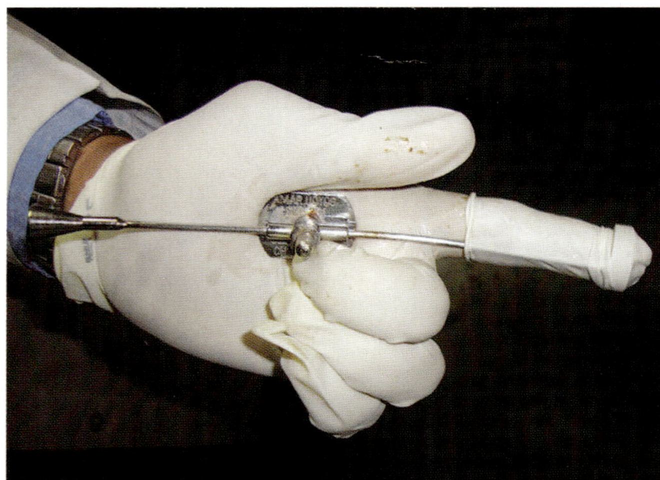

Fig. 15.16: Franzen's guide fixed with the finger.

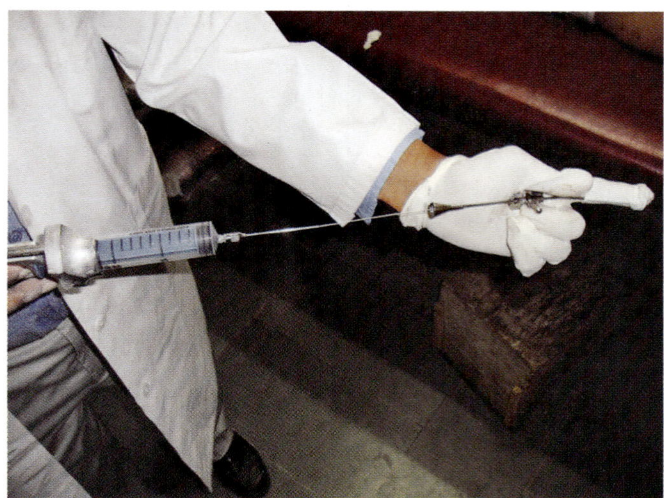

Fig. 15.17: Franzen's needle is introduced within the hole of the guide for fine needle aspiration cytology (FNAC) of the prostate.

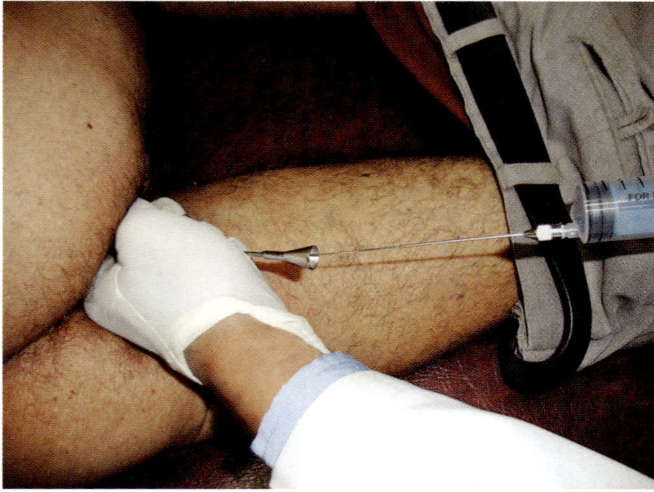

Fig. 15.18: Franzen's guide along with the needle is introduced gently through the rectum.

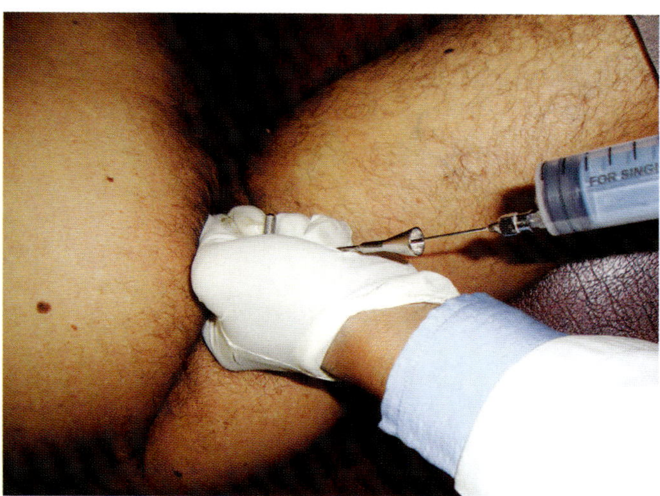

Fig. 15.19: The needle traverses through the glove. It is moved to and fro and negative suction is applied by syringe.

Box 15.10: Nonrepresentative material.

- Excessive blood
- Insufficient material
  - Wrong technique of fine needle aspiration cytology (FNAC)
  - Scarred tissue
- Crushing artifact
- Air drying artifact
- Thick smear

suction. Alternatively, FNS can grossly reduce the amount blood in the sample. Insufficient material may be due to the wrong technique of FNAC. The needle may not hit the mass properly or the movement of the needle may not be sufficient to dissociate the tissue. At times the mass may be too much sclerotic or hard and therefore even after adequate negative suction the material may not be obtained. The other causes of suboptimal smear for interpretation are air dried smear and thick smear.

EVALUATION OF FNAC SMEAR

A FNAC smear of each case should always be evaluated along with the clinical history. The clinician should always give feedback to the cytologist. For medicolegal issue and to avoid false-positive cases a repeat FNAC should be done or if necessary tissue biopsy should be advised. For the initial evaluation of FNAC smear, the cytopathologist should always have the checklist of the important features as mentioned in Box 15.11.

Box 15.11: Check list for evaluation of the fine needle aspiration cytology (FNAC) smear.

- *Clinical*:
  - Chief complaints of the patient
  - Sex and age
  - Any pertinent sign
  - Location of the lesion
  - Radiological or ultrasound features
  - Laboratory data
  - Gross appearance of the aspirated material
- *Cytological data*:
  - Cellularity
  - Cell arrangement or distribution
  - Cell population
  - Cell morphology
  - Background noncellular materials

REFERENCES

1. Brown LA, Coghill SB. Cost effectiveness of a fine needle aspiration clinic. Cytopathology. 1992;3(5):275-80.
2. Orell SR. Pitfalls in fine needle aspiration cytology. Cytopathology. 2003;14(4):173-82.
3. Roussel F. Risk of metastasis during fine needle aspiration. J Clin Pathol. 1990;43(10):878-9.
4. Frable WJ. Fine-needle aspiration biopsy: Clinical applications. Surg Rounds. 1982;5:40-52.
5. Lundstedt C, Stridbeck H, Andersson R, et al. Tumor seeding occurring after fine-needle biopsy of abdominal malignancies. Acta Radiol. 1991;32(6):518-20.
6. Malberger E, Edoute Y, Nagler A. Rare complications after transabdominal fine needle aspiration. Am J Gastroenterol. 1984;79:458-60.
7. Coghill SB, Brown LA. Why pathologists should take needle aspiration specimens. Cytopathology. 1995;6(1):1-4.
8. Polacarz SV. Why pathologists should take needle aspirates. Cytopathology. 1995;6(5):358.
9. Dey P, Ray R. Comparison of fine needle sampling by capillary action and fine needle aspiration. Cytopathology. 1993;4(5):299-303.
10. Yang GC, Alvarez II. Ultrafast Papanicolaou stain. An alternative preparation for fine needle aspiration cytology. Acta Cytol. 1995;39(1):55-60.
11. Dey P. Role of ancillary techniques in diagnosing and subclassifying non-Hodgkin'lymphomas on fine needle aspiration cytology. Cytopathology. 2006;17(5):275-87.
12. Sheikh M, Sawhney S, Dey P, et al. Deep-seated thoracic and abdominal masses: usefulness of ultrasound and computed tomography guidance in fine needle aspiration cytology diagnosis. Australas Radiol. 2000;44(2):155-60.

Review Questions

1. **Contraindications of FNAC is:**
   a. Aneurysm
   b. Hemangioma
   c. Kidney tumor
   d. Testicular tumor
2. **All are advantages of fine needle sampling technique (without aspiration) *except*:**
   a. Least painful
   b. Easy to fix the lesion by needle
   c. Completely devoid of blood
   d. Also useful in cystic goiter
3. **Which one is true for CT-guided FNAC?**
   a. Exact localization of the needle possible
   b. Image of the traversing needle visible
   c. Radiation exposure
   d. All of the above
4. **All are true for USG-guided FNAC *except*:**
   a. Position of the patient can be changed
   b. Real time
   c. Radiation exposure
   d. Significant obscuration due to air or bone

Answers

1. a. Aneurysm
2. d. Also useful in cystic goiter
3. d. All of the above
4. c. Radiation exposure

CHAPTER

16 Routine Laboratory Techniques

INTRODUCTION

In the last few decades, there is a massive advancement in laboratory techniques due to the introduction of various newer technologies. In spite of the modern technologies, the simple routine laboratory techniques are very important because basic staining of the smear and its morphological interpretation are essential for diagnosis. The optimum function of a laboratory depends on proper collection of sample, fixation of the material for cellular details, processing, staining, and accurate interpretation of the sample.

SAMPLE COLLECTION

Cervical Cytology

Preparation of the Patient

The sample should be collected 2 weeks after the first day of the last menstrual period. Patient should avoid the use of vaginal cream, jellies or tampons. She also should be refrained from sexual intercourse 48 hours before the test.

Labeling the Sample

The glass slide (frosted slide is preferred) or the vial [for liquid-based cytology (LBC)] must be labeled by unique identifier to prevent any mix up. The marker on the slide should be permanent so that it is not removed during processing of the smear. As frosted sample is costly so in our institution we use a diamond pencil to write the number on the slide.

Collection Devices

To date, no collection device has been universally accepted to get adequate Papanicolaou's (Pap) smear in all patients. The main target area of any collection device is the transformation zone. This is a dynamic area and may move upwards or downwards depending on the patient's age, parity, menstrual cycle, inflammation or premalignant condition of the cervix. The main aim of the cervical device is to collect the material from this transformation zone. The ideal sampling device should have certain advantages such as it should be accessible to both ectocervical and endocervical regions, the material should not stick to the device, it should not traumatize the region too much and the device should be cheap. Various types of cervical spatula and brushes are now available as a collection device (Fig. 16.1).

1. Wooden spatula
2. Plastic spatula

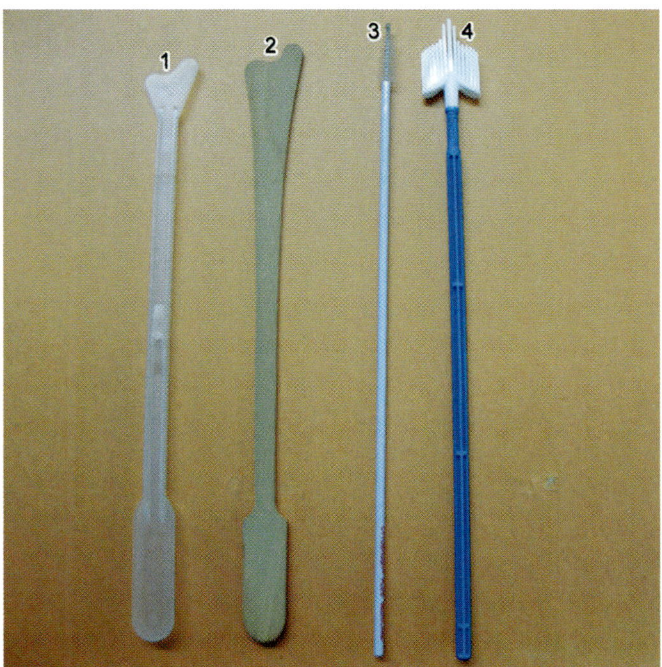

Fig. 16.1: Different sampling devices for the collection of cervical smear: (1) Plastic spatula, (2) Wooden spatula, (3) Endocervical brush, and (4) Cervex-brush.

Table 16.1: Advantages and disadvantages of different collection devices.

Collection device	*Advantages*	*Disadvantages*
Wooden spatula	• Cheap • Easy to use • Relatively atraumatic • Minimal blood contamination	• Cells may be trapped into wood • Endocervical cells are less
Plastic spatula	• Plastic prevents the cells to get trapped	• Costly than wooden spatula
Endocervical brush	• Easy to insert into the endocervical canal • Minimal entrapment of the cells with the brush	• Trauma to the endocervix by stiff bristles so bloody smear • Painful • Chances of air drying
Cotton tip applicator	• Minimum discomfort • Low cost • No trauma • Good amount of endocervical cells	• No ectocervical cells • Cells may be trapped into cotton fibers
Cervix-brush	• Samples of both ectocervix and endocervix on one slide	• Costly • The most widely used • Perfect for liquid-based cytology (LBC)

3. Endocervical brush
4. Cervix-brush.

Each device has certain advantages and disadvantages[1] (Table 16.1). The cervex-brush provides both ectocervix and endocervix on one slide. It is one of the most suitable devices and commonly used in LBC. However, these are costlier than any other sample collection devices.

In a meta-analysis study it has been suggested that the most effective collection device appears to be a combination of the cytobrush with an extended tip spatula.[2]

Box 16.1: Cervical smear collection.

Preparation of the patient:
- Not to use vaginal cream, jellies or tampons at least 2 days prior to the test
- Should not be in menstruation period
- No sexual intercourse within 48 hours

Collection devices:
- Cervex-brush
- Endocervical broom stick
- Plastic spatula
- Wooden spatula

Collection proper:
- Position of the patient: Dorsolithotomy
- Preparation:
  - The vagina is cleaned by wet swab with water
  - No lubricant jellies should be used
  - The plastic spatula is inserted within the vagina
  - The spatula is rotated 360°
  - The sample on the spatula is spread on the glass slide
  - The slide is immediately immersed in 95% ethanol for fixation

Collection Proper (Box 16.1)

The position of the patient: The cervical smear is taken by keeping the patient in dorsolithotomy position. In this position cervix is widely visualized.

Preparation: The vagina is cleaned by wet swab. No lubricant jellies should be used. A speculum is introduced to visualize the cervix. The main focus should be on the transformation zone as most of the preneoplastic lesions develop from this area. Proper inspection of the ectocervix and transformation zone is required and smear should be taken from the abnormal area first. Ectocervix is smooth pink and opaque whereas the endocervix is dark pink.

Collection: For the conventional smear either broom or spatula is used. At first the spatula is inserted within the vagina and the tip of the spatula should be fitted with the contour of the cervix. The spatula is rotated 360° and then it is withdrawn with the material on the one surface. The sample on the spatula is spreaded on the glass slide and the slide is immediately fixed in the 95% ethyl alcohol for 30 minutes. Alternatively spray fixative can be used. Before Papanicolaou's staining the carbowax of the spray fixative must be removed by dipping the slide in alcohol. For LBC preparation usually broom stick-like cervex-brush is used. The broom is introduced in such a way that the central part enters into the endocervical canal and the shorter bristles of the broom touch to the ectocervix (Fig. 16.2). The broom is rotated 4–5 times in a clockwise direction. Then the broom is withdrawn and dipped in the fixative solution provided by the company.

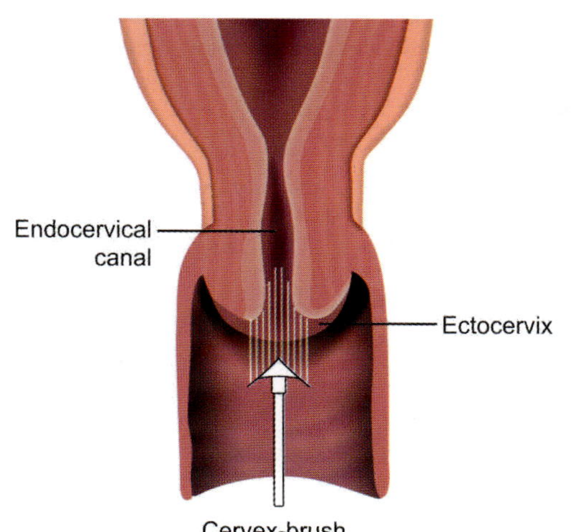

Fig. 16.2: Method of collection of cervical smear with the help of cervix-brush.

Vaginal Smear

The speculum is gently introduced and the lateral vaginal wall is visualized. With the help of a spatula scraping is done from the lateral vaginal wall and the smear is prepared.

Endometrial Aspiration Smear

A sterile canula is inserted into the uterine cavity and with the help of a syringe the material is gently sucked. The aspirated material is spread onto the glass slide and fixed immediately.

Sputum Sample

A morning specimen of sputum should be obtained in a clean wide mouthed container. If necessary, aerosol can be used to get the sputum. Sputum should be sent fresh to the laboratory and no fixative is recommended.

Fluid Sample

Body cavity fluids are collected in a dry clean container as a fresh sample.[3,4] It is preferable to collect the fluid without any fixative and the material should be sent as fresh sample to the laboratory for immediate processing. In our laboratory we collect the fluid in anticoagulant solution to prevent clotting of the fluid. We use 1:9 ratio of ammonium oxalate:fluid. The collected fluid may be kept in a refrigerator if the processing of the fluid is not possible immediately. If a long delay in processing is expected, then an equal amount of 50% ethyl alcohol is mixed with the fluid during the time of collection of the sample.[3] Under no circumstances, fluid for cytological examination is allowed to be frozen.

Urine Sample

The urine sample should be collected 3–4 hours after last micturation. Fresh randomly voided urine specimen should be collected in a clean container and should be sent to the laboratory for immediate processing to avoid any degenerative changes.

Washings

Washing samples are usually sent as fresh without any fixative. The sample should be processed immediately. If a delay in the processing is expected then the fluid is mixed with equal amount of 50% ethanol.

Brushing

Brushing can be submitted in three ways:[4] (1) direct smear, (2) contents of the brush, and (3) tip of the brush.

Direct Smear

The brush is gently rolled over a clean glass slide within 1 inch area. The slide is then immediately fixed by immersing in 95% ethyl alcohol or by spray fixative.

Contents of the Brush and Tip of the Brush

Brush is dipped into the container with a physiologic transport solution and is shaken vigorously. Equal volume of 50% ethyl alcohol is mixed and then the whole container is sent to the laboratory. Alternatively the tip of the brush can be dipped and cut in the liquid supplied by the manufacturer of the liquid-based system. The whole thing is sent to the laboratory. Separate set of fixative should be used for each brush to prevent any contamination.

FIXATION

Preservation of the cellular detail is necessary for studying the cell and to make a diagnosis. It is very much essential to prevent autolysis and to keep the cell as close as possible to the living stage in the body.

Principle of fixation: Fixative prevents the autolytic degradation of the cell by promoting rapid coagulation of the various enzyme proteins. The alcohol removes water

Box 16.2: Fixation.

Desirable properties of fixative:
- Rapid action
- Prevention of cellular distortion
- Maintaining nuclear details
- Facilitation of staining
- Inactivation of microbial organisms
- Fixing the cell on glass slide

Routine fixatives for Papanicolaou and hematoxylin stains:
- 95% ethyl alcohol
- 100% metahnol
- Denatured alcohol

Time of fixation: 15 minutes
Hemorrhagic fluid: Carnoy's fixative
Fixatives for liquid-based preparation:
- ThinPrep system: Methanol-based preservative
- SurePath system: Ethanol-based preservative

Cell block: 10% neutral buffered formalin
Immunocytochemistry: 95% ethanol
Electron microscopy: Glutaraldehyde solution (2.5%)

from the tissue and causing destabilizing of the hydrogen bonds and thereby disruption of the tertiary structure of the enzymatic protein. However, the secondary structure of the protein is maintained.

Essential properties: The cytological fixative should have some essential properties such as rapid action, prevention of cellular distortion, facilitation of staining, and preservation of nuclear detail (Box 16.2).

Common Wet Fixatives for Routine Stain

For Papanicolaou's stain and hematoxylin and eosin stain following fixatives are used:

- *95% ethyl alcohol*: It is the most commonly used fixative. Ethanol causes dehydration of the cell and mild shrinkage.
- *100% methanol*: It is equally effective as 95% ethanol. However it is not cost effective.
- *Denatured alcohol*: This is also equally good. The main advantage of denatured alcohol is that it is unsuitable for human consumption.

Time of Fixation

The smear should be kept in this fixative for at least 15 minutes. Prolonged fixation usually does not alter the morphology of the cells. However it is better to keep the slides in the refrigerator in a closed bottle or jar.

Coating Fixatives

Different varieties of spray fixative are available in the market from different companies. The fixative may be applied as spray or drops to coat the smear (Box 16.3). The main advantage of spray fixative is to avoid bottles with liquid fixative. There are two major functions of spray fixatives: (1) cell fixation and (2) protective covering of thin wax over the smear. The major ingredients of coating fixatives are alcohol and wax. So before staining procedure, the wax should be removed by keeping the smear in 95% ethanol.

The coat fixatives are particularly used for cervical smears. However, the coating fixatives are not recommended for smears prepared from fluid specimen. It is also not recommended for bloody smears as spray fixatives may cause red blood cell (RBC) clumping. The spray fixative should be applied from optimal distance which is considered as 10–12 inches away from the smear.

Box 16.3: Spray fixatives.

Advantage:
- To avoid bottles with liquid fixative

Functions:
- Cell fixation
- Protective covering of thin wax over the smear

Main use:
- Cervical smear

Not recommended:
- Smears prepared from fluid specimen
- Bloody smears

Optimal distance of spray:
- 10–12 inches away from the smear

Special Fixatives

Hemorrhagic Fluid

Carnoy's fixative: It is made of 95% ethanol (60 mL), chloroform (30 mL), and glacial acetic acid (10 mL). This fixative is the most suitable for blood-mixed smear as acetic acid lyses the blood. The nuclear detail of the cell is well preserved. However, Carnoy's fixative may cause remarkable cell shrinkage and overstaining of nucleus by hematoxylin. This fixative should always be used fresh and should be discarded after use.

Fixatives for Liquid-based Preparation

Presently two types of liquid-based systems are available in the market: (1) ThinPrep and (2) SurePath. The ThinPrep system supplies methanol-based preservative and SurePath system supplies ethanol-based preservative for fixation of the cervical samples.

Fixatives for Cell Block

10% neutral buffered formalin: Neutral buffered formaldehyde solution contains 40% formaldehyde (100 mL),

Box 16.4: Preservation of sample prior to processing.

Specimen with high mucus content:
- 24 hours to keep in refrigerator
- Sputum

Specimen with high protein content:
- 24–48 hours to keep in refrigerator
- Peritoneal, pericardial, and pleural fluid

Specimen with low mucus and protein content:
- 1–2 hours
- Urine
- Cerebrospinal fluid (CSF)

Specimen with low pH:
- Immediate processing
- Gastric aspirate

Box 16.6: Receiving the samples.

Slide:
- Slide should be sent in a shock-resistant container
- Slide should be properly labeled
- Paper form should be in a separate bag

Liquid:
- Airtight container
- Proper labeling of the container
- Plastic container is preferable than glass container in case of large amount of liquid sample

water (900 mL), acid sodium phosphate (4 g), and anhydrous disodium phosphate (6.5 g). This is the most suitable solution for cell button fixation to make a cell block.

Fixatives for Immunocytochemistry

95% ethanol: Routine fixative such as 95% ethanol can be used for immunocytochemistry.

Fixatives for Electron Microscopy

Glutaraldehyde solution (2.5%) is most suitable for electron microscopy as it fixes the cell rapidly and preserves the cellular organelles to study.

PRESERVATION OF SAMPLE PRIOR TO PROCESSING

It is expected that the procured sample should be processed immediately. However, it may not always be feasible to process the sample immediately. Specimen with high mucus and protein content can be kept for a few hours to days before processing (Box 16.4). Specimens with no sugar or protein, with extreme pH cannot be kept for a long time.

Box 16.5: Requisition form.

- Name
- Age
- Sex
- Unique identification of the patient (hospital entry number)
- Date of collection
- Site and procedure of collection
- Clinician's name, telephone or fax number
- Tests to be done

Clinical history:
- Chief complaints
- Salient physical findings
- Radiological features
- *Important history*: Surgery, chemotherapy, radiotherapy, exposure of chemicals, history of immunosuppressions, etc.

PROCESSING OF LABORATORY SAMPLES

Processing of a laboratory sample includes several steps of receiving, preparing smear, staining, to final submission of the slide for interpretation.

Receiving the Sample

Requisition form: The sample should always be accompanied with a proper requisition form (Box 16.5).

Glass slides and liquid sample (Box 16.6): The slide should be properly fixed and labeled. It is important to keep the slide in proper container to prevent the breaking of the glass slide. The slide should not be wrapped by requisition form. The paper form should be sent separately. Similarly liquid sample should always be kept in an airtight container with proper labeling.

Unique identification number: It is preferable to check the unique identification number of the sample and requisition form before processing the sample.

Laboratory bar code: A unique laboratory bar code number can be generated by the computer for each sample and this can be sticked on the wall of the container , slides and also on the requisition form.

PROCESSING

Processing of different sample is highlighted in Table 16.2. The common processing techniques are:

- Direct smear
- Centrifuge
- Cytocentrifuge
- Liquid-based preparation
- Millipore technique
- Cell block.

Processing of Sputum

Sputum should be kept in a Petri dish and carefully examined on a black background. Any tissue fragments or gray-white substance or bloody material should be picked up by a clean forceps and smears are prepared on the clean glass slide.

Processing of Fluid

Centrifuge

Fluid specimen should be put in clean airtight centrifuged tube. It is preferable to use a plastic tube than glass tube. The sample is then rotated at 1,500 rounds per minute (RPM) for 10 minutes. The supernatant liquid is discarded and multiple smears are made from the sediments.

Table 16.2: Processing of sample.

Sample	*Processing*
Moderate amount of fluid (40–50 mL effusion fluid, 2–5 mL washing, etc.)	Centrifuge
Large amount (100 mL to 1000 mL) of clear fluid (urine)	Millipore filtration
Small amount of fluid [<1 mL such as cerebrospinal fluid (CSF), vitreous fluid, ureteric sample, etc.]	Cytocentrifuge
Sputum	Pick and process method
Material for immunocytochemistry	Cell block preparation

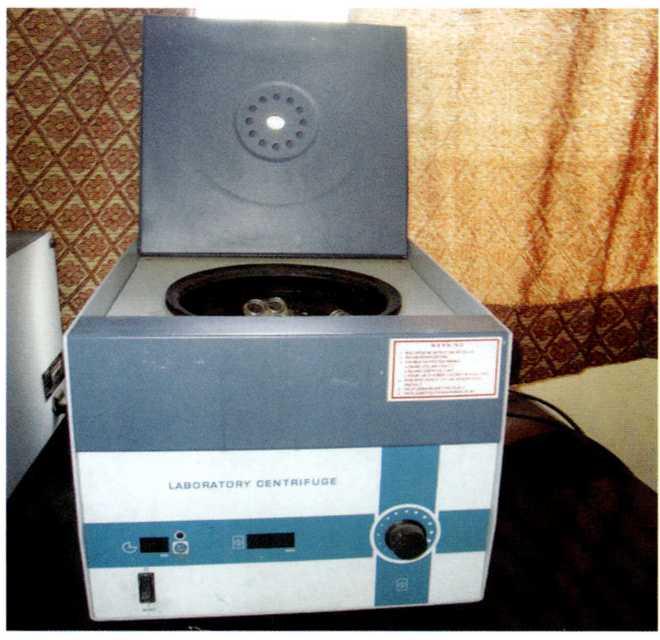

Fig. 16.3: Centrifuge machine.

Cytocentrifuge

If the quantity of the sample is small then cytocentrifugation is done in 1,000 RPM for 5 minutes. A thin layer of smear is formed on the glass slide. The smears are immediately fixed in 95% ethanol for staining.

Centrifugation Technique (Figs. 16.3 and 16.4)

A centrifuge is one of the important separation devices by which the particles in a solution are separated according to their size, shape, density, and viscosity of the suspension medium.

Basic principle: In a liquid suspension, the particles whose density is higher than the liquid sink and the lighter particles float. The movement of the particles in the liquid media greatly depends on the density difference with the suspension liquid. When a particle moves rapidly along the central axis, a centrifugal force is created. This centrifugal force if overcomes the other forces such as byoant force (force to float the particle) and frictional force (the force developed due to friction of the particle in the liquid) then the particle will try to go away from the center (Fig. 16.5). The relative centrifugal force (RCF) depends on the radius of the arm of the centrifuge machine and the rotational rate of the arms. If,

- Relative centrifugal force = RCF
- Rotational radius = r
- Angular velocity in radians per unit time= ω
- Gravitational acceleration = g

$$RCF = \frac{r\omega^2}{g}$$

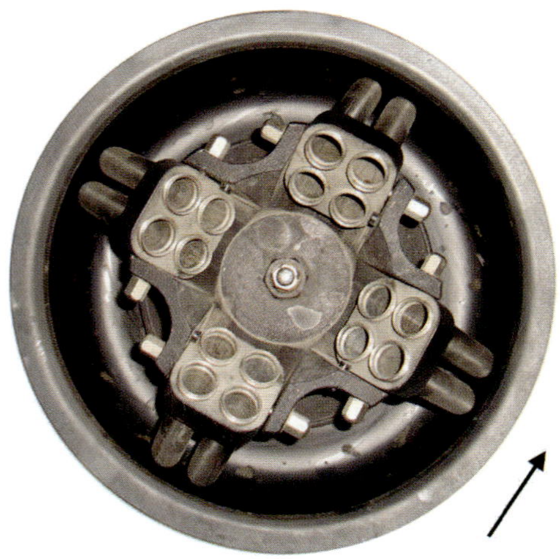

Fig. 16.4: Interior of the centrifuge machine.

The relationship may be expressed as:

$$RCF = 1.11 \times 10^{-5} \times (RPM)^2 \times r$$

The principle of cytocentrifuge is similar to that of the centrifuge. There are two main advantages of cytocentrifuge: (1) small volume of fluid is processed and (2) the smear is directly prepared on the glass slide.

There are two types of commercially available cytocentrifuge: (1) the cytocentrifuge that removes the fluid during the time of sedimentation (Figs. 16.6 to 16.8) and (2) the cytocentrifuge that retains the fluid. When the fluid is removed during the time of sedimentation, the cells experience hydraulic force due to the flow of fluid away from the sample area. The sedimentation velocity should be greater than hydraulic force and a high cell recovery depends on the balance between the centrifugal force and hydraulic force during the machine operation time. In

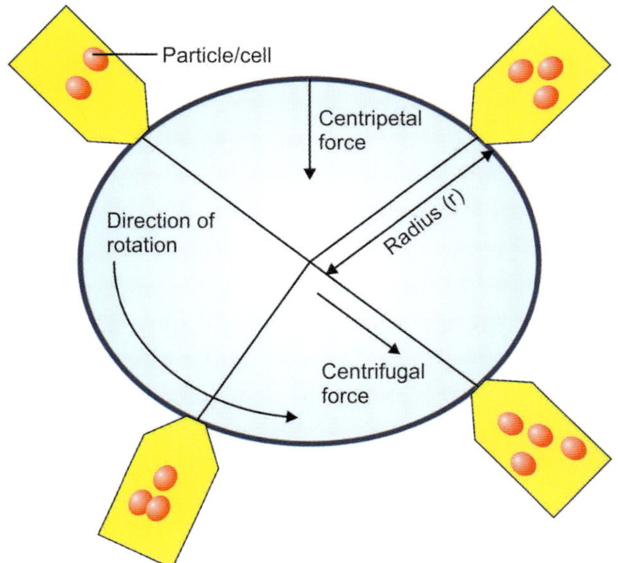

Fig. 16.5: Basic principle of centrifugation is highlighted by this schematic diagram. Centrifugation technique replaces the gravity by a more powerful "centrifugal force" to enhance the rate of sedimentation of suspended particles that are denser than the suspension liquid.

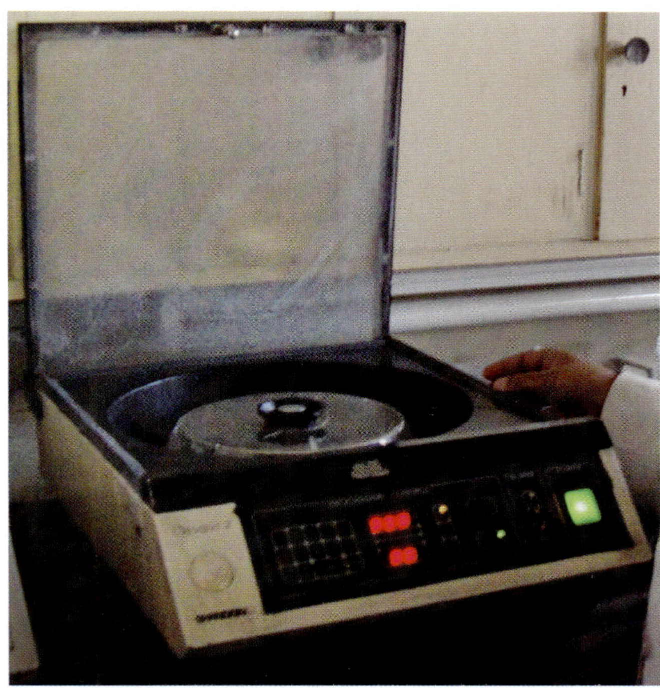

Fig. 16.6: Cytocentrifuge machine.

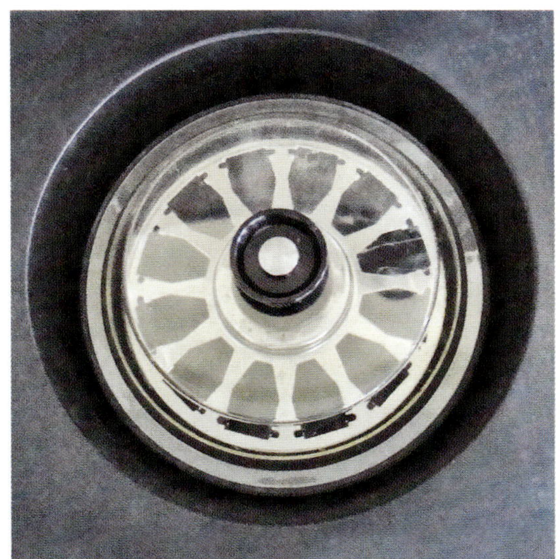

Fig. 16.7: Interior chamber of the cytocentrifuge machine.

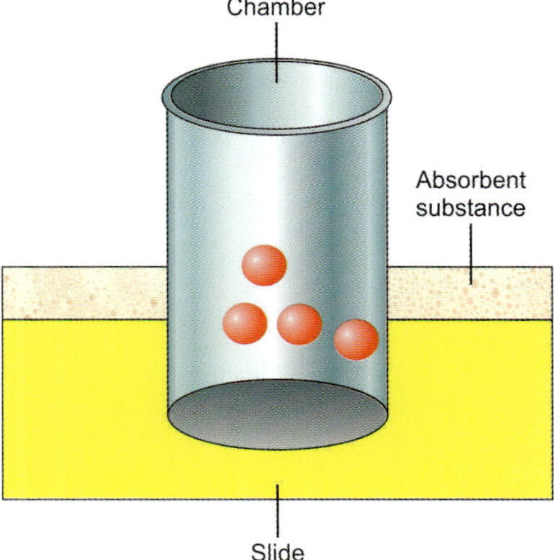

Fig. 16.8: Basic process of the cytocentrifuge technique. Here the liquid suspension medium is absorbed by the absorbent.

another type of centrifugation machine, where the fluid is not removed during sedimentation, the centrifugal force should be adequate to flatten the cells on the glass slide. The supernatant fluid should also be removed carefully. Cytocentrifugation may cause morphological distortion of the cells and careful attention should be given in this aspect. The optimum rotational speed of the machine is the most important factor in this respect.

Millipore Filtration

The Millipore filtration technique is done for processing large quantity of clear urine sample. The Millipore filter paper is moistened with normal saline and the paper is put on the sieve. The filter cup is attached and the sample is put in the filter cup. The negative pressure at 100 mm Hg is created and the fluid is drained into the bottle leaving the cell on the filter paper (Fig. 16.9). Multiple imprint smears on albumin coated slides are made and the slides are fixed immediately in 95% alcohol for 30 minutes.

Processing of Hemorrhagic Fluid

Carony's fixative: This can be used for processing of hemorrhagic fluid.

Buffy coat preparation: This is an alternative way to process bloody samples. The hemorrhagic sample first centrifuged at 2,000 RPM for 10 minutes. The supernatant fluid is discarded. The residual suspension is taken in 2–3 inches long capillary tube. The one end of the tube is sealed and then the capillary tube is centrifuged. The capillary is broken in the buffy coat region and fish tail preparation of smear is made.

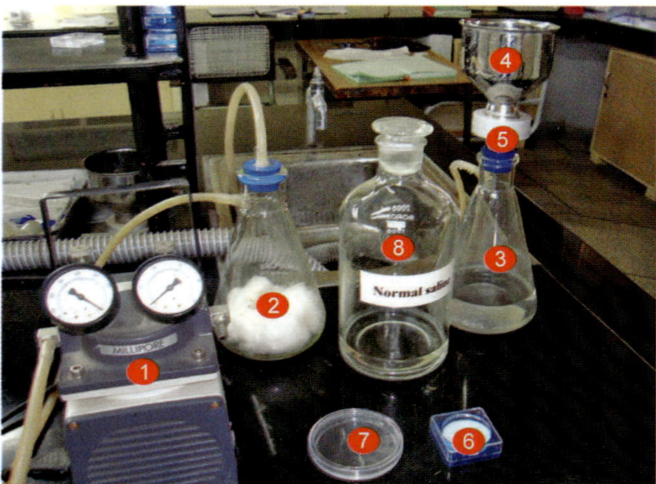

Fig. 16.9: Basic equipments of the Millipore filtration technique are shown: (1) Pump for negative suction, (2) Conical flask, (3) Conical flask attached with filter cup, (4) Filter cup, (5) Sieve, (6) Millipore filter paper, (7) Petri dish, and (8) Normal saline to moisten the filter paper.

Cell Block

The cell block technique helps to get the paraffin-embedded tissue and thus multiple sections can be obtained to do routine hematoxylin and eosin stain, cytochemistry, and immunocytochemistry. Another added advantage of cell block is to keep material for archival use. The cell block is made by the following steps:

1. The specimen is collected in 10% neutral buffered formalin
2. The specimen is kept 4 hours in formalin to fix the cells
3. Centrifuge the sample 1,500 RPM for 10 minutes
4. Wash the sediment twice in PBS by centrifugation
5. Add 100 μL of plasma and 30 μL thrombin
6. The clot is removed and collected on filter paper
7. The clot is processed in the tissue processor.

Compact Cell Block Technique

Yang et al.[5] described compact cell block technique that is in a small area and completely free of RBCs.

Steps:

1. Fluid containing the material is centrifuged.
2. CytoRich solution (designed for hemolysis and gentle fixation of the cell) is added in 1:1 ratio to the sediment and is kept for 2 minutes.
3. Then four drops of plasma and three drops of thrombin (5,000 IU/mL) are added.
4. The mixture is gently agitated to make a cell clot.
5. The clot is transferred to the lens paper.
6. The compact clot is wrapped and then fixed into formalin.
7. The tissue is processed in the tissue processor.

STAINING

Papanicolaou's staining is a worldwide accepted staining method and the staining technique is named as Dr George Papanicolaou, the Father of Cytopathology. This stain is done in all cervical smear and non-gynecologic exfoliative smears. It is a multichromatic staining which helps in the display of cellular maturation, cytoplasmic details and nuclear details. It is a transparent stain so cells with overlapping nuclei can also be studied by this stain.

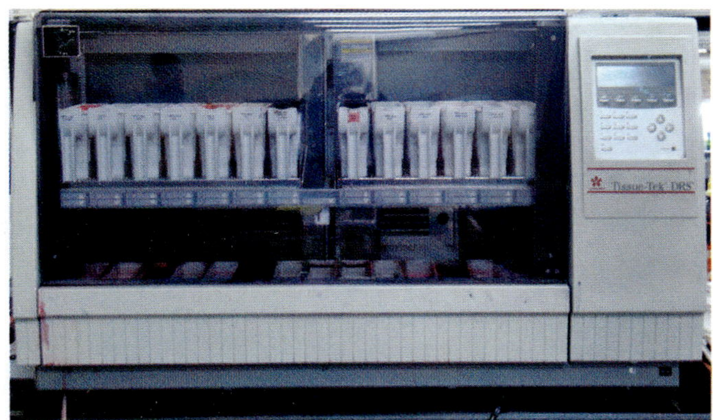

Fig. 16.10: Automatic stainer.

Over the years, various modifications have been done on Papanicolaou's staining in laboratory to laboratory. Presently automated staining technique is available in many laboratories (Fig. 16.10).

Progressive Method

Here the intensity of the nuclear stain is done up to the desired level and the cytoplasm barely takes the dye.

Regressive Method

Here the nuclei are deliberately overstained by hematoxylin dye and then excess stain is removed by diluted hydrochloric acid solution.

Dyes Used in Papanicolaou's Staining

Hematoxylin: Harris hematoxylin is used for nuclear stain.
Orange G (OG): OG-6 is used for cytoplasmic counterstain. This dye specifically stains keratin component of the cytoplasm.

Eosin azure (EA): It is a polychrome stain and consists of three dyes: (1) eosin Y, (2) light-green SF yellowish, and (3) Bismarck brown Y.

Principle of Basic Steps

Basic steps include:

1. *Rehydration of the smear*: By gradual dip of the smear in graded concentration of alcohol.
2. *Nuclear staining by hematoxylin*: Harris hematoxylin is used for the nuclear stain. The excess hematoxyline is removed by 0.25% aqueous solution of hydrochloric acid (0.05% for milipore filter). To make the stain more stable the smear is further treated with a weak alkaline solution.
3. *Cytoplasmic staining by OG*: The smear is again brought into alcohol and stained with OG. OG is an acidic dye and stains keratin as orange color.
4. *Cytoplasmic staining by EA*: EA is a synthetic dye and stains cytoplasm as blue-green color.
5. *Dehydration by absolute alcohol*: Rinsing the smear with absolute alcohol causes dehydration.
6. *Clearing by xylene*: The smear is dipped in xylene. Xylene has the same refractive index as that of glass and mounting medium.
7. *Mounting by dibutylphthalate polystyrene xylene (DPX)*: Mounting medium should be miscible with the clearing agent. It prevents fading of the stain.

Papanicolaou's Staining Steps

These steps include:

1. 70% ethanol: 1 minutes
2. 50% ethanol: 1 minutes
3. Distilled water: 5 dips
4. Harris hematoxylin: Three and half minutes
5. Distilled water: 5 dips
6. 0.25% aqueous solution of hydrochloric acid: Few dips
7. Water: 1 minute
8. Lithium carbonate: One and half minute
9. Water: Few dips
10. 70% ethanol: 2 minute
11. 90% ethanol: 2 minute
12. Orange G: few dips
13. 95% ethanol: 2 minutes
14. EA modified: 2 minutes
15. Absolute ethyl alcohol: Three changes, 2 minutes each
16. Xylene: 5 minutes or till clear
17. Mounting in DPX.

Hematoxylin solution for Papanicolaou's stain:

- Harris hematoxylin: 10 g
- Water: 2 L
- Alum: 200 g
- Absolute alcohol: 100 mL
- Mercuric oxide: 5 g.

Eosin azure solution:

- Eosin: 4 g
- Light green: 0.4 g
- Water: 480 mL
- Alcohol: 500 mL
- Phosphotungstic acid: 2 g
- Glacial acetic acid: 20 mL.

Precautions to be Taken in Papanicolaou's Staining

The following precautions should be taken in Papanicolaou's staining:

- *Staining solutions*:
    - The concentration of stain should be checked regularly. The containers should always be covered to prevent evaporation of fluid. The stain solutions should be periodically replaced to maintain the quality of the stain. Hematoxylin should be changed every day and OG-6 and EA should be changed weekly. Xylene should be changed immediately if it is tinted.
    - The stain solution should be free of stain deposits and should be filtered daily.
- *Containers*: The containers should be washed regularly.
- *Coverslip*:
    - Smears should not dry before placing the coverslip.
    - No air bubbles should be present between the coverslip and smear.
- *Staining proper*: Minor agitation of the slides prevents staining deposit and gives better staining.
- *Too dark nuclear stain*:
    - If the smear is kept in Harris hematoxylin for a long time
    - Too less hydrochloric acid concentration
    - Too less number of dips in hydrochloric acid
- *Too pale nuclear stain*:
    - If hematoxylin is diluted
    - Too less bluing
    - Too much concentration of hydrochloric acid
    - Too much dip in hydrochloric acid
    - Air dried smear prior to fixation
- *Improper cytoplasmic stain*:
    - Smear is air dried prior to fixation
    - If the slides remain in alcohol for too long time then the cytoplasmic stain may be pale
    - If the pH of EA is not optimum
    - If the slide remains in hematoxylin for too long time

Destaining and Restaining of the Smear

For destaining of the smear the following steps are done in our laboratory in Post Graduate Institute of Medical Education and Research, Chandigarh, India:

1. The smear is kept in xylene until the coverslip drops.
2. The smear is then kept in acid alcohol for 20 minutes (80 mL of 95% ethanol and 20 mL of 0.5% hydrochloric acid).
3. The smear is then washed with running water.
4. The smear is restained.

Ultrafast Papanicolaou's Staining

Ultrafast Papanicolaou's staining was first developed by Yang et al. for rapid staining of fine needle aspiration cytology (FNAC). In this technique, the air dried smear is first dipped in normal saline for 30 seconds. The smear is then dipped in alcoholic formalin for 10 seconds. After this the smear is processed as usual for Papanicolaou's stain.[6]

May-Grünwald Giemsa Stain

May-Grünwald Giemsa (MGG) is a Romanowski's stain and is used in addition to Papanicolaou's and hematoxylin and eosin stain in many laboratories. This stain provides excellent cytoplasmic details character. This is a metachromatic stain. MGG is a convenient stain for FNAC smear. Table 16.3 compares the relative advantages and disadvantages of MGG stain over Papanicolaou's stain.

Steps:

1. May-Grünwald Giemsa solution: 5 minutes
2. Running water: 1 minute
3. Giemsa stain: 15 minutes
4. Running water: 1 minute
5. Air drying.

DEHYDRATION AND CLEARING OF THE SMEAR

After performing Papanicolaou's or hematoxyline and eosin stain the smear is dehydrated by a series of increasing concentration of alcohol. Sudden dipping of the slide in absolute alcohol is detrimental for cell morphology. Removal of alcohol or clearing of the sample is done by putting the sample in xylene. The chemical compound of xylene is dimethyl benzene. The clearing agent should be colorless and its refractive index should be close to the mounting media and coverslip (Box 16.7).

Table 16.3: Comparison of Papanicolaou's stain and May-Grünwald Giemsa (MGG) stain.

Parameters	*Papanicolaou's stain*	*MGG stain*
Nuclear detail	Excellent and very good stain for chromatin stain	The chromatin pattern cannot be studied
Keratin demonstration	Orange G stains keratin as bright orange color	Cannot be demonstrated
Metachromasia	Not a metachromatic stain	Metachromatic stain
Transparency	Transparent stain	Not a transparent stain
Background mucin or necrosis	Not good	Good for demonstration of extracellular substance

Box 16.7: Clearing agent.

- Xylene commonly used (dimethyl benzene)

Basic properties:
- Colorless
- Refractive index close to the mounting media and coverslip
- It should render the transparent cytoplasm

Caution: Toxic

Box 16.8: Mounting medium.

- It does bonding between the smear and the coverslip
- It should have same refractive index of coverslip and clearing agent
- Miscible with clearing agent to prevent optical distortion
- Neutral pH
- Low viscosity to prevent air bubbles formation (cornflakes artifact) during putting coverslip

MOUNTING

Mounting medium covers the smear and acts as a permanent bond between the coverslip and the slides. Mounting medium should have the same refractive index of the coverslip and glass slide (Box 16.8). The refractive index of the mounting medium should be 1.52–1.54. Mounting medium should have a neutral pH to prevent the fading of the stain. The viscosity of the mounting medium should be low, otherwise there may be air bubble formation at the time of putting the coverslip. This air bubbles are brownish in color and is known as a *cornflake artifact* (Fig. 16.11).

COVERSLIP

Coverslip should be wide enough to cover the smear properly. No 1 coverslip made up of clear glass of 0.130–0.170 mm thickness is preferable. The surface of the coverslip should be plane and the margins should be straight. Coverslipping should be done once at a time to prevent air drying of the smear. It should always be done in properly ventilated well-lighted area. Plastic coverslip, liquid coverslip, and automated coverslipper are freely available in the market. It is preferable that the mounting medium is dried and the coverslip should be fixed to the slide before examination of the slide (Box 16.9).

STORAGE

After reporting all the positive slide should be stored properly and should not be discarded. However the negative slide should be stored for a minimum of 5 years according to rules and legislation of the country.

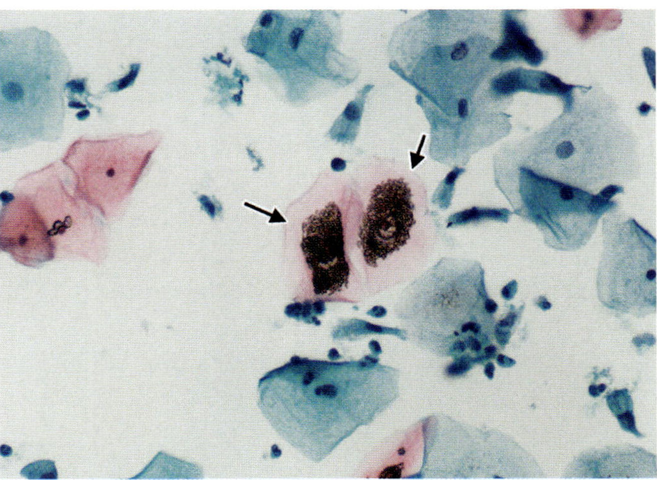

Fig. 16.11: Air bubbles trapped between the coverslip and the glass slide giving rise to cornflakes like cell (Papanicolaou's stain X HP). The arrows indicate the cornflakes like cells.

Box 16.9: Coverslipping.

Coverslip:
- No 1 glass coverslip of 0.130–0.170 mm thickness
- Refractive index: 1.5
- Plane and no irregular surface

Technique:
- Put the mounting medium on the coverslip
- Reverse the coverslip and place it on the glass slide over the smear
- Coverslipping area should be well ventilated and properly lighted
- Mounting medium should be dried before submission of the slide

Comment: Liquid coverslip and automatic coverslipper are also effective

REFERENCES

1. Schumann JL, O'Connor DM, Covell JL, et al. Pap smear collection devices: Technical, clinical, diagnostic, and legal considerations associated with their use. Diagn Cytopathol. 1992;8(5):492-503.
2. Martin-Hirsch P, Jarvis G, Kitchener H, et al. Collection devices for obtaining cervical cytology samples. Cochrane Database Syst Rev. 2000;2:CD001036.
3. NCCLS. Nongynecologic cytologic specimens: Collection and cytopreparatory techniques; approved guideline. NCCLS document GP 23-A[ISBN 1-56238-380-9]. NCCLS, West Valley Road, Suite 14000, Wayne Pennsylvania 19087-1898 USA, 1999.
4. Nongynecologic cytology practice guideline. Acta Cytol. 2004;48(4):521-46.
5. Yang GC, Wan LW, Papellas J, et al. Compact cell blocks. Use for body fluids, fine needle aspirations and endometrial brush biopsies. Acta Cytol. 1998;42(3):703-6.
6. Yang GC, Papellas J, Wu HC, et al. Application of Ultrafast Papanicolaou stain to body fluid cytology. Acta Cytol. 2001;45(2):180-5.

Review Questions

1. **The most suitable fixative for hemorrhagic fluid is:**
   a. Carnoy's fixative b. 95% ethyl alcohol
   c. 100% methanol d. 10% buffered formalin
2. **The best fixative for cell block material is:**
   a. Denatured alcohol b. 95% ethyl alcohol
   c. 100% methanol d. 10% buffered formalin
3. **Small amount (0.5 mL) of vitreous fluid is best processed by:**
   a. Centrifuge b. Cytocentrifuge
   c. Millipore filtration d. Liquid-based cytology
4. **Keratin within the cytoplasm is best stained by:**
   a. Hematoxylin b. Eosin
   c. Orange G d. Schiff's reagent

Identify True/False

5. **For Papanicolaou's stain 10% formalin fixative are also used.** *(True/False)*
6. **Carnoy's fixative contains 95% ethanol, chloroform, and glacial acetic acid.** *(True/False)*
7. **The best fixatives for cell block is 10% neutral buffered formalin.** *(True/False)*
8. **Conventional Papanicolaou staining is a regressive staining technique.** *(True/False)*
9. **May-Grünwald Giemsa stain is a metachromatic stain.** *(True/False)*
10. **The trapped air bubbles under the coverslip causes cornflakes artifact.** *(True/False)*

Answers

1. a. Carnoy's fixative
2. d. 10% buffered formalin
3. b. Cytocentrifuge
4. c. Orange G
5. False
6. True
7. True
8. True
9. True
10. True

CHAPTER

17 Special Stains and Immunocytochemistry

INTRODUCTION

Cytochemistry and immunocytochemistry (IC) are now an integral part of the routine laboratory service. In this chapter, the basic principles, indications, and the significance of these stains have been discussed.

SPECIAL STAINS

Special stains are required in addition to routine cytology for various purposes. This is highlighted in Box 17.1. The preliminary aim of the special stains is the diagnosis and subtyping of the malignant cells by identifying certain cell products and also diagnosis of various infective agent particularly acid fast bacteria and fungi.

PERIODIC ACID-SCHIFF STAIN

Periodic acid-Schiff (PAS) stain demonstrates glycogen. Glycoprotein, sialomucin, and neutral mucin are all positive for PAS stain. PAS positive material takes deep magenta color stain.

Basic Principle

In this staining reaction, the hydroxyl group attached to the carbon atom in carbohydrate is oxidized to two free aldehyde groups by periodic acid. This aldehyde group reacts with Schiff's reagent and produces deep magenta color. PAS positive reaction occurs in glycogen and also monosaccharides, polysaccharides, glycoproteins, mucoproteins, phosphorylated sugars, inositol derivatives, and cerebrosides.

Box 17.1: Applications of special stains in cytology.

- To demonstrate cellular products for confirmation of the type of malignant cells:
  - PAS-Alcian blue with or without diastase in mesothelioma
  - Mucicarmine stains for mucinous adenocarcinoma
  - Melanin for melanoma
  - Oil red O for lipid in renal cell carcinoma
- To demonstrate some extracellular substances with special importance such as amyloid by Congo red stain
- To demonstrate infective organisms such as Gram-positive bacteria, acid fast bacteria, or fungi
- DNA stain for DNA content and ploidy.

Application

Periodic acid-Schiff stain is used to demonstrate glycogen in the cells of adenocarcinoma, demonstration of fungus (capsule) and any mucopolysaccharide substances, basement membrane, and mucin.

Steps

- Alcohol fixed smear to pass through graded lower concentration of alcohol and smear to bring in water
- Periodic acid (1%) for 10 minutes
- Clean with water
- Schiff's reagent for 30 minutes
- Clean in running tap water for 5 minutes
- Counter stain with hematoxylin
- 95% ethyl alcohol
- Absolute alcohol
- Clear in xylene
- Mounting.

MUCICARMINE STAIN

Mucicarmine technique is used to demonstrate mucins particularly acid mucin.

Principle

The active dye molecule in mucicarmine stain is a chelate complex made of cationic aluminum ions and multiring molecule carminic acid. This positively charged chelate complex is known as carmine. Possibly, this positively charged carmine reacts by electrostatic attraction to the anionic groups of acid mucins.

Applications

Mucicarmine stain is applied to demonstrate acid mucin in the malignant cells of adenocarcinoma. It also stains capsule of *Cryptococcus*.

Steps

- Smears to bring in water
- Hematoxylin for 5–10 minutes
- Wash in water
- Mucicarmine solution for 60 minutes
- Wash in water
- Metanil yellow solution for 30 seconds
- Rinse in water
- 95% ethyl alcohol
- Absolute alcohol
- Xylene
- Mount.

Interpretation

Positive mucicarmine stain shows dark red color.

ALCIAN BLUE

Alcian blue stains acid mucin. Acid mucin is sulfated tissue mucin and reacts with a cationic dye.

Basic Principle

Alcian blue is a group of water soluble polyvalent basic dye. The dye is made of a copper-containing phthalocyanine ring with copper atom in its center. Phthalocyanine ring is also attached with four isothiouronium groups that are positively charged. This positively charged Alcian blue dye complex has an attraction with anionic sites of the mucin. Copper imparts the blue color of the dye-mucin complex.

Application

To stain acid mucin present in mesothelioma cells in pleural fluid.

Method

- Rehydration of smear by graded alcohol
- Rinse in water
- Keep the smear in Alcian blue for 30 minutes
- Rinse in water
- Counter stain with hematoxyline for 5 minutes
- 95% ethyl alcohol
- Absolute alcohol
- Xylene
- Mount.

OIL RED O

Oil red O stain is used for demonstration of lipid material. The lipid material takes deep red color in this stain.

Application

Oil red O is particularly useful to demonstrate lipid in renal cell carcinoma. The lipoblasts are also oil red O positive.

Steps

- Put the slides directly into oil red O solution for 20–30 minutes
- Rinse with running water
- Counterstain with hematoxyline for 30 seconds
- Rinse in water
- Mounting in glycerin.

Preparation of Oil Red O Stain

- *Oil red O*: 1.2 g
- *Alcohol, 70%*: 50 mL
- *Acetone*: 50 mL.

FEULGEN STAIN

This stain is specific for DNA and it demonstrates sugar deoxyribose. This is particularly helpful for DNA ploidy examination.

Basic Principle

With the help of hydrochloric acid the purine-deoxyribose bond is broken and then the exposed aldehyde group is demonstrated by Schiff's reagent. DNA is stained as deep red in color.

Application

Feulgen stain is particularly helpful for DNA ploidy examination.

Steps

- Rehydration of smear by graded alcohol
- Rinse in water
- 1(M) hydrochloric acid (preheated at 60°C) for 10 minutes
- Keep in Schiff's reagent for 10 minutes
- Immerse in 0.05 M metabisulfite for 2 minutes for three times
- Counter stain by 0.01% fast-green
- Dehydrate in absolute alcohol
- Xylene
- Mount.

CONGO RED STAIN

Congo red stain is specific for demonstration of amyloid material.

Principle

Congo red is an acidic diazo dye which consists of two molecules of napthionic acid attached to one molecule of Benzedrine. The dye molecules bind to amyloid by hydrogen bond and have an oriented arrangement on the amyloid fibrils. This binding of dye-amyloid complex causes absorption of certain wavelengths of light and produces greenish birefringence under polarized light.

Application

Congo red is used to demonstrate amyloid material particularly in abdominal fat pad and medullary carcinoma of thyroid.

Steps

- Slides bring in water
- Hematoxylin stain for 5 minutes
- Alkaline sodium chloride solution for 20 minutes
- Alkaline Congo red for 20 minutes
- Rinse in alcohol
- Dried and mount.

MYCOBACTERIAL STAINING

Mycobacterial group of organisms are all stained by Ziehl Neelsen staining.

Basic Principle

Mycobacterial cell wall contains mycolic acid. Mycolic acid greatly influences the penetration and removal of any dye. Phenolic acid and high temperature increase the porosity of the membrane and helps in the penetration of the dye. Mycolic acid resists the removal of the stain by acid and alcohol.

Application

Demonstration of *Mycobacterium tubercle* and *Lepra bacilli.*

Steps

- Bring the slide in water by treating it with graded alcohol
- Hot carbol fuchsin for 30 minutes
- Two to three dips in acid alcohol for differentiation
- Counter stain with methyline blue for 1 minute
- Clean with water
- Dry.

Acid Alcohol

- *Concentrated hydrochloric acid*: 3 mL
- *Alcohol 95%*: 97 mL.

Carbol Fuchsin

- *Basic fuchsin*: 0.5 g
- *Absolute alcohol*: 5 mL
- *5% aqueous phenol*: 100 mL.

Methyline Blue Stock Solution

- *Methyline blue*: 1.4 g
- *95% Ethanol*: 100 mL.

Methyline Blue Working Solution

- *Methyline blue stock solution*: 10 mL
- *Water*: 90 mL.

IMMUNOCYTOCHEMISTRY

Basic Principles

The basic principle of IC is to sharp visual recognition of antigen in the cell by applying antigen antibody reaction. The antigen is the substance that is recognized by a particular immunoglobulin or T cell receptor to produce an immune response. The specific set of unique chemical features of antigen is responsible for immune response and it is called as epitope or antigenic determinant site. Antibody combines with the epitope or antigenic determinant site

Box 17.2: Major application of immunocytochemistry in cytology.

- Diagnosis of malignancy particularly in effusion sample
- Subclassification of lung carcinomas
- Diagnosis of malignant round cell tumors
- Subtyping of lymphomas
- Typing of tumor such as carcinoma, sarcoma, melanoma, etc.
- Hormone or receptor expression such as estrogen, progesterone receptors, Her-2 receptor in breast carcinoma
- Diagnosis of infective organisms
- Cell proliferation analysis.

Box 17.4: Different cytological preparations.

- Direct smear
  - Advantages
    - » No extra sampling
    - » No wet preparation
  - Disadvantages
    - » Background staining artifact
    - » Limited antibody panel
- Cytospin
  - Advantages
    - » Multiple smears can be made
    - » Panel of antibodies possible
    - » Overall good result
  - Disadvantages
    - » Specimen not fit for bloody and mucoid materials
    - » Difficult on scanty cellularity
    - » Best choice for lymphoid neoplasm
- Cell block
  - Advantages
    - » Multiple smears can be made
    - » Clean background
    - » Monolayered cells in limited area so cost effective
  - Disadvantages
    - » Costly and limited access.

of the antigen and this is visualized because these two molecules have complementary three-dimensional (3D) structure. So antigen and antibody mirrors each other. Ordinarily the antigen and antibody reaction can not be visualized by the light microscope. Therefore, certain label or flags are attached to the primary antibody or secondary antibody.

APPLICATIONS

Application of IC in cytology material has opened a new horizon in this filed. The demonstration of various antigenic markers of the cell with the help of monoclonal antibodies reveals the additional character of a cell. IC on the cytology material provides us all necessary information that is available from histology sample. IC technique has been widely used in different areas of cytology (Box 17.2).

The cytology samples are easily obtainable and inexpensive to get (Box 17.3). However, cytology material is usually not abundant to apply large panel of antibodies until a cell block is used. Presently, IC is an indispensable ancillary technology in the field of cytology.

Box 17.3: Pros and cons of immunocytochemistry on cytology.

- *Sample*: easily obtained, safe, inexpensive.
- All the immunological markers can be applied on cytology
- Antigen retrieval not necessary.
- Result depends on sample such as cell block provides best result.
- Scanty cellularity may not allow to use large panel of antibodies.

SAMPLING TECHNIQUES FOR IMMUNOCYTOCHEMISTRY

Sample Collection

Different types of specimen can be used for IC such as direct smears, cytospin preparations, cell blocks, and liquid-based cytology (LBC) preparations (Box 17.4).

Direct Smear

The quality of the immunostain is poor in this type of preparation as there may be severe background artifact after immunostain. A panel of antibodies cannot be used in direct smear. Overall it is unsuitable for IC.

Cytospin Preparations

Specimens collected in nonfixative fluid such as fine needle aspiration cytology (FNAC) material or fluid specimen such as effusion sample or cerebrospinal fluid (CSF) is used for cytospin centrifugation. Gross blood-mixed or mucus-mixed materials cannot be used for cytospin. Multiple wet fixed slides can be prepared from cytospin for application of a panel of antibodies for IC. Background artifact may be seen but overall cytospin preparation gives good result for IC.

Cell Block

Cell block material is considered as the best preparation for IC. Any specimen can be used for cell block except the specimen with very low cellularity such as ureteric urine sample or CSF. There should be the proper standardized practice of making a cell block for IC. The major advantages of cell block are:

- To make multiple sections for a panel of IC,
- To have proper control sections for IC,

- To keep the material for archival use, and
- To have a minimum background staining.

Liquid-based Cytology

Liquid-based cytology (LBC) has been now widely used in different laboratories. Multiple smears can be made by LBC. Other advantages of LBC are clean background and concentrated cells in a small area. LBC preparation provides good result for IC.[1]

FIXATION

It is very important to use appropriate fixative for IC. In fact, the choice of proper fixation plays a crucial role in IC. Buffered neutral formalin (10%) is probably best fixative for IC in cytospin, air-dried smear, and cell block. Commercially available fixatives are used in LBC preparations and they give equally good results. Various other fixatives are ethanol, methanol, and acetone. Overall 95% ethanol is a good fixative for FNAC, brush cytology, or cytospin preparations and most of the antibodies work in this fixative.[2] Alcohol fixative is not suitable for the demonstration of HER-2 neu oncoprotein, estrogen, and progesterone receptors, and buffered formalin solution is the most desirable fixative in this context.

CONTROL

Proper positive and negative controls are mandatory in the interpretation of IC staining. Ideally each laboratory should have proper control of positive slides for each antibody. In case of IC on cytospin preparation the laboratory should have a good number of positive cytospin slides in the store. The laboratories who work on cell block only should have adequate sections from cell block of each positive case. Paraffin embedded sections should not be kept as a control for smear preparation.

IMMUNOCYTOCHEMISTRY TECHNIQUE

Steps

The basic steps of IC are (Fig. 17.1):

- *Antigen retrieval*: This is the process to recover the antigens that may have been changed during the fixation.
- *Blocking the background staining*: Primary antibodies are highly charged molecules and therefore may be attached with other reciprocally charged molecules such as collagen or other antibodies present in the serum. Preincubation with normal serum will reduce the unwanted nonspecific binding.
- It is also important to block the endogenous peroxidase enzyme that is present in blood and tissue by using hydrogen peroxide solution prior to incubation by primary antibody.
- *Incubation with primary antibody*: Optimal dilution of primary antibody is needed.
- *Incubation with labeled secondary antibody*: Secondary antibody is usually labeled and directed against the primary antibody.
- *Visualization*: Appropriate chromogen is applied to visualize the reaction.
- *Counter staining*: Light counterstain is applied to visualize the nuclei and tissue architecture.
- Dehydration and mounting are done.

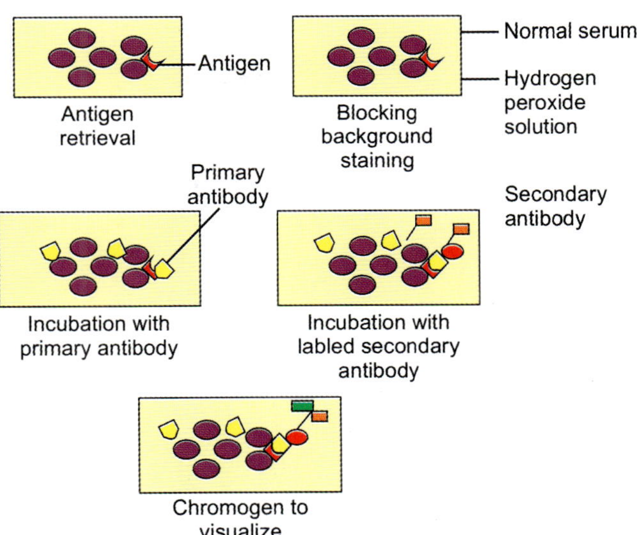

Fig. 17.1: Schematic diagram shows the basic steps of immunocytochemistry.

Detection System

Various types of detection system are used to demonstrate the antigen-antibody reaction (Fig. 17.2).

Direct Method

Primary antibody is directly labeled with an enzyme or fluorescence. This is rapid and easy. However, the antibody should be specific otherwise nonspecific staining may occur. The greatest disadvantage is for each antigen a separate antibody has to be labeled.

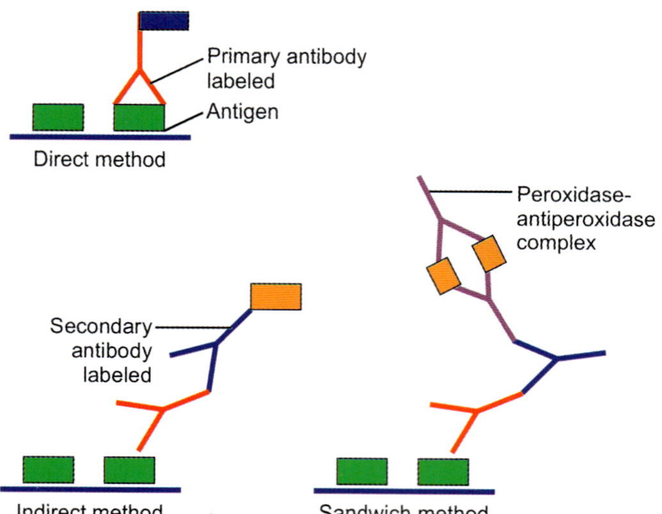

Fig. 17.2: Schematic diagram shows the different methods of visualization of immunocytochemistry stain.

Indirect Method

This is also known as indirect or sandwich conjugate method. Here, the secondary antibody is labeled and it is directed against the primary unconjugated antibody. The advantage of indirect method is that: (1) A single conjugated secondary antibody can be used against different primary antibodies, (2) Higher dilution of primary antibody can be used, (3) Large amount of secondary antibody can be easily produced against the primary antibody, and (4) For negative control, the primary antibody can be omitted.

Peroxidase-antiperoxidase method: In this method peroxidase-antiperoxidase (PAP) reagent is used. PAP is a small and stable immune complex substance. It consists of antibody against horseradish peroxidase and horseradish peroxidase antigen. The primary antibody and PAP reagent are from the same species, whereas the secondary bridging antibody is from a different species with high affinity against the primary antibody. This method is widely used for high degree of sensitivity.

Others: The other popular systems are biotin-avidin conjugate procedure, biotin-streptavidin systems, and alkaline phosfatase–antialkaline phosfatase method.

TROUBLE SHOOTING IN IMMUNOCYTOCHEMISTRY

The common problems of IC are:

- No staining at all
- Weak staining
- Background stain.

These problems have been highlighted in Table 17.1.

INTERPRETATION

Adequate precautions should be taken during the interpretation of IC. It should be always remembered that no immunostain can confirm the presence or absence of malignancy. Cytomorphology and clinical correlation is mandatory for the diagnosis of malignant lesions. It is always advisable to use a panel of antibody for diagnosis. Certain things such as clinical history, cytomorphology, and other biochemical and radiological features should be kept in mind before ordering a panel (Box 17.5).

There are certain causes of false positive interpretation of IC such as poorly fixed cells, too high antibody titer, acute inflammation in the background, insufficient blocking of endogenous peroxide, less specific antibody, and necrotic or cell debris in the background (Box 17.6).

Similarly one should be careful about false negative IC. The predominant causes of false negative IC are highlighted in Box 17.7.

DIAGNOSTIC IMMUNOCYTOCHEMISTRY

Mesothelial Cells versus Adenocarcinoma

The most common problem in any cytology laboratory is to differentiate mesothelial cells from metastatic adenocarcinoma. Reactive mesothelial cells often show significant pleomorphism and the classical two cell populations may not be evident in distinguishing mesothelial cells from adenocarcinoma. A panel of antibodies is always recommended to resolve the issue.[3,4]

Some important mesothelial markers are discussed first.

Mesothelial Markers

Calretinin: This is a 29 kD calcium-binding protein and is present in the mesothelial cells and also in a wide variety of other cells including steroid producing cells of ovary and testis, renal tubular cells, and lipocytes. It is considered as a mesothelial-specific marker and stains both reactive and malignant mesothelial cells. The sensitivity and specificity of calretinin are about 100% and 80%, respectively.[5] Occasionally the cells of adenocarcinoma may also show calretinin positivity.[6] However, calretinin positivity pattern is less intense and focal in adenocarcinoma cells.

Table 17.1: Trouble shooting in immunocytochemistry.

Result	*Possible cause*
No stain	• Any vital steps may have been omitted such as primary antibody, secondary antibody, or substrate material • The correct order of primary antibody and secondary antibody • Optimal dilution of primary antibody • Reagents should not be beyond the expiry date • Proper storage of antibody.
Weak stain	• Too much fixation or improper fixation • Too much diluted primary antibody • Inadequate antigen retrieval.
Background staining	Both negative and positive controls are stained • Secondary antibody is cross reacting with the background substance • Section or smear is dried during staining • Chromogen is incompletely dissolved • The blocking serum is not done properly. *Positive control and test samples are showing background staining but negative control is free from background stain* • Primary antibody is over concentrated • The test sample contains naturally occurring contaminating antibody. *Only test sample showing background stain* • Overfixation and possibly the test sample and controls are differently fixed.

Box 17.5: Factors to be considered before ordering panel of immunocytochemistry.

- Clinical history
  - Age and sex
  - Chief complaints
  - Past history of any disease
  - Radiological features
- Cytomorphological features
- Provisional diagnosis
- Determination of panel.

Box 17.6: Causes of false positive immunocytochemistry.

- Poorly fixed cells
- Too high antibody titer
- Acute inflammation in the background
- Crushed cells
- Insufficient blocking of endogenous peroxide
- Less specific antibody
- Necrotic or cell debris in the background
- Various technical problems such as
  - Omission of steps,
  - Use of wrong antibody
  - Drying of smear.

Box 17.7: Causes of false negative immunocytochemistry.

- Too low antibody titer
- Fragile cell cytoplasm
- Poorly fixed cells
- Alcohol-fixed smear for nuclear antigen
- Insufficient retrieval of antigen.

HBME-1: This monoclonal antibody is raised against the cell surface microvillus of the mesothelial cells. HBME-1 stains intensely around the periphery of the mesothelial cells. The specificity of HBME-1 is about 80% and the majority of the mesothelial cells show strong positivity. However, it is also true that a significant population of adenocarcinoma cells also shows HBME-1 positivity. Therefore, the utility of HBME-1 is a bit debatable.[7]

Wilms' tumor gene 1 (WT-1): Wilms' tumor gene is present in chromosome 11 and acts as a tumor suppressor. This is a transcription factor isolated in the cells of the kidney. It is expressed in the cytoplasm and nucleus of the mesothelial cells. The WT-1 gene product is also present in desmoplastic small round cell tumors and ovarian serous carcinoma.[8] Therefore, the usefulness of WT1 is to some extent restricted to differentiate adenocarcinoma from mesothelioma.

D2-40: D2-40 was initially used as a marker of lymphatic endothelial cells. However, it is a relatively sensitive (85%) and specific (95%) marker of mesothelial cells.[9,10]

Cytokeratin 5 and 6: Cytokeratin 5/6 (CK 5/6) shows diffuse cytoplasmic positivity in both benign and malignant mesothelial cells. CK 5/6 also stains other tumors such as squamous cell carcinoma, breast carcinomas, thymoma, and salivary gland tumors.[11]

Adenocarcinoma Markers in Effusion Fluid

BER EP4: This antibody reacts with the cell surface glycoprotein of the epithelial cells. This antibody is considered as highly specific and sensitive for adenocarcinoma.[12,13]

Table 17.2: Expression of CK and probable origin of tumors.

Cytokeratin 7	*Cytokeratin 20*	*Tumors*
Positive	Positive	Pancreatic carcinoma, transitional carcinoma of bladder
Positive	Negative	Lung, breast, ovary, mesothelioma
Negative	Positive	Colonic, gastric, markel cell carcinoma
Negative	Negative	Prostatic carcinoma, hepatocellular carcinoma, renal cell carcinoma, adrenocortical carcinoma

Carcinoembryonic antigen: This is a glycoprotein detected in fetal epithelial cells. It is usually present in a scanty amount in normal epithelial cells and large amount in gastrointestinal adenocarcinoma and lung adenocarcinoma. Specificity of carcinoembryonic antigen (CEA) is very high (100%) and it is considered as a useful marker to differentiate mesothelial cells from adenocarcinoma.[3]

MOC-31: This is a transmembrane glycoprotein present on the epithelial membrane. MOC-31 is positive in all the cases of adenocarcinoma of the lung and many nonpulmonary adenocarcinomas. Reactive mesothelial cells rarely show MOC-31 positivity. MOC-31 is considered as an effective antibody to distinguish mesothelial cells from adenocarcinoma.[14]

Leu M1 (CD 15): Monoclonal antibody to Leu M1 (CD 15) specifically demonstrates carcinoma cells. Sensitivity of Leu M1 is low (29%), and it may also show false positivity as a result of high hyaluronic acid content.[15]

BENIGN VERSUS MALIGNANT MESOTHELIAL CELLS

This is already discussed in effusion cytology chapter.

Epithelial Markers

Cytokeratin

There are three types of cytoskeletal filaments in the cell, namely microfilaments, intermediate filaments (IFs), and microtubules. The intermediate filaments are intermediate in size and organize the internal 3D structure of the cell. There are seven varieties of IF and cytokeratin is one of them (*see* Chapter 1). CK is expressed in all types of epithelial cells. Depending on their molecular weights cytokeratin is classified into 20 different types. The demonstration of specific cytokeratin is immensely helpful in pointing out the origin of an unknown metastatic tumor. Cytokeratin 7 (CK 7) and cytokeratin 20 (CK 20) phenotyping are particularly helpful to find out the primary tumor in metastasis.[16,17] Table 17.2 illustrates the expression of CK and probable origin of tumors. Stable and consistent expression of CK is very important for diagnosis. Loss or gain of antigen during metastasis or development of the tumor may hamper their potential use. CK 20 is stably expressed in colorectal carcinoma, ductal and lobular carcinoma of breast, transitional carcinoma, endometrial, prostate, and renal cell carcinoma. CK 7 positivity is consistently noted in transitional carcinoma of bladder, biliary adenocarcinomas, lung, ovarian, endometrial, breast, and pancreatic adenocarcinomas. Therefore, combined use of CK 7 and CK 20 immunostain may indicate the probable origin of metastatic tumor of unknown primary cases (Table 17.2). Figures 17.3A to D show a case of metastatic carcinoma in pleural effusion where the combined use of CK and TTF1 solved the issue of possible source of origin.

Epithelial membrane antigen: This epithelial marker has been discussed previously.

Carcinoembryonic antigen: This epithelial marker has been discussed previously.

Mesenchymal Markers

Vimentin

Vimentin is an intermediate filament which is usually expressed in mesenchymal cells such as fibroblast, endothelial cells, smooth muscle, etc. However, it has been demonstrated in epithelial neoplasms such as renal cell carcinoma and also mesothelial cells. Therefore, vimentin has limited specificity in the diagnosis of mesenchymal tumors.

Desmin

This is also a variety of intermediate filament and present in smooth muscle, skeletal muscle, and cardiac muscle.

Actin

Actin is a contractile protein and is present in smooth muscle cells and myofibroblasts.

Figures 17.4A and B show the use of mesenchymal marker in a childhood malignant tumor.

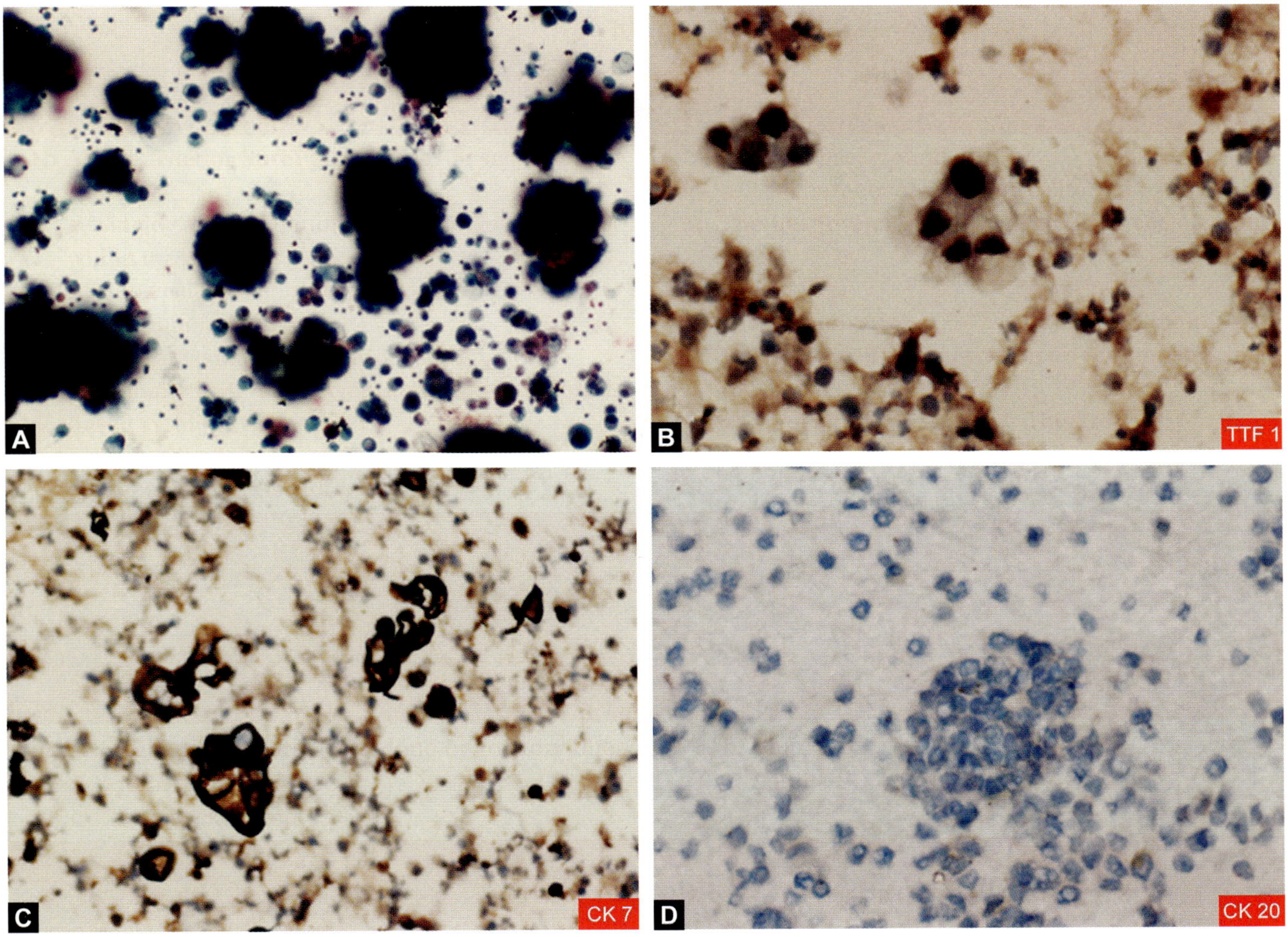

Figs. 17.3A to D: (A) A case of pleural effusion of unknown primary. Judicious use of TTF 1 (B), CK 7 (C), and CK 20 (D) were used. The positive TTF 1 and CK 7 with negative CK 20 indicate primary lung origin.

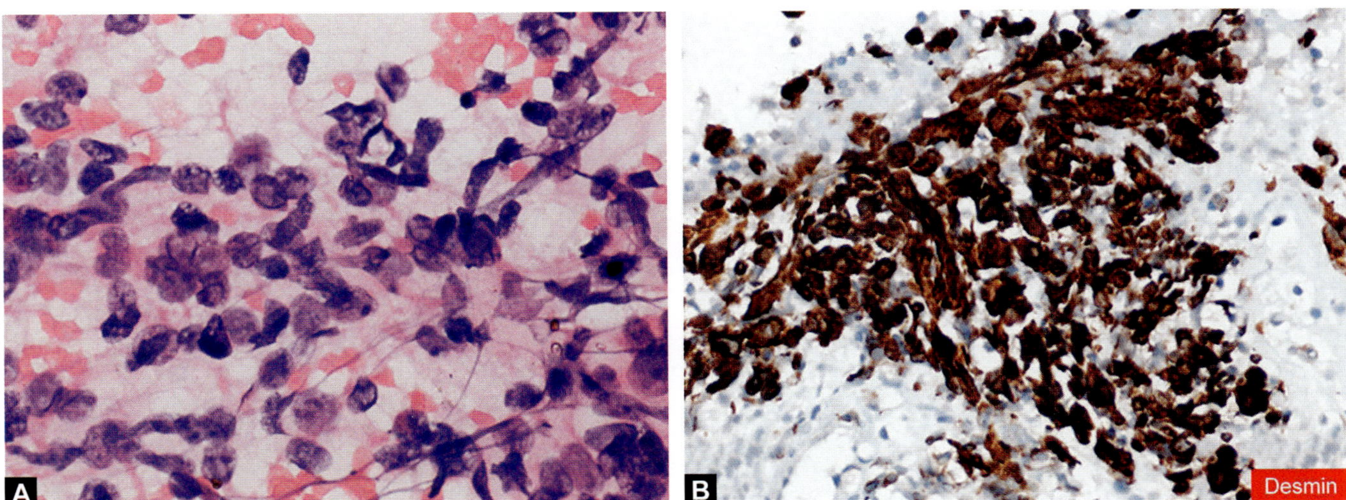

Figs. 17.4A and B: Thigh swelling in a 12-year-old female. Aspiration cytology smear (A) along with desmin stain (B) indicates the diagnosis of rhabdomyosarcoma.

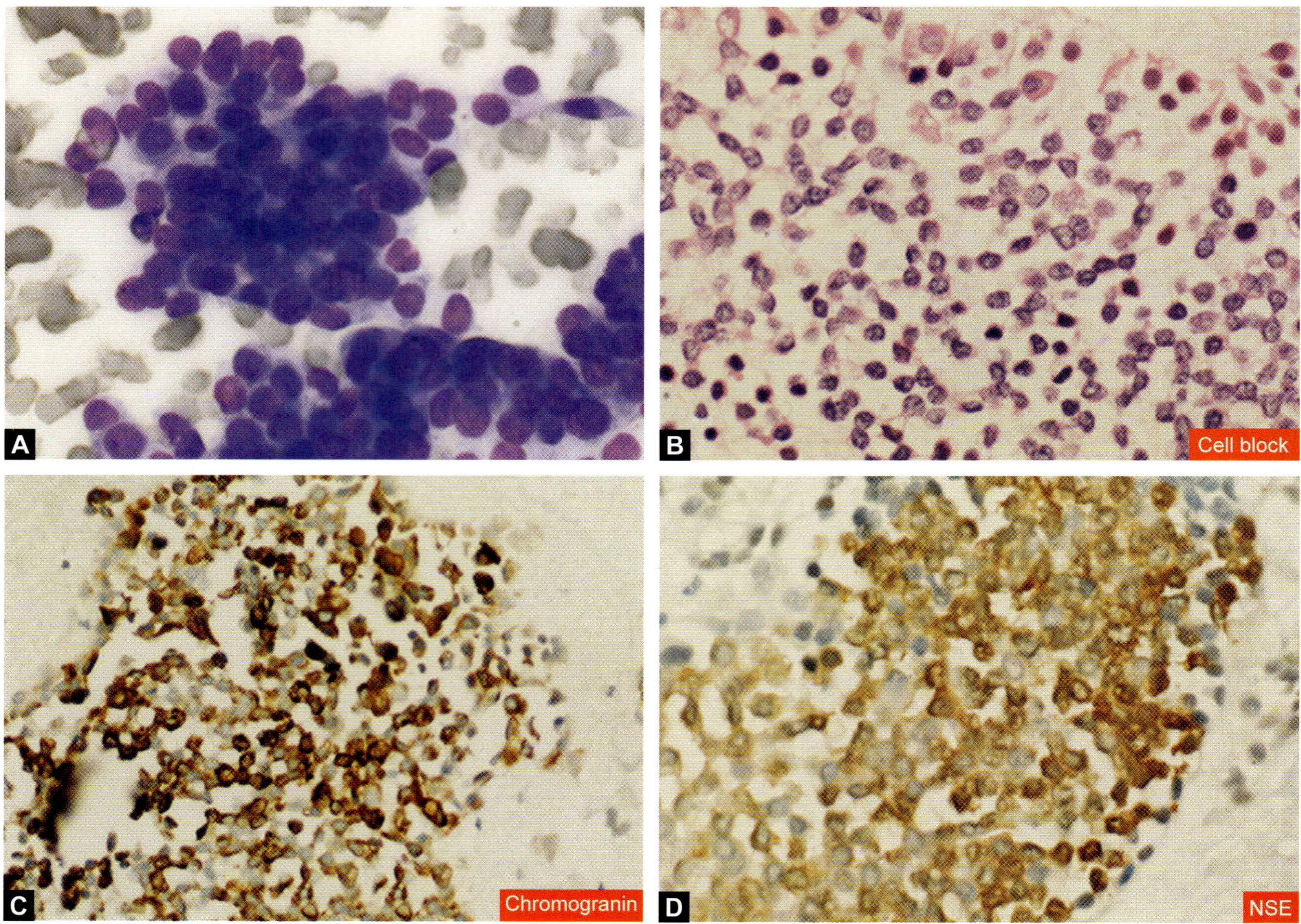

Figs. 17.5A to D: Cytology (A) and cell block (B) of a pancreatic tumor with positive chromogranin (C) and NSE (D) indicate a diagnosis of neuroendocrine tumor.

Neuroendocrine Markers

Chromogranin

Chromogranin is present in the neurosecretory granules in the neuroendocrine cells. It is a reliable marker in all types of neuroendocrine tumors.

Synaptophysin

This is a transmembrane glycoprotein and is present in the presynaptic vesicles of neurons. Synaptophysin is a marker of neuroendocrine and neuroectodermal tumors.

S-100 Protein

This is a calcium-binding protein and is present in the nucleus and cytoplasm of glial and Schwann cells. Other than the cells of neural origin, S-100 protein is also demonstrated in melanocytes, Langerhan's cells, and myoepithelial cells and the neoplasm derived from those cells.

Figures 17.5A to D highlight the diagnostic utility of neuroendocrine markers in a case of pancreatic tumor.

Lymphoid Markers

The detailed immunophenotyping of lymphoid markers is very useful for identification of lymphoid cells and subclassification of lymphomas. The IC should be done either on cell block sections and if not possible then on cytospin smear (Figs. 17.6 to 17.8). Presently, flow cytometric immunophenotyping has largely replaced IC.

CD45 or leukocyte common antigen is the common marker of lymphoid cells (Box 17.8). The majority of the cases of non-Hodgkin's lymphomas is positive for CD45 except anaplastic large cell lymphoma and plasmacytic lymphoma.

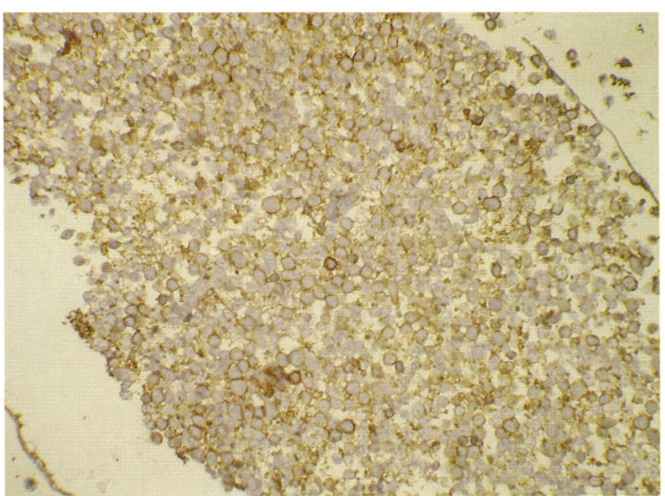

Fig. 17.6: CD45 (leucocyte common antigen) positivity in a case of non-Hodgkin's lymphoma in cell block section (immunocytochemistry × MP).

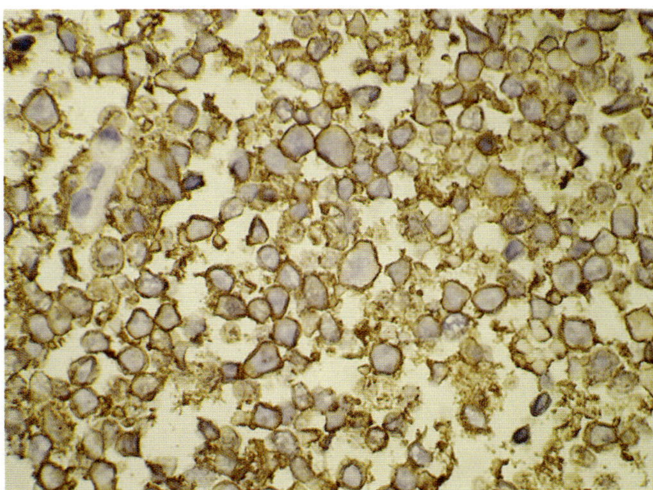

Fig. 17.7: CD20 (B cell marker) positivity in a case of B cell type of non-Hodgkin's lymphoma in cell block preparation (immunocytochemistry × HP).

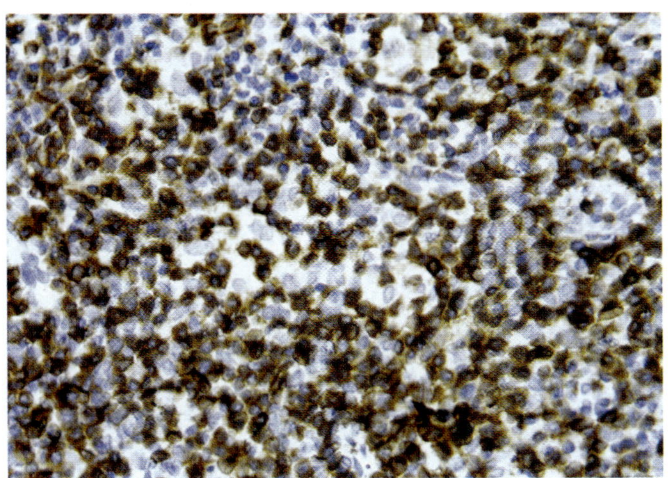

Fig. 17.8: CD3 (T cell marker) positivity in a case of T cell type of non-Hodgkin's lymphoma in cell block preparation (immunocytochemistry × MP).

Melanoma Markers

HMB-45

HMB-45 identifies an oncofetal glycoconjugate associated with immature melanosomes. This is a highly specific marker of melanoma. However, it also identifies neural crest-derived tumors, occasional carcinomas, and immunoblastic lymphomas.[18,19]

Melan A (Mart-1)

This is a melanocyte-associated marker with high sensitivity for detection of melanoma. However, Melan A is also positive in peripheral nerve sheath tumor, angiomyolipoma, and steroid-producing cells of adrenal cortex.[20]

Box 17.8: Panel of antibodies for lymphoma subtyping.

Common lymphoid marker: CD45 (leukocyte common antigen)
Monoclonality
- *Light chain restriction*: Predominant Kappa or Lambda chain restriction for B cell clonality.

B cell markers: CD19, 20, 23, 10
T cell markers: CD3, 5, 4, 8
Hodgkin's lymphoma: CD15, CD30
NK cell: CD3+, CD56+, and CD19, CD10, CD23 negative.

Germ Cell Markers

Placental Alkaline Phosphatase

Placental alkaline phosphatase (PLAP) is expressed in normal placenta. This is an oncofetal antigen and is expressed in all germ cell tumors.[21] PLAP positivity is seen on the cell membrane and occasionally in the cytoplasm. Therefore, PLAP stain is used to differentiate germ cell tumor and any other undifferentiated malignancy.

Human Chorionic Gonadotropin

Human chorionic gonadotropin (HCG) is normally secreted by the syncytiotrophoblast cell of the placenta. The beta subunit of HCG is hormone specific. HCG usually shows intense positivity in choriocarcinoma.

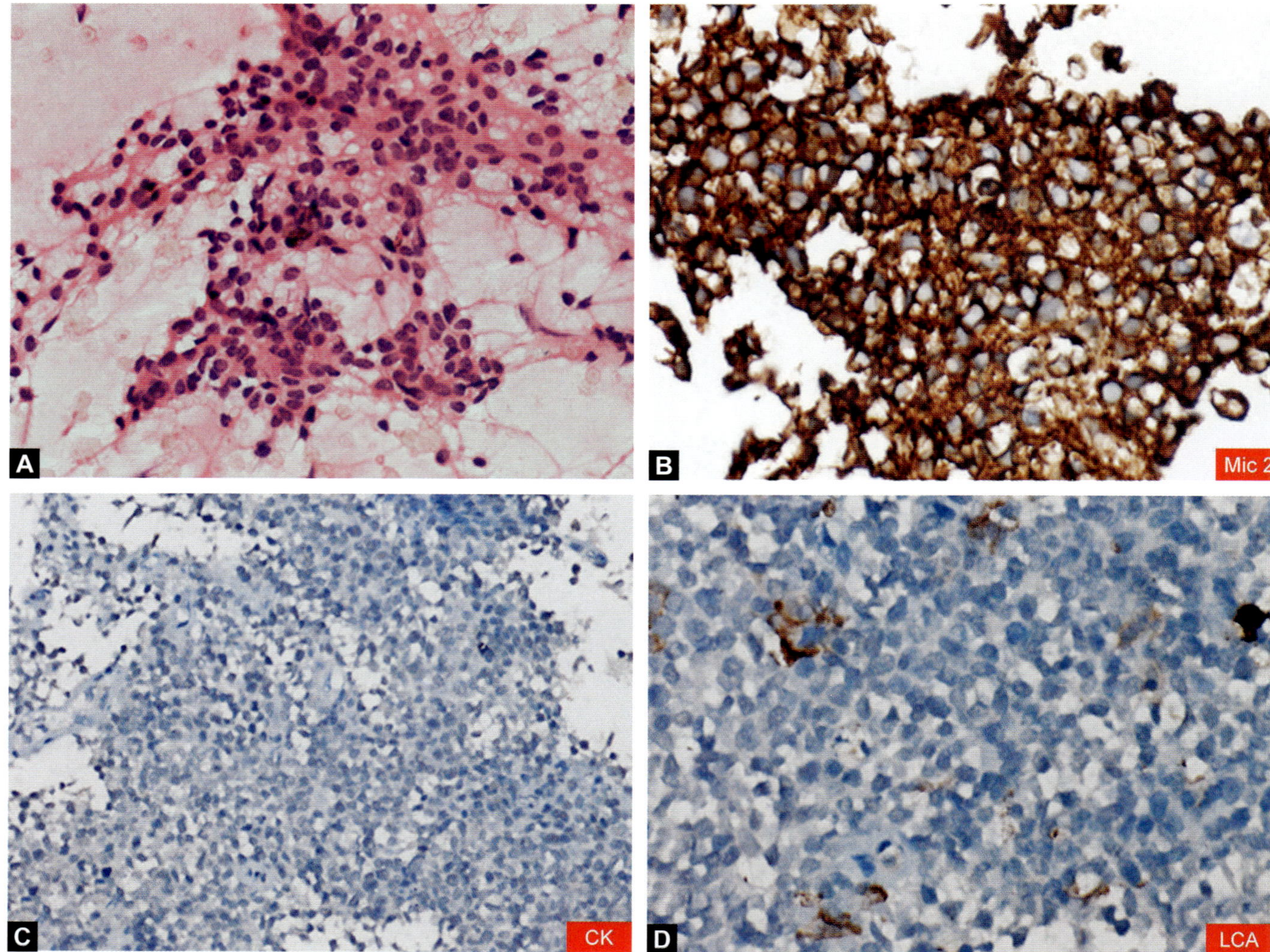

Figs. 17.9A to D: Malignant round cell tumor of the chest wall. Cytology smear (A) along with immunocytochemistry of Mic-2 (B), CK, (C), and LCA or CD45 (D) indicates peripheral neuroectodermal tumor.

DIAGNOSIS OF UNDIFFERENTIATED MALIGNANCIES

Immunocytochemistry is a great help in diagnosis of an undifferentiated malignancy. A judicious panel of IC should be used for determination of the type of the tumor.

A panel of CK, CD45, vimentin, HMB-45, and chromogranin could be used for initial determination of a broad category of the tumor. Once the tumor is classified in broad category then a further detailed IC could be done for more accurate subtyping and subclassification.

ROUND CELL MALIGNANCIES

Malignant small round cell tumor is a great diagnostic problem in routine cytology sample. IC is of great help in distinguishing different malignant round cell tumor (MRCT) (Figs. 17.9A to D). Table 17.3 shows the IC pattern of different MRCT.

It is important to remember that there is a lack of specificity in IC and there is also overlapping positive reaction of different monoclonal antibodies. Moreover, some MRCTs may be so poorly differentiated that they may not show any antigenic expression.[22,23] It is always preferable to apply a panel of monoclonal antibodies for accurate diagnosis.

PROBLEMS IN LUNG CARCINOMA

It is very essential to differentiate small cell carcinoma of lung from nonsmall cell carcinoma. The detailed IC has been described in Chapter 12.

Table 17.3: Malignant round cell tumor.

	Immunocytochemistry						
	CD45	*NB-84*	*MyoD1*	*CK*	*Desmin*	*WT1*	*Mic-2 (CD99)*
NHL	+	–	–		–	–	–
NB	–	+	–	–	–	–	+
EWS/PNET	–	Occasional	–		–	+	+
WT	–	+	–	+	+	Focal	–
RMS	–		+		+	+	–
DSRCT	–		–	+	+	+	
Synovial sarcoma	–	No data	No data	+	–	–	Occasional

(NHL: Non-Hodgkin's lymphoma; NB: Neuroblastoma; EWS: Ewing's sarcoma; PNET: Peripheral neuroectodermal tumor; WT: Wilms' tumor; RMS: Rhabdomyosarcoma; DSRCT: Desmoplastic small round cell tumor).

SITE-SPECIFIC ANTIBODY IN DIFFERENT EPITHELIAL MALIGNANCIES (TABLE 17.4)

It is often essential to diagnose primary malignancy from a metastatic site or ascertain the exact character of two simultaneously evolved malignancies. IC is a great help to resolve these problems.

CK 7 and CK 20

The combined use of these two antibodies is very helpful for assessment of the probable site of origin of the epithelial malignancies (*see* Table 17.2).

Table 17.4: Site-specific antibody.

Organ or cell type	*Antibodies*
Thyroid	TTF, thyroglobulin
Breast	Estrogen and progesterone receptors, EMA
Lung	TTF, CK 7 positive, and CK 20 negative
Pancreas	CK 7 and CK 20 positive, CA 19-9
Liver	Hep Par, alpha-fetoprotein, CK 7, and CK 20 negative
Colon	CEA, CK 7 negative, CK 20 positive
Mesothelial cells	Calretinin, WT 1, CK 5 and 6 positive
Prostate	PSA, AR, CK 7, and CK 20 negative
Bladder	CK 7 and 20 positive

(EMA: Epithelial membrane antigen; CEA: Carcinoembryonic antigen; PAS: Prostate-specific antigen; AR: Androgen receptor).

Prostate-specific Antigen and Androgen Receptor

Prostate-specific antigen (PSA) and androgen receptor (AR) are helpful in diagnosis of prostate carcinoma. PSA is positive in normal, hyperplastic, and neoplastic prostate tissue. However, PSA is also positive in breast carcinoma and salivary gland tumors.[24,25]

Androgen Receptor

Androgen receptor is also demonstrated in the nucleus of the prostate epithelial cells and it is considered as a reliable indicator of prostate origin of cells. However, salivary gland tumor also shows AR positivity.[26]

Thyroid Transcription Factor

Thyroid transcription factor (TTF) is a tissue-specific transcription factor and is expressed in follicular epithelial cells of the thyroid, bronchial epithelial cells of lung, and adenocarcinomas developed from those cells. TTF is occasionally expressed in ovarian neuroendocrine carcinomas and carcinoid of lung.[27]

Estrogen and Progesterone Receptors

These two hormonal receptors present in the nucleus of the breast (Fig. 17.10) and endometrial adenocarcinomas. They may help in identification of metastatic carcinoma of the breast in selective condition.

IMMUNOCYTOCHEMISTRY FOR THERAPY AND MANAGEMENT

Molecular-targeted therapy is a type of therapy where the drugs or other chemicals block the growth and progression

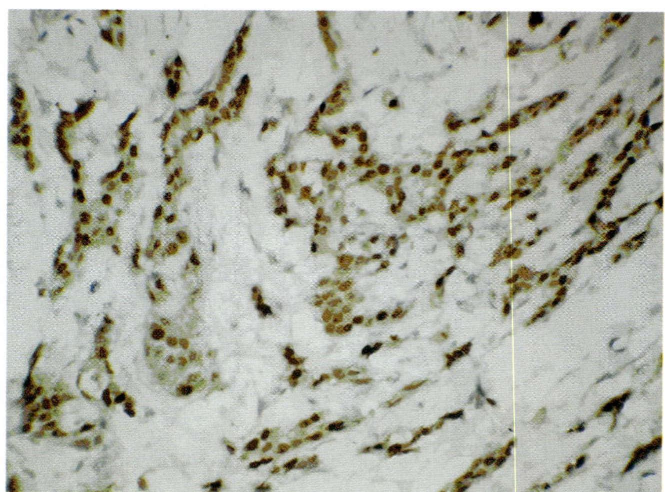

Fig. 17.10: Estrogen receptor positivity in a carcinoma of breast in cell block section. The cell block is made from cell scrape of the cytology smear (immunostain × MP).

of cancer cells by interfering with the specific molecules related to the growth and progression of cancer cells.[28]

The different antigen receptor can be accurately assessed in the cytology specimen.[29]

Estrogen and Progesterone Receptors

Estrogen and progesterone receptors (ER and PR) are nuclear receptors and can be successfully assessed on cytology specimen. ER/PR nuclear positivity is related to antiestrogen hormone therapy of breast cancer.

Her 2/Neu

This oncogene is overexpressed in a certain fraction of breast carcinoma. Overexpression of Her 2/Neu is manifested as intense staining of cell membranes. The status of Her 2/Neu overexpression in breast cancer is needed to know for administering anti Her 2/Neu antibody.

CD117 (c-Kit)

CD117 is also known as c-Kit. It is a cell membrane protein and is expressed in gastrointestinal stromal tumor (GIST), primitive neuroectodermal tumor, seminomas, and melanomas. The demonstration of the CD117 expression is necessary for the diagnosis of GIST.[30]

The GIST often shows the mutation of c-Kit or CD117. This results in high surface level of CD117 expression. GIST with c-Kit mutation is responsive to tyrosine kinase inhibiting agent (imatinib) therapy.[31]

Antibodies Directed to Anti-infective Agent

Various antibodies can be used to identify the infective organisms on cytology smear. Antibodies to cytomegalovirus, Chlamydia, herpes simplex virus, and human papillomavirus are available. Epstein-Barr virus (EBV)-related antigen is useful to detect the presence of EBV.

REFERENCES

1. Dey P, Luthra UK, George J, et al. A comparison of thin prep and conventional preparation of fine needle aspiration cytology material. Acta Cytol. 2000:44;46-50.
2. Osamura RY. Applications of immunocytochemistry to diagnostic cytopathology. Diagn Cytopathol. 1989;5:55-63.
3. Delahaye M, van der Ham F, van der Kwast TH. Complementary value of five carcinoma markers for the diagnosis of malignant mesothelioma, adenocarcinoma metastasis, and reactive mesothelium in serous effusions. Diagn Cytopathol. 1997;17:115-20.
4. Davidson B. The diagnostic and molecular characteristics of malignant mesothelioma and ovarian/peritoneal serous carcinoma. Cytopathology. 2011;22:5-21.
5. Yaziji H, Battifora H, Barry TS, et al. Evaluation of 12 antibodies for distinguishing epithelioid mesothelioma from adenocarcinoma: identification of a three-antibody immunohistochemical panel with maximal sensitivity and specificity. Mod Pathol. 2006;19:514-23.
6. Doglioni C, Dei Tos AP, Laurino L, et al. A novel immunocytochemical marker for mesothelioma. Am J Surg Pathol. 1996;20:1037-46.
7. Politi E, Kandaraki C, Apostolopoulou C, et al. Immunocytochemical panel for distinguishing between carcinoma and reactive mesothelial cells in body cavity fluids. Diagn Cytopathol. 2005;32:151-5.
8. Hecht JL, Lee BH, Pinkus GS. The value of Wilms tumor susceptibility gene 1 in cytologic preparations as a marker for malignant mesothelioma. Cancer. 2002;96:105-9.
9. Bassarova AV, Nesland JM, Davidson B. D2-40 is not a specific marker for cells of mesothelial origin in serous effusions. Am J Surg Pathol. 2006;30:878-82.
10. Saad RS, Lindner JL, Lin X, et al. The diagnostic utility of D2-40 for malignant mesothelioma versus pulmonary carcinoma with pleural involvement. Diagn Cytopathol. 2006; 34: 801-6.
11. Chu PG, Weiss LM. Expression of cytokeratin 5/6 in epithelial neoplasms: an immunohistochemical study of 509 cases. Mod Pathol. 2002;15:6-10.
12. Singh HK, Silverman JF, Berns L, et al. Significance of epithelial membrane antigen in the work-up of problematic serous effusions. Diagn Cytopathol. 1995;13:3-7.
13. Gaffey MJ, Mills SE, Swanson PE, et al. Immunoreactivity for Ber-EP4 in adenocarcinomas, adenomatoid tumors and malignant mesotheliomas. Am J Surg Pathol. 1992;16:3-9.

14. Robb JA. Mesothelioma versus adenocarcinoma: false-positive CEA and LeuM1 staining due to hyaluronic acid (letter to the editor). Hum Pathol. 1989;20:400.
15. Su XY, Li GD, Liu WP, et al. Cytological differential diagnois among adenocarcinoma, epithelial mesothelioma, and reactive mesothelial cells in serous effusions by immuno-cytochemistry. Diagn Cytopathol. 2011;39(12):900-8.
16. Tot T. Cytokeratins 20 and 7 as biomarkers: usefulness in discriminating primary from metastatic adenocarcinoma. Eur J Cancer. 2002;38:758-63
17. Chu P, Wu E, Weiss LM, et al. Cytokeratin 7 and cytokeratin 20 expression in epithelial neoplasms: a survey of 435 cases. Mod Pathol. 2000;13(9):962-72.
18. Friedman HD, Tatum AH. HMB-45-positive malignant lymphoma. A case report with literature review of aberrant HMB-45 reactivity. Arch Pathol Lab Med. 1991;115: 826-30.
19. Hancock C, Allen BC, Herrera GA. HMB-45 detection in adenocarcinomas. Arch Pathol Lab Med. 1991;115:886-90.
20. Busam KJ, Iversen K, Coplan KA, et al. Immunoreactivity for A103, and antibody to melan-A (Mart-1), in adreno-cortical and other steroid tumors. Am J Surg Pathol. 1998; 22:57-63.
21. Niehans GA, Manivel JC, Copland GT, et al. Immunohisto-chemistry of germ cell and trophoblastic neoplasms. Cancer. 1988;62:1113-23.
22. Pohar-Marinsˇek Z, Difficulties in diagnosing small round cell tumours of childhood from fine needle aspiration cytology samples. Cytopathology. 2008;19:67-79.
23. Rekhtman N. Immunohistochemical algorithm for differentiation of lung adenocarcinoma and squamous cell carcinoma based on large series of whole-tissue sections with validation in small specimens. Modern Pathol. 2011;24: 1348-59.
24. Bodey B, Bodey B Jr, Kaiser HE. Immunocytochemical detection of prostate specific antigen expression in human breast carcinoma cells. Anticancer Res. 1997;17:2577-81.
25. Fan CY, Wang J, Barnes EL. Expression of androgen receptor and prostate specific markers in salivary duct carcinoma. An immunochemical analysis of 13 cases and review of the literature. Am J Surg Pathol. 2000;24;579-86.
26. Nasser SM, Faquin WC, Dayal Y. Expression of androgen, estrogen, and progesterone receptors in salivary gland tumors. Am J Clin Pathol. 2003;119:801-6.
27. Hecht JL, Pinkus JL, Weinstein LJ, et al. The value of thyroid transcription factor-1 in cytologic preparations as a marker for metastatic adenocarcinoma of lung origin. Am J Clin Pathol. 2001;116:483-8.
28. Scott AM, Wolchok JD, Old LJ. Antibody therapy of cancer. Nat Rev Cancer. 2012;12(4):278-87.
29. Suthipintawong C. Immunostaining of estrogen receptor, progesterone receptor, MIB1 antigen, and c-erbB-2 onco-protein in cytologic specimens: a simplified method with formalin fixation. Diagn Cytopathol. 1997;17:127-33.
30. Tsuura Y, Hiraki H, Watanabe K, et al. Preferential localization of c-kit product in tissue mast cells, basal cells of skin, epithelial cells of breast, small cell lung carcinoma and seminoma/dysgerminoma in humans: immunohisto-chemical study on formalin-fixed, paraffinembedded tissues. Virchows Arch. 1994;424:135-41.
31. Saleem TB, Ahmed I. Gastrointestinal stromal tumour—evolving concepts. Surgeon. 2009;7(1):36-41.

Review Questions

1. **The stain demonstrates acid mucin:**
   a. Alcian blue
   b. PAS
   c. Oil red O
   d. Sudan black
2. **The best choice for immunocytochemistry on aspiration cytology material:**
   a. Direct smear fixed on 95% ethanol
   b. Cytospin
   c. Cell block section
   d. Destain the Papanicolao's stain
3. **All are the markers of mesothelial cells except:**
   a. HBME-1
   b. Calretinin
   c. Wilms' tumor gene product (WT1)
   d. Leu M1 (CD15)
4. **All are the causes of false negative immunostain except:**
   a. Too high antibody titer
   b. Fragile cell cytoplasm
   c. Poorly fixed cells
   d. Insufficient retrieval of antigen
5. **The tumor that is strongly positive for CK 7 and negative for CK 20:**
   a. Ovary
   b. Colon
   c. Markel cell carcinoma
   d Prostatic carcinoma
6. **A childhood malignancy which is positive for CK, desmin, WT1 and negative for Mic 2 and CD45:**
   a. Peripheral neuroectodermal tumor
   b. Desmoplastic small round cell tumor
   c. Rhabdomyosarcoma
   d. Neuroblastoma
7. **A lung tumor that is positive for CK5/6 and p63 but are negative for TTF 1, and CK7:**
   a. Adenocarcinoma
   b. Squamous cell carcinoma
   c. Small cell carcinoma
   d. Carcinoid
8. **In the immunostaining, both negative and positive controls are stained in the background. The possible cause:**
   a. Secondary antibody is cross reacting with the background substance
   b. Primary antibody is over concentrated
   c. Too much fixation
   d. Primary antibody is over concentrated

Answers

1. a. Alcian blue
2. c. Cell block section
3. d. Leu M1 (CD15)
4. a. Too high antibody titer
5. a. Ovary
6. b. Desmoplastic small round cell tumor
7. b. Squamous cell carcinoma
8. a. Secondary antibody is cross reacting with the background substance

CHAPTER

18 Light Microscope

VISIBLE LIGHT

Visible light covers the narrow range of the electromagnetic spectrum extending from deep violet to red that means 400–750 nanometer wavelength of light. Ordinary white light is the combination of light of different wavelengths, whereas the monochromatic light is the light of a single wavelength.

IMAGE FORMATION IN HUMAN EYE

Light travels from the object to the iris, cornea, and lens. Ultimately the light is focused on the retina and through the optical nerve the image is transmitted to the brain for final interpretation (Fig. 18.1).

LENS

Human eye is not able to magnify the image of the object. Simple convex lens as glass magnifiers can magnify the image of an object. The convex lens if kept between the object and the eye and is focused properly then the magnified virtual image is formed toward the object side (Fig. 18.2). In fact, this was the basic principle of early light microscope.

HISTORY

Long back about 3,000 years ago, lens was used by the Assyrians as burning glass. Egyptian and Greeks have also used biconvex lenses about 800–400 years BC. History says that the famous Roman Emperor, Nero, used emerald lenses to watch the gladiator games. In the year 1590, two Dutch opticians Hans and Zacharias Janssen (father and son) invented microscope. This was further improved by Anton von Leeuwenhoek from Holland in the 17th century. He noted blood cells, sperm, amoeba, and other various microorganisms in detail. Today microscopy system is much more advanced and much more complicated. Modern microscope can not only

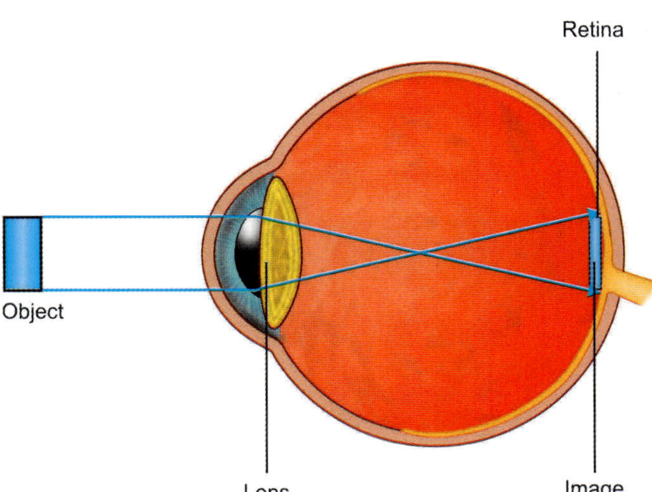

Fig. 18.1: Schematic diagram shows how the image is formed in the eye.

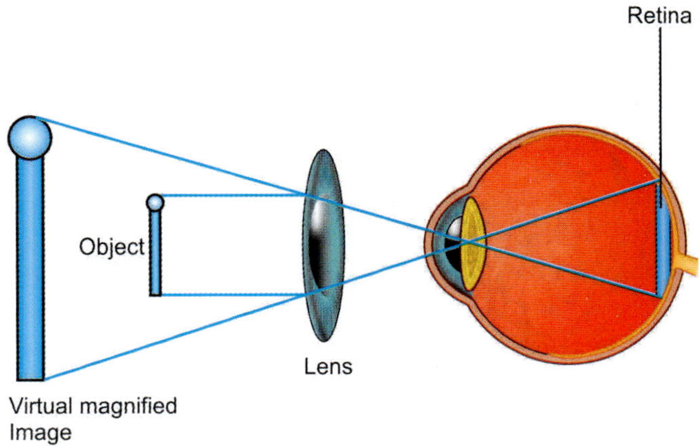

Fig. 18.2: Schematic diagram shows how the image is magnified if a convex lens is kept between the object and eye. A magnified virtual image is formed toward the side of the object.

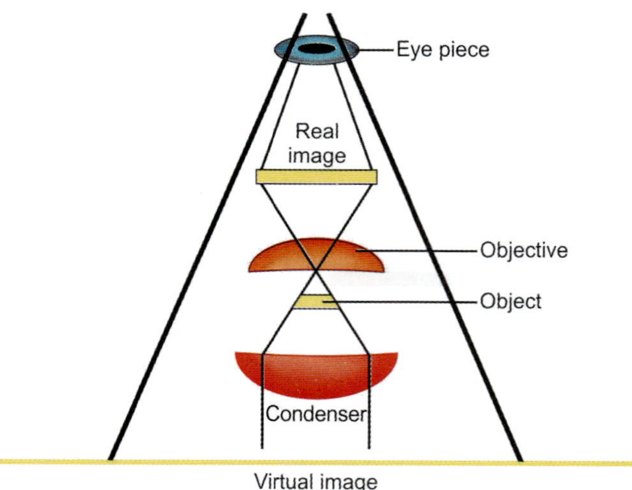

Fig. 18.3: Schematic diagram explains the basic principle of the light microscope. Final magnified virtual image is formed beyond the condenser.

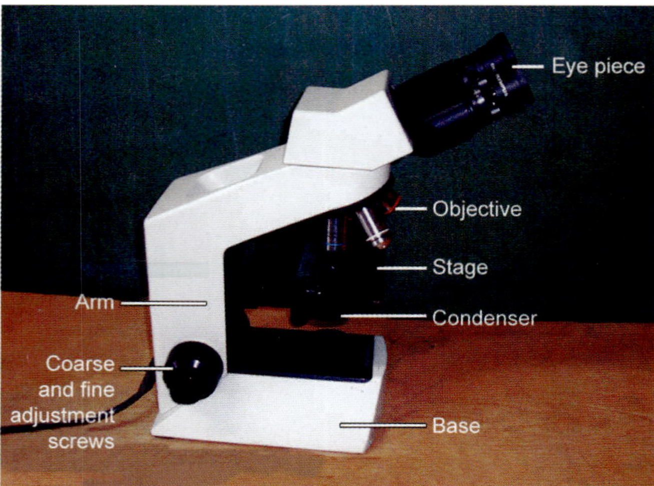

Fig. 18.4: Simple light microscope and its parts.

use light but can also use electron beam to produce a magnified image with very high resolution.

LIGHT MICROSCOPE

Light microscope uses visible light for the source of light so it is named as light microscope. The light microscope performs three basic tasks: (1) magnification, (2) resolution, and (3) contrast.

Magnification

It is one of the basic tasks of a light microscope. In most of the microscope, the first magnification is done with the objective and this image is further magnified by an ocular lens. Therefore, the total magnification is: magnification done by the objectives multiplied by magnification done by ocular lens.

Resolution

Resolution means the finer details of the object and it is defined as the ability to distinguish two closely spaced objects. The resolution of a microscope depends on two factors: (1) wavelength of light and (2) the light accumulating power of the objective and condenser lenses. This light gathering capability of the lens is mathematically represented as numerical aperture (NA). NA value is usually written on the objective. If the resolution is expressed as the smallest distance separating the two closely spaced very small objects (d_{min}), then $d_{min} = 0.61\sigma/NA$. Sigma (σ) is the wavelength of light.

IMAGE FORMATION IN A COMPOUND MICROSCOPE (FIG. 18.3)

The microscope is the simple collection of lenses to magnify the image of an object. The first lens is the objective which creates a real image in the body tube of the microscope and the second lens is the eye piece that further magnifies the first image. At first light passes through the condenser that concentrates the light in a collection of parallel beams onto the object placed on the stage. The light subsequently passes through the objective which projects a real inverted image within the body tube of the microscope. The eye piece second time magnifies the real image and produces a virtual image that appears to be 250 mm away from the eye.

Mechanical and Electrical Components (Fig. 18.4)

Base: This is the bottom support of the microscope.

Stage: This is the flat movable platform like area where the object is kept. The stage can be moved side-by-side also up and down.

Tube: It is the part that connects the eyepiece to the objective of the microscope.

Arm: It is the connecting part between the tube and the base of the microscope.

Revolving nose-piece: This is the part that holds the different objectives of the microscope for different magnification of the image of the object.

Coarse and fine adjustment knobs: These knobs help to move the stage up and down.

Diaphragm: It is situated just below that stage and it regulates the amount of light on the specimen.

Light source: Light is projected below and goes upwards through the diaphragm and the object and lenses up to the eye.

Optical Components

The optical components of the light microscope are:

Condensers: The principal function of the condenser is to focus light on the object placed on the stage. This is particularly helpful when the higher objective lens is used.

Objectives: There are multiple objectives attached to the rotating nose piece. The main function of the objective is to magnify the image and to produce a real inverted image in the body tube of the microscope.

Eye piece: It contains the ocular lens. This ocular lens further magnifies the real image when it is focused on it. A virtual image is produced at 250 mm away from the eye.

CARE AND HANDLING OF THE MICROSCOPE

- During transport the stage of the microscope should be parallel to the ground. One hand should always support the base and the other arm should grasp the arm of the microscope.
- The lens of the microscope should not be touched with the hand. The oil immersion lens should always be cleaned by the lens paper after use.
- Lens are delicate so over cleaning may damage the lens. If it is necessary to clean, then compressed air can be used for cleaning the lens.
- After the work, the nose piece should always be rotated to keep in low power objective and far away from the stage.
- The microscope should always be covered by a dust cover plastic sheet.

FLUORESCENCE MICROSCOPE

The fluorescence microscopy uses light of much higher intensity instead of ordinary light. This high intensity light stimulates the fluorescent in the object of interest and emits lower energy light that forms an image detected by the observer.

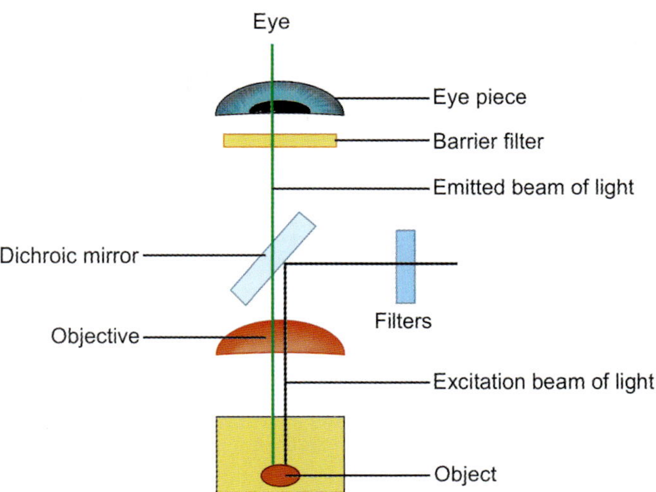

Fig. 18.5: The schematic figure explains the basic working principle of incident fluorescence microscopy.

Principles of Fluorescence

When light of high energy hits the atom then the electron shifts from lower orbit to higher orbit and immediately the electron again jumps back to the ground state and releases photon or packet of light. This makes the atom fluorescing.

Principle of Fluorescence Microscopy

The basic principles of fluorescence microscopy are described below:

- The specimen or object is stained with a fluorescent dye.
- The light of the high energy excitation beam is directed through the filter to the object.
- The fluorescent dye bound object is hit by the excitation beam of light and emits light of longer wavelength (low energy light).
- This emitted light travels through the filter to the observer and the image is visualized.

Incident Fluorescent Light

Figure 18.5 explains the basic working principles of fluorescence microscopy. In the incident fluorescent light microscopy, the high energy light beam passes directly through the filters and then with the help of a dichroic mirror it is directed toward the objective followed by the object. This excitation light beam hits the fluorescent dye bound object and low energy light is liberated.

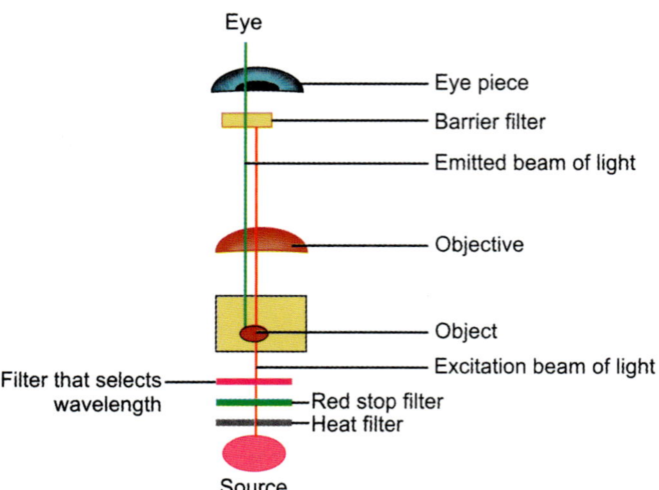

Fig. 18.6: The schematic figure explains the basic working principle of transmitted light fluorescence microscopy.

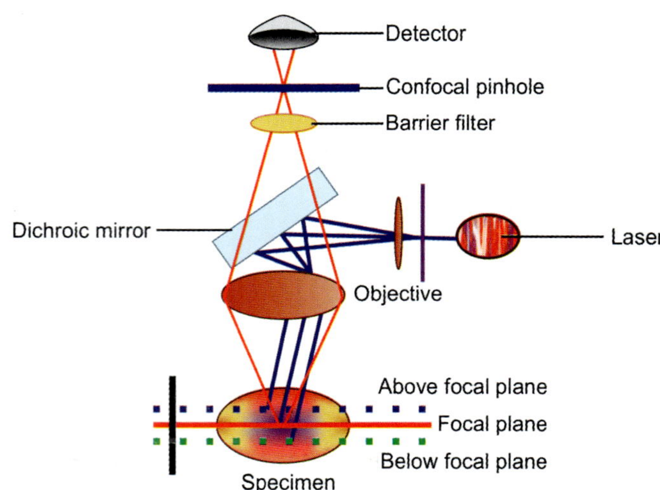

Fig. 18.7: Schematic diagram showing the basic principles of confocal microscopy.scope with attached polarizer.

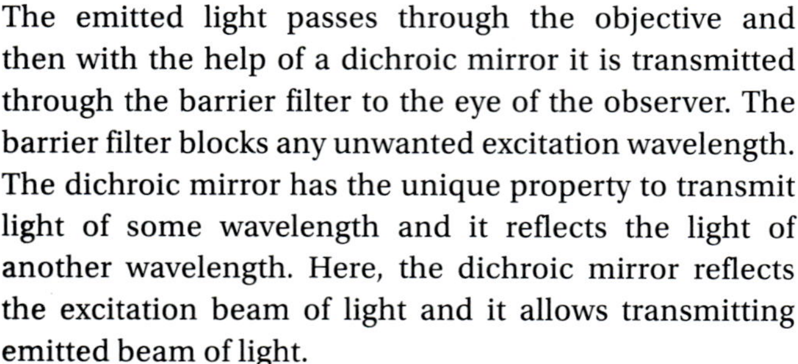

The emitted light passes through the objective and then with the help of a dichroic mirror it is transmitted through the barrier filter to the eye of the observer. The barrier filter blocks any unwanted excitation wavelength. The dichroic mirror has the unique property to transmit light of some wavelength and it reflects the light of another wavelength. Here, the dichroic mirror reflects the excitation beam of light and it allows transmitting emitted beam of light.

Transmitted Light Fluorescent (Fig. 18.6)

Here, light from the source passes through the heat-absorbing filter followed by red light removing filter that stops the red light and then through the other filter that selects the only excitation light beam. The excitation beam passes through the condenser to the object of interest. The objective collects both the excitation and emitted wavelength. The barrier filter allows only the emitted beam to pass through to the eye of the observer.

Applications

- Fluorescent microscope is used for the detection and imaging of the specific component of the cell or an object.
- It is also used for DNA or RNA study.
- Fluorescent in situ hybridization technique can show cytogenetic abnormalities of the cell.

CONFOCAL MICROSCOPY

Confocal microscopy (CFM) is a remarkable development in the field of image analysis. In a light microscope, the entire object is illuminated by light to see it directly. In contrast, in a CFM the image in particular depth is visualized at one point of time. The images can be reconstructed in the computer to get three dimensional (3D) images of the object.

Principle

In CFM illumination is done by scanning single or multiple focused beam of light derived from a laser source. The high intensity laser light is reflected from a dichroic mirror, i.e. the mirror which has the selected property to transmit and reflect the light of a particular wavelength) and is focused by the objective lens at the labeled "plane of focus" (Fig. 18.7). Emitted fluorescence from the point of focus of the specimen comes back through the dichroic mirror and the confocal aperture to the photomultiplier detector. The fluorescence are also emitted from planes above and below the plane of focus. However, this light cannot reach to the detector because of the pinhole/confocal aperture. Ultimately, the computer attached to the photomultiplier tube detector builds the whole image. Therefore, by scanning of multiple sections one can get a 3-D image of the object with the help of CFM.

Advantages

- The rapid assessment of the spatial distribution of various macromolecules, including proteins and nucleic acids is possible with the help of confocal microscope.[1]
- Clear visible image with high resolution.
- The fixation of tissue is not needed in CFM as it can work on living tissue.
- It is now also possible to record images around living cells in thick tissue slices.[2]

Applications

- *The detection of colocalization*: When two different fluorophores combine with closely spaced substances then their fluorescence may overlap which is known as colocalization. With the help of advanced CFM it is possible to assess the exact localization of such closely spaced substance.
- *Epitope tagging*: The gene of the antigenic determinant site (epitope) of the protein can be tagged by green fluorescence protein (GFP) and it is possible to track the distribution and function of this epitope.
- *Green fluorescence protein*: The gene of GFP, a bio-luminescent protein, can be inserted into a protein and it is possible to track the distribution and function of the tagged protein with the help of CFM.
- *Diagnosis*: (1) Corneal thickness measurement, (2) Screen and surveillance of colorectal cancer by using CFM, etc.
- *Functions of cytoplasmic organelles*: With the help of GFP in CFM it is possible to have detailed study of the various cytoplasmic organelles such as endoplasmic reticulum, Golgi apparatus, etc. The study of tissue changes in neoplasms can also be done by CFM.
- *Nuclear study*: Localization of genes and also chromosomal domain and telomere can be studied.
- Analysis of cell signaling pathway and cell division can be done by CFM with GFP.
- *Morphometry*: The two-dimensional (2D) structures measured can be reconstructed as 3D structure.
- Study of ionic influx and membrane potential can be done.

REFERENCES

1. Weichselbaum M, Everett AW, Sparrow MP. Mapping the innervation of the bronchial tree in fetal and postnatal pig lung using antibodies to PGP 9.5 and SV2. Am J Respir Cell Mol Biol. 1996;15(6):703-10.
2. Cook RJ, Azzopardi A, Thompson ID, et al. Real-time confocal imaging, during active air abrasion—substrate cutting. J Microsc. 2001;203(Pt 2):199-207.

Review Questions

1. **Which statement is true about the enlarged images in the light microscope?**
   a. The first image is real, and the final image is virtual
   b. Both the first and final images are real
   c. Both the images are virtual
   d. The first image is virtual, and the final image is real
2. **It is possible to track the distribution and function of the tagged protein by:**
   a. Simple fluorescence microscope
   b. By tagging the protein by green fluorescence protein and then observing in cone focal microscopy
   c. By simply tagging the protein by green fluorescence protein and then observing in light microscope
   d. None of the above is true
3. **All are true about the handling of light microscope *except*:**
   a. During transport the stage of the microscope should be parallel to the ground
   b. Xylene can be used for cleaning the lens
   c. The oil immersion lens should always be cleaned by the lens paper after use
   d. Compressed air can be used for cleaning the lens
4. **A three-dimensional image of an object is obtained in:**
   a. Light microscope with attached polarizer
   b. Fluorescence microscope
   c. Electron microscope
   d. Confocal microscope

Answers

1. a. The first image is real and the final image is virtual
2. b. By tagging the protein by green fluorescence protein and then observing in cone focal microscopy
3. b. Xylene can be used for cleaning the lens.
4. d. Confocal microscope.

CHAPTER

19 Digital Image Analysis

INTRODUCTION

Perception of human being is subjective. However, we need objective and quantitative assessment in our day-to-day cytology practice. Image analysis helps us to have quantitative cytology. The term image analysis means acquiring and then further analyzing the quantitative data from any image of an object. In the last two decades, there is a massive development in the field of image analysis. This is due to significant computational capability for data accumulation and storage. The other factor is rapid development of knowledge-based systems for data analysis and diagnostic decision-making. Presently, image analysis is used not only as a major research tool in the field of cytology but also has been applied routinely in various fields such as in automated screening technology of cervical cancer screening.

PRINCIPLES OF IMAGE ANALYSIS (BOX 19.1)

The knowledge of principles of image analysis is very essential for understanding and further application of this field. The basic principles and steps are described below:

- *Image digitalization (Fig. 19.1)*: In this step, the image is stored in the computer as digital image. The smallest unit of the image is known as a pixel. Each pixel is located in particular X- and Y-axis. Now depending on the gray intensity of the pixel of the black-and-white image, the pixel is given a particular numerical value. So, every pixel of the image in each particular location (X, Y) is stored in the computer as a numeric value. Now from the stored gray value data the computer can generate the whole image again. In case of colored image, each pixel is given three values for red, green, and blue depending on the relative intensity of the image.
- *Image detection (Fig. 19.2)*: Now from the digital image stored in the computer one can detect the area or object of interest by manipulating or adjusting the gray value or color code of the image.
- *Image editing*: Image editing is needed to process the detected object of interest so that it is free of background noise. The detected object should also be free of any overlapping objects. Different mathematical algorithms can be used to separate or segregate the objects.

Box 19.1: Image analysis: Few basic points.

Steps
- *Digitalization*: Image is converted into digits depending on gray value
- *Detection*: Objects of interest is selected by adjusting gray value or color code
- *Editing*: Detected image is processed to extract data
- *Feature extraction*: The data are extracted from the identified object

Performing image analysis: Interactive and automated
Basic requirements: Microscope, digital camera and computer
Types: Morphometry, cytometry and pattern recognition.

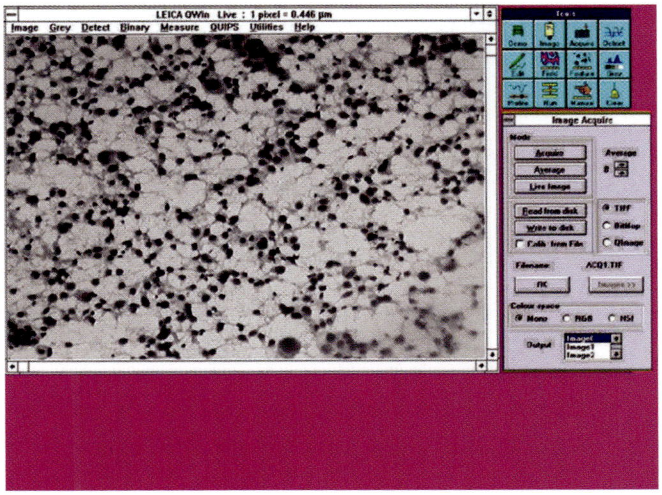

Fig. 19.1: At first the image is digitized. This digitized image may be black and white or in color.

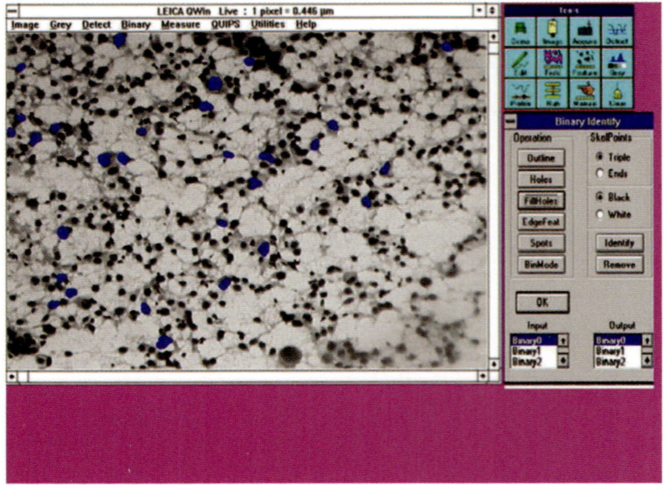

Fig. 19.2: Object of interest is detected by adjusting gray value.

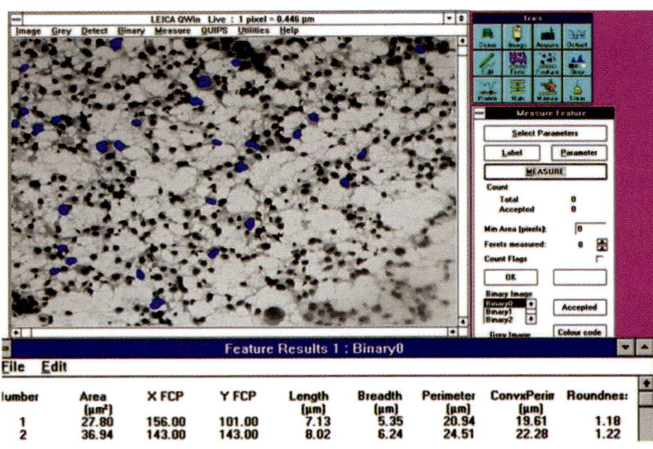

Fig. 19.3: Data are extracted from the detected image.

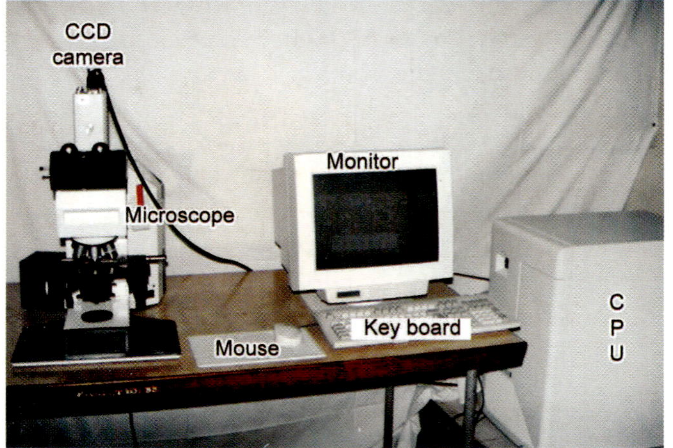

Fig. 19.4: Basic instruments of image cytometry are highlighted in this photograph.

- *Feature extraction (Fig. 19.3)*: Feature extraction means extraction of different geometric data from the object such as size, shape, texture, etc. In each case, hundreds of different features can be measured.

INSTRUMENT REQUIREMENTS (FIG. 19.4)

The basic instruments required are: (1) microscope, (2) attached digital camera, (3) central processing unit, (4) keyboard, (5) mouse pointer, and (6) a suitable software program.

A digital camera is attached to the microscope. The image is transferred from the digital camera to the computer processing unit and is shown directly into the monitor. Now this digitized image is manipulated for data extraction and analysis.

IMAGE ANALYSIS: AUTOMATED OR INTERACTIVE

An automated image analysis system has automated control of different functions of the microscope controlled by a microcomputer. The interactive image analysis features a user friendly mode wherein the user can select the cell of interest and obtain various cell parameters required. The system is equipped with a microscope and video camera for acquisition of cell images. The image processing hardware accepts the video data from the camera and converts the image into the digital image and then into signals for displaying the image on the monitor. Now with the help of mouse the object of interest is selected, edited, and feature is extracted.

Types of Image Analysis

It can be arbitrarily classified as:

- Morphometry
- Cytometry
- Chromatin pattern recognition.

Morphometry

This means a quantitative description of geometric features of structures of any dimensions. The stereologic or three-dimensional information is obtained from the two-dimensional (2D) data by assumptions from the data of 2D objects or directly by calculating the third dimension.

The targets of application of image morphometry are (Box 19.2):

Box 19.2: Areas of application of image analysis.

- *Morphometry*
  - Linear distance measurement: Distance between two objects
  - Object counting: Number of objects in a field area is counted
  - Form factor: Area, diameter, perimeter, etc.
  - Area fraction: Relative area of the substance
  - Mean nuclear volume: Nuclear volume from two dimensional image
  - Fractal dimension measurement
  - Complex measurement: Cell-to-cell relation, roundness, etc.
- *Cytometry*
  - Relative DNA content
  - Quantitative estimation of antigen
- Chromatin pattern recognition

- *Linear distance measurement*: Linear distance between two objects such as cell-to-cell distance or basement membrane to cell distance, etc. is measured.
- *Object counting*: It means to count the number of objects such as mitotic figures or any other particular object in a particular field area.
- *Form factor*: This means measurement of area, diameter, perimeter, and other geometric features of the object.
- *Area fraction*: This indicates the measurement of particular areas in the total field area such as the measurement of argyrophilic nucleolar organizer region (AgNOR) area occupied in the nucleus[1] or measurement of the area of reticulin fiber in trephine biopsy.[2]
- *Complex measurement*: With the help of image morphometry, complex measurements such as cell-to-cell relation or measurement of roundness can be done.
- *Mean nuclear volume*: Mean nuclear volume can be estimated in 2D planes with the help of stereotactic method.[3,4]
- *Fractal dimension*: Fractal geometry is a relatively new area of the morphometry. Unlike Euclidean geometry, fractal geometry deals with noninteger dimensions.[5] The fractal dimension of an object describe the irregularity of the object. Measurement of fractal dimension may help in assessment of chromatin distribution, nuclear margin irregularity, tumor angiogenesis, and collagen distribution in the section.[5] With the help of image morphometry, fractal dimension can be measured.

Nuclear morphometry may be used to do tumor grading, subtyping, diagnosis, and prognosis.

Cytometry

In case of cytometry, the amount of dye within a certain tissue or cell or nuclei is measured with the help of image analysis. DNA cytometry measures the relative amount of DNA within the nucleus. The principle of DNA cytometry is using a stoichiometrically bound DNA-specific dye and then the optical density of the nucleus is measured to assess the relative amount of DNA. Finally, the optical density of the test and the control nuclei are compared. Commonly normal human peripheral lymphocytes are used for diploid control. For the successful DNA cytometry, two things are needed: (1) the nuclei should be total, and (2) each nucleus should be discrete as overlapping nuclei may give wrong results. DNA image cytometry may help in identification of aneuploid tumor cells in effusion fluid or bladder wash cytology sample. Aneuploidy in these samples usually indicates malignancy. It can also be used for tumor grading on the basis of ploidy.[6]

Image cytometry is also used to measure the amount of immunohistochemically stained proteins in cells such as estrogen receptors or p53 antigens.[7] The amount of stained material in immunohistochemistry is not stoichiometric. So, stringent calibration of the immunohistochemistry staining is required for quantitative assessment of antigen.

Box 19.3: Limitations and difficulties of image analysis.

- *Disease identification*: Exact identification of disease difficult.
- *Decision on individual patient*: Overall classification of cases possible but difficult to decide on individual cases.
- *Selection of images of interest*: Objects of interest are difficult to identify by automated analysis.
- Large amount of data handling is problematic
- *Other technical challenges*: Rapid panning, zooming, focusing, data storage.

Chromatin Pattern Recognition

With the help of image analyzer, it is possible to assess the chromatin pattern recognition of the nuclei. Recently, fractal geometry is also used for chromatin pattern recognition.[8] The assessment of chromatin pattern may help to classify the different cells.

DIGITAL IMAGE ANALYSIS: CERTAIN PROBLEMS (BOX 19.3)

Disease Identification

With the help of visual microscopic examination, we reach to diagnostic identification of the disease. In this identification process, we collect the information and assessed the diagnosis with certainty. The adequate amount of information on a particular entity makes us more certain.

In contrast, a classification procedure operates in a closed feature space. The statistical classification procedure is dependent on a certain number of features to discriminate the member of different classes. A class member should have the typical values of the certain features. In an unknown case, the classification is done based on the different features of the objects. Traditional image analysis may be efficient in classification, but not so much reliable for diagnostic identification.

Decision on Individual Patient

Till now the various analytical methods deal with the population as a whole. There is not much methodology on individual case-based decision. Massive database of the patients for a particular diagnostic condition is needed to solve this issue. The exact clinical outcomes of the patients are also needed. Data mining technique with the help of artificial neural network (ANN) may be helpful in such condition.[9]

Selection of Images of Interest

Selection of images for interpretation is a challenge to the automated image analysis. A successful automated image analyzer should have the capability of processing the scene, segmentation, and feature extraction. Montironi et al.[10] applied a machine vision-based system in histopathology sections of the prostate to resolve this issue.

Large Amount of Data Handling

First and foremost, to automate pathology, it is essential to digitize slide data. For interpretation of any slide, large amount of data has to be captured and processed rapidly. This is still a challenge to the image analyzer.

Other Technical Challenges

There are other challenges of image analysis and interpretation such as rapid panning and zooming of the microscope, focusing to the point of interest, database storage for metadata, visualization, and pattern recognition.

OTHER DEVELOPMENTS IN IMAGE ANALYSIS

Laser Scanning Cytometry

It is a relatively new area of image cytometry with significant advantages (Box 19.4) over the routine image cytometry.[11,12]

Principle (Fig. 19.5)

In laser scanning cytometry (LSC), the object on the glass slide is automatically scanned by laser beam. The slide position and laser beam are moved automatically under the control of a computer. The cells are stained with antibody tagged with fluorescence dye. Fluorescent labeling does not need any enzyme amplification so the measurement of intensity of fluorescence helps in the accurate quantification of antigen in this fluorescence-based study. The emitted fluorescence of the object or cell is measured in multiple wavelengths. A fluorescence value for each object or cell is recorded along with the X-Y position of the individual cells. So it is possible to correlate directly the result of immunofluorescence and cytomorphology of each cell. The various other features of

Box 19.4: Laser scanning cytometry.

Principle
- Fluorescent labeled cells on the smear are hit by laser beam
- Intensity of fluorescence measured
- Cell image is also stored for correlation

Advantages
- Rapid technique
- No single cell preparation or special processing
- Cell loss negligible so can be done on scanty cellular smear
- Cell can be stored for long time
- Morphologic correlation with fluorescence data possible

Applications
- DNA ploidy estimation
- Immunophenotyping
- Cell proliferation fraction
- Apoptotic cell counting
- Quantification of antigenic substance

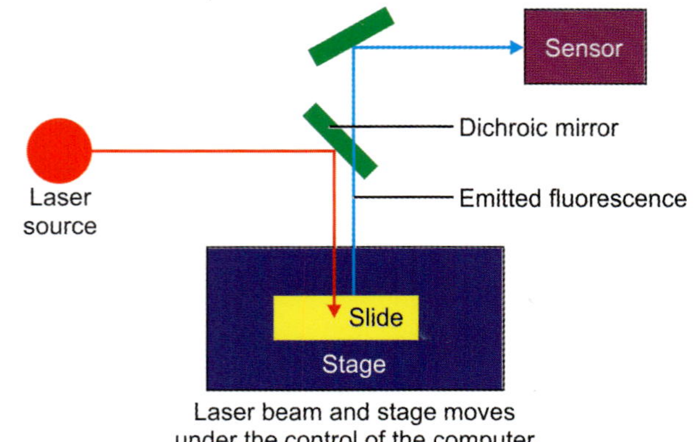

Fig. 19.5: The basic principles of laser scanning cytometry.

objects such as area, diameter, perimeter, etc. can also be measured simultaneously.

Advantages of Laser Scanning Cytometry

There are various advantages of LSC:[13]

- This is a very *rapid technique* in comparison to simple image cytometry done by light microscope.
- In LSC, the *cells are on a solid support* as they are placed on a glass slide. It is not necessary to have single cell or nuclei preparation as that is required for flow cytometry. Touch preparation or fine needle aspiration cytology (FNAC) smears can also be used for LSC.
- There is *no need for* centrifugation or *special processing* for LSC so cell loss is negligible.
- The cells are permanently fixed on glass slides and cytomorphology can be correlated with the functional studies.
- The archival preservation of the object or cell is possible.

Applications

There are various applications of LSC.

- With the help of LSC, the measurement of DNA content is possible and the ploidy status of the cell can be correlated with the morphology
- Immunophenotyping of cells
- LSC is helpful in demonstration of apoptotic cells by staining of propidium iodide, Rh 123 or FITC-tagged annexin V.
- Quantification of estrogen and progesterone receptors in breast carcinoma.
- Quantification of actively proliferating cells with the help of Ki-67 immunostain.

KNOWLEDGE-BASED EXPERT SYSTEM FOR DATA INTERPRETATION OF IMAGE ANALYSIS

Data analysis and interpretation is a very important aspect of image analysis. There is a major advancement in this area. Various computer-based expert systems are available now for the data interpretation. These systems are based on a Bayesian belief network (BBN), ANN works, and logistic regression analysis.[14,15]

Bayesian Belief Network (Fig. 19.6)

Bayesian belief network is a knowledge-based decision support system.[14] The network is comprised of multiple nodes that means multiple evidences or features with multiple outcomes. Such as for diagnosis of carcinoma of the breast, the various cytological features are the nodes. Each cytological feature may have various outcomes such as nuclear enlargement may be mild, moderate or marked. Therefore, the nuclear enlargement (node) has three outcomes: (1) mild, (2) moderate, and (3) severe. Belief in various outcomes is stored in each node and is expressed as a probability. Each node is connected with other by links. Links between the nodes are quantified by conditional probability (CP) matrix. When the descendant or evidence nodes are connected to the parent node or final outcome node, the CP matrix in between the nodes expresses the probability of getting a particular outcome. Such as in the diagnosis of breast carcinoma, the final outcome may be benign or malignant or in urine cytology the outcome may be benign, atypia, or malignant.

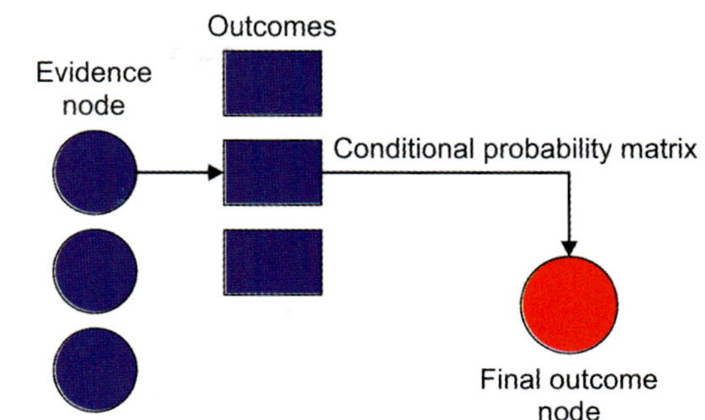

Fig. 19.6: The basic principles of Bayesian belief network.

Bayesian belief network has been applied in cytology for diagnosis and grading of carcinomas. It is a promising field expert-based knowledge system.[16]

Artificial Neural Network (Box 19.5)

Artificial neural network is a powerful nonlinear statistical classifier whose architecture is designed on the basis of human brain.[9]

How Does Artificial Neural Network Work (Fig. 19.7)?

Artificial neural network is made up of many simple processing units, which are bundled together in a complex communication network. Each of this processing unit is known as "node" which simulates "neuron" of the brain. Each node receives signal from other nodes or from external stimuli. The receiving node then sends signals to other nodes via connection. The end node receives signal from all other neurons and then it produces the final decision.

Box 19.5: Artificial neural network.

Basis: Artificial neural network simulates human brain. Here instead of neurons there are multiple interconnecting nodes. Each node receives signal from other nodes or from external stimuli. Ultimately final outcome node sends the result.

Layers
- Input layer
- Hidden layer
- Output layer

Training: Three sets of data
1. Training set
2. Validation set
3. Test set

Advantages
- Robust and can tolerate missing data
- Can analyze nonlinear complex data
- Can take decision on individual cases
- Faster and can process parallel data
- Learn from example rather than logic

Applications
- In automated analysis of cases particularly in cervical cancer
- Analysis of complex data in gene microarray
- Diagnosis of difficult or complex cases.

The layers of ANN consist of (1) an input layer, (2) single or multiple hidden layers, and (3) an output layer. The nodes of input layer receive input signals from the external stimuli. The nodes of the output layer communicate with the external environment. The single to multiple hidden layers exist in between the input and output layers. The signal is received by input nodes and produces an output signal. Ultimately the output layer finally processes its signal for the exact decision.[9] To provide training to ANN, three nonoverlapping sets of data are used: (1) training set, (2) validation set, and (3) test set. The training set helps in the adjustment of weights of various nodes and validation set helps to maintain the topology of the network. The results of the test set can be considered as a true prediction of ANN performance on new data.

Advantages and Disadvantages

Artificial neural network has certain advantages. It learns by example rather than the specific logic. ANN is a robust system and can adjust the missing data. There are certain problems in ANN implementation. ANN lacks transparency and no one knows how the hidden layer functions. There is also ambiguity of the optimal architecture of ANN and the risk of overtraining of ANN cannot be ignored.

Application

The ANN can be used to identify malignancy in urine cytology, pleural effusion, breast cytology, etc.[17-19] In future, ANN will be a powerful tool in routine cytology practice.

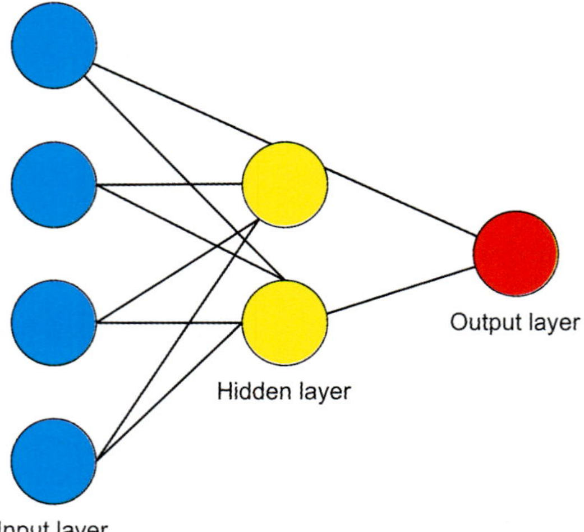

Fig. 19.7: The basic principles of artificial neural network.

REFERENCES

1. Mohanty SK, Dey P, Rana P. Manual and automated AgNOR count in differentiating reactive mesothelial cells from metastatic malignant cells in serous effusion. Anal Quant Cytol Histol. 2003;25(5):273-6.
2. Lamba A, Dey P, Savita K, et al. Prognostic significance of the histomorphometric features of bone marrow trephine biopsies in patients with chronic myeloid leukemia. Anal Quant Cytol Histol. 2007;29(6):370-6.
3. Mohanty SK, Dey P. Mean nuclear volume in squamous cell carcinoma of the vulva. Anal Quant Cytol Histol. 2004;26: 84-6.
4. Mohanty SK, Dey P, Saha SC. Mean nuclear volume in ovarian papillary serous cystadenocarcinoma. Anal Quant Cytol Histol. 2004;26(1):28-30.
5. Dey P. Fractal geometry: basic principles and applications in pathology. Anal Quant Cytol Histol. 2005;27(5):284-90.
6. Dey P, Luthra UK, Prasad A, et al. Cytological grading and DNA image cytometry of breast carcinomas on fine needle aspiration cytology smears. Anal Quant Cytol Histol. 1999:21;17-20.
7. Aziz DC, Barathur RB. Quantitation and morphometric analysis of tumors by image analysis. J Cell Biochem Suppl. 1994;19:120-5.
8. Dey P, Banik T. Fractal dimension of chromatin texture of squamous intraepithelial. Diagn Cytopathol. 2012;40(2): 152-4.
9. Dey P, Dey R. Artificial neural network–mechanism and application in pathology. Indian J Pathol Microbiol. 2002;45:371-4.
10. Montironi R, Bartels PH, Thompson D, et al. Prostatic intraepithelial neoplasia. Quantitation of the basal cell layer with machine vision system. Path Res Pract. 1995;191:917-23.
11. Clatch RJ, Foreman JR, Walloch JL. Simplified immunophenotypic analysis by laser scanning cytometry. Cytometry. 1998;34:3-16.

12. Clatch RJ, Walloch JL, Zutter MM, et al. Immunophenotypic analysis of hematologic malignancies by laser scanning cytometry. Am J Clin Pathol. 1996;105:744-55.
13. Kamentsky LA, Burger DE, Gershman RJ, et al. Slide-based laser scanning cytometry. Acta Cytol. 1997;41(1):123-43.
14. Whimster WF, Hamilton PW, Anderson NA, et al. Reproducibility of Bayesian belief network assessment of breast fine needle aspirates. Anal Quant Cytol Histol. 1996;18(4):267-74.
15. Karakitsos P, Cochand-Priollet B, Guillausseau PJ, et al. A potential of the back propagation neural network in the morphologic examination of thyroid lesions. Anal Quant Cytol Histol. 1996;18(6):494-500.
16. Bibbo M, Bartels PH, Pfeifer T, et al. Belief network for grading prostate lesions. Anal Quant Cytol Histol. 1993;15: 124-35.
17. Muralidaran C, Dey P, Nijhawan R, et al. Artificial neural network in diagnosis of urothelial cell carcinoma in urine cytology. Diagn Cytopathol. 2015;43(6):443-9.
18. Dey P, Rajesh L, Joshi K. Artificial neural network in diagnosis of lobular carcinoma of breast in fine needle aspiration cytology. Diagn Cytopathol. 2013;41(2):102-6.
19. Barwad A, Dey P, Susheilia S. Artificial neural network in diagnosis of metastatic carcinoma in effusion cytology. Cytometry B Clin Cytom. 2012;82(2):107-11.

Review Questions

1. **When the objects of interest are selected by adjusting gray value or color code, it is known as:**
   a. Digitalization
   b. Detection
   c. Editing
   d. Feature extraction
2. **All are true about laser scanning cytometry *except*:**
   a. Rapid technique
   b. No single cell preparation or special processing
   c. Cell loss is considerable and cannot be done on scanty cellular smear
   d. Morphologic correlation with fluorescence data possible
3. **Which one is true for artificial neural network?**
   a. Cannot analyze nonlinear complex data
   b. Can take decision on individual cases
   c. Cannot process parallel data
   d. Learn from logic rather than example

Identify True/False

4. **With the help of image analyzer it is possible to assess the chromatin pattern recognition of the nuclei.** *(True/false)*
5. **Morphologic correlation with fluorescence data is possible in laser scanning cytometry.** *(True/false)*
6. **Artificial neural network (ANN) is a powerful linear statistical classifier.** *(True/false)*

Answers

1. b. Detection
2. c. Cell loss is considerable and cannot be done on scanty cellular smear
3. b. Can take decision on individual cases
4. True
5. True
6. False

CHAPTER

20

Flow Cytometry

INTRODUCTION

Flow cytometry (FCM) is the study of different characteristics of the single cell in the fluid stream. This technology was developed rapidly in the past few decades. Unlike the older instrument, the modern flow cytometer is now smaller, user-friendly, versatile, and less costly. The instrument is now used not only for research but also for routine clinical activities.[1-3]

PRINCIPLES OF FLOW CYTOMETRY

Single cells in fluid suspension are needed to do FCM. These cells are stained with a fluorescent dye. The fluorescent dye binds with the specific components of the cell. DNA-specific dye binds with DNA stoichiometrically and similarly antibody tagged with the fluorescent dye binds with the cell surface antigen or receptors. The fluorochrome-stained cells flow singly in front of a laser beam. When the laser beam of particular wavelength hits the cell, then the cell absorbs light and emits fluorescence. In case of multiple fluorochrome dyes, the excitation beam of light may be of same wavelength but the emission beam of light from different fluorochrome dye will have different wavelengths. With the help of appropriate filter, the simultaneous evaluation of multiple colors (parameters) for each cell can be recorded. The flow cytometer receives the emitted light signal with the help of the photodetectors and then converts it into digital signals for storage on the computer. The intensity of this digital signal is graded on a relative scale known as channel. The results are then displayed as histogram or two-dimensional dot plots.

CYTOLOGY SAMPLES

Different types of cytology specimen can be processed for FCM:

- *Fine needle aspiration cytology materials*: Lymph node, breast, lung, prostate, etc.
- *Exfoliative samples*: Effusion fluid, cerebrospinal fluid (CSF), bladder wash, etc.

Cytology specimen has some special *advantages* over the histopathology tissue. These are:

- Cytology sample is easy to process and requires less disaggregation and thereby single cell preparation is easier to make for FCM.
- It is relatively easy to procure cytology sample.
- Multiple areas of the tumor or lymph nodes can be collected for processing.
- As the cells are viable so functional studies can be done.

Collection

The cytology samples can be collected in 1 mL of citrate buffer solution (Box 20.1). The sample can be processed immediately or may be kept at –70°C to process later on.

Control

Lymphocytes from the peripheral blood samples of healthy individuals may be kept as an external control for DNA FCM. Certain general requirements are needed for instrument control such as optics, fluidics, and electronics. This is usually done with commercially available fluorescein-labeled beads. The individual laboratories should always follow the recommendations of the manufacturers of the instruments on daily, weekly, or monthly basis.

For flow cytometric immunophenotyping (FCI), both positive and negative controls should be used. Negative

Box 20.1: Citrate buffer.

- 85.3 g sucrose
- 11.8 g trisodium citrate (Sigma)
- 50 mL of dimethyl sulfoxide in 100 mL of water pH adjusted at 7.6.

control is needed to eliminate background autofluorescence and nonspecific staining. Positive control is needed to verify the working condition of the reagents. The fresh normal blood sample is ideal for the control sample. Commercially available preparations may be more convenient as these preparations are stable and more reproducible.

Dye Used

Propidium iodide, ethidium bromide, Hoechst 33342, and diamidinophenylindole (DAPI), etc. are used for DNA content measurement. The presence and quantity of surface receptors or intracellular antigens are measured with fluorescein isothiocyanate (FITC), phycoerythrin (PE), allophycocyanin (APC), and Texas red (Box 20.2). Most of the fluorochrome dyes are excited in same wavelength (488 nm) and they emit light of different wavelengths. RNA content is measured with acridine orange, pyronin Y, and oxazine 1. Intracellular enzyme activity is detected with the help of chromogenic or fluorogenic substances.

Sample Processing

DNA flow cytometry: The aspirated material should be centrifuged and resuspended in citrate buffer. The single cell suspension is done either mechanically by repeated syringing through nylon mesh or by trypsinization.[3] The cell concentration in the buffer is kept as at least 2×10^6 cells per mL. The cells are permeabilized and stained with a DNA-specific dye such as propidium iodide.[2]

FLOW CYTOMETRIC IMMUNOPHENOTYPING

Direct Stain

The fresh effusion fluid sample of 100 µL will be incubated with 10 µL of labeled antibodies for 25 minutes in the dark place at room temperature. The cell will be further treated with a lysing solution for 10 minutes followed by centrifugation. The supernatant fluid will be discarded and the cells will be resuspended in 0.5 mL phosphate buffered saline (PBS) for analysis.

Indirect Staining Procedure (Box 20.3)[4,5]

At first, the nonspecific staining will be blocked by incubating the cells with 100 µL mouse myeloma IgG1 protein (1:50) for 25 minutes at room temperature. The cells will be washed with few drops of PBS. The sample of 100 µL of effusion will be incubated with 50 µL of primary nonconjugated antibody for 25 minute at room temperature in dark. The cell will be washed by few drops of PBS by centrifugation for 10 minutes. Next, 50 µL of a conjugated secondary antibody will be added for another 25 minute and will be kept at room temperature. A few drops of PBS will be added and centrifugation will be done. Finally, supernatant will be decanted and 500 µL FACS-flow solutions will be added and the sample will be examined.

TARGET OF APPLICATIONS

Flow cytometry can be used for quantitative measurement of various cellular characteristics (Box 20.4). Many of the targets of application of FCM are research oriented.

Most common applications of FCM in clinical laboratory are immunophenotyping, DNA content analysis, and cell cycle analysis (Box 20.5). In addition, FCM is used also for histocompatibility cross matching, HLA-B27 detection, cluster of differentiation (CD4), and CD8 counting for immunodeficiency, reticulocyte enumeration, and paroxysmal nocturnal hemoglobinuria (PNH) detection.

Box 20.2: Dyes used for flow cytometry.

- DNA content measurement
  - Propidium iodide, ethidium bromide, Hoechst 33342, diamidinophenylindole (DAPI), mithramycin, chromomycin
- RNA content measurement
  - Acridine orange, thiazole orange, pyronin Y, thioflavin T, and oxazine 1
- Surface receptors or intracellular antigens
  - Fluorescein isothiocyanate (FITC), phycoerythrin (PE), peridinin-chlorophyll-protein and allophycocyanin (APC), Texas red.

Box 20.3: Flow cytometric immunophenotyping processing: indirect method.

- Sample collected in citrate buffer
- Samples are washed in PBS
- Resuspended and kept 1.5×10^6 cells/mL into multiple small aliquots
- Incubated with 50 µL of primary nonconjugated antibody for 25 minutes at room temperature in dark.
- Cells are washed in PBS
- 50 µL of a conjugated secondary antibody will be added
- Keep for 25 minute at room temperature
- A few drops of PBS will be added and centrifugation will be done, specimen is then centrifuged, and supernatant solution is discarded
- Finally supernatant will be decanted and 500 µL flow solutions will be added to fix the cells.
- FCI is performed.

(FCI: Flow cytometric immunophenotyping; PBS: Phosphate buffered saline).

Box 20.4: Measurement of cellular features.

- Cell size
- Cell shape
- DNA content and cell cycle analysis
- RNA content
- Mitochondrial function
- Cellular protein, lipid, hemoglobin, calcium
- Intracellular and surface receptors
- Apoptotic cells.

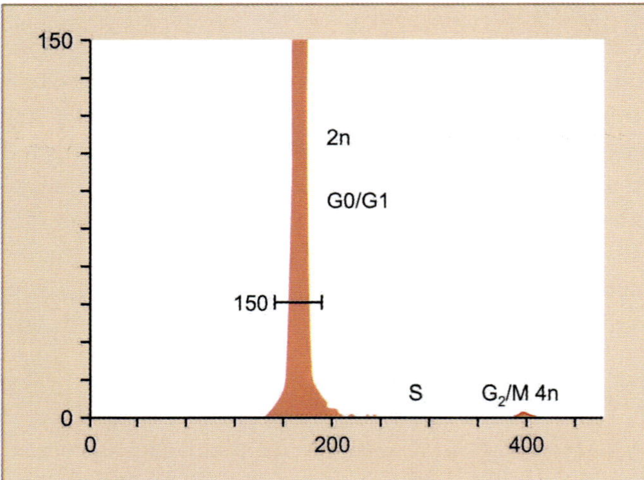

Fig. 20.1: Diploid DNA peak in DNA flow cytometry.

DNA CONTENT AND PLOIDY ANALYSIS

Deoxyribonucleic acid content measurement is based on the stoichiometric binding of the DNA-specific dye with the DNA of the nucleus and subsequent measurement of emitted fluorescence form the dye-DNA complex. The emitted fluorescence is supposed to be proportional to the DNA content of the cells and is represented as channel number which is an arbitrary value depending on the initial set up of the machine in a particular day. The data are displayed as DNA histogram. As the majority of the normal cells contain diploid (2n) chromosome, therefore they emit a certain amount of fluorescence represented by a channel number. This forms a single peak known as the diploid peak in DNA histogram (Fig. 20.1). As the cells in G_2M phase contain the double amount of DNA (4n), so they emit the double amount of fluorescence and are present in double channel number in the DNA histogram forming a small tetraploid peak. In between these two peaks the cells have varying amount of DNA from 2n to 4n and they are in synthetic (S) phase. Any peak, other than these two peaks should be considered as an aneuploid peak.

Box 20.5: Common clinical applications of flow cytometry.

- Immunophenotyping of lymphoma and leukemia by various CD markers
- Malignancy detection in body fluid
- DNA ploidy analysis by measuring DNA content
- Cell cycle analysis by S phase estimation and Ki-67 measurement
- Histocompatibility cross matching by IgG and IgM antibody
- HLA-B27 detection
- CD4 and CD8 counting for immunodeficiency
- Reticulocyte enumeration
- Paroxysmal nocturnal hemoglobinuria (PNH) detection by CD55 and CD59 estimation.

Following information is obtained from DNA FCM:

- Identification of aneuploid cell population
- DNA index
- Proliferative cell fraction (% of S-phase).

DNA Ploidy

During proliferation of the cells in malignant tumor there may be a generation of clone of malignant cells that contain a specific amount of DNA other than diploid DNA content. This clone of cells containing the abnormal amount of DNA is known as aneuploid cells. In DNA histogram, the aneuploid population will form a peak somewhere other than diploid peak.

The relative DNA content of the aneuploid population of cells is calculated by DNA index.

$$\text{DNA index} = \frac{\text{Mean channel number of aneuploid peak}}{\text{Mean channel number of normal diploid peak}}$$

The different types of aneuploidy are:

Hyperdiploid Aneuploidy (Fig. 20.2)

If the aneuploid peak is in between diploid or tetraploid (DNA index more than 1 and less than 2).

Hypodiploid Aneuploidy

Aneuploid cell population contains less than the 2n amount of DNA and form a peak left of the diploid peak (DNA index less than 1).

Tetraploid Aneuploidy

Aneuploid population forms a peak that overlaps with G_2M or tetraploid peak. This is difficult to distinguish from G_2M cells. However, the aneuploid G_2M peak contains more than 20% cell population (DNA index is 2).

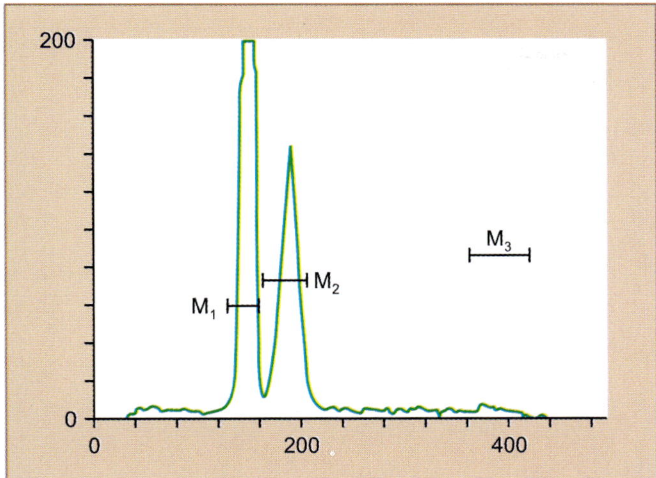

Fig. 20.2: DNA histogram showing hyperdiploid aneuploidy.

Hypertetraploid Aneuploidy

Aneuploid population of cells contains more than 4n amount of DNA and forms a peak right to the G_2M peak (DNA index more than 2).

S phase

S-phase fraction of cells is calculated as the population of cells in between G_0G_1 and G_2M peak. This is easily calculated from the DNA histogram.

CLINICAL RELEVANCE

DNA FCM is considered as useful for diagnosis and prognosis of tumors. DNA aneuploidy and high S-phase (proliferative fraction) percentage are commonly noted in malignant tumors and may be used for diagnosis of malignancies.[1-3] However, false negative or positive cases may occur because many malignant tumors are diploid and rare benign tumor may show DNA aneuploidy.[6]

DIAGNOSIS

Effusions

There is a variable success rate of DNA FCM in the diagnosis of malignancy in effusion fluid. The false-negative rate of FCM is as high as 41% and false-positive rate of FCM is only 2–3% FCM.[6] DNA FCM alone is not cost-effective and dual color FCM is more helpful in diagnosis of malignancy.[7]

Bladder Washings

DNA FCM of bladder wash specimen is a helpful ancillary technique for detection of malignancy of the bladder. DNA FCM shows 78–93% sensitivity.[8] DNA FCM is especially helpful in follow-up cases of urothelial carcinoma of the bladder. DNA ploidy estimation of gated population of cytokeratin positive cell is more helpful to detect malignancy in urine.[9]

Cerebrospinal Fluid (CSF)

DNA FCM is not very helpful in the detection of malignancy in CSF because of low cellularity in CSF. However, combined use of immunophenotyping and DNA FCM may be useful in the diagnosis of lymphoma in CSF.[10]

Prognosis

It is considered that DNA aneuploidy and high S-phase is a poor prognostic factor in solid tumors such as bladder, prostate, ovarian, and endometrial carcinomas.[11]

IMMUNOPHENOTYPING

Presently, FCI is widely used in the detection of various antigen or receptor markers on the surface of the cells. CD indicates the specific receptor or ligand on the cell surface. More than 300 CDs are listed till now.[12] Similarly, a large number of monoclonal antibodies against various CD markers are also commercially available for FCM. Demonstration of various CD markers on the lymphoid cell surface has great impact in the subclassification of lymphomas and leukemia.

Diagnosis

Flow cytometry can demonstrate kappa and lambda chain on the cell surface of lymphoid cells. As non-Hodgkin lymphoma (NHL) is monoclonal in origin so in B-NHL, the neoplastic cells show light chain restriction and they show either lambda or kappa light chains (Figs. 20.3A and B). Therefore, the presence of light chain restriction indicates lymphoma. In FCM the kappa/lambda ratio more than 4:1 or more than 1:2 is usually considered as an evidence of monoclonality. It is difficult to determine clonality of the T-cell NHL. Predominant expression of CD4 or CD8 expression may be considered as surrogate markers of clonality of T-NHL. However, the aberrant expression of CD2, CD5, and CD7 expression may suggest

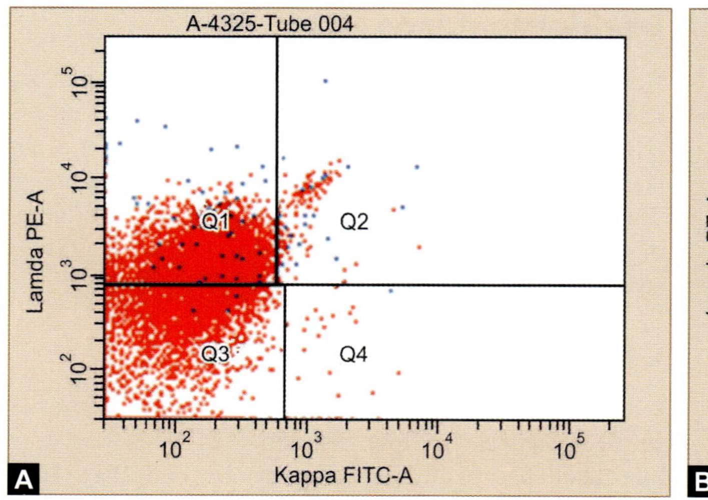

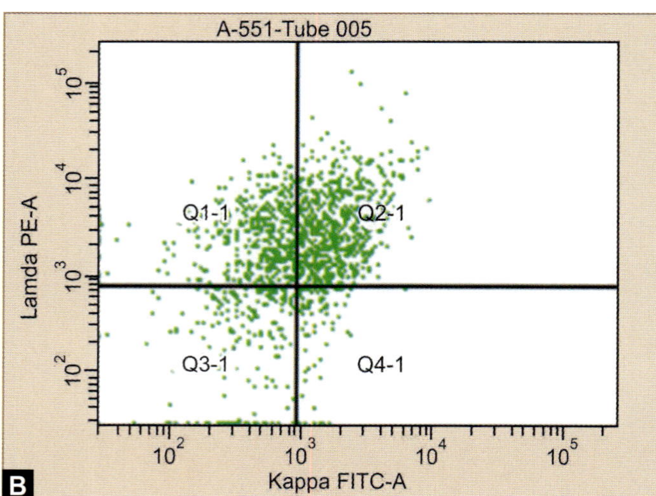

Figs 20.3A and B: (A) Light chain restriction as only lambda chain is expressed; (B) No light chain restriction as both kappa and lambda chains are expressed.

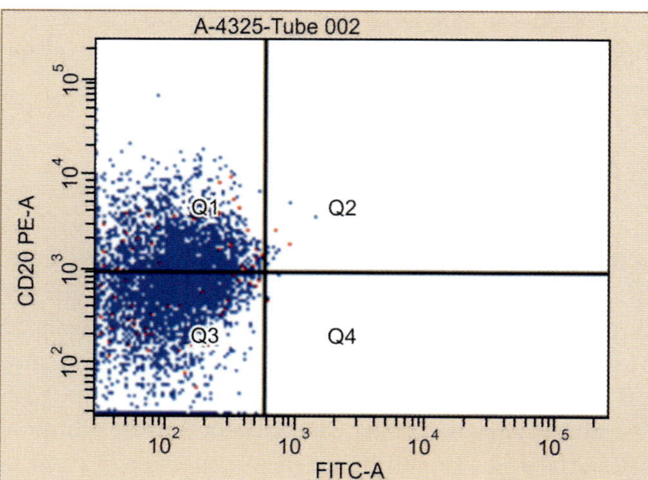

Fig. 20.4: CD20 positivity in a case of lymphoma.

T-NHL.[13] There is no doubt that the only way to diagnose T-cell clonality is by demonstration of T-cell receptor gene arrangement of molecular methods.

Subclassification

B-cell NHL shows a specific pattern of CD marker expression on their surface and the use of a panel of markers along with cytomorphology is very helpful in subclassification of NHL (Figs. 20.4 and 20.5).[13] In fact, FCM is especially useful for lymphoma phenotyping of fine needle aspiration cytology (FNAC) material as the cells are discrete. FCM has certain unique *advantages* over routine immunocytochemistry (Table 20.1). These are:

- It is a relatively fast technique and large number of cells can be analyzed rapidly.
- A large panel of CD markers can be used in the FCM.
- Dual expression of CD markers can be demonstrated.
- Many other additional features such as DNA ploidy, cell cycle analysis, etc. can be done simultaneously along with immunophenotyping.
- FCM is helpful to measure the percentage of positive cells along with the intensity of antigen expression in individual cells.

Limitations of Flow Cytometric Immunophenotyping (Box 20.6)

Flow cytometric immunophenotyping (FCI) has certain limitations:

- Inability to correlate morphological findings with the FCI data is one of the major defects of FCI. Newer technology such as laser scanning cytometry (LSC) may overcome this problem.
- Admixture of benign reactive components of the lymph node such as vascular or stromal material.
- Inability to identify Hodgkin's lymphoma because of scanty Reed-Sternberg (R-S) cells in the specimen.
- Necrosis, blood mixed sample, etc. may produce faulty reporting and gated population of lymphoid cells are needed.
- All cases of B-NHL may not always show light chain restriction. This may be due to absence of expression of light chain on the surface of the cell.
- FCM is overall a costly technique and needs good skill.

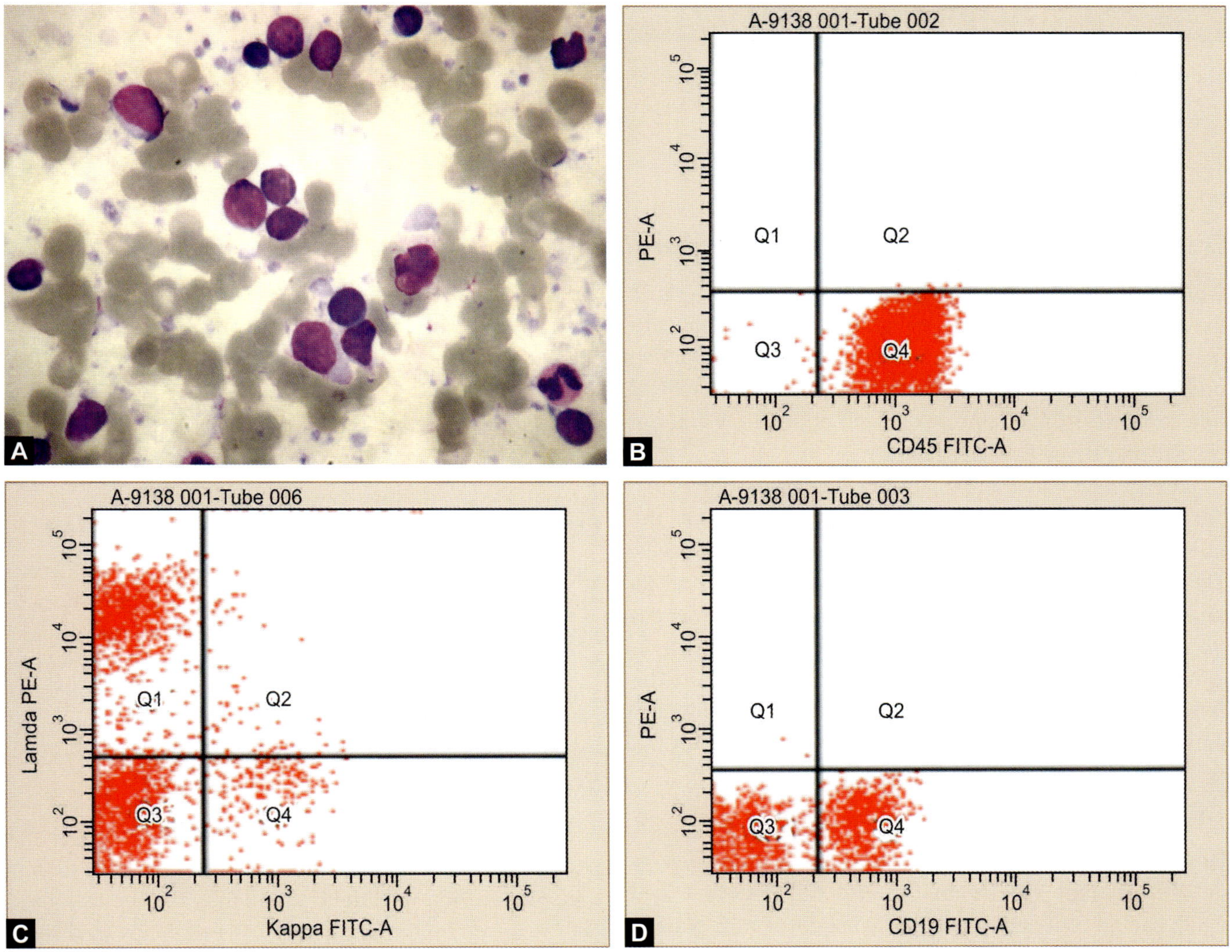

Figs. 20.5A to D: (A) Fine needle aspiration cytology smear of an orbital lymphoma showing discrete lymphoid cells. Individual cells show round nuclei and scanty cytoplasm. Background of the smear shows lymphoglandular bodies (May-Grünwald Giemsa stain × HP); (B) Predominant cells are CD45 positive; (C) Cells show predominantly lambda light chain expression indicating monoclonality of the cells; and (D) Majority of the cells are CD19 positive indicating B-cell origin.

Table 20.1: Comparison of flow cytometry immunophenotyping and immunocytochemistry.

	Flow cytometry immunophenotyping	*Immunocytochemistry*
Processing speed	Very rapid	Slow
Subjectivity	Objective	Interpretation is more or less subjective
Antibody panel	Wide variety of cluster of differentiation (CD) markers can be used	Limited CD markers are used in cytology material
Dual expression of CD markers	Possible	Not feasible
Additional features	Possible to estimate multiple other features	Not feasible
Quantitation of CD-positive cells	Possible and easy	Laborious process to estimate manually
Quantitation of intensity of antigen positivity	Possible and easy to do	Not possible
Morphology of the cells	Not possible to visualize	Possible to visualize
Archival preservation	Not possible	Possible to preserve for a long time

Box 20.6: Limitations of flow cytometric immunophenotyping.

- No morphologic correlation
- Admixture of benign cells
- Costly and sophisticated technique
- Inability to identify HL
- No evidence of light chain restriction in certain number of cases.

Detection of Malignancy in Effusion Fluid

Flow cytometric immunophenotyping of effusion fluid may be helpful to detect malignant cells hidden with mesothelial cells and inflammatory cells. By applying multiple antigens in a single setting in multicolor FCM one can assess the character of a cell population in more precise manner with high accuracy.

Ber-EP4 is an epithelial cell adhesion molecule. Ber-EP4 is a monoclonal antibody directed against the protein moiety of the glycopeptides of the epithelial cells. This molecule is expressed in the epithelial cell and its malignancies. As epithelial cells are not normally present in the effusion fluid so the presence of Ber-EP4 positive cells in effusion usually indicates metastatic epithelial tumor. The sensitivity and specificity of Ber-EP4 in detection of malignancies in effusion are about 80% and 90%, respectively.[14]

Apoptosis

Flow cytometry is one of the important technologies to detect apoptotic cell death because the apoptotic cell death can be assessed with the help of light scatter, plasma membrane changes, and DNA content. Apoptotic cell shrinks and produces a loss in forward light scatter (FSC).

Flow Cytometry in HIV Infection

Monitoring of CD4 and CD8 count in the blood sample of HIV-infected patients is a mainstay of clinical FCM. During the progression of HIV the blood CD4 count decreases, therefore the measurement of absolute CD4 count provides a valuable tool for monitoring disease progression or treatment response to HIV-infected patients.

Reticulocyte Count

Flow cytometry analysis of reticulocyte is a standard and preferred method. Auramine O and thiazole orange are Food and Drug Administration (FDA) approved reagents for reticulocyte analysis using FCM. Reticulocyte count by FCM is precise and sensitive over the manual method.

Predicting Response to Monoclonal Therapy

Monoclonal antibodies are targeted against the specific receptors on cancer cells. Her-2 is a growth receptor that is present in the cells of the breast cancer patients. Monoclonal antibody trastuzumab is developed against the extracellular domain of Her-2 for treatment of breast cancer.[15] Presently, monoclonal antibodies are used for treatment of NHL. Rituximab, a monoclonal antibody directed against CD20 on B cells, is used in follicular or low-grade NHL.[16] Similarly anti-CD33 is used against myeloid cells and anti-CD52 is used against lymphoid cells. The measurement of monoclonal antibody CD20 with the help of FCM is helpful in follow-up of cases after rituximab therapy (anti-CD20 antibody).[17]

Detection of Minimal Residual Disease

Flow cytometry is also very useful for the detection of leukemia or lymphoma-associated immunophenotype of the neoplastic cells for the assessment of minimal residual disease. It is time-saving and cost-effective technique. It has been shown that FCM is almost equally effective as quantitative PCR in the detection of minimal residual disease.[18]

Soluble Antigen Assessment for Transplant Patient Monitoring

OKT3 is a mouse antihuman antibody and is used to treat transplant rejection patient. Circulating concentrations of OKT3 can be quantified with FCM that helps in disease monitoring.[19]

FUTURE OF FLOW CYTOMETRY

The FCM instrument is developed significantly in last few decades and there are also vast numbers of monoclonal antibodies commercially available for FCM. Therefore, multiple characteristics of single cells can be assessed by single cells. Presently, FCM is used in clinical laboratories for immunophenotyping of lymphomas or leukemias, DNA content measurement, cell cycle assessment, reticulocyte count, HIV patient monitoring, and follow-up of monoclonal antibody-based therapy. In future, FCM will be an integral part of routine laboratory techniques for diagnosis and disease monitoring.

REFERENCES

1. O'Leary TJ. Flow cytometry in diagnostic cytology. Diagn Cytopathol. 1998;18:41-6.

2. Saha I, Dey P, Vohra H, et al. Role of DNA flow cytometry and image cytometry on effusion fluid. Diagn Cytopathol. 2000;22:81-5.
3. Saikia UN, Dey P, Vohra H, et al. DNA flow cytometry of non-Hodgkin's Lymphomas: correlation with cytologic grade and clinical relapse. Diagn Cytopathol. 2000;22:153-6.
4. Kentrou NA, Tsagarakis NJ, Tzanetou K, et al. An improved flow cytometric assay for detection and discrimination between malignant cells and atypical mesothelial cells, in serous cavity effusions. Cytometry B Clin Cytom. 2011;80(5):324-34.
5. Dey P, Amir T, Al Jassar A, et al. Combined applications of fine needle aspiration cytology and flow cytometric immunphenotyping for diagnosis and classification of non-Hodgkin lymphoma. Cytojournal. 2006;3:24.
6. Joensuu H, Klemi PJ, Eerola E. Diagnostic value of flow cytometric DNA determination combined with fine needle aspiration biopsy in thyroid tumors. Anal Quant Cytol Histol. 1987;9:328-34.
7. Davidson B, Dong HP, Holth A, et al. Flow cytometric immunophenotyping of cancer cells in effusion specimens: diagnostic and research applications. Diagn Cytopathol. 2007;35(9):568-78.
8. Kumar UN, Dey P, Mondal AK, et al. DNA flow cytometry and bladder irrigation cytology in detection of bladder carcinoma. Diagn Cytopathol. 2001;24(3):153-6.
9. Sánchez-Carbayo M, Ciudad J, Urrutia M, et al. Diagnostic performance of the urinary bladder carcinoma antigen ELISA test and multiparametric DNA/cytokeratin flow cytometry in urine voided samples from patients with bladder carcinoma. Cancer. 2001;92(11):2811-9.
10. Bromberg JE, Breems DA, Kraan J, et al. CSF flow cytometry greatly improves diagnostic accuracy in CNS hematologic malignancies. Neurology. 2007;68(20):1674-9.
11. Coon JS, Landay AL, Weinstein RS. Advances in flow cytometry for diagnostic pathology. Lab Invest. 1987;57:453-79.
12. Zola H, Swart B, Nicholson I, et al. CD molecules 2005: human cell differentiation molecules. Blood. 2005;106:3123-6.
13. Dey P. The role of ancillary techniques to diagnose and sub-classifiy non-hodgkin lymphomas on fine needle aspiration cytology. Cytopathology. 2006;17(5):275-87.
14. Diaz-Arias AA, Loy TS, Bickel JT, et al. Utility of Ber-EP4 in the diagnosis of adenocarcinoma in effusions:an immunocytochemical study of 232 cases. Diagn Cytopathol. 1993; 9:516-21.
15. Seal MD, Speers CH, O'Reilly S, et al. Outcomes of women with early-stage breast cancer receiving adjuvant trastuzumab. Curr Oncol. 2012;19(4):197-201.
16. Hagenbeek A, Czuczman MS, Ghielmini M, et al. Rituximab therapy for indolent non-Hodgkin's lymphoma. Anticancer Drugs. 2002;13(Suppl 2):S11-7.
17. Miyoshi H, Arakawa F, Sato K, et al. Comparison of CD20 expression in B-cell lymphoma between newly diagnosed, untreated cases and those after rituximab treatment. Cancer Sci. 2012;103(8):1567-73.
18. Gaipa G, Cazzaniga G, Valsecchi MG, et al. Time point-dependent concordance of flow cytometry and RQ-PCR inminimal residual disease detection in childhood acute lymphoblasticleukemia. Haematologica. 2012;97(10):1582-93.
19. Cinti P, Cocciolo P, Evangelista B, et al. OKT3 prophylaxis in kidney transplant recipients: drug monitoring by flow cytometry. Transplant Proc. 1996;28:3214-6.

Review Questions

1. **All are true of flow cytometry *except*:**
   a. Wide variety of CD markers can be used
   b. Quantitation of CD-positive cells possible
   c. Dual expression of CD markers not possible
   d. Morphology of the cells not possible to visualize
2. **DNA index 1.2 indicates:**
   a. Hypodiploid aneuploidy
   b. Diploid
   c. Hyperdiploid aneuploidy
   d. Tetraploidy
3. **The main limitation of flow cytometric immunophenotyping is:**
   a. Slow
   b. Subjective
   c. Morphologic correlation not possible
   d. Complicated procedure
4. **Either lambda or kappa light chains expression in flow cytometry of lymph node indicates:**
   a. Reactive lymphoid hyperplasia
   b. Possibly B-cell monoclonality
   c. Possibly T-cell monoclonality
   d. Metastatic carcinoma

Identify True/False

5. **Clone of cells containing the abnormal amount of DNA is known as aneuploid cells.** *(True or False)*
6. **Quantitation of CD-positive cells is not possible in flow cytometry.** *(True or False)*
7. **All cases of B-NHL may not always show light chain restriction.** *(True or False)*

Answers

1. c. Dual expression of CD markers not possible
2. c. Hyperdiploid aneuploidy
3. c. Morphologic correlation not possible
4. b. Possibly B-cell monoclonality
5. True
6. False
7. True

CHAPTER

21 Liquid-based Cytology and Automation

INTRODUCTION

Computer science has progressed remarkably in the last few decades and like every other field it has also a significant impact on cervical cytology. Now automated devices have been applied in the field of cervical cytology with the intention to have a more efficient system in smear preparation, recognition and interpretation of the slide.

The reduction of false negative cytology is the major aim of automation. There may be two types of errors in a case of false negative cytology:

1. *Sampling error*: This means that the lesion is present in the body but is not properly sampled. Sampling error is one of the major sources of error.
   Remedies: It is not entirely possible to avoid the sampling error, but with the help of liquid-based cytology (LBC), we can get the maximum number of cells on the smear.
2. *Screening errors*: Screening error may be due to failure to find out the representative cells on the smear or it may be due to interpretation errors.
   I. *Recognition errors*: It is just like finding out the "needle in the haystack". The representative cells may be too few to find out even after a laborious search or they may be obscured within the blood, mucus or inflammatory cells and necrotic debris. Cytoscreener may overlook these cells due to fatigue or due to the above-mentioned technical difficulties.
   Remedies:
   » LBC may provide a clean background of the smear, which is free of mucus or blood. Moreover, the proportionate amounts of cells are concentrated in a small part of the slide as a monolayer form. This may help to find out the abnormal cell more easily.
   » The automated adjunctive technique helps the manual screening by locating the path of the screening on the computer screen. Automated screening may also help to find out the abnormal cells.
   II. *Interpretation errors*: Another possible source of errors is nonrecognition of abnormal cells. This may be because of professional incompetence or inadequate training.
   Remedies: Automated screening devices may initially help to find out the abnormal cells. However, a trained cytopathologist is needed for further confirmation of the abnormal cells detected by automated machines.

AUTOMATION IN SPECIMEN COLLECTION AND PREPARATION

Liquid-based Cytology

For the last few decades, cervical cancer screening is based on conventional preparation (CP) of cervical smear. Conventional cervical smear is a quick, relatively cheap technique and so far it has helped to reduce the incidence of cervical cancer significantly in many developed countries. However, the false negative rate of conventional cervical smear is as high as 29% and sensitivity of this test varies from 47% to 62%.[1] Samples taken by CP may often be inadequate, nonrepresentative and may be obscured by blood, debris or may show air-drying artifact. LBC technique is an important step in the preparation of cervical smear. It has overcome many limitations of conventional cervical cytology. Presently, LBC is widely accepted in many laboratories despite the high cost of this technique.[2,3]

Collection Procedure of Liquid-based Cytology

The cervical sample is obtained using a combination of plastic spatula and cervical broom-type device in the same manner of conventional screening. Alternatively, a sample is collected by cervix-brush supplied by the company. The sample is then rinsed into a vial containing preservative solution. The head of the device is kept in the vial containing preservative solution and the handle is removed. The sample is sent to the cytology laboratory for further processing. The cells are made discrete and a monolayer is prepared.

Different Company Products

Presently, only two commercially available liquid-based technologies are approved by US Federation of Drug Administration (FDA): (1) ThinPrep® Pap test, and (2) SurePath™. ThinPrep® was approved in 1996 and SurePath™ in 1999. The preparation techniques of the ThinPrep® Pap test and SurePath™ have been compared in Table 21.1.

ThinPrep® (Cytic, UK) (Fig. 21.1)

Here the cells are collected by a plastic spatula or cytobrush and then transferred to the transport media provided by the company. Presently, ThinPrep® 5000 processor is available in the market that can automatically process up to 20 samples in 45 minutes' time period. The steps of ThiPrep® processing are:

1. *Dispersion*: The sample is collected in 20 mL of PreservCyt® solution for fixation. A cylindrical tube with attached filter in one end is dipped within the vial containing the specimen in PreservCyt® solution. The cylinder is rotated within the vial rapidly and this rotatory movement disperses the cells singly. The filter rotates within the vial which contains the cells in liquid. The cells are dispersed mechanically by rotation of the filter.
2. *Cell collection*: A continuous negative suction pressure is applied through the cylinder to drain the fluid in the vial. The cells are stuck on the surface of the filter. The flow of fluid through the filter is constantly monitored to get an optimal quantity of cells by adjusting the negative pressure with the help of in-built software in the ThinPrep® processor.
3. *Cell transfer*: The cells are now trapped over the outer surface of the filter. The ThinPrep® filter now automatically transfers the cells on the circular area of the glass slides. The slide is immediately dipped within a fixative.

Table 21.1: Comparison of Pap test and SurePath™ techniques.

Features	*ThinPrep® Pap test*	*SurePath™*
Collection	PreservCyt® fluid, methanol-based	Cytorich fluid, ethanol-based
Single cell preparation	By rotatory filter within the vial	By vortexing
Cell concentration	By negative suction	By density gradient
Monolayered cells	Present, good	No monolayered cells
Cell concentration	Relatively less	Good cell concentration

SurePath™ Test (AutoCyt Prep, Cytorich Prep) (Figs. 21.2 to 21.4)

The cells are collected with the help of a plastic device and transferred to a transport fluid.

Vortexing: The cells are mechanically dispersed by vortexing.

Cell enrichment: Subsequently, the sample, mixed with PrepStain® Density Reagent and is centrifuged to enrich the cells. The supernatant unwanted elements, such as blood, mucus and necrotic debris are decanted by using vacuum suction. The reaming fluid is again centrifuged to get a cell-rich pellet.

Resuspension: The cell pellet is revortexed to resuspend the cellular material within the fluid and then transferred into the PrepStain® slide processor.

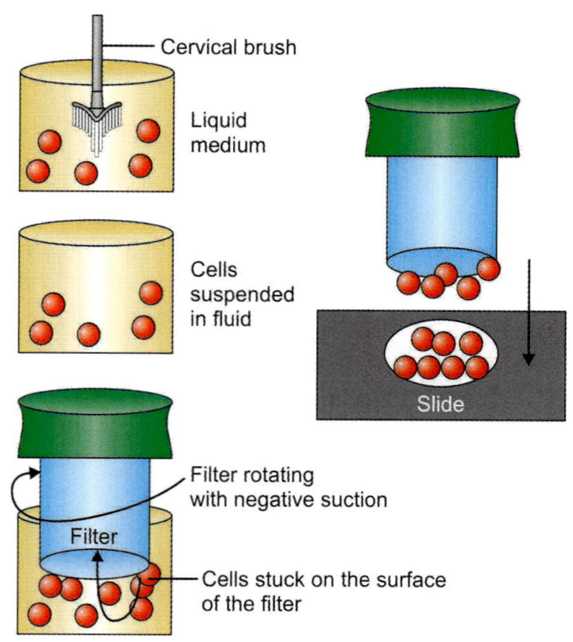

Fig. 21.1: Schematic diagram showing the basic principles of ThinPrep® technique.

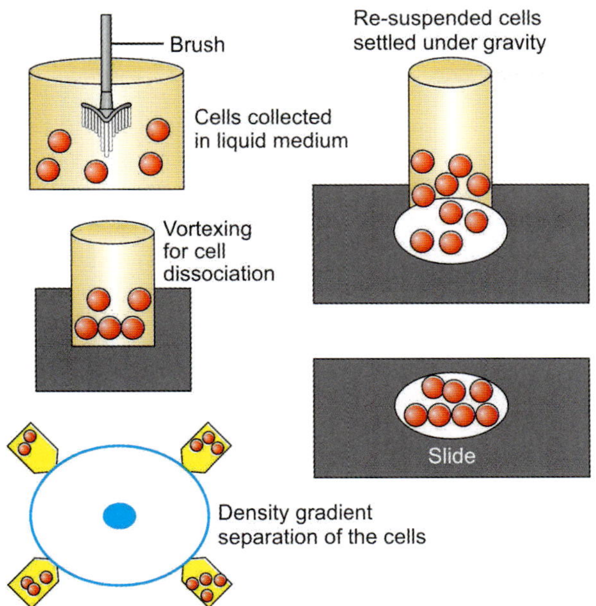

Fig. 21.2: Schematic diagram showing the basic principles of SurePath™ technique.

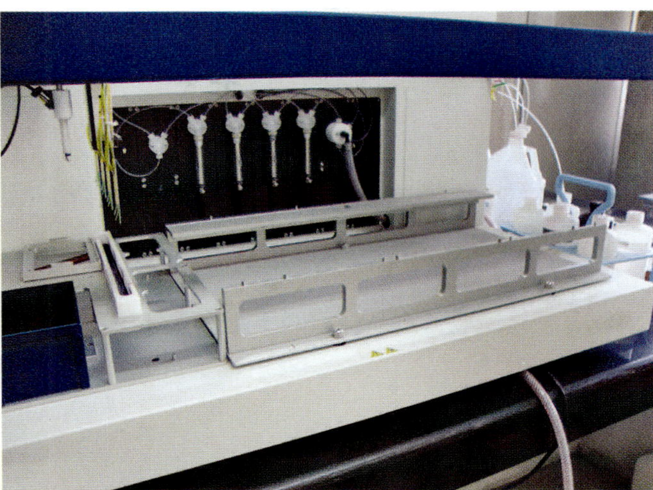

Fig. 21.3: Photograph of SurePath™ machine in the laboratory of PGIMER, Chandigarh, India.

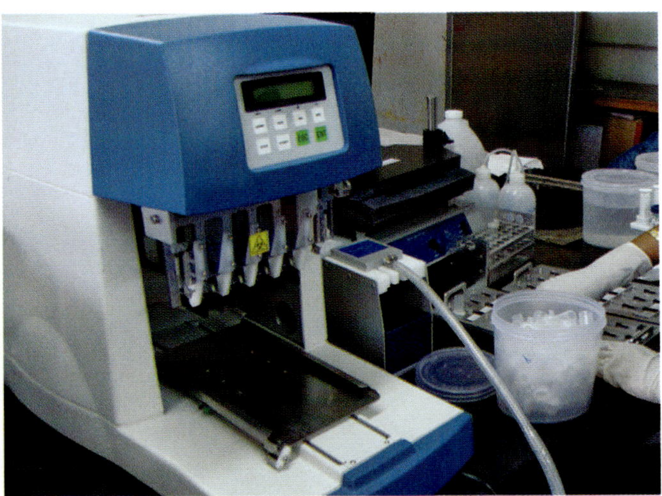

Fig. 21.4: Photograph showing preliminary preparation of sample in SurePath™ technique.

Table 21.2: Comparison of liquid-based cytology (LBC) and conventional preparation.

Criteria	*LBC*	*Conventional preparation*
Sample collection	Liquid preservative	On glass slide
Air-drying	No	Yes, at times
Number of cells	Much more and adequate	Less
Screening time	Less	More
Background	Clean	May be obscured by blood, polymorphs or mucus
Sensitivity	High	Low
Further ancillary test	Possible	Not possible
Cost of equipment	High	No cost
Cost to the patient	High	Low
Training	Needs adequate training	Routinely trained technician
Monolayer	Yes, in ThinPrep®	No
Automation	Easy to implement	Difficult

Density gradient sedimentation: In PrepStain® settling chamber with the help of gravitational force, the cells are sedimented on a precoated slide.

Advantages and Disadvantages of LBC over Conventional Pap Smears

Both LBC and conventional smear have certain advantages and disadvantages (Table 21.2). The main advantages of LBC are adequate representative material, complete avoidance of air-drying, monolayered preparation and clean background (Figs. 21.5 and 21.6). The background is clean from necrotic debris in LBC smear. However, it is still possible to recognize the tumor diathesis in case of squamous cell carcinoma of cervix. Infective organisms can also be identified in LBC smear. In fact, adequate training is needed for proper interpretation of LBC smear. One major advantage of LBC is that the residual sample can be kept for human papillomavirus (HPV) testing or any other ancillary tests. Moreover, the monolayered cellular smear is of great help in studying individual cells for automation.

LBC instrument is costly. The overall processing cost of LBC is also much more than conventional preparation. As mentioned before, the laboratory technical staff also needs adequate training for interpreting LBC smear.

Comparison of Overall Efficiency of Conventional Preparation versus LBC

A large number of studies compared CP and LBC on cervical smear.[3-5]

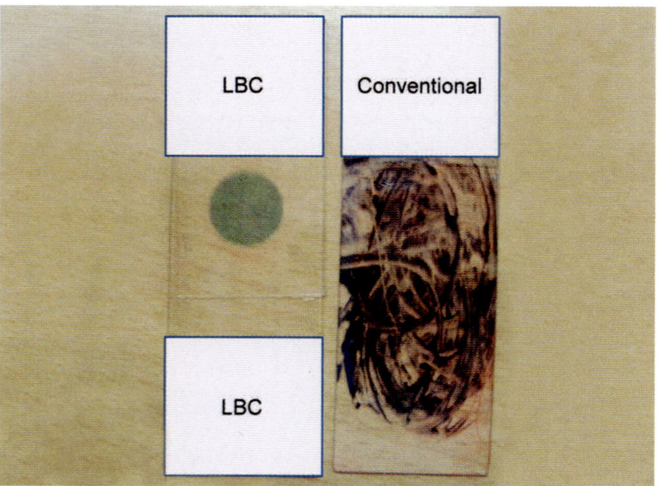

Fig. 21.5: Gross smears of liquid-based cytology preparation (SurePath™) and conventional preparation.

Most of these studies claim that LBC reduces the inadequacy rate of cervical smear and it also increases sensitivity and specificity of the cervical smear compared to CP. Most of the studies were not randomized control trial. A large meta-analysis study claimed that LBC does not have any better performance than CP.[6] However, there is no doubt that LBC significantly reduces the load of unsatisfactory sample. LBC sample is easy to screen and the remaining material in the vial can be used for HPV test. Therefore, many laboratories are shifted from CP to LBC.

ADJUNCTIVE DEVICES TO MANUAL SCREENING

Pathfinder

It is an adjunctive device for manual screening to keep a record of screening by a cytotechnologist. The pathfinder is now obsolete and out of the market.

Trac Cell 2000 System

Trac Cell 2000 system (AccuMed) is a fully automated prescreening system that supports the screener in respect of speed of screening, map of areas which are screened, etc. The company claims that Trac Cell 2000 system increases the productivity of the screener and also contributes strict vigilance over the cytoscreener.

AUTOMATED SCREENING

Automated screening procedure should be designed in such a way that—(1) no dysplastic or malignant cells

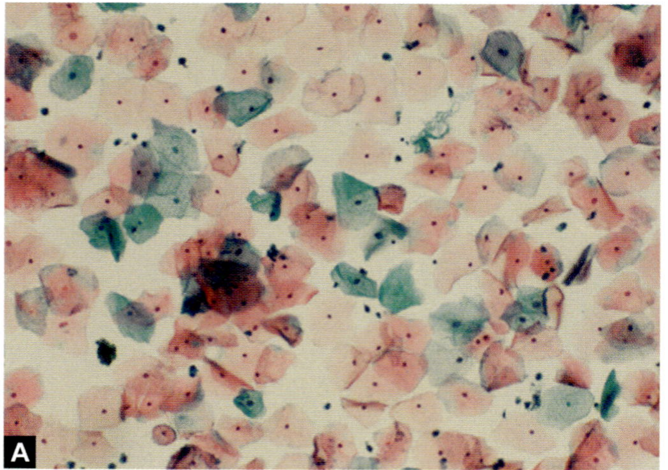

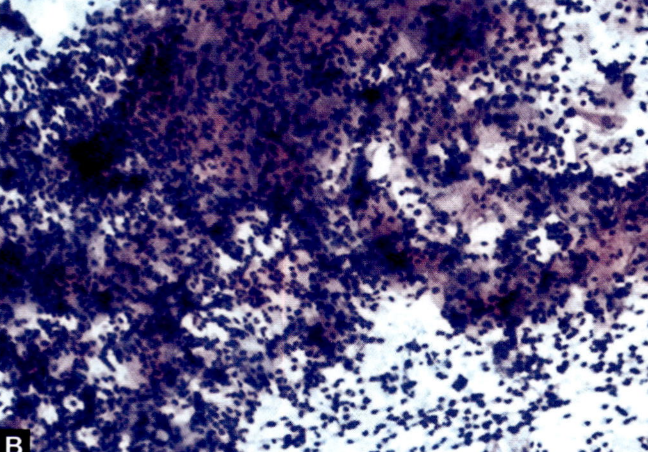

Figs. 21.6A and B: (A) Clean background of liquid-based cytology preparation (SurePath™) (Papanicolaou stain X MP). (B) Dirty background and cell-clumping of cells in conventional smear preparation (Papanicolaou stain X MP).

should be passed as normal or negative; and (2) it should not label the normal cell as malignant cells. In addition, the automated screening technique should be economically cost-effective and it should shorten the period of screening. Therefore, the two main goals of automated screening are—to increase the accuracy and productivity of the cervical screening.

Automated Screening Devices

Till date, there is no fully automated system available in the market. Presently, only two semiautomated systems are available—(1) BD FocalPoint GS Imaging System (previously known as TriPath AutoPap System), and (2) HOLOGIC ThinPrep Imaging System (formerly known as Cytyc ThinPrep Imaging System).

Redundant systems: Both PAPNET and AutoPap 300 QC systems were popular once upon a time. Presently, both the systems are out of market.

Available Automated Screening Devices

BD FocalPoint™ GS Imaging System

BD FocalPoint GS is FDA approved automated device. It is used for primary screening of SurePath™ and conventional smear.

This system includes:

- BD FocalPoint™ Slide Profiler
- BD FocalPoint™ GS Review Station.

BD FocalPoint™ Slide Profiler: It is a computer-based automated screening device that scans the slide in low and high magnification. The system studies several cytological features, such as nuclear size, nucleo-cytoplasmic ratio, etc. and the images are interpreted by an image analyzer software program and each slide is given a "device score" according to the probability of abnormality. The slide is categorized as no further review and review group. Subsequently, the slide-processing data is transferred to the review station.

BD FocalPoint™ GS Review Station: Here the slides "for review" group are reviewed by the cytotechnologists. The slides for specimen adequacy are also reviewed. If no abnormality is detected by manual screening, then the slides are labeled as normal and can be kept in archives. If any abnormality is detected, then the slides are reviewed further by cytopathologists for final interpretation.

HOLOGIC ThinPrep Imaging System

This system includes:

- ThinPrep imaging system
- ThinPrep review system.

ThinPrep image processor: Here the system acquires and processes data from the ThinPrep test slides. This computer-based system scans slides to find out the abnormal nuclei (largest and darkest). The imaging system always excludes the overlapping cell or the objects other than nuclei. The system screens the slide and records the locations of 22 microscopic fields that contain the potential abnormal cells.

Review scope: Review scope is an automated microscope with a motorized stage. It guides the cytotechnologist to review 22 microscopic fields of interest. If there are no abnormal cells in the 22 fields of view, then the slides are passed as normal. However, if there is any abnormal cell present, then the whole slide is screened thoroughly.

COMPARISON OF MANUAL AND AUTOMATED DEVICES

Several studies claimed that automated screening done by either of these two techniques is more sensitive than routine manual screening.[7,8] However, these studies were not randomized and done in a small number of patients. Moreover, the studies are often sponsored by the company itself. In a large randomized control study,[9] the automation-assisted reading of cervical cytology was compared with manual report of cervical cytology smear considering histology as an end-point. Both BD FocalPoint GS Imaging System and ThinPrep Imaging System were applied in two groups of patients and in both groups, manual screenings were also done. It was noted, that automation-assisted reading was 8% less sensitive compared to manual report. Cervical smear categorized as "no further review" by automated screening was very reliable. Kitchener et al.[9] also noted that automated screening and manual screening were almost similar in cost-effectiveness issue. However, there was 60–80% increase in productivity for automated screening. It was concluded that there is no justification to introduce an automated screening technique in relation to sensitivity and cost-effectiveness of cervical screening.

PROBLEMS OF IMPLEMENTING AUTOMATION

There are certain problems in automated screening devices.

Table 21.3: Comparison of the automated screening versus manual screening.

Criteria	*Automated screening*	*Manual screening*
Fatigue	The machine does not feel fatigue	A man may feel fatigue
Logic	The device follows the standard direction of logic consistently	A man may not be uniform in approach
Time	The machine takes a fixed time and usually shorter period	Man takes longer time to screen
Interpretation	The machine cannot take final interpretation	Man can take meaningful interpretation
Training	The machine does not need training	Man needs training
Cost	The machine is very costly	Manual screening is less costly

Technical

- *Data*: Present-generation computer technology can handle large amount of data. However, it is difficult for a computer to handle the immense amount of data gathered during the screening of the individual slides till date.
- *Autofocus*: Continuous focusing of the cells, particularly overlapping cells, is a challenge.

Diagnostic

It is still very difficult for an automated system to make individual decisions in single cases.

Financial

Automated systems are commercially available but they are very costly for routine laboratories for daily use. This is particularly true for the developing countries.

Medicolegal

It is still not settled about the medicolegal issues related to the machine-given report in primary screening.

AUTOMATION: ADVANTAGES AND DISADVANTAGES

Automation of cervical smears has several advantages such as higher number of false negative detection rate, no fatigability, consistency and relatively decreased turn-around time (Table 21.3).

However, the automated screening techniques are costly and this may make the cervical screen program unpopular. Moreover, recent trends in high-risk HPV screening may have negative influence on automated screening.

REFERENCES

1. Nanda K, McCrory DC, Myers ER, et al. Accuracy of the Papanicolaou test in screening for and follow-up of cervical cytologic abnormalities: a systemic review. Ann Intern Med. 2000;132:810-9.
2. Luthra UK, Chishti M, Dey P, et al. Performance of ThinPrep smear method in a gynaecology outpatient setting in Kuwait. Acta Cytol. 2002;46:303-10.
3. Moseley RP, Paget S. Liquid-based cytology: is the way forward? Cytopathology. 2002;13:71-82.
4. Weintraub J, Morabia A. Efficacy of a liquid-based thin layer method for cervical cancer screening in a population with a low incidence of cervical cancer. Diagn Cytopathol. 2000;22:52-9.
5. Cheung AN, Szeto EF, Leung BS, et al. Liquid-based cytology and conventional cervical smears: a comparison study in an Asian screening population. Cancer. 2003;99:331-5.
6. Davey E, Barratt A, Irwig L, et al. Effect of study design and quality on unsatisfactory rates, cytology classifications, and accuracy in liquid-based versus conventional cervical cytology: a systematic review. Lancet. 2006;367(9505):122-32.
7. Halford JA, Batty T, Boost T, et al. Comparison of the sensitivity of conventional cytology and the ThinPrep Imaging System for 1,083 biopsy confirmed highgrade squamous lesions. Diagn Cytopathol. 2010;38:318-26.
8. Wilbur DC, Black-Schaffer WS, Luff RD, et al. The Becton Dickinson FocalPoint GS Imaging System: clinical trials demonstrate significantly improved sensitivity for the detection of important cervical lesions. Am J Clin Pathol. 2009;132:767-75.
9. Kitchener HC, Blanks R, Cubie H, et al. MAVARIC Trial Study Group. MAVARIC—a comparison of automation-assisted and manual cervical screening: a randomised controlled trial. Health Technol Assess. 2011;15(3):iii-iv, ix-xi, 1-170.

Review Questions

1. **All are true for SurePath™ liquid-based cytology except:**
   a. Single cell preparation is done by rotatory filter within the vial
   b. Good cell concentration
   c. No monolayered cells
   d. Cells are concentrated by density gradient
2. **In comparison to conventional smear, liquid-based cytology shows:**
   a. High specificity
   b. Screening time is more
   c. Clean background
   d. Less number of adequate cells
3. **The best preparation of monolayer cells is done by:**
   a. SurePath™ b. ThinPrep®
   c. Cytocentrifuge d. Millipore filtration
4. **Very good cell concentration on the smear is seen in:**
   a. SurePath™ b. ThinPrep®
   c. Cytocentrifuge d. Millipore filtration

Answers

1. a. Single cell preparation is done by rotatory filter within the vial
2. c. Clean background
3. b. ThinPrep®
4. a. SurePath™

CHAPTER

22 Polymerase Chain Reaction and DNA Sequencing

INTRODUCTION

Polymerase chain reaction (PCR) is one of the important developments in molecular pathology. With the help of PCR, the specific target portion of the DNA (deoxyribonucleic acid) can be amplified. PCR is now widely used in both diagnosis and also in research.

PRINCIPLE

The basic principles of PCR are (Fig. 22.1):

- By applying heat double-stranded DNA is made to single stranded
- Two oligonucleotide strands or primers are used that are complementary to the 3′ ends of each strand of DNA
- The primers attach to the 3′ end of the DNA strand
- Taq polymerase helps to extend the DNA strand by incorporating nucleotides.

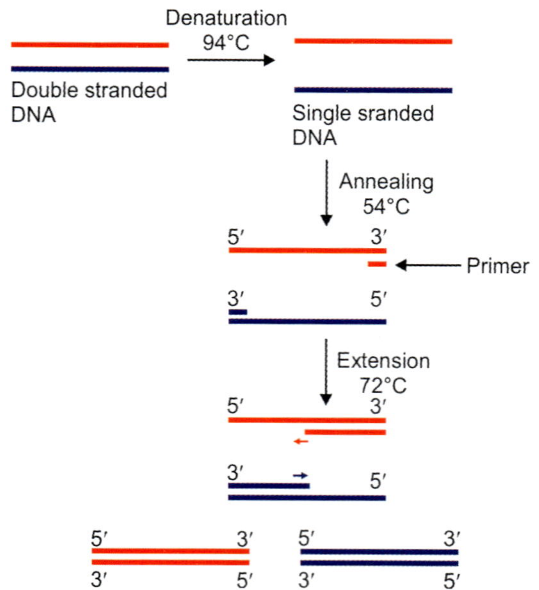

Fig. 22.1: Schematic diagram showing the basic principle of polymerase chain reaction.

COMPONENTS OF POLYMERASE CHAIN REACTION

- *Primers*: The primers are artificially made short DNA strands consisting of 20–25 nucleotides. The DNA strands of the primers are the complementary strand of the 3′ end of each strand of target DNA.
- *DNA polymerase (Taq polymerase)*: DNA polymerase enzyme extends the new DNA strand. It attaches near the end of the primer and then sequentially adds complimentary nucleotides to the new DNA strand at 3′ end. High temperature (94°C) is needed to separate the double-stranded DNA. Ordinary DNA polymerase breaks down in this temperature. In PCR, we use Taq DNA polymerase which is extracted from *Thermus aquaticus*. The unique property of Taq polymerase is that it is stable and can work in high temperature.
- *Deoxynucleotide triphosphate*: Deoxynucleotide triphosphates (dNTPs) are the basic "building blocks" to make new DNA strands. dNTPs are: deoxyadenosine triphosphate (dATP), deoxycytidine triphosphate (dCTP), deoxyguanosine triphosphate (dGTP), and deoxythymidine triphosphate (dTTP).
- *DNA template from the sample*: This is the target DNA. The double-stranded DNA is separated to single-stranded DNA by high temperature.
- *Others*: Buffer solution, $MgCl_2$.

STEPS OF POLYMERASE CHAIN REACTION (BOX 22.1)

The steps of PCR are:

- *Denaturation*: 94°C: DNA is heated to 94°C to make it single stranded. Only 1–2 minutes are given to this heating process in each cycle.
- *Annealing*: 54°C: The temperature is rapidly cooled. In this lowered temperature, the primer quickly anneals

with the respective site of DNA. With the help of Taq polymerase, the reaction starts at the primer-DNA template site.

- *Extension*: 72°C: The complementary nucleotides are attached from the 3′ end to 5′ end of DNA. There is an exponential increment in the number of genes in each cycle. At least 30 cycles of denaturation-annealing-extension is done in each PCR.

TYPES OF POLYMERASE CHAIN REACTION

There are different types of PCR methods for diagnostic purposes. These are:

- *Direct PCR*: This is the standard PCR method described earlier.
- *Reverse transcriptase PCR (RT-PCR)*: In this method, complementary DNA (cDNA) is made from RNA and then cDNA is amplified by PCR technique. RT-PCR is used for RNA targets.[1]
- *Asymmetric PCR*: In this process, unequal molar concentration of primer is used and single-stranded DNA is made. This is used for DNA sequencing.[2]
- *Inverse PCR*: Inverse PCR amplifies DNA outside the boundary of the known target sequence. This is particularly employed to find out the clonality of lymphoma and the insertion site of viral DNA.[3]
- *Single-strand conformation polymorphism (SSCP)*: This method is used to detect single base change mutation in DNA or RNA and uses the property of different mobility of DNA strand having a different base pair.[4]
- *In situ PCR*: This technique is used to amplify the nucleic acid in the fixed tissue and cell instead in solution. As the cells are intact, so the PCR can be correlated with the morphology.[5]
- *Real-time PCR*: Real-time quantitative PCR helps in specific and reproducible quantitation of nucleic acids.[6] In the case of original PCR, the same quantity of the product is generated after the end of the process. In real-time PCR, the amount of product can be monitored during each cycle of PCR with the help of a fluorescent dye and therefore it is possible to calculate the number of DNA molecules of the amplified sequence that were initially present in the sample.
- *Nested PCR*: In case of nested PCR, more than two pairs of primers are used for DNA amplification. The first pair of primer is used as the standard PCR practice and the second pair of primer is used to bind within the first PCR product. This prevents the contamination or wrong amplification of DNA because if any wrong locus is amplified by error then the second time it will not be amplified again by the second PCR primer.

Box 22.1: Polymerase chain reaction: Principle and steps.

Principle: The target gene is amplified with the help of a pair of primer, Taq polymerase, and nucleotides.

Steps

- *Denaturation*: Single-stranded DNA is made by heating double-stranded DNA.
- *Annealing*: Primer binds with the complementary DNA strand in 3′ region.
- *Extension*: With the help of Taq polymerase and in presence of nucleotides, new DNA strand is formed from 3′ to 5′ direction.
- At least 30 such cycles occur.

APPLICATIONS OF POLYMERASE CHAIN REACTION (BOX 22.2)[7,8]

Diagnosis of Infection

- *Viral*: Polymerase chain reaction is able to diagnose a long list of viruses such as herpes virus, human papilloma virus (Fig. 22.2), cytomegalovirus, hepatitis virus, human immunodeficiency virus, Epstein-Barr virus,[9] etc.
- *Bacterial*: Detection of tuberculosis—conventional diagnosis of the culture of *Mycobacterium tubercle* takes about 6 weeks. However, PCR can diagnose tuberculosis within few hours. It also can diagnose the infection in early and latent phase which is not possible with the conventional laboratory techniques. Other bacterial infections such as *Borrelia burgdorferi, Legionella pneumophila, Listeria monocytogenes, Chlamydia trachomatis* can also be diagnosed by PCR.[9]
- *Parasitic infection*: PCR has been used to detect parasitic infection such as *Toxoplasma gondii* and *Plasmodium falciparum*.[9]

Box 22.2: Polymerase chain reaction: Applications.

- *Diagnosis of infection*
  - Viral
  - Bacterial
  - Parasitic
- *Cancer*
  - To detect base pair mutation
  - To detect chromosomal translocation
  - To detect minimal residual diseases
  - To detect monoclonality of B and T cell in non-Hodgkin's lymphoma (NHL)
- *Genetic*
  - Intrauterine detection of genetic disorder such as Down's syndrome, cystic fibrosis, sickle cell anemia, Gaucher's disease, thalassemia, hemophilia
  - *Parental detection*: By detection of tandem repeat in non-coding DNA.

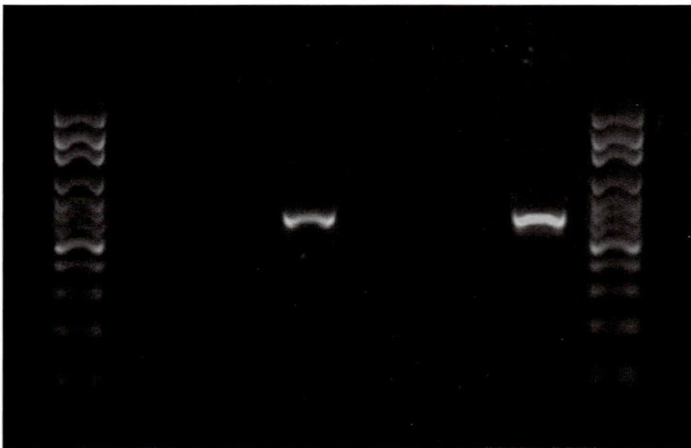

Fig. 22.2: Agarose gel electrophoresis (1.5%) from fine needle aspiration cytology of lung carcinoma to demonstrate human papilloma virus. Lane 1 and 8: Molecular weight marker (100 bp); Lane 2: Negative control; Lane 3, 4, 5, and 6: Expression of human papilloma virus subtype 16 in patients; and Lane 7: Positive control (690 bp).
Courtesy: Dr Ritu Aggarwal, Professor, Department of Immunopathology, PGIMER, Chandigarh.

Cancer

Polymerase chain reaction has been used widely in cancer genetics. It is used:

- *To detect mutation in oncogenes and tumor suppressor gene*: p53, c-Myc, ras gene.[8]
- *To detect diagnostic chromosomal translocation in various malignancies*: With the help of highly specific primers, various chromosomal translocations can be detected by PCR.[8]
- To detect monoclonality of non-Hodgkin's lymphoma (NHL) such as T-cell receptor gene analysis.[10]
- To detect minimal residual disease during follow-up of a patient.[11]

Genetic Diseases

With the help of PCR technique, various genetic diseases can be diagnosed such as Down's syndrome, cystic fibrosis, sickle cell anemia, Gaucher's disease, thalassemia, hemophilia, etc. PCR technique helps in diagnosis of many intrauterine genetic diseases of fetus much early without any aggressive placental bed biopsy. Fetal cell can be isolated either from blood or from cervical mucosa of the mother. PCR of DNA of the fetal cell can be amplified to detect these chromosomal abnormalities.[12]

Polymerase chain reaction (PCR) may also be helpful to detect tandem repeats in noncoding DNA part of the chromosome and therefore to help in parental identity of the fetus.[13]

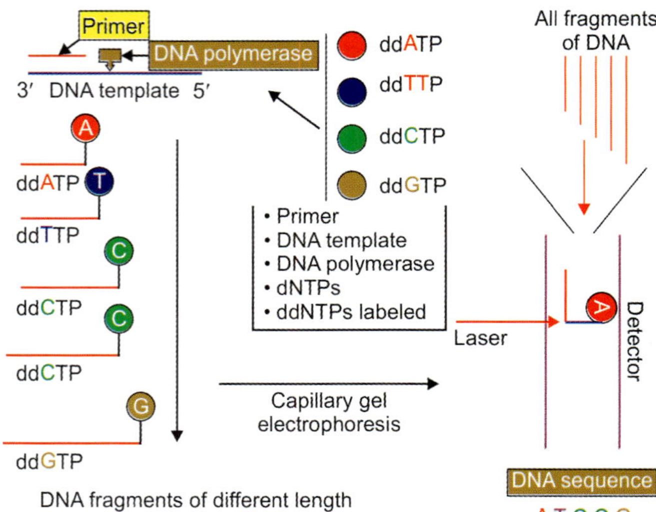

Fig. 22.3: Schematic diagram of Sanger sequencing.

SANGER SEQUENCING

Sanger sequencing is the most commonly used commercial DNA sequencing which is named on Sanger F.[14]

Basic Principle

Here the DNA replication by DNA polymerase enzyme is selectively terminated by using 2′, 3′-dideoxynucleotides (ddNTP) and each DNA fragment is recorded at the terminal end to assess the DNA sequence.

Reagents Used

- Primers
- DNA template
- DNA polymerase enzyme
- dNTPs
- ddNTP (fluorescent labeled).

Basic Steps (Fig. 22.3)

- The reagents (primers, DNA template, DNA polymerase enzyme, dNTPs, and fluorescent-labeled ddNTP) are mixed.
- Heated at 96°C to separate the complementary strands of DNA template.
- The temperature is lowered (50°C) to combine the primer DNA with the complementary strand of the template DNA.
- The temperature is raised (60°C) again so that DNA polymerase acts to elongate the chain of DNA.

- The enzyme incorporates both dNTP and fluorescent-labeled ddNTP. However, when it incorporates ddNTP, the DNA chain elongation is terminated as ddNTP lacks 3′-OH group and therefore two nucleotides cannot be joined by the phosphodiester bond.
- This DNA chain has the terminal ddNTP and the base A, T, C, and G are labeled with a specific fluorescent dye.
- The cycle of DNA chain elongation is continued repeatedly till each base position of the target DNA is terminated by ddNTP labeled with fluorescent base.
- Ultimately, we get DNA chain of the target DNA in many fragments of different length terminated by unique fluorescence-labeled base.
- These DNA chains are then run in capillary gel electrophoresis which is hit by a laser beam. The terminal base tagged with fluorochrome dye emits fluorescence when it is hit by laser beam and four color emission spectra from the four different bases (A, T, C, and G) are recorded.
- The software finally translates the sequence of terminal bases in the DNA target chain based on DNA spectrum of each terminal base in each small fragments of the terminated chain.

Pros and Cons of Sanger Sequencing

- This is highly specific (error rate: 0.001–1%)
- It is clumsy, cumbersome, and time-consuming
- High cost.

NEXT-GENERATION SEQUENCING

Next-generation sequencing (NGS) is also known as high-throughput sequencing. NGS can be divided into following broad categories:[15]

- Microelectrophoretic methods
- Hybridization sequencing
- Real-time observation of single molecules
- Cyclic-array sequencing.

Microelectrophoretic Methods

In this method, microfabricated technical device is used instead of conventional electrophoretic separation. This technique has integrated sample processing, DNA amplification, isolation, and concentration of DNA fragments and sequencing.

Hybridization Sequencing

In this technique, differential hybridization of oligonucleotide probes are applied to identify the target DNA sequence. The DNA is at first immobilized on a membrane and then serially hybridized with many short length oligonucleotide probes.

Real-time Observation of Single Molecules

In this technique, DNA is driven through a nanopore. The different base pair of nucleic acid obstructs the pore in different degrees and thereby generates fluctuation of electrical conductance. Measuring the fluctuation of pore conductance, the DNA sequence is measured.

Cyclic-Array Sequencing

In this technique, multiple cycles of enzymatic manipulation of the oligonucleotide probes are done to know the sequence of each base pair. Many million such features are processed in parallel.

Pros and Cons of Next-generation Sequencing

- Conventional Sanger sequencing is very slow, and it gives limited data on small segment of DNA. In comparison, NGS provides full spectrum of genomic variation in a single experiment.
- All novel mutational changes noted in NGS should be further reconfirmed by Sanger sequencing.
- NGS is completely unselective and is able to detect any novel mutation.
- NGS is very sensitive and can identify the variants that are present in small percentage of cells.
- NGS can be used to track the circulating tumor cells in blood.
- By studying the cancer genome completely it may be possible to diagnose and classify the cancer at molecular level.
- NGS may help in the personalized drug treatment of cancer.

REFERENCES

1. Tse WT, Forget BG. Reverse transcriptase and direct amplification of cellular RNA transcripts by Taq polymerase. Gene. 1990;88:293-6.

2. Gyllensten UB, Erlich HA. Generation of single stranded DNA by the polymerase chain reaction and its application to direct sequencing of the HLA-DQA locus. Proc Natl Acad Sci USA. 1988;85:7652-6.
3. Triglia T, Peterson MG, Kemp DJ. A procedure for in vitro amplification of DNA segments that lie outside the boundaries of unknown sequences. Nucleic Acid Res. 1988;16:8186.
4. Orita M, Iwahana H, Kanazawa H, et al. Detection of polymorphisms of human DNA by gel electrophoresis as single-strand conformation polymorphisms. Proc Natl Acad Sci USA. 1989;86:2766-70.
5. O'Leary JJ, Chetty R, Graham AK, et al. In situ PCR: pathologist's dream or nightmare? J Pathol. 1996;178:11-20.
6. Higuchi R, Dollinger G, Walsh PS, et al. Simultaneous amplification and detection of specific DNA-sequences. Biotechnology. 1992;10(4):413-7.
7. Greiner TC. Polymerase chain reaction: uses and potential applications in cytology. Diagn Cytopathol. 1992;8(1):61-4.
8. O'Leary JJ, Engels K, Dada MA. The polymerase chain reaction in pathology. J Clin Pathol. 1997;50(10):805-10.
9. Ronai Z, Yakubovskaya M. PCR in clinical diagnosis. J Clin Lab Anal. 1995;9(4):269-83.
10. Wan JH, Trainor KJ, Brisco MJ, et al. Monoclonality in B cell lymphoma detected in paraffin wax embedded sections using the polymerase chain reaction. J Clin Pathol. 1990;43: 888-90.
11. Lee MS, Chang KS, Cabanillas F, et al. Detection of minimal residual cells carrying the T(14:18) by DNA sequence amplification. Science. 1987;237:175-8.
12. Tutschek B, Sherlock J, Halder A, et al. Isolation of fetal cells from transcervical samples by micromanipulation: molecular confirmation of their fetal origin and diagnosis of fetal aneuploidy. Prenat Diagn. 1995;15:951-60.
13. Sullivan KM. Forensic applications of DNA fingerprinting. Mol Biotechnol. 1994;1:13-27.
14. Sanger F, Nicklen S, Coulson AR. DNA sequencing with chain-terminating inhibitors. Proc Natl Acad Sci USA. 1977;74(12):5463-7.
15. Shendure J, Mitra RD, Varma C, et al. Advanced sequencing technologies: methods and goals. Nat Rev Genet. 2004; 5(5):335-44.

Review Questions

1. Which one is true for polymerase chain reaction?
   a. The primer anneals with the respective site of DNA at 94°C
   b. The complementary nucleotides are attached from the 5′ end to 3′ end of DNA
   c. With the help of Taq polymerase, the reaction starts at the primer-DNA template site
   d. Taq polymerase is heat-sensitive and cannot work at high temperature

2. In what type of polymerase chain reaction (PCR) the amount of product can be monitored during each cycle of PCR with the help of a fluorescent dye:
   a. Nested PCR
   b. Real-time PCR
   c. Single-strand conformation polymorphism
   d. Reverse transcriptase PCR

3. Annealing in polymerase chain reaction is carried out at:
   a. Room temperature
   b. Freezing point
   c. 94°C
   d. 54°C

4. In this technique the nucleic acid is amplified in the fixed tissue and cell instead in solution:
   a. Nested PCR
   b. Real-time PCR
   c. In situ PCR
   d. Reverse transcriptase PCR

5. In this technique, DNA replication by DNA polymerase enzyme is selectively terminated by using 2′,3′-dideoxynucleotides:
   a. Next-generation sequencing
   b. Sanger sequencing
   c. Reverse transcriptase PCR
   d. Direct PCR

6. In this method of next-generation sequencing microfabricated technical device is used instead of conventional electrophoretic separation:
   a. Microelectrophoretic methods
   b. Hybridization sequencing
   c. Real-time observation of single molecules
   d. Cyclic-array sequencing

Answers

1. c. With the help of Taq polymerase, the reaction starts at the primer-DNA template site
2. b. Real time PCR
3. d. 54°C
4. c. In situ PCR
5. b. Sanger sequencing
6. a. Microelectrophoretic methods

CHAPTER

23 Quality Control and Laboratory Organization

INTRODUCTION

Quality control (QC) is defined as a bunch of measures for verifying and maintaining a desired level of quality in an individual test or process.[1] Whereas, the quality assurance is defined by college of American pathologists as "systematic monitoring of quality control results and quality practice parameters to assure that all systems are functioning in a manner appropriate to excellence in healthcare delivery".[2] It is in fact the dynamic process by which the QC is built up in a laboratory.

Quality control starts from the receiving of the sample to the final delivery of reports and further storage and follow-up of the cases. QC can be divided as

- Preanalytical phase: Before interpretation of slide
- Analytical phase: At the time of interpretation of slide
- Postanalytical phase: After the interpretation of slide.

All these stages are part of internal quality control (IQC) program.

PREANALYTICAL PHASE

Quality control in this stage includes specimen collection, receiving, processing and staining of the sample, maintenance of all the records, instrument and instrument calibration records.[1] Overall the essential components of preanalytical quality control include the following:

Receiving the Specimen

This is the first and preliminary part of the QC. The receptionist should follow the certain duties:

- Always match the slide and requisition form
- Fully filled up form should be received
- All essential data should be entered in the computer
- Unique specification number should be allotted to the specimen.

The essential measures to maintain the QC in this step are:

- There should be a laboratory standard operating protocol (SOP) for specimen collection and processing
- Unique bar code or number should be issued for each specimen.

Laboratory Processing of the Specimen

To maintain the QC in the laboratory processing, the following measures can be taken:

- Laboratory SOP for processing and staining
- Senior laboratory personnel should keep a thorough check of daily smear quality including smear preparation, staining, mounting and cover slipping. A log book should be maintained about the quality of the smear
- The complete data record of staining material, chemicals and fixatives
- Laboratory supervisor should check about health and safety requirements of the laboratory staffs.

ANALYTICAL PHASE

Microscopic Analysis

Cervical Smears

- The primary screener may be the cytotechnologist who should screen every slide thoroughly
- The primary screener should not screen more than 100 slides in 24 hours' time period[3] and should not screen slides more than 8 hours in a day.
- All the positive slides must be reported by the cytopathologist.[4] Any discordance in the interpretation of cytoscreener and cytopathologists should be noted and this may be used in future for continuous medical education.

Nongynecological Smears

In case of nongynecological sample the laboratory should follow the norms as:[5]

- Every case should be reported by the cytopathologist[6]
- In case of difficulty in particular cases the reporting cytopathologist should discuss with the fellow colleague to reach to a consensus diagnosis.

Reporting

This is one of the important stages in laboratory service.

Cervical Smears

Rescreening of negative smear: To decrease the false negative rate in cervical smear screening various rescreening techniques have been recommended.[7] These have been discussed in chapter 9 also. In brief, the method of rescreening includes:

- *Proportional rescreening*: In proportional rescreening, 10% of all negative cervical smears should be rescreened by the senior cytotechnologists or cytopathologist.
- *Selected rescreening*: In this type of rescreening, the smears of selected group (of the patients with abnormal bleeding, suspicious cervix on visual examination, HIV-infected patients, etc.) are rescreened.
- *Rapid review*: In this technique, all the cervical cytology smears are rapidly screened by a trained cytoscreener after the initial screening by primary screener. This is currently considered as the most efficient technique in detection of false negative cases.
- *Automated rescreening*: Automated rescreening is done by the computerized automated system and this has been described in Chapter 21.

Others Nongynecological Lesions

- During reporting the cases the cytopathologists should follow the consistent reporting format used in that laboratory.
- One should be careful about using terminology such as "suspicious", "highly suspicious", "suggestive", "consistent with", etc.

POSTANALYTICAL PHASE

It is very important to have further follow-up result of the reported cases as far as possible. For IQC of the laboratory the following measures should be taken.

Cytology-Histology Correlation

- *Cytohistology correlation*: Cytological diagnosis should always be correlated either with histology or clinical follow-up or autopsy.
- All the discordant cases should be reviewed carefully and both cytology and histology slides should be seen.
- During review of the discrepant cases one should avoid bias. This can be done by:
  - A third person should screen the slide without any knowledge of clinical outcome
  - The discrepant cases could be introduced among the routine slides.

Computerized Record

There should be complete computerized record of all the cytology and histology cases. The data and slides should be kept for at least 10 years.[8]

Statistical Analysis and Performance Measurement

Periodic statistical analysis of the cytohistology correlation is mandatory for QC. There are various ways to measure the performance of the test.

False Positive

It is defined as a diagnostic test that is reported as malignant, however, the patient or the person shows a benign tumor.

Sensitivity

It means the percentage of actual (true) positive cases reported among all the positive cases.

$$\text{Sensitivity} = \frac{\text{True positive}}{\text{True positive} + \text{False negative}} \times 100\%$$

Specificity

It means the percentage of truly negative cases reported among all the negative cases.

$$\text{Specificity} = \frac{\text{True negative}}{\text{True negative} + \text{False positive}} \times 100\%$$

False Positive

It is defined as a diagnostic test that is reported as malignant, however, the patient shows a benign tumor or no tumor at all. The false positive report is described differently by different persons and there is a lack of uniformity in definition.

False Negative

False negative diagnosis means that in a diseased individual the diagnosis is either completely missed in the report or the severity of the disease process is underestimated.

False Negative Proportion

It is defined as the fraction of the patients missed among the total number of abnormal cases.

$$\text{False negative proportion} = \frac{\text{False negative report}}{\text{True positive + False negative}}$$

Record Keeping

This is also a part of the IQC. All the slides should be kept at least for 10 years for future review.[8] Slides should be arranged numerically and so that any slide could be retrieved as quickly as possible. In some laboratories, the negative report is kept only for 3 years for shortage of space.

EXTERNAL QUALITY ASSURANCE

Interlaboratory Comparison

The laboratory should take part in the interlaboratory QC program. The smear is circulated by the accrediting agency for the diagnosis. Alternatively the sample is sent for the preparation of the smear and interpretation. The diagnosis offered by the laboratory is compared with the final diagnosis. The overall performance of the laboratory is assessed by the accrediting agency and this is discussed with the laboratory staff. The error or faults are corrected by taking the appropriate measures.

Proficiency Test

The proficiency test is not mandatory for the laboratory personnel who examine gynecological samples. However, it is preferable that all the cytotechnologists should appear in proficiency evaluation test. There should be option for retraining and retesting the laboratory staff.

Continuing Medical Education Program

There should be adequate facilities or option for laboratory staffs to take part in continuing medical education, workshop, and symposium so that they are able to improve their knowledge and efficiency.

Overview of the quality assurance procedures are highlighted in Box 23.1.

Box 23.1: Quality assurance procedure.

Internal Quality Control
- Preanalytical phase
  - Sample receiving:
    - » Match slide with the requisition form
    - » Duly filled-up form
    - » Unique bar code
    - » Standard operating protocol (SOP)
  - Sample processing:
    - » SOP
    - » Daily checking of the smear preparation and stain by laboratory supervisor
    - » Log book of reagents, and necessary materials
- Analytic phase
  - All the positive slides of cervical smear should be reported by cytopathologists
  - All the nongynecological sample should be reported by cytopathologists
  - *Rescreening*: To reduce false negative cases the rescreening of the cervical cytology can be done by—rapid review/selective rescreening/automated screening
  - Thorough review of the abnormal smear and discussion for continuous medical education
  - Maintaining standard reporting format
- Postanalytic phase
  - Histology-cytology correlation
  - Review all the smears of invasive carcinoma on histology
  - Seeding the abnormal smear in the routine cytology reporting cases
  - Statistical monitoring of the overall performance of reporting at periodic interval
  - Proper preservation of slides and reports
  - Maintaining annual audit report

External Quality Control
- Interlaboratory comparison
- Proficiency test and continuing medical education
- Continuing medical education
- Accreditation and certification

Accreditation and Certification

Accreditation is a process by which the group of the experts of the accrediting agency verify whether a laboratory has fulfilled the required standard criteria that are already mentioned in the manual of the agency. If the laboratory fulfills the standard requirement then the agency awards an accreditation certificate. This gives the users of the laboratory the assurance of the quality of the laboratory. The accreditation certificate has to be renewed annually by the agency. The accreditation agency should have proper printed guidelines and the experts should be unbiased. The agency should collect the quality manual from the laboratory which should include:

- Standard operating protocol
- Laboratory organization
- Job description of all the staffs
- QC policy
- Annual audit.

LABORATORY ORGANIZATION

Laboratory organization of a cytology laboratory has the following components:

- Laboratory personnel
- Building, instrument and safety precautions
- Organization infrastructure and system protocol.

Laboratory Personnel

In each cytology laboratory the following staffs are needed to maintain the smooth quality work:

- Consultant cytopathologist
- Senior cytotechnologist or biomedical scientist
- Cytology screeners
- Technical laboratory personnel
- Clerical staff.

Consultant Cytopathologist

The consultant cytopathologist should be qualified pathologist with adequate experience in cytology. The duties of the cytopathologist are:

1. *Final reporting*: He/she is the final reporting authority and should assess and sign all the cases.
2. *Screening*: The consultant cytopathologist should examine all the abnormal cases and certain proportion of negative cases to maintain the accuracy and quality of the work in the laboratory.
3. *Cytohistology correlation*: He/she should try to correlate cytology-histology and review all the discrepant cases. He/she should maintain a regular audit of the laboratory cases.
4. *Communication with clinicians*: He/she should maintain communication between the clinician and the laboratory staff. He/she should take part in clinicopathological meeting, and inform the clinician about the discrepant cases, give an opinion on individual cases regarding further investigations or management.
5. *Teaching and training*: The consultant cytopathologist should educate the laboratory technologists by regular teaching and training and arrange continuing medical education program. Cytopathologist should also teach and train the postgraduate medical students in cytology. He/she should also encourage the nonmedical clerical staff for further training.

Senior Cytotechnologist or Biomedical Scientist

The senior cytotechnologist should have adequate experience in gynecological cytology. The duties and responsibilities of senior cytotechnologist are:

1. Management and supervision of all the junior cytotechnologists.
2. Screening certain proportion of negative cases and should review all abnormal cases.
3. He/she should act as a communication link between the other junior cytotechnologists and consultant cytopathologist.
4. Senior cytotechnologist may have to manage daily laboratory services and also personal affairs of all the staff.

Cytology Screeners

The cytology screener should have:

- Adequate training on screening cytology slides
- Cytology screener can screen both gynecological and nongynecological smears. However, all the cases of nongynecological smears should be re-examined by the cytopathologist for final reporting.
- In addition, the cytology screeners should also do routine cytology laboratory work, if needed.

Technical Laboratory Personnel

There should be an adequate number of trained technical personnel in the laboratory. The laboratory technical staff should be able to do the routine laboratory work. They should take part in a QC program.

Secretarial and Clerical Staff

The secretarial and clerical staff should be efficient enough to receive the sample, enter the data and dispatch the report. All the staff should be computer literate and should be acquainted in medical terminologies.

Laboratory Building and Instrument

Location

Proper location of the laboratory is very important. So the laboratory should be located and built in such a way that its function can be performed properly.

Rooms

There should be separate rooms for reception and secretarial staffs, processing and staining, and screening or reporting.

Specimen processing and staining area: This area should be spacious and well lighted and well ventilated. The sinks for handwash should be separated from the sink used for laboratory samples. There should be proper place or racks to store chemicals, particularly toxic chemicals should be in separate places.

Specimen preparation area: This room should have a Class I microbiological safety cabinet for processing of nongynecological samples. In addition, this room must contain centrifuge machine, cytocentrifuge, refrigerator and autoclave machine.

The benches for slide preparation should be in proper height to prevent excessive bending.

Screening room: The screening room or reporting room should be properly ventilated, spacious and pleasant. There should be comfortable chairs and tables for screening or reporting slides. This room should be free from noise as much as possible. The cytoscreener should have proper privacy in this room.

Secretarial and office room: This room should have adequate light and enough space for computer, printer and other necessary equipment. The staff should have comfortable furniture and comfortable area for work.

Organization Infrastructure and System Protocol

Infrastructural organization of a laboratory is important for smooth workflow and overall quality work. Flowchart 23.1 shows the workflow of a laboratory. All specimens should be received by the clerical staff and should be transferred to the laboratory staff after entering the data and giving a specific unique bar code. The sample should be processed and stained according to the standard laboratory protocol by the medical laboratory assistant. The stained smears should be screened by the cytoscreener. All the abnormal smears and a certain proportion of negative smears should be checked by the senior cytotechnologist. In case of rapid review of negative cases the senior cytotechnologist should screen all the cases rapidly. Finally the cytopathologist should examine and report all the abnormal smears. In case of nongynecological cases the consultant cytopathologist should report all the cases. The computerized typed report should be signed manually or electronically by the consultant cytopathologist and delivered to the patient.

Flowchart 23.1: An algorithmic approach showing workflow of the cytology laboratory.

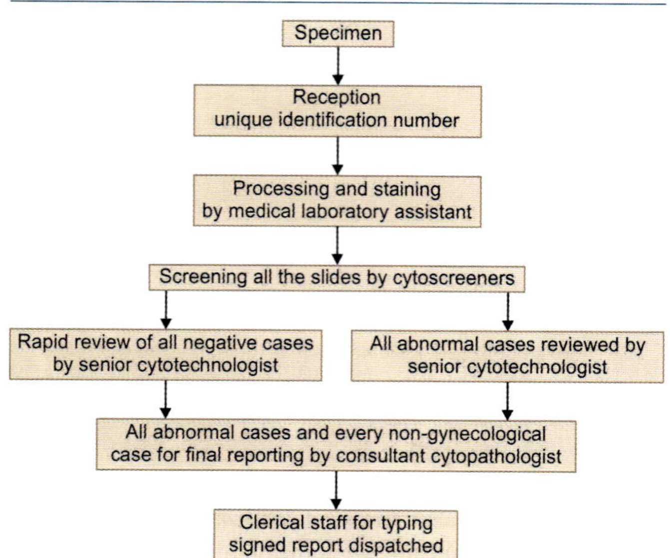

LABORATORY SAFETY

Laboratory safety should be the prime importance for all the staff working in the laboratory. Following matters should be kept in mind for the proper safety of the laboratory:

- Security
- Fire hazards
- Chemical
- Infective
- Waste disposal.

Security

- Proper security of the laboratory staff, chemicals and valuable equipment are mandatory
- Entry of unauthorized person should be restricted to the laboratory.

Fire Hazards

- All the laboratories should have fire extinguishers and smoke alarm
- The staff should know how to use the fire extinguishers
- Explosive or inflammable chemicals should handle with adequate precautions.

Chemical Hazards

- All the chemicals should be kept in proper place particularly inflammable chemicals and they should be kept in a fireproof metal cabinet
- All the chemicals should be kept in respective original bottles. Suction by mouth to draw material should not be allowed

- Laboratory staff should wear proper gloves, laboratory coat, etc. during handling of chemicals
- During the preparation of diluted solution, the concentrated acid or alkali should be added in water.

Infective

In this era of HIV infection, every laboratory sample should be handled cautiously and unless specified the sample should be considered as a potential source of infection. The laboratory staff should follow "universal precautionary measures".[9]

Barrier Precautions

- *Gown*: All healthcare personnel should wear proper laboratory gowns. The gown should cover the full arms and the front of the body from neck to mid-thigh.
- *Mask*: Mask may be used in combination with goggles to protect the face and eyes and also to prevent droplets or aerosol infection.
- *Gloves*: Gloves are used to prevent infection contamination by hands. Hygienic measures of the hand after removal of the gloves further help to prevent contamination particularly if the person has cut in hand.
- *Goggles*: To prevent eye infection.

Precautions from the Sharp Objects

Following precautions should be taken to prevent injury by sharp objects such as needles, scalpel etc.

- The needles should not be recapped or manipulated by hand
- Sharp objects should be placed in appropriate containers
- Needle cutter should be used to destroy the needle.

Hand Hygiene

If hands are contaminated with blood or other body products then they should be washed immediately with the antiseptic soap and water. Alcohol-based products such as gel or foam is better to wash as they do not require any water.

Prevention from Mucus Membrane Contact

Exposure to the mucus membrane of eyes, mouth or nose should be avoided. In addition to wearing protective barrier such as mask, gloves, etc. one should always avoid mouth to mouth resuscitation during emergencies and other mechanical ventilation devices should be used.

Duty of the Sick Person

Healthcare workers with weeping dermatitis or wound in the hand should not work for direct healthcare.

Common Norms in the Laboratory

In addition, the laboratory workers should follow certain norms to prevent infection:

- Eating, drinking or smoking should not be allowed in the laboratory
- Contaminated material, syringes, fluids, etc. should always be placed in proper containers
- Specimen preparation of high risk substances should always be done in biological safety cabinet
- Laboratory personnel should always wash their hands and face after laboratory duty.

Waste Disposal

Laboratory waste material may be of two broad types: (1) general waste material, and (2) biohazardous waste.

- *Label*: All waste material should be kept in properly labeled waste disposal container in a proper colored container as mentioned here.
- *Storage of waste*: Closable, puncture resistant, leak proof container should be used.
- *Accumulation of laboratory waste*: Only one container is used for each kind of waste material. The waste material should be disposed before it completely fills the container.
- *Container*: The container for sharper objects should be closable, puncture resistant and leak proof.
- The colors of the containers and their contents (Fig. 23.1) have been described here.
  - *Biological contaminated wastes*: This includes microbiological wastes and contaminated body fluids such as urine, sputum, blood, etc.
    - Color of container: *Yellow*
    - Type of container: *Plastic bag*
    - Treatment: This should be treated with disinfectant followed by autoclaving.
  - *Sharp objects*: This includes needles, scalpel, broken glasses, etc.
    - Color of container: *Blue*
    - Type of container: It should be closable, puncture resistant and *leak proof hard plastic container*
    - Treatment: Incineration.

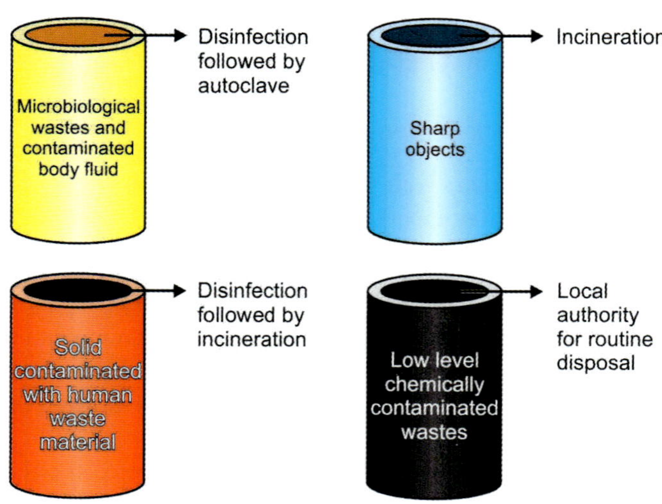

Fig. 23.1: Schematic diagram showing color of the bags and methods of waste disposal.

- *Solid contaminated with human waste materials*: This includes syringes, catheters, etc.
  - » Color of container: *Red*
  - » Type of container: *Plastic bag*
  - » Treatment: Disinfected followed by incineration.
- *Low level chemically contaminated waste*: Unused medicines, papers, various chemicals used for disinfection.
  - » Color of container: *Black*
  - » Type of container: *Plastic bag*
  - » Treatment: Local authority for routine waste disposal.

Disinfectant Used in the Contaminants

Sodium Hypochlorite

This is a fast acting oxidant and a broad spectrum chemical disinfectant. It is diluted with water to get optimal strength. An aqueous solution 1:10 dilution of sodium hypochlorite may serve the purpose of disinfection in the laboratory. The solution should be prepared daily. Chlorine is liberated from the solution that is highly corrosive. Therefore the solution should not be kept in metal containers.

Many other chemical germicides such as quaternary ammonium compounds (cetrimide, Savlon®, etc.), iodine and iodophors, hydrogen peroxide, etc. can also be used for laboratory disinfection.

REFERENCES

1. Cortese C. Cervical cytology practice guidelines. Acta Cytol. 2001;45:201-26.
2. College of American Pathologists. Quality Improvement Manual in Anatomic Pathology. Chicago: College of American Pathologists; 1993.
3. Department of Health and Human Services. Clinical laboratory improvement amendments of 1988 (Final rule federal register). 1992;57:493.1257(b).
4. Royal College of Pathologists. Medical and Scientific Staffing of NHS Pathology Departments. London: Royal College of Pathologists; 1992.
5. Nongynecologic cytology practice guidelines. Acta Cytol. 2004;48:521-46.
6. Department of Health and Human Services. Clinical laboratory improvement amendments of 1988 (Final rule federal register). 2003;68:493.1274(e)(3).
7. Krieger P, Naryshkin S. Random rescreening of cytologic smears: a practical and effective component of quality assurance programs in both large and small cytology laboratories. Acta Cytol. 1994;38(3):291-8.
8. Report of Working Party on internal quality control for cervical cytopathology laboratories—summary and recommendations. Cytopathology. 1996;7:4-9.
9. Siegel JD, Rhinehart E, Jackson M, et al. Health Care Infection Control Practices Advisory Committee. 2007 guideline for isolation precautions: preventing transmission of infectious agents in health care settings. Am J Infect Control. 2007;35(10 Suppl 2):S65-164.

Review Questions

1. **The percentage of actual (true) positive cases reported among all the positive cases is known as:**
   a. Sensitivity
   b. Specificity
   c. Positive predictive value
   d. Negative predictive value
2. **Barrier precaution includes all *except*:**
   a. Wearing gown
   b. Wearing mask
   c. Using biological safety cabinet
   d. Wearing gloves
3. **Sharp objects such as needles, scalpel, and broken glasses should be thrown in:**
   a. Red container
   b. Blue container
   c. Black container
   d. Yellow container
4. **Which will be the *best* screening test?**
   a. The test that shows 40% sensitivity and 90% specificity
   b. The test that shows 90% sensitivity and 80% specificity
   c. The test that shows 60% sensitivity and 50% specificity
   d. The test that shows 80% sensitivity and 20% specificity
5. **Proficiency test and continuing medical education is part of:**
   a. Internal quality assurance
   b. External quality assurance
   c. Preanalytical phase
   d. Analytical phase

Answers

1. a. Sensitivity
2. c. Using biological safety cabinet
3. b. Blue container
4. b. The test that shows 90% sensitivity and 80% specificity
5. b. External quality assurance

Section 4

Fine Needle Aspiration Cytology

Chapter Outline

CHAPTER

24 Head, Neck and Orbit

HEAD AND NECK

INTRODUCTION

Large varieties of primary and metastatic tumors from the different tissues may occur in the head and neck region. Fine needle aspiration cytology (FNAC) is often used to detect the primary and recurrent tumors in this region. It can be taken from the multiple sites and also from the distorted scar sites after radiation of the primary malignancies. It is also important to have thorough knowledge of the non-neoplastic lesions in this region that may mimic as malignant tumors.

CYSTIC LESIONS

The cysts may be congenital or acquired (Box 24.1). Various neoplastic lesions may also present as cyst such as metastatic squamous cell carcinoma (SQC), papillary carcinoma of thyroid in the lymph node and a large number of parotid tumors are often cystic. There are chances to have false positive or negative diagnosis and adequate cares must be taken to avoid the mistake.

Box 24.1: Cysts in head and neck region.

- **Congenital**
  - Branchial cyst
  - Thyroglossal cyst
  - Cystic hygroma
- **Acquired**
  - Non neoplastic
    - » Dermoid cyst
    - » Cysts of the jaw
    - » Salivary gland retention cyst
    - » Mucocele
  - Neoplastic
    - » Metastatic squamous cell carcinoma
    - » Warthin's tumor
    - » Acinic cell carcinoma
    - » Pleomorphic adenoma

Branchial Cyst[1]

The branchial cyst is one of the common non-neoplastic cysts in the lateral neck region. They are usually noted along the medial border of the sternocleidomastoid muscle. This cyst possibly develops from the congenital remnants of the branchial cleft.

Cytology (Fig. 24.1)

Aspiration of the cyst usually yields turbid fluid. The smears from the centrifuged fluid specimen show many discrete squamous cells, occasional clusters of columnar cells and

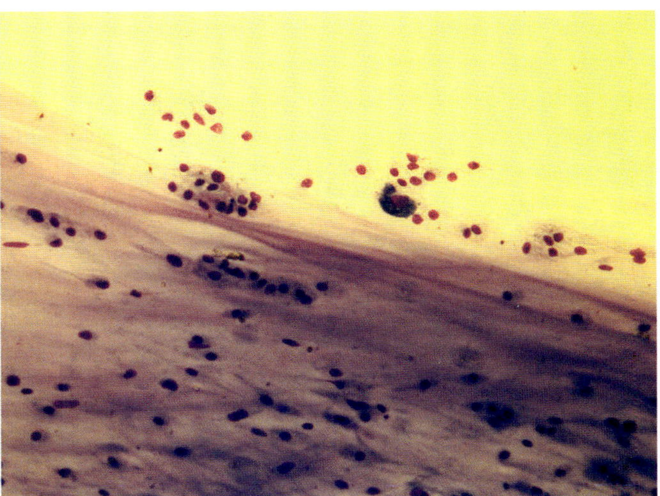

Fig. 24.1: Branchial cyst: Columnar cells and foamy histiocytes in the background of mucinous material (MGGX MP).

foamy histiocytes (Box 24.2). Squamous cells often show reactive changes such as nuclear enlargement and mild degree of pleomorphism. Background of the smear shows mucinous material and cholesterol crystals.

Metastatic SQC in the lymph node often shows cystic changes. FNAC of such lesions yield brownish fluid and smears of which show mature looking squamous cells and polymorphs in a thin necrotic background (Fig. 24.2). Cytology smears of such cases are the potential sources of misdiagnosis. The following features may be helpful in diagnosis of branchial cyst:

- Young patient
- Long history
- Bland looking nuclear chromatin
- Minimal nuclear pleomorphism.

Differential Diagnosis

- Metastatic SQC.[2]

Thyroglossal Cysts

Thyroglossal cysts are commonly present as midline neck cysts. During embryogenesis the thyroid comes down from the foramen of caecum of the tongue and thyroglossal duct is formed. Later on this duct obliterates. Dilatation of the persistent thyroglossal duct causes the formation of the thyroglossal cyst.

Cytology

Fine needle aspiration cytology of the thyroglossal cyst yields colloid (Box 24.3). The smear shows many ciliated columnar cells and occasional squamous cells. In addition, thyroid follicular cells may be present. Without the precise location of the tumor, it may be difficult to differentiate thyroglossal cyst from the colloid goiter.

Epidermal Inclusion Cyst

Epidermal inclusion cysts are often present in the head and neck region. FNAC yields thick whitish material. The smears show many discrete benign squamous cells and anucleated squames (Fig. 24.3). At times these cells may show nuclear enlargement and pleomorphism. This type of reactive changes should always be distinguished from the metastatic SQC. Occasional multinucleated giant cells are also seen.

Box 24.2: Branchial cyst.

- Turbid fluid
- Benign squamous cells
- Columnar cells
- Foamy macrophages
- Cholesterol crystals

Box 24.3: Thyroglossal cyst.

- Ciliated columnar cells
- Squamous cells
- Occasional thyroid follicular cells
- Background colloid

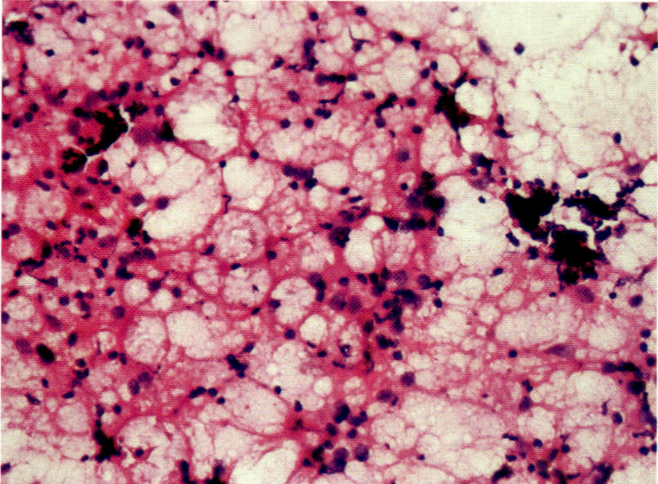

Fig. 24.2: Cytology smear of cystic squamous cell carcinoma showing multiple foamy histiocytes and scattered malignant squamous cells (H & E X HP).

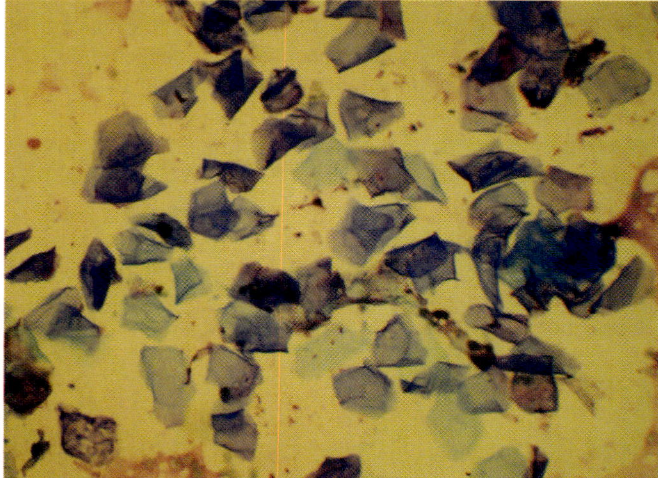

Fig. 24.3: Fine needle aspiration cytology (FNAC) smear of epidermal inclusion cyst showing abundant anucleated squamous cells (Papanicolaou's stain X HP).

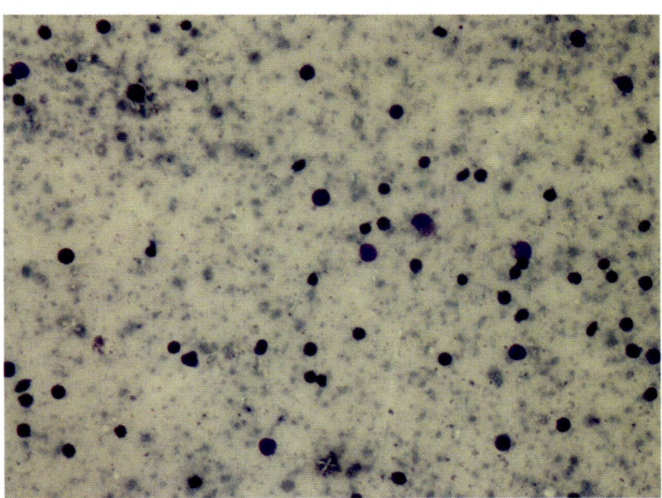

Fig. 24.4: Cystic hygroma: Lymphocytes and foamy macrophages (MGGX MP).

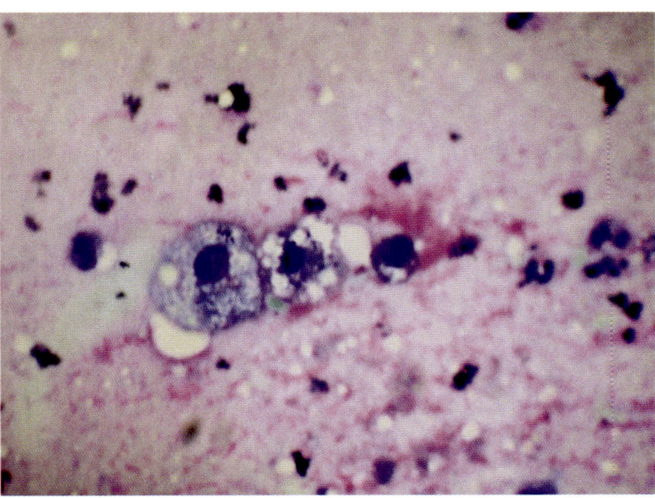

Fig. 24.5: Fine needle aspiration cytology (FNAC) smear of mucocele showing abundant mucoid material and foamy vacuolated histiocytes (MGGX HP).

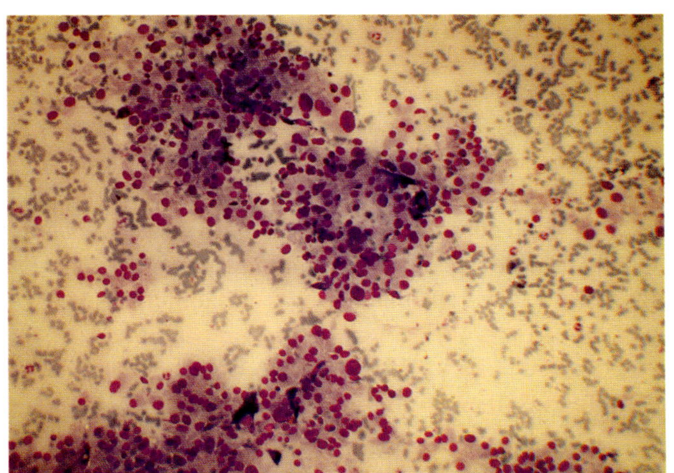

Fig.24.6: Loose clusters and dissociated cells in fine needle aspiration cytology (FNAC) smear of paraganglioma (MGGX MP).

Cystic Hygroma

Cystic hygroma is large diffuse lymphangioma that predominantly occurs in the infant and young adults. FNAC usually yields thin fluid. The smears show many discrete lymphocytes (Fig. 24.4).

Mucocele

This is due to the extravasations of fluid from the retention cyst of the minor salivary gland to the neighboring soft tissues. FNAC yields thick mucinous fluid and the smears of which show many histiocytes (Fig. 24.5).

NEOPLASTIC LESIONS

Paraganglioma[3]

Carotid body paraganglioma is a neuroendocrine tumor that originates from the glomus jugulare of the neck. It is also known as carotid body tumor. The tumor locates in the bifurcation of the common carotid artery. The patient presents as a slow growing mass under the sternocleidomastoid muscle. The swelling is pulsatile and moves from side to side but not vertically. It is often recommended that FNAC should not be done from this tumor as there is a chance of local hemorrhage and cerebral catastrophe after FNAC. However, we have not seen in such complications so far.

Cytology (Figs. 24.6 to 24.8)

Fine needle aspiration cytology yields predominantly blood mixed material. The smear shows small loosely cohesive clusters and dissociated tumor cells (Box 24.4). Occasional rosette-like arrangement may be seen. The individual cells show moderate amount of cytoplasm with ill-defined cell border. The nuclei are round to spindle shaped and are relatively monomorphic in shape. Salt and pepper like nuclear chromatin is seen. Occasional cells show nuclear pleomorphism among the monomorphic nuclei. The presence of intranuclear inclusions has also been described in paraganglioma.

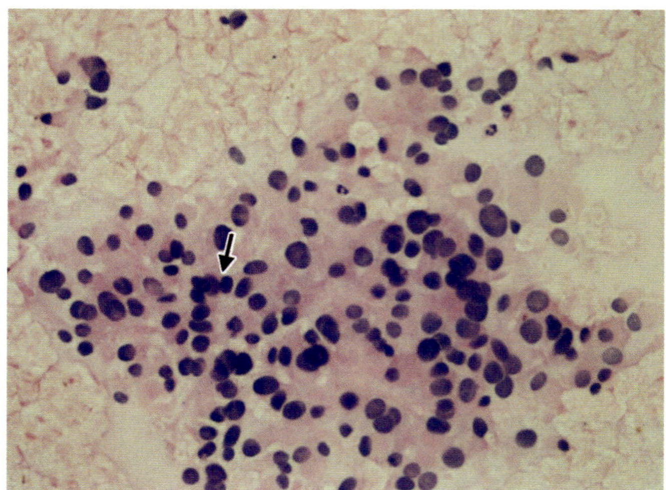

Fig. 24.7: Round to oval cells with indistinct cytoplasmic margin in paraganglioma. Occasional vague rosette-like structure is also seen (arrow) (H & E X MP).

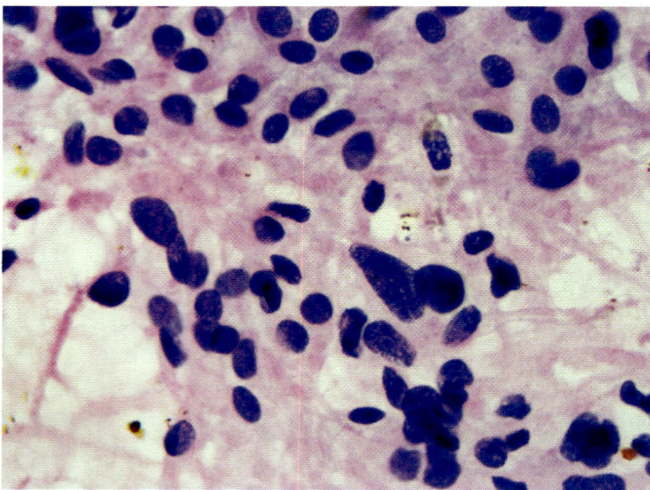

Fig. 24.8: Pleomorphic cells with bland chromatin in paraganglioma (H & E X HP).

Box 24.4: Paraganglioma.

- Syncytial clusters and dissociated cells
- Round to spindle cells.
- Cells with indistinct cytoplasmic margin
- Monomorphic nucleus
- Occasional cell shows nuclear atypia
- Bland nuclear chromatin
- Intranuclear inclusion
- Rosette-like structures

Immunocytochemistry: Positive for synaptophysin, NSE and Chromogranin and negative for cytokeratin, carcinoembryonic antigen, S-100 protein and calcitonin

Differential diagnosis: Medullary carcinoma, metastatic carcinoma, carcinoid

Immunocytochemistry

It is positive for synaptophysin, NSE and chromogranin; and is negative for cytokeratin, carcinoembryonic antigen, S-100 protein, and calcitonin.

Differential Diagnosis

- *Medullary carcinoma*: Both medullary carcinoma and paraganglioma have overlapping cytological features. However, medullary carcinomas are positive for calcitonin.
- *Carcinoid*: Metastatic carcinoid tumors may simulate as paraganglioma.
- *Metastatic carcinoma*: Marked nuclear pleomorphism in occasional cells of paraganglioma may simulate metastatic carcinoma. However, the nuclear chromatin is bland in paraganglioma.

NASOPHARYNGEAL CARCINOMA[4]

Nasopharyngeal carcinoma (NPC) develops from the nasopharyngeal mucosa. It is also known as lymphoepithelioma. It includes nonkeratinizing SQC and basaloid SQC. NPC is closely related with Epstein-Barr virus (EBV) infection. NPC commonly presents with metastatic lymph nodal mass. The patients may also have postnasal blood stained drip, serous otitis media and headache. The tumor has a bimodal age incidence.

Cytology (Figs. 24.9 and 24.10)

Fine needle aspiration cytology is usually done from the lymph nodal neck mass of the nasopharyngeal carcinoma. The smears show abundant reactive lymphoid cells admixed with syncytial or dissociated malignant cells (Box 24.5). The tumor cells contain moderate amount of cytoplasm with ill-defined border. Nuclei of the cells are round with mild pleomorphism, fine chromatin and single to multiple prominent nucleoli. Prominent macronucleoli are also noted. At times, binucleated cells with macronucleoli may simulate Reed-Sternberg cell.

Differential Diagnosis

- *Non-Hodgkin lymphoma (NHL)*: Abundant lymphocytes along with the dispersed round malignant cells may simulate NHL.
- *Hodgkin lymphoma (HL)*: Large binucleated cells with prominent nucleoli may resemble Reed-Sternberg cells of HL.

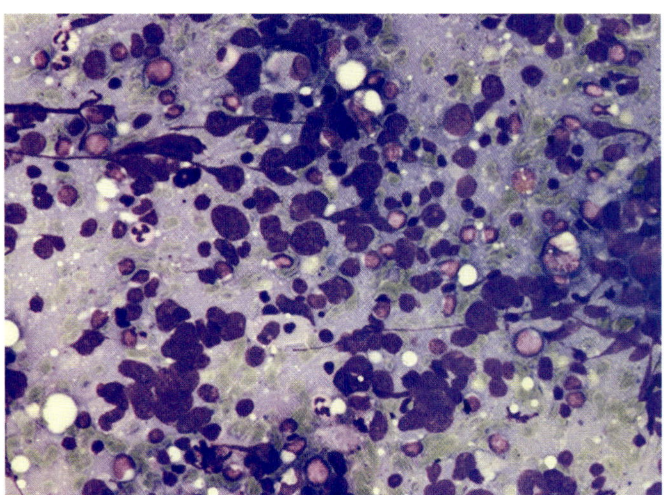

Fig. 24.9: The smears show reactive lymphoid cells admixed with dissociated malignant cells in nasopharyngeal carcinoma (MGGX MP).

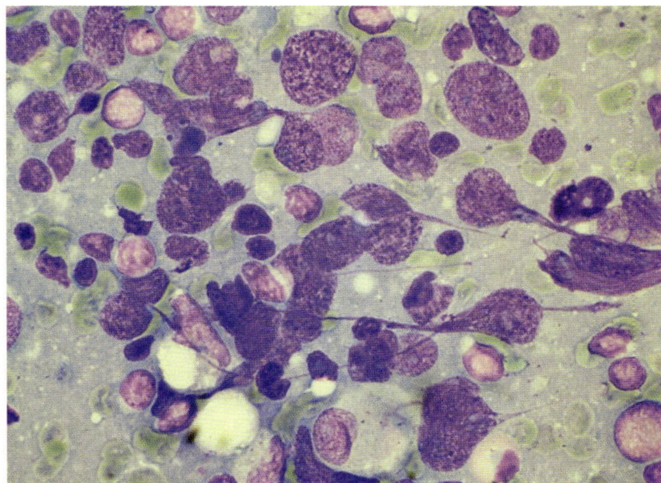

Fig. 24.10: Large cells with fine chromatin and prominent nucleoli in nasopharyngeal carcinoma (MGGX HP).

Box 24.5: Nasopharyngeal carcinoma.

- Syncytial or dissociated cells
- Abundant lymphoid cells in the background
- Round to oval cells
- Indistinct cytoplasmic boarder
- Mild nuclear pleomorphism, fine nuclear chromatin and single to multiple prominent nucleoli

Immunochemistry: Positive for pan-Cytokeratin (AE1/AE3), CK 5, and 6

Differential diagnosis: NHL, HL, metastatic small cell carcinoma

(NHL: Non-Hodgkin lymphoma; HL: Hodgkin lymphoma).

- *Metastatic small cell carcinoma*: Small cell carcinoma shows cells with scanty cytoplasm, hyperchromatic nuclei, nuclear molding and crushing artifact.

AMELOBLASTOMA[5]

Ameloblastoma develops from the odontogenic epithelium of the maxilla. It is a locally aggressive neoplasm and usually occurs in the 3rd to 5th decades of life. The overall incidence of ameloblastoma is less than 1% of all cystic lesions of jaw.

Cytology (Figs. 24.11 and 24.12)

Fine needle aspiration cytology smears show predominantly two types of cells: (1) Basaloid cells, and (2) squamous cells. The basaloid cells are commonly present in tight clusters and cords (Box 24.6). The cells are arranged in peripheral palisading manner. Individual cells show scanty cytoplasm and round to oval monomorphic nuclei. Discrete squamous cells are also seen along with occasional squamous pearls. The squamous cells show abundant cytoplasm and centrally placed nuclei. The background of the smear shows loose spindle cells and eosinophilic granular material.

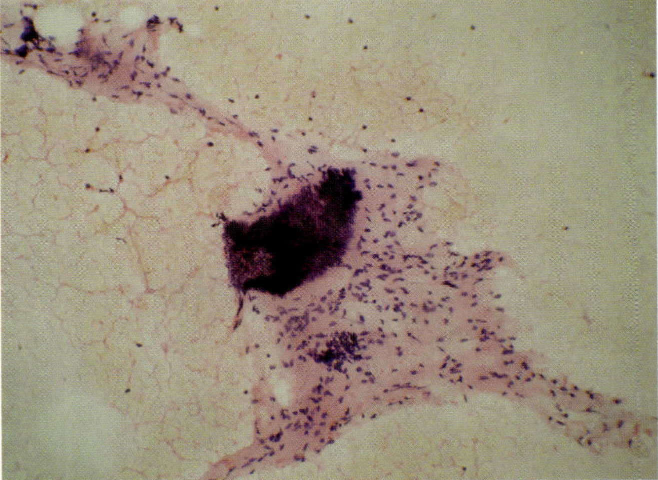

Fig. 24.11: Tight cohesive cluster of basal cells surrounded by loose connective tissue stroma in ameloblastoma (H & E X MP).

PARATHYROID TUMORS[6,7]

Parathyroid glands are located behind the thyroid gland. They are total four in number. Parathyroid tumors are nonpalpable and ultrasound (USG) or computed tomography (CT) scan is needed for their demonstrations. Parathyroid adenomas may develop in any age but commonly occurs in the 4th decade of life. The cases of parathyroid adenomas are usually present with the features of hyperparathyroidism. The clinical presentations of hyperparathyroidism are the presence of brown tumor, renal problems, and increased serum calcium and parathormone level.

Box 24.6: Ameloblastoma.

- Basaloid cells
  - Tight clusters and cords
  - Palisading arrangement
  - Scanty cytoplasm
  - Round to oval monomorphic nuclei
- Squamous cells
- Squamous pearls

Cytology (Figs. 24.13 to 24.16)

Fine needle aspiration cytology smears of parathyroid neoplasm show loosely cohesive clusters, papillary structures and microfollicular pattern (Box 24.7). The tumor cells are round with moderate amount of pale vacuolated cytoplasm. The cell shows mildly pleomorphic nuclei and inconspicuous nucleoli. The nuclear chromatin is finely granular. Occasional cells show marked nuclear pleomorphism. In fact, the absence of colloid and abundant eosinophilic or clear cytoplasm should raise the suspicion of parathyroid adenoma.

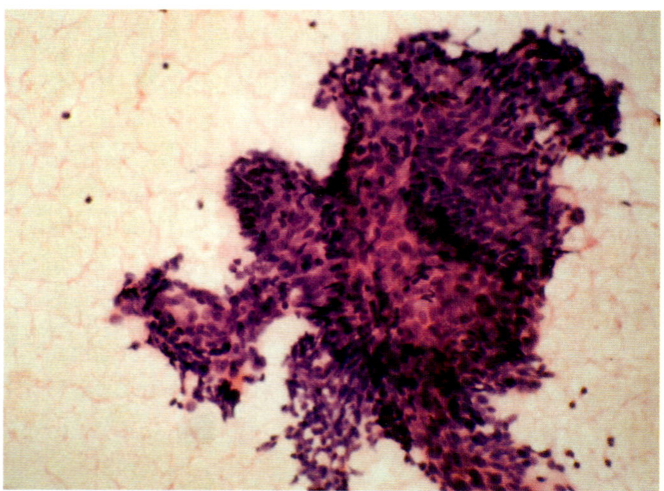

Fig. 24.12: Basaloid cells are arranged in peripheral palisading manner in ameloblastoma (H & E X MP).

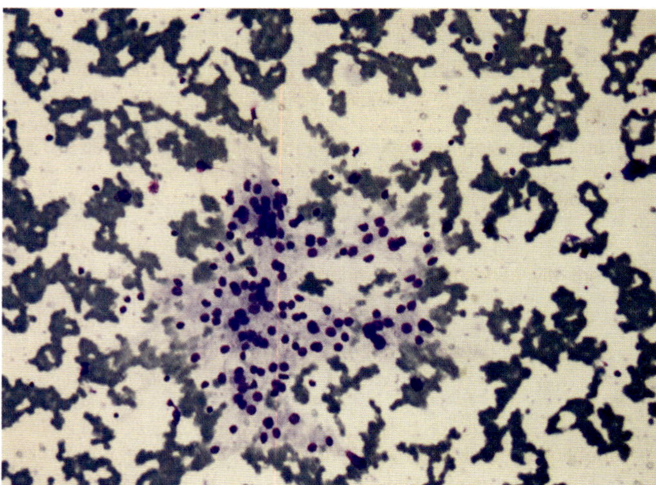

Fig. 24.13: Fine needle aspiration cytology (FNAC) smear of parathyroid neoplasm show loosely cohesive clusters of cells (MGGX LP).

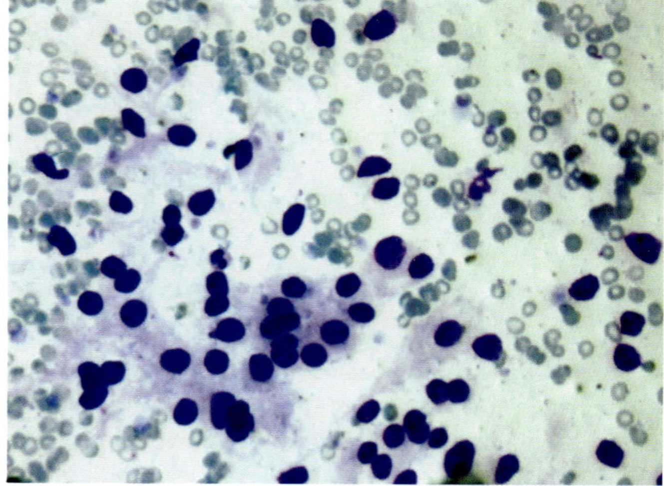

Fig. 24.14: The cell shows mildly pleomorphic nuclei and inconspicuous nucleoli in parathyroid neoplasm (MGGX MP).

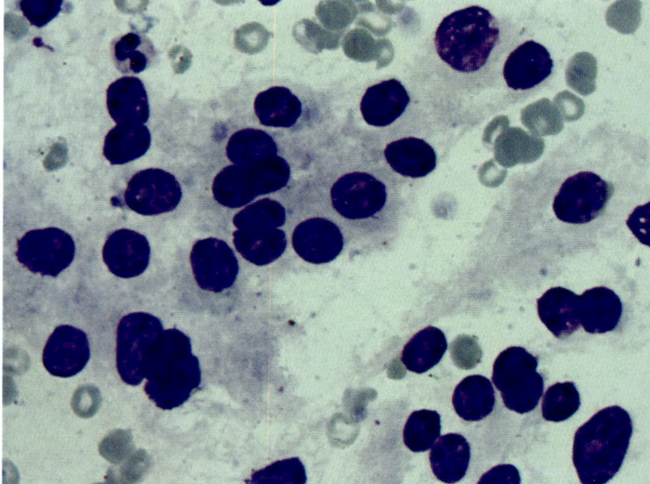

Fig. 24.15: Vague follicle-like arrangement in parathyroid neoplasm (MGGX HP).

Predominant population of dissociated cells with marked nuclear pleomorphism, frequent mitosis and the presence of necrosis should raise the suspicion of malignant parathyroid tumor.

Differential Diagnosis

- *Thyroid tumors*: Without proper clinical history, it is often difficult to suspect parathyroid neoplasm.

MENINGIOMA[8]

Meningioma is rarely noted in the nasal cavity as a protruding mass in the superior part of the nasal cavity and also in the posterior-superior orbital region.

Cytology (Figs. 24.17 to 24.20)

Fine needle aspiration cytology smears show predominantly tight clusters and dissociated cells. The tumor cells show syncytial pattern and whorling appearance (Box 24.8). The peripheral cells of the whorls are flattened, having more

Box 24.7: Parathyroid neoplasm.

- Loose aggregates and microfollicular pattern
- Small cells
- Vacuolated clear cytoplasm
- Monomorphic nuclei with salt and pepper chromatin
- Marked nuclear pleomorphism in occasional cells

Immunocytochemistry: Parathyroid hormone (PTH) positive
Differential diagnosis: Thyroid tumor

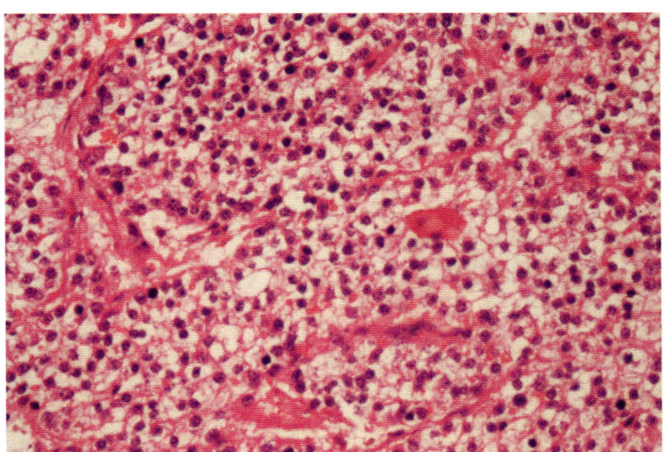

Fig. 24.16: Histopathology section of a parathyroid adenoma showing cells with clear cytoplasm and monomorphic nuclei (H & E X MP).

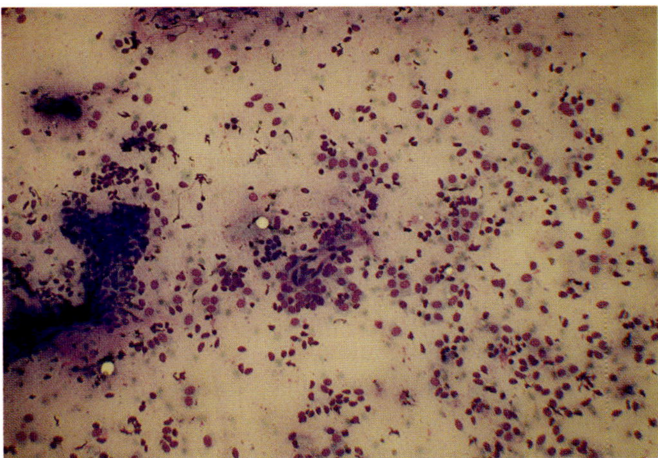

Fig. 24.17: Fine needle aspiration cytology (FNAC) smear showing tight clusters and dissociated cells in meningioma (MGGX MP).

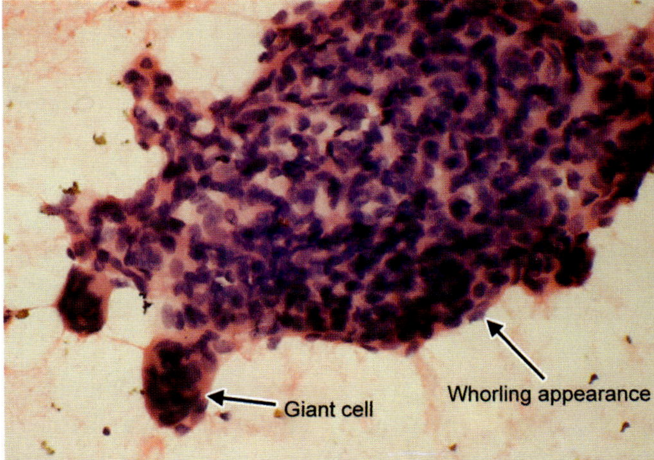

Fig. 24.18: Whorling arrangement of cells and multinucleated cells in meningioma (H & E X MP).

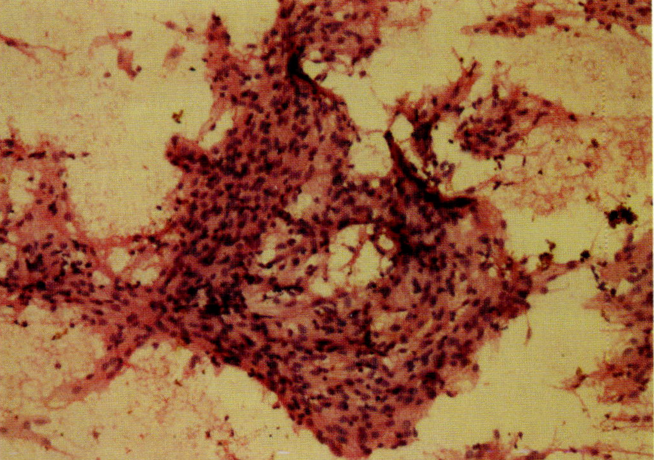

Fig. 24.19: Syncytial arrangement of cells in meningioma (H & E X MP).

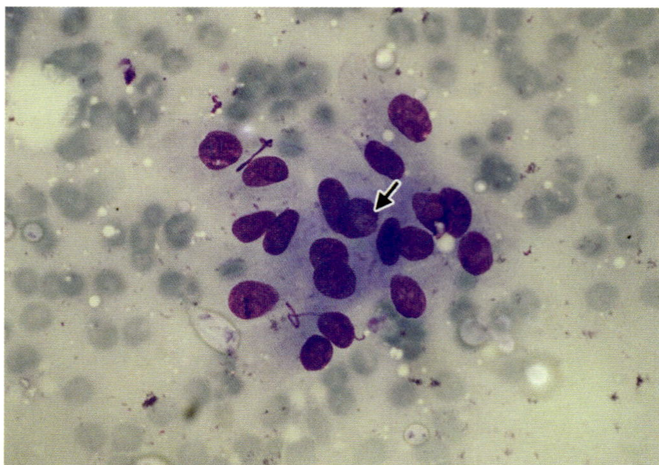

Fig. 24.20: Intranuclear inclusion in meningioma (arrow) (MGGX HP).

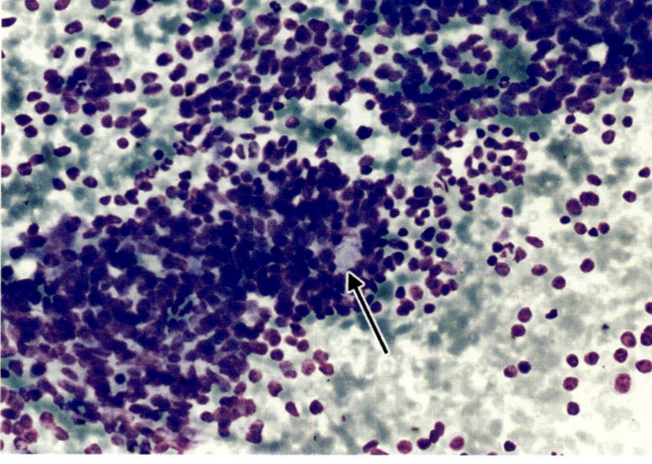

Fig. 24.21: Abundant discrete round to oval small cells with scanty cytoplasm in esthesioneuroblastoma. Occasional rosette is also seen (arrow) (MGGX MP).

Box 24.8: Meningioma.

- Tight clusters and dissociated cells
- Whorling appearance
- Oval to spindle cells with scanty cytoplasm
- Nuclear grooves and intranuclear inclusions
- Psammoma body
- Multinucleated cells

Differential diagnosis: Soft tissue tumor of spindle cell origin

Box 24.9: Olfactory neuroblastoma.

- Discrete round to oval small cells
- Scanty deep blue cytoplasm
- Round monomorphic nuclei
- Indistinct to small nucleoli
- Fine to granular chromatin
- Homer Wright rosettes

spindly nuclei. The tumor cells contain moderate amount of pale cytoplasm with mildly pleomorphic nuclei. The nuclear chromatin is bland. Occasional nuclear grooving, intranuclear inclusions and psammoma bodies are noted.

Differential Diagnosis

- Soft tissue tumor of spindle cell origin.

OLFACTORY NEUROBLASTOMA[9]

This is also known as esthesioneuroblastoma. This tumor develops from the neuroepithelial cells in the olfactory mucosa. Olfactory neuroblastoma may occur in any age group. This tumor presents as soft mass in the roof of the nasal cavity.

Cytology (Fig. 24.21)

Fine needle aspiration cytology smears show abundant discrete round to oval small cells. The cells have scanty deep blue cytoplasm with round monomorphic nuclei. Nuclear contour of the cell is regular with indistinct to small nucleoli and fine to granular chromatin (Box 24.9). Homer Wright rosettes are frequently seen in olfactory neuroblastoma. The background of the smear shows numerous naked nuclei.

ORBIT

ORBITAL LESIONS

Fine needle aspiration cytology is a safe and simple and reliable technique to diagnose various orbital lesions.[10-16] It is important in the diagnosis of non-resectable retrobulbar lesions and in recurrence of malignancy or metastasis. FNAC also prevents any unnecessary surgical exploration in leukemia and lymphomas. The diagnostic accuracy of orbital FNAC ranges from 72 to 100%.[16-24]

Techniques of Orbital FNAC

In our institution, FNAC of orbital and eyelid lesion is a team work that includes cytologist, ophthalmologist and radiologist. Superficial and easily approachable lesions are done directly and deep seated lesions are done under USG or CT guidance. The patients are kept in supine position. With the help of the USG probe the orbit is scanned to visualize the lesion. The eyeball is properly fixed by applying firm pressure. The patient is also requested to fix his eye away from the needle path. The aspiration needle is put from the opposite side of the USG probe and the needle is kept near the bony wall of the orbit. The needle track is closely supervised by USG visualization. The needle is gently moved in the lesion with applying suction. The suction is released and the needle is withdrawn gently.[25] Multiple wet fixed and air dried smears are made and the material is also processed for the cell block preparation. If needed, a repeat FNAC could be done for the collection of material for ancillary investigations or from the residual material in the needle hub.

Complications

Fine needle aspiration cytology may give rise to various complications such as retrobulbar hemorrhage, hematoma, bleeding and infections. The more serious complications such as perforation of the globe and intracranial injury have also been described in literature.[16,17]

MALIGNANT NEOPLASM OF EYELID

Basal Cell Carcinoma

It is a common tumor of the eyelid and represents almost 80–90% of all eyelid carcinomas.[26-28] These lesions are readily diagnosed by clinical examination and surgical excision are done without doing any FNAC.

Cytology

Detailed cytological features have been described in the skin section. The scrapping or FNAC smears of basal cell carcinoma (BCC) show tight cohesive clusters of basaloid cells. Palisading like nuclear arrangement at the periphery of the clusters is also noted. The tumor cells show round monomorphic nuclei with high nuclear-cytoplasmic (N/C) ratio and uniform coarse chromatin.

Squamous Cell Carcinoma

Fine needle aspiration cytology smears of SQC show clusters of malignant epithelial cells. The cells are polyhedral with hyperchromatic and pleomorphic nuclei having cytoplasmic orangeophilia (Papanicolaou-stained smears).

Sebaceous Carcinoma (Meibomian Carcinoma)

Sebaceous carcinoma commonly presents as swelling in eyelid. It has high morbidity and mortality and early diagnosis by FNAC is helpful for the management of the patient.

Cytology (Figs. 24.22 and 24.23)

The cytology smear shows clusters and discrete malignant cells containing moderate to abundant vacuolated cytoplasm. The nuclei are centrally in location, moderately pleomorphic with coarse chromatin and prominent nucleoli. The tumor cells are positive for Oil red O.

LESIONS OF LACRIMAL GLAND

The tumors of the lacrimal gland include pleomorphic adenoma, adenoid cystic carcinoma and mucoepidermoid carcinoma. Pleomorphic adenoma is a common tumor of the lacrimal gland. The cytological features of these tumors have been described elaborately in Chapter 25.

INTRAORBITAL TUMORS

Retinoblastoma

Retinoblastoma is a common intraocular neoplasm in children. Usually clinical presentation and indirect

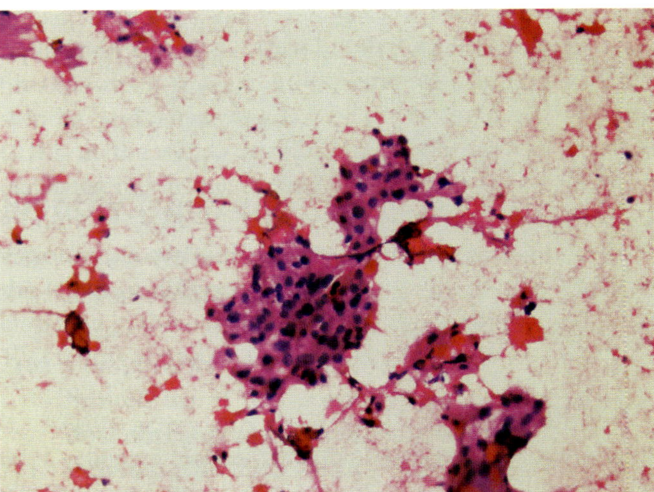

Fig. 24.22: Clusters of malignant cells in meibomian carcinoma (H & E X MP).

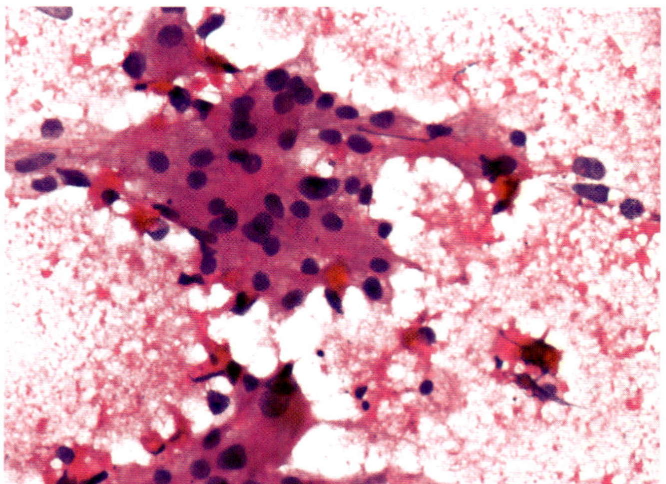

Fig. 24.23: Cells with abundant cytoplasm and centrally placed mildly pleomorphic nuclei in meibomian carcinoma (H & E X HP).

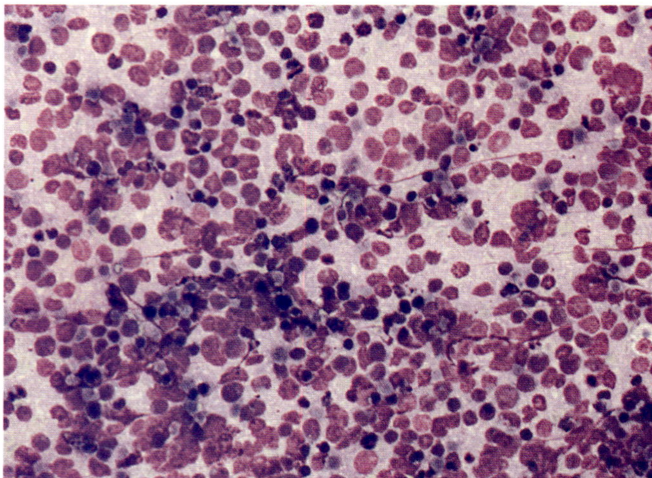

Fig. 24.24: Predominantly discrete population of small round cells in retinoblastoma (MGGX MP).

ophthalmoscopic examination are adequate for the diagnosis of retinoblastoma. FNAC is helpful only in doubtful cases. The patient usually has progressive loss of vision and/or proptosis.

Cytology (Fig. 24.24)

Fine needle aspiration cytology smears show predominantly discrete population of small round cells. Occasional rosette-like structures are also present. Two types of rosettes are seen: (1) Flexner-Wintersteiner rosettes, and (2) Homer-Wright rosettes.[21,29] In Flexner-Wintersteiner rosettes the cells are encircled around the lumen, whereas, in case of Homer-Wright rosettes the cells are arranged around cobweb like material.

The tumor cells are round with scanty cytoplasm. The nuclei are round, monomorphic and hyperchromatic with fine nuclear chromatin (Box 24.10). Occasional prominent nucleoli are also seen. Cohesive clusters and nuclear molding are the distinct cytological features of retinoblastoma.[29-32]

The differential diagnosis of retinoblastoma includes various small round cell tumors. Immunocytochemistry is helpful in doubtful cases.[26,31]

Box 24.10: Retinoblastoma.

- Small round to oval cells in clusters and rosettes
- Round cells
- Scanty cytoplasm
- Hyperchromatic nuclei
- Inconspicuous nucleoli

Rhabdomyosarcoma

Rhabdomyosarcoma is the most common sarcoma of the orbit in children. FNAC smears show clusters and single cells. The tumor cells are small and round with moderate amount of cytoplasm. The nuclei are round, central to eccentric in position with fine nuclear chromatin and prominent nucleoli. Frequent bi- and multinucleation are also seen.

Rhabdomyosarcomas are positive for desmin, MyoD and myogenin. Expression of these antigens is helpful to distinguish this tumor from retinoblastoma and neuroblastoma.[33]

Malignant Melanoma

Malignant melanoma of the orbit develops from the uveal tract. FNAC smears of the orbital melanoma shows discrete and small clusters of cells. The cells show moderate amount of cytoplasm and moderately pleomorphic nuclei. Large prominent macronucleoli is often seen in melanoma cases. Majority of malignant melanoma cases show intracytoplasmic melanin pigment. In case of amelanotic melanoma, immunocytochemistry particularly HMB45 is helpful.

Lymphoma

Near about one-tenth of all orbital tumors are lymphomas. On the other hand, 1.3% of the cases of systemic lymphomas may also secondarily affect the orbit.[34,35] Majority of the orbital lymphomas are well-differentiated lymphocytic, lymphoplasmacytoid or centrocytic/centroblastic lymphomas of the extranodal marginal type.[36] Burkitt's lymphomas also involve the orbit. The cytology smears of the lymphoma depend on the type of NHL (Figs. 24.25 to 24.27).

Detailed immunocytochemistry and flow cytometric immunophenotyping are helpful in the diagnosis and subtyping of lymphomas.[37]

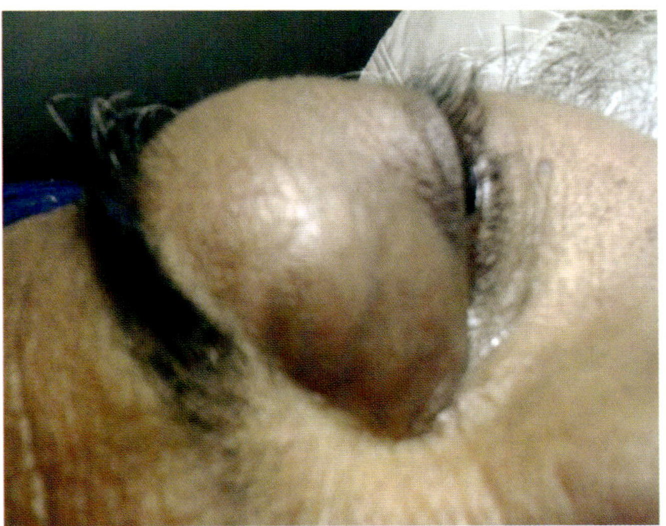

Fig. 24.25: Slow growing intraorbital swelling in a case of orbital lymphoma.

Leukemic Infiltration

The patients with leukemic infiltration of the orbit may often present as proptosis. In myeloid leukemia, the cytology smears show abundant myeloblasts, myelocytes and metamyelocytes. The demonstration of Auer rods helps in the recognition of the myeloblasts.

Meningioma

These are benign tumors originated from the arachnoid cells of the meninges. Meningiomas in the orbit usually present with proptosis and progressive loss of eye sight. The cytological features are same as described in the previous section of this chapter.

Optic Glioma (Figs. 24.28 and 24.29)

Optic glioma presents as retro-orbital space occupying lesion. The cytology smear shows spindle cells embedded the fibrillary pinkish substance.

Metastatic Malignancy[22]

A large variety of malignancies may metastasize in the orbit. The common primary sites are head and neck carcinomas, lung, breast and colon. Cytological features of such metastatic masses depend on the exact type of primary carcinomas.

Fig. 24.26: Round discrete monomorphic cells in MALToma of orbit (MGGX MP).

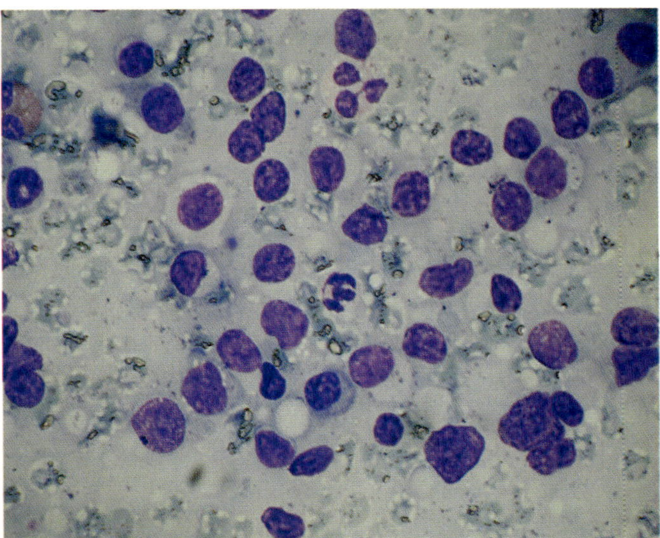

Fig. 24.27: Round cells with scanty cytoplasm and monomorphic nuclei with clumped chromatin MALToma of orbit (MGGX OI).

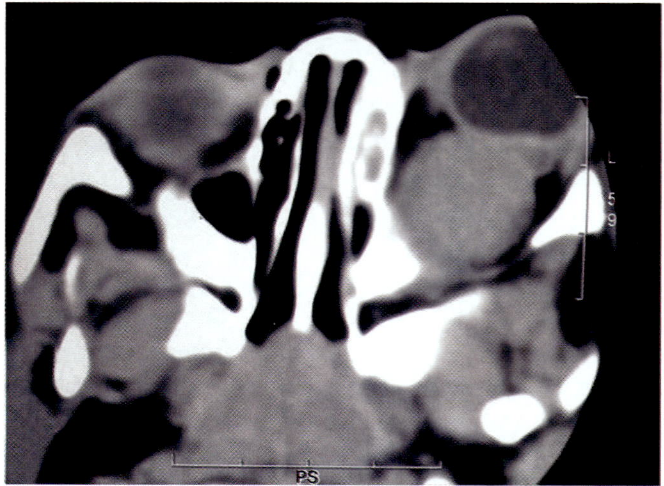

Fig. 24.28: Computed tomographic scanning photograph of optic glioma.
Courtesy: Dr Anupam Lal, Additional Professor, Department of Radiodiagnosis, PGIMER, Chandigarh, India.

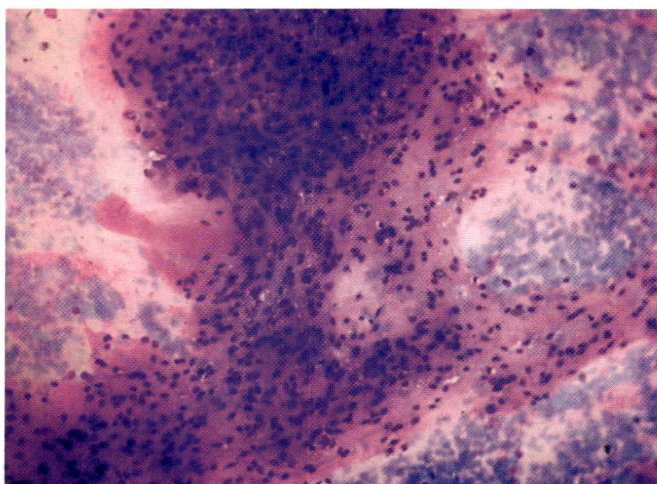

Fig. 24.29: Oval to elongated cells embedded in pink fibrillary background (MGGX MP).

REFERENCES

1. Firat P, Ersoz C, Uguz A, et al. Cystic lesions of the head and neck: cytohistological correlation in 63 cases. Cytopathology. 2007;18(3):184-90.
2. Ustün M, Risberg B, Davidson B, et al. Cystic change in metastatic lymph nodes: a common diagnostic pitfall in fine-needle aspiration cytology. Diagn Cytopathol. 2002;27(6):387-92.
3. Rana R, Dey P, Das A. Fine needle aspiration cytology of extra-adrenal paragangliomas. Cytopathol. 1997:8;108-13.
4. Mohanty SK, Dey P, Ghoshal S, et al. Cytologic features of metastatic nasopharyngeal carcinoma. Diagn Cytopathol. 2002;27(6):340-2.
5. Radhika S, Nijhawan R, Das A, et al. Ameloblastoma of the mandible: diagnosis by fine-needle aspiration cytology. Diagn Cytopathol. 1993;9(3):310-3.
6. Saikia UN, Saikia B, Dey P, et al. Fine needle aspiration cytology of parathyroid neoplasms. J Cytol. 2004;21(3):140-3.
7. Agarwal AM, Bentz JS, Hungerford R, et al. Parathyroid fine-needle aspiration cytology in the evaluation of parathyroid adenoma: cytologic findings from 53 patients. Diagn Cytopathol. 2009;37(6):407-10.
8. Agrawal P, Dey P, Saikia UN, et al. Fine-needle aspiration cytology of orbital meningiomas. Diagn Cytopathol. 2012;40(11):967-9.
9. Bellizzi AM, Bourne TD, Mills SE, et al. The cytologic features of sinonasal undifferentiated carcinoma and olfactory neuroblastoma. Am J Clin Pathol. 2008;129(3):367-76.
10. Jakobiec FA, Bilyk JR, Font RL. Orbit. In: Spencer WH (Ed). Ophthalmic Pathology: an Atlas and Textbook, 4th edition. Philadelphia: WB Saunders; 1996. pp. 2686-719.
11. Shields JA, Bakewell B, Augsburger JJ, et al. Classification and incidence of space-occupying lesions of the orbit. A survey of 645 biopsies. Arch Ophthalmol. 1984;102:1606-11.
12. Rootman J. Diseases of the orbit: a multidisciplinary approach. Philadelphia: JB Lippincott; 1988. pp. 119-39.
13. Wilson MW, Buggage RR, Grossniklaus HE. Orbital lesions in the southeastern United States. Orbit. 1996;15:17-24.
14. Seregard S, Sahlin S. Panorama of orbital space-occupying lesions. The 24-year experience of a referral centre. Acta Ophthalmol Scand. 1999;77:91-8.
15. Henderson JW, Campbell RJ, Farrow GM, et al. Orbital tumors, 3rd edition. New York: Raven Press; 1994. pp. 43-52.
16. Solo S, Siddaraju N, Srinivasan R. Use of fine needle cytology in the diagnosis of orbital and eyelid mass lesions. Acta Cytol. 2009;53:41-52.
17. Dey P, Radhika S, Rajwanshi A, et al. Fine needle aspiration of orbital and eyelid lesions. Acta Cytol. 1993;37:903-7.
18. Cangiarella JF, Cajigas A, Savala E, et al. Fine needle aspiration cytology of orbital masses. Acta Cytol. 1996;40:1205-11.
19. Zeppa P, Tranfa F, Errico ME, et al. Fine needle aspiration biopsy of orbital masses. A critical review of 51 cases. Cytopathol. 1997;8:366-72.
20. Gupta N, Kaur J, Rajwanshi A, et al. Spectrum of orbital and ocular adnexal lesions: an analysis of 389 cases diagnosed by fine needle aspiration cytology. Diagn Cytopathol. 2012;40:582-5.
21. Arora R, Rewari R, Betharia SM. Fine needle aspiration cytology of orbital and adenexal masses. Acta Cytol. 1992;36:483-91.
22. Glasgow BJ, Layfield LJ. Fine needle aspiration biopsy of orbital and periorbital masses. Diagn Cytopathol. 1991;7:132-41.
23. Zajdela A, Schlienger P, Haye C. Fine needle cytology of 292 palpable orbital and eyelid tumors. Am J Clin Pathol. 1990;93:100-4.
24. Das DK, Das J, Bhatt NC, et al. Orbital lesions: diagnosis by fine needle aspiration cytology. Acta Cytologica. 1994;38;158-64.

25. Gupta S, Sood B, Gulati M, et al. Orbital Mass lesions: US-Guided Fine needle aspiration Biopsy-Experience in 37 patients. Radiology. 1999;213:568-72.
26. Abdi U, Tyagi N, Mahesgwari V, et al. Tumors of the eyelid. A clinicopathologic study. J Indian Med Assoc. 1996;94:405-18.
27. Lee SB, Saw SM, Eong KG, et al. Incidence of eyelid cancers in Singapore from 1968 to 1995. Br J Ophthalmol. 1999;83:595-7.
28. Margo CE, Waltz K. Basal cell carcinoma of the eyelid and periocular skin. Surv Ophthalmol. 1993;38:169-92.
29. Das DK, Das JC, Chachra KL, et al. Diagnosis of retinoblastoma by fine needle aspiration and aqueous cytology. Diagn Cytopathol. 1989;5:203-6.
30. Rodriguez A. Diagnosis of retinoblastoma by cytologic examination of aqueous and the vitreous. Mod Probl Ophthalmol. 1977;18:142-8.
31. Sen S, Singha U, Kumar H, et al. Diagnostic intraocular fine-needle aspiration biopsy—an experience in three cases of retinoblastoma. Diagn Cytopathol. 1999;21(5):331-4.
32. Karcioglu ZA. Retina. Fine needle aspiration biopsy (FNAB) for retinoblastoma. 2002;22(6):707-10.
33. Morotti RA, Nicol KK, Parham DM, et al. An immunohistochemical algorithm to facilitate diagnosis and subtyping of rhabdomyosarcoma: the Children's Oncology Group experience. Am J Surg Pathol. 2006; 30:962-8.
34. Rubin PA, Kent CJ, Jakobiec FA. Orbital and ocular adnexal lymphoid tumors. In: Albert DM, JaKobiec FA (Eds). Principles and Practice of Ophthalmology, 2nd edition. Philadelphia: WB Saunders; 1999. pp. 3182-97.
35. Jakobiec FA, Bilyk JR, Font RL. Orbit. In: Spencer WH (Eds). Ophthalmic Pathology: an Atlas and Textbook, 4th edition. Philadelphia: WB Saunders; 1996. pp. 2686-719.
36. Curling M. The eye. In: Grey W, McKee GT (Eds). Diagnostic Cytopathology, 2nd edition. London: Churchill Livingstone; 2003. pp. 977-94.
37. Tani E, Seregard S, Rupp G, et al. Fine-needle aspiration cytology and immunocytochemistry of orbital masses. Diagn Cytopathol. 2006;34(1):1-5.

Review Questions

1. **A 3-year-old boy presented with proptosis of left eye.**
   a. What is your provisional diagnosis from the cytology smear of this space occupying lesion of the eye (Fig. 24.30)?
   b. What is your differential diagnosis?
   c. What immunocytochemistry markers can be used to confirm the diagnosis or eliminate the differential diagnosis?
2. **A 35-year-female presented with proptosis of left eye for 20 days. Figures 24.31A and B show the representative microphotographs of FNAC of the eye. What is your diagnosis?**

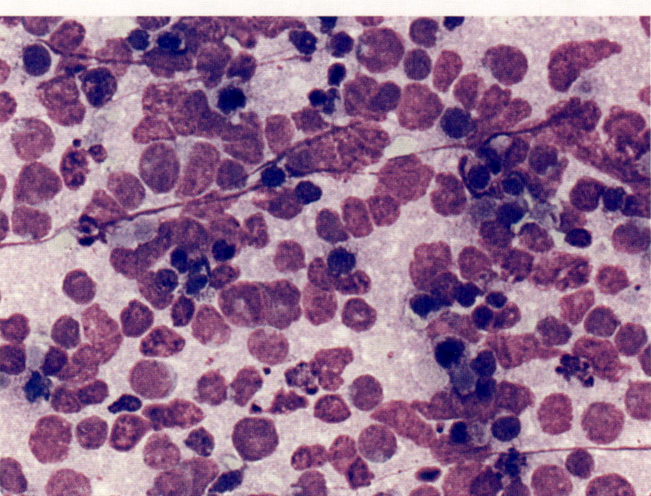

Fig. 24.30: Cytology smears of space occupying lesion of the eye.

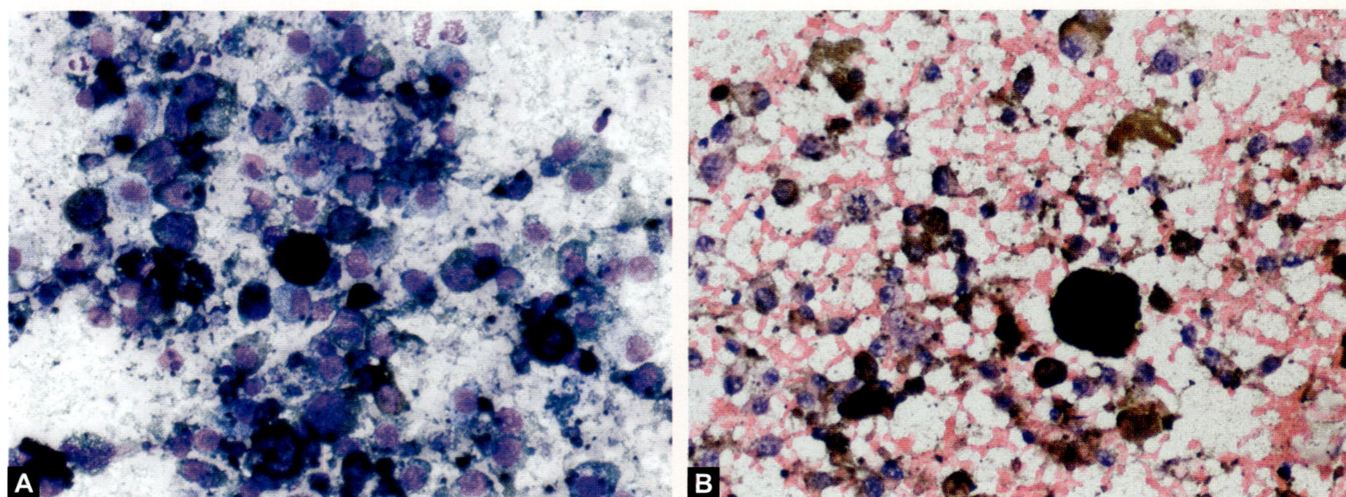

Figs. 24.31A and B: Representative microphotographs of FNAC of the eye.

Answers

1. a. Retinoblastoma
   b. Non-Hodgkin lymphoma (NHL), Neuroblastoma, Acute leukemic deposit
   c. CD 45 to rule out NHL, NB 40 for neuroblastoma

   Note: The cytology smear shows a malignant round cell tumor and with the clinical history of proptosis the most likely diagnosis is retinoblastoma.

2. Malignant melanoma

   Note: The malignant cells containing the dark brown melanin pigment indicates the diagnosis of melanoma.

CHAPTER

25 Salivary Gland

ANATOMY AND HISTOLOGY

Salivary glands are the exocrine glands that are responsible for secretion of the saliva. There are two groups of salivary glands:

1. *Major salivary glands*: Major salivary glands include pair of parotid glands, submandibular glands and sublingual salivary glands.
2. *Minor salivary glands*: Large numbers of minor salivary glands are present in the mucosa of the oral cavity, nasal sinuses, larynx and bronchial tree.

Parotid Glands

Parotid glands are mainly serous glands. Each gland weighs about 15–25 g. The parotid gland is situated in the angle of mandible. Anatomically the gland is bounded anteriorly by masseter muscle, superiorly by zygomaticus arch, posteriorly by the external auditory canal, and inferiorly by styloid process, internal carotid artery and jugular vein. The Stensen's duct is the main secretory duct of the parotid gland. This is about 6 cm long and 5 mm in diameter. The duct travels along the masseter muscle and then it passes through the buccinator muscle to open near the upper 2nd molar tooth within the oral cavity. During the embryological development of the parotid gland lymphoid tissue is incorporated within it and in future this lymphoid tissue may be the source of origin of Warthin's tumor. The parotid gland has two components: superficial and deep. The facial nerve with its braches passes in between these two compartments. Majority of the tumor arises from the superficial lobe of the parotid gland and form superficial bulging whereas the tumors of the deeper lobe of the parotid gland may have parapharyngeal swelling. Therefore, fine needle aspiration cytology (FNAC) of the parotid gland tumor is easy to perform and the subsequent surgical resection of the tumor is not difficult.

Submandibular Salivary Glands

Submandibular salivary glands are located in the submandibular triangle, which is bounded anteriorly by anterior belly of digastrics, posteriorly by posterior belly of digastrics and superiorly by mandible. This is a seromucinous gland and weighs 7–8 g. The gland has two lobes: superficial and deep lobes. The secretion of the gland flows through the Wharton's duct that opens into the floor of the mouth.

Sublingual Glands

These are the smallest salivary glands and weigh only 3 g. These are mucinous gland. The glands are present in the sublingual fossa and the secretion of the gland flows through multiple excretory ducts to open into the floor of the mouth.

Histology

The major salivary gland is composed of secretory part and duct part. The secretory part is made of acini which are lined by serous, mucinous or mixed (seromucinous) type of cells. The cells in acini are arranged as lobules encircled by myoepithelial cells. Each acini opens into the intercalated ducts that further joins with each other and forms larger excretory duct.

FNAC OF THE SALIVARY GLANDS

Indications

Fine needle aspiration cytology is indicated in any space occupying lesion of the salivary glands. The patients usually present with the complaints of swelling, pain, facial nerve palsy, palatal palsy and paresthesia. FNAC of salivary gland is especially helpful as incision biopsy may lead to fistula formation, potential infection in the plane of

Box 25.1: Indications and advantages of fine needle aspiration cytology (FNAC).

Indications: Any palpable swelling of the salivary gland.
Advantages:
- Rapid
- Safe
- High sensitivity and specificity
- Cheap
- Avoids any unnecessary surgery
- Helps in planning of surgery in case of neoplasm
- Various ancillary investigations can be done: Microbiological examination, flow cytometry, cell block

Box 25.3: Technical and clinical considerations of fine needle aspiration cytology (FNAC) of the salivary gland.

Technical
- FNAC from multiple sites
- Cyst should be reaspirated after drainage of fluid
- MGG and Papanicolaou's stain to do
- Tests for ancillary investigations: Microbial culture, flow cytometry (FCM), cell block

Clinical indications of malignancy
- Rapid enlargement
- Swelling fixed into skin or deeper structure
- Facial nerve palsy
- Pain in the ear

surgery and facial nerve palsy. Besides that, FNAC has high sensitivity and specificity. It is a rapid and safe technique and devoid of any serious complications[1-3]

Fine needle aspiration cytology helps to differentiate a neoplastic from a nonneoplastic lesion with confidence (Box 25.1). In case of nonneoplastic inflammatory lesion a conservative treatment may be helpful. Moreover, the aspirated material can be send to microbiological or other ancillary tests. FNAC diagnosis of the neoplastic lesion helps the surgeon to plan surgery according to the nature of the tumor.

Contraindications

There are no absolute contraindications of FNAC of the salivary gland. However, it is better to avoid FNAC in case of bleeding diathesis (Box 25.2). FNAC should not be done in absence of any swelling of the salivary gland or if there is infection over the skin of the gland.

Complications

There is no serious complication reported after FNAC of the salivary gland. The needle tract seeding of the malignant cell is a myth.[4]

Rarely there may be local hemorrhage, short-term facial nerve pain, or infection. Careful FNAC procedure

Box 25.2: Complications and contraindications of fine needle aspiration cytology (FNAC) of the salivary gland.

Complications:
- Hemorrhage
- Facial pain
- Infection

Contraindications:
- Bleeding diathesis
- Severe skin infection
- No swelling

such as local compression after FNAC avoids local hemorrhage. Similarly strict maintenance of sterility avoids any possibility of infection.

FNAC: TECHNICAL CONSIDERATION

Fine needle aspiration cytology of the salivary gland is done preferably by thin needle with 23 gauge diameter. It should be done from multiple sites to have adequate sampling (Box 25.3). Cystic lesions are the potential source of mistakes. Therefore, in case of cystic lesion a repeat FNAC should be done from the residual swelling after drainage of the cyst fluid. The repeat FNAC may help to avoid missing of the neoplasm with cystic changes. Gross appearance of the aspirated material may also provide important information. Aspiration of thick gelatinous material often indicates pleomorphic adenoma. Drops of dirty fluid are aspirated in case of Warthin's tumor. Aspiration of pus like material usually indicates suppurative inflammation. In every FNAC, both May-Grünwald Giemsa (MGG) and Papanicolaou's stains should be done. MGG stain is the metachromatic stain and it is helpful to demonstrate stromal material. This is particularly useful in pleomorphic adenoma (PA) and adenoid cystic carcinoma (ACC). Papanicolaou's stain is particularly helpful to demonstrate the squamoid component of the mucoepidermoid carcinoma (MEC). In addition, depending on the situation the material should be kept for Gram stain and microbiological culture. There is limited scope of immunocytochemistry in case of salivary gland tumors. However, cell block may be helpful for cytochemistry and histological features.

Clinical Evaluation

Detailed clinical history is helpful in demonstrating the nature and exact type of the lesion. The triads of pain, fever and local sign of inflammation indicate an inflammatory lesion. Most of the low grade salivary gland tumors present as a slowly enlarging painless mass. Clinically, there

Box 25.4: Cystic lesions in the salivary gland.

Non-neoplastic cyst:
- Retention cyst due to obstruction of the salivary duct
- Lymphoepithelial cyst
- Salivary duct cyst

Comments: Does not pose much problem except nuclear atypia due to inflammation.

Neoplastic cyst:
- Warthin's tumor
- Mucoepidermoid carcinoma
- Pleomorphic adenoma
- Cyst adenocarcinoma

Comments: Inadequate sampling may cause false negative diagnosis.

may not be any distinctive features between a benign and a malignant tumor. However, a rapidly increasing mass, facial palsy, paresthesia, fixation of the swelling with adjacent skin and deeper structure and lymph nodal enlargement indicate the malignant nature of the lesion.

OVERVIEW OF THE DIAGNOSTIC CHALLENGES

Fine needle aspiration cytology diagnosis of the salivary gland tumors often poses diagnostic challenges to the cytologist. The various facets of the diagnostic problems are:

- *Varied and heterogeneous nature of salivary gland neoplasia*: Large varieties of the epithelial and nonepithelial tumors are present in the salivary gland.[5] The cell of origin of these tumors is common and they differ only by architectural pattern. Therefore, it is difficult to diagnose them with certainty on FNAC.
- *Cystic lesions (Box 25.4)*: Many lesions of salivary gland are cystic. The non-neoplastic cysts develop due to obstruction of the excretory ducts of the salivary gland. Many neoplasms of the salivary gland show cystic changes such as Warthin's tumor, MEC, pleomorphic adenoma and cyst adenocarcinoma. Inadequate sampling from the cystic tumor is the common source of false negative diagnosis.
- *Low grade tumor*: Many salivary gland tumors are low grade and are often mistaken as normal aspirate such as benign salivary acinar cells often simulate acinic cell carcinoma. Similarly low grade mucoepidermoid tumor may be misdiagnosed as benign lesion.
- *Benign versus malignant tumor of the same type*: Occasionally, it is very difficult to distinguish the benign and the malignant counterpart of a tumor such as myoepithelioma is difficult to distinguish from malignant myoepithelioma.

Box 25.5: Lymphoid rich lesions.

Non-neoplastic
- Chronic sialadenitis
- Lymphoepithelial lesions
- Granulomatous sialadenitis

Neoplastic
- Lymphoma
- Warthin's tumor
- Mucoepdermoid carcinoma
- Acinic cell tumor

- *Lymphoid rich lesion (Box 25.5)*: Lymphoid cell rich aspirate of the salivary gland lesion may also pose diagnostic challenge. Aspirated material rich in lymphoid cells may be noted in non-neoplastic lesions such as chronic sialadenitis or lymphoepithelial lesions. Similarly, neoplastic conditions such as Warthin's tumor, MEC and acinic cell tumor may show good amount of lymphoid cells. At times the distinction between a low-grade non-Hodgkin lymphoma (NHL) from the lymphoepithelial lesions is difficult.
- *Squamoid differentiation*: FNAC of the salivary gland may often show epithelial cells with squamoid differentiation. Metaplastic benign squamous cells may be present in chronic sialadenitis, Warthin's tumor and pleomorphic adenoma. The individual cells do not show any nuclear enlargement and pleomorphism and therefore they usually do not create any problem. However, inadequate sample containing only the metaplastic squamous cells may be misinterpreted as MEC. Malignant squamous cells are seen in MEC, and primary or metastatic squamous cell carcinoma of the salivary gland.
- *Oncocytic changes*: Many neoplastic and non-neoplastic lesions of the salivary gland may show oncocytic changes and thereby may create diagnostic confusion. Oncocytoma and Warthin's tumor are two benign tumors that show good amount of oncocytic changes. Whereas the malignant tumor with oncocytic changes are oncocytic carcinoma and MEC.

NORMAL SALIVARY GLAND CELLS

Fine needle aspiration cytology of the normal salivary gland usually yields scanty material.

Benign Ductal Cells (Fig. 25.1)

Ductal cells are usually present in tight small clusters or honeycombed like monolayered sheets. The individual cells are round with scanty cytoplasm having monomorphic round nuclei.

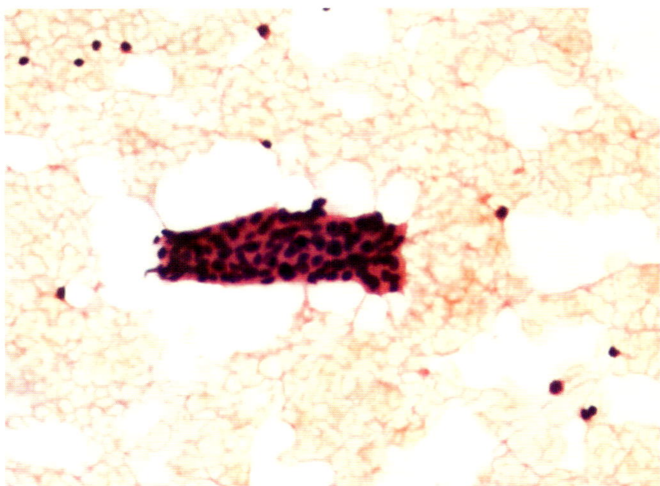

Fig. 25.1: Round to oval monomorphic benign ductal cells (MGG stain X MP).

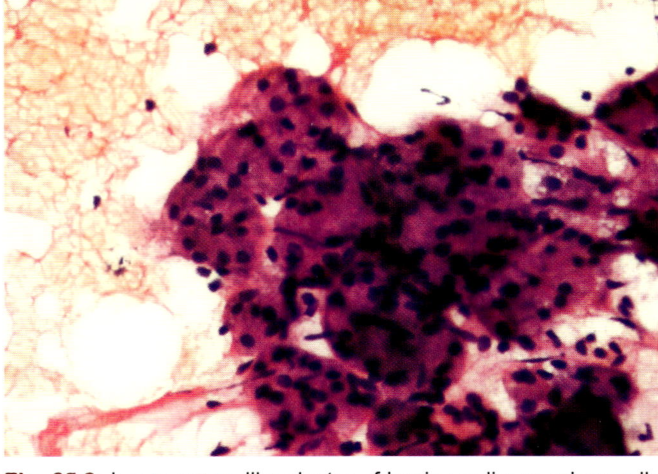

Fig. 25.2: Loose grape-like cluster of benign salivary acinar cells (H & E stain X MP).

Acinar Cells (Fig. 25.2)

These cells are commonly present as loose grape-like clusters or discretely. The individual cells are pyramid in shape with abundant foamy cytoplasm and small eccentrically placed round nuclei. Due to cytoplasmic fragility, the acinar cells often present as bare nuclei and these cells should be distinguished from the background lymphocytes.

Myoepithelial Cells

Myoepithelial cells are oval to spindle shaped with scanty cytoplasm. Oval plasmacytoid myoepithelial cells may also be seen.

Other Components

Fragments of fibrous and adipose tissue may also be seen in the background of the normal salivary aspirate. Due to the presence of intraparotid lymph node, lymphoid cells are often noted in the normal salivary aspirate.

It is important to note that FNAC smears containing only normal salivary gland cells in a swelling is mainly caused by sampling error. The common causes of finding normal salivary gland cells in FNAC smears are:

- Sampling error in a neoplastic lesion
- Sialadenitis
- Sialolithiasis
- Idiopathic enlargement of parotid gland
- Acinic cell carcinoma mistaken as normal acinar cells. Therefore, in case of any suspicion, a repeat FNAC should always be performed.

Box 25.6: Retention cyst.

- Watery or mucoid fluid
- Macrophages
- Cuboidal, columnar or squamous cells
- Polymorphs and lymphocytes

SALIVARY GLAND LESIONS

Non-neoplastic Conditions

Cystic Lesions of the Salivary Gland

Approximate 5% of the salivary gland lesions are cystic in nature.[6] Box 25.4 highlights different types of cystic lesions of the salivary gland.

Retention cyst (Box 25.6): The deep seated retention cysts are firm in consistency and may be mistaken as neoplastic lesion. The retention cyst develops due to obstruction of the salivary duct. FNAC yields clear watery to mucoid fluid. Smears from the fluid show macrophages along with degenerated epithelial cells. The epithelial cells may be cuboidal, columnar or squamous. The cysts may show variable number of polymorphs and lymphocytes depending on superadded infection.

Simple cyst: These are mostly superficial and clinically recognizable as benign lesion. FNAC smear usually shows scanty benign squamous cells.

Mucocele: This is due to the extravasations of the mucus filled cyst of the minor salivary gland to the adjacent soft tissue. FNAC smears show histiocytes in the background of mucinous material.

Lymphoepithelial cyst (Box 25.7): Lymphoepithelial cysts are seen in adult. These cysts are unilateral and mainly involve the parotid gland. Lymphoepithelial cysts are also noted in human immunodeficiency virus (HIV) patients.[7] HIV-related lymphoepithelial cysts are usually bilateral.

FNAC of the cyst shows foamy macrophages, reactive lymphocytes along with squamous cells. Multinucleated giant cells may also be seen.

Box 25.7: Lymphoepithelial cyst.

- Foamy macrophages
- Reactive lymphocytes
- Squamous cells
- Multinucleated giant cells

Sialadenosis

Sialadenosis is an uncommon entity. It is a non-neoplastic and noninflammatory lesion. It usually involves bilateral parotid gland. The swelling is diffuse and doughy in feel. Sialadenosis is commonly associated with diabetes mellitus, obesity, chronic alcohol intake and cirrhosis.

Cytology (Fig. 25.3): FNAC smears show scattered clusters of ductal and abundant acinar cells. Background of the smear is free from lymphocytes. The acinar cell may show mild nuclear enlargement. In long standing case, the gland becomes atrophic and is replaced with fibrofatty tissue and FNAC may show scanty cellularity.

Sialadenitis

Acute sialadenitis: Acute sialadenitis usually occurs in older patients, postoperative patients with poor oral hygiene, sialolithiasis or in case of obstruction of the salivary duct. In younger patient and child it may occur due to viral infection such as mumps. The patient of acute sialadenitis presents with pain, swelling of the salivary gland and fever. Both parotid and submandibular gland may be involved by acute sialadenitis. However, parotid gland involvement is more common because serous secretion of this gland has less antimicrobial property. The underlying factors in any acute sialadenitis are poor oral hygiene, dehydration and immunodeficiency.

Cytology: FNAC smears show abundant polymorphs, and necrotic cellular debris. In addition, many clusters and dissociated benign ductular and acinar cells are seen.

Chronic sialadenitis:[8] The cases of chronic sialadenitis usually presents with recurrent enlargement of the salivary gland along with pain during chewing food. This is usually due to obstruction of the ducts of salivary glands by stone. The proximal to the obstruction of the glands may be affected by infection. Near about 80% of chronic sialadenitis occurs in the parotid gland and the remaining 20% occurs in the submandibular gland. The sublingual gland is infrequently involved by chronic sialadenitis.

Cytology (Fig. 25.4): FNAC smears show many clusters of ductal cells, scanty acinar cells and lymphocytes in a background of mucinous material. The sparse amount of acinar cells is usually due to chronic destruction of such cells.

Lymphoepithelial sialadenitis (LESA):[9] This disease is also known as benign lymphoepithelial lesion and Mikulicz's disease and myoepithelial sialadenitis. This is an autoimmune condition and no age is exempted. The patients are usually female with unilateral or bilateral

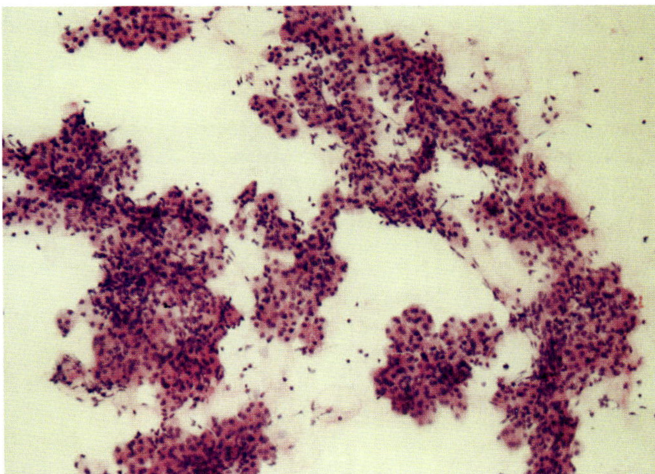

Fig. 25.3: Abundant clusters of benign salivary acini in sialadenosis (H & E stain X MP).

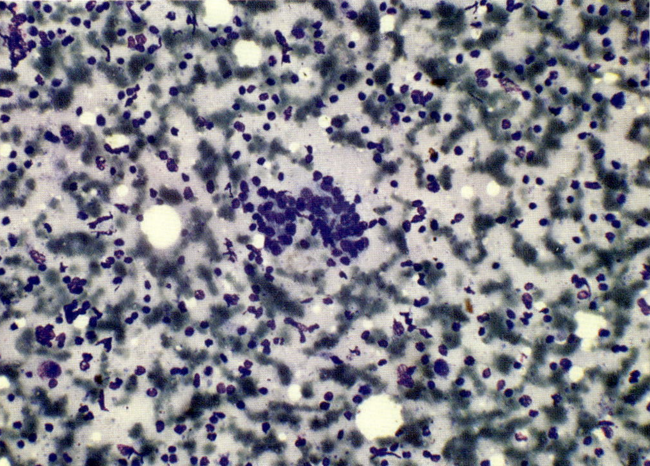

Fig. 25.4: Abundant lymphocytes and ductal cells in chronic sialadenitis (MGG stain X MP).

enlargement of the parotid gland. The submandibular gland is uncommonly involved. In 50% of the cases, LESA is associated with Sjögren's syndrome. The patients with LESA have higher risk to develop NHL particularly B cell type. Therefore, the cases of LESA should always be followed up by FNAC.

Cytology (Fig. 25.5): The cytology smears show abundant reactive lymphoid cells consisting of mature lymphocytes, centroblasts, follicular center cells and plasma cells (Box 25.8). In addition, occasional loose clusters of ductal epithelial cells along with lymphocytic infiltrate may also be seen. It is necessary to exclude the possibility of a low-grade NHL.

Differential diagnosis:

- *Lymphoma*: Low grade mucosa associated lymphoma is often difficult to distinguish from the LESA. Monomorphic population of immature lymphoid cells is noted in lymphoma, whereas in case of LESA the lymphoid cell population is polymorphic. Demonstration of monoclonal nature of the lymphoid cells may be necessary for the diagnosis of low grade NHL.
- *Warthin's tumor*: Warthin's tumor may also show large amount of reactive lymphoid cells and may simulate LESA. However, Warthin's tumor shows good number of oncocytic cells.
- *Lymphoepithelial cyst*: Lymphoepithelial cyst may yield fluid with predominant lymphocytes.
- *Intraparotid reactive lymph node*: Intraparotid reactive lymph node may also show identical cytological features.

Box 25.8: Lymphoepithelial sialadenitis.

- Associated with autoimmune disease (Sjögren's syndrome)
- Mature lymphocytes and follicular center cells
- Clusters of ductal cells with lymphocytic infiltration

- *Chronic sialadenitis*: It may pose diagnostic difficulty because of similar cytological features. However, the amount of reactive lymphoid cells is usually less in chronic sialadenitis.

Granulomatous sialadenitis: It is caused by tuberculosis, sarcoidosis, fungal infections etc.[10] FNAC smears show epithelioid cell granulomas, multinucleated giant cells, lymphocytes and histiocytes. In addition, salivary ductal cells may be seen. Epithelioid cells should not be mistaken as component of epithelial tumor. Ziehl-Neelsen stain should always be done to exclude the possibility of tuberculosis.

Neoplastic Lesions

The World Health Organization (WHO) classification of the salivary gland lesions have been highlighted in Table 25.1.[5]

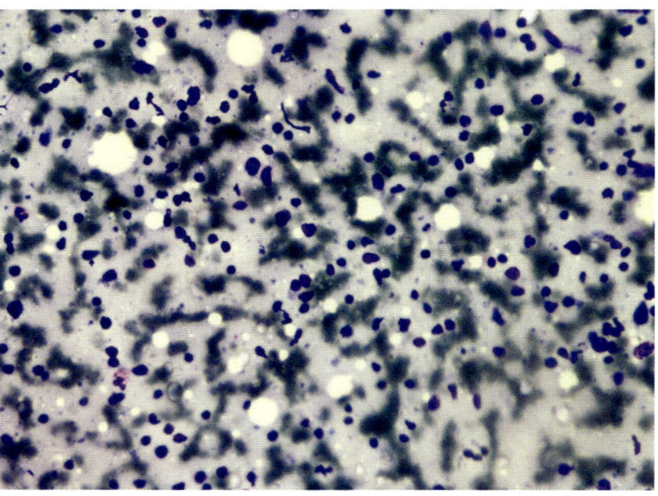

Fig. 25.5: Abundant reactive lymphoid cells in lymphoepithelial sialadenitis (MGG stain X MP).

Table 25.1: Classification of salivary gland tumors (modified from the World Health Organization classification).[5]

Benign epithelial tumor	*Malignant epithelial tumor*	*Soft tissue tumors*	*Hematolymphoid tumor*	*Metastatic tumor*
• Pleomorphic adenoma • Myoepithelioma • Basal cell adenoma • Warthin's tumor • Oncocytoma • Canalicular adenoma • Lymphadenoma • Duct papilloma	• Adenoid cystic carcinoma • Mucoepidermoid carcinoma • Acinic cell carcinoma • Epithelial myoepithelial carcinoma • Polymorphous low grade adenocarcinoma • Basal cell adenocarcinoma • Squamous cell carcinoma • Carcinoma expleomorphic adenoma • Adenocarcinoma • Myoepithelial carcinoma • Carcinosarcoma • Sebaceous carcinoma	• Hemangioma	• Extranodal marginal zone lymphoma • Diffuse large B cell lymphoma • Hodgkin lymphoma	• Metastatic tumor

Benign Neoplasm

Pleomorphic adenoma:[11,12] Pleomorphic adenoma (PA) is the most common tumor of the salivary gland represents about 60% of all tumors of the salivary gland. About 80% cases of PA develop in parotid gland, 10% in submandibular gland and the rest 10% cases in the paranasal sinuses, oral cavity, upper respiratory tract and skin.[13] PA commonly presents as a solitary well-defined, slow growing, and painless swelling. Mean age of the patient is around 46 years and females are commonly affected than male.[13] About 90% of PA in parotid gland arises in the superficial lobe and small number of cases of PA arises in the deep lobe of the parotid gland. The involvement of the tail of the parotid gland may mimic as lymph nodal swelling.

PA is also known as mixed tumor as it contains both epithelial and also mesenchymal or stromal material. The tumor possibly develops from the pluripotent reserve cells of the intercalated duct.

Cytology (Figs. 25.6 to 25.10): FNAC of the PA yields thick mucoid like material that is often difficult to spread. MGG smears show abundant deep magenta colored fibrillar

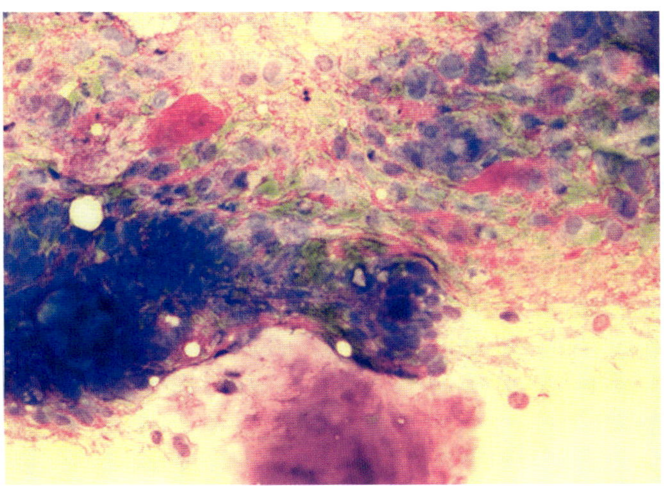

Fig. 25.6: Discrete and clusters of cells embedded in magenta colored chondromyxoid material in pleomorphic adenoma (MGG stain X LP).

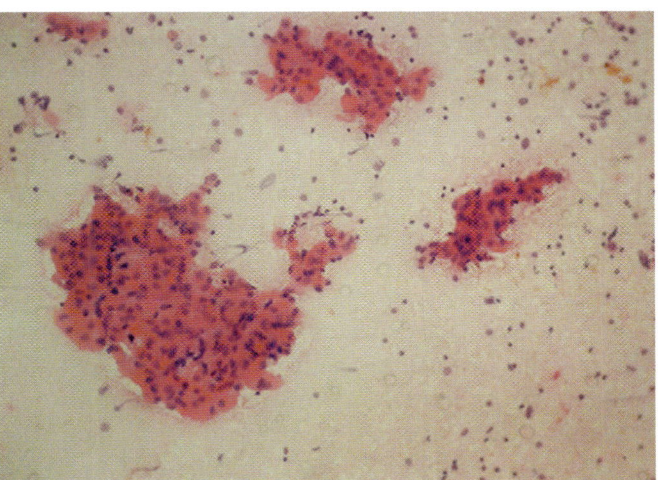

Fig. 25.7: Multiple clusters of epithelial cells along with many discrete myoepithelial cells in pleomorphic adenoma (H & E stain X MP).

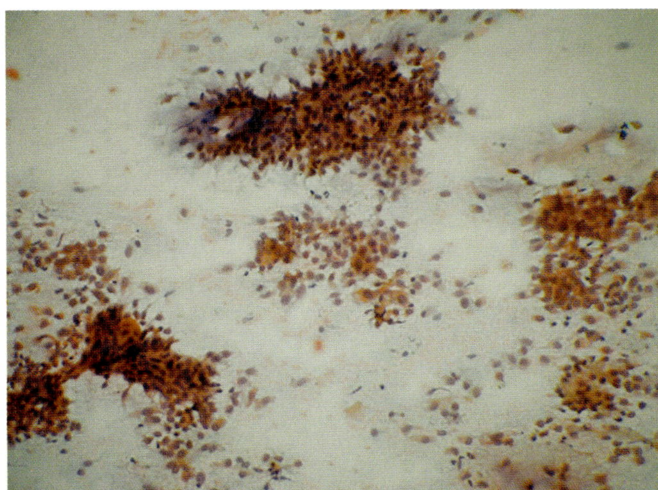

Fig. 25.8: Round to oval cells with moderate amount of cytoplasm in pleomorphic adenoma. The cells are embedded in the stromal material (Papanicolaou's stain X HP).

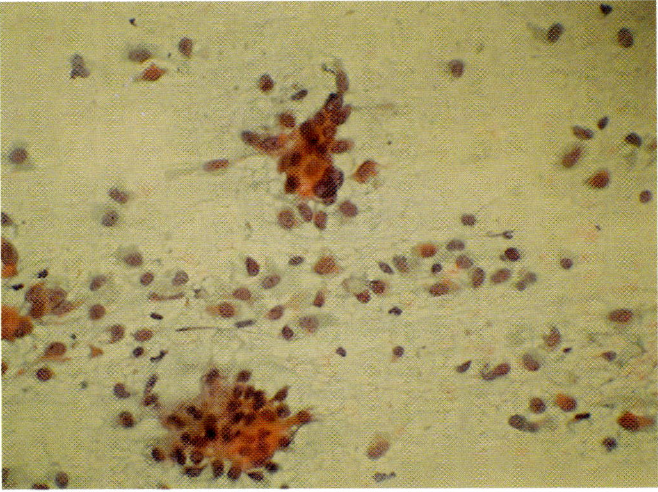

Fig. 25.9: Fine needle aspiration cytology (FNAC) smear of pleomorphic adenoma showing discrete oval to elongated myoepithelial cells with moderate amount of cytoplasm. Nuclei are central to eccentric in position (H & E stain X MP).

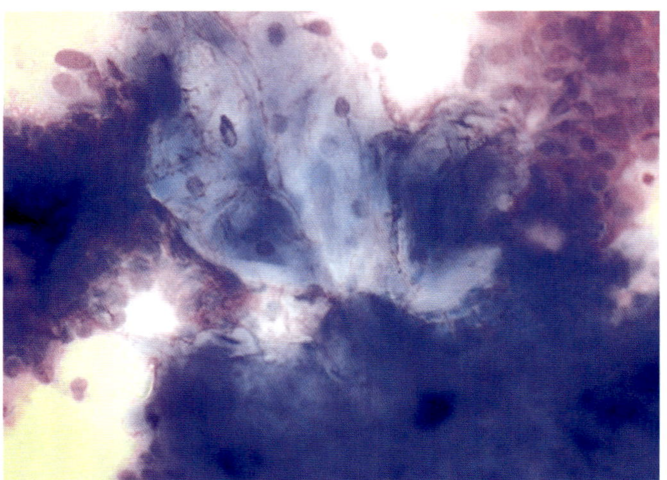

Fig. 25.10: Metaplastic squamous cells in pleomorphic adenoma (MGG stain X MP).

chondromyxoid stromal material (Box 25.9). This stromal material is pale grayish color in Papanicolaou's stain and difficult to recognize. Therefore, MGG stain is mandatory for proper recognition of PA as this demonstrates the detailed character of stromal material. The epithelial cells are present predominantly in cohesive clusters with honeycomb-like pattern and also singly. The individual cells are round to oval with moderate to scanty cytoplasm having distinct cell border. Myoepithelial cells of PA are usually embedded in the myxoid stroma. These cells are oval with moderate cytoplasm and eccentric nuclei simulating plasma cells. Other than the plasmacytoid appearance, myoepithelial cells may be spindle shaped polygonal, epithelioid or clear appearance. The proportion of cellular and stromal component is extremely variable in PA. At times, epithelial component may form the main tumor mass and the smears may show predominantly cellular component. This variety of cellular PA has no separate prognostic importance. However, cellular PA may pose diagnostic problem. On contrary, some cases of pleomorphic adenoma may show abundant myxoid stromal material and scanty cellular component. Matrix material in PA is characteristic with certain important features:

- Chondromyxoid and myxoid
- Fibrillar
- Fraying margins
- Cellular: Spindle cells are embedded in the matrix material
- Metachromatic and magenta colored in Romanowsky stain.

Box 25.9: Pleomorphic adenoma.

Cytology
- Pinkish fibrillar chondromyxoid matrix material with frayed indistinct margins
- Clusters of round, ovoid or plasmacytoid epithelial cells
- Moderate amount of dense cytoplasm
- Central to eccentric monomorphic nucleus
- Bland chromatin
- Clusters and discrete spindle shaped myoepithelial cells embedded in mesenchymal stroma

Immunochemistry
Epithelial cells are positive for cytokeratin (CK) and myoepithelial cells are positive for CK and vimentin (co expressed), S-100, Glilal fibrillary acid protein (GFAP) and Calponin.

Genetics
PLAG1 gene often shows translocation with CTNNB1 and LIFR.

Various changes in pleomorphic adenoma:

Atypical cells: PA may show mild atypical cells in one-fifth of the cases. In absence of necrosis and significant changes in nuclear size, shape and chromatin pattern, these atypical cells should be ignored. However, the presence of necrosis should raise the possibility of carcinoma in PA.

Metaplastic change: PA often shows metaplastic changes such as

- Squamous metaplasia
- Mucinous metaplasia
- Sebaceous metaplasia
- Oncocytic metaplasia.

Squamous metaplasia is noted about one-fourth cases of PA. The squamous cells are present in small clusters (Fig. 25.10). The cells are polyhedral with well-defined cell border. The nuclei of the cells are bland. The keratin pearls may also be seen. At times PA with extensive metaplastic squamous cells may be mistaken as epidermoid component of MEC. A careful sampling from multiple sites of the tumor is helpful in this condition.

Cystic degeneration: Cystic changes may also be seen in PA. This is due to the degeneration of the tumor mass. The cyst fluid shows cellular debris and histiocytes. Aspiration from multiple sites may avoid any false negative report in such cases.

Differential diagnosis:

- *Adenoid cystic carcinoma*: The matrix material and the individual cell morphology of the tumor are the most important clues to differentiate ACC from PA. The matrix material is usually in small globules in ACC. The round hyaline globules are surrounded by cells of ACC. These globules are homogenous, well circumscribed and acellular. The individual cells of

ACC show scanty cytoplasm, high nucleocytoplasmic (N/C) ratio, hyperchromatic nuclei and coarse chromatin, whereas, the cells of pleomorphic adenoma show moderate cytoplasm and finely granular nuclear chromatin (Table 25.2).

- *Basal cell adenoma*: Discussed in basal cell adenoma section.
- *Mucoepidermoid carcinoma*: As mentioned earlier, the presence of metaplastic squamous cells in PA may mimic low-grade MEC. The squamous cells in PA are usually scanty and show mild nuclear atypia.

Warthin's Tumor[14]

Warthin's tumor is first described by Aldred Warthin in the year 1929. This tumor is also known as adenolymphoma and cystadenolymphoma and papillary cystadenoma lymphomatosum. It is the second most common tumor of the salivary gland and it accounts for almost 15% of the salivary gland neoplasm. No monoclonality has been demonstrated in this tumor and probably Warthin's tumor is developmental in origin rather than neoplastic.

Table 25.2: Differentiating features between pleomorphic adenoma (PA) and adenoid cystic carcinoma (ACC).

	Type of tumor	
Cytology features	*PA*	*ACC*
Cell arrangement	Loose cluster and dissociated	Tight cohesive cluster
Cells		
Shape	Round and spindle cells	Round
Cytoplasm	Moderate	Scanty
Matrix material		
Appearance	Fibrillary pink material	Amorphous homogenous material
Cells within the matrix	Matrix contains cells	Acellular Matrix

Male and female both are almost equally affected by this tumor. The mean age of the tumor is 62 years. The tumors may be bilateral (5–20%) and is mainly seen in the parotid gland. The tumor commonly presents as a soft, painless mass with ill-defined margins. On palpation the mass shows doughy feel.

Cytology (Figs. 25.11 to 25.13): Aspiration of Warthin's tumor yields thick greenish-brown dirty fluid. The smears show reactive lymphocytes and oncocytic cells in the background of amorphous and granular debris. Oncocytic cells are commonly seen in loose sheets (Box 25.10).

The individual cells show abundant granular eosinophilic cytoplasm with well-defined cell border. The nuclei are round, monomorphic and eccentrically placed. There may be variable amount of reactive lymphoid cells consisting of mature lymphocytes, follicular center cells and tangible body macrophages. Mast cells are also noted. Squamous metaplasia may occur in one-third cases of Warthin's tumor and FNAC smear shows many mature squamous cells along with parakeratotic cells.[15] In addition, the smear may also show inflammatory cells and degenerated cells and may falsely be interpreted as squamous cell carcinoma. Mucinous metaplasia of Warthin's tumors shows many mucin secreting cells and is often misinterpreted as MEC.

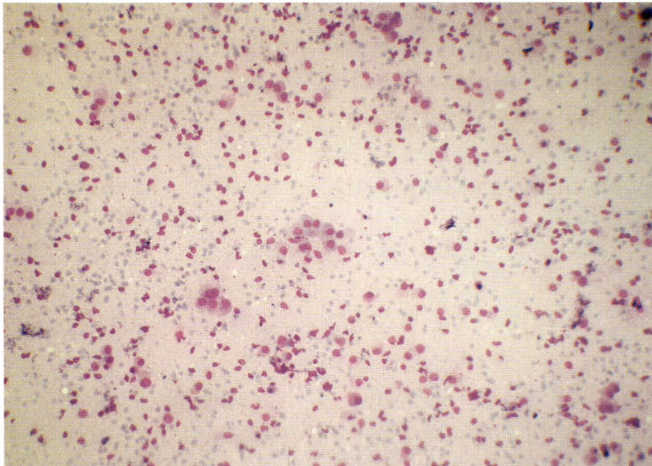

Fig. 25.11: Warthin's tumor: Abundant reactive lymphoid cells and oncocytic cells (MGG stain X LP).

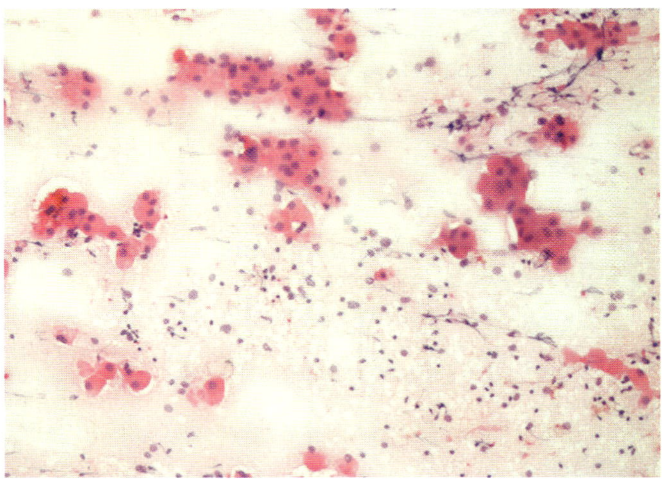

Fig. 25.12: Warthin's tumor: Clusters of oncocytic cells (H & E stain X MP).

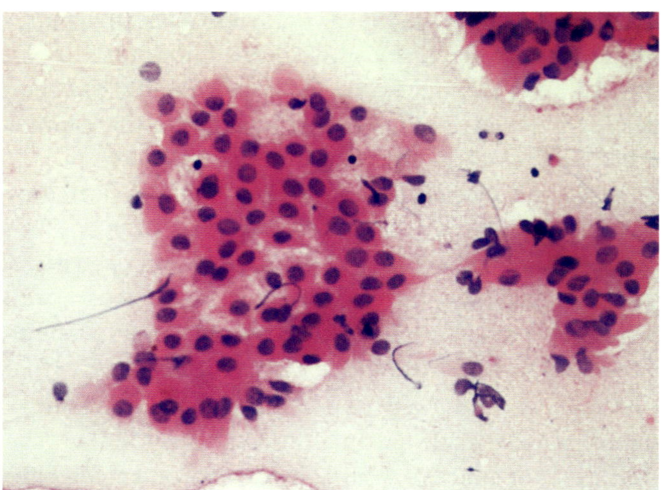

Fig. 25.13: High powered view of the oncocytic cells. The cells have abundant cytoplasm with eccentric nuclei. The nuclei are round and monomorphic (H & E stain X HP).

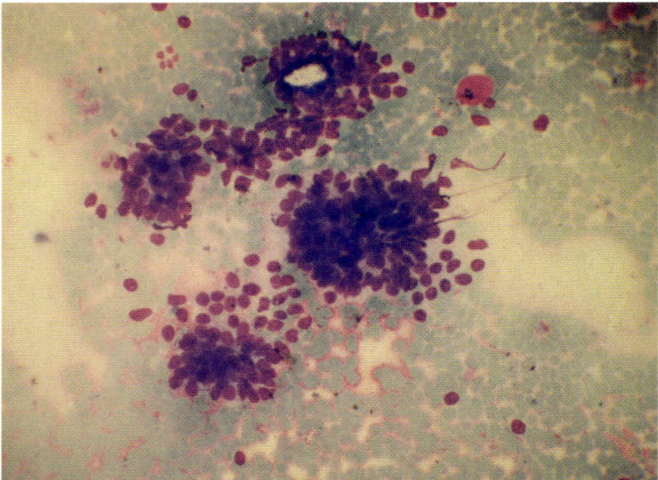

Fig. 25.14: Multiple clusters of basaloid cells with scanty cytoplasm and round monomorphic nuclei in basal cell adenoma (MGG stain X MP).

Box 25.10: Warthin's tumor.

Clinical
- Second common tumors of salivary gland tumors
- Mean age 62 years
- Exclusively within the parotid gland
- One-fifth cases are bilateral
- Doughy feel on palpation
- Probably developmental, not neoplastic

Cytology
- Thin dirty mucoid or greenish-brown fluid
- Many cohesive sheets of oncocytes
- Reactive lymphoid cells
- Squamous and mucinous metaplasia

Differential diagnosis:
- *Mucoepidermoid carcinoma*: Mucoid material along with metaplastic squamous and mucinous cells in Warthin's tumor may simulate cystic low grade MEC. Bland nuclear morphology, presence of oncocytes and reactive lymphoid cells favor a diagnosis of Warthin's tumor.
- *Squamous cell carcinoma*: Metaplastic squamous cells, nuclear debris and dirty background in Warthin's tumor may simulate cystic squamous cell carcinoma. A careful search may reveal oncocytic cells and lymphoid cells in Warthin's tumor.
- *Oncocytoma*: Abundant oncocytes may pose diagnostic difficulty with oncocytoma.

Basal Cell Adenoma[16]

Basal cell adenomas (BCA) are rare tumors of the salivary gland. Previously, it was named as monomorphic adenoma. This tumor is characterized by basaloid type of tumor cells and lack of chondromyxoid stroma. Basal cell adenoma accounts for 1–3% of all salivary gland tumors. It predominantly affects older individuals. Majority of the BCAs (more than 75%) are seen in the parotid gland and rarely other salivary glands are involved. This tumor usually presents as solitary, firm, well-defined, mobile nodules. They are usually firm but occasionally cystic.

Box 25.11: Basal cell adenoma.
- Cohesive groups of cells
- Peripheral palisading arrangement
- Round nucleus, bland nuclear chromatin and scanty cytoplasm
- Squamous morules
- Scanty homogenous acellular stromal material

Cytology (Fig. 25.14): Four histological variants of basal cell adenoma are present: (1) solid, (2) trabecular, (3) tubular, and (4) membranous patterns. Occasionally there may be admixture of these subtypes. FNAC smear of BCA shows sheets and irregular geographical shaped cords of cells. The cells are often arranged as peripheral palisading manner (Box 25.11). There may be sparse metachromatic stained small dense, nonfibrillar intercellular globules of matrix material in between the cell. This matrix material is devoid of any cells. Individual cells in BCA are small, with scanty, pale, basophilic cytoplasm, and bland, monomorphic nuclei. The nuclei show granular chromatin with inconspicuous nucleoli. Many naked cells are also seen in the background. In addition, the solid variants of BCA may show squamous morules.

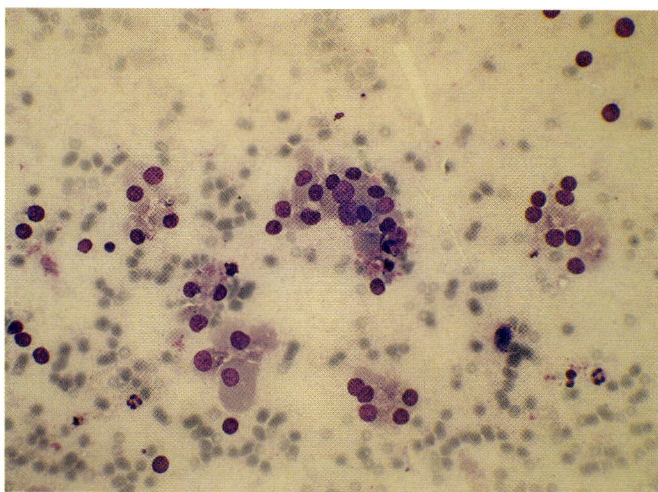

Fig. 25.15: Multiple clusters and discrete oncocytic cells in oncocytoma (MGG stain X MP).

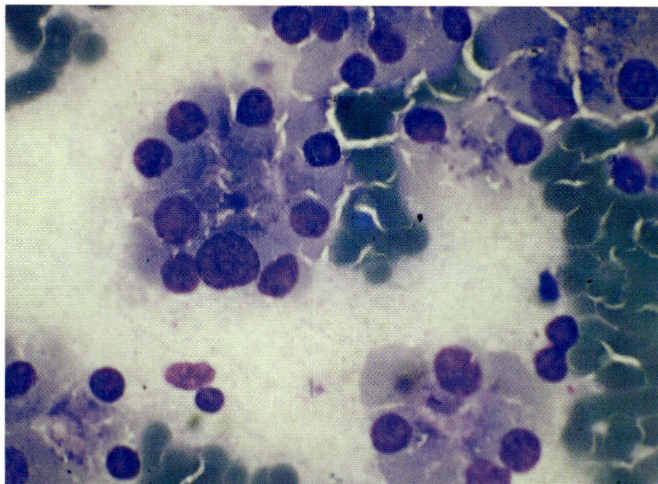

Fig. 25.16: Large, polygonal cells with abundant densely granular eosinophilic cytoplasm and well defined cell border of oncocytes in oncocytoma (MGG stain X oil immersion).

Differential diagnosis:

- *ACC*: It is the most important differential diagnosis of BCA and at times it is difficult to differentiate BCA and ACC particularly in solid type of ACC. Compared to small uniform globules in BCA, the globules are large and varying sized in ACC. These globules are typically surrounded by cells in PA. In addition, the cells show bland nuclear chromatin in BCA compared to hyperchromatic coarse nuclear chromatin in ACC.
- *PA*: The stromal material is sparse in BCA. In comparison, PA shows abundant chondromyxoid stromal material. Cellular PAs have scanty stromal material and therefore is difficult to differentiate from BCA.

Oncocytoma

Oncocytoma represents 1% of all salivary gland neoplasms.[17] The mean age of the tumor is 58 years. This tumor is rarely seen below the age of 50 years. Male and female are equally affected by this tumor. More than 80% of the tumor arises from the parotid gland and the rest of the tumor develops from the submandibular gland.[18] The tumor predominantly presents as well-circumscribed painless mobile mass.

This is a benign salivary gland neoplasm that predominantly involves parotid gland (about 75%) as a painless mobile mass.

Cytology (Figs. 25.15 and 25.16): Cytology smears show sheets, cords, 3D clusters and dyscohesive abundant oncocytic cells. The individual oncocytic cells are large and polygonal with well-defined cell border. The cell contains abundant densely granular eosinophilic cytoplasm (Box 25.12). On MGG stained smear cytoplasm looks deep blue and on Papanicolaou's stain the cytoplasm appears eosinophilic granular. This dense granular cytoplasm is due to the presence of abundant mitochondria in the oncocytes. Nuclei of the cells are enlarged, monomorphic, round and central in position. Nuclear chromatin is fine with small prominent nucleoli. Unlike Warthin's tumor, the background of the smear is clean and free of any lymphocytes. Oncocytoma is difficult to differentiate from the oncocytic hyperplasia on cytology.

Box 25.12: Oncocytoma.

- Three-dimensional clusters of oncocytes
- Polygonal cells
- Abundant eosinophilic cytoplasm
- Monomorphic round nucleus
- Fine chromatin
- Small nucleoli

Differential diagnosis:

- *Warthin's tumor*: See earlier.
- *Acinic cell carcinoma*: Acinic cells in acinic cell carcinoma may be mistaken as oncocytes. The cytoplasm of the acinic cell is pale, delicate and often vacuolated. The vacuoles contain zymogen granules and are positive for PAS stain. Whereas, the oncocytes have waxy, granular cytoplasm. The cytoplasm is rich in mitochondria and is positive for PTAH stain (Table 25.3).

- *Tumors with oncocytic changes*: Oncocytic metaplasia is noted in PA, MEC and Warthin's tumor. However, they usually do not pose significant problem as these tumors also contain other components.

Myoepithelial Tumors[19,20]

Myoepithelial tumor is a rare benign neoplasm and comprises only 1.5% of salivary gland tumors. Both male and female are affected equally by myoepithelioma.[20] The age range of the patient is from 1st to 9th decade and the mean age of the patient is 44 years. Myoepithelioma may occur both in major and minor salivary gland. However, parotid and minor salivary glands of palate are the most common sites of involvement. The patients usually present with a slow growing painless mass.

Histological types of myoepithelioma are spindle, plasmacytoid or hyaline, epithelioid, and clear cell.[21] Occasionally, there may be combination of more than one type.

Table 25.3: Cytological features to differentiate oncocytoma and acinic cell carcinoma.

Features	*Oncocytoma*	*Acinic cell carcinoma*
Background	Clean	Naked nuclei
Cytoplasm	Waxy, granular	Pale
Cytoplasmic vacuoles	Absent	Present
PAS	Negative	Positive
PTAH	Positive	Negative

Cytology (Box 25.13): Cytology smear of myoepithelioma depends on the variant of myoepithelioma. In spindle cell type of the tumor, the FNAC smears show abundant cohesive groups and isolated spindle cells. The smear shows striking absence of chondromyxoid material. Individual cells are elongated with ovoid to fusiform nuclei. The nuclear ends are more rounded than pointed. The chromatin is fine and nucleoli are indistinct. Occasional cells show nuclear groove. Cytoplasm of the cell is pale and scanty.

The smears of plasmacytoid variant (Figs. 25.17 and 25.18) show dissociated plasmacytoid cells with abundant cytoplasm and eccentric nucleus. These cells are much larger than the plasma cells and they have fine chromatin. The nuclei lack typical cartwheel appearance and perinuclear hof of plasma cells.

Box 25.13: Myoepithelial tumors.

Cytology
- Rich in cells
- Lack of chondromyxoid stroma

Spindle cell type
- Cohesive clusters and dissociated spindle cells
- Elongated nuclei, fine nuclear chromatin and inconspicuous nucleoli
- Nuclear grooves
- Scanty pale cytoplasm

Plasmacytoid (hyaline) myoepithelial cells
- Dissociated round to oval cells
- Plasmacytoid cells with abundant cytoplasm and eccentric nucleus
- Fine nuclear chromatin, no perinuclear hof

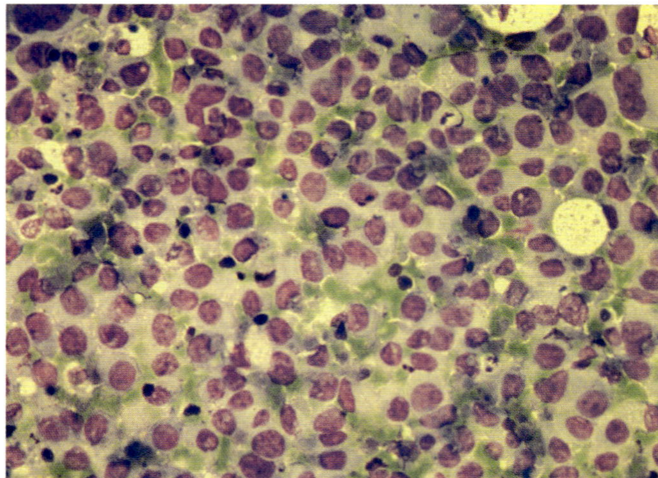

Fig. 25.17: Plasmacytoid variant of myoepithelial tumor showing dissociated plasmacytoid cells with abundant cytoplasm and eccentric nucleus (MGG stain X MP).

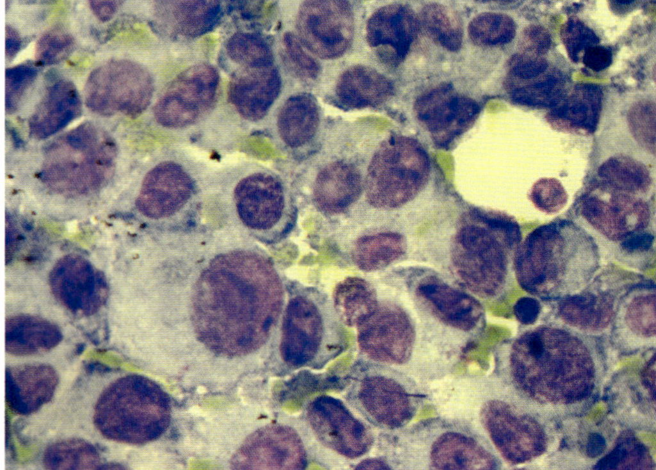

Fig. 25.18: Individual cell morphology of myoepithelial cells is better viewed in higher magnification in myoepithelial tumor (H & E stain X HP).

Immunocytochemistry: The tumor is positive for cytokeratin (CK) 7 and CK14. The spindle cells in myoepithelioma are also positive for alpha smooth muscle actin, calponin, muscle specific actin, glial fibrillary acidic protein (GFAP) and S-100. In addition myoepithelial cells are also positive for p63.

Differential diagnosis:

- *Schwannoma*: Spindle cell variants of myoepithelioma closely mimic schwannoma. Cells of schwannoma have spindle shaped nuclei with wavy pointed ends compared to round ends in cells of myoepithelioma. At times, rows of palisaded nuclei in hypocellular fibrillar stroma, called as Verocay bodies, may also be seen. In case of difficulty, a panel of immunocytochemistry particularly myoepithelial markers may be helpful. Table 25.4 shows differential diagnosis of spindle cell lesions of the salivary gland.

Table 25.4: Differential diagnosis of spindle cell lesions in salivary glands.

Features	*Myoepithelioma (spindle cell type)*	*Pleomorphic adenoma*	*Schwannoma*
Verocay bodies	Absent	Absent	Present
Chondromyxoid stroma	Scanty to absent	Abundant	Absent
Nucleus	Elongated with rounded ends	Elongated with rounded ends	Wavy and pointed
Immunostaining			
S-100	Weak	Weak	Strong
Keratin	Positive	Positive	Negative
Calponin	Positive	Positive	Negative
Smooth muscle actin	Positive	Positive	Negative

- *Plasma cell tumor*: Plasma cell tumor is the close differential diagnosis of plasmacytoid type of myoepithelioma. However, the myoepithelioma cells show lack of nuclear characters of plasma cells such as cart wheel chromatin and perinuclear hof.
- *PA with predominantly spindle cells (Fig. 25.19)*: PA with scanty epithelial cell may pose diagnostic difficulty.[22] This may happen due to improper sampling from the predominant myoepithelial rich area of PA. The stromal cells of PA are almost similar in morphology as that of myoepithelioma and in absence of chondromyxoid material it is very difficult to distinguish PA with spindle cell rich aspirate from myoepithelioma.

Adenoid Cystic Carcinoma[23,24]

It is a slow growing tumor and represents 5–10% of salivary gland tumors. It comprises about 10–20% of salivary gland malignancies. ACC commonly affects parotid, submandibular gland and minor salivary glands in the palate. ACC may also occur in nasal cavity and sinuses, tongue, buccal mucosa and lip. Uncommonly ACC may also affect other sites such as skin, lung, prostate, breast, and the lower part of the female genital tract. Females are slightly more affected than male. The peak incidence of the tumor is in the 4th to 6th decade of life. The patient commonly presents as slow growing swelling followed by pain in the ear as the tumor often infiltrates local nerves.

Cytology (Figs. 25.20 to 25.23): There are histologic subtypes of ACC—cribriform, tubular, and solid. The solid form is considered as high grade type of ACC because it often follows an

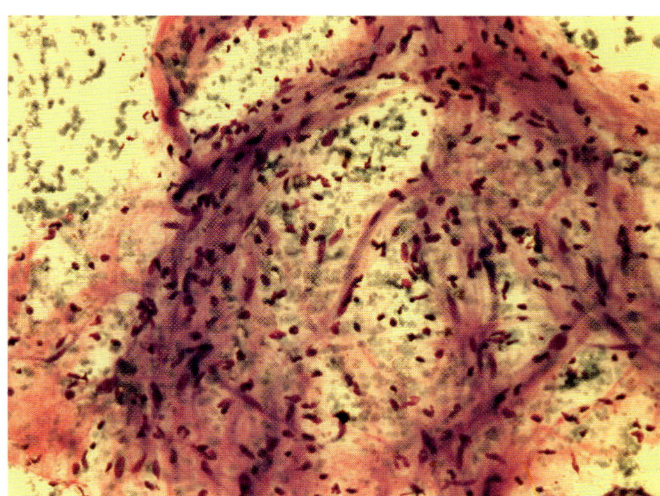

Fig. 25.19: Spindle cell type of pleomorphic adenoma showing elongated spindle cells in pinkish connective tissue stroma (MGG stain X HP).

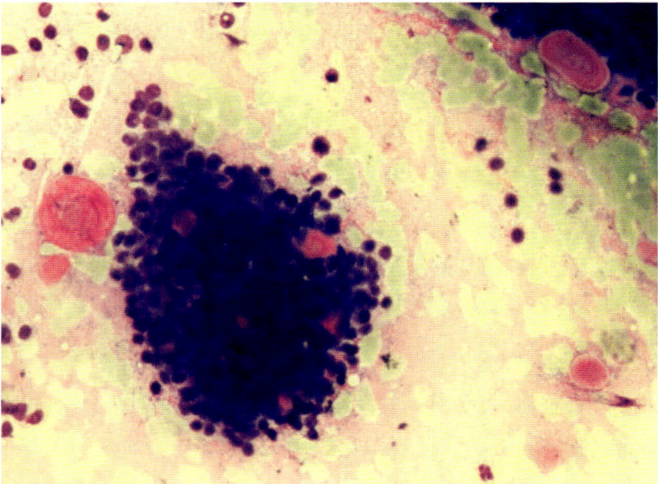

Fig. 25.20: Cribriform appearance of adenoid cystic carcinoma on cytology smear (MGG stain X MP).

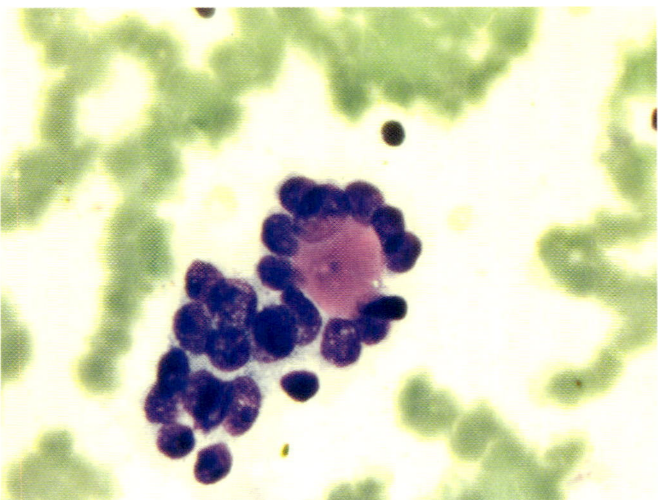

Fig. 25.21: Pinkish homogenous globules surrounded by round mildly pleomorphic cells in cribriform variant of adenoid cystic carcinoma (MGG stain X MP).

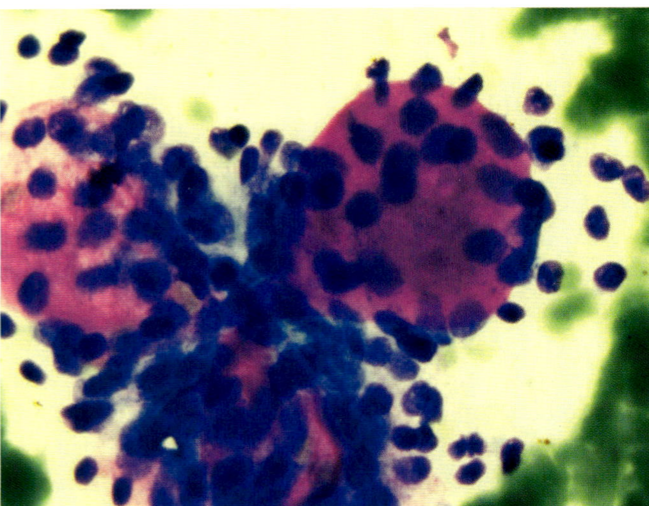

Fig. 25.22: Adenoid cystic carcinoma: Higher magnification of pinkish globule surrounded by cells (MGG stain X HP).

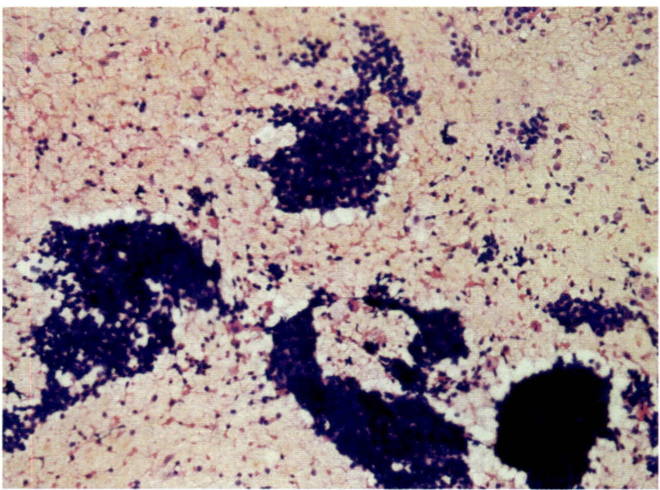

Fig. 25.23: Clusters and dissociated round cells in solid variant of adenoid cystic carcinoma (H & E stain X MP).

Box 25.14: Adenoid cystic carcinoma.

- Multiple variables sized globular, spherical or tubular homogenous, acellular magenta colored matrix material
- Globules are surrounded by cells
- Clusters and dissociated small cells
- Scanty cytoplasm
- Round monomorphic nuclei
- Hyperchromatic nuclei
- Coarse chromatin

Immunocytochemistry: Ki67—high Ki67 index, c-Kit over expression.

Box 25.15: Important features of matrix in adenoid cystic carcinoma (ACC).

- Homogenous
- Globular or branching tubular
- Sharp margin
- Acellular: Inside matrix—no cells
- Surrounded by basaloid cells

aggressive course. However, the solid variety of ACC is more difficult to diagnose in FNAC than the other two subtypes (Box 25.14). The cribriform and tubular subtypes of ACC show characteristic matrix material. On MGG smear the matrix material looks deep, homogenous, magenta color globules, or branching tubules with sharp outline and devoid of any cells (Box 25.15). On Papanicolaou's stain this matrix material appears as colorless area. The globular material is surrounded by basaloid cells. The individual basaloid cells are round with scanty clear cytoplasm. The nuclei are monomorphic, hyperchromatic with angulated margin.

In histological solid variant of ACC the characteristic metachromatic matrix material is scanty to absent. The cytology smears show 3D clusters of basaloid cells with scanty cytoplasm and dark angulated nuclei. Nuclei are hyperchromatic and show mild to moderate pleomorphism. In addition, variable degree of mitotic activities and apoptosis may also be noted.

Differential diagnosis:

- Pleomorphic adenoma
- Basal cell adenoma
- Polymorphous low grade adenocarcinoma (PLGA)

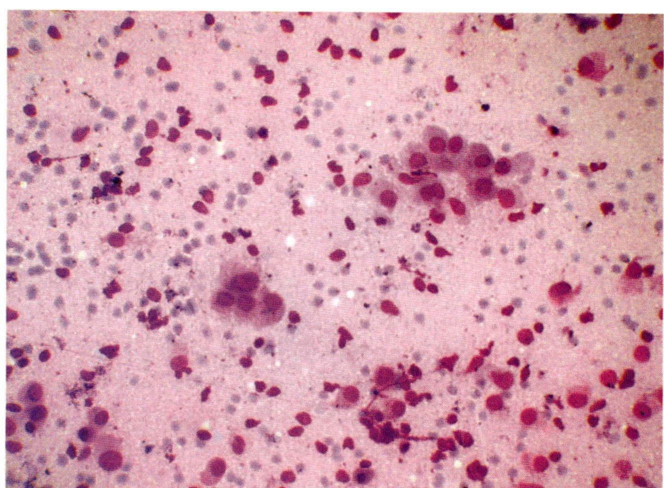

Fig. 25.24: Small aggregates and discrete acinar cells in acinic cell carcinoma. Background of the smear shows many naked nuclei (MGG stain X MP).

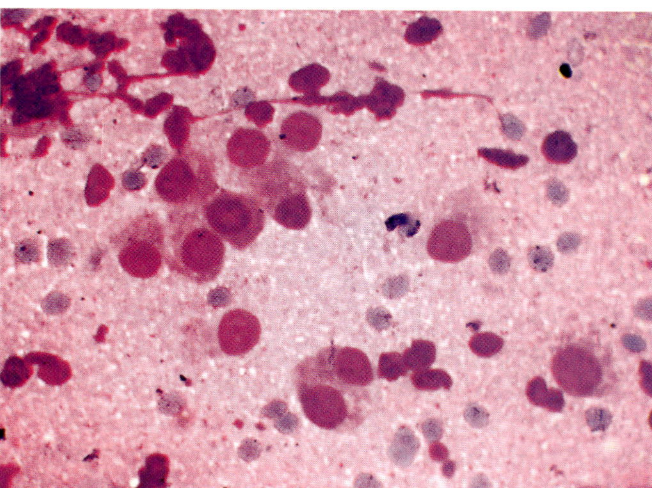

Fig. 25.25: Higher magnification of the acinic cell carcinoma showing abundant eosinophilic cytoplasm and round central to eccentric nuclei (MGG stain X oil immersion).

Acinic Cell Carcinoma[25,26]

Acinic cell carcinoma is the malignant neoplasm of the epithelial cell with serous acinar cell differentiation. It represents only 1–3% of the malignant tumors of the salivary gland. Females are slightly more affected by acinic cell carcinoma than male and no age group is exempted by this tumor. The peak incidence of the tumor is in 3rd decade of life. About 80–90% of tumor develops in the parotid gland and a small group of tumor arises from the minor salivary glands. The patients classically presents as a single, mobile and painless mass in short duration. However, some patient may give the history of swelling for 10 years or more. About one-third of the cases may have vague pain and about 10% patients may also show facial paralysis at the time of presentation.[27]

Cytology (Figs. 25.24 and 25.25): Several histopathological subtypes of acinic cell carcinoma are recognized:

- Solid/lobular
- Microcystic
- Papillary-cystic
- Follicular growth patterns

The tumor also contains various types of cells such as:

- Serous acinar
- Nonspecific glandular
- Intercalated ductal
- Vacuolated
- Clear

Therefore, the FNAC smears may show variable features depending on the primary architectural and cell type of the tumor. However, all the tumors show predominant acinar cell differentiation.

Box 25.16: Acinic cell carcinoma.

- Abundant cohesive clusters of acinar cells
- Acinar like arrangement
- Large polygonal cells
- Abundant finely vacuolated cytoplasm
- Naked tumor nuclei
- Occasionally lymphocytes and psammoma bodies
- Clean background

FNAC smear is usually rich in cells. The cells are present in three-dimensional (3D) clusters and sheets in a clean background (Box 25.16). Occasionally, follicular or micropapillary structures may be noted. The cells may also be arranged around thin capillaries. The tumor cells are polygonal with abundant cytoplasm. Nuclei are round, monomorphic, centrally placed with a small distinct nucleoli. The cytoplasmic vacuole is subtle and better seen in MGG stain. The vacuoles contain zymogen granules which are PAS positive and diastase-resistant. The cytoplasmic vacuole is one of the important findings and should not be overlooked. Careful observations help to differentiate the acinic cell from oncocytes (Table 25.3). The acinic cells are delicate so they may breakdown and the background often shows many bare naked nuclei. About 10% cases of acinic cell carcinoma may also background lymphocytes.

In case of papillary cystic variety of acinic cell carcinoma, the aspirate may yield fluid and smears of which shows foamy vacuolated hemosiderin laden macrophages and granular debris (Box 25.17). A complex architecture of branching papillary structure is also noted in such cases. Papillary cystic variant of acinic cell carcinoma may also show psammoma bodies. These findings may mislead to the false diagnosis of MEC or Warthin's tumor.[28]

Differential diagnosis:

- *Benign salivary gland aspirate*: The presence of benign looking acinar cells in acinic cell carcinoma may give the false impression of benign salivary gland aspirate and vice versa. However, the normal acinar cells are polarized in lobular groups unlike 3D clusters of cells in acinic cell carcinoma.
- *Mucoepidermoid carcinoma*: Papillary cystic variant of acinic cell carcinoma may mimic as MEC. The presence of malignant squamous cell indicates MEC.
- *Warthin's tumor*: As mentioned earlier, occasional lymphoid cells in the background of acinic cells may simulate Warthin's tumor. Oncocytes in Warthin's tumor show abundant granular cytoplasm and no vacuoles are demonstrated within the cytoplasm. If necessary, PAS positive diastase resistant material can be shown in the acinic cells.
- *Oncocyoma*: Abundant acinic cells in acinic cell carcinoma may simulate oncocytes and this may be mistaken as oncocyoma.

Box 25.17: Cytological features of papillary cystic acinic cell carcinoma.

- Cystic with cellular debris
- Paucicellular
- Small papillary structures and flat sheets
- Vacuolated histiocyte-like cells
- Monotonous polygonal neoplastic cells with enlarged nuclei
- Rare oncocytic cells

Differential Diagnosis: Mucoepidermoid carcinoma, pleomorphic adenoma (PA), Warthin's tumor, retention cyst and metastatic renal cell carcinoma

Table 25.5: Oncocytes versus acinic cells of acinic cell carcinoma.

Features	*Acinic cell*	*Oncocytes*
Cell margin	Indistinct	Well-defined
Cytoplasm character	Fine vacuolations	Eosinophilic granular
Cytoplasm: quantity	Abundant	Moderate
PAS with diastase	Positive	Negative
PTAH	Negative	Positive
Electron microscopy	Zymogen granules	Mitochondria

(PAS: Periodic acid–Schiff; PTAH: Phosphotungstic acid hematoxylin).

The differential diagnoses of acinic cell carcinoma are highlighted in Table 25.5.

Mucoepidermoid Carcinoma

Mucoepidermoid carcinoma is the most common malignant tumors of the salivary gland and represents 10–15% of salivary gland tumors. MEC occurs in age groups from children to old, and mean age of the patient is 45 year. There is mild female predilection of this tumor. About 50% of MEC arises from the major salivary gland and rest of the tumor arises from buccal mucosa and palate.[29]

The patients usually present with painless, firm and fixed mass.

Cytology (Figs. 25.26 to 25.29; Box 25.18): MEC is divided on histology as low, intermediate and high grade tumor. The high-grade MEC is aggressive compared to low-grade MEC.[30,31] The cytological features of different grades of MEC show considerable differences. Low-grade MEC is usually cystic and often gives rise to false negative diagnosis.

FNAC smears show predominantly three types of cells: (1) squamoid cells, (2) intermediate cells, and (3) mucus secreting cells. The background of the tumor is dirty with mucus and debris.

The squamoid or epidermoid cells are polygonal in shape with orangeophilic cytoplasm in Papanicolaou's stain. The intermediate cells are smaller in size, columnar to polygonal and have enlarged hyperchromatic nuclei with high N/C ratio. The mucus secreting cells are round with abundant vacuolated cytoplasm. The nuclei

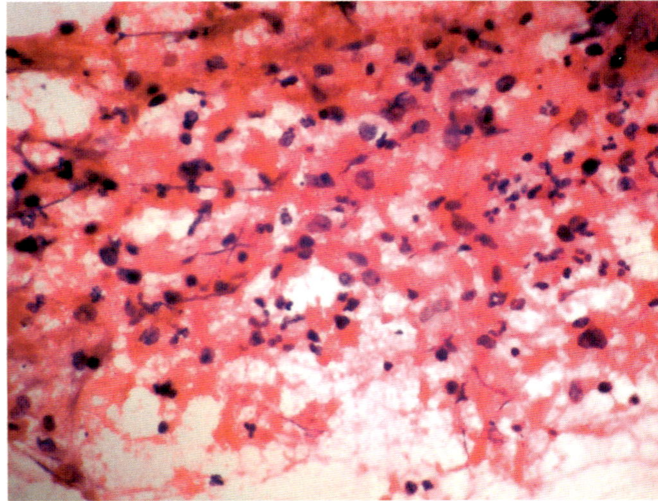

Fig. 25.26: Dirty background in mucoepidermoid carcinoma. Smear shows many tumor cells and polymorphs (H & E stain X MP).

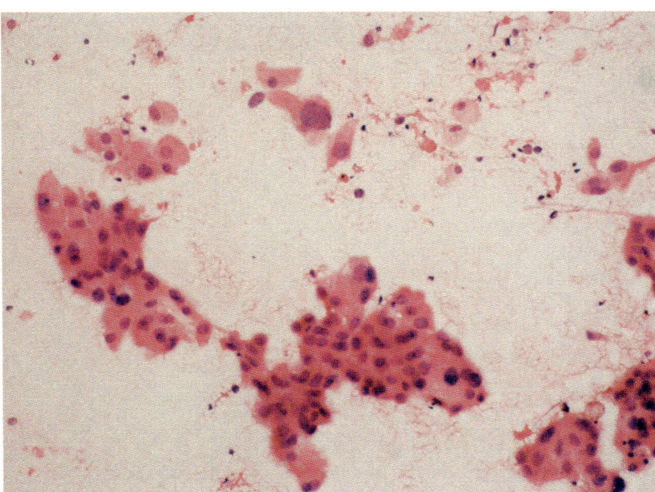

Fig. 25.27: Mucoepidermoid carcinoma: Both squamoid cells and mucus secreting cells (H & E stain X MP).

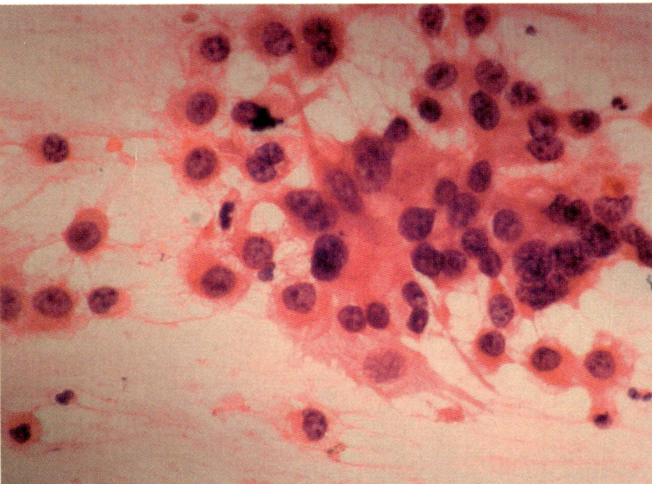

Fig. 25.28: Malignant cells with vacuolated cytoplasm along with intermediate type of squamoid cells in mucoepidermoid carcinoma (H & E stain X HP).

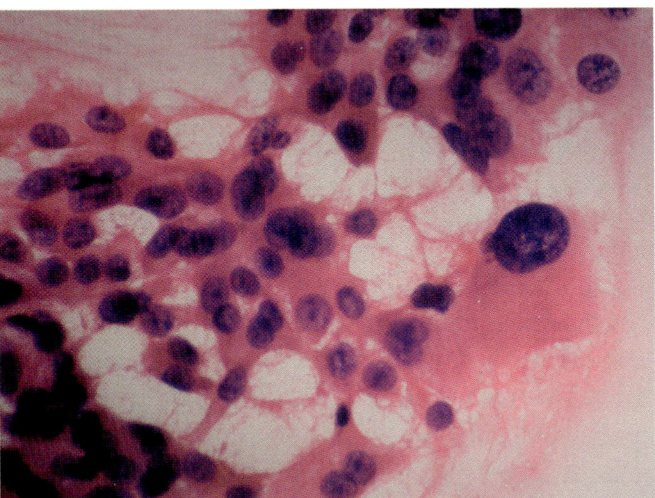

Fig. 25.29: Epidermoid cells with enlarged hyperchromatic nuclei in mucoepidermoid carcinoma (H & E stain X HP).

are eccentrically placed and indented and often give signet ring-like appearance. The nuclei of mucus secreting cells of MEC show low N/C ratio and almost no nuclear enlargement. These cells are easily mistaken as histiocytes. However, the histiocytes show multiple vacuoles, phagocytosed material and often centrally placed nuclei. In addition, there may be clear cell or oncocytic cells. Oncocytic variant of MEC show relatively large amount of oncocytes admixed with mucus secreting cells. The cytology smear may be misinterpreted as oncocytoma. However, the presence of mucus secreting cells is the key feature of correct diagnosis.

Box 25.18: Mucoepidermoid carcinoma.

- Clusters and dissociated cells with vacuolated cytoplasm
- Intermediate squamous cells
- Gradual transition of squamoid to mucus producing cells
- Dirty background produced by debris and mucus
- Histiocytes and background lymphocytes
- Mucus secreting cells are positive for mucicarmine or Alcian blue

In case of low-grade MEC, considerable cystic changes are seen and FNAC may yield fluid. The smears show mucus secreting cells and many histiocytes in a background of mucus. About one-fifth of MEC shows background lymphocytes. Malignant squamous and intermediate cells are usually less in low-grade tumor and these cells show mild nuclear enlargement and pleomorphism. The low-grade MEC is often underdiagnosed as benign lesion such as retention cyst, Warthin's tumor and cystic PA. In high-grade MEC, the malignant epidermoid cells are more in amount and these cells show moderate to marked nuclear enlargement and pleomorphism. The high-grade MEC is easily recognizable malignant tumor in the salivary gland.

Differential diagnosis:

- *Acinic cell carcinoma*: See earlier.
- *Warthin's tumor*: See earlier.
- *Retention cyst*: Mucus and cellular debris along with inflammatory cells may cause diagnostic confusion with retention cysts of the salivary gland.
- *Metastatic squamous cell carcinoma with cystic changes*: Metastatic squamous cell carcinoma in an intraparotid lymph node may often simulate MEC. A careful history may avoid this mistake.

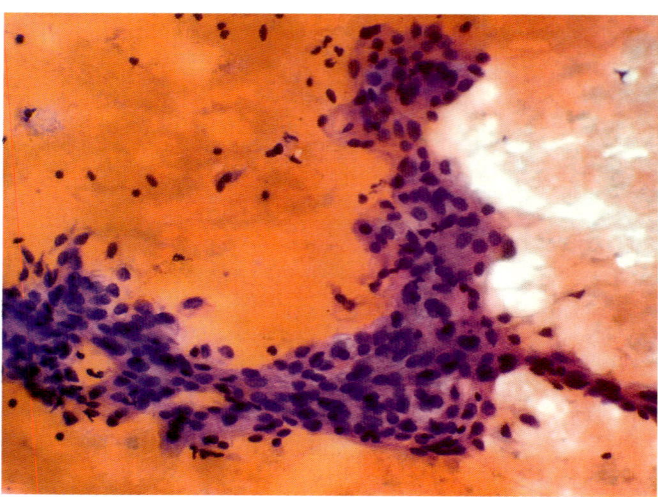

Fig. 25.30: Long papillary like cluster in polymorphous low-grade adenocarcinoma (MGG stain X MP).

Box 25.19: Polymorphous low grade adenocarcinoma.

Cell arrangement
- Papillary
- Ductal
- Trabecular
- Discrete

Morphology
- Scanty to moderate pale cytoplasm
- Round to oval nucleus
- Fine stippled nuclear chromatin
- Inconspicuous nucleoli
- Scanty matrix material

Differential diagnosis: PA, ACC

(PA: Pleomorphic adenoma; ACC: Adenoid cystic carcinoma).

Polymorphous Low Grade Adenocarcinoma[32,33]

It represents about 26% of all intraoral carcinomas.[32] The tumor is more common in female than male. The age range of the patient varies from 2nd to 9th decade. However, majority of the patients are in between 50 years and 70 years of age. Mean age of the patient is 59 years. PLGA commonly affects the minor salivary glands and 60% of the tumor develops in palate.[33] It is a less aggressive malignant tumor with better prognosis. The patient usually presents as painless mass in the palate.

Cytology (Fig. 25.30)[34]: FNAC smears of PLGA show clusters, papillary, trabecular and discrete arrangement of cells. The tumor cells are cuboidal to columnar rather than basaloid cells of ACC. The individual cells are monomorphic cuboidal to columnar with moderate amount of eosinophilic pale cytoplasm (Box 25.19). The nuclei of the cells are relatively monomorphic having fine stippled nuclear chromatin and inconspicuous nucleoli. The extracellular matrix material of PLGA is scanty and is fibrillar in appearance similar to that of PA. However, spherical acellular homogenous globules like stromal material similar to ACC are also seen in PLGA. There are overlapping cytomorphological features of PA, ACC and PLGA. Therefore, it is very difficult to diagnose PLGA in FNAC. However, the presence of papillary and trabecular pattern of cells are helpful features to diagnose PLGA in FNAC.

Differential diagnosis:

ACC: The presence of hyaline stromal globules and the small monomorphic cells may simulate ACC. However, the cells of PLGA are more cuboidal to columnar and contains relatively more eosinophilic cytoplasm.

Epithelial-myoepithelial Carcinoma

Epithelial-myoepithelial carcinoma shows both ductal and myoepithelial malignant cells and it gives a biphasic pattern. It is an uncommon tumor and represents only 1% of salivary gland tumors. It occurs in a wide range of age, however, the peak incidence of the tumor is 6th to 7th decade. Epithelial-myoepithelial carcinoma occurs twice in females than males. The epithelial-myoepithelial carcinoma mainly (60–80%) develops in the parotid glands (60–80%) and occasionally arises in the minor salivary glands of the oral cavity. The patient usually presents as painless slowly growing swelling in the parotid gland for months to even years.

Cytology:[35] Cytology of the epithelial-myoepithelial carcinoma usually gives a bland outlook. However, a possibility of malignancy is considered in most of the studies.[35] The cytology smears usually show a biphasic pattern consisting of small ductal epithelial and myoepithelial cells (Box 25.20). The myoepithelial cells are present in loose cohesive sheets and 3D spherical clusters. The tumor cells are large polygonal with abundant clear vacuolated cytoplasm. The nuclei are monomorphic, round and enlarged. The nuclear chromatin is finely dispersed chromatin with distinct nucleoli.

The other population of cells is ductal. These cells form cohesive sheets or tubular structures. The ductal cells are small, cuboidal with well-defined border. The nuclei are round hyperchromatic with high N/C ratio. The nuclear chromatin is granular with prominent nucleoli. In some cases the biphasic pattern may be lost and the smears show apparently one population of cells. This may

Box 25.20: Epithelial myoepithelial carcinoma.

- Biphasic pattern
- Myoepithelial cells
    - Loose cohesive cluster
    - Large polygonal clear cell
    - Round, monomorphic nuclei
    - Mild nuclear enlargement
    - Fine chromatin
- Epithelial cells
    - Scanty
    - Small cuboidal
    - High N/C ratio
- Stromal material
    - Spherical hyaline globules
    - Acellular

Differential diagnosis: PA, ACC

(PA: Pleomorphic adenoma; ACC: Adenoid cystic carcinoma).

be due to the breakdown of the cytoplasm of the cell and dispersed naked nuclei on the background of the smear.[36] In addition, the FNAC smear of the tumor also shows background stromal material. The hyaline globules may be tight and spherical and surrounded by the small cuboidal cells. At times, these may closely mimic ACC.

Carcinoma Ex Pleomorphic Adenoma

Carcinoma ex pleomorphic adenoma (Ca Ex PA) develops from the previously existing PA. It is also known as malignant mixed tumor. Ca Ex PA represents 12% of malignant salivary gland tumors. The tumor commonly occurs in 6th and 7th decade of life.[37] Ca Ex PA commonly involves the parotid gland. The patient usually presents with history of a sudden rapid enlargement of a longstanding swelling of the parotid gland.

Cytology: Cytology smear is usually cellular. The smear shows a high-grade carcinoma usually adenocarcinoma of ductal type. The background shows metachromatic fibrillar matrix material. Myoepithelial cells are embedded in this material (Box 25.21). The malignant nature of the tumor is easy to identify. However, for the diagnosis of Ca Ex PA, a preexisting diagnosis of PA is required. On cytology alone it is difficult to distinguish the tumor from high-grade MEC and metastatic adenocarcinoma.[38]

Myoepithelial Carcinoma

Myoepithelial carcinoma is the rare malignant counterpart of myoepithelioma. This represents less than 2% of all salivary gland carcinoma. Both males and females are equally affected by myoepithelial carcinoma. About 75% myoepithelial carcinoma arises in the parotid gland.[39]

Box 25.21: Carcinoma ex pleomorphic adenoma.

- History of pre-existing PA
- High-grade carcinoma of ductal type
- Metachromatic fibrillar matrix with myoepithelial cells
- *Differential diagnosis*: High-grade MEC, metastatic carcinoma

(PA: Pleomorphic adenoma; MEC: Mucoepidermoid carcinoma).

Cytology: The presence of pleomorphism, coarse chromatin, mitosis and necrosis in a myoepitheioma suggest myoepithelial carcinoma.

Salivary Duct Carcinoma

Salivary duct carcinoma is a rare malignancy of the salivary gland and comprises 9% of salivary malignancies. The males are four times more affected than females.[40] The parotid gland is commonly involved by this tumor and the patient presents with a rapidly growing mass. This is an aggressive adenocarcinoma.

Cytology: FNAC smears show sheets and papillary group of cells. The individual cells are large, polygonal with abundant vacuolated cytoplasm. The nuclei show marked pleomorphism, hyperchromasia and prominent nucleoli. In addition, there may be atypical mitosis, increased mitotic activity and necrosis. Salivary duct carcinoma simulates high-grade malignant tumor and the malignant nature of the tumor is easily detectable.[41]

Adenocarcinoma not Otherwise Specified

This tumor represents 17% of all salivary gland malignancies and predominantly involves the parotid gland. The tumor cells exhibits ductal differentiation.[42] FNAC smears show recognizable malignant cells with features of adenocarcinoma but there is lack of definitive evidence of other specific subtypes.

NEWLY DESCRIBED SALIVARY GLAND TUMORS

The relatively newer entities of the salivary glands include: mammary analog secretory carcinoma (MASC), sclerosing polycystic adenoma (SPA) and cribriform adenocarcinoma of tongue.[43]

Mammary Analog Secretory Carcinoma

It is a rare salivary gland carcinoma with distinctive chromosomal translocation, t(12;15) (p13;q25) that produces

Box 25.22: Mammary analog secretory carcinoma (MASC).

- Characteristic chromosomal translocation, t(12;15) (p13;q25) that gives rise an ETV6–NTRK3 fusion
- Similar to secretory carcinoma of breast
- Extremely uncommon

Cytology

- Clusters, sheets of tumor cells, acinar and papillary arrangements
- Background mucin
- Polygonal in shape with abundant vacuolated cytoplasm
- Nuclei: Central in position and monomorphic bland

Differential diagnosis:

- Acinic cell carcinoma
- Mucoepidermoid carcinoma

an ETV6–NTRK3 fusion. This fusion gene ETV6–NTRK3 is responsible for encoding a chimeric tyrosine kinase enzyme that stimulate neoplastic proliferation of ductal and myoepithelial cells. The histopathology of the tumor is identical with secretory carcinoma of breast.

Cytology[44,45]

Fine needle aspiration cytology smears of MASC simulate acinic cell carcinoma. The smears show multiple clusters and sheets of tumor cells (Box 25.22). Acinar and papillary arrangements are also noted. The individual cells are polygonal in shape with abundant vacuolated cytoplasm containing mucin. The nuclei are central in position and monomorphic bland in appearance. Occasional cases show abundant extracellular mucinous material.

Immunocytochemistry

The tumor is positive for epithelial membrane antigen (EMA), pan-cytokeratin, CK7, CK8, CK18, CK19, S100 protein and vimentin.

Differential Diagnosis

- *Acinic cell carcinoma*: Abundant cytoplasm and central bland nuclei of MASC may simulate acinic cell carcinoma. The differentiating points are:
  - Cytoplasmic basophilia is absent in MASC
  - Completely different immunocytochemistry: MASC is positive for S100 protein, mammaglobin, vimentin, STAT5 and MUC4
  - Translocation, t(12;15) (p13;q25) that gives rise an ETV6–NTRK3 fusion
- MEC: Cells with abundant vacuolated cytoplasm containing mucin may simulate MEC.

Sclerosing Polycystic Adenoma

It is also a rare sclerosing tumor of salivary gland that simulates fibrocystic changes and sclerosing adenosis of the breast. The tumors are mostly described in major salivary glands.

Cytology

Fine needle aspiration cytology of SPA is rarely described.[46] The smears show syncytial clusters of ductal cells along with foamy histiocytes and oncocytes. Background of the smear shows proteinaceous material. In addition apocrine cells, sebaceous cells and lymphocytes are also seen in the smear. The cells show round to oval bland nuclei.

Cribriform Adenocarcinoma of Minor Salivary Glands

This tumor mainly occurs in the minor salivary gland of the tongue. Histologically the tumor shows cribriform, solid and glomeruloid structures. The nuclei of the cells often show "Orphan Annie eye-like nuclei". The tumor at times may simulate papillary carcinoma of thyroid.

Immunocytochemistry

The tumor cells are positive for CAM5.2, CK7, CK8, CK18, S100 protein, SOX10, calponin and vimentin.

Lymphoma of the Salivary Gland

Primary NHL of the salivary gland is uncommon and represents only 5% of all extranodal lymphoma.[47] For the definition of primary NHL of the salivary gland, two essential features are required:

1. The main tumor mass of the lymphoma should be in the salivary gland.
2. The parenchyma of the salivary gland should be involved.

The most of NHL are B-cell type and the *common subtypes* are:[48]

- Extranodal marginal zone lymphoma of the MALT type
- Follicular lymphoma, and
- Diffuse large B-cell lymphoma

All the B-cell NHL cases are positive for CD 45 and CD 20. In addition the lymphoid cells show light chain restriction.

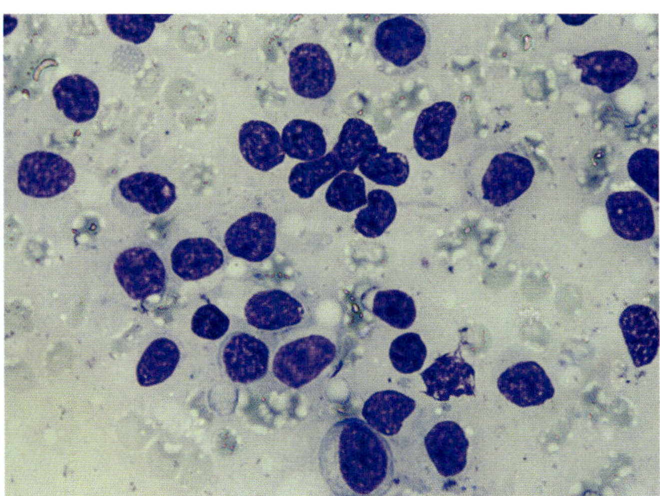

Fig. 25.31: MALToma in salivary gland. The lymphoid cells are round with scanty cytoplasm and mildly pleomorphic nuclei with condensed chromatin (MGG stain X oil immersion).

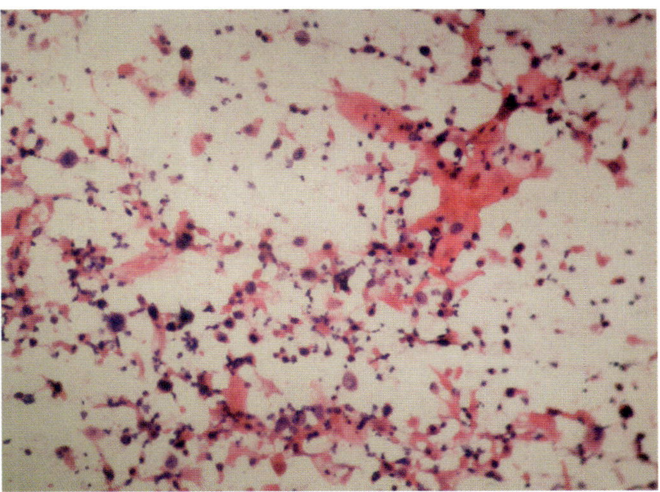

Fig. 25.32: Fine needle aspiration cytology (FNAC) smear of metastatic squamous cell carcinoma of parotid gland (H & E stain X HP).

Extranodal marginal zone lymphoma of the MALT type is a low-grade NHL. Cytology smears show discrete monomorphic small to intermediate sized lymphoid cells (Fig. 25.31). The cytoplasm of the cells is scanty. Nuclei are small round, hyperchromatic with indented nuclear margin and indistinct nucleoli.

Diffuse large B cell lymphoma shows discrete large immature lymphoid cells. The nuclei show fine nuclear chromatin with prominent nucleoli.

Differential Diagnosis

The common differential diagnoses of MALT NHL of the salivary gland are:

- LESA
- Chronic sialadenitis
- Intraparotid reactive lymph node.

FNAC smear of MALT NHL shows monomorphic population of lymphoid cells in contrast to lymphoid cells in variable stage of maturation in LESA. The demonstration of the light chain restriction may be necessary to confirm NHL in certain cases. In all cases of NHL, a detailed immunocytochemistry in cell block or flow cytometry (FCM) from the aspirate is required for further subtyping.

Metastatic Carcinoma

Various other malignancies may metastasize in the salivary gland. The common malignant tumors are NHL, squamous cell carcinoma (Fig. 25.32), renal cell carcinoma and malignant melanoma.

REFERENCES

1. Lim CM, They J, Loh KS, et al. Role of fine-needle aspiration cytology in the evaluation of parotid tumours. ANZ J Surg. 2007;77(9):742-4.
2. Rajwanshi A, Gupta K, Gupta N, et al. Fine-needle aspiration cytology of salivary glands: diagnostic pitfalls—revisited. Diagn Cytopathol. 2006;34(8):580-4.
3. Tyagi R, Dey P. Diagnostic problems of salivary gland tumors. Diagn Cytopathol. 2015;43(6):495-509.
4. Tyagi R, Dey P. Needle tract seeding: an avoidable complication. Diagn Cytopathol. 2014;42(7):636-40.
5. Barnes L, Eveson JW, Reichart P, et al. World Health Organization Classification of tumours. Pathology and Genetics of head and neck tumours. Lyon, France: IARC Press; 2005.
6. Wong DS, Wong LY. "Cystic" parotid swelling on FNA: significance on clinical management. Otolaryngol Head Neck Surg. 2004;130:593-6.
7. Gupta N, Gupta R, Rajwanshi A, et al. Multinucleated giant cells in HIV-associated benign lymphoepithelial cyst-like lesions of the parotid gland on FNAC. Diagn Cytopathol. 2009;37(3):203-4.
8. Allen EA, Ali SZ, Mathew S. Lymphoid lesions of the parotid. Diagn Cytopathol. 1999;21:170-3.
9. Harris NL. Lymphoid proliferations of the salivary glands. Am J Clin Pathol. 1999;111:S94-S103.
10. Singh B, Maharaj TJ. Tuberculosis of the parotid gland. Clinically indistinguishable from a neoplasm. J Laryngol Otol. 1992;106:929-31.
11. Handa U, Dhingra N, Chopra R, et al. Pleomorphic adenoma: cytologic variations and potential diagnostic pitfalls. Diagn Cytopathol. 2009;37(1):11-5.
12. Kapila K, Mathur S, Verma K. Schwannomas: a pitfall in the diagnosis of pleomorphic adenomas on fine needle aspiration cytology. Diagn Cytopathol. 2002;27:53-9.

13. Eveson JW, Cawson RA. Salivary gland tumours. A review of 2410 cases with particular reference to histological types, site, age and sex distribution. J Pathol. 1985;146:51-8.
14. Raymond MR, Yoo JH, Heathcote JG, et al. Accuracy of fine-needle aspiration biopsy for Warthin's tumours. J Otolaryngol. 2002;31(5):263-70.
15. Mooney EE, Dodd LG, Layfield LJ. Squamous cells in fine needle aspiration biopsies of salivary gland lesions: Potential pitfalls in cytologic diagnosis. Diagn Cytopathol. 1996;15:447-52.
16. Hood IC, Qizilbash AH, Salama SS, et al. Basal cell adenoma of parotid: difficulty of differentiation from adenoid cystic carcinoma on aspiration biopsy. Acta Cytol. 1983;27:515-20.
17. Brandwein MS, Huvos AG. Oncocytic tumors of major salivary glands. A study of 68 cases with follow-up of 44 patients. Am J Surg Pathol. 1991;15:514-28.
18. Thompson LD, Wenig BM, Ellis GL. Oncocytomas of the submandibular gland. A series of 22 cases and a review of the literature. Cancer. 1996;78:2281-7.
19. Kirti G, Dey P, Das A. Cytomorphological features of a metastatic myoepithelial carcinoma arising in a minor salivary gland. Diagn Cytopathol. 2005 ;33(1):56-7.
20. Barnes L, Appel BN, Perez H, et al. Myoepithelioma of the head and neck: case report and review. J Surg Oncol. 1985;28:21-8.
21. Dardick I, Thomas MJ, van Nostrand AW. Myoepithelioma—new concepts of histology and classification: a light and electron microscopic study. Ultrastruct Pathol. 1983;13: 187-224.
22. Elsheikh TM, Bernacki EG. Fine needle aspiration cytology of cellular pleomorphic adenoma. Acta Cytol. 1996;40:1165-75.
23. Shin SJ, Rosen PP. Solid variant of mammary adenoid cystic carcinoma with basaloid features: a study of nine cases. Am J Surg Pathol. 2002;26(4):413-20.
24. Zhang S, Bao R, Bagby J, et al. Fine needle aspiration of salivary glands: 5-year experience from a single academic center. Acta Cytol. 2009;53(4):375-82.
25. Jayaram G, Othman MA, Kumar M, et al. Papillary cystic type of acinic cell carcinoma of parotid: fine needle aspiration cytological features of a high grade variant with oncocytic metaplasia. Malays J Pathol. 2002;24:107-12.
26. Ali SZ. Acinic-cell carcinoma, papillary-cystic variant: a diagnostic dilemma in salivary gland aspiration. Diagn Cytopathol. 2002;27:244-50.
27. Laskawi R, Rodel R, Zirk A, et al. Retrospective analysis of 35 patients with acinic cell carcinoma of the parotid gland. J Oral Maxillofac Surg. 1998;56:440-3.
28. Shet T, Ghodke R, Kane S, et al. Cytomorphologic patterns in papillary cystic variant of acinic cell carcinoma of the salivary gland. Acta Cytol. 2006;50(4):388-92.
29. Auclair PL, Goode RK, Ellis GL. Mucoepidermoid carcinoma of intraoral salivary glands. Evaluation and application of grading criteria in 143 cases. Cancer. 1992;69:2021-30.
30. Guzzo M, Andreola S, Sirizzotti G, et al. Mucoepidermoid carcinoma of the salivary glands: clinicopathologic review of 108 patients treated at the National Cancer Institute of Milan. Ann Surg Oncol. 2002;9:688-95.
31. Klijanienko J, Vielh P. Fine-needle sampling of salivary gland lesions. IV. Review of 50 cases of mucoepidermoid carcinoma with histologic correlation. Diagn Cytopathol. 1997;17:92-8.
32. Gibbons D, Saboorian MH, Vuitch F, et al. Fine needle aspiration findings in patients with polymorphous low grade adenocarcinoma of the salivary glands. Cancer. 1999;87:31-6.
33. Evans HL, Luna MA. Polymorphous low-grade adenocarcinoma: a study of 40 cases with long-term follow up and an evaluation of the importance of papillary areas. Am J Surg Pathol. 2000;24:1319-28.
34. Arora SK, Sreedharanunni S, Dey P. Cytomorphological features of an aggressive variant of polymorphous low-grade adenocarcinoma in adolescence with lymph node metastasis. Diagn Cytopathol. 2013;41(2):186-8.
35. Arora VK, Misra K, Bhatia A. Cytomorphologic features of the rare epithelial-myoepithelial carcinoma of the salivary gland. Acta Cytol. 1990;34:239-42.
36. Miliauskas JR, Orell SR. Fine-needle aspiration cytological findings in five cases of epithelial-myoepithelial carcinoma of salivary glands. Diagn Cytopathol. 2003;28(3):163-7.
37. Gnepp DR. Malignant mixed tumors of the salivary glands: a review. Pathol Annu. 1993;28(Pt 1):279-328.
38. Heintz PW, Schmidt WA, Pommier RF, et al. Submandibular gland carcinoma ex pleomorphic adenoma. Report of a case with cytologic features and diagnostic pitfalls. Acta Cytol. 1998;42:1431-6.
39. Savera AT, Sloman A, Huvos AG, et al. Myoepithelial carcinoma of the salivary glands: a clinicopathologic study of 25 patients. Am J Surg Pathol. 2000;4:761-74.
40. Barnes L, Rao U, Krause J, et al. Salivary duct carcinoma. Part I. A clinicopathologic evaluation and DNA image analysis of 13 cases with review of the literature. Oral Surg Oral Med Oral Pathol. 1994;78:64-73.
41. Fyrat P, Cramer H, Feczko JD, et al. Fine-needle aspiration biopsy of salivary duct carcinoma: Report of five cases. Diagn Cytopathol. 1997;16:526-30.
42. Auclair P, van der Wall JE. Adenocarcinoma not otherwise specified. In: Barnes L, Eveson JW, Reichart P (Eds). WHO Classification of Tumours. Head and Neck Tumours. Lyon: IARC Press; 2005. pp. 238-9.
43. Skalova A, Michal M, Simpson RH. Newly described salivary gland tumors. Mod Pathol. 2017;30(s1):S27-S43.
44. Jung MJ, Kim SY, Nam SY, et al. Aspiration cytology of mammary analogue secretory carcinoma of the salivary gland. Diagn Cytopathol. 2015;43:287-93.
45. Bishop JA, Yonescu R, Batista DA, et al. Cytopathologic features of mammary analogue secretory carcinoma. Cancer Cytopathol. 2013;121:228-33.
46. Imamura Y, Morishita T, Kawakami M, et al. Sclerosing polycystic adenosis of the left parotid gland: report of a case with fine needle aspiration cytology. Acta Cytol. 2004;48:569-73.
47. Freeman C, Berg JW, Cutler SJ. Occurrence and prognosis of extranodal lymphomas. Cancer. 1972;29:252-60.
48. Harris NL. Lymphoid proliferations of the salivary glands. Am J Clin Pathol. 1999;111:S94-S103.

Review Questions

1. **A 38-year-male presented with 5 cm diameter right parotid swelling for 3 months. Fine needle cytology was done (Figs. 25.33A to D):**
   a. **What is your possible diagnosis?**
      a. Mucoepidermoid carcinoma
      b. Benign salivary gland aspirate
      c. Warthin's tumor
      d. Acinic cell carcinoma
   b. **What are the differential diagnoses?**
2. **A 29-year-male had 4 cm dimeter left parotid gland swelling for 25 days. Fine needle cytology was done (Figs. 25.34A to D):**
   a. **What is your possible diagnosis?**
      a. Mucoepidermoid carcinoma
      b. Warthin's tumor
      c. Squamous cell carcinoma
      d. Acinic cell carcinoma
   b. **What are the differential diagnoses?**
3. **Which is true for mammary analog secretory carcinoma?**
   a. Fairly common tumor but they are missed in routine reporting
   b. Resembles adenoid cystic carcinoma
   c. Characteristic chromosomal translocation, t(12;15)(p13;q25)
   d. Positive for for S100 protein but negative for mammaglobin, STAT5 and MUC4
4. **Magenta colored hyaline globules are seen in all *except*:**
   a. Adenoid cystic carcinoma
   b. Pleomorphic adenoma
   c. Polymorphous low grade adenocarcinoma
   d. Mucoepidermoid carcinoma
5. **A 26-year-old lady presented with 5 cm diameter firm right parotid swelling for 6 months. Aspiration yielded brownish fluid material. Figures 25.35A and B represent the FNAC smears:**
   What is your diagnosis?
   a. Mucoepidermoid carcinoma
   b. Warthin's tumor
   c. Chronic sialadenitis
   d. Acinic cell carcinoma

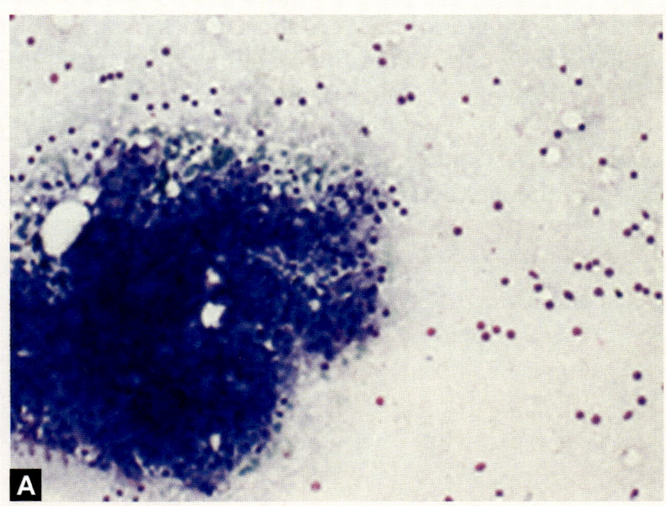

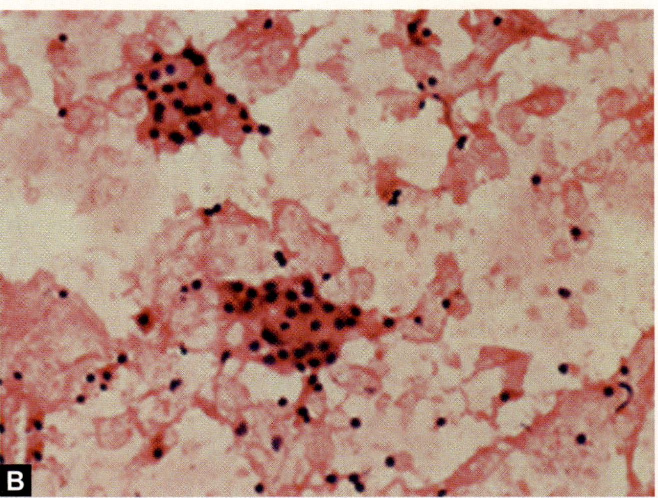

Figs. 25.33A and B

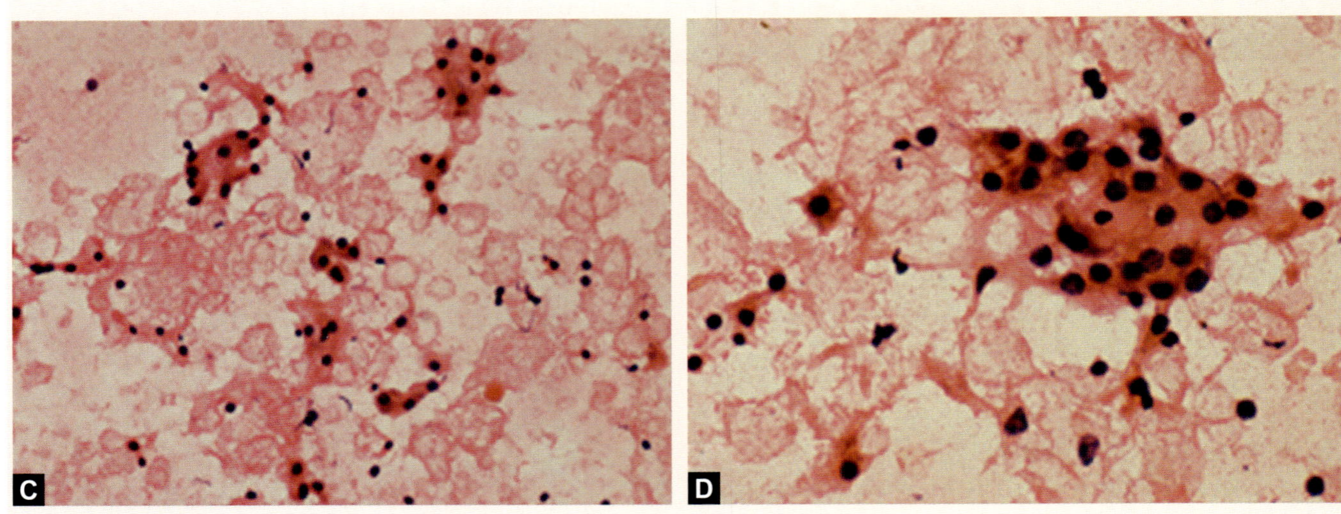

Figs. 25.33A to D: Fine needle aspiration cytology smear of salivary gland of question 1.

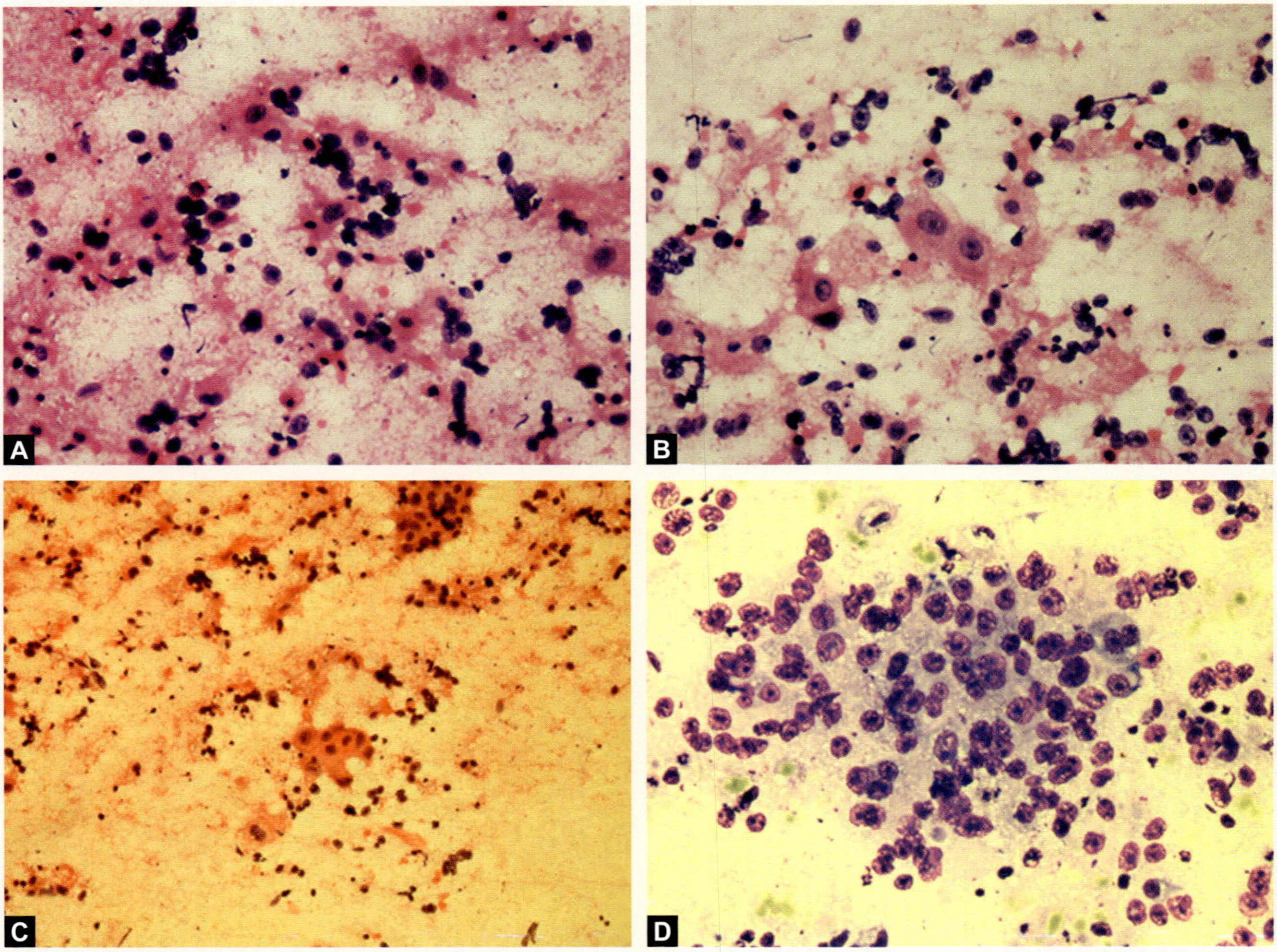

Figs. 25.34A to D: Fine needle aspiration cytology smear of salivary gland of question 2.

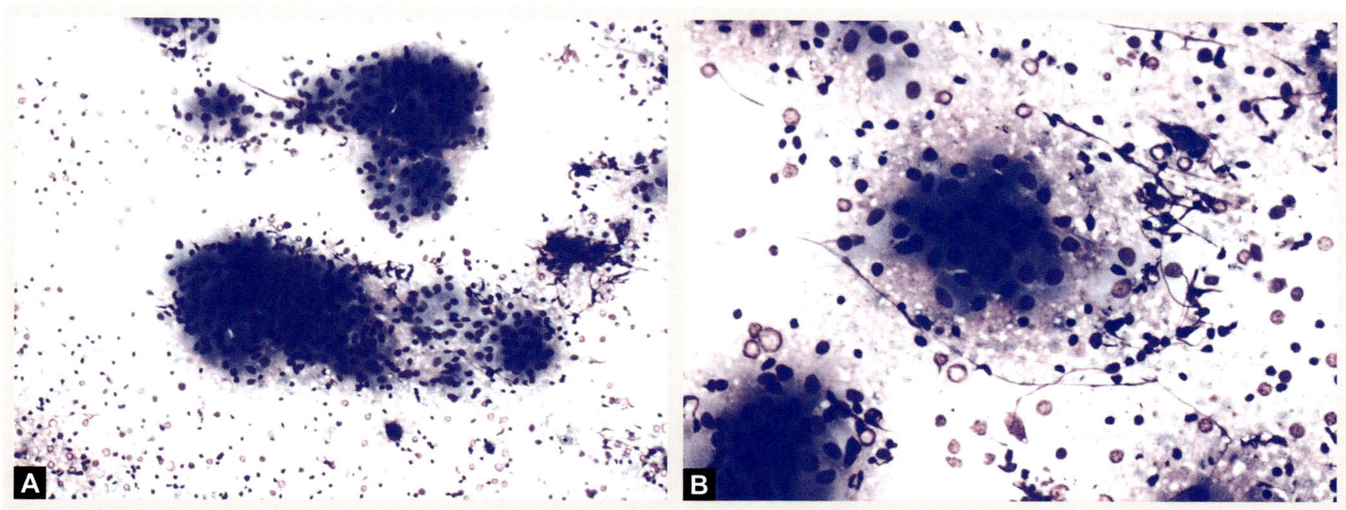

Figs. 25.35A and B: Fine needle aspiration cytology smear of salivary gland of question 5.

Answers

1. a. Answer is (d) Acinic cell carcinoma
   b. Possible differential diagnoses are:
   - Benign salivary acini
   - Warthin's tumor

   Note: Abundant discrete and loose clusters of acinar cell indicate the diagnosis of acinic cell carcinoma. This tumor is often mistaken as benign acinic cell.
2. a. Answer is (a) Mucoepidermoid carcinoma
   b. Squamous cell carcinoma and acinic cell carcinoma

   Note: The smears show both mucus secreting cells and malignant squamous cells indicating the diagnosis of mucoepidermoid carcinoma.
3. c. Characteristic chromosomal translocation, t(12;15) (p13;q25)
4. d. Mucoepidermoid carcinoma
5. b. Warthin's tumor

   Note: The tumor shows abundant oncocytic cells and lymphocytes indicating the diagnosis of Warthin's tumor.

CHAPTER

26

Thyroid

INTRODUCTION

Fine needle aspiration cytology (FNAC) of thyroid has been reported long back in history. Martin and Ellis in New York in 1930 first time reported the usefulness of FNAC of thyroid.[1] Later on, FNAC of thyroid was reported by Söderström from Sweden.[2] In Karolinka, Sweden FNAC of thyroid lesions was routinely used and slowly it was popular in USA and other countries.

Fine needle aspiration of cytology is a very helpful and relatively noninvasive technique in the diagnosis of various thyroid lesions.[3] Any palpable thyroid nodule can be aspirated for diagnosis. The main aim of thyroid FNAC is to distinguish benign form malignant lesions and to determine the cases that require surgery. It may also be used in certain high-risk patients for follow-up. FNAC is a safe, cost-effective, and reliable technique. Due to introduction of this technique, the incidence of surgery in thyroid has been reduced considerably. The endocrine surgeons have widely accepted FNAC of thyroid. The common indications of FNAC of the thyroid lesions have been highlighted in Box 26.1.

APPROACH TO FINE NEEDLE ASPIRATION CYTOLOGY OF THE THYROID

Clinical History and Physical Examination

Clinical details and physical findings of the patient are helpful in the interpretation of the cytology smear. Rapidly enlarged swelling, hoarseness of the voice, hard consistency, and fixation with the deeper structure usually indicate malignancy (Box 26.2). History of irradiation or any history of carcinoma is needed. A detailed family history of thyroid carcinoma is also helpful. Clinical features of hypo- or hyperthyroid should also be recorded.

Other Investigations

Following other investigations are preferable before doing FNAC:

- Thyroid-stimulating hormone (TSH) level
- Thyroid scan
- Ultrasonography (USG) findings.

Before performing FNAC of the thyroid, serum TSH should be measured. If the patient has decreased serum TSH, then thyroid scan is recommended. All the cold nodules of thyroid should have FNAC. In case of normal or increased TSH level, an USG of the thyroid should be performed and USG-guided FNAC should be done.

TECHNIQUES

The patient should be kept in supine position with a small pillow under his neck to make the thyroid region prominent. The technique of FNAC in the thyroid gland is essentially same. After cleaning the area of thyroid, the gland is hold in between the two fingers so that the thyroid will be prominent. Depending on the aspirator's choice,

Box 26.1: Indications of Fine needle aspiration cytology (FNAC) of thyroid.

- Any palpable nodule of thyroid.
- Thyroid nodule of less than 10 mm diameter with clinical or suspicious features in ultrasonography (USG).
- Predominantly solid nodule in USG.
- USG-guided FNAC could be done in solid area of a cystic nodule and from a nonpalpable nodule.

Box 26.2: Clinical features suspicious for malignancy.

- Extreme age group
- Single dominant nodule
- Hoarseness of the voice
- History of irradiation of neck
- Family history of thyroid malignancy
- History of multiple endocrine neoplasia
- Hard and fixed nodule
- Enlarged cervical lymph node.

Box 26.3: Fine needle aspiration cytology-induced changes in histology section.

- Infarction
- Hemorrhage
- Cystic degeneration
- Vascular proliferation
- Fibrosis
- Atypia

FNAC or nonsuction Fine needle sampling (FNS) can be done. As the thyroid is a vascular organ so FNS is preferable in small swelling of the thyroid gland. However, in case of a cystic lesion, FNAC is preferable as there is a chance of spillage by FNS technique. It is recommended to do three to five passes of needle in each nodule.[4]

Multiple smears should be made immediately from the aspirated material and both air-dried smear and alcohol-fixed smears should be kept. If necessary, the material should be taken for cell block and other ancillary investigations.

The thyroid nodule is hold in between two fingers and gentle suction is done. FNS is preferable in thyroid as the material is free from blood.[5,6] Thyroid swelling is hold tightly in between the two fingers so that the thyroid will be prominent. Now the needle is moved gently to and from within the lesion. Material comes to the needle hub with the help of capillary pressure. The needle is gently withdrawn and the syringe is attached with the hub. The material in the needle is spread on the slide. The FNAC material can also be collected for cell block and flow cytometry to do ancillary technique.

Fine needle aspiration cytology can produce various preoperative artifacts. The common changes include infarction, hemorrhage, cystic degeneration, vascular proliferation, fibrosis, and FNAC-induced atypia (Box 26.3).[7] Linear artifactual changes occur along the needle track and this may be relatively easily identifiable.

Ultrasound Guidance Fine Needle Aspiration Cytology

Recently, USG localization of thyroid lesions followed by USG-guided FNAC of palpable thyroid nodule has been advocated to reduce the rate of the nondiagnostic material and subsequently to reduce the false negative interpretation.[8,9]

In fact, USG guidance significantly helps in diagnosis, and it gives proper guidance to target the palpable thyroid nodule. USG-guided FNAC is not mandatory, but the pathologists should be encouraged to do USG guidance FNAC of thyroid lesions as far as possible. National Cancer Institute (NCI) sponsored Bethesda recommended USG FNAC in case of nonpalpable nodule or nodule that has more than 25% cystic component.[10] Other indication of USG FNAC is failure to get adequate material in prior aspiration (Box 26.4).

Box 26.4: Ultrasonograph-guided Fine needle aspiration cytology of thyroid.

Indications
- Nonpalpable nodule
- Nodule with more than 25% cystic component
- Failure to get adequate material in prior aspiration

Advantages
- Less nondiagnostic material
- Reduction of false negative cases
- Nodule of interest is aspirated
- Puncture of the critical structure can be avoided.

Complications

Fine needle aspiration cytology of thyroid is almost free of any complications. Rarely needle tract seeding, hemorrhage, infection, and recurrent laryngeal nerve injury have been described. These complications are mainly encountered if thick bore needle is used for FNAC.[11,12]

Optimal Material

Adequacy of the material in thyroid FNAC sample is a controversial issue. The various criteria have been proposed:

- Six groups of thyroid follicular cells with at least 10 cells in each group[13,14]
- Ten groups each with 20 or more cells[15]
- Six groups of cells on at least two aspirates[16]
- Eight groups on at least two slides.[17]

However, these criteria should not be strictly applied in thyroid FNAC because aspirates of colloid goiter may yield abundant colloid material with minimal number of cells. Cystic goiter may not yield thyroid follicular cells and ideally the aspiration should be repeated from the solid area (if any) under USG guidance. FNAC smear should be considered as suboptimal in case of extensive drying artifact, blood or thick ill spread.

ANATOMY AND HISTOLOGY

The thyroid glands are located in the anterior part of neck in front of trachea and inferior to larynx. The gland is composed of two lobes, which are connected by central part known as isthmus. The thyroid gland is covered by thick fibrous septae. The fibroconnective tissue has divided the lobes into multiple smaller lobules.

Follicles are the basic structural unit of thyroid gland. Each follicle contains homogenous eosinophilic colloid material. Follicles are lined by low cuboidal to columnar cells. Thyroid follicular cells liberate triiodothyronine (T_3) and thyroxine (T_4) hormone. Due to some unknown reason, thyroid follicular cell may undergo Hürthle cell change. These are large cells with abundant eosinophilic cytoplasm and central round nuclei. Electron microscopy of such cells show abundant mitochondria.

Parafollicular cells are present in the periphery of the follicles as small cluster. These cells are three to four times larger than the follicular cells. They have pale moderate amount of cytoplasm with central spherical nuclei. Parafollicular cells secrete calcitonin hormone that takes important role in calcium homeostasis. Calcitonin hormone inhibits bone resorption by osteoclasts and thereby helps to lower the calcium concentrations in blood.

DIAGNOSTIC ACCURACY

It is difficult to assess the sensitivity and specificity of FNAC of thyroid because vast majority of the benign lesions of thyroid do not have any surgical intervention and therefore no histological correlations are available in such cases. Moreover, only selected patients with clinical symptoms and signs are operated.

False negative rate of thyroid FNAC varies from 1% to 11%.[18,19] False negative report of cytology is mainly due to inadequate sampling of thyroid. The false positive rate of FNAC of thyroid is about 3% and it largely depends on diagnostic category.[20] The major causes of false positive cytology are hyalinizing trabecular adenoma and follicular neoplasia. The error in FNAC of thyroid depends both on sampling error and interpretation error. Overall sensitivity and specificity of thyroid FNAC is 83% and 92%, respectively.[21,22]

In a large meta-analysis study by Tee et al., the sensitivity and specificity of FNAC of thyroid were measured by a statistically designed model excluding the significant bias in previous study designs. Only those studies were selected that have histopathological outcome in every case. They noted that the sensitivity of FNA may be as low as 66%. It was also noted that the specificity of FNA has a consistently high value of 93%.[23] The authors concluded that FNAC may miss a significant fraction of patients with thyroid malignancy. All the patients should be followed up either conservatively or with repeat FNAC biopsy to exclude malignancy.

TERMINOLOGY

There are various reporting terminologies of FNAC smear of thyroid lesions. Papanicolaou Society of Cytopathology Task Force on Standards of Practice, 1997, recommended following terminology system:[24]

- Inadequate or unsatisfactory
- Benign
- Atypical cells present
- Suspicious for malignancy
- Malignant.

However, NCI sponsored the conference on thyroid FNAC on October 22–23, 2007 in Bethesda[25] and recommended this updated terminology:

BETHESDA TERMINOLOGY

- *Benign lesions*: Colloid goiter, lymphocytic thyroiditis, hyperplastic nodule, etc.
    - *Risk of malignancy*: Less than 1%
    - *Management*: Clinical follow-up
- *Follicular lesions of undetermined significance/atypia of undetermined significance*: The smear pattern is not convincingly either benign or follicular neoplasm.
    - *Risk of malignancy*: 5–10% risk of malignancy.
    - *Management*: Repeat FNAC should be done along with clinical and radiological correlation.
- *Follicular neoplasm or suspicious of follicular neoplasm*: Follicular and Hürthle cell neoplasm. The other diagnostic terms in this category include follicular lesions, micropapillary proliferation, and suggestive of neoplasm.
    - *Risk of malignancy*: 20–30%.
    - *Management*: The patients should have definitive surgery such as lobectomy or hemithyroidectomy.
- *Suspicious for malignancy*: Suspicious for follicular variant of papillary carcinoma of thyroid, medullary carcinoma, certain cases of anaplastic carcinoma of thyroid, non-Hodgkin's lymphoma (NHL), and metastatic carcinoma.
    - *Risk of malignancy*: 50–75% risk of malignancy.
    - *Management*: Thyroidectomy is advised.

- *Malignancy*: Specify the type of malignancy
    - *Risk of malignancy*: 97–99% risk of malignancy.
    - *Management*: Thyroidectomy is advised.
- *Nondiagnostic*: Here the specimen is inadequate due to
  Low cellularity
  Lack of follicular cells
  Poor fixation
- *Management*: Repeat FNAC is advised.

NORMAL ASPIRATED MATERIAL

Colloid (Fig. 26.1): Gross appearance of colloid is thick to thin brownish material. The May-Grünwald Giemsa (MGG)-stained cytology smear shows a pale blue acellular material.

Thyroid follicular cells (Figs. 26.2A and B): Follicular cells are present in small clusters and follicles. The cells are round with scanty cytoplasm and round monomorphic nucleus. Nuclear chromatin is homogeneously spread.

Foam cells (Fig. 26.3): The foam cells show abundant foamy cytoplasm with small monomorphic nucleus.

DISEASES OF THYROID

The classification of commonly encountered lesions on FNAC of the thyroid hsas been given in Table 26.1.

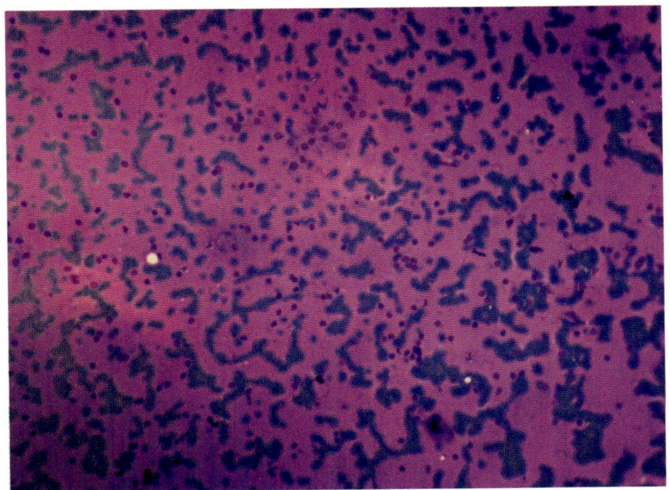

Fig. 26.1: Pale blue thin colloid material (MGG × MP).

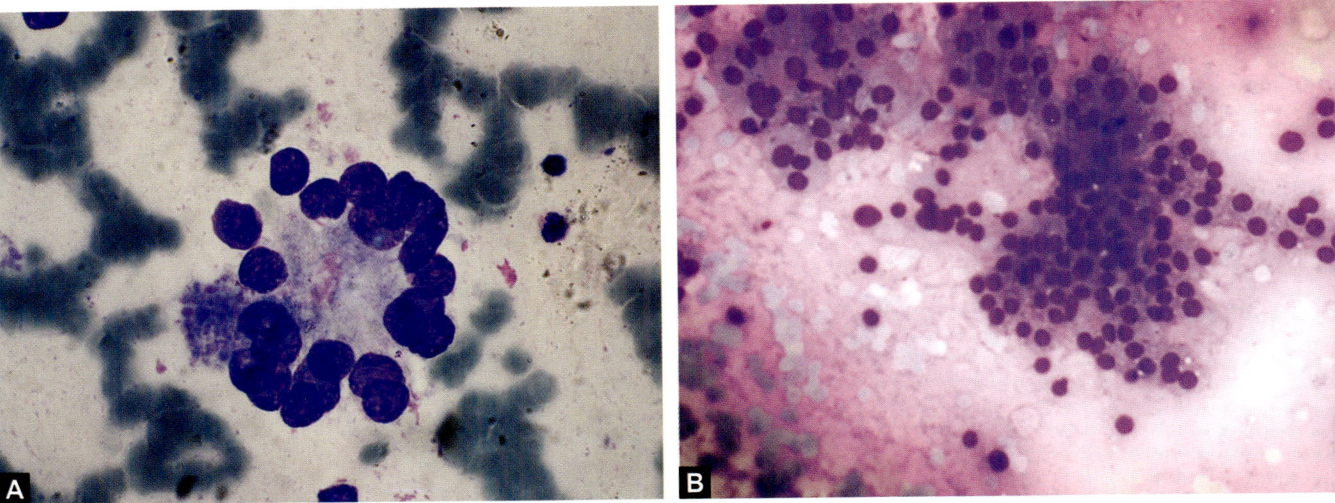

Figs. 26.2A and B: (A) Thyroid follicle lined by round monomorphic follicular cells (MGG × HP) and (B) Small cluster of thyroid follicular cells with round monomorphic nuclei and moderate amount of cytoplasm (MGG × HP).

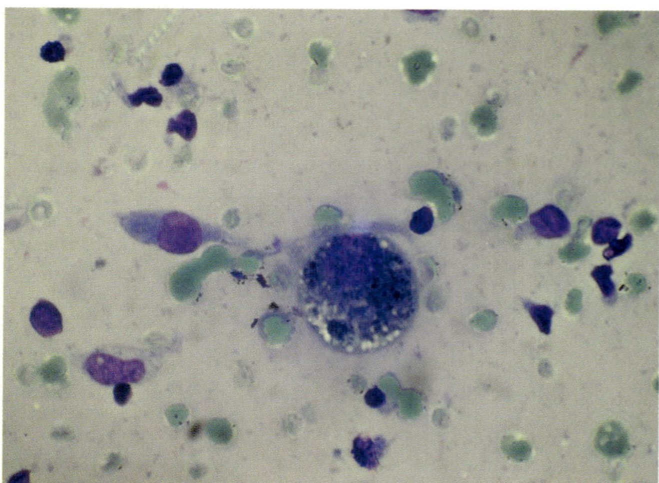

Fig. 26.3: Cytology smear of foam cell showing abundant foamy cytoplasm with phagocytosed material in the cytoplasm (MGG × HP).

Table 26.1: Classification of thyroid lesion.

Nonneoplastic	*Neoplastic*
• Colloid goiter • Thyroiditis - Acute - Chronic - Subacute - Riedel's struma	• Follicular tumor - Follicular adenoma - Follicular carcinoma • Hürthle cell tumor - Hürthle cell adenoma - Hürthle cell carcinoma • Papillary carcinoma • Medullary carcinoma • Anaplastic carcinoma • Insular carcinoma • Non-Hodgkin's lymphoma • Sarcoma • Metastatic carcinoma

Box 26.5: Cytology of nodular goiter.

- Abundant colloid
- Discrete or flat sheet of thyroid follicular cells
- Macrophages.

Colloid Goiter

Nodular colloid goiter is the most common disease of thyroid. The patients have iodine deficiency due to low iodine in water and soil. The deficient iodine leads to decreased production of thyroid hormone from thyroid gland. The deficient thyroid hormone induces stimulation of TSH secretion from pituitary gland. Excess TSH hormone causes thyroid follicular hyperplasia with massive storage of colloid. The thyroid may have single or multiple nodules (Fig. 26.4). Uncommonly, the thyroid may be massively enlarged causing tracheal obstruction. Salient cytological features are highlighted in Box 26.5.

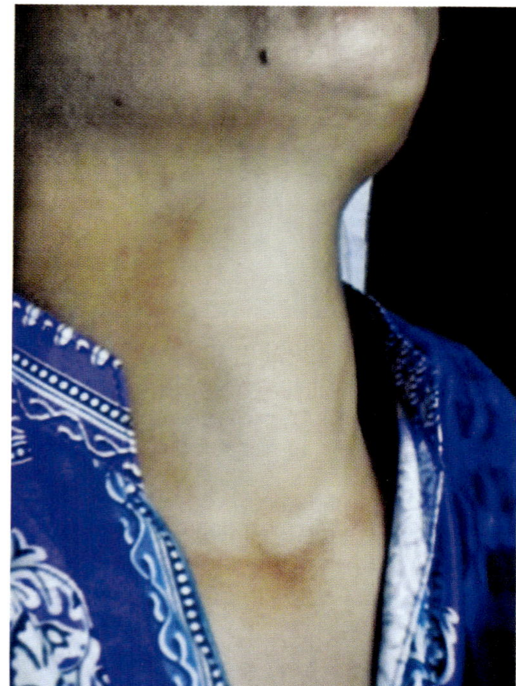

Fig. 26.4: Nodular goiter in a young female.

Cytology (Figs. 26.5A and B)

The aspirate yields thick to thin brownish material on gross examination. In MGG-stained smear the colloid material looks like pale blue to dark blue material. In Papanicolaou's stained smear it is difficult to appreciate water clear colloid and it looks like pink homogenous material. Varying amount of thyroid follicular cells is embedded in the colloid. The cells are present in flat small sheets, in small clusters, and discretely. The individual cells are small cuboidal with round monomorphic nuclei and fine chromatin. Many follicular cells are naked with stripped of cytoplasm. These cells may resemble lymphocytes. Nodular goiter often shows cystic degeneration and in that case the smears show abundant foamy macrophages-containing dark brown hemosiderin-laden pigments. Longstanding goiter may show multinucleated giant cells due to reaction of colloid. Occasionally, fibrosis occurs in the nodular goiter and the smear may show young active fibroblasts. The large atypical active fibroblast may be misinterpreted as malignant cell.

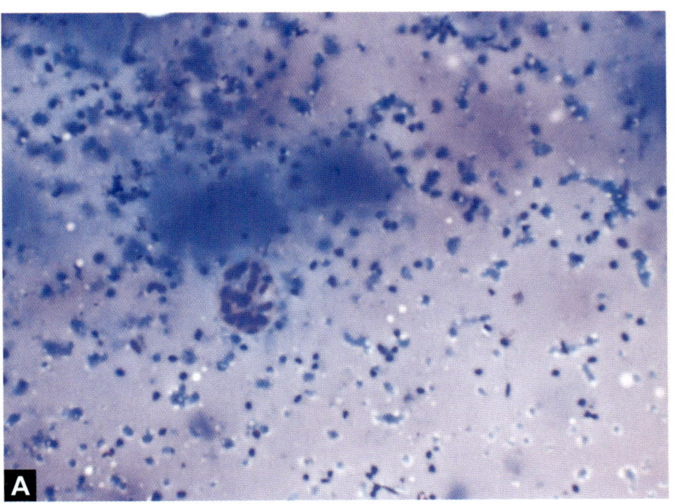

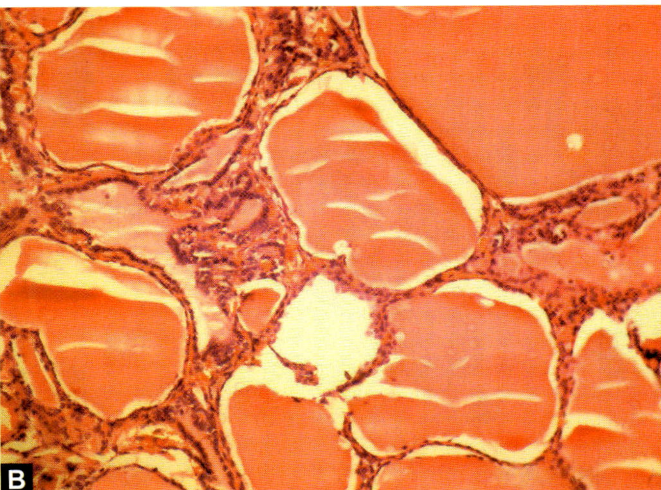

Figs. 26.5A and B: (A) Abundant thick and thin colloid along with scattered benign thyroid follicular cells in colloid goiter (MGG × MP) and (B) Histopathology of the same showing variable sized thyroid follicles filled with colloid (H & E × MP).

Box 26.6: Adenomatoid hyperplasia or hyperplastic nodules.

- Cellular smear
- Dissociated and microfollicular arrangement
- Hürthle cells
- Foamy macrophages
- Scanty colloid.

Differential Diagnosis

- *Colloid goiter versus hyperplastic nodules*: At times the amount of thyroid follicular cells may be relatively more and there may be difficulties to differentiate a colloid goiter from a hyperplastic or adenomatoid nodule. The relative excess of colloid is a helpful diagnostic feature of colloid goiter.
- Atypical large cells.

Adenomatoid Nodule or Hyperplastic Nodule

This is mainly a cytological terminology. Smears show good number of thyroid follicular cells and scanty colloid. The follicular cells are arranged in flat sheet, macrofollicles, microfollicles, and singly (Box 26.6). The follicular cells are monomorphic with regular nuclear margin. However, occasional cells may show nuclear atypia. Hürthle cells and foamy macrophages may be seen in the background. At times, the microfollicles may be relatively abundant and the differentiation of hyperplastic nodules versus follicular neoplasm (FN) is very difficult (Fig. 26.6). The neoplastic lesions are usually cold nodule. There may be variable types of cells such as follicular cells, Hürthle cells, and foam cells in adenomatoid nodule.

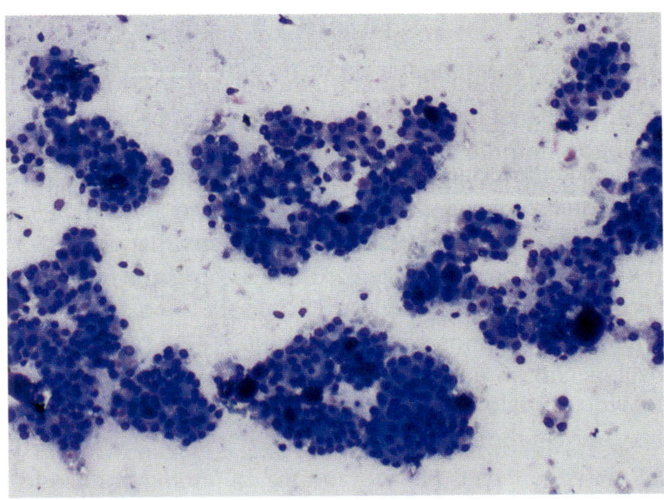

Fig. 26.6: Multiple follicles and thin colloid in adenomatoid nodule (MGG × MP).

Diagnostic Difficulties

- Follicular neoplasm.

Diffuse Toxic Goiter (Graves' Disease)

This is an autoimmune disorder characterized by diffuse enlargement of thyroid along with features of toxicity such as tachycardia, exophthalmos, weakness, weight loss, dermatopathy, and irritability. The patients have IgG immunoglobulin [thyroid-stimulating immunoglobulin (TSI)] directed

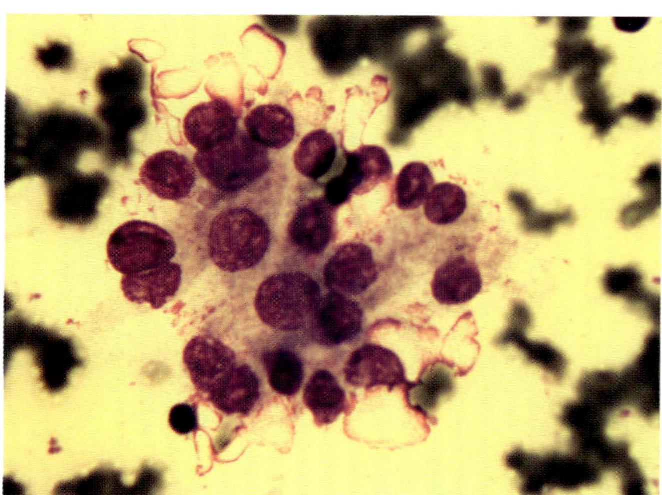

Fig. 26.7: Fire flare appearance in Graves' disease of thyroid (MGG × HP).

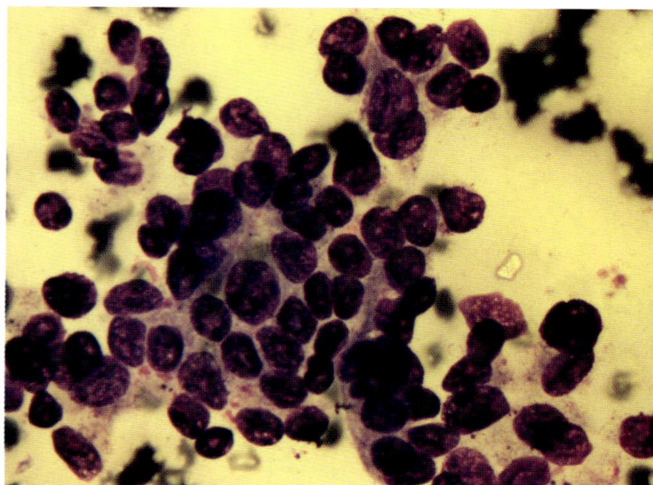

Fig. 26.8: Graves' disease of thyroid: Nuclear enlargement and pleomorphism along with occasional nuclear grove (MGG × HP).

Box 26.7: Diffuse toxic goiter (Graves' disease).

- Cellular
- Scanty watery colloid
- Enlarged cell with vacuolated cytoplasm
- Prominent nucleoli
- Fire flares appearance.

Box 26.8: Acute thyroiditis.

- Polymorphs and lymphocytes
- Necrosis
- Degenerated thyroid follicular cells.

against the TSH receptor of the thyroid follicular cells. The antibody functions as agonist of TSH receptors and stimulates thyroid hormone synthesis. FNAC is not indicated in Graves' disease except the nodular swelling in thyroid.

Cytology (Figs. 26.7 and 26.8)

Aspirates of the Graves' disease show good amount of cells and scanty colloid (Box 26.7). The follicular cells are in clusters and scattered. The cells have moderate to abundant eosinophilic cytoplasm and centrally placed round nuclei with prominent nucleoli. Nuclear atypia is often noted particularly in longstanding Graves' disease. The nuclei may show nuclear grooving and chromatin clearing simulating papillary carcinoma of thyroid. Cluster of cells with peripheral red granules known as fire flare appearance is a common finding.[26]

Thyroiditis

Acute Thyroiditis

Acute thyroiditis patient presents with fever, tachycardia, and sudden painful enlargement of thyroid. The thyroid is diffusely enlarged and tender on palpation. FNAC is rarely done in acute thyroiditis.

Cytology: Smears show abundant acute inflammatory cells consisting of polymorphs, lymphocytes, and necrotic tissue fragments (Box 26.8). Scattered degenerated thyroid follicular cells may also be seen on the background. The follicular cells may exhibit reparative changes and nuclear atypia. Necrosis and polymorphs infiltration are also seen in anaplastic carcinoma of thyroid. A careful examination is needed to exclude the possibility of anaplastic carcinoma. If required, a repeat FNAC should be done from multiple sites of thyroid.

Differential Diagnosis

- Anaplastic carcinoma.

Subacute Granulomatous Thyroiditis

This is probably related with viral infection. The patient is usually a young woman and presents with painful swelling of thyroid, fever and myalgia, sore throat, and high erythrocyte sedimentation rate. The thyroid is diffusely enlarged. In the initial phase of the disease the patient may have hyperthyroidism. This disease is usually self limiting. Subacute thyroiditis may be mistaken as neoplasm due to firm thyroid swelling.

Cytology (Fig. 26.9): The destruction of thyroid follicular cell releases colloid in the neighboring tissue causing

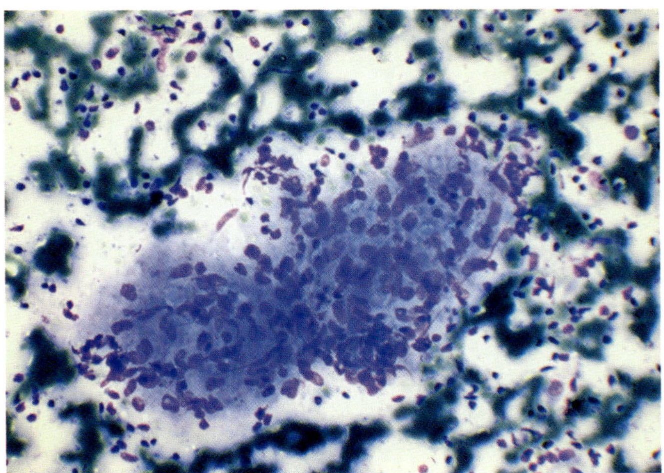

Fig. 26.9: Epithelioid cell granuloma and reactive lymphoid cells in subacute granulomatous thyroiditis (MGG × MP).

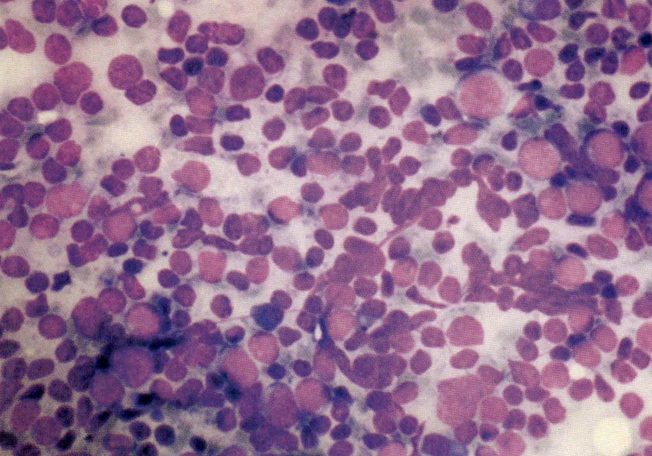

Fig. 26.10: Abundant reactive lymphoid cells in lymphocytic thyroiditis (MGG × HP).

Box 26.9: Subacute granulomatous thyroiditis.

- Dirty background formed by cellular debris and scanty colloid
- Epithelioid cell granulomas
- Multinucleated giant cells
- Lymphocytes and plasma cells
- Benign thyroid follicular cells with paravacuolar granulations.

granulomatous reaction. The FNAC smears show many multinucleated giant cells (Box 26.9). These cells are large with 50–100 nuclei. Ill-formed epithelioid cell granulomas along with polymorphs and lymphocyte and plasma cells are also noted. Background of the smear shows cellular debris and colloid. In addition, clusters and discrete thyroid follicular cells with prominent intracytoplasmic paravacuolar granules of lipofuscin and lysosomal debris are seen.

The presence of multinucleated giant cells is an important finding in granulomatous thyroiditis. However, similar cells are also noted in lymphocytic thyroiditis (LT) and papillary carcinoma of thyroid. It is important to mention that in early or late stage of subacute thyroiditis the typical cytological features may be absent.

Differential Diagnosis

- Chronic lymphocytic thyroiditis
- *Tuberculosis*: It shows almost similar features. However, tuberculosis is very uncommon in thyroid.

Chronic Lymphocytic Thyroiditis (Hashimoto's Thyroiditis)

Chronic LT is an autoimmune thyroiditis and is much more common in women than men. It can occur in any age group; however, it is more common in fourth to six decade. Thyroid antimicrosomal antibody and antithyroglobulin antibodies are elevated in the patient and destroy the thyroid follicle. The damage of thyroid gland may release thyroid hormone in early phase causing hyperthyroidism. Later on, the patient goes to hypothyroid phase.

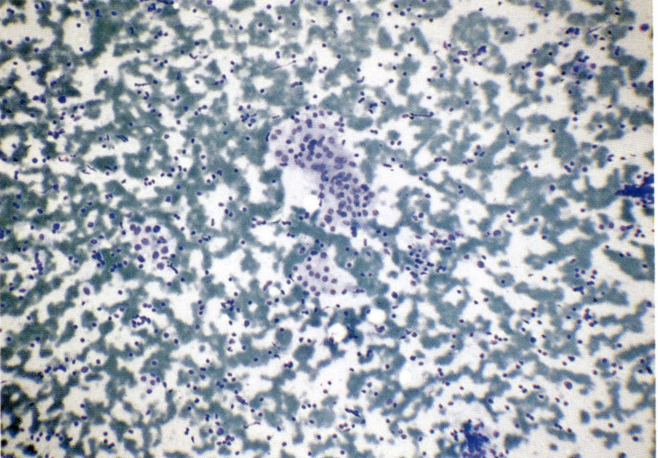

Fig. 26.11: Excess reactive lymphoid cells in the background along with the thyroid follicles in lymphocytic thyroiditis (MGG × LP).

Cytology (Figs. 26.10 to 26.16): In early stage of LT the thyroid gland is infiltrated by florid reactive lymphoid cells. There is little destruction of thyroid follicles and the patients are usually euthyroid. In the advanced stage of LT, there is considerable destruction of thyroid follicles by lymphoid cells and the patients are mostly hypothyroid in this phase (Box 26.10). In the initial phase of LT, the

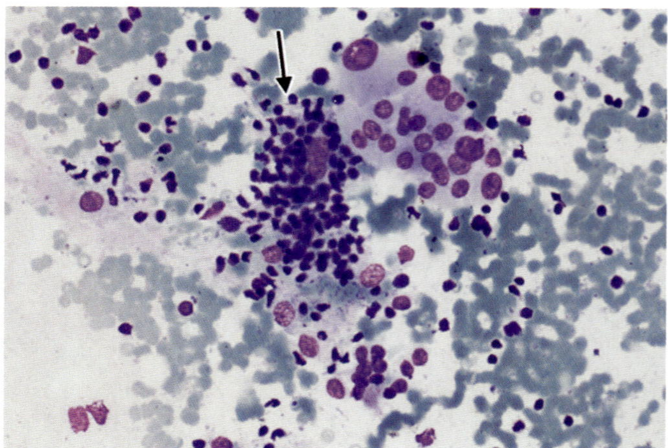

Fig. 26.12: Lymphoid cells infiltration in the thyroid follicular cells in lymphocytic thyroiditis (*see* arrow) (MGG × MP).

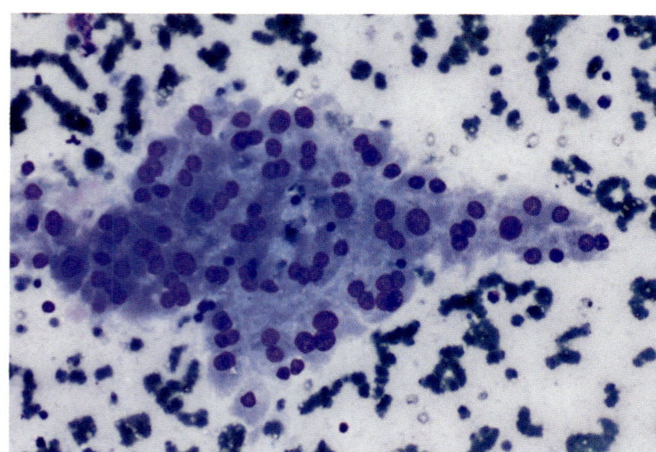

Fig. 26.13: Hürthle cell changes in lymphocytic thyroiditis (MGG × MP).

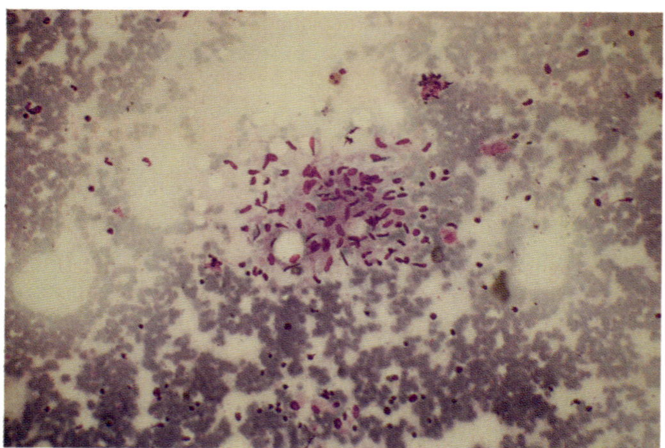

Fig. 26.14: Ill-formed epithelioid cell granuloma in lymphocytic thyroiditis (MGG × HP).

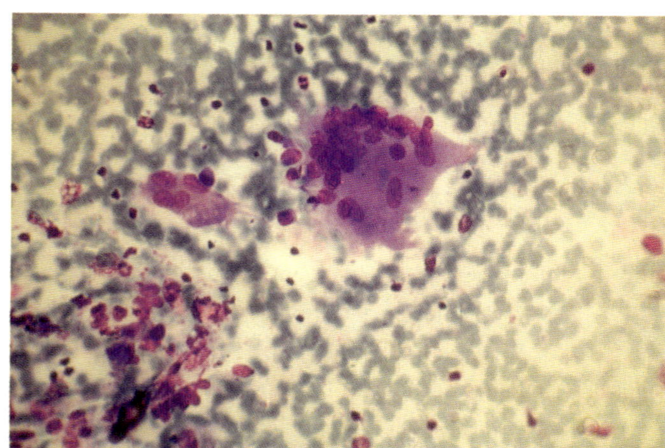

Fig. 26.15: Multinucleated giant cells in lymphocytic thyroiditis (MGG × MP).

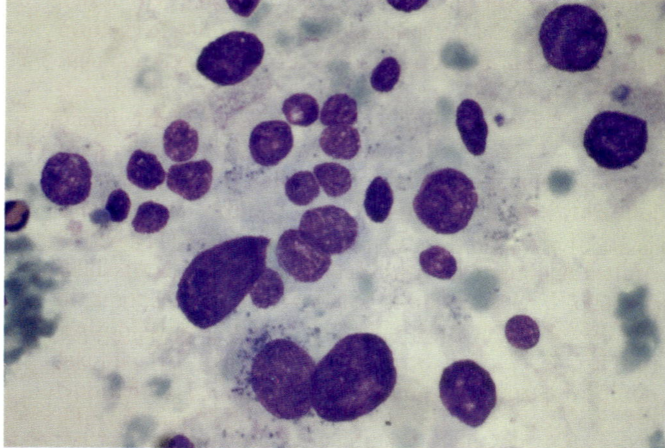

Fig. 26.16: Marked nuclear enlargement and pleomorphism in lymphocytic thyroiditis (MGG × HP).

Box 26.10: Chronic lymphocytic thyroiditis.

- Lymphocytic infiltration in thyroid follicular cells.
- Lymphocytes and plasma cells
- Scanty colloid
- Hürthle cells
- Multinucleated giant cells
- Ill-formed epithelioid cell granuloma
- Elevated thyroid antimicrosomal antibody and antithyroglobulin antibodies.

aspirate shows florid germinal center cells consisting of immunoblasts, small cleaved and large cleaved mature lymphocytes, and plasma cells. Occasional clusters of thyroid follicular cells are noted in the background. The smears may be mistaken as reactive lymph node if the follicular cells are overlooked.

In the advanced or late stage, there is too some extent fibrosis of the gland and the smear shows sparse lymphocytes associated with adjacent follicular cells. There is infiltration of lymphoid cells within the follicles and evidence of destruction of thyroid follicles.[27,28] In addition, the smears also show Hürthle cells. These cells are present in loose clusters. The Hürthle cells have abundant eosinophilic cytoplasm with centrally placed regular nuclei. Nuclei may show crowding and overlapping. At times, considerable nuclear pleomorphism of the Hürthle cells may give false impression of malignancy, particularly Hurtle cell neoplasm.

The smears of LT show scanty colloid. There may be ill-formed epithelioid granulomas, multinucleated giant cells, and foamy histiocytes in the aspirate. Epithelioid cell granulomas may give rise to the differential diagnosis of subacute granulomatous thyroiditis. However, the clinical findings of painful swelling of thyroid, fever, and myalgia along with multiple giant cells and epithelioid cell granulomas favor subacute granulomatous thyroiditis.

Diagnostic Difficulties

- *Hürthle cell neoplasm*: Discussed later.
- *Non-Hodgkin's lymphoma*: Florid LT should be distinguished from NHL particularly low-grade lymphoma of thyroid. Demonstration of light chain restriction in B-NHL or aberrant expression of T cell markers in T-NHL on flow cytometry indicates monoclonality and suggests the possibility of NHL.
- Subacute granulomatous thyroiditis.

Follicular Neoplasm

Thyroid nodule with predominant follicular pattern in the smear is the diagnostic challenge to the cytopathologist. The various benign and malignant entities of thyroid may simulate this pattern. This includes nodular hyperplasia, follicular adenoma (FA), follicular carcinoma (FCa), and follicular variant of papillary carcinoma of thyroid (FVPCT). Differentiating the cases of FA from FCa in FNAC smear is not possible. Probably FNAC just helps to identify the nodule that needs surgical excision. FA is a well-encapsulated benign neoplasm with predominant follicular cell differentiation. The tumor does not show any capsular or vascular invasion and follicular cells do not have the nuclear characteristics of papillary carcinoma. FA is a monoclonal tumor and commonly affects female (female: male ratio is 3:1). The tumor presents as a solitary well-encapsulated nodule with variant histological pattern such as normofollicular, macrofollicular, microfollicular, and trabecular or solid.

Follicular carcinoma (FCa) of thyroid represents 10–15% of the thyroid cancers. They show typical follicular differentiation, lack of nuclear features of papillary carcinoma of thyroid, and capsular or vascular invasion. Capsular and vascular invasion are the two most important characteristics of FCa. Depending on the extent of such invasion FCa is divided into:

- Minimally invasive FCa
- Invasive FCa.

Minimally invasive FCa is a well-encapsulated tumor with partial infiltration of tumor cells in the capsule. In case of invasive FCa, the tumor extends entirely through the capsule and shows vascular invasion. The surrounding soft tissue may also be involved in invasive FCa.

Cytology (Figs. 26.17 to 26.19): FNAC smears show abundant cellularity with scanty colloid (Box 26.11). The cells are arranged in three-dimensional (3D) crowded groups, microfollicles, and trabeculae.[29] Colloid is thin and often present focally as dense droplets. The less the amount of colloid more should be the suspicion for FN. Macrofollicles always break down in small fragments in the aspirated material. However, architectural pattern of microfollicles are usually preserved in FNAC and its presence suggests the diagnosis of FN. In FNAC material, microfollicles are defined as small follicles composed of near about 15 cells and at least two-thirds of the circumference of them are covered by follicular cells.[30] Microfollicular pattern are also demonstrated in the hyperplastic nodular goiter and therefore the

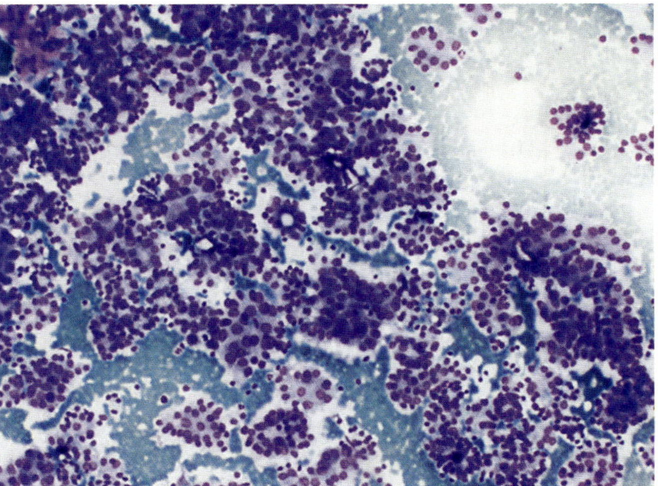

Fig. 26.17: Abundant discrete cells and follicles in follicular neoplasm (MGG × LP).

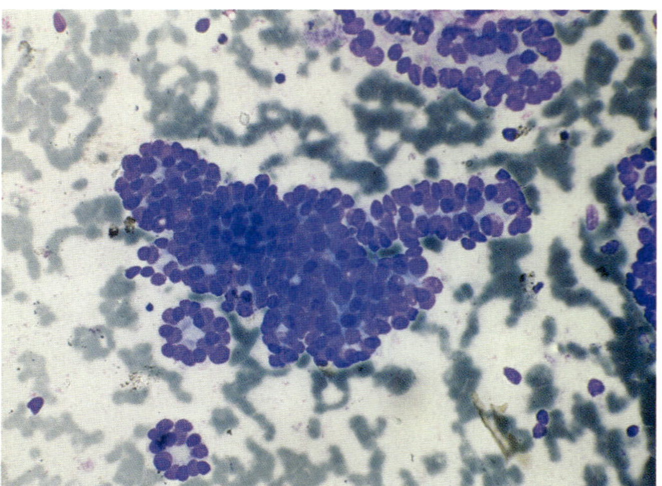

Fig. 26.18: Multiple microfollicles and solid sheets of cells in follicular neoplasm (MGG × MP).

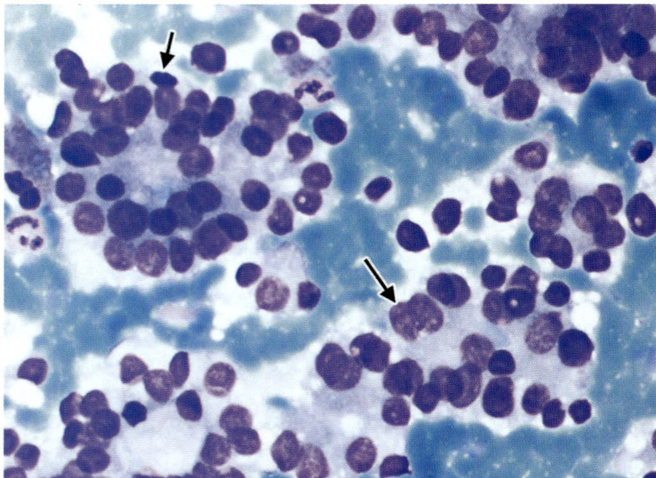

Fig. 26.19: Higher magnification showing microfollicles in follicular neoplasm of thyroid (*see* arrows) (MGG × HP).

Box 26.11: Follicular neoplasm.

- Abundant cellularity
- Scanty droplet-like dense colloid
- Microfollicles
- Three-dimensional crowded groups
- Trabeculae
- Cold nodule on scan
- Usually solitary nodule.

smear of FN should be carefully interpreted. In fact, as mentioned before colloid in FN is denser than that of nodular hyperplastic goiter. FN shows significant proportion of microfollicles with nuclear crowding and overlapping. Aspirate may show different types of changes such as:

- Cells with bizarre nuclei,
- Prominent Hürthle cell change,
- Papillary structures, and
- Signet ring cells.

It is truly not possible to differentiate FA and carcinoma on FNAC smears. However, high nucleocytoplasmic ratio, nuclear atypia, and coarse granular chromatin are suggestive of FCa.[24,27,31]

Without proper clinical history, aspirates of parathyroid adenoma can be mistakenly considered as FN. On cytomorphology alone it is very difficult to diagnose parathyroid adenoma. However, absence of colloid, abundant clear cells, and history of hypercalcemia should raise the suspicion of parathyroid adenoma. In doubtful situation immunocytochemistry may be helpful to confirm the diagnosis of parathyroid adenoma. The cells of parathyroid adenomas are thyroglobulin negative, parathormone positive, and chromogranin positive.

Table 26.2: Distinguishing features of follicular neoplasm and follicular variant of papillary carcinoma.

Features	*Follicular neoplasm*	*Follicular variant of papillary carcinoma*
Colloid	Scanty dense droplet like	Thick ropy colloid
Thyroid cells arrangement	Abundant microfollicles, 3D clusters, trabeculae	Microfollicles and discrete cells
Nuclear grooving	Absent	Present
Chromatin	Evenly dispersed fine nuclear chromatin in adenoma to coarse chromatin	Fine powdery chromatin; nuclear clearing present
Intranuclear inclusion	Absent	Present
Psammoma body and multinucleated giant cells	Absent	Present
RET-PTC oncogenic transformation	Absent	Present

Follicular variant of papillary carcinoma also shows multiple microfollicles and may pose diagnostic problem with FN. The diagnostic clues of follicular variant of papillary carcinoma in aspirates are chewing gum-like colloid, nuclear grooving, and intranuclear pseudoinclusion (Table 26.2).[32]

Diagnostic Difficulties

- Follicular hyperplasia versus neoplasm
- Follicular adenoma versus carcinoma
- Parathyroid adenoma
- Follicular variant of papillary carcinoma.

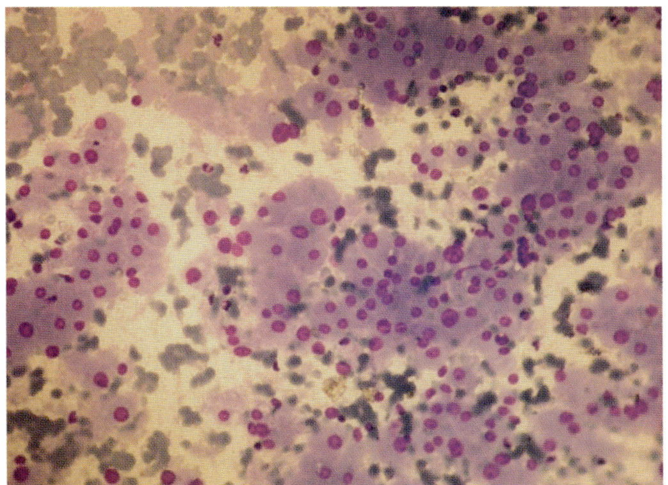

Fig. 26.20: Abundant discrete Hürthle cells in Hürthle cell neoplasm of thyroid (MGG × MP).

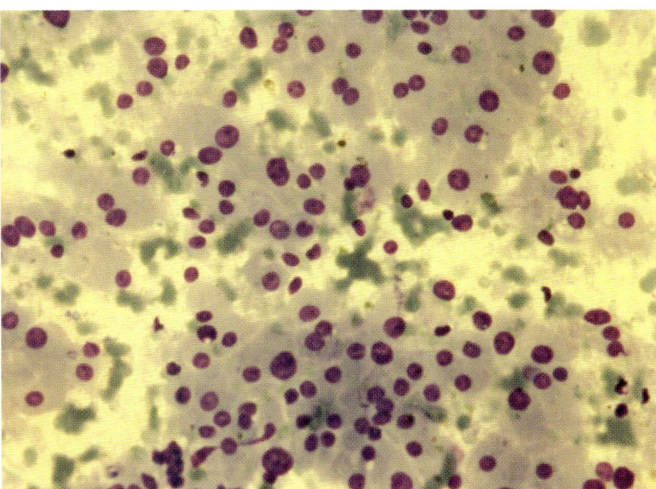

Fig. 26.21: Large cells with abundant eosinophilic granular cytoplasm in Hürthle cell neoplasm of thyroid (MGG × HP).

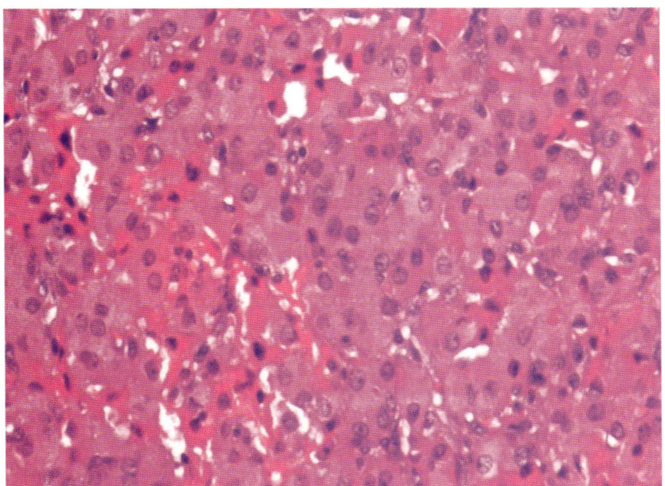

Fig. 26.22: Histopathology of the above case of Hürthle cell adenoma (H & E × MP).

Box 26.12: Oncocytes (Hürthle cell) in thyroid.

- Large cells with abundant deeply eosinophilic granular cytoplasm
- Enlarged round to oval nucleus with a prominent nucleolus
- Rich in mitochondria
- Positive for GLUT-4, CK14, thyroglobulin.

Noted in:

- Hürthle cell neoplasm
- Lymphocytic thyroiditis
- Nodular goiter.

Box 26.13: Hürthle cell neoplasm.

- Multiple clusters and dissociated Hürthle cells
- Enlarged nuclei with prominent macronucleoli
- Colloid is scanty to absent.

Hürthle Cell Neoplasm

Hürthle cell tumor as a distinct separate entity is controversial. WHO recognized this entity only as oncocytic subset of FNs.[33]

Hürthle cell tumor represents 3–5% of all thyroid tumors and is classified as Hürthle cell adenoma and carcinoma. The mean age of the patient is about 50 years. The same histological criteria of FCa are also applied for Hürthle cell carcinoma. The term oncocytes are preferable than "Hürthle cell". These are large cells with abundant deeply eosinophilic granular cytoplasm. This granularity of the cytoplasm is due to accumulation of mitochondria. The oncocytes are positive for thyroglobulin, CK14, and glucose transporter-4 (GLUT-4).[34-36]

Cytology (Figs. 26.20 to 26.22): Aspirates of Hürthle cell neoplasm show abundant dissociated oncocytes (Box 26.12). The cells are polygonal, large with abundant eosinophilic cytoplasm having centrally placed enlarged nuclei. The nuclei of the cell show prominent nucleoli and macronucleoli. The Hürthle cells are polygonal, large cells with abundant eosinophilic granular cytoplasm.[37,38] The nuclei are eccentric in position, enlarged with prominent nucleoli (Box 26.13). Variable degree of cellular atypia may be noted in Hürthle cells in the form of nuclear enlargement, binucleation, and multinucleation. Colloid is scanty to absent. Chronic LT may often show marked Hürthle cell changes. Markedly pleomorphic Hürthle cells with background lymphocytes should always raise the possibility of

Table 26.3: Differential diagnosis of Hürthle cell tumor and lymphocytic thyroiditis.

Features	*Hürthle cell tumor*	*Lymphocytic thyroiditis*
• Lesion • Hormonal status • Antithyroid antibodies	• Solitary nodule • Euthyroid • Absent	• Diffuse • Hypothyroid • Present
• Colloid • Hürthle cell • Pleomorphism • Nucleoli • Normal follicular cells • Lymphocytes and plasma cells	• Absent • Abundant • Monomorphic • Macronucleoli • Scanty to absent • Scanty to none	• Scanty • Variable • Pleomorphic • Nucleoli present • Present • Present

LT (Table 26.3). It has been suggested that intracytoplasmic lumen and transgressing vessels are also diagnostic features of Hürthle cell neoplasm.[39] Hürthle cell neoplasm often mimic as medullary carcinoma because both the tumors show dissociated cells with plasmacytoid appearance. However, the cells of medullary carcinoma show reddish granular cytoplasm and they usually do not have prominent nucleoli (Table 26.4). Moreover, Hürthle cell neoplasm is negative for calcitonin stain.

Immunocytochemistry: The Hürthle cells are positive for thyroglobulin, CK14, TTF, GLUT-4 and negative for calcitonin.

Diagnostic Difficulties

- Lymphocytic thyroiditis
- Hürthle cells in colloid goiter
- *Medullary thyroid carcinoma*: Both medullary thyroid carcinoma and Hürthle cell neoplasm show the presence of single cells and plasmacytoid appearance. Prominent nucleoli are the important distinguishing feature of Hürthle cell neoplasm.

Hyalinizing Trabecular Adenoma

Hyalinizing trabecular adenoma is a type of follicular cell neoplasm that exhibits trabecular arrangement of cells and prominent hyaline appearance. The hyaline is accumulated both intra- and extracellularly.

Cytology[40]

Fine needle aspiration cytology smears show cohesive clusters and dissociated tumor cells. The tumor cells are arranged radially in cohesive groups around hyaline material. The cells are round and monomorphic in appearance with abundant cytoplasm. The cytoplasm contains round paranuclear spherical body that stains purple-gray with MGG stain. Nuclei of the cells are single, moderately large, and round, oval, polygonal, or spindled. The nucleocytoplasmic ratio is low. The intranuclear inclusions are seen frequently. Multiple intranuclear inclusions may cause nuclear enlargement and distortion. Intranuclear longitudinal grooves are also noted and may simulate papillary thyroid carcinoma (PTC).

Table 26.4: Medullary carcinoma versus Hürthle cell tumor.

Feature	*Hürthle cell tumor*	*Medullary carcinoma*
Cytoplasmic granularity	Bluish granules	Reddish granules
Nucleoli	Large, prominent	Indistinct
Calcitonin	Negative	Positive
CK14	Positive	Negative

Background of the smear shows abundant extracellular, dense, lumpy, and usually structureless material. The material stains pink with MGG and turquoise blue with Papanicolaou stain. This hyaline material may simulate amyloid material.

Differential Diagnosis

- Papillary carcinoma of thyroid.

Papillary Carcinoma

Papillary thyroid carcinoma is the most common thyroid tumor and represents about 60–80% of thyroid cancers. PTC is commonly noted in the age group of 30–50 years; however, no age is exempted from this tumor and this is the most common malignancy of thyroid in the pediatric age. Females are more often affected than male, and female:male ratio is 4:1. This tumor commonly spreads to the cervical lymph node. Occasionally the patient may present with palpable cervical lymph node as the only initial manifestation of the tumor. The prognosis of PTC is excellent and overall 5 year survival rate is 80%.[41] The exact etiology of PTC is unknown. However, it has been noted that excess iodine intake in the diet increased the risk of PTC. External radiation of neck region also increases the chance of PTC. The incidence of PTC was 100-folds greater in the atom bomb survivors and after Chernobyl accident of the atomic reactor in Ukraine.

Somatic *RET/PTC* gene rearrangements occurs in 20–40% cases of PTC and creates a chimeric RET/PTC fusion oncogene. Here, entire RET tyrosine domain fuses with other genes to form this fusion gene.[42] Till now a total of 17 chimeric fusion genes have been identified with fusion of RET and other 12 genes. RET/PTC rearrangements can be demonstrated by reverse transcriptase-polymerase chain reaction (RT-PCR) or fluorescence in situ hybridization (FISH). The point mutation of BRAF gene is detected in 30–70% of PTC.[43] This particular mutation is associated with aggressive clinical behavior of PTC. RAS mutation is infrequent in PTC and is commonly noted in FN.[44]

Cytology (Figs. 26.23 to 26.29)

Arrangement: PTC shows multiple papillary structures, 3D clusters, and occasional discrete cells (Box 26.14). The papillae with central fibrovascular core are uncommonly seen[45] because the structures may be too big to come in the aspiration needle. The peripheral arrangement of cells in a papillary cluster is perpendicular to the inner layer of cells. Most of the time, the fragments or tip of the papillae is seen as 3D clusters of cells. The nuclei of the cells show crowding and overlapping.

Colloid: Colloid is scanty and round to oval dense hyperchromatic. In MGG smear the colloid is seen as dark magenta colored material. At times colloid is present as ropy streaks connecting clusters of cells. This is also mentioned as "bubble gum" colloid.[17]

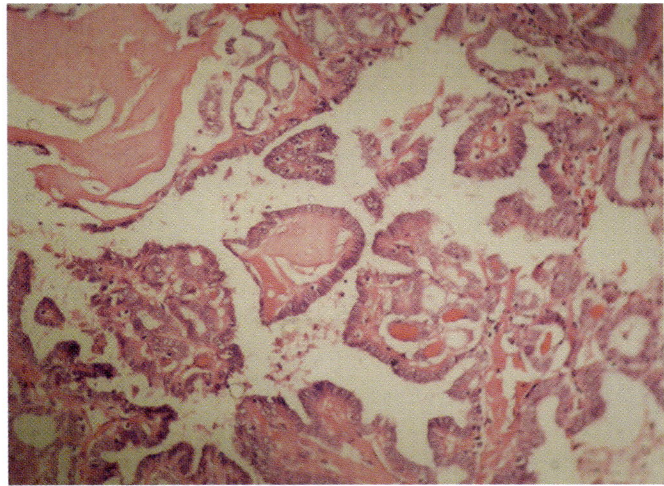

Fig. 26.23: Papillary carcinoma of thyroid: Histopathology section shows multiple papillae with fibrovascular core (H & E × MP).

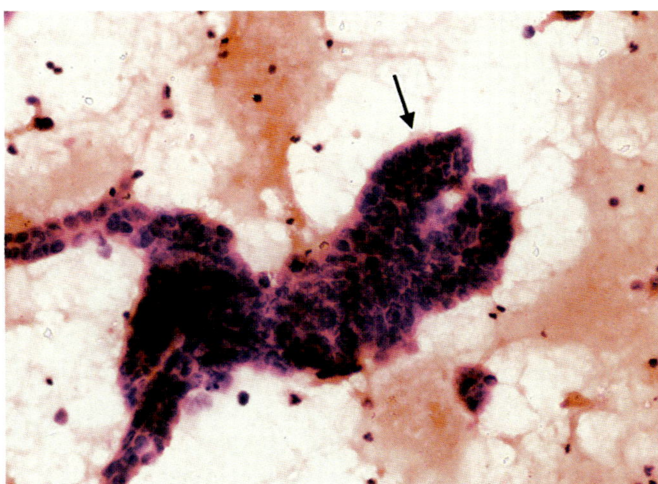

Fig. 26.24: Papillary carcinoma of thyroid: Papillary cluster of cells (*see* arrow) (H & E × MP).

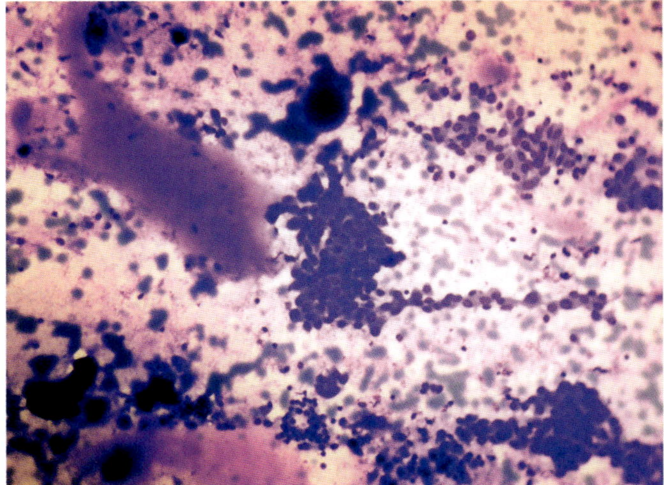

Fig. 26.25: Papillary carcinoma of thyroid: Clusters and dissociated cells in the background of chewing gum-like thick colloid (MGG × MP).

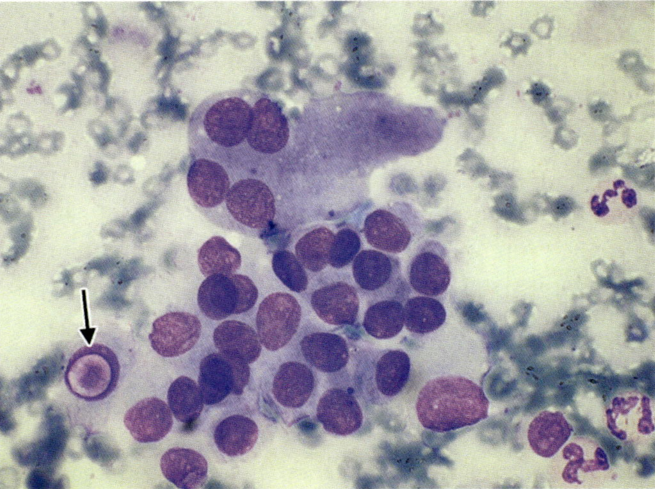

Fig. 26.26: Papillary carcinoma of thyroid: Prominent intranuclear pseudoinclusion (MGG × HP). The arrow indicates intranuclear pseudoinclusion.

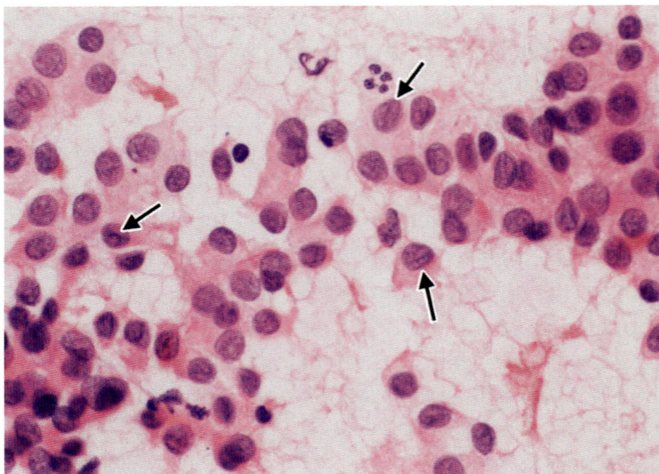

Fig. 26.27: Nuclear groove in papillary carcinoma of thyroid (H & E × HP). The arrows indicate nuclear grooves.

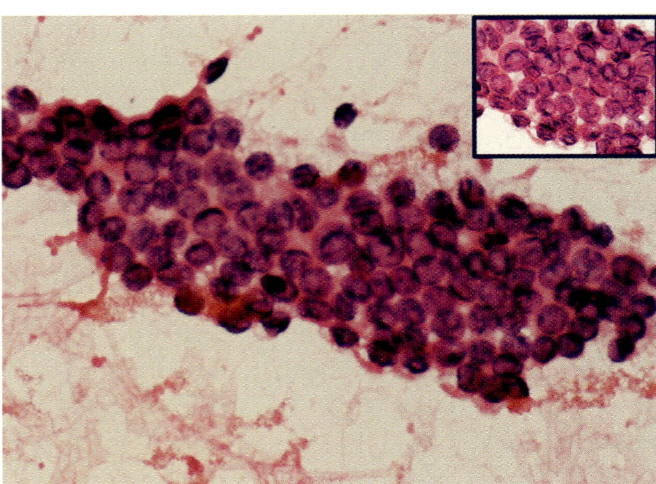

Fig. 26.28: Papillary carcinoma of thyroid: Nuclear clearing (inset showing higher magnification) (H & E × HP).

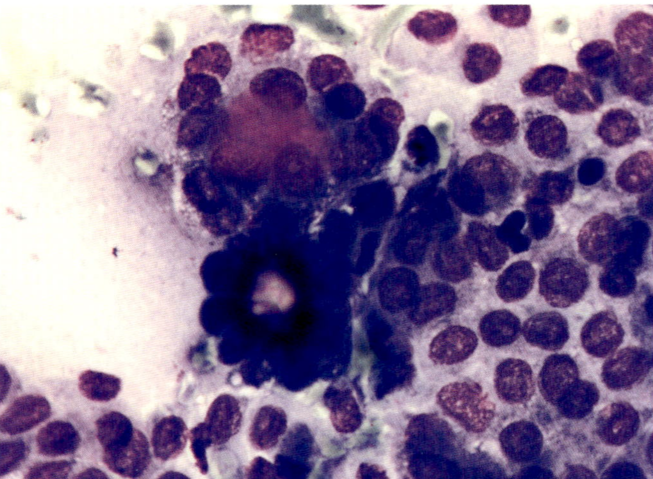

Fig. 26.29: Concentric lamellated psammoma body in papillary carcinoma of thyroid (MGG × HP).

Cell cytoplasm: Individual cells in PTC are oval with moderate amount of cytoplasm and well-defined cell border. The cytoplasm of the cell is often dense granular and appears like squamous cell. Cytoplasm with fine granularity resembles oncocytes. In case of cystic PTC, there may be significant clearing of the cytoplasm giving rise to clear cell appearance. These cells may be confused with histiocytes in cystic goiter.

Nucleus: Nuclei of the cells in PTC are enlarged and mild pleomorphic. The nuclei show pale chromatin and small eccentric nucleoli. The characteristics nuclear morphology of PTC is:

Box 26.14: Papillary carcinoma.

- Papillary arrangement
- Intranuclear grooves
- Intranuclear pseudoinclusions
- Optically clear nucleus
- Thick chewing gum-like ropy colloid
- Psammoma bodies
- Multinucleated giant cells
- Histiocytes and lymphocytes.

- *Optically clear nucleus*: The nucleus of PTC shows pale, fine, and powdery chromatin. This type of nucleus in alcohol-fixed smear gives the so called "Orphan Annie-eye" or optically clear appearance. Exact molecular etiology of the optically clear nucleus is not known. Probably RET oncogene expression is responsible for this change.
- *Intranuclear groove*: It is due to the deep longitudinal folding of the nuclear membrane parallel to the long axis of the nuclei. This is well appreciated in Papanicolaou's stained smear. Nuclear groove is a nonspecific finding but it is a useful diagnostic feature when detected in an enlarged nucleus with pale chromatin.
- *Intranuclear pseudoinclusion*: The intranuclear pseudoinclusions represent the cytoplasmic invaginations within the nucleus. They are also seen in more than 90% of PTC. Intranuclear inclusions are best seen in Papanicolaou's or H & E (hematoxylin and eosin) stained smear. The major characteristics of intranuclear pseudoinclusion are:
  - Large membrane bound structure
  - Condensed outer rim of chromatin

Box 26.15: Psammoma body.

Appearance: Round, concentric, lamellated, and calcified structures.
Pathogenesis:
- Dystrophic calcification
- Thrombosis and focal necrosis of tips of papillae followed by calcification

Incidence in papillary thyroid carcinoma: 10–35% cases
Other thyroid lesions with psammoma bodies: Nodular goiter and Hashimoto's thyroiditis
Differential diagnosis:
- Thick colloid
- Calcified material.

Psammoma bodies noted in diseases other than thyroid:
- Meningioma
- Papillary cystic adenocarcinoma of ovary
- Chromophobe renal cell carcinoma
- Psammoma carcinoma of the peritoneum
- Cholangiocarcinoma.

- Clear than the surrounding chromatin
- Identical tinctorial color of the cytoplasm.

The other structures which can be mistaken as intranuclear pseudoinclusions are: (1) nucleoli and (2) overlapping RBC on the nucleus.[46] Intranuclear inclusions are not specific for PTC and can be seen in other neoplastic and nonneoplastic conditions of thyroid such as hyalinizing trabecular adenoma, medullary carcinoma, Hürthle cell tumor, LT, and nodular goiter.

Giant cells: Multinucleated giant cells are frequently noted in PTC. These cells are huge with homogenous cytoplasm and contain multiple nuclei. Multinucleated giant cells in PTC are positive for CD68 immunostaining. These are histiocytes and not tumor cell.[47]

Psammoma bodies (Box 26.15): Psammoma bodies (PBs) are round, concentric, lamellated, and calcified structures. In cytology smear they are 50–70 micron size, round shaped, glassy in look and take dark blue to black color in MGG staining and brown to black color in Papanicolaou's stained smear.

There are many theories of pathogenesis of PB formation. It was considered that in the process of dystrophic calcification, the necrotic tumor cells act as seed around which minerals are deposited in a concentric manner.[48] LiVolsi et al. suggested that true PBs are formed due to focal areas of infraction in tips of the papillae because of thrombosis of the small vessels. However, these are different from dystrophic calcification as they are irregular or jagged and rarely show lamellations.[49] Based on detailed ultrastructural studies of PB, Johannessen and Sobrinho-simoes[50] suggested that PB may be due to: (1) thickening of the basal lamina of the small vessels leading to thrombosis, calcification, and necrosis; and (2) necrosis and calcification of the intralymphatic tumor thrombi in adjacent nontumor thyroid areas.

The presence of PBs in the aspirate is pathognomonic for PTC. FNAC smears of 11–35% cases of PTC show PBs.[51] PBs are particularly helpful in the diagnosis of cystic papillary carcinoma. It has been recommended that the presence of PBs in FNAC of solitary thyroid nodule should have surgical excision of the thyroid due to high risk of malignancy.[52]

Psammoma bodies should be distinguished from the inspissated colloid and calcified material due to degenerative changes in thyroid. It is important to note that PBs are also found in nodular goiter and LT.[53]

Macrophages and lymphocytes: These cells are also noted in the aspirates of PTC in variable amount. Macrophages are usually abundant in PTC with cystic changes. Lymphocytes and occasional plasma cells may also be seen in PTC and their presence may lead to the false negative diagnosis of lymphocytic thyroiditis.

A combination of cytological features is needed to diagnose a case of PTC. The nuclear features are the most important among all the other diagnostic criteria of PTC. In the NCI sponsored symposium on cytology, in 2007 some major diagnostic criteria of PTC have been recommended as:[25]

The *major diagnostic criteria of PTC* include:
- Enlarged, oval "irregular" nucleus
- Eccentric and often multiple micronucleoli
- Fine, pale chromatin
- Longitudinal nuclear grooves
- Intranuclear pseudoinclusions.

Similarly, the *minor diagnostic criteria of PTC* include:
- Papillary cytoarchitecture
- Syncytial monolayers
- Squamoid cytoplasm
- Psammoma bodies
- Multinucleated giant cells
- Histiocytoid cells and cellular swirls.

Variants of Papillary Carcinoma of Thyroid

There are several variants of papillary carcinoma of thyroid which are often encountered in routine reporting. These cases are difficult to diagnose on cytology alone. The salient cytological features of these variants are described below:[32,54-58]

Follicular variant of papillary carcinoma of thyroid (FVPCT)[32,55] *(Figs. 26.30 to 26.32)*: This is one of the common

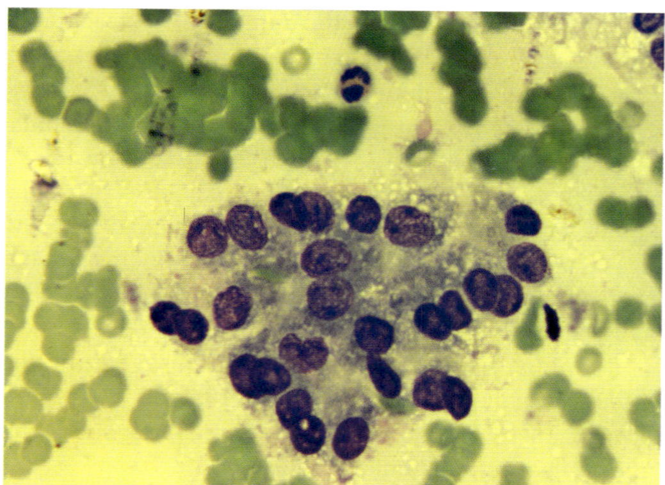

Fig. 26.30: Follicular variant of papillary carcinoma of thyroid: Follicles lined by cells with nuclear groove (MGG × HP).

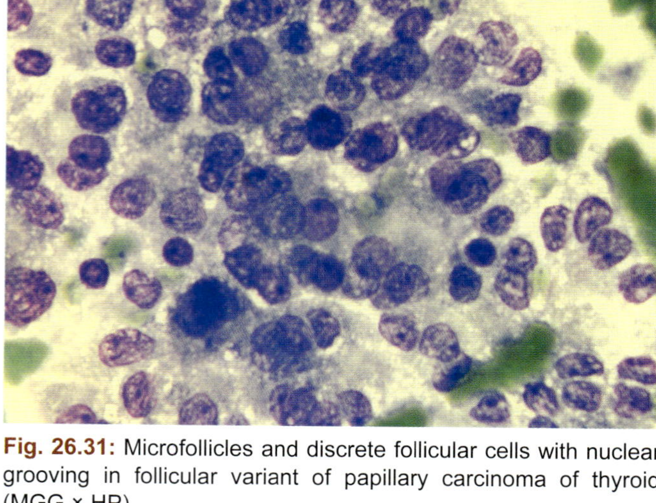

Fig. 26.31: Microfollicles and discrete follicular cells with nuclear grooving in follicular variant of papillary carcinoma of thyroid (MGG × HP).

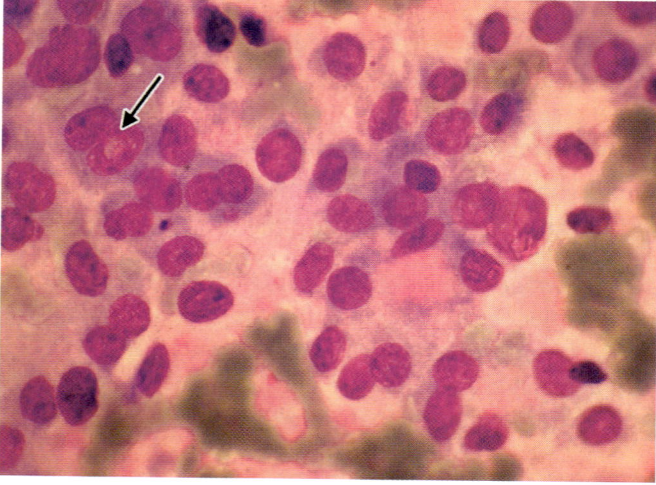

Fig. 26.32: Higher magnification showing intranuclear inclusion and grooving in follicular variant of papillary carcinoma of thyroid (MGG × OI).

variants of PTC. Typical papillary arrangement of the cells is missing in this variety and the smears show large number of microfollicles. The exact diagnosis largely depends on the identification of the nuclear features. Cytology smears of FVPCT are often misdiagnosed as follicular neoplasia and this tumor is the most common cause of false negative diagnosis of PTC. Characteristically the aspirate shows multiple follicles and also syncytial-like cells (Box 26.16). Individual cells usually show nuclear features of PTC which is very important to recognize. Chewing gum-like thick colloid is seen in the background. Rarely multinucleated giant cells and PB are noted.

Box 26.16: Follicular variant of papillary carcinoma of thyroid.

- Large number of microfollicles
- Nuclear features of papillary thyroid carcinoma
- Chewing gum-like thick colloid
- Rarely multinucleated giant cells and psammoma body.

Differential diagnosis: Follicular neoplasia.

Cystic papillary carcinoma: It is not in fact a true variant of PTC. PTC often undergoes extensive cystic changes and aspirate yields fluid. The smears show occasional papillae. Large number of foamy histiocytes is seen along with loose clusters and discrete tumor cells. The individual cells show characteristic nuclear features of PTC. Cystic PTC is one of the common sources of false negative diagnosis.

Tall cell variant[54] *(Figs. 26.33 and 26.34)*: This is an aggressive variant of PTC with poor clinical outcome. The tumor commonly affects older patient. The cytology smear shows large number of tall columnar looking cells with abundant eosinophilic cytoplasm resembling oncocytic cells. The cell in tall cell variant should be three times tall as they are wide. Nuclei of the cells are basally placed and show features of papillary carcinoma of thyroid (Box 26.17). Moderate amount of lymphocytes may be seen in the background of the smear. Tall cell variant of PTC is difficult to recognize on the cytology smears.

Columnar cell variant: In case of columnar cell variant the smears show crowded, stratified clusters of elongated cells with cigar-shaped nuclei. The cells are tall columnar with scanty cytoplasm. The nuclei are cigar shaped, hyperchromatic, monomorphic in appearance with indistinct

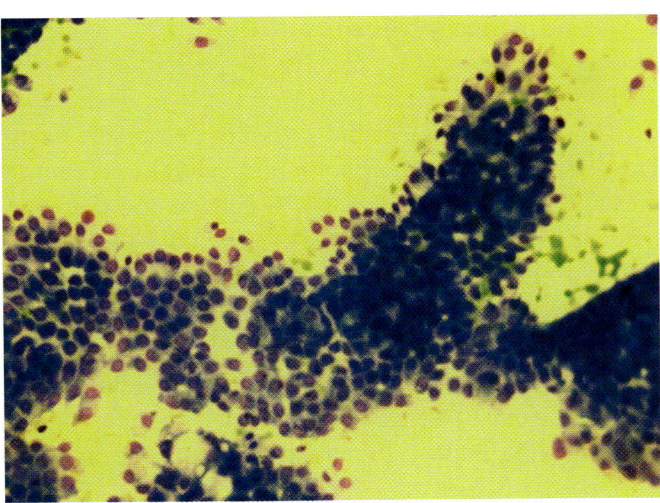

Fig. 26.33: Tall cell variant of papillary carcinoma of thyroid: Papillary clusters of tall cells (MGG × MP).

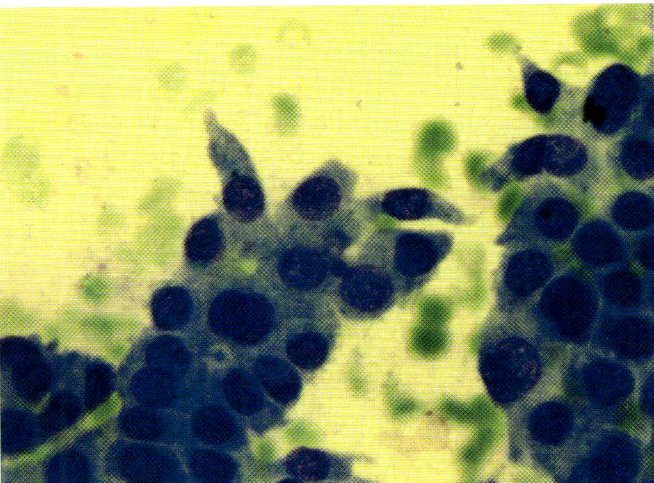

Fig. 26.34: Tall cell variant of papillary carcinoma of thyroid: Higher magnification showing tall cell (MGG × OI).

Box 26.17: Tall cell variant.

- Large numbers of tall columnar cells
- Abundant eosinophilic cytoplasm
- Are basally placed nuclei
- Lymphocytes
- Nuclear features of papillary thyroid carcinoma.

Box 26.18: Diffuse sclerosing variants.

- Syncytial clusters of cells having typical nuclear features of papillary thyroid carcinoma
- Abundant psammoma bodies
- Metaplastic squamous cells.
- Dense lymphocytic infiltrate.

nucleoli. Unlike tall cell variant, these cells are taller; cytoplasm is scanty, and lack classical nuclear features of PTC.

Diffuse sclerosing variants:[58] This is a relatively uncommon variant of PTC and usually occurs in younger patients. PTC is noted within the dense fibrous stroma. The smears characteristically show syncytial clusters of tumor cells in the background of scattered lymphocytes (Box 26.18). Squamous metaplastic cells and abundant PBs are also noted.

Oncocytic variant: This is also a relatively uncommon variant of PTC. FNAC smears show abundant oncocyte-like cells in clusters, follicular, and papillary arrangement (Box 26.19). The individual cells show abundant eosinophilic granular cytoplasm. This granularity is caused by mitochondrial proliferation. The nuclei of the cells show features of PTC. This variant comes in differential diagnosis of oncocytic variant of PTC, Hürthle cell tumor, and medullary carcinoma.

Warthin-like papillary thyroid carcinoma: In this tumor, the cytology smear shows papillary clusters of oncocyte-like cells along with discrete lymphocytes and plasma cells. The tumor cells show classical nuclear features of malignancy. The FNAC smears of this entity may often be misdiagnosed as lymphocytic thyroiditis. However, the nuclear features of PTC are helpful in diagnosis.

Box 26.19: Oncocytic variant.

- Cell in clusters, papillae, and discrete
- Abundant eosinophilic granular cytoplasm
- Nuclear features of papillary thyroid carcinoma.

Differential Diagnosis

- Chronic lymphocytic thyroiditis
- *Hyalinizing trabecular adenoma*: The frequent nuclear grooves and intranuclear pseudoinclusion in hyalinizing trabecular adenoma may be misinterpreted as PTC.

Differential Diagnosis of Variants of Papillary Carcinomas

- FN versus FVPCT
- Lymphocytic thyroiditis versus diffuse sclerosing variants of PTC.

Medullary Carcinoma

Medullary carcinoma (MC) represents almost 10% of thyroid carcinomas. The tumor is composed of parafollicular or C cell of thyroid and shows neuroendocrine morphology. The majority of the MC is sporadic and do not show any association with age or sex. Approximately one-fourth of MC is inherited and is related with multiple endocrine neoplasia (MEN) syndrome 2A and 2B. Majority of MC (90%) secretes calcitonin hormone and therefore serum estimation of calcitonin may be used as a screening test of MC. The tumor metastasizes to the regional cervical lymph node and occasionally the patient first time presents with an enlarged lymph node. Therefore, MC may come in the differential diagnosis of positive lymph nodal mass with unknown primary.

Cytology[59-62] *(Figs. 26.35 to 26.42)*: Aspirates of MC show predominantly dissociated cell population (Box 26.20). Occasional loose syncytial aggregates or follicular pattern may be present. Three types of cells are present:

1. Round plasmacytoid cells
2. Spindle cells
3. Polygonal cells.

The round plasmacytoid cells are commonly seen. The cells have monomorphic round central to eccentric nuclei. Cytoplasmic border is well defined and there are reddish granules in the cytoplasm. The nuclei have stippled chromatin giving salt and pepper appearance like that of neuroendocrine tumor. Polygonal angulated cells have well-defined reddish cytoplasm. These cells resemble oncocytes. The third cell types are spindle-shaped cells with elongated cigar-shaped nuclei. The presence of predominant spindle cells may create diagnostic difficulty

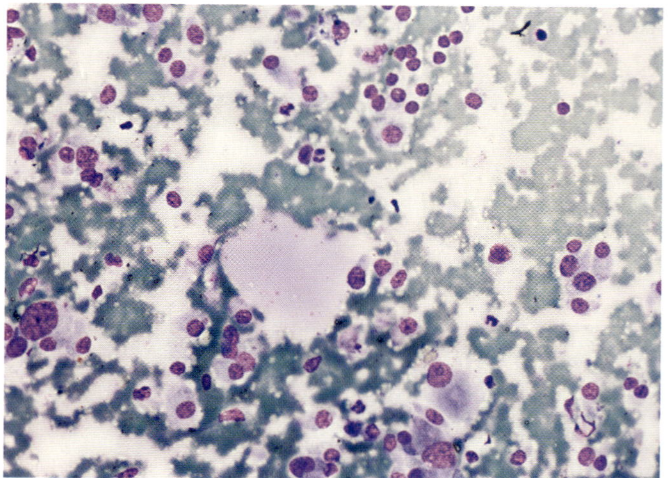

Fig. 26.35: Discrete cells in medullary carcinoma of thyroid (MGG × MP).

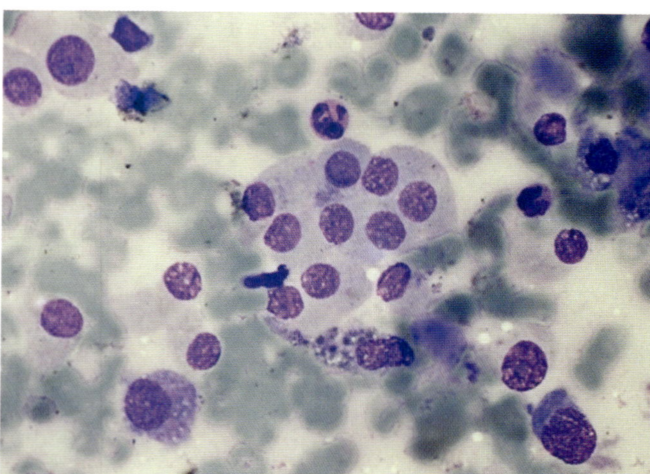

Fig. 26.36: Round cells with moderate amount of cytoplasm having eccentric nuclei in medullary carcinoma of thyroid (MGG × MP).

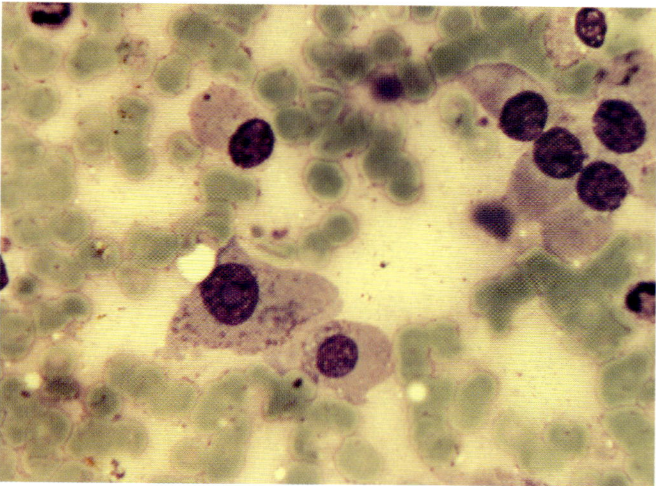

Fig. 26.37: Medullary carcinoma of thyroid: Large polygonal cells (MGG × HP).

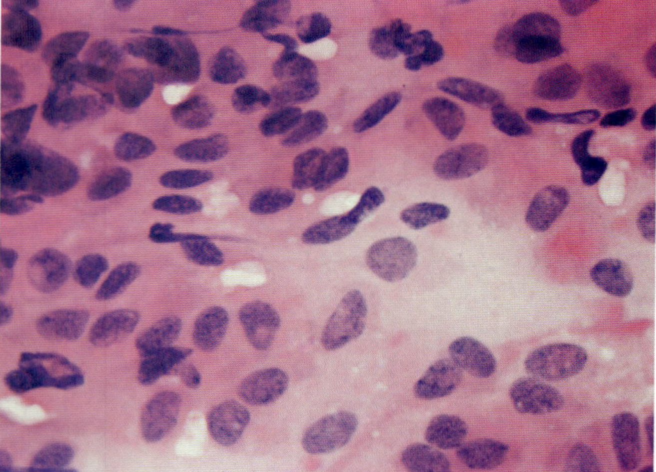

Fig. 26.38: Medullary carcinoma of thyroid: Many spindle cells (H & E × MP).

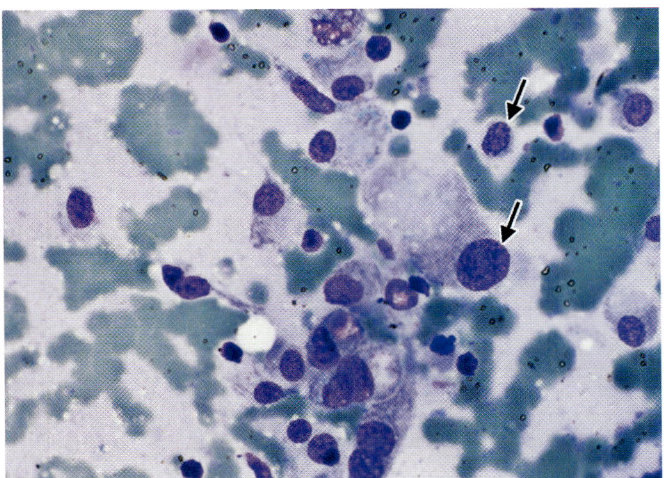

Fig. 26.39: Medullary carcinoma of thyroid: Cells with stippled nuclear chromatin are indicated by arrows (MGG × HP).

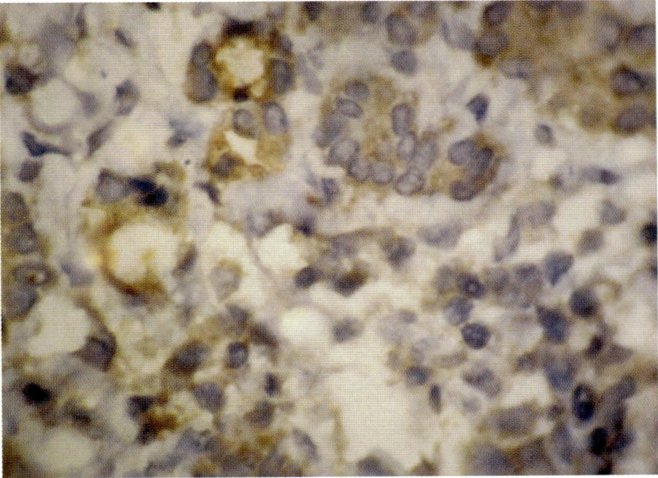

Fig. 26.40: Calcitonin positivity in medullary carcinoma of thyroid (immunostain × HP).

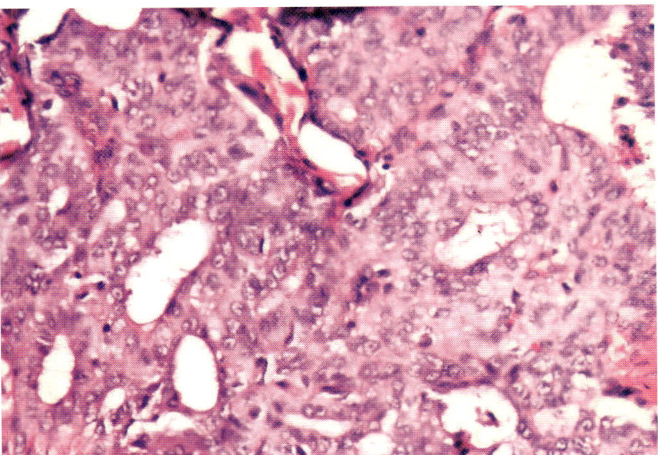

Fig. 26.41: Histopathology section of medullary carcinoma of thyroid (H & E × HP).

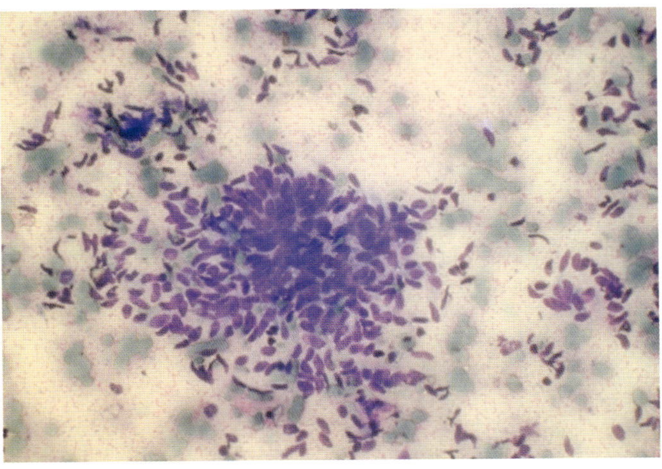

Fig. 26.42: Predominantly spindle cells in medullary carcinoma of thyroid (MGG × HP).

Box 26.20: Cytological features of medullary carcinoma.

- Predominantly dissociated cells.
- Cells
  - Round plasmacytoid cells
  - Spindle cells
  - Polygonal cells
    - Reddish granular cytoplasm
    - Salt and pepper chromatin
    - Amorphous acellular pinkish amyloid material
    - Squamous cells, small cells, clear cells.

Immunocytochemistry: Positive for calcitonin, chromogranin, and synaptophysin.

with fibroblastic tumor. These cells show less nuclear pleomorphism and rarely may have small nucleoli. In addition, uncommonly squamous cells, small cells, and clear cells may also be seen. Majority of times, mixed population of cells or plasmacytoid cells are present. Occasional intranuclear pseudoinclusion and multinucleated giant cells in MC may be noted.

Pale blue amorphous and acellular amyloid material is seen in 80% of MC cases. Amyloid is round or string like with smooth edged and fibrillar in appearance. This amyloid is present discretely in the smear or may be surrounded by tumor cells. At times, it is difficult to differentiate amyloid from colloid on routine MGG smear. However, amyloid is round with smooth demarcated margin and fibrillar in contrast to cracking artifact and sharp angulated edges of colloid. Special stain such as Congo red stain may be needed to confirm the presence of amyloid. Amyloid shows apple green birefringence in polarized light when stained by alkaline Congo red.

Immunocytochemistry

- Calcitonin positivity is specific of MC.
- Cells of MC are also positive for neuroendocrine markers such as chromogranin, NSE, and synaptophysin.
- Positive for CEA.
- Negative for thyroglobulin.

Differential Diagnosis

- Hürthle cell neoplasm
- Papillary carcinoma of thyroid
- Follicular neoplasm
- Metastatic tumors such as malignant melanoma, plasmacytoma, neuroendocrine carcinoma.

Anaplastic Carcinoma

This is a highly aggressive malignant tumor of thyroid and represents less than 5% of thyroid carcinoma.[33] This is commonly found in the elderly patient (average age 65 year) and is very uncommon under the age of 50 year. In majority of the cases the patient gives a history of preexisting colloid goiter, FCa, or PTC.

Cytology (Figs. 26.43 and 26.44)

On histology anaplastic carcinoma is of two types. The first type is totally undifferentiated without any follicular, trabecular, or nest. However, the epithelial nature of this tumor is evident. The tumor shows squamoid differentiation sand keratinization. In other type, the tumor gives sarcomatoid appearance and is composed of spindle cells and giant cells. There are large areas of polymorphonuclear leucocytic infiltration in the tumor. Osteoid, cartilaginous and skeletal muscle differentiation is seen.

Cytology picture of anaplastic carcinoma mainly depends on its histological subtype.

Anaplastic carcinoma of thyroid shows necrosis along with loose clusters and discrete malignant cells and polymorphonuclear leucocytes (Box 26.21). The tumor cells are large with markedly pleomorphic bizarre nuclei having irregular nuclear margin and single to multiple nucleoli. Many multinucleated cells are seen. The tumor cells may show neutrophilic cannibalism. Occasionally the smear may show predominant spindle cell population with moderate pleomorphism. Osteoclast-like giant cells, chondroid, and osseous material may also be noted.[63] Marked background necrosis and leucocytes infiltration may obscure the malignant cells and the

Box 26.21: Cytological features of anaplastic carcinoma.

- Necrosis
- Polymorphs
- Discrete large pleomorphic tumor cell
- Prominent nucleoli, irregular membrane
- Neutrophil cannibalism
- Spindle cells
- Squamous cells
- Multinucleated giant cells.

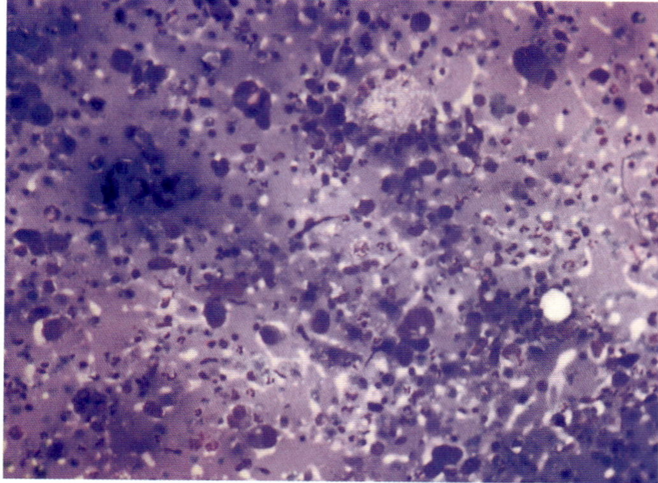

Fig. 26.43: Many discrete malignant cells in a necrotic background in anaplastic carcinoma of thyroid (MGG × MP).

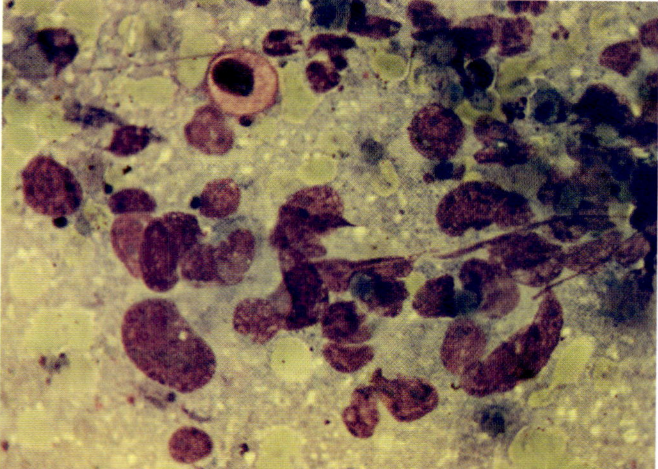

Fig. 26.44: Malignant cells have enlarged moderately pleomorphic nuclei in anaplastic carcinoma of thyroid (MGG × HP).

tumor may rarely be missed as acute thyroiditis. If there is any suspicion of underlying tumor, then a repeat FNAC is mandatory. Predominant population of spindle cells in anaplastic carcinoma may pose diagnostic difficulty with MC, fibrosarcoma, or hemangioendothelioma. The associated large bizarre cells and background necrosis may be helpful in the diagnosis of anaplastic carcinoma. In difficult situation, immunocytochemistry in the cell block preparation is always helpful.

Immunocytochemistry

The cells are negative for thyroglobulin and positive for vimentin.

Differential Diagnosis

- Acute thyroiditis
- Spindle cell variant of medullary carcinoma
- *Other sarcomas*: Fibrosarcoma, malignant hemangio-endothelioma, etc.
- Metastatic giant cell tumors from lung.

Insular Carcinoma

Insular carcinoma (IC) is a poorly differentiated carcinoma and represents 4–7% of all thyroid carcinoma.[64] The cell of origin of insular carcinoma is follicular cells of thyroid. It commonly occurs in elderly patient. The biological behavior of insular carcinoma is intermediate between well-differentiated carcinoma and undifferentiated carcinoma. Distant metastasis of this tumor is common at the time of first presentation. The 5 year survival rate is 50%.

Cytology (Figs. 26.45 to 26.48)

On histology insular carcinoma shows insular pattern of growth and solid to microfollicular arrangement. In insular type of growth, the small round tumor cells are arranged as nests surrounded by thin fibrovascular septae. The tumor cell may also be arranged in solid sheets to varying amount of small microfollicles.

Cytology smears of insular carcinoma shows predominantly discrete cells. Depending on histological type variable amount of microfollicles and clusters of cells are seen. The tumor cells are round to oval with scanty to moderate cytoplasm and often give rise to plasmacytoid appearance (Box 26.22).[65-67] The nuclei are monomorphic, round with regular nuclear margin and inconspicuous nucleoli. Nuclear grooves and intranuclear pseudoinclusions are also noted and may simulate PTC. On cytology smear, it is difficult to diagnose insular carcinoma with confidence. Microfollicular pattern present in insular carcinoma may simulate FN.

Immunocytochemistry

Insular carcinoma is positive for thyroglobulin and TTF-1 and negative for calcitonin.

Differential Diagnosis

- Papillary thyroid carcinoma
- Follicular neoplasm.

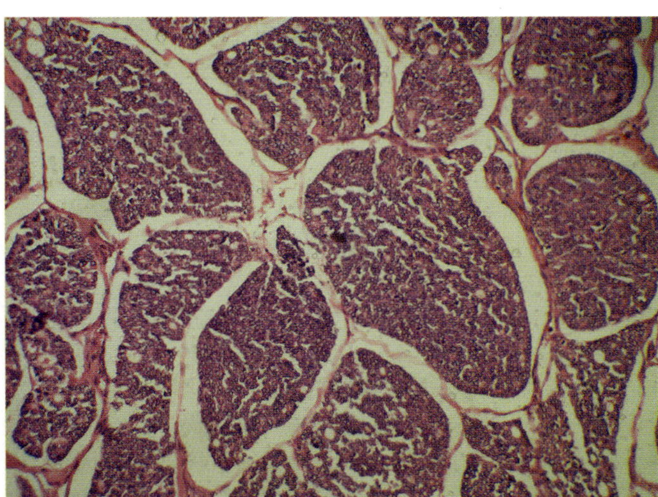

Fig. 26.45: Histopathology of insular carcinoma of thyroid showing large nests of cells separated by fibrous septae (H & E × MP).

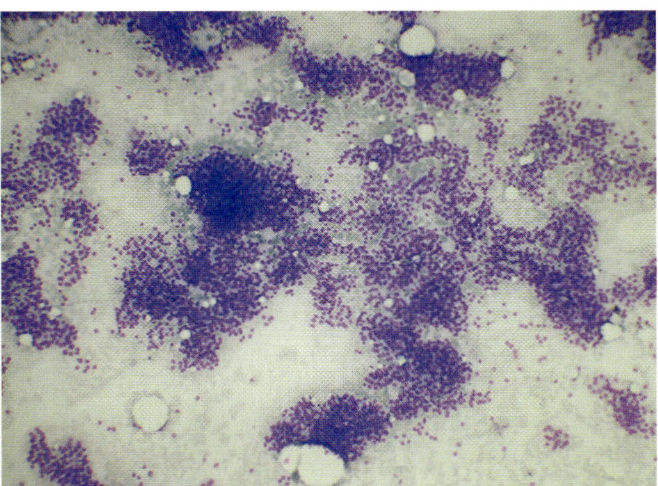

Fig. 26.46: Abundant cells in sheets and discretely placed in insular carcinoma of thyroid (MGG × LP).

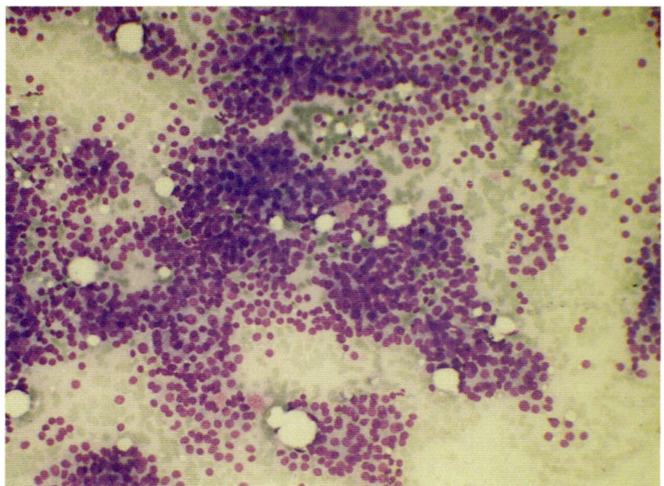

Fig. 26.47: Mainly solid sheets and occasional microfollicles in insular carcinoma of thyroid (MGG × MP).

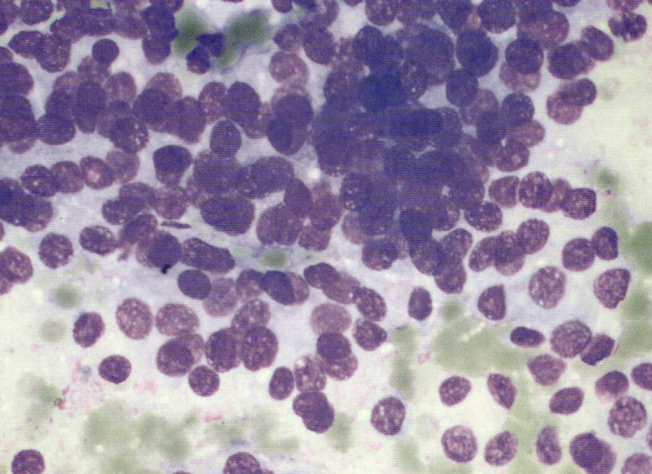

Fig. 26.48: Insular carcinoma: Higher magnification showing round monomorphic cells with occasional nuclear grooves (MGG × HP).

Box 26.22: Cytology of insular carcinoma.

- Dissociated cells
- Occasional microfollicles
- Small round cells
- Monomorphic round nuclei and inconspicuous nucleoli.

Lymphomas[68-71]

Primary thyroid lymphoma, labeled as mucosa-associated lymphoma (MALToma), represents less than 5% of all thyroid malignancies and constitutes less than 2% of all extranodal lymphomas. As thyroid involvement is common in any systemic NHL, so this possibility should always be excluded before the diagnosis of primary NHL. Primary thyroid NHL usually occurs in elderly patient with a female predilection. Hashimoto's thyroiditis is a risk factor of NHL of thyroid.

Cytology

The morphology of thyroid NHL is essentially same as that of NHL in other body sites. Most of the cases of thyroid lymphomas are B cell type. Three histological subtypes of B-NHL are seen:

1. Diffuse large B-cell lymphoma (DLBCL)
2. Marginal zone B-cell lymphoma (MZL)
3. Mixed MZL and DLBCL type.

Diffuse large B-cell lymphoma (DLBCL): Cytology smear shows discrete large lymphoid cells with scanty to moderate amount of basophilic cytoplasm. The nuclei show coarse chromatin pattern with prominent nucleoli (Fig. 26.49).

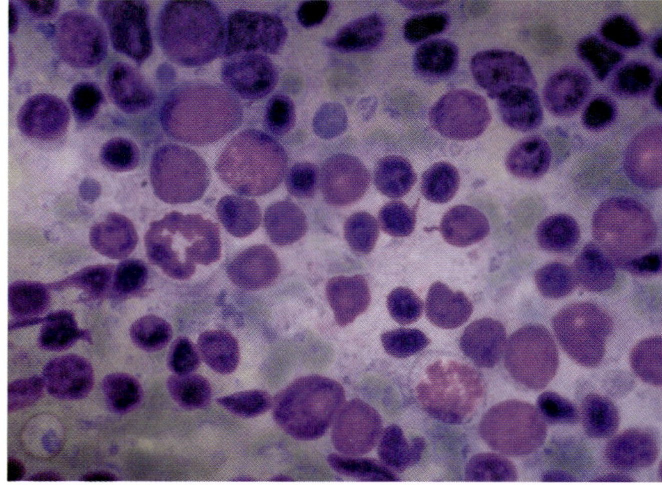

Fig. 26.49: Large discrete cells in diffuse large B-cell lymphoma of thyroid (MGG × HP).

Marginal zone B-cell lymphoma (MZL): FNAC of MZL shows lymphoid cells that are twice the size of small lymphocytes. Cells show scanty basophilic cytoplasm and irregular nuclear margin with small inconspicuous nucleoli (Fig. 26.50).[70] Variable amount of normal thyroid follicular cells may be admixed with the lymphoid cells. Florid lymphoid cell population in LT may be difficult to distinguish from MALToma. At times, LT may coexist with thyroid lymphoma. Immunocytochemistry or flow cytometry may be needed to establish the monoclonality of lymphoma to resolve the diagnostic confusion.

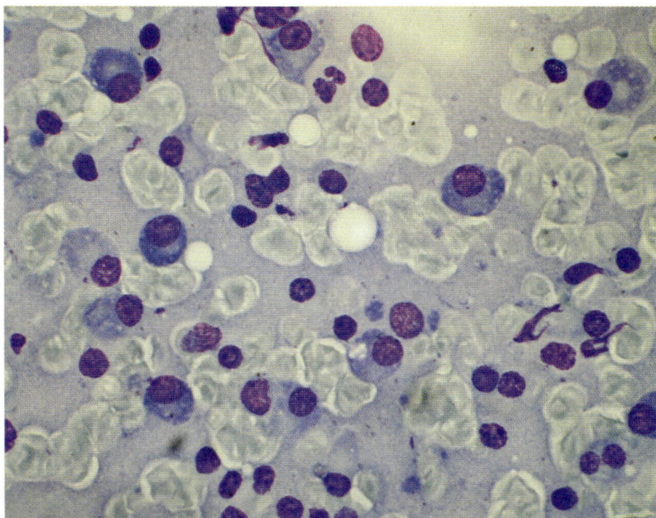

Fig. 26.50: MALTOMA of thyroid: Immature lymphoid cells and plasmacytoid cells with eccentric nuclei in MALTOMA of thyroid (MGG × HP).

Differential Diagnosis

- Chronic lymphocytic thyroiditis.

Metastatic Malignant Tumors

Metastatic malignant tumor of thyroid represents about 0.1% of all thyroid cancers.[72] However, the incidence is reported more in autopsy cases (about 25%).[73] The majority of the cases of thyroid metastasis are due to direct extension of the malignancy from the adjacent structures such as larynx or esophagus. The other distant common sources of the primary tumors are kidney, lung, and breast.[74-76] Metastatic tumors in thyroid is suspected if (1) thyroid nodule associated with a history of known primary malignant tumors, (2) cytology smears show benign thyroid follicular cells along with malignant cells. In one half of the cases no prior history of malignancy is available and the patients present with nodule in thyroid with an occult malignancy.[77] The cases of medullary carcinoma with predominant spindle cell component may simulate a metastatic fibrosarcoma. Hürthle cell tumor or FN may often mimic as metastatic renal cell carcinoma and vice versa. Metastatic giant cell carcinoma from lung or malignant melanoma may mimic anaplastic carcinoma of thyroid.

Differential Diagnosis

- Hürthle cell and follicular cell tumor
- Anaplastic carcinoma
- Spindle cell variant of medullary carcinoma.

ANCILLARY TECHNIQUES

Majority of the thyroid lesions can be diagnosed on the basis of the cytomorphological characteristics particularly PTC, medullary carcinoma, and anaplastic carcinoma. In certain thyroid tumors such as follicular and Hürthle cell neoplasm it is not possible to distinguish adenoma from carcinoma. Ancillary techniques in thyroid are unable to differentiate benign from malignant tumors. However, the ancillary techniques may help in confirmation of specific subtypes of thyroid carcinomas. The special techniques also help in the assessment of the prognosis of thyroid malignancies.

The common ancillary techniques used in thyroid tumors are:

- Special stains
- Immunocytochemistry
- Flow cytometry
- Molecular genetics.

The common indications for ancillary technique to apply in the thyroid tumors are:

- Diagnosis of primary thyroid malignancy
  - Medullary carcinoma
  - Anaplastic carcinoma
  - NHL
- Diagnosis of metastatic carcinoma
- Diagnosis of parathyroid lesions.

Special Stains

Congo red stain is commonly used in thyroid FNAC to detect amyloid material.

Immunocytochemistry

The panel of immunocytochemistry helps in the identification of different primary and secondary malignancies of thyroid (Table 26.5). Immunocytochemistry should be preferably done on cell block preparation. Calcitonin positivity in case of MC and parathormone positivity along with TTF negativity in parathyroid neoplasm are diagnostic of these tumors. Anaplastic carcinomas are positive for vimentin and negative for thyroglobulin. To differentiate chronic LT and NHL, the demonstration of light chain restriction is helpful. However, this is necessary in selected cases only.

Table 26.5: Immunocytochemistry in thyroid aspirate.

	Antibody	
Tumors	*Positive*	*Negative*
Medullary carcinoma	Calcitonin is specific, chromogranin, NSE synaptophysin, and CEA	Thyroglobulin
Anaplastic carcinoma	Vimentin	Thyroglobulin
Papillary thyroid carcinoma	Thyroglobulin, TTF-1, CK7, CK19, EMA	CK20
Insular carcinoma	Thyroglobulin, TTF-1	Calcitonin
Undifferentiated carcinoma	Vimentin, Pan cytokeratin, Focal positivity for CEA and EMA	TTF-1, thyroglobulin (usually negative)
Non-Hodgkin's lymphoma (NHL)	Light chain restriction (either kappa or lambda expression), CD19, CD20, CD3, CD5, CD23, CD10 (depending on the type of NHL)	
Parathyroid tumors	Parathyroid hormone	Calcitonin, TTF-1
Metastatic carcinoma	Cytokeratin, EMA	TTF-1, thyroglobulin

(EMA: Epithelial membrane antigen; TTF: Thyroid transcription factor; CK: Cytokeratin).

Table 26.6: Management of thyroid swelling after FNAC report.

Diagnostic category	*Management*
Group 1: Benign lesions such as colloid goiter	Clinical follow-up should be done at 6 monthly to 1 year interval. USG in case of poorly palpable lesion
Group 2: Follicular lesions of undetermined significance or atypia of undetermined significance	• Serum TSH should be measured. • If serum TSH is low, thyroid scan. • If cold nodule, then surgical resection. • Or FNAC should be repeated after 3–6 months. If repeat FNAC is also reported as atypical then surgical excision is advised.
Group 3: Follicular neoplasm or Hürthle cell neoplasm	Surgical consultation for lobectomy or hemithyroidectomy
Group 4: Suspicious for malignancy	Surgical consultation for lobectomy
Group 5: Specific malignancy	Surgical consultation for lobectomy or hemithyroidectomy
Group 6: Inadequate	Re-aspirate under USG guidance, Repeat FNAC after 3 months

(FNAC: Fine needle aspiration cytology; USG: Ultrasonography; TSH: Thyroid-stimulating hormone).

Flow Cytometry

This is useful in the diagnosis of NHL. To differentiate a florid Hashimoto's thyroiditis and MALToma is a challenge to the cytopathologist. The demonstration of the light chain restriction is helpful in the diagnosis of B-NHL. Aberrant expression of T cell markers suggests a case of T-NHL.

Molecular Genetics

RET/PTC chromosomal rearrangements are commonly found in PTC. The demonstration of RET/PTC chromosomal rearrangement by RT-PCR for the diagnosis of PTC especially in the cases of difficult situation is fascinating.[78]

BRAF point mutations are the genetic hallmarks of PTC and the demonstration of these mutations is also helpful in the confirmation of PTC.[79]

MANAGEMENT OF POST FNAC DIAGNOSIS OF THYROID LESION

The treatment and management of the thyroid nodule largely depend on the FNAC diagnosis of thyroid lesions and the broad category of the thyroid swelling.

Table 26.6 summarizes the post FNAC management outline in brief as suggested by NCI-sponsored group.[80]

REFERENCES

1. Martin HE, Ellis EB. Biopsy by needle puncture and aspiration. Ann Surg. 1930;92:169-81.
2. Söderström N. Puncture of goiters for aspiration biopsy. A preliminary report. Acta Med Scand. 1952;144:237-44.
3. Jogai S, Jassar A, Adisena A, et al. Fine needle aspiration cytology of thyroid lesions. Acta Cytol. 2005;49(5):483-8.
4. Pitman MB, Abele J, Ali S, et al. Techniques for thyroid FNA: a synopsis of the National Cancer Institute Thyroid Fine Needle Aspiration State of the Science Conference. Diagn Cytopathol. 2008;36:407-24.
5. Dey P, Ray R. Comparison of fine needle sampling by capillary action and fine needle aspiration. Cytopathology. 1993;4:299-303.
6. Baloch ZW, LiVolsi VA. Post Fine needle aspiration histologic alterations of thyroid revisited. Am J Clin Pathol. 1999; 112(3):311-6.
7. LiVolsi VA, Merino MJ. Worrisome histologic alterations following Fine needle aspiration of the thyroid (WHAFFT). Pathol Annu. 1994;Part 2:99-120.
8. Alexander EK, Heering JP, Benson CB, et al. Assessment of nondiagnostic ultrasound-guided fine needle aspirations of thyroid nodules. J Clin Endocrinol Metab. 2002;87: 4924-7.
9. Bellantone R, Lombardi CP, Raffaelli M, et al. Management of cystic or predominantly cystic thyroid nodules: the role of ultrasound-guided Fine needle aspiration biopsy. Thyroid. 2004;14:43-7.
10. Cibas ES, Alexander EK, Benson CB, et al. Indications for thyroid FNA and pre-FNA requirements: a synopsis of the National Cancer Institute Thyroid Fine needle Aspiration State of the Science Conference. Diagn Cytopathol. 2008; 36:390-9.
11. Ashcraft MW, Van Herle AJ. Management of thyroid nodules. II: scanning techniques, thyroid suppressive therapy, and fine needle aspiration. Head Neck Surg. 1981;3:297-322.
12. Wang C, Vickery AL Jr, Maloof F. Needle biopsy of the thyroid. Surg Gynecol Obstet. 1976;143:365-8.
13. Goellner JR, Gharib H, Grant CS, et al. Fine needle aspiration cytology of the thyroid, 1980-1986. Acta Cytol. 1987; 31:587-90.
14. Grant CS, Hay ID, Gough IR, et al. Long term follow up of patients with benign thyroid fine needle aspiration cytologic diagnoses. Surgery. 1989;106:980-6.
15. Nguyen GK, Ginsberg J, Crockford PM. Fine needle aspiration biopsy cytology of the thyroid: its value and limitations in the diagnosis and management of solitary thyroid nodules. Pathol Annu. 1991;23:63-80.
16. Hamburger JI, Hussain M. Semiquantitative criteria for fineneedle biopsy diagnosis: reduced false negative diagnoses. Diagn Cytopathol. 1988;4:14-17.
17. Kini SR. Guides to Clinical Aspiration Biopsy: Thyroid, 2nd edition. New York, NY: Igaku-Shoin Ltd.; 1996.
18. Yassa L, Cibas ES, Benson CB, et al. Long-term assessment of a multidisciplinary approach to thyroid nodule diagnostic evaluation. Cancer. 2007;111(6):508-16.
19. Bakhos R, Selvaggi SM, DeJong S, et al. Fine needle aspiration of the thyroid: rate and causes of cytohistopathologic discordance. Diagn Cytopathol. 2000;23:233-7.
20. Khurana KK, Baloch ZW, LiVolsi VA. Aspiration cytology of pediatric solitary papillary hyperplastic thyroid nodule. Arch Pathol Lab Med. 2001;125(12):1575-8.
21. Morgan JL, Serpell JW, Cheng MS. Fine needle aspiration cytology of thyroid nodules: how useful is it? ANZ J Surg. 2003;73:480-3.
22. Dwarakanathan AA, Ryan WG, Staren ED, et al. Fine needle aspiration biopsy of the thyroid. Diagnostic accuracy when performing a moderate number of such procedures. Arch Intern Med. 1989;149:2007-9.
23. Tee YY, Lowe AJ, Brand CA, et al. Fine needle aspiration may miss a third of all malignancy in palpable thyroid nodules: a comprehensive literature review. Ann Surg. 2007; 246:714-20.
24. The Papanicolaou Society of Cytopathology Task Force on Standards of Practice. Guidelines of the Papanicolaou Society of Cytopathology for the examination of Fine needle aspiration specimens from thyroid nodules. Diagn Cytopathol. 1996;15:84-89.
25. Baloch ZW, LiVolsi VA, Asa SL, et al. Diagnostic terminology and morphologic criteria for cytologic diagnosis of thyroid lesions: a synopsis of the National Cancer Institute Thyroid Fine needle Aspiration State of the Science Conference. Diagn Cytopathol. 2008;36(6):425-37.
26. Centeno BA, Szyfelbein WM, Daniels GH, et al. Fine needle aspiration biopsy of the thyroid gland in patients with prior Graves' disease treated with radioactive iodine. Morphologic findings and potential pitfalls. Acta Cytol. 1996;40: 1189-97.
27. Singh N, Kumar S, Negi VS, et al. Cytomorphologic study of Hashimoto's thyroiditis and its serologic correlation: a study of 150 cases. Acta Cytol. 2009;53(5):507-16.
28. Poropatich C, Marcus D, Oertel YC. Hashimoto's thyroiditis: Fine needle aspirations of 50 asymptomatic cases. Diagn Cytopathol. 1994;11(2):141-5.
29. Maruta J, Hashimoto H, Suehisa Y, et al. Improving the diagnostic accuracy of thyroid follicular neoplasms: cytological features in Fine needle aspiration cytology. Diagn Cytopathol. 2010;39(1):28-34.
30. Renshaw AA, Wang E, Wilbur D, et al. Interobserver agreement on microfollicules in thyroid Fine needle aspirates. Arch Pathol Lab Med. 2006;130:148-52.
31. Goldstein RE, Netterville JL, Burkey B, et al. Implications of follicular neoplasms, atypia, and lesions suspicious for malignancy diagnosed by Fine needle aspiration of thyroid nodules. Ann Surg. 2002;235:656-64.
32. Powari M, Dey P, Saikia UN. Fine needle aspiration cytology of follicular variant of papillary carcinoma of thyroid. Cytopathology. 2003;14:212-5.
33. DeLellis RA, Williams ED. Thyroid and parathyroid tumors: introduction. In: DeLelis RA, Lloyd RV, Heit PU, et al. (Eds). World Health Organization Classification of Tumours. Pathology and Genetics of Tumours of Endocrine Organs. Lyon: IARC Press; 2004. pp. 51-6.

34. Muller-Hocker J, Schafer A, Strowitzki T. Glucose transporter 4 (GLUT 4) is highly expressed in mitochondria-rich oxyphil cells. Appl Immunohistochem. 1998;6:224-7.
35. Papotti M, Gugliotta P, Forte G, et al. Immunocytochemical identification of oxyphilic mitochondrion-rich cells. Appl Immunohistochem. 1994;2:261-67.
36. Santeusanio G, D'Alfonso V, Iafrate E, et al. Antibodies to cytokeratin 14 specifically identify oncocytes (Hürthle cells) in thyroid lesions and tumors. Appl Immunohistochem. 1997;5:223-8.
37. Hemachandran M, Rajwanshi A, Srinivasan R, et al. Cytology of Hürthle cell neoplasms of thyroid gland. Indian J Pathol Microbiol. 2007;50(4):859-61.
38. Wu HH, Clouse J, Ren R. Fine needle aspiration cytology of Hürthle cell carcinoma of the thyroid. Diagn Cytopathol. 2008;36(3):149-54.
39. Elliott DD, Pitman MB, Bloom L, et al. Fine needle aspiration biopsy of Hurthle cell lesions of the thyroid gland: a cytomorphologic study of 139 cases with statistical analysis. Cancer. 2006;108:102-9.
40. Casey MB, Sebo TJ, Carney A. Hyalinizing trabecular adenoma of thyroid gland. Cytologic features in 29 cases. Am J Surg Pathol. 2004;28:859-67.
41. LiVolsi VA, Albores-Saavedra J, Asa SL, et al. Papilary carcinoma. In: DeLelis RA, Lloyd RV, Heit PU, et al. (Eds). World Health Organization Classification of Tumours. Pathology and Genetics of Tumours of Endocrine Organs. Lyon: IARC Press; 2004. pp. 57-66.
42. Castellone MD, Santoro M. Dysregulated RET signaling in thyroid cancer. Endocrinol Metab Clin North Am. 2008; 37:363-74.
43. Adeniran AJ, Zhu Z, Gandhi M, et al. Correlation between genetic alterations and microscopic features, clinical manifestations, and prognostic characteristics of thyroid papillary carcinomas. Am J Surg Pathol. 2006;30:216-22.
44. Kondo T, Ezzat S, Asa SL. Pathogenetic mechanisms in thyroid follicular-cell neoplasia. Nat Rev Cancer. 2006;6: 292-306.
45. Kaur A, Jayaram G. Thyroid tumors: cytomorphology of papillary carcinoma. Diagn Cytopathol. 1991;7(5):462-8.
46. Arora SK, Dey P. Intranuclear peudoinclusions: morphology, pathogenesis, and significance. Diagn Cytopathol. 2012;40 (8):741-4.
47. Tabbara SO, Acoury N, Sidawy MK. Multinucleated giant cells in thyroid neoplasms: a cytologic, histologic and immunohistochemical study. Acta Cytol. 1996;40(6):1184-8.
48. Cotran RS, Kumar V, Collins T. Robbins Pathologic basis of Disease, 6th ed., Vol. 44. Noida, India: W.B. Saunders Co., Harcourt Asia Pte Ltd; 1999, pp. 1143-4.
49. Li Volsi VA. Surgical pathology of the thyroid. Philadelphia: W.B. Saunders Co; 1990. p. 138.
50. Johannessen JV, Sobrinho-Simoes M. The origin and significance of thyroid psammoma bodies. Lab Invest. 1980;43: 287-29.
51. Das DK, Mallik MK, Haji BE, et al. Psammoma body and its precursors in papillary thyroid carcinoma: a study by fine needle aspiration cytology. Diagn Cytopathol. 2004;31: 380-6.
52. Das DK. Psammoma body: a product of dystrophic calcification or of a biologically active process that aims at limiting the growth and spread of tumor?. Diagn Cytopathol. 2009;37:534-41.
53. Cooper DS, Tiamson E, Ladenson PW. Psammoma bodies in fine needle aspiration biopsies of benign thyroid nodules. Thyroidology. 1988;1:55-59.
54. Urano M, Kiriyama Y, Takakuwa Y, et al. Tall cell variant of papillary thyroid carcinoma: its characteristic features demonstrated by Fine needle aspiration cytology and immunohistochemical study. Diagn Cytopathol. 2009;37 (10):732-7.
55. Nair M, Kapila K, Karak AK, et al. Papillary carcinoma of the thyroid and its variants: a cytohistological correlation. Diagn Cytopathol. 2001;24(3):167-73.
56. Baloch ZW, LiVolsi VA. Cytologic and architectural mimics of papillary thyroid carcinoma. Diagnostic challenges in Fine needle aspiration and surgical pathology specimens. Am J Clin Pathol. 2006;125(Suppl):S135-44.
57. Albores-Saavedra J, Wu J. The many faces and mimics of papillary thyroid carcinoma. Endocr Pathol. 2006;17:1-18.
58. Bongiovanni M, Triponez F, McKee TA, et al. Fine needle aspiration of the diffuse sclerosing variant of papillary thyroid carcinoma masked by florid lymphocytic thyroiditis; a potential pitfall: a case report and review of the literature. Diagn Cytopathol. 2009;37(9):671-5.
59. Zeppa P, Vetrani A, Marino M, et al. Fine needle aspiration cytology of medullary thyroid carcinoma: a review of 18 cases. Cytopathology. 1990;1(1):35-44.
60. Bose S, Kapila K, Verma K. Medullary carcinoma of the thyroid: a cytological, immunocytochemical, and ultrastructural study. Diagn Cytopathol. 1992;8(1):28-32.
61. Bugalho MJ, Santos JR, Sobrinho L. Preoperative diagnosis of medullary thyroid carcinoma: fine needle aspiration cytology as compared with serum calcitonin measurement. J Surg Oncol. 2005;91(1):56-60.
62. Das A, Gupta SK, Banerjee AK, et al. Atypical cytologic features of medullary carcinoma of the thyroid: a review of 12 cases. Acta Cytol. 1992:36;137-41.
63. Berry B, MacFarlane J, Chan N. Osteoclastoma-like anaplastic carcinoma of the thyroid. Acta Cytol. 1990;34: 248-50.
64. Pietribiasi F, Sapino A, Papotti M, et al. Cytologic features of poorly differentiated "insular" carcinoma of the thyroid, as revealed by Fine needle aspiration biopsy. Am J Clin Pathol. 1990;94:687-92.
65. Oertel YC, Miyahara-Felipe L. Cytologic features of insular carcinoma of the thyroid: a case report. Diagn Cytopathol. 2006;34(8):572-5.
66. Gong Y, Krishnamurthy S. Fine needle aspiration of an unusual case of poorly differentiated insular carcinoma of the thyroid. Diagn Cytopathol. 2005;32(2):103-7.
67. Barwad A, Dey P, Saikia UN, et al. Fine needle aspiration cytology of Insular carcinoma of thyroid. Diagn Cytopathol. 2012;40 Suppl 1:E43-7.

68. Gospodarowicz MK, Sutcliffe SB. The extranodal lymphomas. Sem Rad Oncol. 1995;5:281-300.
69. Sangalli G, Serio G, Zampatti C, et al. Fine needle aspiration cytology of primary lymphoma of the thyroid: a report of 17 cases. Cytopathology. 2001;12(4):257-63.
70. Kaba S, Hirokawa M, Kuma S, et al. Cytologic findings of primary thyroid MALT lymphoma with extreme plasma cell differentiation: FNA cytology of two case. Diagn Cytopathol. 2009;37(11):815-9.
71. Gupta N, Nijhawan R, Srinivasan R, et al. Fine needle aspiration cytology of primary thyroid lymphoma: a report of ten cases. Cytojournal. 2005;2:21.
72. Schmid KW, Hittmair A, Ofner C, et al. Metastatic tumors in fine needle aspiration biopsy of the thyroid. Acta Cytol. 1991;35:722-4.
73. Berge T, Lundberg S. Cancer in Mälmo 1958-1969. An autopsy study. Acta Pathol Microbiol Scand Supp. 1977;260: 1-235.
74. Chen H, Nicol TL, Udelsman R. Clinically significant, isolated metastatic disease to the thyroid gland. World J Surg. 1999;23:177-80.
75. Owens CL, Basaria S, Nicol TL. Metastatic breast carcinoma involving the thyroid gland diagnosed by Fine needle aspiration: a case report. Diagn Cytopathol. 2005;33(2): 110-5.
76. Cozzolino I, Malapelle U, Carlomagno C, et al. Metastasis of colon cancer to the thyroid gland: a case diagnosed on Fine needle aspirate by a combined cytological, immunocytochemical, and molecular approach. Diagn Cytopathol. 2010;38(12):932-5.
77. Smith SA, Gharib H, Goellner JR. Fine needle aspiration: usefulness for diagnosis and management of metastaticcarcinoma to the thyroid. Arch Intern Med. 1987;147: 311-2.
78. Cheung CC, Carydis B, Ezzat S, et al. Molecular genetic analysis refines the fine needle aspiration diagnosis of thyroid cancer. J Clin Endocrinol Metab. 2001;86:2187-90.
79. Salvatore G, Giannini R, Faviana P, et al. Analysis of BRAF point mutation and RET/PTC rearrangement refines the Fine needle aspiration diagnosis of papillary thyroid carcinoma. J Clin Endocrinol Metab. 2004;89(10):5175-80.
80. Layfield LJ, Abrams J, Cochand-Priollet B, et al. Post-thyroid FNA testing and treatment options: a synopsis of the National Cancer Institute Thyroid Fine Needle Aspiration State of the Science Conference. Diagn Cytopathol. 2008;36 (6):442-8.

Review Questions

1. **A 42-year-old male presented with 5-cm diameter isthmic nodule. Fine needle aspiration cytology was done (Figs. 26.51A and B).**
   What is your possible diagnosis?
   a. Lymphocytic thyroiditis
   b. Medullary carcinoma of thyroid
   c. Hürthle cell neoplasm
   d. Plasma cell neoplasm
2. **An 8-year-old girl with macroglossia and facial deformity with mental retardation presented with 3-cm diameter isthmic swelling of thyroid gland since birth. The patient is hypothyroid. Fine needle aspiration cytology of thyroid was done (Figs. 26.52A to D).**
   The most likely diagnosis is:
   a. Dyshormonogenetic goiter
   b. Papillary carcinoma of thyroid
   c. Follicular neoplasm
   d. Parathyroid neoplasm
3. **A 31-year-old female presented with 4-cm diameter enlarged right lobe of thyroid. Figures. 26.53A to D represents the Fine needle aspiration cytology smear of the swelling.**
   What is your diagnosis?
   a. Papillary carcinoma of thyroid
   b. Medullary carcinoma
   c. Lymphocytic thyroiditis
   d. Colloid goiter

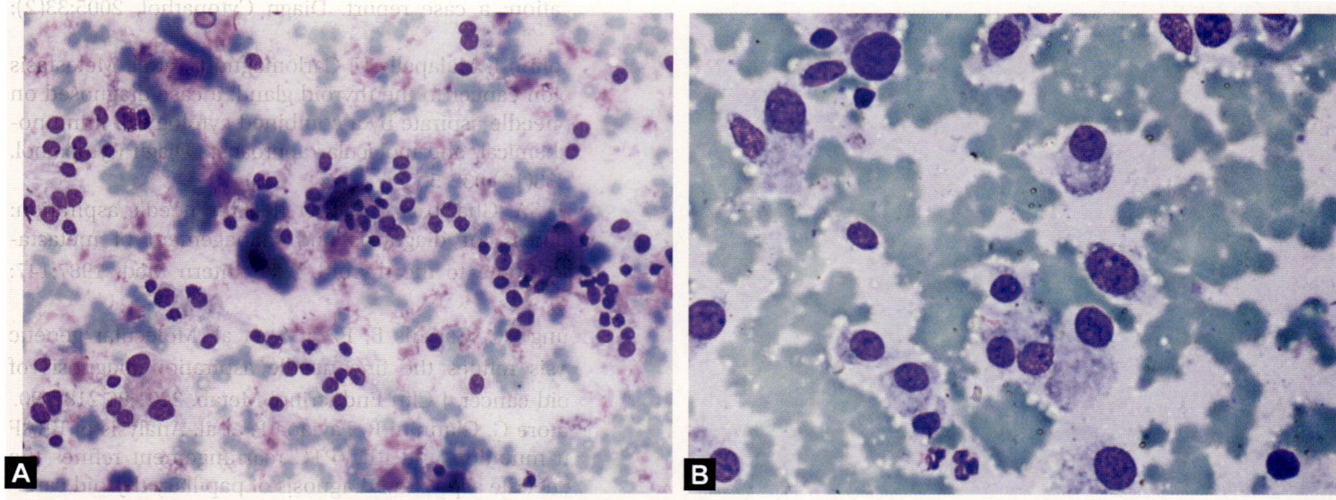

Figs. 26.51A and B: Cytology smears of thyroid swelling in question 1.

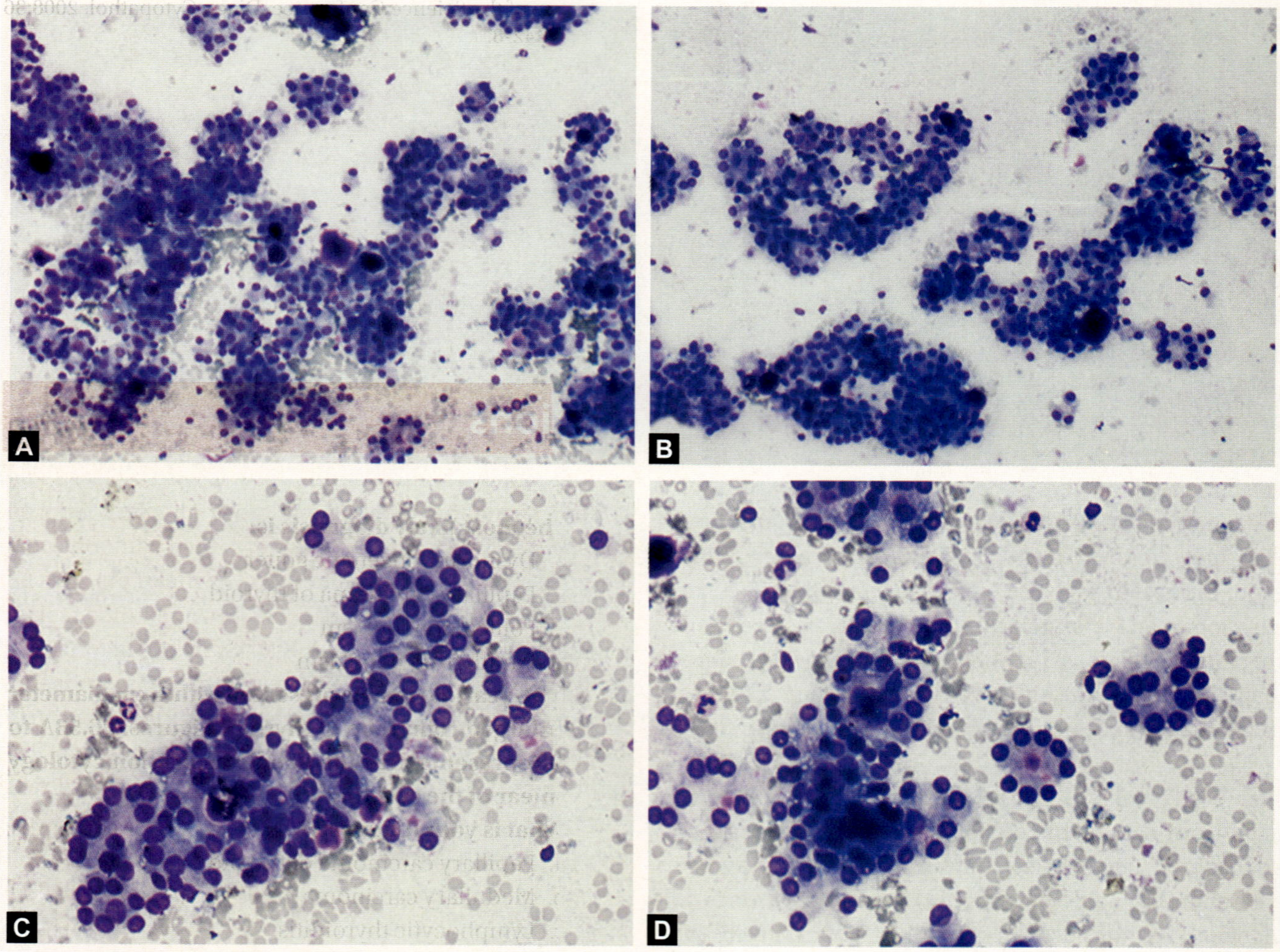

Figs. 26.52A to D: Cytology smears of thyroid swelling in question 2.

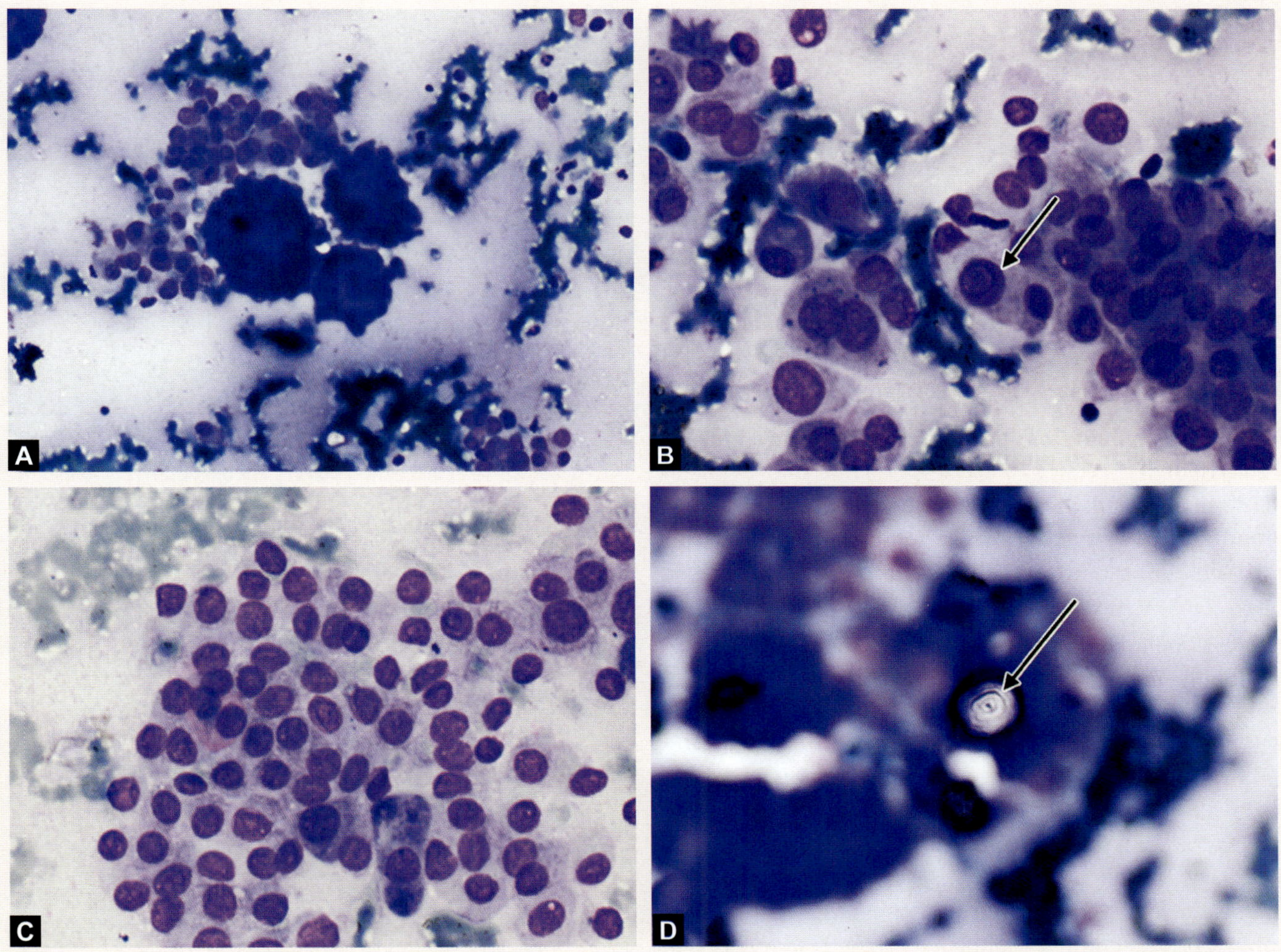

Figs. 26.53A to D: Cytology smears of thyroid in question 3.

Answers

1. b. Medullary carcinoma of thyroid
   Note: The discrete cells with moderate amount of reddish cytoplasm and eccentrically placed mildly pleomorphic nuclei indicate the diagnosis of medullary carcinoma of thyroid. Further confirmation can be done by doing calcitonin-immune stain.
2. a. Dyshormonogenetic goiter
   Note: Classical history of the swelling since birth, other congenital anomalies along with the abundant microfollicles indicate the dyshormonogenic tumor. The tumor is commonly mistaken as follicular neoplasm.
3. a. Papillary carcinoma of thyroid
   Note: The tumor cells with intranuclear pseudoinclusion, longitudinal nuclear groove and psammoma bodies. These cytological features confirm the diagnosis of papillary carcinoma of thyroid.

CHAPTER 27 Breast

INTRODUCTION

Breast cancer is one of the most important public health problems in the world. It is one of the major causes of death due to cancer. It has been shown that the invasive carcinoma of breast passes through in situ carcinoma. There is considerable higher mortality and morbidity in the higher stage of invasive carcinoma of the breast. However, only 16% of breast carcinoma cases are diagnosed in stage I and majority of the women (54%) are diagnosed in stage II.[1] The palpable breast lesions are easily detected by the physicians. With the help of USG and mammogram, the nonpalpable breast lesions are also detectable and early stages of breast cancer can be recognized. However, in a meta-analysis study, Gøtzsche and Olsen did not notice any effect of mammographic screening on breast cancer mortality and they raised the validity of mammography as a screening test of breast cancer.[2] Other workers have highlighted the importance of mammographic test in breast cancer screening and till now it is considered as the best screening technique.[3] Newer other modalities particularly fine needle aspiration cytology (FNAC) is also very useful for the definitive diagnosis of breast cancer. Presently, FNAC is a popular technique and it is also a part of "triple test" for the diagnosis of breast lesions particularly breast carcinomas. FNAC has good diagnostic accuracy and has reduced the rate of the excision biopsy.[4]

INDICATIONS OF FINE NEEDLE ASPIRATION CYTOLOGY OF BREAST

Fine needle aspiration cytology is indicated almost all the palpable breast lesions and mammographically abnormal nonpalpable breast lesions. The major indications of FNAC of the breast lesion have been mentioned in Box 27.1.

There are several advantages of FNAC of breast lesion. These include (1) rapid diagnosis, (2) economically cost effective, (3) high diagnostic accuracy, (4) multiple sampling from the multiple areas of the breast, (5) avoids open surgery in nonoperable malignancies, (6) performing ancillary techniques, and (7) preoperative planning in malignant tumors. In addition, cytological diagnosis of benign lesion provides a rapid psychological relief to the patient.

Box 27.1: Indications of fine needle aspiration cytology of breast.

Diagnostic
- Benign versus malignant lesions of the breast
- Preoperative grading of breast carcinoma
- Hormone (estrogen and progesterone) and growth receptor (HER2/neu) evaluation
- Nonpalpable breast lesion with abnormal mammogram
- Inflammatory diseases of breast
- Recurrent tumor.

Therapeutic
- Evacuation of cyst.

CONTRAINDICATIONS

Truly speaking, there is no contraindication of FNAC of the breast. It is a safe procedure and the patient encounters minimal trauma. Needle tract seeding does not occur after FNAC technique. If adequate sterility is maintained then there is no chance of secondary infection. Hematoma after FNAC procedure may occur if adequate precaution is not taken after FNAC procedure. Pneumothorax may occur in case of FNAC of the axillary swelling. However, the conservative management is enough to manage such cases.

DIAGNOSTIC ACCURACY

Fine needle aspiration cytology of the breast is a good diagnostic technique because of high sensitivity and specificity. The diagnostic accuracy is too some extent operator dependent. However, the sensitivity of the technique ranges from 68% to 99%. The specificity of FNAC is as

Box 27.2: Limitations of fine needle aspiration cytology (FNAC) of breast.

- Inability to distinguish
  - Ductal carcinoma in situ (DCIS) from infiltrating duct carcinoma (IDC)
  - Atypical ductal hyperplasia (ADH) from DCIS.
  - Atypical cell in breast FNAC with indeterminate/gray zone area needs to have histopathology.
  - Inability to identify various low-grade carcinoma with certainty.
- Certain benign breast lesions are difficult to subtype.

Box 27.3: False negative diagnosis of breast fine needle aspiration cytology.

Sampling Error
- Cystic lesion or necrosis
- Poor preservation and drying artifact
- Small focus of carcinoma in a benign lesion
- Scanty cellularity in deep seated lesion or fibrotic lesion
- Inadequate sampling from a large mass

Interpretation Error
- *Certain types of carcinoma*: Tubular carcinoma, mucinous or colloid carcinoma, lobular carcinoma
- Well-differentiated carcinoma
- Carcinoma arising from papillary tumor or fibrocystic disease.

Box 27.4: False positive diagnosis of breast fine needle aspiration cytology.

- Fibroadenoma with reactive atypia
- Regenerative cells particularly histiocytes in inflammation
- Papilloma
- Fat necrosis
- Atypical ductal hyperplasia
- Sclerosing duct adenosis
- Pregnancy-induced changes
- Gynecomastia with atypia
- Radiation-induced changes
- Skin adnexal tumors.

Table 27.1: Clinical comparison of malignant and benign breast lesions.

Features	*Malignant*	*Benign*
Age	More than 45 years are suspicious	Younger patients
Duration	Recent origin	Long duration
Rapidity	Rapidly growing	Slowly growing
Swelling	Hard, fixed	Soft, mobile
Skin	Inflamed, ulcerated	Normal
Nipple	Recent retraction	Normal
Family history of breast cancer	May be present	Absent
Mammogram	Microcalcification	Normal

high as 99%.[5-7] The diagnostic accuracy of FNAC of breast increases if the cytopathologist performs FNAC and reports the same case. The false negative rate of FNAC is about 3–5%; however, it has been reported as high as 30%.[8]

These false negative cases can be easily avoided if the FNAC is done by an experienced cytologist and multiple sampling is done. Clinical history should also be considered and any clinically suspicious mass that are negative on cytology should be repeated. False positive rate in breast is near about 4%.[6,9]

In many centers, definitive surgery is done on the basis of FNAC report. Therefore, extreme care should be taken to avoid a false positive diagnosis. Medicolegal aspects of the false positive cases are also serious. Majority of the medicolegal cases are related with breast and mostly due to over diagnosis than under diagnosis.

LIMITATIONS OF FINE NEEDLE ASPIRATION CYTOLOGY

The cytologist should have adequate experience of FNAC technique. There may be many technical problems related to this procedure that can be easily avoided such as air drying of the smear, poor cellularity, and improper sampling. However, there are certain inherent limitations of breast FNAC (Box 27.2). The major such limitation is inability to distinguish atypical ductal hyperplasia (ADH) from ductal carcinoma in situ (DCIS) of the breast. Similarly, it is very difficult to distinguish DCIS from infiltrating duct carcinoma (IDC) on the cytology smear.

The false negative FNAC diagnosis of the breast may be due to sampling or interpretative error.[10] The major causes of sampling error may be due to necrosis, cystic change of the lesion or may be due to heterogeneous distribution of the tumor tissue such as small focal carcinomas in a large fibrocystic disease (Box 27.3). Low-grade carcinoma of breast and certain type of carcinomas such as lobular carcinoma, tubular carcinoma and papillary carcinomas are often difficult to diagnose on FNAC and may produce false negative diagnosis due to error in the interpretation.

The other major concerns are false positive diagnosis of breast FNAC that may give rise to medicolegal problems. The major reasons of false positive diagnosis are atypical cells in various reactive inflammatory lesions, fibroadenomas with atypia, pregnancy- and lactation-induced changes in breast and ADH[11] (Box 27.4).

CLINICAL HISTORY

The detailed clinical history is helpful for diagnosis of cytology smear (Table 27.1). Malignancy is extremely

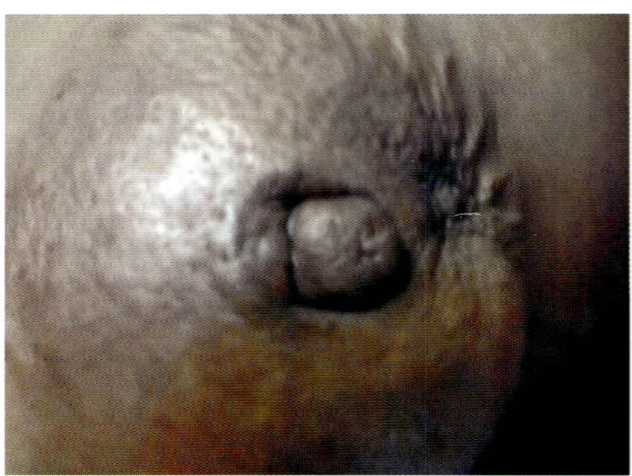

Fig. 27.1: Retracted nipple and puckered skin of the breast in a patient of carcinoma of breast.

uncommon in younger patients. Whereas the presence of breast lump in any patient older than 45 years needs careful evaluation. Any hard, fixed lump with skin indurations is suspicious for cancer. Recent history of nipple retraction also indicates an underlying malignancy (Fig. 27.1 and Table 27.1). Any rapidly growing mass within a short period of time suggests a malignant neoplasm. However, mucinous carcinoma may have long history of the swelling. Family history of breast carcinoma is informative because certain breast carcinomas are hereditary. Treatment history of carcinoma of the breast is also helpful for proper interpretation of cytology smear.

TRIPLE TEST

The triple test was introduced by Johansen in 1975 for the diagnostic evaluation of breast lump in elderly woman (more than 40 years). This test was introduced to avoid unnecessary open biopsy or frozen section.[12] This triple test includes mammogram, physical examination, and FNAC. When all the three tests are positive then the lump should be considered as malignant. Similarly, when all the components of the triple test are negative then the lump is considered as benign. Triple test is highly accurate, and it can avoid the necessity for open biopsy. However, frozen section or histopathological examination may be required if any of the components of the triad of triple test is negative.[13,14]

CORE NEEDLE BIOPSY VERSUS FINE NEEDLE ASPIRATION CYTOLOGY

Fine needle aspiration cytology is a simple, fast, cost effective, and less invasive method for evaluation of breast lesions. However, despite its indisputable merit, FNAC has its own limitations such as high false negative rates and equivocal results particularly to distinguish ADH from DCIS. To combat these limitations, core needle biopsy (CNB) has been introduced. CNB is becoming a popular technique among the pathologists for the diagnosis of breast lesions.[15] It is believed that CNB technique avoids FN cases and increases the diagnostic accuracy. However, Park et al. showed that the false negative rate is marginally different in FNAC (6.2%) versus CNB (9%). The sensitivity and specificity of FNAC in breast lesions are 93.8% and 80.8%, whereas the sensitivity and specificity of CNB are 92.1% and 90.9%, respectively.[16] Other studies also showed marginal increase in sensitivity and specificity in CNB versus FNAC.[17,18]

Table 27.2: Comparison of FNAC and CNB.

Features	*FNAC*	*CNB*
Time to take	Rapid	Time consuming
Anesthesia	Not required	Required
Multiple sampling	Possible	Not possible
Cost	Cheap	Costly
Sensitivity and specificity	Low	Slightly high
Gray zone lesion (ADH, DCIS)	Not easily detectable	Detectable

(FNAC: Fine needle aspiration cytology; CNB: Core needle biopsy; ADH: Atypical ductal hyperplasia; DCIS: Ductal carcinoma in situ).

Core needle biopsy has also certain disadvantages. It is a time-consuming procedure and requires anesthesia. The result of CNB may show considerable variation depending on the needle size, number of cores, and operator experience. Table 27.2 has compared CNB and FNAC technique.

In fact, the choice between CNB versus FNAC depends to some extent on the experience of the cytopathologist. Radiological guided FNAC may reduce the inadequacy and false negativity rate. A combined use of CNB and FNAC gives much better result and many people suggest that CNB and FNAC is complementary to each other.[19,20]

ADEQUACY OF THE SAMPLE

Adequacy criteria of FNAC of breast sample are too some extent depends on the laboratory and the operators who perform FNAC. The National Cancer Institute-sponsored conference in Bethesda on uniform approach of breast did not recommend any specific number of cells for adequacy of breast FNAC.[21] They considered a sample adequate that leads to resolution of a problem presented by a lesion in a

Box 27.5: Adequacy of breast fine needle aspiration cytology.

- No specific minimal cell number
- Aspirator should judge whether the FNAC report is consistent with the clinical or radiological findings.
- Cytologists should judge the smear quality such as air drying, artifact, etc.
- Cytologists should mention the amount of epithelial cells.
- Individual laboratories may decide their own guidelines about the number of cells for adequacy.

Layefield's proposal of adequacy criterion

Six or more cell clusters (cumulative total) or the presence more than 10 intact bipolar cells per 10 medium-power fields (× 200).

particular patient's breast and no minimal quantity of cells is required for adequacy. The cytologists should determine the adequacy of the sample based on the cytologic and clinical findings of individual cases. The pathologists should also judge the smear regarding any significant distortion and artifact. According to NCI conference, the cytopathologist should always mention about the quantity of the epithelial cells on the smear such as:

- *Scanty cellularity*: Only occasional epithelial cell clusters present
- *Moderate cellularity*: Readily identifiable clusters on the smear
- *Abundant cellularity*: Multiple clusters of epithelial cells in every field.

Layfield et al. believes that the stringent criterion on adequacy is required to reduce the number of false negative diagnosis because majority of the false negative sample is due to inadequate cellularity.[22] They suggested a cut-off point for satisfactory smears at a level of 6 or more cell clusters (cumulative total) or the presence more than 10 intact bipolar cells per 10 medium-power fields (×200) (Box 27.5).

In case of cystic lesions of breast there is no strict criterion about the number of epithelial cells on the smear. However, after evacuation of the cyst any residual solid mass should be reaspirated.

HISTOLOGY OF BREAST

Breasts are modified apocrine sweat glands. Breasts develop embryologically along the milk line that extends from the thorax to groin. Therefore, accessory breast may be found anywhere along the milk line. Each breast consists of 15–20 lobes radiating out from the nipple. These lobes are separated by collagenous septae. Each lobe has its own duct and before opening on the surface, the duct is dilated to form the lactiferous sinus. The main duct divides within each lobe of the breast and ultimately forms multiple terminal ducts. Each terminal duct is connected with lobule and each lobule consists of multiple acini. The combined terminal duct and lobule is known as terminal duct lobular unit. The duct and acini of the breast are lined by luminal layer of columnar to cuboidal epithelium and basal layer of myoepithelial cells.

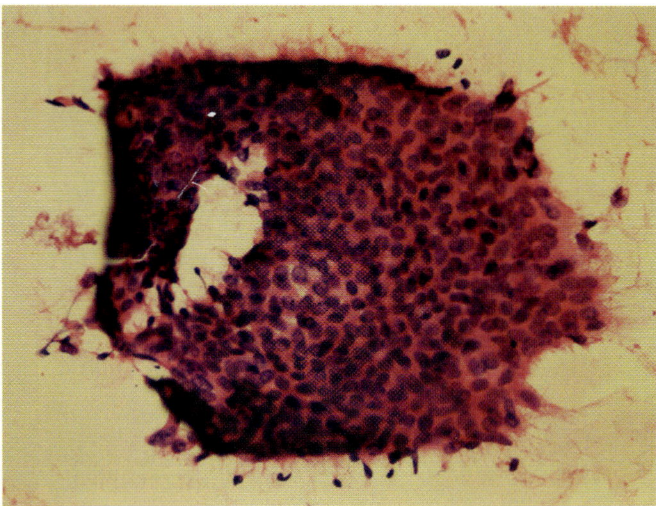

Fig. 27.2: Benign ductal cells in tight cluster (H & E × MP).

NORMAL CYTOLOGY OF BREAST

Fine needle aspiration cytology of the normal breast usually yields scanty cellularity. The following cells are seen in FNAC of a nonneoplastic breast.

Ductal Cells (Fig. 27.2)

These are found singly or honeycomb-like flat cluster. Ductal cells are small round cells with monomorphic nuclei. The individual cells have regular nuclear margin with homogenous chromatin and inconspicuous nucleoli.

Myoepithelial Cells

These are easily identifiable bipolar naked cells. Occasional cells may have scanty preserved cytoplasm.

Apocrine Cells (Fig. 27.3)

These are large cells with abundant granular eosinophilic cytoplasm. The nucleus of the cell is central to eccentric in position, round, and monomorphic.

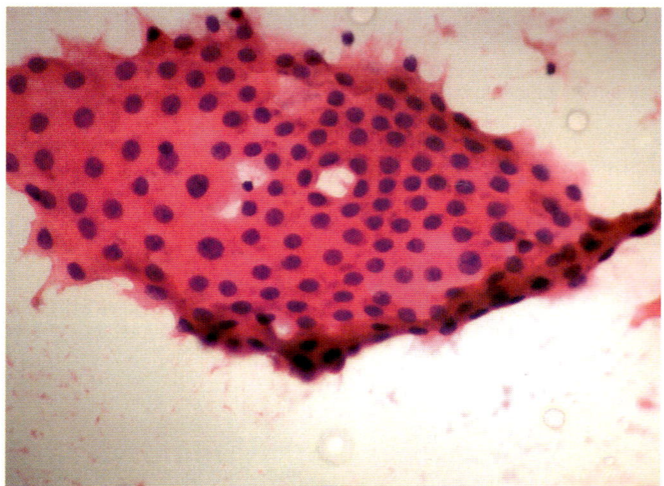

Fig. 27.3: Large cluster of apocrine cells with moderate to abundant cytoplasm and centrally placed monomorphic nuclei (H & E × HP).

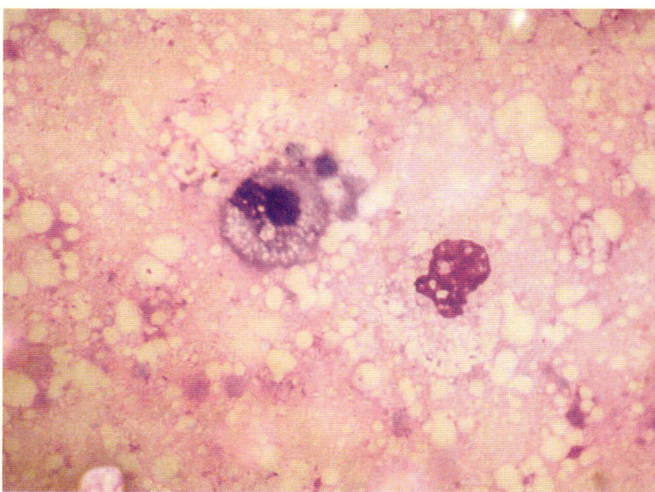

Fig. 27.4: Foamy histiocytes indicating degenerative changes (MGG × HP).

Foam Cells (Fig. 27.4)

The foam cells have abundant vacuolated cytoplasm and centrally placed monomorphic round nucleus. Phagocytosed material may be found in the cytoplasm. The presence of foam cells usually indicates cystic degeneration.

In addition, FNAC of the breast may also yield fat and stromal fragment.

BENIGN LESIONS OF THE BREAST

Box 27.6 shows the classification of the benign lesions of breast.

Box 27.6: Benign breast lesions.

- Inflammatory lesions
  - Acute inflammation
  - Chronic inflammation
  - Granulomatous mastitis
- Lesions caused by trauma
  - Fat necrosis
  - Lesions caused by breast augmentation or reduction surgery
- Benign proliferative breast disease
  - Fibroadenoma
  - Fibrocystic disease
  - Lactating adenoma
  - Granular cell tumor
  - Intraductal papilloma
  - Atypical ductal hyperplasia.

Benign Inflammatory Lesions

Mastitis

It is the inflammation of breast. Mastitis usually occurs in postpartum lactating woman. The bacteria invade the breast through small cracks of the nipple. The common organisms are staphylococci and streptococci. The patient presents with swelling, pain, and tender mass in the breast. Mastitis may mimic clinically as inflammatory carcinoma.

Cytology: Fine needle aspiration cytology of the cases of mastitis usually yields pus. The cytological picture depends on the chronicity of the inflammation. In acute mastitis the smears show abundant polymorphs, necrotic debris, and occasional ductular cells. In subacute and chronic mastitis the smears show increased proportion of lymphocytes, plasma cells, histiocytes, and clusters of ductular cells. The ductal cells may show reactive nuclear atypia due to chronic inflammation.

Differential diagnosis:

Inflammatory carcinoma: Reactive nuclear atypia of ductal cells may mimic carcinoma.

Granulomatous Mastitis

Granulomatous mastitis (GM) is an uncommon breast lesion. The clinical and radiological features of GM often mimic malignancy. The patients usually present as hard breast lump. The patients are in reproductive age period and are often lactating. The etiology of GM is mainly idiopathic of unknown etiology. The specific causes of GM are tuberculosis, sarcoidosis, fungal infections, or foreign body granulomas such as due to leakage of silicone implant or suture granuloma.[23]

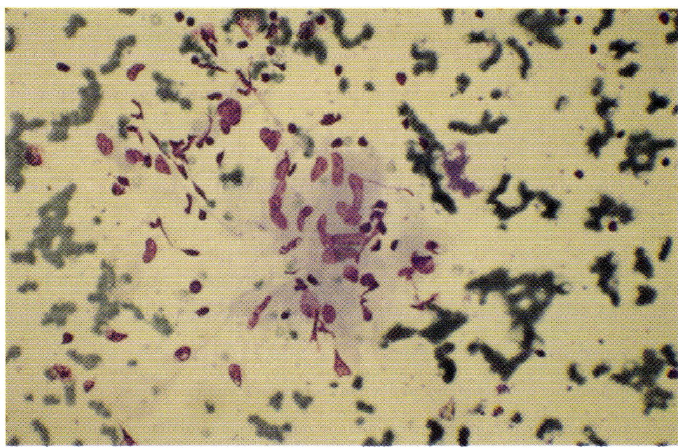

Fig. 27.5: Epithelioid cell granuloma in a case of granulomatous mastitis (MGG × MP).

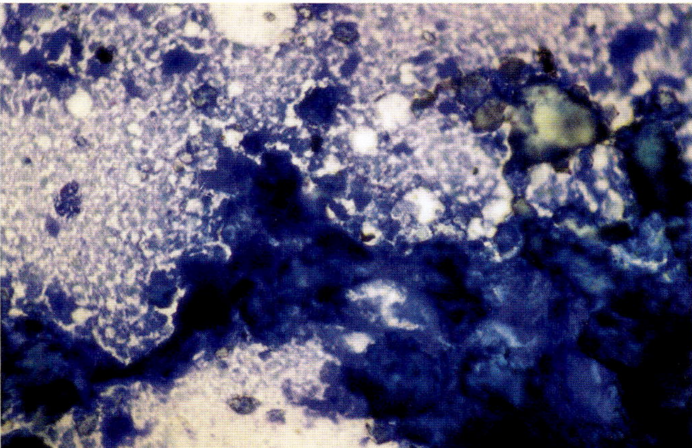

Fig. 27.6: Degenerated necrotic fat and calcification in fat necrosis of breast (MGG × MP).

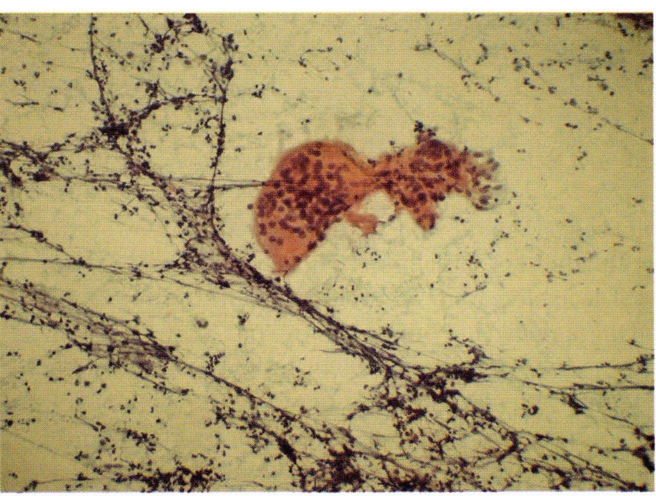

Fig. 27.7: Inflammatory cells and multinucleated giant cells in fat necrosis (Papanicolaou's stain × MP).

Box 27.7: Granulomatous mastitis.

- Multiple epithelioid cell granulomas
- Lymphocytes and capillary fragments
- Multinucleated giant cells
- Necrosis
- Reactive ductal epithelial cells.

Cytology (Fig. 27.5): Fine needle aspiration cytology of GM shows multiple epithelioid cell granulomas, reactive lymphoid cells, multinucleated giant cells, necrosis, and occasional clusters of ductular cells (Box 27.7). In addition there may be specific causes of GM such as suture material, fungal profiles, or AFB in Z-N stain.

Differential diagnosis: Low-grade IDC is the main differential diagnosis of GM.

Box 27.8: Fat necrosis.

- Neutrophils and lymphocytes
- Multinucleated giant cells
- Necrotic fatty background.
- Epithelioid cell granuloma

Differential Diagnosis: Carcinoma.

Chronic Subareolar Abscess

This is a specific clinical condition characterized by chronic infection of the lactiferous sinus or duct and the formation of subareolar abscess. The chronic inflammatory reaction often causes squamous metaplasia of the duct lining epithelium and blockage of the duct lumen due to keratin plugging. This abscess often bursts out on the surface and forms fistula in the nipple.

Cytology: Fine needle aspiration cytology of the subareolar abscess shows abundant polymorphs, lymphocytes, histiocytes, multinucleated giant cells, and metaplastic squamous cells. In addition, the smears also show reactive atypical ductal cells.[24,25]

Fat Necrosis

Fat necrosis clinically mimics malignancy. It may occur due to direct trauma to the breast or as an effect of local radiation in a carcinoma of breast. The presence of fat necrosis does not exclude the possibility of an underlying malignancy. The patient typically presents as hard lump in the breast fixed to the adjacent tissue.

The salient diagnostic points of fat necrosis are highlighted in Box 27.8.

Cytology (Figs. 27.6 and 27.7): Fine needle aspiration cytology of the fat necrosis yields amorphous material.

The smears show dirty degenerated fat (Box 27.8). The nuclei of the fat cells are often enlarged. In addition, the smear shows mixed inflammatory cells and large atypical histiocytes. The enlarged and mildly pleomorphic histiocytes may mimic malignant cells. Occasional ductal cells show mild nuclear enlargement.

Benign Noninflammatory Lesions

Fibroadenoma

Fibroadenoma (FAd) is the most common benign breast tumor of the breast. FAd may occur in any age group. However, it is typically noted between 20 years to 35 years of age. The presence of FAd in prepubertal and postmenopausal women is rare. The patient usually presents with a well circumscribed, firm to soft, mobile mass in the breast.

Cytology (Figs. 27.8 to 27.11): Fine needle aspiration cytology of the FAd yields thick sticky material. The cytology smears show abundant cellularity (Box 27.9). Striking biphasic pattern is seen in most of the cases. The smears show both round to oval ductal cells and spindle bipolar cells. The ductal cells are present in multiple tight clusters, and in three-dimensional antler horns like arrangement. Single dissociated duct cells are also seen. Individual cells have round monomorphic nuclei with fine granular chromatin and small nucleoli. Chondromyxoid stromal material is also noted. This gives bright magenta-colored appearance in May-Grünwald Giemsa (MGG) stain. Clusters of stromal cells are embedded in the pinkish connective tissue stroma. The stromal cell shows scanty cytoplasm and spindle-shaped nuclei. Naked bipolar myoepithelial cells are easily recognizable in Papanicolaou's staining.

There may be various changes in FAd such as:

- Nuclear atypia
- Apocrine metaplasia
- Foam cells
- Mucinous metaplasia
- Bony metaplasia
- Cartilaginous metaplasia.

Out of these, the most significant change is nuclear atypia of ductal cells. This atypia in FAd may be due to hormonal stimulation or inflammation. Atypia is one of the causes of false positive diagnosis in breast FNAC. In most of the times histopathology of such cases reveal benign lesion. Well-maintained polarity of the cells, abundant naked bipolar cells in the background, and essentially normal chromatin pattern of the atypical cells are suggestive of fibroadenoma. Mild atypia in a smear of fibroadenoma should be overlooked.[26,27]

The presence of tight papillary clusters of ductal cells in FAd may simulate papillary tumors. However, FAd does not show typical fibrovascular core as noted in papillary tumors. In addition, the multiple stromal fragments are more often seen in fibroadenoma. It is very difficult to distinguish FAd and cystosarcoma phylloides (CP) in FNAC smear. In CP, there is relative abundance of stromal component over the epithelial component. The stroma is also more cellular in CP than in FAd. FNAC smear of CP also

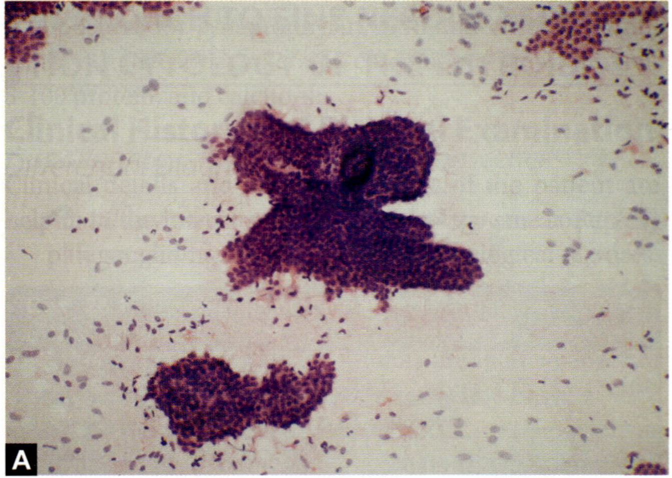

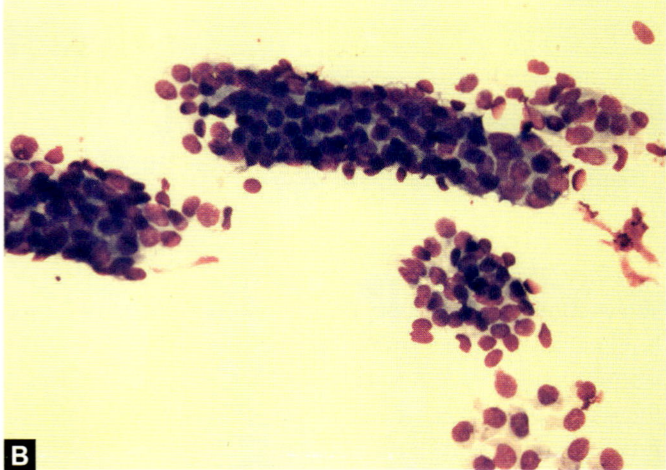

Figs. 27.8A and B: (A) Stag horn-like clusters of ductular cells in fibroadenomas of breast (H & E × MP); (B) Fibroadenomas of breast: ductular cells in tight clusters along with bipolar cells (MGG × MP).

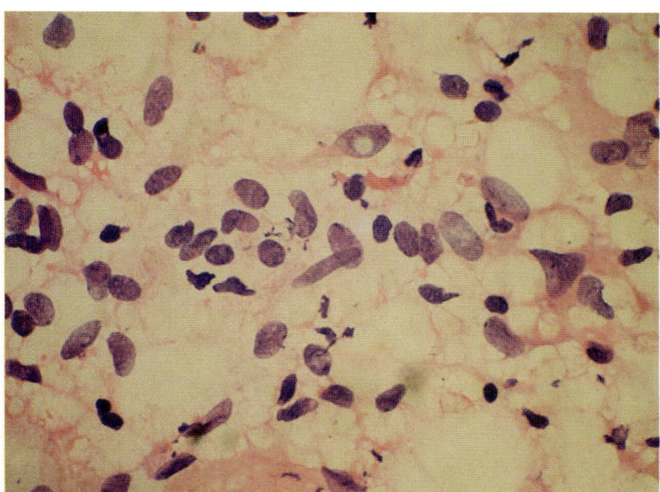

Fig. 27.9: Discrete ductular cells and many bipolar stromal cells in fibroadenomas of breast (H & E × HP).

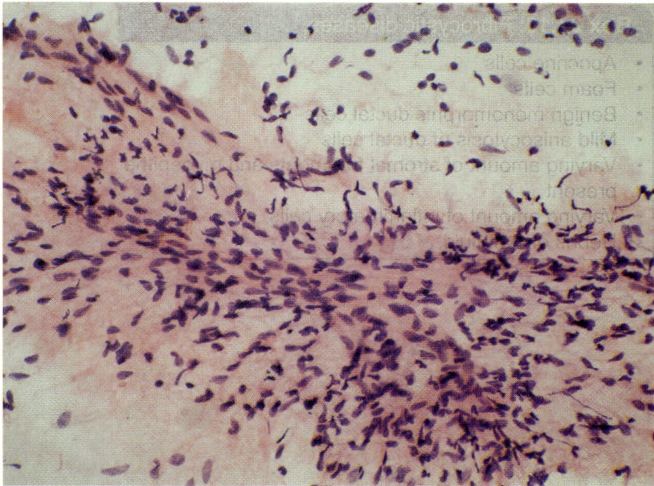

Fig. 27.10: Oval- to spindle-shaped stromal cells embedded in connective tissue stroma in fibroadenomas of breast (H & E × HP).

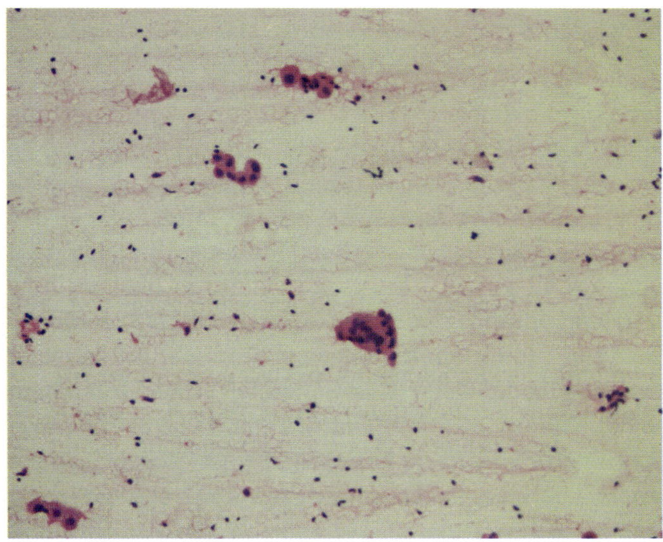

Fig. 27.11: Fibroadenoma: Apocrine cells and multinucleated giant cells (H & E × LP).

shows numerous long plump spindle-shaped cells along with large folded sheets of epithelium.[28,29] However, at times FAd may show large stromal fragments and may be difficult to distinguish from CP on the basis of cytological features.[30]

Differential diagnosis:

- Phyllodes tumor
- Low-grade IDC
- Atypical ductal hyperplasia
- Papillary neoplasm.

Box 27.9: Fibroadenoma.

- Abundant cellularity
- Sheets of cells
- Antler horns like tight clusters
- Biphasic pattern
- Ductal cells
  - Round, monomorphic
  - Fine granular chromatin
  - Small nucleoli
- Bright magenta-colored stromal material
- Many bipolar spindle-shaped cells
- Naked nuclei
- Occasional foam cells and apocrine cells.

Fibrocystic Diseases

Fibrocystic disease (FD) is extremely common lesion in adult female and about 60–90% women are affected by FD in their life time. This disease is most frequently seen in the patients of 25–45 years age. The FD is usually bilateral and multifocal, however one breast may be affected more than the other one. The patient presents with breast lump that shows variation in size and symptoms according to hormonal fluctuation of the menstrual cycle. The clinical and radiological features of FD may simulate carcinoma and the presence of FD makes the detection of carcinoma by mammography more difficult.

Cytology (Figs. 27.12 and 27.13): Fine needle aspiration cytology in predominant fibrous type of FD yields scanty material. However, in cystic type of FD, FNAC yields clear to turbid fluid. Discrete and large monolayer clusters of apocrine cells are often seen (Box 27.10). These cells have abundant granular eosinophilic cytoplasm. The nuclei

Box 27.10: Fibrocystic diseases.

- Apocrine cells
- Foam cells
- Benign monomorphic ductal cells
- Mild anisocytosis of ductal cells
- Varying amount of stromal fragments and myoepithelial cells present
- Varying amount of inflammatory cells
- Debris of cyst fluid.

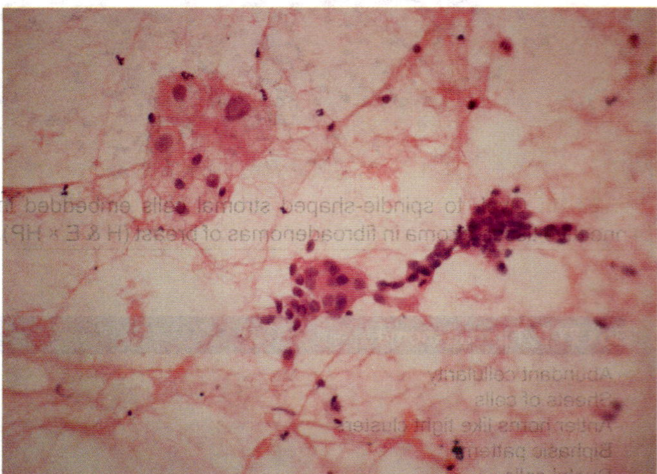

Fig. 27.13: Fibrocystic disease of breast: Foamy histiocytes and benign ductal cells (H & E × HP).

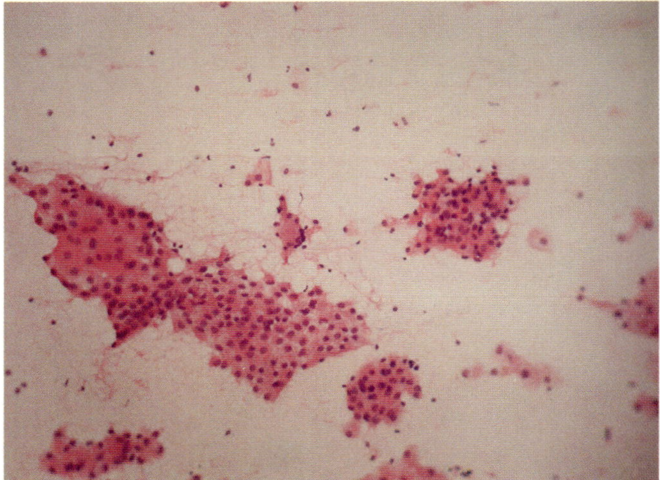

Fig. 27.12: Fibrocystic disease of breast: Clusters of apocrine cells and foamy histiocytes (H & E × MP).

of the apocrine cells are in central position. Nuclei may show mild enlargement and pleomorphism. The smears also show many foamy histiocytes, and small clusters of benign ductal cells. The ductal cells are usually in monolayer sheets. The cells have monomorphic nuclei with fine granular chromatin and inconspicuous nucleoli. The smear also shows scattered naked bipolar cells, stromal fragments, and adipose tissue. Occasionally, it is difficult to distinguish FAd from FD due to the relative abundance of ductal cells in the fibrocystic disease. However, large fragments of stromal cells, abundant bipolar spindle cells, and antler horn-like cells are characteristically seen in FAd (Table 27.3). Mild degree of nuclear enlargement may be noted in ductal cells due to fluid effect. At times, the atypical ductal cells may create diagnostic difficulty with a low-grade carcinoma. Chromatin pattern of the cell is helpful in this condition.

Differential diagnosis:

- FAd
- ADH
- Carcinoma.

Table 27.3: Distinguishing points between fibroadenoma and fibrocystic change.

	Fibroadenoma	*Fibrocystic disease*
Swelling	Well circumscribed, mobile	Ill-defined, diffuse, firm area
Location	Usually unilateral	Bilateral, multifocal
Hormonal dependency	No	Variation of size and symptoms depending on menstrual cycle
Aspirate	Particulate	Usually clear or turbid fluid
Ductal cells	Abundant	Relatively scanty
Ductal cell arrangement	Antler horn-like 3D clusters	Monolayer sheets
Naked bipolar myoepithelial cells	Abundant	Scanty
Chondromyxoid stromal fragments	Abundant	Scanty to absent
Apocrine cells	Scanty	Relatively more

Galactocele

Glactoceles are small cysts filled with milk due to occlusion of the lactiferous duct. Aspirate yields milky fluid. FNAC smear shows (Fig. 27.14) large cells with abundant vacuolated cytoplasm in a milky background.[31,32]

Lactating Adenoma and Lactational Breast

Lactating adenoma is well-circumscribed freely mobile solitary or multiple mass and characteristically seen in pregnant or lactating patients. This is actually the localized area of hyperplasia in the lactating breast.

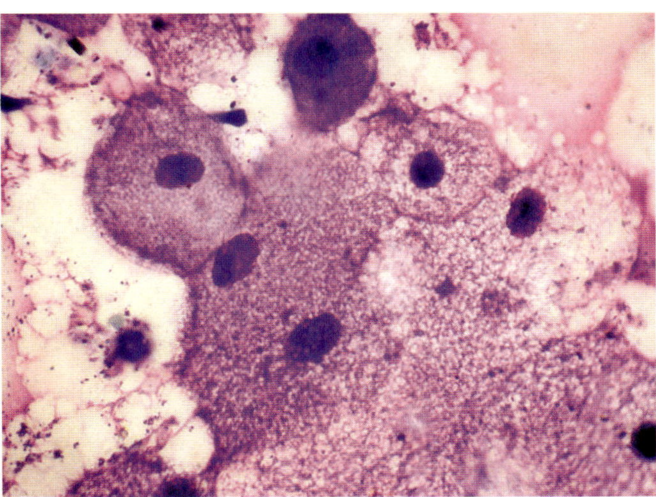

Fig. 27.14: Large cells with abundant vacuolated cytoplasm in a milky background in a case of galactocele of breast (MGG × HP).

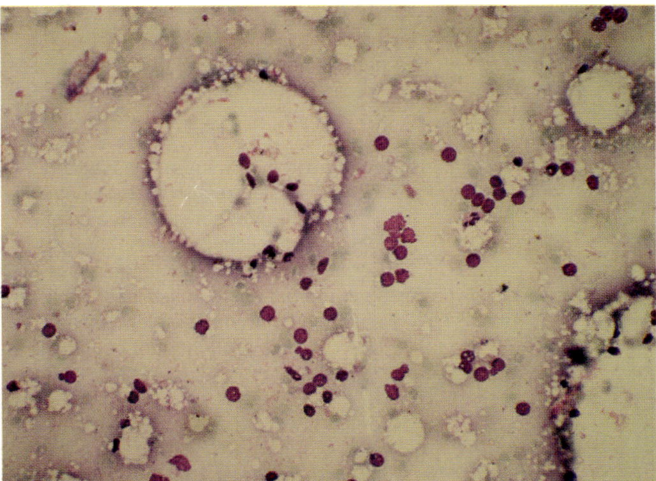

Fig. 27.15: Lactating adenoma: Many discrete cells in a milky background (MGG × MP).

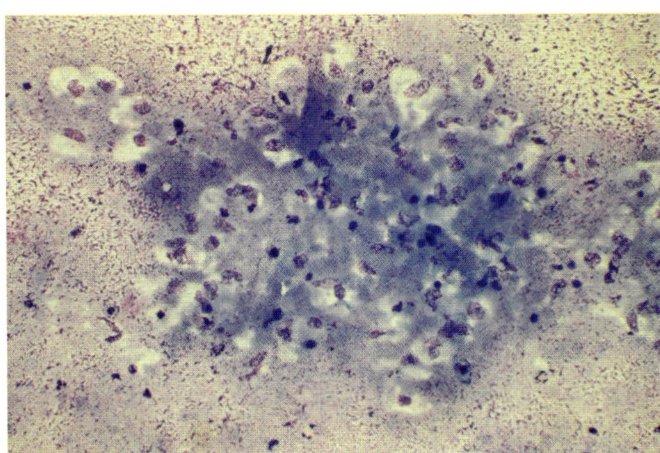

Fig. 27.16: Lactating adenoma: Abundant foamy galactophages in a milky fatty background (MGG × HP).

Cytology (Figs. 27.15 and 27.16): To distinguish lactating adenoma and lactational changes in breast is difficult in FNAC smear as both the lesions show similar cytomorphological features. FNAC yields milky white fluid. Smears show discrete or loosely cohesive ductal epithelial cells in a proteinaceous dirty background (Box 27.11). Individual cells are large and filled with multiple vacuoles. The nuclei are round, monomorphic, and hyperchromatic with single prominent nucleoli. Due to the breakdown of the fragile cytoplasm of the cells, the smear may show many naked nuclei. In addition, the smears may also show many polymorphs, lymphocytes, and macrophages. The proteinaceous and frothy dirty background of the smear may obscure the detailed cytomorphology of the individual cells.

Box 27.11: Lactational adenoma or lactating breast.

- Milky white fluid
- Discrete or loosely cohesive ductal epithelial cells
- Large cells filled with multiple vacuoles
- Enlarge round hyperchromatic nuclei with single prominent nucleoli
- Numerous naked nuclei
- Many polymorphs, lymphocytes, and macrophages
- Proteinaceous dirty background.

Discrete cells with nuclear pleomorphism and prominent nucleoli may mislead the cytologists to a wrong diagnosis of carcinoma. This wrong diagnosis can be avoided if the history of lactation is known. The nuclear abnormality of carcinoma is much greater than that of lactating breast.

Differential diagnosis: Carcinoma in pregnancy or lactation: It is often very difficult to distinguish carcinoma in pregnancy or lactation with pregnancy associated changes. However, nuclear characters such as nuclear pleomorphism and angulated irregular thickened nuclear margin indicate malignancy.

- Fibroadenoma
- Galactocele.

PROLIFERATIVE BREAST DISEASE

Benign epithelial lesions of the breast are classified on the basis of relative risk to develop carcinoma. The lesions, those are not associated with the risk of development of cancer, are known as *nonproliferative* breast disease

Box 27.12: Traditional classification of epithelial hyperplasia.

- Usual ductal hyperplasia
- Flat epithelial atypia
- Atypical ductal hyperplasia
- Ductal carcinoma in situ grade 1
- Ductal carcinoma in situ grade 2
- Ductal carcinoma in situ grade 3.

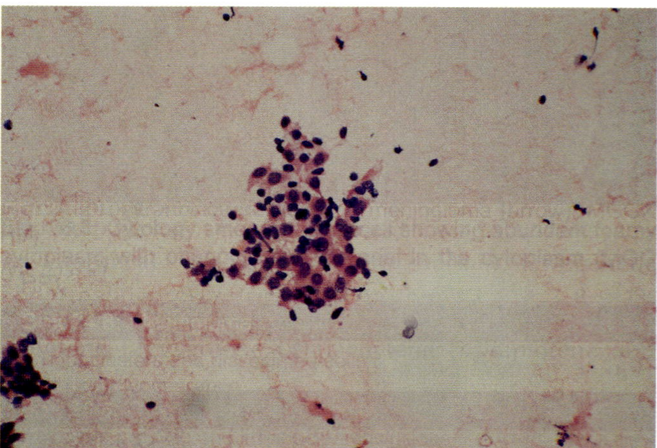

Fig. 27.17: Monlayered cluster of ductular cells with mild nuclear atypia in proliferative breast disease with mild atypia (H & E × MP).

and rest of the lesions are known as *proliferative* breast disease. The proliferative breast disease without atypia is associated with 1.5- to 2-fold relative risk of developing carcinoma, whereas proliferative breast disease with atypia is associated with almost 4- to 5-folds higher risk of developing carcinoma.[33] Proliferative breast disease without atypia includes sclerosing adenosis, collagenous spherulosis, papillomatosis, and ductal hyperplasia.

The World Health Organization (WHO) working group favors to maintain the traditional classification of epithelial hyperplasia as such given in Box 27.12:

It is often difficult to distinguish these lesions on FNAC material. Proliferative breast disease shows large number of cohesive ductal cells along with naked nuclei. Here, the ductal cells are predominantly arranged in monolayer sheets. Occasional clusters of cells with mild nuclear crowding and pleomorphism are also seen. Cells show fine granular nuclear chromatin and inconspicuous nucleoli.

Proliferative Breast Disease with Atypia

As already mentioned, proliferative breast disease is divided into three grades (1) mild, (2) moderate, and (3) severe hyperplasia.[34]

Box 27.13: Hall marks of proliferative breast disease with atypia or atypical ductal hyperplasia.

- Large complex multilayered clusters
- Crowding and loss of polarity of nuclei
- Cellular pleomorphism
- Nuclear anisocytosis
- Irregular coarse chromatin and prominent nucleoli
- Presence of myoepithelial cells.

Grade 1: No or mild hyperplasia: There is no risk for carcinoma.

Grade 2: Moderate or florid hyperplasia: 1.5–2 times risk for carcinoma.

Grade 3: Atypical ductal or lobular hyperplasia: 4–5 times risk for carcinoma.

In addition, another group was included in this category:

Grade 4: Ductal or lobular carcinoma in situ.[35]

Diagnosis of proliferative breast disease with atypia or ADH is primarily based on following criteria:

- Cellularity
- Cell arrangement
- Cellular pleomorphism
- Myoepithelial cells
- Nuclear pleomorphism
- Nucleoli
- Chromatin clumping.

Salient cytological features to proliterative breast disease are given in Box 27.13.[34, 36-40]

Cytology (Figs. 27.17 to 27.19): Fine needle aspiration cytology smear of ADH is rich in cellularity. The cells are arranged in large, complex, and multilayered sheets. The myoepithelial cells are closely intermingled with the cluster of ductal cells. Pseudopapillary arrangement of ductal cells is often seen. Occasionally the cells are arranged as cribriform-like pattern with slit-like spaces in between. There is nuclear crowding and loss of polarity of the cells. The cells show distinct cytoplasmic borders and pleomorphism. The nuclei are enlarged, pleomorphic with coarse chromatin, and prominent nucleoli. Loosely cohesive small clusters of cells and occasional dispersed ductal cells are also seen. These cytological features of ADH may be mistaken as IDC. However, the presence of myoepithelial cells, clustering and cohesion of cells, and lack of significant number of isolated single cells are the important features to distinguish ADH from IDC.

The diagnosis of ADH is a challenge to the cytopathologist as the cytomorphology of this lesion is intermediate between IDC and benign lesion. The distinction of these

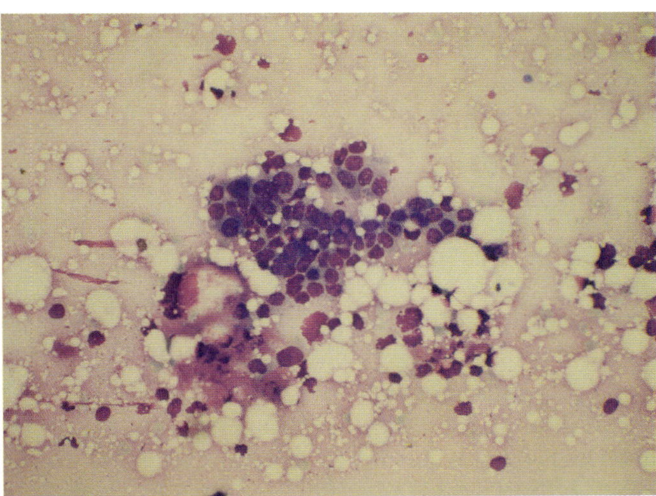

Fig. 27.18: Cluster and discrete ductal cells with nuclear overlapping and moderate nuclear pleomorphism (MGG × MP).

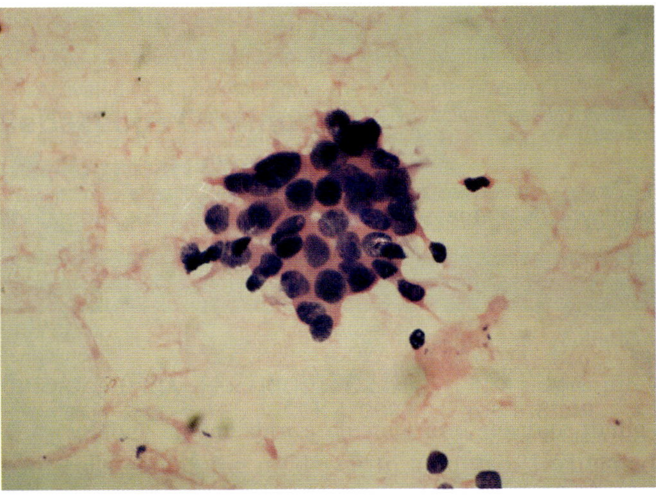

Fig. 27.19: Proliferative breast disease with atypia showing nuclear overlapping and pleomorphism (H & E × MP).

Table 27.4: Cytologic features of proliferative breast disease without atypia and atypical ductal hyperplasia of breast.

Cytology	*Proliferative breast disease without atypia*	*Atypical ductal hyperplasia*
Cellularity	Moderate	Abundant
Cell arrangement	Crowded sheets with regular nuclear spacing	Three-dimensional crowded sheets with nuclear overlapping
Nuclear pleomorphism	Absent	Present, mild to moderate
Nucleoli	Inconspicuous	Prominent
Hyperchromasia	Absent	Present
Chromatin	Fine	Coarse

lesions has important clinical implications. To combat the challenge Masood et al. proposed a scoring system based on cellular arrangement, cellular pleomorphism, anisonucleosis, nucleoli, nuclear chromatin, and the presence of myoepithelial cells. Each feature is scored from 1 to 4 and the final diagnosis depends on total scoring.[41]

Differential Diagnosis

- *Fibroadenoma*: Cellular fibroadenoma may be difficult to distinguish from proliferative breast disease. The key cytological features of FAd are:
  - Antler horn clusters
  - Flat or monolayered sheets, and
  - Fragments of fibromyxoid stroma.
- Ductal carcinoma in situ: Discussed here.
- *Proliferative breast disease without atypia*: It is important to distinguish proliferative breast disease without atypia from ADH. Table 27.4 highlights the salient points.

DUCTAL CARCINOMA IN SITU[36,42]

Ductal carcinoma in situ (DCIS) is a heterogeneous group of lesion with variable architectural, histological, and natural history. DCIS is characterized by marked epithelial proliferation with mild to marked nuclear atypia. The chance of progression of DCIS to invasive cancer depends on several factors such as histological subtype, grade, and also extent of the tumor. Due to increasing use of mammography the incidence of DCIS has increased significantly. DCIS represents almost 25% of breast cancer in screened population.[42] The vast majority of DCIS is detected by screening mammography and only a few cases present with clinical symptoms such as palpable swelling, nipple discharge, and nipple retraction.

Cytology (Figs. 27.20 and 27.21)

It is extremely difficult to recognize this entity on cytology smear. The cytological features depend on noncomedo versus comedo variety of DCIS (Box 27.14). FNAC smears of comedocarcinoma show predominantly cohesive clusters and also discrete malignant cells with background necrotic cell debris and calcified material. Individual cells show moderate nuclear enlargement and pleomorphism

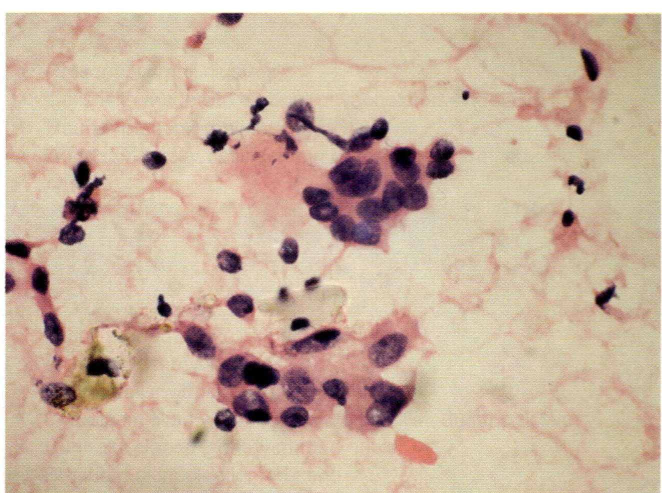

Fig. 27.20: Loose clusters of cells with marked nuclear pleomorphism in carcinoma in situ. Note the clean background (H & E × MP).

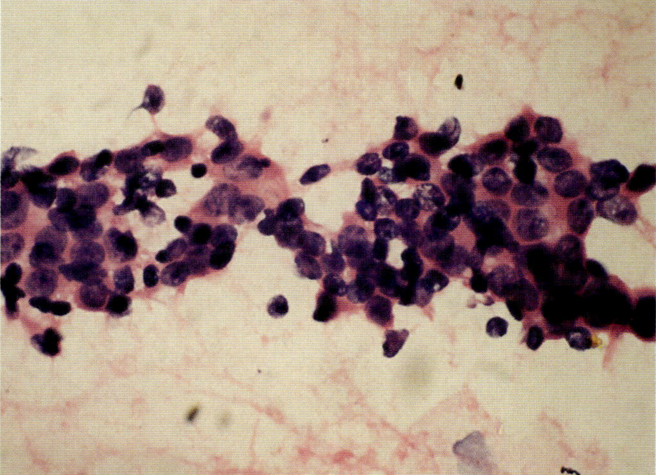

Fig. 27.21: Cluster of cells showing nuclear pleomorphism and irregular clumped chromatin in carcinoma in situ (H & E × MP).

Box 27.14: Ductal carcinoma in situ.

Comedo type
- Cohesive clusters and also discrete malignant cells
- Necrotic cell debris
- Calcified material
- Moderate nuclear enlargement
- Nuclear pleomorphism
- Mitotic activity

Noncomedo type
- Solid, papillary and cribriform clusters
- Relatively monomorphic, small to intermediate in sized cells
- Round nuclei and small nucleoli
- No myoepithelial cells.

along with mitotic activity. Individual cell morphology of comedocarcinoma and IDC is not different. Therefore, to distinguish these two entities in FNAC smear is a controversial issue. Lilleng and Hagmar suggested that cohesive tumor cells in the background of necrotic cellular debris favor DCIS of comedo type, whereas numerous dissociated tumor cells along with occasional clusters of cells in a background of minimal or absent necrosis indicate IDC.[43] FNAC smears of noncomedo type of DCIS show solid, papillary, and cribriform clusters of cells (Box 27.14). The individual cell is small to intermediate in size and monomorphic in appearance. The cells look oval to polygonal with round nuclei and small nucleoli. Myoepithelial cells are absent in the smear. In addition, foamy histiocytes, apocrine cells, and calcified material may also be seen in the background.[44] In FNAC smear, the noncomedo type of DCIS is difficult to categorize exactly and the lesion may be labeled as suspicious for malignancy.

Differential Diagnosis

- *Atypical ductal hyperplasia versus DCIS*: Differentiating ADH from DCIS is difficult. Smear of ADH is usually moderately cellular. The epithelial cells are arranged in cribriform and micropapillary pattern along with admixture of benign monolayered fragments. The myoepithelial cells are also present in ADH that are absent in DCIS. In comedo type of DCIS, the background necrotic debris and calcification are helpful in diagnosis. However at time, noncomedo type DCIS is difficult to distinguish from ADH as both lesions may display similar cytomorphologic features.

PHYLLODES TUMOR[45]

Phyllodes tumor (PT) represents about 0.3–1% of all primary tumors of breast. The older terminology "cystosarcoma phyllodes" is inappropriate because it gives a wrong impression about malignant nature of the tumor, whereas the majority of PTs are benign. This tumor occurs in middle-aged women and the patients are about 20 years older than the age group of fibroadenoma. The patient usually presents as a slow growing solitary well-circumscribed mass in the breast and the average size is about 5 cm at the time of presentation. The tumor may often be mistaken clinically as carcinoma due to the massive size of PT. Recurrence of PT is common and about 15–20% tumors recur after excision. On histology, PTs are classified as benign, borderline, and malignant type.

Cytology (Figs. 27.22 and 27.23)

Cytology of the PT is more like FAd and the smear shows a biphasic cellular tumor composed of both stromal and epithelial cells with relative abundance of stromal component (Box 27.15). There are abundant spindle-shaped cells embedded in the fibromyxoid stroma. The spindle cells with plump fusiform nuclei are also present discretely. The nuclei are usually monomorphic; however, mild degree of atypia may also be noted. In addition, there are multiple large folded sheets of benign monomorphic ductal cells. The smear may also show apocrine cells, foam cells, and multinucleated giant cells. Benign PT does not show increased mitotic activity or any necrosis. Occasionally, the needle may pick up the myxoid stromal material only and the smear may show low cellularity. This hypocellular smear of PT is difficult to diagnose. Therefore, a thorough sampling is always needed. Occasionally, PT may show predominantly epithelial hyperplasia with nuclear pleomorphism. Selective sampling of these areas may lead to a false positive diagnosis of carcinoma of breast.[31]

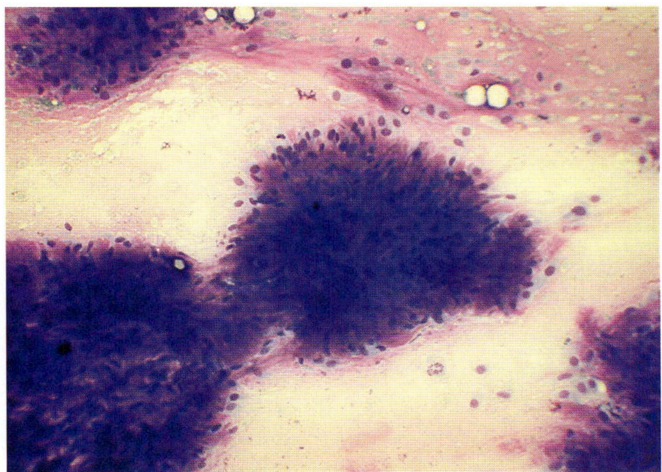

Fig. 27.22: Phyllodes tumor: Multiple clusters and discrete oval- to spindle-shaped stromal cells embedded in abundant pinkish stroma (MGG × MP).

Malignant PT shows large fragment of atypical stromal cells with significant nuclear pleomorphism that often simulates fibrosarcoma (Figs. 27.24 and 27.25). In addition, the smear may also show high mitotic activity and necrosis.[30,46,47]

The stromal overgrowth in malignant PT may be so significant that there may be almost complete absence of epithelial cells and this may make difficult to distinguish these lesions from the pure sarcoma. However, pure sarcoma such as dermatofibrosarcomas and malignant fibrous histiocytomas are exceedingly rare in breast.[48]

Differential Diagnosis

- *Fibroadnoma versus phyllodes tumor*: PT shows relative abundance of stromal component over the epithelial component.

Box 27.15: Phyllodes tumor.

- Biphasic cellular tumor
- Both stromal and epithelial cells
- Abundant stromal component
- Abundant plump spindle-shaped cells
- Large-folded sheets of benign monomorphic ductal cells.

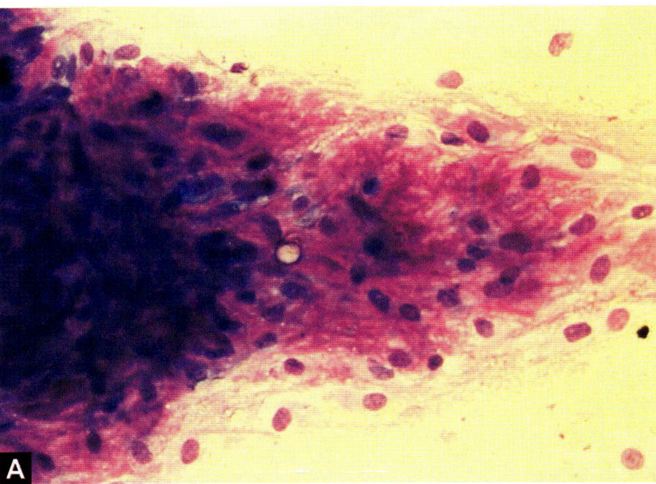

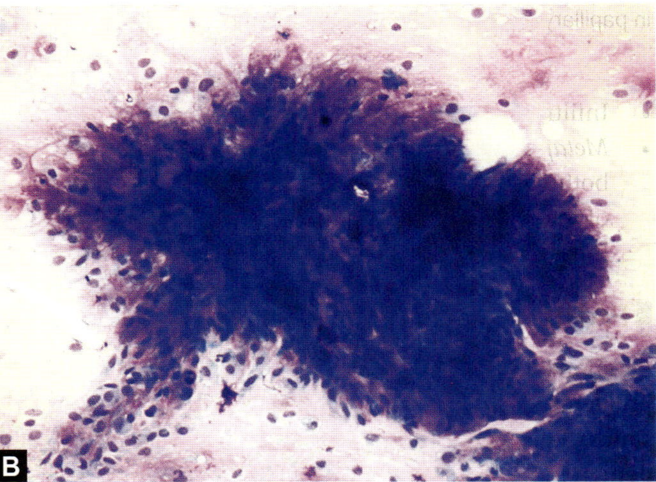

Figs. 27.23A and B: (A) Phyllodes tumor: Large clusters of spindle cells embedded in deep magenta-colored material (MGG × HP); (B) Phyllodes tumor: Individual cells are oval- to spindle-shaped with blunt ended nuclei (MGG × HP).

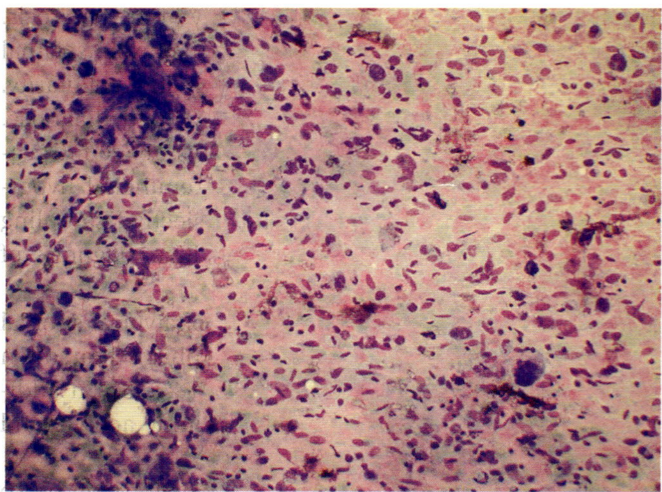

Fig. 27.24: Abundant discrete spindle cells with moderate nuclear pleomorphism in a case of malignant phyllodes tumor (MGG × MP).

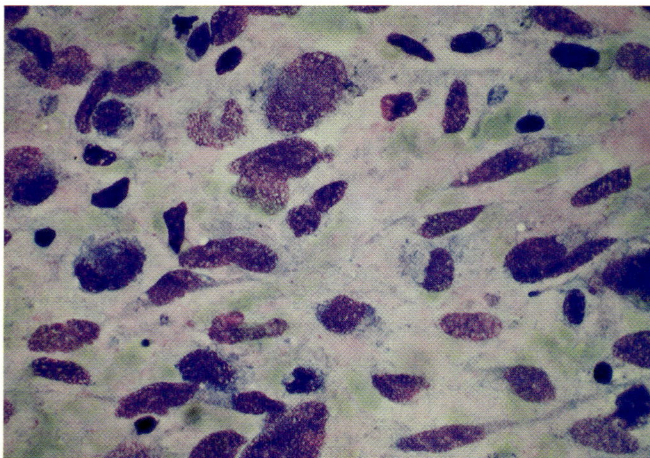

Fig. 27.25: Higher magnification showing large oval to spindle cells with markedly pleomorphic nuclei and irregular coarse chromatin in malignant phyllodes tumor (MGG × HP).

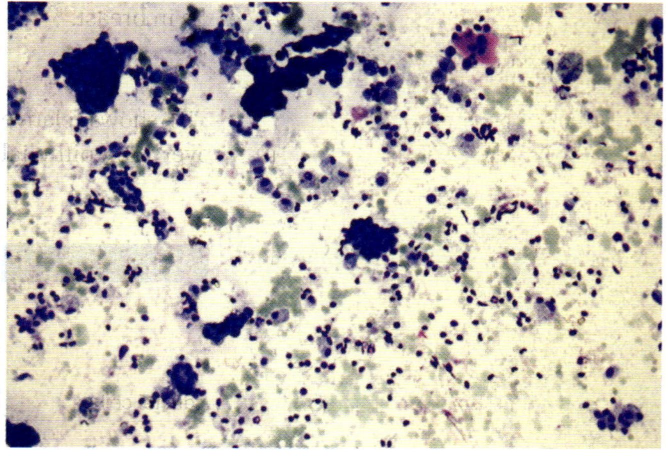

Fig. 27.26: Small papillae-like structures and many macrophages in papillary neoplasm of breast (MGG × MP).

- Infiltrating duct carcinoma.
- *Metaplastic carcinoma*: Here, the epithelial and stromal both components are malignant. A careful observation of the benign epithelial component of PT may resolve the issue.

PAPILLARY NEOPLASM

Papilloma is a benign neoplasm characterized by the proliferation of the epithelial cells around the fibrovascular stalks. Recognizable myoepithelial cells are present in benign intraductal papilloma. It may arise from anywhere in the duct of the breast and most commonly seen near the areola. Papilloma mostly occurs in older woman; however, it may also affect the younger female. The tumor is usually solitary and obstructs the duct causing blood-stained nipple discharge. Cytological evaluation of the nipple discharge is usually the method of detection of papilloma and FNAC is uncommonly needed as the lesion is small and subareolar in majority of times.

Papillary carcinoma accounts for 1–2% of all breast carcinomas. This tumor may be cystic or solid and invasive or noninvasive. The overall prognosis of papillary carcinoma is better than IDC. In case of intraductal papillary carcinoma, the fibrovasuclar stalks are lined by epithelial cells and are almost totally (more than 90%) devoid of any myoepithelial cells. The important histological features of papillary carcinoma are:

- Absence of myoepithelial cells around the fibrovascular core
- Absence of apocrine cells
- Monomorphic cells with hyperchromatic nuclei
- Positive for smooth muscle action (SMA) and high molecular weight-cytokeratins (HMW-CK), the markers of myoepithelial cells.

Cytology[49] (Figs. 27.26 and 27.27)

The cytology smears are usually hypercellular and shows multiple papillary structures with fibrovascular core (Box 27.16). Smaller fragments of the tip of the papillae may also be seen. The ductal cells are arranged as palisading manner at the edge of the papillae. The individual cells are cuboidal to columnar with round nuclei and fine granular chromatin. The nuclei may show varying degree

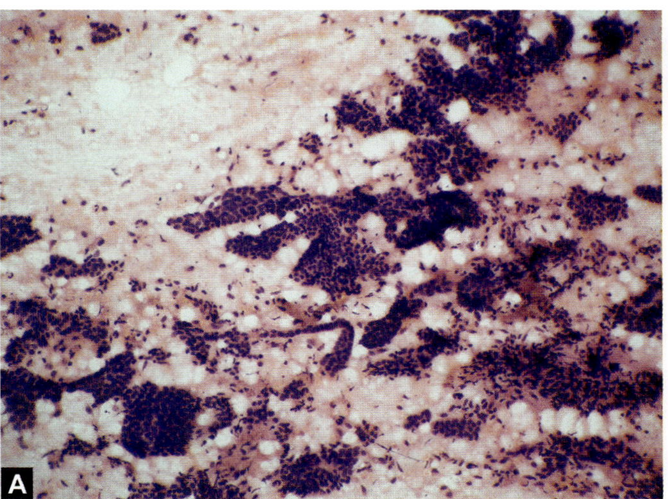
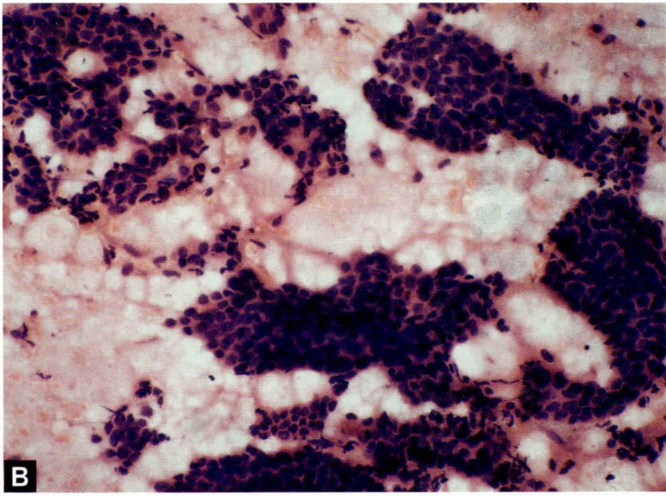

Figs. 27.27A and B: (A) Abundant avascular papillary structures and occasional bipolar myoepithelial cells in papillary neoplasm of breast (H & E × MP); (B) Higher magnification showing better morphology in papillary neoplasm of breast. Note the sharp margin of the clusters of cells. Individual cells are round with mildly pleomorphic nuclei (H & E × HP).

Box 27.16: Papillary tumor of the breast.

- Multiple papillae-like clusters of ductular cells with central stromal material.
- Cuboidal to columnar cells arranged in regular manner at the edge of papillae.
- Occasional discrete cell with intact cytoplasm.
- Background shows foamy macrophages.
- Varying amount of naked bipolar cells.
- Varying degrees of nuclear atypia.

Box 27.17: Cytology features suggestive of papillary carcinoma.

- Monomorphic nuclei
- Nuclear hyperchromasia
- Abundant discrete columnar cells
- Complete absence of myoepithelial cells
- Hemorrhagic background.

of nuclear enlargement and pleomorphism. Naked bipolar myoepithelial cells are seen. In addition, the background shows hemosiderin-laden macrophages and apocrine cells. In FNAC, it is almost impossible to differentiate an intraductal papilloma from a papillary carcinoma. Therefore, it is better to label it as "papillary lesion" only. However, certain cytological features such as monomorphic nuclei, nuclear hyperchromasia, abundant discrete columnar cells, complete absence of myoepithelial cells, and hemorrhagic background are the indicators of papillary carcinoma (Box 27.17).

Differential Diagnosis

- Fibroadenoma
- Papillary carcinoma versus papilloma.

CARCINOMA

Infiltrating Duct Carcinoma

Infiltrating ductal carcinoma, not otherwise specified, is the most common malignant tumor of the breast and represents about 70–80% of all breast cancers. IDC is a heterogeneous group of tumor and lack specific or characteristic histologic pattern. It occurs predominantly in older women and is uncommon in the female younger than 35 years of age. The risk factors of the breast carcinoma include early menarche, late menopause, high intake of saturated fat in diet, nulliparity, and history of first-degree relative with breast cancer. Most of the IDC have characteristic mammographic pattern such as spiculated mass with microcalcification. USG of the IDC shows hypoechoic mass with altered echotexture and ill-defined border. The patient usually presents with hard fixed palpable mass. The overlying skin may be ulcerated and nipple may show retraction.

Cytology (Figs. 27.28 to 27.30)

Fine needle aspiration cytology smears of IDC are highly cellular. The smears show multiple clusters and dissociated ductal cells with nuclear overlapping or crowding (Box 27.18). The ductal cells have enlarged pleomorphic and hyperchromatic nuclei with thickened and irregular membrane. Nucleoli are multiple and prominent. The chromatin shows irregular clumping. Smears show the

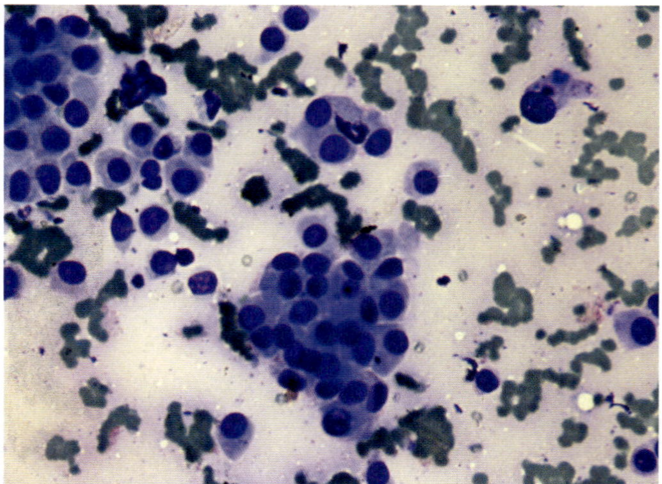

Fig. 27.28: Infiltrating duct carcinoma: Loose clusters and discrete malignant cells in infiltrating duct carcinoma of breast (MGG × HP).

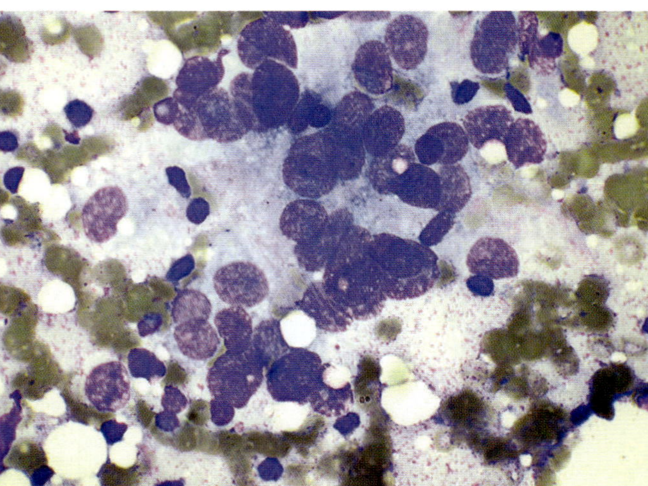

Fig. 27.29: Infiltrating duct carcinoma: Malignant cells with gland formation in infiltrating duct carcinoma of breast (MGG × HP).

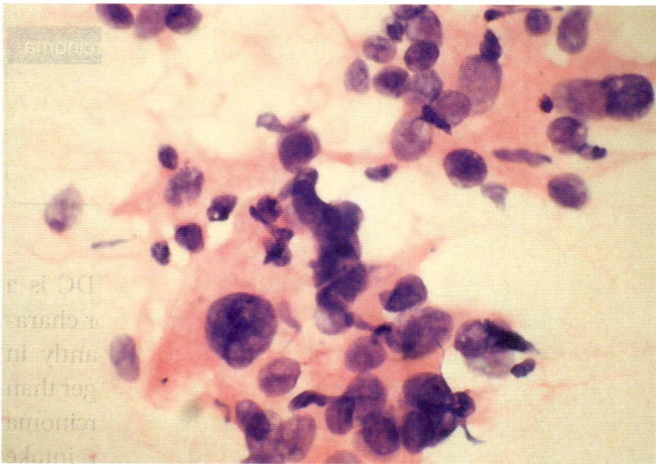

Fig. 27.30: Infiltrating duct carcinoma: Malignant cells showing irregular clumped chromatin in infiltrating duct carcinoma of breast (H & E × HP).

complete absence of naked bipolar cells. It is important to give attention on the single isolated malignant cells. Without their presence, the diagnosis of malignancy should be given with caution. Similarly, the presence of bipolar cells should be taken as serious evidence against the malignant nature of the tumor. At time, it may be difficult to distinguish a low-grade ductal carcinoma versus proliferative breast lesion with atypia. Granular to vesicular nuclear chromatin and thickened irregular nuclear membrane are useful cytological features of low-grade carcinoma.

About 70–80% of breast carcinomas are positive for estrogen receptor and 15–30% cases are positive for HER2/neu.

Box 27.18: Infiltrating duct carcinoma.

- Hypercellular
- Clusters and dissociated ductal cells
- Nuclear crowding
- Often eccentric nucleus protruding out from the cytoplasm giving a plasmacytoid appearance
- Enlarged, pleomorphic, hyperchromatic nuclei
- Nuclear margin thickened and irregular
- Fine to coarse clumped chromatin and prominent nucleoli
- Myoepithelial cell absent
- Tumor diathesis.

Diagnostic Difficulties

- Low-grade carcinoma versus proliferative breast lesion with atypia.
- Usual ductal carcinoma of low-grade versus lobular carcinoma.
- Pregnancy and lactational changes.

Other Types

Medullary Carcinoma

Medullary carcinoma accounts for 1–7% of all breast carcinomas. It is more common in the younger females. Clinically, the tumor may simulate as a fibroadenomas or cyst in the breast. The patient presents as well circumscribed, solitary, soft, and mobile mass. As this carcinoma is well circumscribed so it may be mistaken as FA. It is important to identify this subtype of breast carcinoma because the tumor simulates the cytological features of high-grade carcinoma; however, the prognosis of medullary carcinoma is far better than high-grade IDC. The cytologic features are[50] described in Box 27.19.

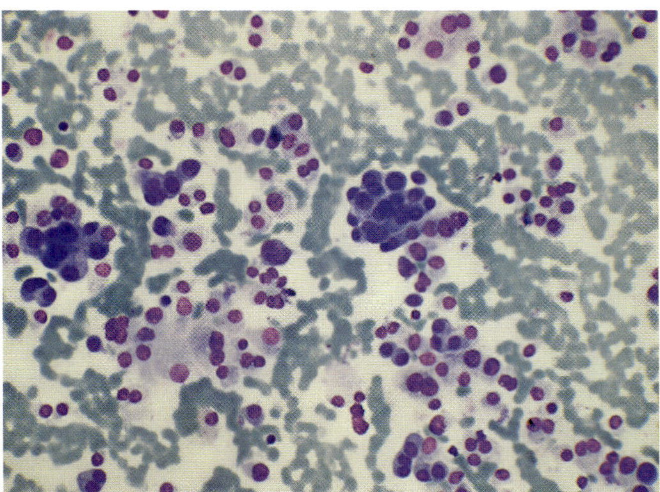

Fig. 27.31: Predominantly discrete cells in medullary carcinoma of breast (MGG × MP).

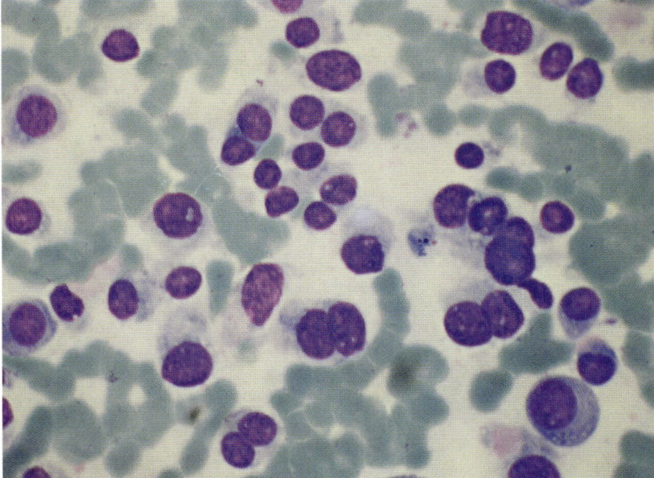

Fig. 27.32: Higher magnification showing pleomorphic nuclei and prominent nucleoli in medullary carcinoma of breast (MGG × HP).

Box 27.19: Medullary carcinoma.

- Abundant dissociated cells
- Syncytial clusters of malignant cells
- Large cells with moderate nuclear pleomorphism
- Multiple prominent nucleoli
- Naked nuclei with macronucleoli
- Lymphocytes and plasma cells
- Tumor necrosis.

Cytology (Figs. 27.31 and 27.32): Medullary carcinoma of the breast shows usually abundant dissociated malignant cells (Box 27.19). The cells are often seen as syncytial clusters. The tumor cells are large and undifferentiated with moderately pleomorphic nuclei having large prominent nucleoli. Many malignant naked nuclei are present. Background of the smear shows moderate lymphocytes and plasma cell infiltration. This is an important diagnostic feature of medullary carcinoma of breast. At times, the presence of the bare nuclei may simulate pregnancy and lactational-induced changes in the breast and vice versa. The presence of large amount lymphoid cells in the aspirates of medullary carcinoma may be confused with metastatic carcinoma in the intramammary lymph node. This tumor often lacks ER/PR and HER2/neu expression.

Differential diagnosis:

- Poorly differentiated high-grade ductal carcinoma
- Metastatic breast carcinoma in an intramammary lymph node
- Chronic mastitis
- Lymphoma.

Mucinous Carcinoma (Colloid Carcinoma)[51]

Mucinous carcinoma is also labeled as colloid, mucoid, or gelatinous carcinoma. Pure mucinous carcinoma represents 2% of breast carcinomas. The tumor occurs in all age groups; however, the mean age of occurrence of mucinous carcinoma is higher than that of IDC. It is important to diagnose mucinous carcinoma because the tumor carries an excellent prognosis with 10-year survival in excess of 80%.[52] The patient presents as large slowly growing well-circumscribed lump in the breast. On mammography, the tumor may appear as a benign neoplasm.

Cytology (Figs. 27.33 and 27.34): FNAC of mucinous carcinoma yields thick mucoid material. The smears show abundant pale blue acellular mucinous material (Box 27.20). The loose clusters and discrete malignant cells float in the pool of mucin. The cells are blunt looking and may be mistaken as benign cells. Individual cells are monomorphic with moderate to abundant cytoplasm and round monomorphic nuclei. The chromatin of the nuclei is bland. Nucleoli are usually absent. Occasional cells show moderate nuclear enlargement and pleomorphic. Thin endothelial-lined vessels within the mucin are also described in mucinous carcinoma.[51] Mucinous material may also be noted in IDC, not otherwise specified. However, the amount of mucinous material is less in that case and cells show more nuclear atypia.

Mucinous material may be aspirated in different benign and malignant lesions of the breast and this should be remembered before the diagnosis of mucinous carcinoma (Box 27.21).

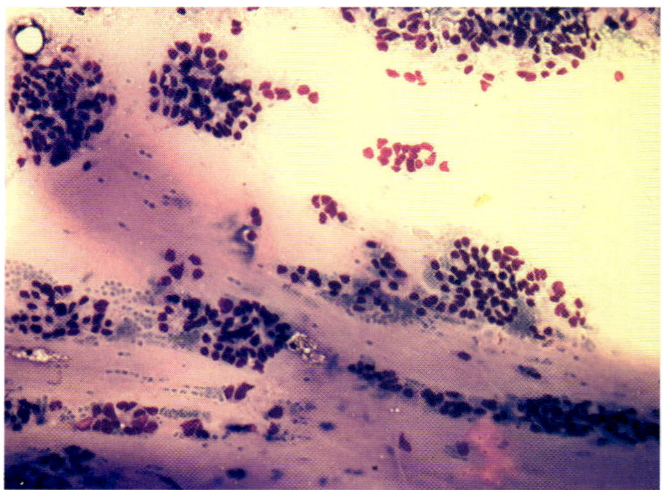

Fig. 27.33: Mucinous carcinoma of breast: Malignant cells embedded within the pool of mucin (MGG × MP).

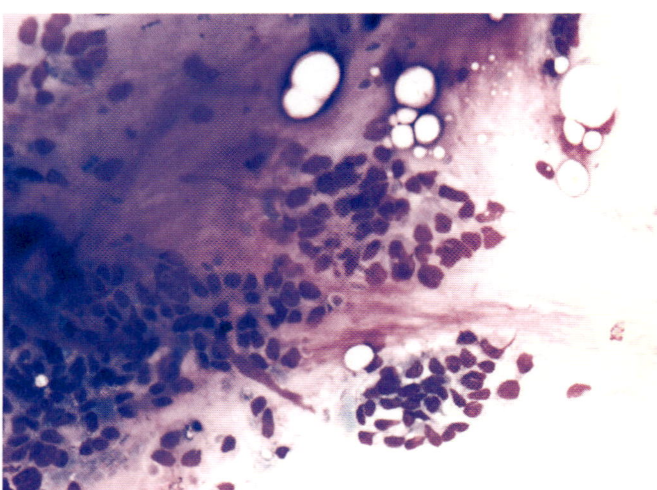

Fig. 27.34: Mucinous carcinoma of breast: Higher magnification showing round to oval pleomorphic cells in reddish bluish material (MGG × MP).

Box 27.20: Mucinous carcinoma.

- Abundant mucinous material
- Floating malignant cells in the pool of mucin
- Cells with abundant cytoplasm and mild to moderately pleomorphic nuclei
- Bland nuclear chromatin.

Box 27.21: Mucinous material in breast fine needle aspiration cytology.

- Mucocele
- Mucinous adenocarcinoma of breast
- Mixed mucinous and ductal carcinoma
- Mucinous papillary neoplasm
- Secretory carcinoma.

Table 27.5: Distinguishing features between mucinous carcinoma and mucocele.

Features	*Mucinous carcinoma*	*Mucocele*
Cellularity	Mild to moderate	Scanty
Cell arrangement	Loose clusters and discrete	Discrete
Nuclear atypia	Mild to moderate	Nil
Background cell	Thin wire like capillaries	Macrophages, apocrine cells, and benign ductular cells

Differential diagnosis:

- *Mucocele of the breast*: Mucocele of the breast lesion may also yield abundant mucoid material. Mucocele-like lesions of the breast usually show sheets of benign ductular cells with scanty cytoplasm and monomorphic nuclei.[53] In addition, background may show histiocytes and apocrine cells (Table 27.5).
- *Myxoid change in FAd*: Myxoid change in FAd may be confused with colloid carcinoma. FAd is usually cellular and show large tight clusters of cells along with many bipolar cells in the background. If it is not possible to distinguish myxoid fibroadenoma from colloid carcinoma then the tumor should be excised for histopathology.[51]

Ductal Carcinoma with Mucinous Metaplasia

Apocrine Carcinoma

Apocrine carcinoma is a relatively uncommon malignancy and represents 0.3–4% of all breast cancers. This tumor is characterized by a malignant tumor with predominant population of apocrine cells (more than 90%). It usually affects the women of older age group. There is no special clinical feature of apocrine carcinoma to distinguish it from IDC.

Cytology (Figs. 27.35 and 27.36): Cytology smear of apocrine carcinoma is cellular. The cells are predominantly arranged as sheets, cords, tubules, and discretely (Box 27.22). The individual cells are morphologically recognizable as apocrine cells. The cells are large with abundant granular eosinophilic cytoplasm. The nuclei are centrally placed

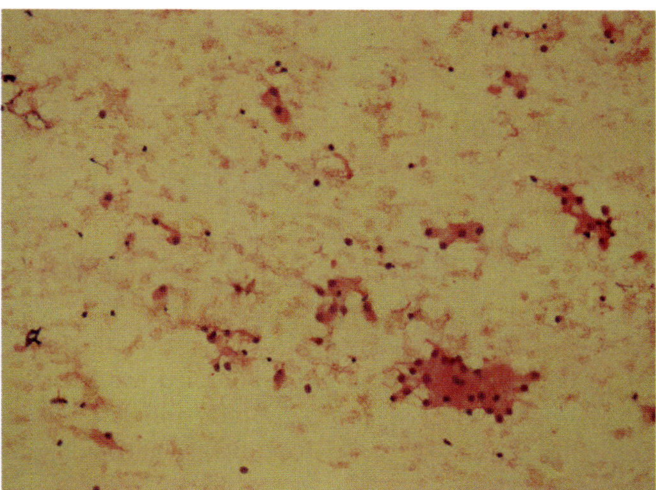

Fig. 27.35: Loose clusters and discrete apocrine cells in apocrine carcinoma of breast (H & E × MP).

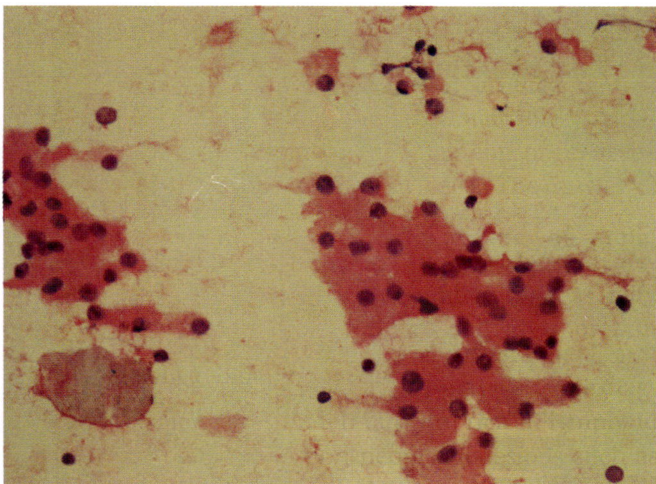

Fig. 27.36: The cells show mild nuclear enlargement and pleomorphism in apocrine carcinoma of breast (H & E × MP).

Box 27.22: Apocrine carcinoma.

- Clusters and sheets of cells
- Abundant apocrine cells with moderate to abundant granular cytoplasm.
- Centrally placed large vesicular nucleus.
- Mild to moderate nuclear pleomorphism and prominent nucleoli
- Comet-shaped cells with protruding nuclei
- *Immunostain*: Positive for GCDFP-15, a marker of apocrine cells and negative for ER/PR.

large and pleomorphic having prominent nucleoli. Frequent binucleation and multinucleation are also noted. At times, the nuclei are eccentric in position and give a comet-like appearance. Background necrosis may also be seen.

Apocrine change is common in fibrocystic disease, and it usually indicates benign nature of the lesion. Mild degree of nuclear enlargement is also common in apocrine cells. So, cytologist should be careful to report an apocrine carcinoma. In fact, apocrine carcinoma is the gray zone tumor and often be mistaken as benign apocrine changes or vice versa (Table 27.6).

It is important to remember that apocrine changes are noted in IDC. Therefore, mere presence of apocrine cells may not indicate apocrine carcinoma and significant amount of apocrine cells is needed to diagnose apocrine carcinoma.

Differential diagnosis:

- Apocrine metaplasia
- Apocrine changes in other carcinomas.

Table 27.6: Differentiating metaplastic apocrine cells and apocrine carcinoma.

Features	*Benign metaplastic apocrine cells*	*Apocrine carcinoma*
Age	Younger	Older
Nuclei	Normal	Mild to moderate enlargement
Nucleoli	Single	Multiple prominent
Comet-shaped cells	Absent	Present

Box 27.23: Tubular carcinoma.

- Usually scanty cellularity
- Small tubular structures
- Cohesive cells arranged in comma-shaped manner
- The cells with monomorphic nuclei, finely granular chromatin, and small nucleoli
- Absence of bipolar naked cells in the background
- Densely collagenized fibrous tissue fragments.

Tubular Carcinoma

Tubular carcinoma represents 1–2% of all breast carcinomas. This is a special type of breast carcinoma with well-differentiated tubular structures. Tubular carcinoma occurs in older patients compared to IDC and usually bilateral, smaller in size at the time of presentation with less incidence of lymph nodal involvement.

Cytology: Aspirates of tubular carcinoma of the breast usually show scanty cellularity due to stromal fibrosis. The smears show many small well-defined tubular structures and tight cohesive clusters of cells (Box 27.23).

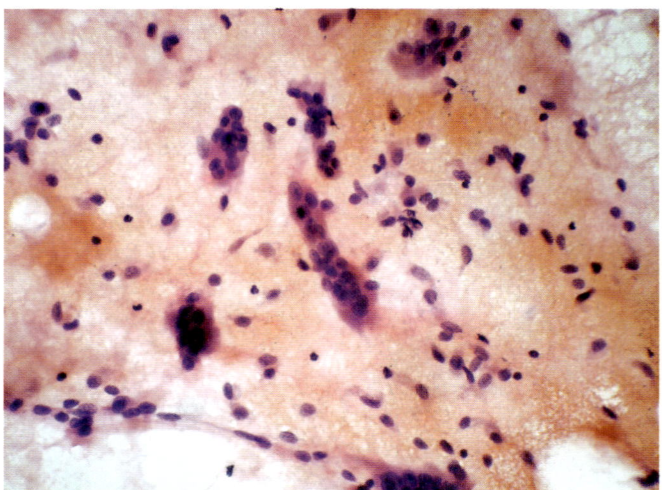

Fig. 27.37: Metaplastic carcinoma: Many multinucleated giant cells and scattered oval to spindle cells (H & E × MP).

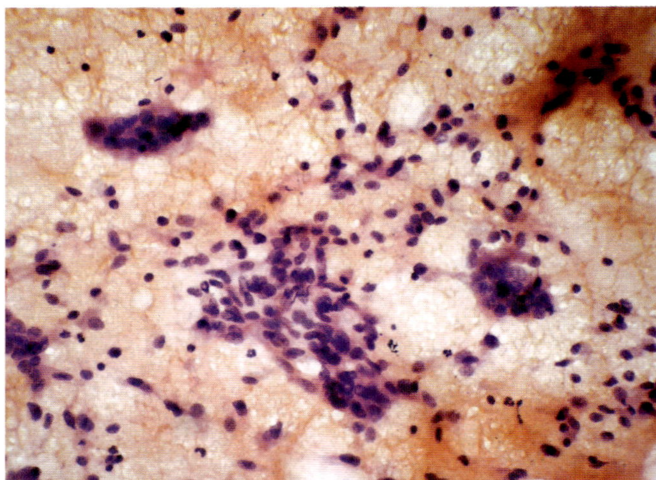

Fig. 27.38: Metaplastic carcinoma: Multinucleated osteoclast-like giant cells and malignant spindle cells (H & E × HP).

Box 27.24: Cytology of metaplastic carcinoma.

- Epithelial cells with moderately pleomorphic nuclei
- Large clusters of spindle cells
- Multinucleated giant cells
- Squamous cells
- Malignant heterologous or homologous mesenchymal elements.

The tubular wall is lined by small round to oval cells. The long cord of cells with angular comma-shaped division is seen. The individual cells have monomorphic nuclei with granular chromatin and small nucleoli. There is scanty to complete absence of bipolar naked cell in the background. At times, dense collagenized tissue fragments are also noted in the background. Scanty amount of cells with monomorphic nuclei may often give rise to a false negative diagnosis of tubular carcinoma. However, the absence of bipolar naked cells should raise the suspicion of carcinoma.

Diagnostic difficulties:

- Fibroadenoma
- Lobular carcinoma.

Metaplastic Carcinoma

This is a very uncommon malignancy of breast and accounts for less than 1% of breast carcinoma. This is a heterogeneous group of tumor characterized by adenocarcinoma along with dominant areas of spindle cell, squamous cells, or mesenchymal differentiation. The average age of the patient is 55 years and clinical presentation is not different from IDC. This is an aggressive tumor with poor prognosis.

Cytology (Figs. 27.37 and 27.38): Cytology of this malignancy depends on the various component of the metaplastic carcinoma. The tumor may show adenocarcinoma with squamous cells. There may be prominent clusters of spindle cells, multinucleated tumor giant cells, or malignant heterologous mesenchymal elements (Box 27.24).

Differential diagnosis:

- Sarcoma
- CP
- Fibromatosis.

Adenoid Cystic Carcinoma of Breast

This is an extremely uncommon tumor of breast and represents 0.1% of breast carcinomas. This tumor has very good prognosis. Cytology features of adenoid cystic carcinoma of breast are similar to that of breast. The smear shows many deep magenta-colored globules surrounded by round to oval cells. Individual cells are small, round to oval with scanty cytoplasm, and regular, hyperchromatic nuclei.

Differential diagnosis:

- Benign collagenous spherulosis.

Signet Ring Carcinoma

This represents 2–4% of all breast carcinomas. The signet ring carcinoma usually occurs in higher age group. This is

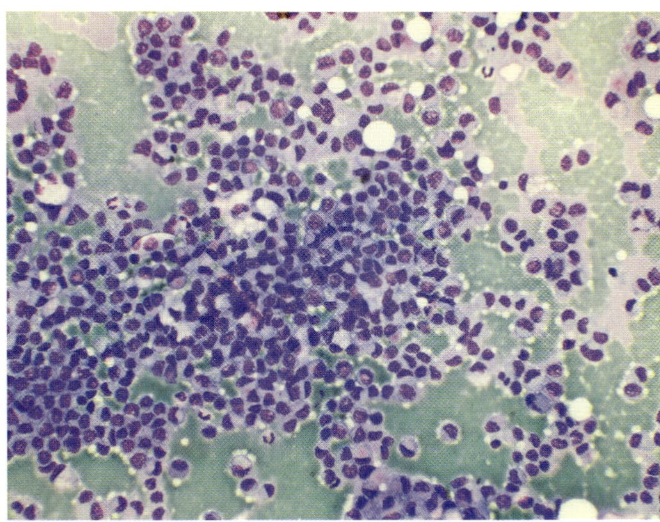

Fig. 27.39: Abundant discrete round mildly pleomorphic cells in lobular carcinoma of breast (MGG × MP).

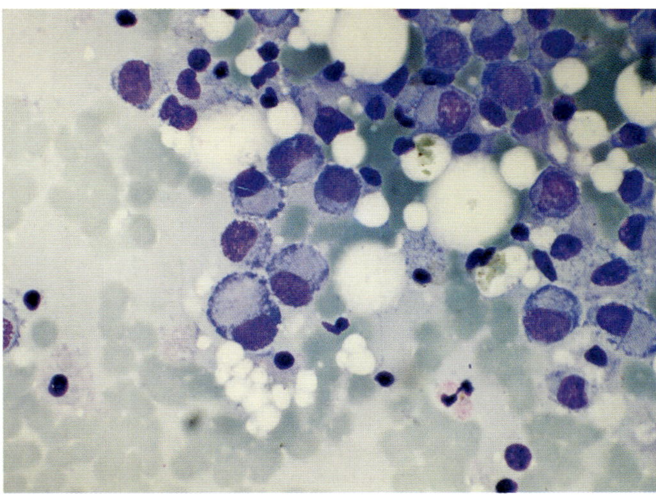

Fig. 27.40: Lobular carcinoma of breast: Discrete cells with moderate cytoplasm having eccentric nuclei in lobular carcinoma of breast (MGG × HP).

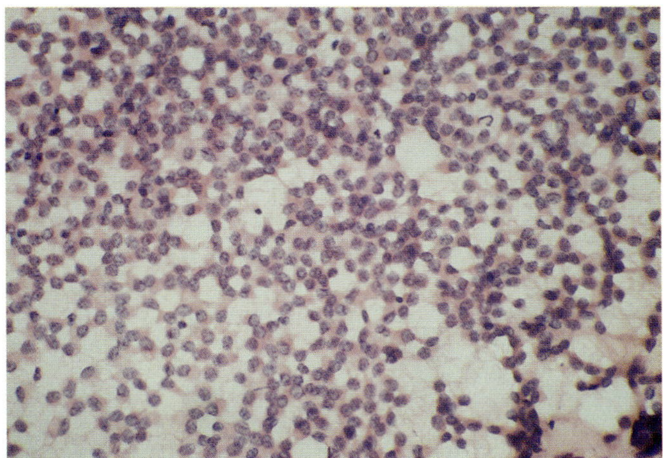

Fig. 27.41: Discrete monomorphic cells with bland nuclear chromatin in lobular carcinoma of breast (H & E × MP).

an aggressive carcinoma and more often involves the axillary lymph nodes.

Cytology: FNAC smears show loose clusters and dissociated malignant cells. Individual cells have abundant cytoplasm. The nucleus of the cell is pushed to the periphery and gives a signet ring-like appearance (Box 27.25). Unlike mucinous carcinoma, this tumor shows intracellular mucin. The mucin within the cell is positive for mucicarmine and PAS stain.

Box 27.25: Signet ring carcinoma.

- Rich in cells
- Loose clusters and dissociated malignant cells
- *Signet ring cells*: Abundant cytoplasm and eccentric nucleus
- Positive for mucicarmine and PAS stain.

Invasive Lobular Carcinoma[54,55]

Invasive lobular carcinoma (ILC) accounts for 5–15% of all breast cancers.[55] ILC occurs in all age groups from 3rd to 9th decade. The lobular carcinomas are usually ill-defined and multicentric (Box 27.26). At mammography, architectural distortion is commonly noted and microcalcification is less frequently seen.

Cytology (Figs. 27.39 to 27.41): The FNAC smears of lobular carcinoma of breast shows variable cellularity. There may be scanty cellularity due to stromal fibrosis.

The tumor cells are often arranged in cords, small clusters, and discretely. The cells often are arranged in small rows giving rise to Indian file-like arrangement. The individual cells are small with scanty cytoplasm having hyperchromatic mildly pleomorphic nuclei with inconspicuous nucleoli. Occasionally, the cells may compress with each other and may show nuclear molding. Cytoplasm of the cells may be filled with mucin and nucleus may be pushed to the periphery-giving rise to signet ring cells. The intracytoplasmic lumen within the cell is one of the characteristics features of ILC.

Diagnostic difficulties:

- *Benign lesion*: ILC shows lack of myoepithelial cells and may show several other characteristic cytological features.

Table 27.7: The differentiating points between lobular carcinoma and infiltrating duct carcinoma.

	Lobular carcinoma	Ductal carcinoma
Indian file arrangement	Present	Absent
Cell size	Small sized cell	Relatively larger size
Nucleus	Monomorphic	Pleomorphic
Nuclear molding	Present	Absent
Intracytoplasmic lumina	Present	Absent
Signet ring cells	Present	Absent

Box 27.27: Paget's disease.

- Dissociated and occasional clusters of cells
- Large cells with clear cytoplasm and centrally placed large pleomorphic nuclei
- Inflammatory cells and squamous cells
- *Immunostain*: Positive for CEA, EMA and negative for S-100 and HMB-45.

- *Ductal carcinoma*: Monomorphic cells in ILC may simulate a low-grade IDC. However, the presence of Indian file-like cells, nuclear molding, and signet ring type of cells favor the diagnosis of lobular carcinoma. Table 27.7 highlights the differentiating points between lobular carcinoma and IDC.

Paget's Disease

Paget's disease typically presents as ulcerated eczematous lesion around the nipple and areola. In majority of the cases, an underlying breast carcinoma is also present.

Paget's disease is diagnosed by scraping of the ulcerated lesion.

Cytology

- The cytology smears show dissociated and occasional clusters of large cells. Individual cells have clear cytoplasm and centrally placed moderately pleomorphic nuclei (Box 27.27). Occasional cell may contain melanin pigments that probably have been transferred from adjacent melanocytes. Background of the smears may show inflammatory cells and squamous cells. The presence of melanin pigment may mislead the cytologists to diagnose the lesion as malignant melanoma. Immunocytochemistry is helpful in this aspect as Paget's cells are positive for CEA, EMA, and ER, whereas malignant melanomas are positive for HMB45 and S-100 protein.

Box 27.26: Lobular carcinoma.

- Sparse to moderately rich cellularity
- Dissociated cells
- Small rows of cells known as Indian file arrangement
- Signet ring-like cells with small intracytoplasmic lumina
- Small cells with scanty cytoplasm having minimal nuclear pleomorphism
- Nuclear molding.

Differential Diagnosis

- Malignant melanoma
- *Inflammatory atypia*: Nonspecific inflammation in areola or nipple may also produce reactive atypia. Nuclear features may be helpful in diagnosis of malignancy.

Inflammatory Carcinoma

This is an uncommon aggressive tumor and represents 2–4% of all breast carcinomas. Clinically, the breast is erythematous, diffusely enlarged, edematous, and tender. This is due to lymphatic obstruction by the tumor emboli. As there is no definite swelling, so FNAC may not yield any representative material and aspiration from the multiple sites are recommended. Cytology smear shows discrete and clusters of large pleomorphic cells with prominent macronucleoli. Contrary to its name as "inflammatory carcinoma" no inflammatory cells are seen in the background.

Other Uncommon Malignancies

Carcinoma with Neuroendocrine Differentiation (Figs. 27.42 and 27.43)

Neuroendocrine carcinomas are rare breast cancer and accounts for 2–5% of all breast cancers. Most patients are in 6th to 7th decade of life. There is no special clinical feature of neuroendocrine carcinomas. These tumors are argyrophilic but not argentaffin and show dense core granules. In true sense, these tumors are not carcinoid and they should be better designated as a type of IDC with neuroendocrine differentiation.

Cytology: The tumor shows abundant discrete cells. The cells are round, monomorphic with scanty to moderate cytoplasm. The nuclei are mildly pleomorphic with finely granular chromatin and inconspicuous nucleoli. The cells are positive for chromogranin and synaptophysin.

Metastatic Tumors (Fig. 27.44)

Breast is the uncommon site of the metastatic tumor, and it represents 0.5–6% of all malignancies of the breast.

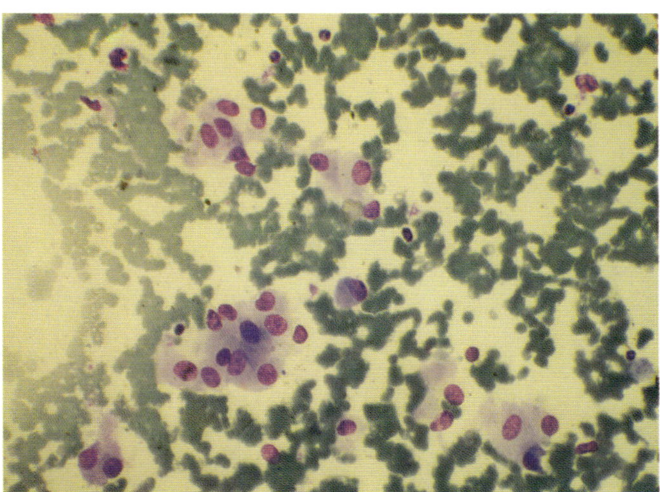

Fig. 27.42: Cytology smear of neuroendocrine carcinoma of breast showing discrete cells with moderate amount of cytoplasm and eccentric nuclei (MGG × MP).

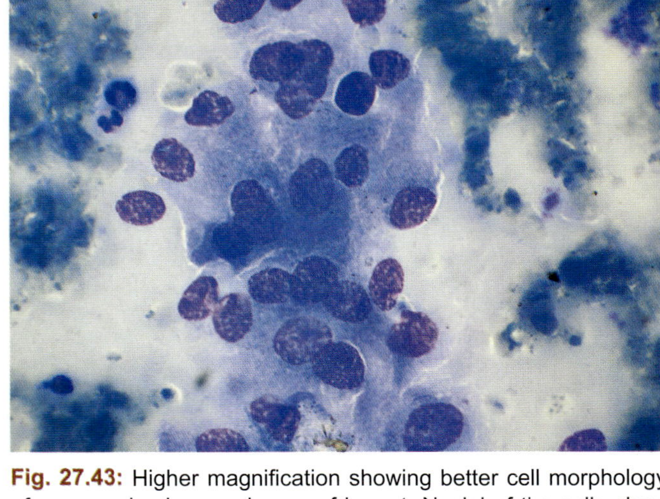

Fig. 27.43: Higher magnification showing better cell morphology of neuroendocrine carcinoma of breast. Nuclei of the cells show fine stippled chromatin and inconspicuous nucleoli (MGG × OI).

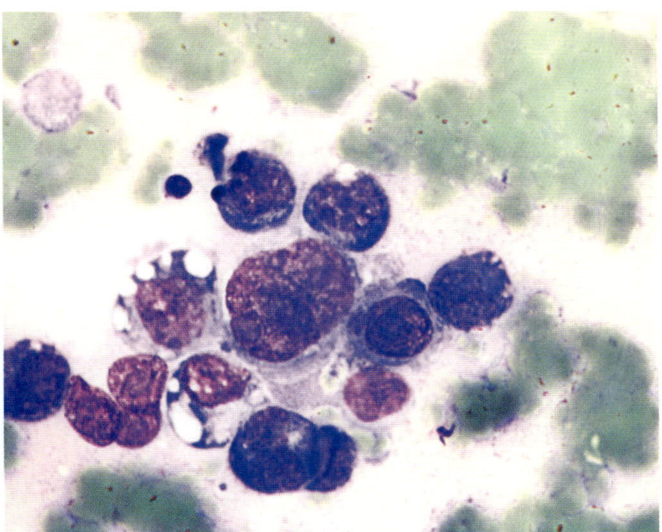

Fig. 27.44: Fine needle aspiration cytology smears of metastatic rhabdomyosarcoma in breast from a thigh swelling in a 7-year-old child (MGG × OI).

The contralateral breast is the most common source of the metastasis in breast carcinoma. The other common sources of metastasis in adults are lung, kidney, and gastrointestinal tract. In case of children, rhabdomyosarcoma is the most common metastatic tumors. In adult male, prostatic carcinoma is the common source of metastasis in male breast.

On the basis of cytology features, it is not always possible to distinguish a primary from a metastatic tumor of breast. However, if the cytomorphology of the tumor does not fit with any known primary malignancy of the breast, then one should think about the possibility of a secondary tumor. Clinical history may be helpful in certain situations.

Non-Hodgkin Lymphoma

Non-Hodgkin lymphomas (NHLs) of the breast, both primary and secondary, are rare. Most of the NHL affects the breast as a manifestation of generalized involvement. The clinical presentation of the primary NHL may mimic as breast cancer. The patient usually presents as a painless lump in the breast. In one-tenth of the cases, the lump is bilateral. For the diagnosis of primary NHL of the breast, the following histological criteria are mandatory.[56]

- No prior history of lymphoma
- No nodal involvement of lymphoma at the time of presentation
- The presence of breast tissue in adjacent lymphoid tissue
- Histological confirmation of the case.

The common types of lymphomas in the breast are (1) diffuse large B-cell lymphoma, (2) MALT lymphoma, and (3) follicular lymphoma.

The cytomorphology of NHL depends on the subtype of NHL.

Differential diagnosis:

- Chronic mastitis
- Intramammary lymph node.

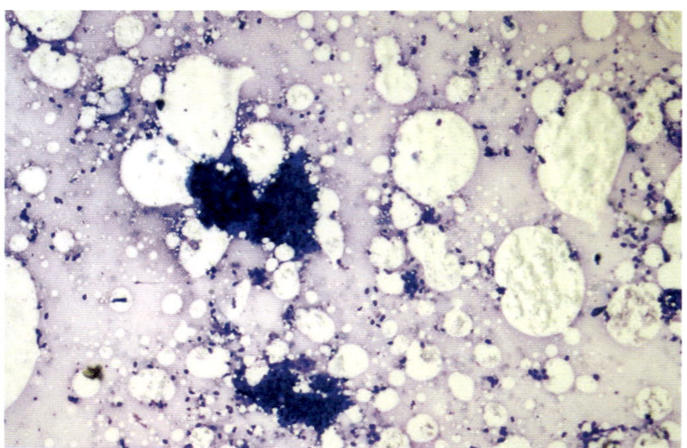

Fig. 27.45: Tight clusters of benign ductular cells in a case of gynecomastia (MGG × MP).

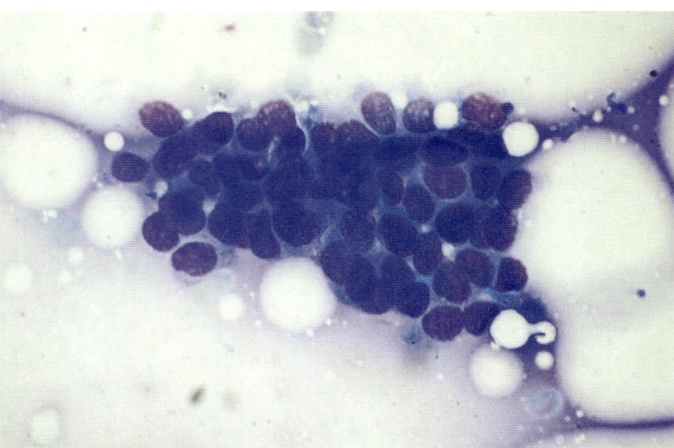

Fig. 27.46: Mild nuclear enlargement and pleomorphism in gynecomastia (MGG × HP).

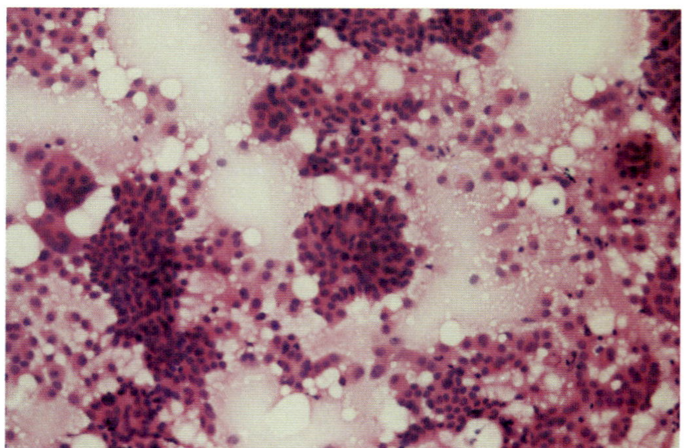

Fig. 27.47: Male breast carcinoma: Abundant discrete malignant cells (H & E × MP).

MALE BREAST LESIONS

Gynecomastia[57] (Figs. 27.45 and 27.46)

The gynecomastia is the most common breast lesions in male and is caused by hypertrophy and hyperplasia of the ductal and stromal component of the breast. The main cause of gynecomastia is due to decreased androgenic hormone and increased estrogen. The gynecomastia is commonly associated with cirrhosis of liver, hyperthyroidism, renal failure, chronic lung disease, germ cell tumor of the testis, and various drugs such as spironolactone, digitalis, cimetidine, marijuana, and tricyclic antidepressants.

Cytology

The cytology smears of gynecomastia usually show sparse cellularity. The ductal cells are arranged in dissociation and occasionally in monolayer sheets. The individual cells show round nuclei with mild nuclear atypia. Discrete ductal cells do not show significant atypia. Nuclear crowding, significant dyscohesive cells, and marked nuclear pleomorphism are the characteristic cytological features of malignancy. Bipolar myoepithelial cells are noted in the background.

Differential Diagnosis

- *Ductal carcinoma*: Nuclear atypia in gynecomastia may cause diagnostic difficulties with invasive duct carcinoma.

Carcinoma in Male Breast (Fig. 27.47)

Male breast carcinoma is a rare carcinoma and represents less than 1% of all carcinoma of the breast. It is more aggressive than female breast carcinoma. Almost all male breast carcinomas are ductal type. The cytomorphology of the male breast carcinoma is similar to that of female breast IDC. However, male breast carcinoma shows dyscohesive cells with marked nuclear enlargement and pleomorphism. Bipolar cells are absent in the smear.

ANCILLARY INVESTIGATIONS ON BREAST ASPIRATION MATERIAL

Aspiration cytology material of the breast lesions can be used for various ancillary investigations such as immunocytochemistry, flow cytometry, and microbial culture.

Immunocytochemistry

Direct smear, cytospin smear, or section from the cell block could be used for immunocytochemistry of the breast lesions. Section from the cell block is preferable as it gives consistent and good result. Estrogen, progesterone, and HER2/neu receptors can be demonstrated on the aspirate material for the further management of carcinoma of breast.

Flow cytometry and image cytometry: Information on DNA ploidy and S-phase fraction can be assessed by flow cytometry and image cytometry.

Reporting of Breast Fine needle Aspiration Cytology

In the symposium conducted by National Cancer Institute of Bethesda, Maryland, USA,[21] a uniform reporting system of the breast was proposed:

- *Benign*: No evidence of malignancy.
- *Atypical or indeterminate*: Mild atypia present, possibly benign lesion. However, clinical and radiologic correlation is advised. In this category, triple test is strongly recommended.
- *Suspicious or probably malignant*: Cytology smear shows many atypical cells and is highly suggestive of malignancy, however for a more definitive opinion histopathology should be advised.
- *Malignant*: Cytomorphological features are diagnostic of malignancy and further subcategorization should be mentioned, if possible.
- *Unsatisfactory*: The smear quality is substandard because of scant cellularity, air drying artifact, obscuration by blood or inflammation, etc.

National Cancer Institute (NCI)-sponsored symposium[21] also suggested that the cytology report should mention certain information in the reporting format such as:

Reporting Format of Fine needle Aspiration Cytology of Breast

- *Precise location of the lesion*: Distance from the nipple and exact clock position.
- *Type of specimen*: Whether solid or cystic lesion, scrapping, nipple discharge or FNAC material.
- *Localization technique*: Whether palpable mass or image-guided FNAC.
- *Diagnostic terminology*: As mentioned above.
- *Adequacy of the aspirated material*: Adequate number of ductal cells, air drying artifact, etc.
- Comments on the specimen findings.
- *Recommendations*: Comments on requirement of any other clinical and radiological correlations.

Table 27.8: Robinson's criteria for grading of breast cancer on fine needle aspiration cytology (FNAC) smears.

Parameter	*Score 1*	*Score 2*	*Score 3*
Cell dissociation	Mostly in cluster	Mixture of single cell and cluster	Mostly single cell
Cell size	1–2 times of RBC	3–4 times of RBC	>5 times of RBC
Cell uniformity	Monomorphic	Mildly pleomorphic	Pleomorphic
Nucleoli	Indistinct	Noticeable	Prominent
Nuclear margin	Smooth	Folds	Clefts
Chromatin	Vesicular	Granular	Clumped

Cytological Grade

Neoadjuvant therapy is now being applied as one of the treatment modalities of breast carcinoma, and therefore grading of breast carcinoma is needed for the management. Histological grading of breast carcinoma is well established. In FNAC material, cytological grading system has been also tried. Cytological grading by Robinson et al. and Idvall et al.[58,59] are well correlated with histological grade. Robinson's et al. included six cytological criteria and each scored separately from 1 to 3. Total score obtained in each sample is used for grading of breast cancer on FNAC smears (Table 27.8). In contrast, Idvall et al.[59] used an ocular micrometer to measure the nuclear diameter of the tumor cells. They used a total of six cytological features to grade the carcinoma. Both the grading systems can be applied on MGG or Papanicolaous' stained smear. However, the later stain is preferable to grade the breast carcinoma.

Grade 1: 6–11 score, *Grade 2*: 12–14 score, and *Grade 3*: 15–18 score.

Ancillary Techniques

Ancillary investigations are helpful to provide some essential information on breast cancer. Following information is mandatory for management of breast carcinoma:

- Estrogen and progesterone receptor status
- HER2/neu oncogene receptor status.

Prognostic parameters:

- DNA ploidy and S-phase fraction
- Proliferation markers such as Ki 67 index.

Intracellular steroid hormone receptors particularly ER and PR have drawn considerable attention. Patients with hormone receptor positivity have higher 5-year survival rate.[60] Studies have shown that the hormone receptor-positive tumors are usually well differentiated, diploid tumor with low proliferation rate. These tumors also show low propensity for visceral recurrence.[61,62]

Assessment of hormone receptors status is very essential for the preoperative management of breast carcinoma. Majority of estrogen and progesterone receptor-positive cases are hormone responsive and only one-tenth of hormone receptor cases are hormone sensitive. The receptor status of breast carcinoma can be provided with the help of immunocytochemistry on cell block preparation (Figs. 27.48A to D).[63] HER2/neu oncogene amplification is one of the common genetic changes in breast carcinoma.[64] About 25–30% of breast cancer shows HER2/neu oncogene over expression.

Carcinoma cases, which are HER2/neu oncogene positive in FISH or by immunohistochemistry, show clinical response to trastuzumab (Herceptin) therapy. Both immunohistochemistry and FISH analysis can be done on FNAC sample.[65,66]

Over expression of HER2/neu is demonstrated by immunocytochemistry using anti-HER2/neu antibody. Similarly, HER2/neu amplification is detected with the help of HER2/neu DNA probe. Due to difficulty in the interpretation of membranous staining of HER2/neu receptor, it is advisable to do FISH on FNAC material.

MOLECULAR CLASSIFICATION OF BREAST CARCINOMA

Based on gene expression profile breast carcinomas are classified into four subtypes:[67-69]

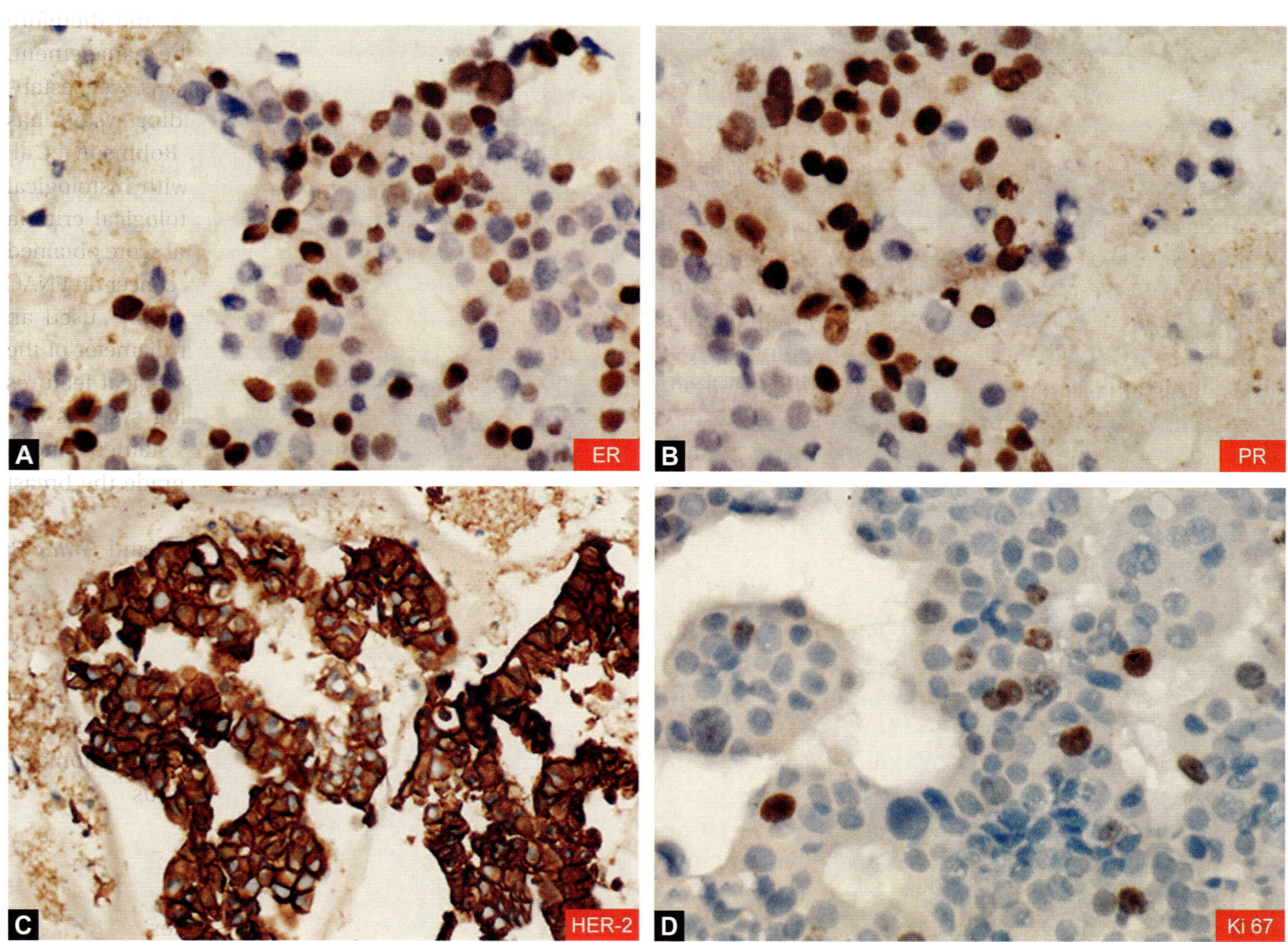

Figs. 27.48A to D: Infiltrating duct carcinoma: (A) Estrogen receptor (ER), (B) Progesterone receptor (PR), (C) HER-2, and (D) Ki 67 immunostaining in cell block preparation.

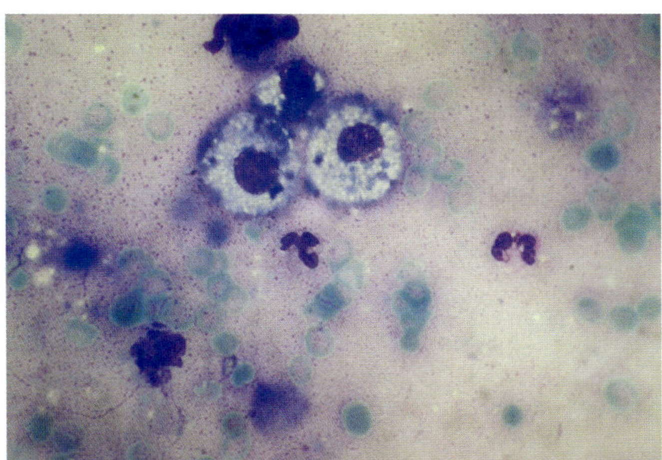

Fig. 27.49: Foamy histiocytes in nipple discharge smear (MGG × HP).

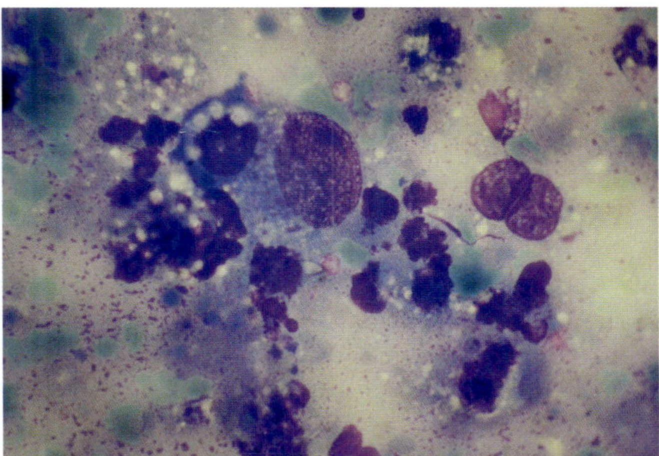

Fig. 27.50: Nipple discharge showing large cells with enlarge nuclei having multiple nucleoli in an infiltrating duct carcinoma (MGG × OI).

1. *Luminal A (50% of carcinoma)*: This group shows higher expression of hormone receptors and related genes. They express luminal low molecular weight cytokeratin.
2. *Luminal B (20% of carcinoma)*: This group shows moderate to weak expression of hormone receptors and related genes. They express luminal low molecular weight cytokeratin.
3. *HER2 (15% of carcinoma)*: (a) High expression of HER2 and other genes in amplicon and (b) Low expression of ER and associated genes.
4. *Basal like (15% of carcinoma)*: (a) High expression of basal epithelial genes, basal cytokeratins, (b) Low expression of ER and associated genes, and (c) Low expression of HER2.

For routine subtyping of breast carcinoma immunohistochemistry is used as surrogate markers. The following markers are necessary for molecular subtyping:

- ER
- PR
- HER2
- CK 5/6
- Ki 67

Luminal A: Positive for ER/PR, negative for HER-2, and Ki 67 less than 14%.

Luminal B: Weak positive for ER/PR, positive or negative for HER-2, and Ki 67 more than 14%.

HER-2: Negative for ER/PR, Positive for HER-2

Basal: Negative for ER/PR and HER-2 and positive for CK 5/6

All these immunostaining can be done on FNAC of breast and therefore molecular classification is possible on FNAC material.[70]

NIPPLE DISCHARGE

Nipple discharge may be due to physiological or pathological causes. Pregnancy and lactation are the physiologic causes of nipple discharge. The various pathological causes of nipple discharge are endocrine disorders such as hyper- and hypothyroidism, pituitary adenoma, and drugs. The primary lesions of breast causing nipple discharges are intraductal papilloma, duct adenosis, and ductal carcinoma. Only 3% of breast carcinoma presents nipple discharge and nipple discharge cytology is not suitable for cancer screening.[71] The nipple discharge is suspicious for malignancy when it is unilateral, bloody, associated with lump and mammography is abnormal. It is highly unlikely to have any malignant cells in milky or purulent nipple discharge.[72]

Cytology

Benign nipple discharge is usually sparsely cellular. Smear shows many foamy cells, occasional loose clusters of ductular cells, red blood cells (RBCs), and ploymorphs (Fig. 27.49).

Cytology smear from the intraductal papilloma shows tight cohesive ductal cells often arranged as papillae. The lining cells of the papillae are columnar to cuboidal with scanty cytoplasm and monomorphic nuclei. In addition, foamy histiocytes are also noted. Exact nature of the papillary neoplasm is difficult to ascertain on cytology smear.

Ductal carcinoma in nipple discharge shows many discrete malignant cells (Fig. 27.50 and Box 27.28). Occasional cluster of cells with nuclear abnormality may also

Box 27.28: Ductal carcinoma in nipple discharge.

- Discrete and loose clusters of cells
- Moderate nuclear enlargement and pleomorphism
- Naked nuclei
- Necrotic debris
- Polymorphs and blood.

be seen. Degenerated ductal cells in nipple discharge may give false impression of malignancy. It is important to give adequate attention on the discrete ductular cells. All cases of positive for malignancy in nipple discharge should have histopathological confirmation.

REFERENCES

1. Schwartsmann G. Breast cancer in South America: challenges to improve early detection and medical management of a public health problem. J Clin Oncol. 2001;19:118-24.
2. Gøtzsche PC, Olsen O. Is screening for breast cancer with mammography justifiable? Lancet. 2000;355(9198):129-34.
3. Elmore JG, Armstrong K, Lehman CD, et al. Screening for breast cancer. JAMA. 2005;293(10):1245-56.
4. Mottahedeh M, Rashid MH, Gateley CA. Final diagnoses following C3 (atypical, probably benign) breast cytology. Breast. 2003;12:276-9.
5. Lieske B, Ravichandran D, Wright D. Role of fine needle aspiration cytology and core biopsy in the preoperative diagnosis of screen-detected breast carcinoma. Br J Cancer. 2006;95(1):62-6.
6. Silverman JF. Diagnostic accuracy, cost-effectiveness, and triage role of fine needle aspiration biopsy in the diagnosis of palpable breast lesions. Breast J. 1995;1:3-8.
7. Collaco LM, de Lima RS, Werner B, et al. Value of fine needle aspiration in the diagnosis of breast lesions. Acta Cytol. 1999;43(4):587-92.
8. Wang HH, Ducatman BS, Eick D. Comparative features of ductal carcinoma in situ and infiltrating ductal carcinoma of the breast on fine needle aspiration biopsy. Am J Clin Pathol. 1989;92:736-40.
9. Al-Kaisi N. The spectrum of the "gray zone" in breast cytology: A review of 186 cases of atypical and suspicious cytology. Acta Cytol. 1994;38:898-908.
10. Dey P, Luthra UK. False negative cytological diagnosis of breast carcinomas. Acta Cytol. 1999:43(5);801-5.
11. Silverman JF, Elsheikh TM, Singh HK. The role of fine needle aspiration cytology of the breast in the core biopsy era. Pathol Case Rev. 2007;12:44-8.
12. Johansen C. A clinical study with special reference to diagnostic procedures. Acta Clin Scand. 1975;451(Suppl):1-70.
13. Negri S, Bonetti F, Capitanio A, et al. Preoperative diagnostic accuracy of fine needle aspiration in the management of breast lesions: comparison of specificity and sensitivity with clinical examination, mammography, echography, and thermography in 249 patients. Diagn Cytopathol. 1994;11:4-8.
14. Morris KT, Pommier RF. Usefulness of the triple test score for palpable breast masses. Arch Surg. 2001;136(9):1008-12.
15. Tabbara SO, Frost AR, Stoler MH, et al. Changing trends in breast fine needle aspiration: results of the Papanicolaou Society of Cytopathology Survey. Diagn Cytopathol. 2000; 22:126-30.
16. Park S-M, Lee D-W, Jin S-Y, et al. Fine needle aspiration cytology as the first pathological diagnostic modality in breast lesions: a comparison with core needle biopsy. Basic Appl Pathol. 2010;1:1-6.
17. Berner A, Davidson B, Sigstad E, et al. Fine needle aspiration cytology vs. core biopsy in the diagnosis of breast lesions. Diagn Cytopathol. 2003;29(6):344-8.
18. Westenend PJ. A comparison of aspiration cytology and core needle biopsy in the evaluation of breast lesions. Cancer. 2001;93:146-50.
19. Poole GH, Willsher PC, Pinder PC, et al. Diagnosis of breast cancer with core-biopsy and fine needle aspiration cytology. Aust N Z J Surg. 1996;66:592-4.
20. Cheung PS, Yan KW, Alagaratnam TT. The complementary role of fine needle aspiration cytology and Tru-cut needle biopsy in the management of breast masses. Aust N Z J Surg. 1987;57:615-20.
21. National Cancer Institute Fine needle Aspiration of Breast Workshop Subcommittees. The uniform approach to breast fine needle aspiration biopsy. Diagn. Cytopathol. 1997; 16:295-311.
22. Layfield LJ, Mooney EE, Glasgow B, et al. What constitutes an adequate smear in fine needle aspiaration cytology of the breast? Cancer. 1997;81:16-21.
23. Kumarasinghe MP. Cytology of granulomatous mastitis. Acta Cytol. 1997;41:727-30.
24. Silverman JF, Lannin DR, Unverferth M, et al. Fine needle aspiration cytology of subareolar abscess of the breast. Spectrum of cytomorphologic findings and potential diagnostic pitfalls. Acta Cytol. 1986;30(4):413-9.
25. Galblum LI, Oertel YC. Subareolar abscess of the breast: diagnosis by fine needle aspiration. Am J Clin Pathol. 1983; 80(4):496-9.
26. Mori I, Han B, Wang X, et al. Mastopathic fibroadenoma of the breast: a pitfall of aspiration cytology. Cytopathology. 2006;17(5):233-8.
27. Lopez-Ferrer P, Jimenez-Heffernan JA, Vicandi B, et al. Fine needle aspiration cytology of breast fibroadenoma: A cytohistologic correlation study of 405 cases. Acta Cytol. 1999;43:579-86.
28. Veneti S, Manek S. Benign phyllodes tumour vs. fibroadenoma: FNA cytological differentiation. Cytopathology. 2001;12(5):321-8.
29. Jayaram G, Sthaneshwar P. Fine needle aspiration cytology of phyllodes tumors. Diagn Cytopathol. 2002;26(4):222-7.
30. Dusenbery D, Frable WL. Fine needle aspiration cytology of phyllodes tumor: Potential diagnostic pitfalls. Acta Cytol. 1992;36:215-21.
31. Novotny DB, Maygarden SJ, Shermer RW, et al. Fine needle aspiration of benign and malignant breast masses associated with pregnancy. Acta Cytol. 1991;35(6):676-86.

32. Bottles K, Taylor RN. Diagnosis of breast masses in pregnant and lactating women by aspiration cytology. Obstet Gynecol. 1985;66(3 Suppl):76S-78.
33. Fitzgibbons PL, Henson DE, Hutter RV. Benign breast changes and the risk for subsequent breast cancer: an update of the 1985 consensus statement. Cancer Committee of the College of American Pathologists. Arch Pathol Lab Med. 1998;122(12):1053-5.
34. Hutter RVP. Consensus meeting: Is 'fibrocystic disease' of the breast precancerous? Arch Pathol Lab Med. 1986;110: 171-3.
35. Page DL. Cancer risk assessment in benign breast biopsies. Hum Pathol. 1986;17:871-4.
36. Zhao C, Raza A, Martin SE, et al. Breast fine needle aspiration samples reported as "proliferative breast lesion": clinical utility of the subcategory "proliferative breast lesion with atypia". Cancer. 2009;117(2):137-47.
37. Gangopadhyay M, Nijhawan R, Joshi K, et al. Cytology of "significant" breast ductal proliferations. Acta Cytol. 1997; 41(4):1112-20.
38. Frost AR, Aksu A, Kurstin R, et al. Can nonproliferative breast disease and proliferative breast disease without atypia be distinguished by fine needle aspiration cytology? Cancer. 1997;81(1):22-8.
39. Silverman JF, Masood S, Ducatman BS, et al. Can FNA biopsy separate atypical hyperplasia, carcinoma in situ, and invasive carcinoma of the breast? Cytomorphologic criteria and limitations in diagnosis. Diagn Cytopathol. 1993;9: 713-28.
40. Thomas PA, Raab SS, Cohen MB. Is the fine needle aspiration biopsy diagnosis of proliferative breast disease feasible? Diagn Cytopathol. 1994;11:301-6.
41. Masood S, Frykberg ER, McLellan G, et al. Cytologic differentiation between proliferative and nonproliferative breast disease in mammographically guided fine needle aspirates. Diagn Cytopathol. 1991;7:581-90.
42. Silverstein MJ, Gamagami P, Rosser RJ, et al. Hooked-wire-directed breast biopsy and overpenetrated mammography. Cancer. 1987;59(4):715-22.
43. Lilleng R, Hagmar B. The comedo subtype of intraductal carcinoma: Cytologic characteristics. Acta Cytol. 1992;36: 345-52.
44. Lilleng R, Hagmar BM, Farrants G. Low-grade cribriform ductal carcinoma in situ of the breast: Fine needle aspiration cytology in three cases. Acta Cytol. 1992;36:48-54.
45. El Hag IA, Aodah A, Kollur SM, et al. Cytological clues in the distinction between phyllodes tumor and fibroadenoma. Cancer. 2010;118(1):33-40.
46. Stanley MW, Tani EM, Rutqvist LE, et al. Cystosarcoma phyllodes of the breast: a cytologic and clinicopathologic study of 23 cases. Diagn Cytopathol. 1989;8:29-34.
47. Vladescu T, Klijanienko J, Caillaud JM, et al. Fine needle sampling in malignant phyllodes tumors: clinicopathologic study of 22 cases seen at the Institut Curie. Diagn Cytopathol. 2004;31(2):71-6.
48. Shabb N. Phyllodes tumor-fine needle aspiration cytology of eight cases. Acta Cytol. 1997;41:321-6.
49. Bhatia A, Dey P, Saikia UN, et al. Letter to the editor: fine needle aspiration cytology of papillary carcinoma of breast. Cytopathology. 2007;18(5):321-4.
50. Haji BE, Das DK, Al-Ayadhy B, et al. Fine needle aspiration cytologic features of four special types of breast cancers: mucinous, medullary, apocrine, and papillary. Diagn Cytopathol. 2007;35(7):408-16.
51. Ventura K, Cangiarella J, Lee I, et al. Aspiration biopsy of mammary lesions with abundant extracellular mucinous material: Review of 43 cases with surgical follow-up. Am J Clin Pathol. 2003;120:194-202.
52. Ellis IO, Galea M, Broughton N, et al. Pathological prognostic factors in breast cancer. II. Histological type. Relationship with survival in a large study with long-term follow-up. Histopathology. 1992;20:479-89.
53. Sohn JH, Kim LS, Chae SW, et al. Fine needle aspiration findings of breast mucinous neoplasms: differential diagnosis between mucocele like tumor and mucinous carcinoma. Acta Cytol. 2001;45:723-9.
54. Rajesh L, Dey P, Joshi K. Fine needle aspiration cytology of lobular carcinoma: comparison with other breast lesions. Acta Cytol. 2003;47(2):177-82.
55. Tavassoli FA, Devilee P. Tumours of the Breast and Female Genital Organs. Lyon, France: IARC Press; 2003.
56. Wiseman C, Liao KT. Primary lymphoma of the breast. Cancer. 1972;29(6):1705-12.
57. Siddiqui MT, Zakowski MF, Ashfaq R, et al. Breast masses in males: multi-institutional experience on fine needle aspiration. Diagn Cytopathol. 2002;26(2):87-91.
58. Robinson JA, McKee G, Nichols A, et al. Prognostic value of cytological grading of fine needle aspirates from breast carcinomas. Lancet. 1994;343:947-9.
59. Idvall I, Ferno M, Sigurdsson H, et al. Fine needle aspiration cytology of breast carcinoma: a pre-operative prognostic tool? Breast. 1995;4:189-95.
60. Osborne CK, Yochmowitz MG, Knight WA III, et al. The value of estrogen and progesterone receptors in the treatment of breast cancer. Cancer. 1980;46(suppl 12):2884-8.
61. Fisher ER, Osborne CR, McGuire WL, et al. Correlation of primary breast cancer histopathology and estrogen receptor content. Breast Cancer Res Treat. 1981;1:37-41.
62. Dressler LG, Seamer LC, Owens MA, et al. DNA flow cytometry and prognostic factors in 1331 frozen breast cancer specimens. Cancer. 1988;61:420-7.
63. Masood S. Estrogen and progesterone receptors in cytology: a comprehensive review. Diagn Cytopathol. 1992;8:475-91.
64. Ross JS, Fletcher JA. The Her-2/neu oncogene: prognostic factor, predictive factor and target for therapy. Semin Cancer Biol. 1999;9:125-38.
65. Nizzoli R, Bozzetti C, Crafa P, et al. Immunocytochemical evaluation of HER-2/neu on fine needle aspirates from primary breast carcinomas. Diagn Cytopathol. 2003;28: 142-6.
66. Bozzetti C, Nizzoli R, Guazzi A, et al. HER2/neu amplification detected by fluorescence in situ hybridization in fine needle aspirates from primary breast cancer. Ann Oncol. 2002;13:1398-403.

67. Sørlie T, Perou CM, Tibshirani R, et al. Gene expression patterns of breast carcinomas distinguish tumor subclasses with clinical implications. Proc Natl Acad Sci. U S A. 2001; 98(19):10869-74.
68. Schnitt SJ. Will molecular classification replace traditional breast pathology? Int J Surg Pathol. 2010;18:162S-6S;
69. Correa Geyer F, Reis-Filho JS. Microarray-based gene expression profiling as a clinical tool for breast cancer management: are we there yet? Int J Surg Pathol. 2009;17: 285-302.
70. Ferguson J, Chamberlain P, Cramer HM, et al. ER, PR, HER2 immunocytochemistry on cell-transferred cytologic smears of primary and metastatic breast carcinomas: a comparison study with formalin-fixed cell blocks and surgical biopsies. Diagn Cytopathol. 2013;41(7):575-81.
71. Takeda T, Matsui A, Sato Y, et al. Nipple discharge cytology in mass screening for breast cancer. Acta Cytol. 1990;34:161-4.
72. Dey P, Dhar KK. Cytologic evaluation of nipple discharge in relation to mammary dysplasia. J Assoc Physicians India. 1994:42;369-70.

Review Questions

1. **Bloody nipple discharge in a 57-year-old female (Figs. 27.51A and B). What is your diagnosis?**
2. **A 35-year-old female with 24 cm diameter swelling in breast. She also had 2 cm diameter two left cervical lymph nodes for 2 months. Fine needle aspiration cytology (FNAC) of the breast was done (Figs. 27.52A to D).**
   What is your most likely diagnosis?
   How do you want to confirm your diagnosis on FNAC material?
3. **A 28-year-old female presented with 15 cm diameter swelling in the upper quadrant of left breast for last 3 years. Figures 27.53A to D show the fine needle aspiration cytology smear of the swelling. What is your most likely diagnosis?**

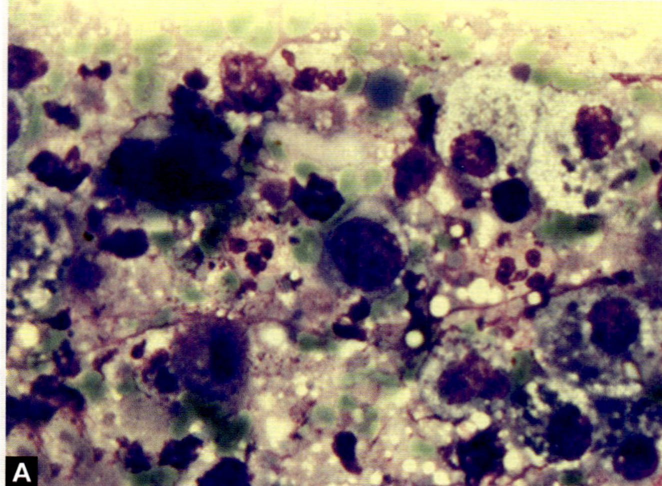

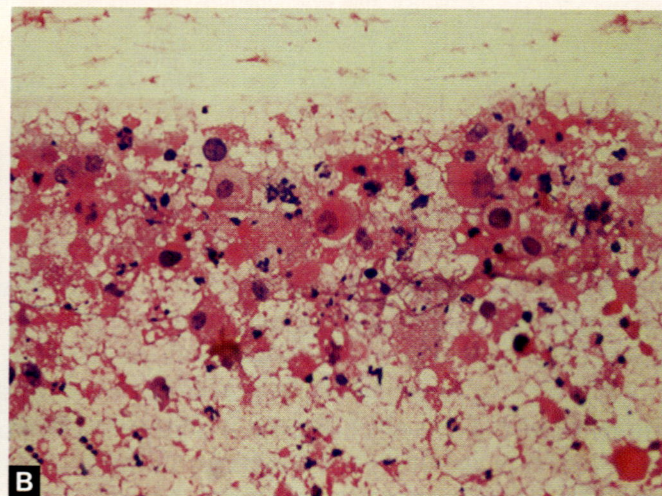

Figs. 27.51A and B: The microphotographs of the cytology smears of nipple discharge in question 1.

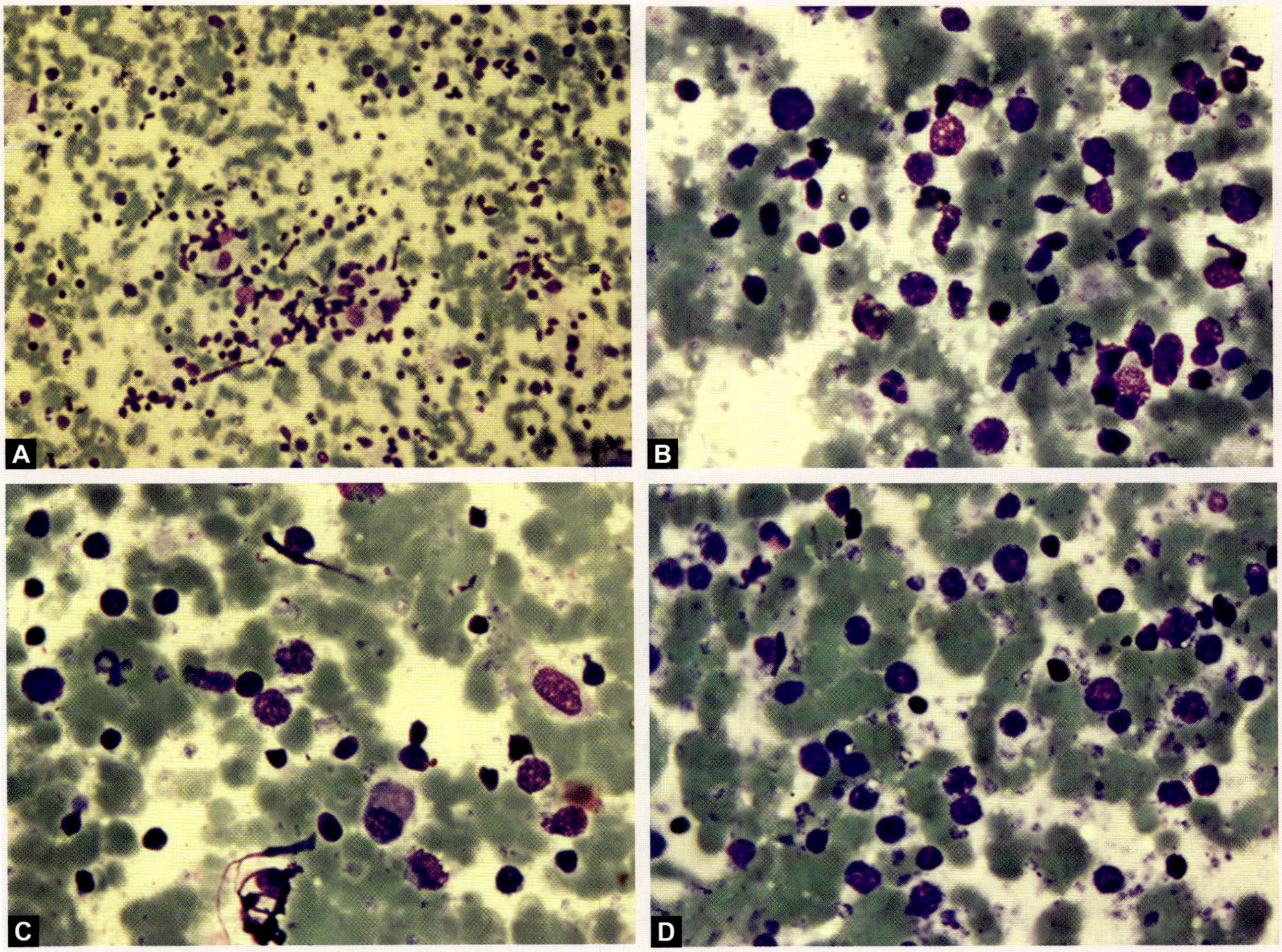

Figs. 27.52A to D: The microphotographs of the aspiration cytology smears of question 2.

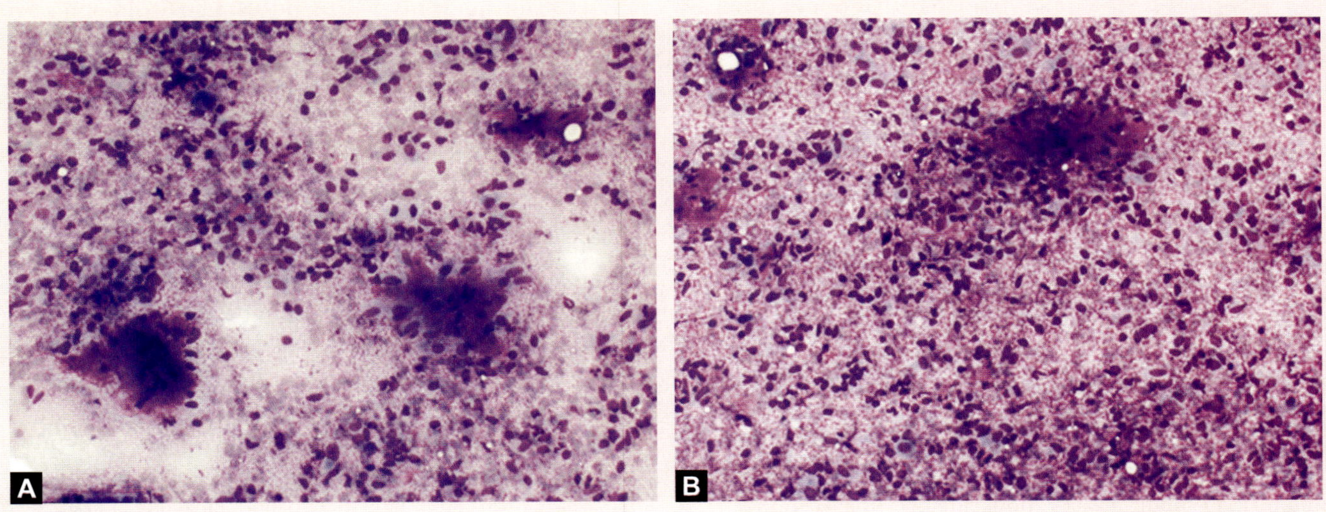

Figs. 27.53A and B

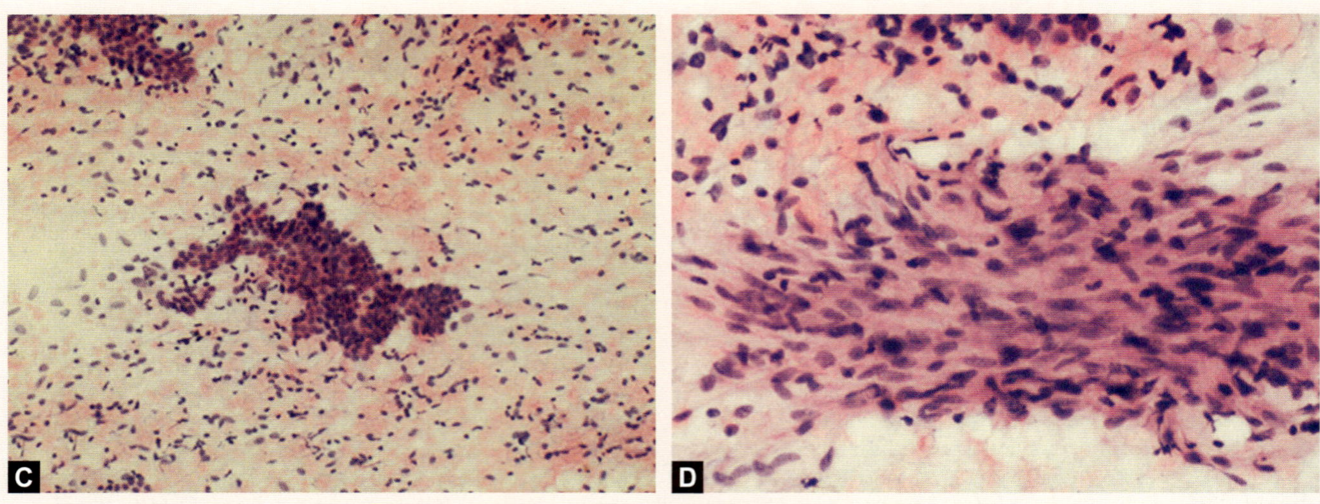

Figs. 27.53A to D: The microphotographs of the aspiration cytology smears of question 3.

Answers

1. Positive for malignant cells
   Note: The smears show large cells with moderate nuclear enlargement and pleomorphism in an inflammatory background. The cells are malignant. In such cases a thorough examination of the breast is mandatory.
2. a. NHL of breast
   b. Immunocytochemistry CD45 and CK
   Note: The smears show many immature lymphoid cells and scattered lymphoglandular bodies indicating the diagnosis of non-Hodgkin lymphoma. Complete panel of immunocytochemistry panel on cell block material is helpful:
   Confirmation of NHL: CD45
   Immunophenotyping: CD19, CD20 for B cell, CD3, CD5, CD7, CD4/ CD8 for T cell along with CD23, Tdt, CD10.
3. Phyllodes tumor
   Note: Microphotographs show abundant discrete spindle cells, stromal fragments and benign ductular cells. The features are that of a phyllodes tumor. The further subtyping of the tumor will depend upon the mitotic activity, pleomorphism and necrosis.

CHAPTER

28 Lymph Node

INTRODUCTION

Fine needle aspiration cytology (FNAC) of the lymph node is now a widely applied technique for rapid and accurate diagnosis of various lesions. Peripheral lymph nodes are easily approachable and safe to aspirate. The *common indications* of FNAC of the lymph node are:

- Diagnosis and confirmation of clinically suspicious reactive lymphoid hyperplasia
- Diagnosis of infective lymphadenopathy
- Diagnosis of metastatic malignancies
- Diagnosis, classification, and staging of lymphomas
- Confirmation of the transformation of low to high grade of lymphoma in course of disease process.

Fine needle aspiration cytology is widely accepted to both the children and adult. It is a more or less painless procedure and does not need any anesthesia. The FNAC diagnosis is accurate and reliable. Presently various ancillary investigations are possible from the FNAC material of the lymph node and these include microbiological culture, cell block for immunocytochemistry, flow cytometry, molecular genetics, etc.[1] Moreover, if necessary, lymph node can be excised for histopathological examination after FNAC report (Box 28.1).

There is no absolute contraindication of FNAC of lymph node. Local hematoma can be easily prevented by putting pressure on the aspiration site.

There are a few limitations of FNAC (Box 28.2). FNAC may not yield adequate or optimal material due to small size, fibrosis of the node, large areas of necrosis, and deep-seated lymph node. The other major limitation of FNAC of lymph node is the loss of architectural pattern. Lymph nodal architecture is helpful in diagnosis of certain lesions such as Castleman's disease, diffuse large B-cell lymphoma arising from the follicular lymphoma, vascular transformation of lymph nodal sinuses, progressively transformed germinal center (GC), etc. Moreover, in a large research institute tissue section of the lymph node may be required to do correlative study and future research.

Box 28.1: Advantages of lymph node Fine needle aspiration cytology.

- Rapid
- Economical
- Flow cytometric immunophenotyping
- Microbial and fungal culture
- Molecular genetics study
- Safe procedure.

NORMAL ANATOMY AND HISTOLOGY OF THE LYMPH NODE

Lymph node is a small bean-shaped encapsulated structure situated in the neck, axilla, inguinal region, body cavity, and along the blood vessels. The outer part of the lymph node is covered by capsule. The fibrous trabeculae of the capsule divide the lymph node into several small incomplete compartments. The afferent lymph vessels enter into the convex side of the lymph node and efferent lymph vessels emerge through the concave side where the hilum of the lymph node is situated.

Anatomically the lymph node is divided into three regions: cortex, paracortex, and medulla (Fig. 28.1).

Box 28.2: Limitations of lymph node Fine needle aspiration cytology.

- Suboptimal material:
  - Due to small size
  - Fibrosis of the node
  - Large areas of necrosis
- Loss of architectural detail:
  - Castleman's disease
  - Diffuse large B cell lymphoma arising from the follicular lymphoma
  - Vascular transformation of lymph nodal sinuses
  - Progressively transformed germinal center, etc.
- Tissue material may be needed for further research.

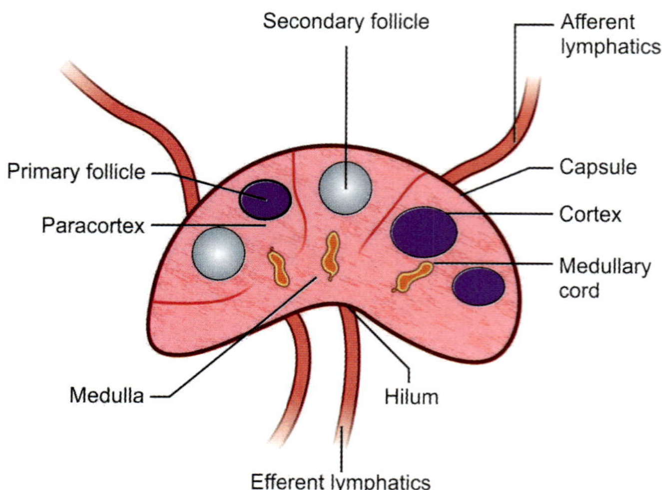

Fig. 28.1: Schematic diagram showing anatomy of the lymph node.

Cortex

This is the subcapsular outer convex region of the lymph node. There are multiple lymphoid nodules (follicles) in the cortex. Two types of lymphoid nodules are seen: primary and secondary lymphoid nodules. The secondary lymphoid nodule contains pale GC. The lymphoid nodules contain B lymphocytes.

Paracortex

Paracortex is situated in between the cortex and medulla. T lymphocytes remain in the paracortex. Many high endothelial venules are located in this region.

Medulla

There are large tortuous lymphatic sinuses in the medulla. These sinuses are surrounded by cords of lymphoid cell known as medullary cords. The lymphocytes from the cortex often migrate from the cortex and enter the sinuses in medulla. From the medulla they enter the efferent lymphatic vessels and ultimately leave the lymph node.

Lymphoid Cells

The ontogenic differentiation of B lymphoid cells has been described in detail in Chapter 6, Section 1 of this book (*see* Fig. 6.8).

B Lymphocyte

B lymphocytes originally develop from pluripotential stem cells of bone marrow and pass through the several stages such as pro-B cell, pre-B cell, immature B cell, and the mature B cells. The mature B cells migrate to the primary lymphoid follicle or nodule. During antigenic stimulation these mature B cells transform into centroblasts and form the GC into the secondary lymphoid follicles.

Morphologically B cell undergoes a series of changes within the GC. The GC is a highly dynamic area and recently multiphoton laser scanning microscopy is used to visualize the events in the GC.[2] B cells constantly move in the GC and dynamically interact with antigen and also T lymphocytes. The resting B cells undergo transformation to blasts to produce clones of plasma cells and memory B cells. The B cells transform from centroblasts, centrocytes, immunoblasts to plasma cells. The various populations of cells in the GC are follicular center cells, immunoblasts, plasma cells, and T lymphocytes.

Follicular Center Cells

Follicular center cells (Fig. 28.2) are categorized as follows:

- *Small non-cleaved cell (lymphoblast)*:
  - Small lymphocytes
  - Regular nuclear margin
  - Fine chromatin
  - Inconspicuous nucleoli
- *Large non-cleaved cell (centroblast)*:
  - Twice the size of the small lymphocytes
  - Fine nuclear chromatin
  - Multiple nucleoli
- *Large cleaved cell (centrocytes)*:
  - Large cells with cleaved nuclei
  - Coarse chromatin
  - Small nucleoli
- *Small cleaved cell (centrocytes)*:
  - Small cells
  - Larger than the mature lymphocytes
  - Cleaved nuclear margin
  - Coarse chromatin.

Immunoblasts

Immunoblasts are developed in the GC and then migrate to the medullary cords. Here the cells complete their differentiation into plasma cells to produce antibody. Morphologic characteristic of the cells are:

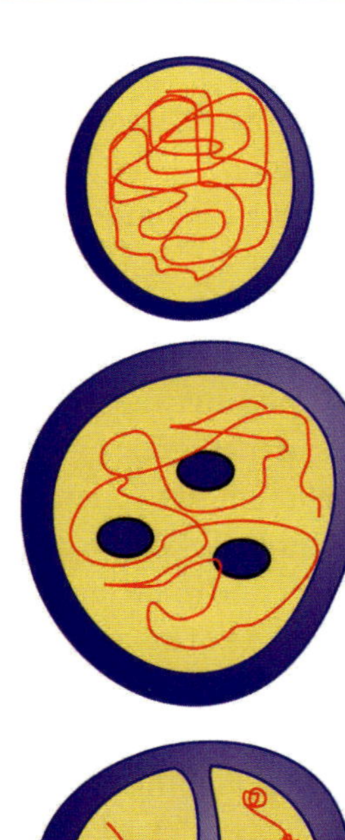

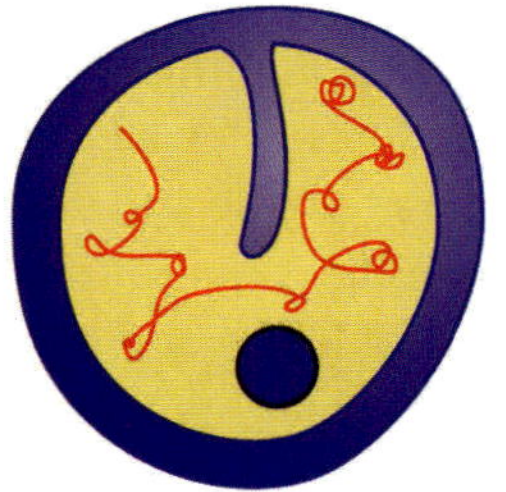

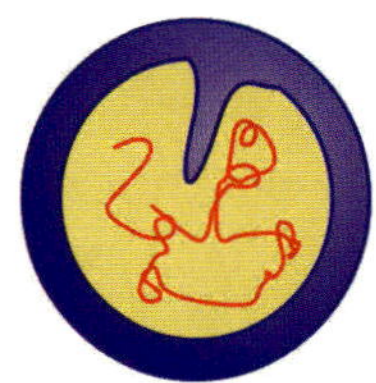

Fig. 28.2: Schematic diagram of different follicular center cells.

- Large cells
- Three times larger than the mature lymphocytes
- Abundant deep basophilic cytoplasm
- Nuclei are round, regular
- Marginally placed prominent nucleoli.

Plasma Cells

These are antibody-producing cells. The morphologic characteristics of the cells are:

- Small cells with eccentric nuclei
- Peripheral clumped chromatin giving rise to cartwheel appearance
- Clear hallo around the nucleus (perinuclear hof).

In addition the lymph node also shows many histiocytes. The morphological characteristics of *histiocytes* are:

- Cells with abundant cytoplasm
- Centrally placed regular nuclei
- Reticular chromatin
- Variable amount of phagocytosed materials such as nuclear debris or pigments.

Large histiocytes with many nuclear fragments are known as tingible body macrophages which are also seen in lymph node.

T Lymphocytes

T lymphocytes are small round cells with scanty light blue cytoplasm having round nuclei with condensed chromatin. Morphologically they are indistinguishable from B lymphocytes.

APPROACH OF LYMPH NODE FNAC

Clinical History

Before doing FNAC, proper clinical history is mandatory in each case. It is preferable to have clinical background of the patient and correlate the FNAC findings in the final interpretation. Most of the metastatic carcinoma occurs in elderly patient, whereas, lymphomas may occur in any age group. Duration of the enlarged lymph node is also important. Lymph nodal enlargement for long duration is unlikely to be a neoplastic process. Majority of the cases of lymphomas and metastatic carcinoma are of recent origin and rapidly progressive. Malaise and significant loss of body weight suggest the possibility of a neoplastic process. Evening rise of temperature and loss of weight are suggestive of tuberculosis. Any history of malignancy is helpful for the proper interpretation of FNAC.

Physical Findings

Site of lymph nodal enlargement is to some extent important. Most of the supraclavicular lymph nodes show metastatic carcinoma. In contrast, posterior cervical lymph nodes are frequently reactive in nature. FNAC of inguinal lymph nodes is usually reactive in nature. Any lymph node more than 2 cm diameter is pathognomonic. Consistency of the lymph node is also very important. India rubber-like consistency is noted in Hodgkin lymphoma (HL). Hard and fixed lymph node is suspicious for metastatic malignancy. Soft and tender lymph node is more commonly seen in inflammatory reaction.

ASPIRATION

Fine needle aspiration cytology of the lymph node can be done by the physician, surgeon, and the pathologists.

However, it is always preferable that cytologists should do FNAC procedure because at the time of FNAC the pathologist may get a brief idea of the possibility of the diagnosis and onsite assessment of the aspiration smear may help to collect more samples for ancillary technique. FNAC of the peripheral lymph nodes does not deserve any local anesthesia. The overlying skin of the lymph node should be properly cleaned. The type of aspirated material may provide a lot of information. Necrotic material usually indicates an inflammatory disease. Thick white caseous material strongly favors the possibility of tuberculosis. Turbid fluid is often aspirated in metastatic squamous cell carcinoma. The aspirated material should be transferred to buffered formalin for cell block to do immunocytochemistry. In case of suspicion of lymphoma the pathologist should always take another pass to put the aspirated material in citrate buffer solution for flow cytometric immunophenotyping (FCI).[1] Similarly one should send the necrotic material for bacterial or fungal culture. In all cases both the air-dried smear and alcohol-fixed wet smear should be made for May-Grünwald Giemsa (MGG) and Papanicolaou's stain, respectively. MGG-stained smear gives better idea in hematolymphoid tumors.

NORMAL COMPONENTS OF A LYMPH NODE

The detailed description of these cells has been discussed earlier in this chapter (Box 28.3). Small bluish cytoplasmic fragments of the lymphoid cell are seen in the background. These bluish fragments are known as lymphoglandular bodies (LG) (Fig. 28.3).

DIAGNOSTIC ACCURACY

The diagnostic accuracy of FNAC of lymph node largely depends on:

- The adequacy of material
- Experience of the cytopathologists
- Type of the malignancy
- Ancillary techniques such as flow cytometry, immunocytochemistry, molecular genetics, etc.

Fine needle aspiration cytology material is limited or suboptimal in case of predominantly necrotic or fibrotic lymph node and accurate diagnosis may be difficult in such conditions. Similarly, in case of subcapsular deposition of the malignant cells, FNAC may give false negative report.

Diagnostic accuracy of FNAC is 95% in metastatic in the lymph node.[3,4] False positive report of metastatic malignancy is also very rare.[3] However, the cytopathologist should be careful regarding the false positive report due to inclusion of skin adnexal glands in axillary lymph node of breast carcinoma cases. Similarly benign salivary epithelial cells may also be included in the lymph node aspirate of neck gland.

The diagnostic accuracy of lymphomas is variable and overall it is near about 80%, if the diagnosis is based only on cytomorphology. FNAC can provide a reliable and conclusive diagnosis in high-grade non-Hodgkin lymphoma (NHL) and HL. However, the diagnosis of low-grade NHL is often difficult. There may be considerable difficulty in cytological diagnosis of low-grade NHL particularly small lymphocytic lymphoma. Similarly, lymphocytic predominant HL is difficult to diagnose on FNAC. In contrast, high-grade NHL such as Burkitt lymphoma (BL) and lymphoblastic lymphomas are relatively easy to diagnose. The appropriate use of ancillary techniques increases the diagnostic accuracy rate. In fact, accurate FCI greatly helps in the subtyping of NHL.[5]

Box 28.3: Normal components of a lymph node.

- Mature lymphocytes
- Centrocytes
- Centroblasts
- Immunoblasts
- Plasma cells
- Polymorphs
- Eosinophils
- Mast cells
- Tingible body macrophages.

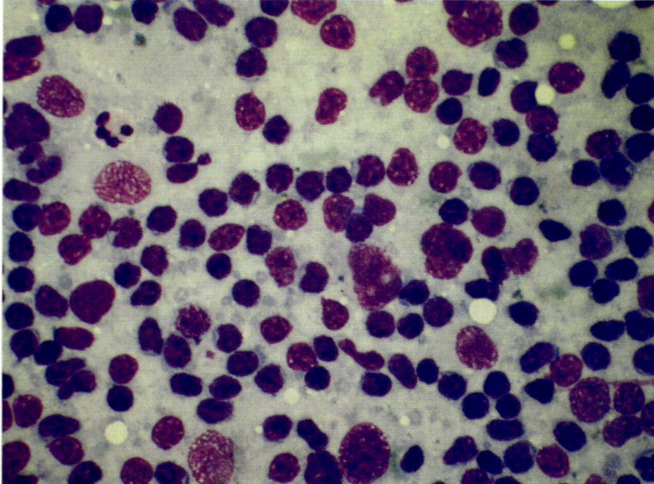

Fig. 28.3: Fine needle aspiration cytology smear of reactive lymphoid hyperplasia. Note the bluish acellular fragments known as lymphoglandular bodies (MGG × OI).

Fine needle aspiration cytology is highly accurate (more than 90%) in diagnosis of metastatic malignant lesions of the lymph node. FNAC can diagnose the broad category of lymphoma cases. However, the accuracy of the classification of lymphoma is variable in aspiration material. The overall accuracy rate of lymphoma is near about 95–99% and subtyping accuracy rate is 96%.[6-8] FNAC can provide a reliable and conclusive diagnosis in high-grade NHL and HL. However, the diagnosis of low-grade NHL is often difficult. Different ancillary techniques are very helpful to help in this aspect.

BENIGN LESIONS IN THE LYMPH NODE

Reactive Lymphoid Hyperplasia

Reactive lymphoid hyperplasia (RLH) is frequently encountered in FNAC of lymph node. Patients may be in any age group but the children more commonly show enlarged reactive lymph node than the elderly population. The neck, axilla, and inguinal regions are more frequently involved. There are various causes of RLH such as viral infection, bacterial infection, drainage area of cancer site, and any sort of antigenic stimulation (Figs. 28.4 to 28.8).

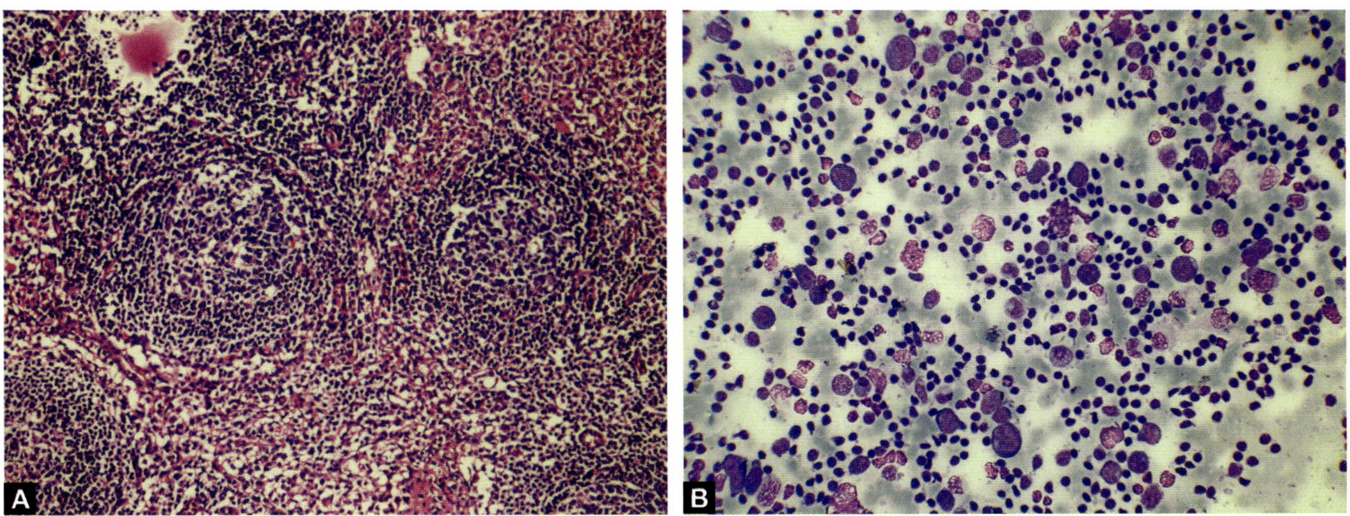

Figs. 28.4A and B: (A) Histopathology section of reactive lymphoid hyperplasia (H & E × MP). (B) Polymorphic population of cells in reactive lymphoid hyperplasia (MGG × HP).

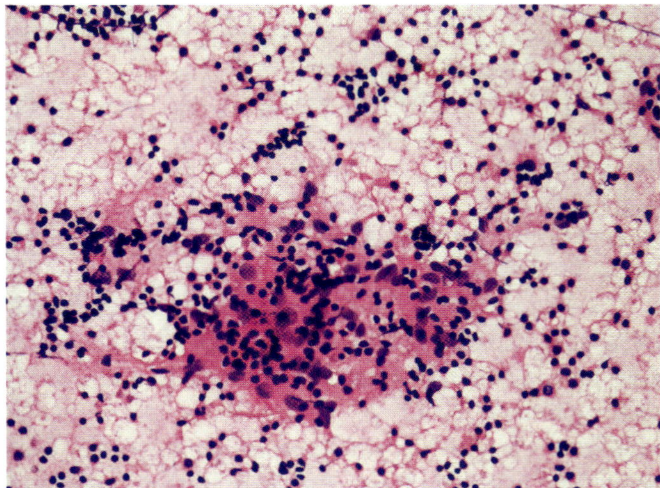

Fig. 28.5: Lymphohistiocytic aggregate in reactive lymphoid hyperplasia (MGG × MP).

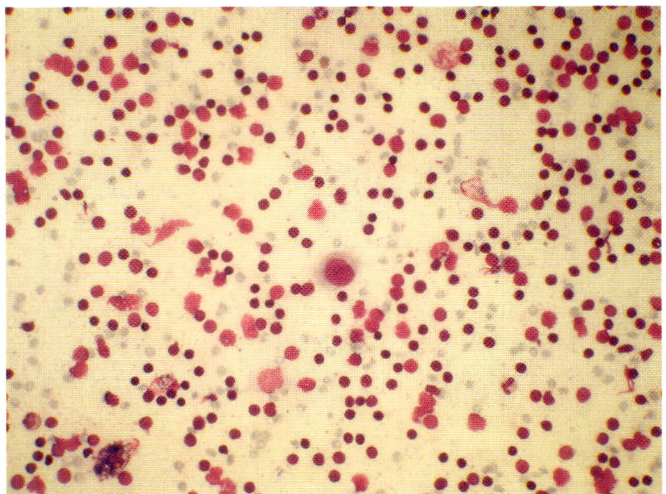

Fig. 28.6: Viral infection—large atypical lymphoid cells (MGG × MP).

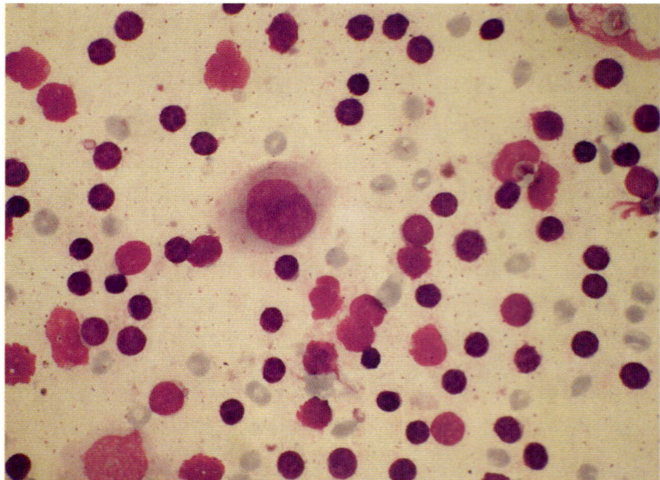

Fig. 28.7: Viral infection—higher magnification shows enlarged lymphoid cell with moderate amount of cytoplasm (MGG × HP).

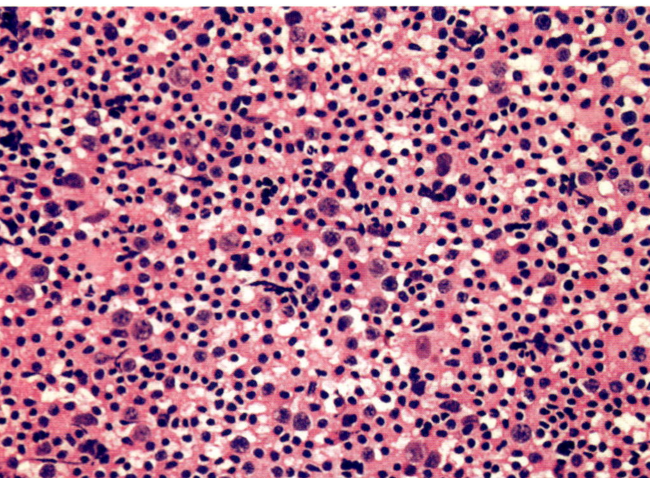

Fig. 28.8: Abundant immunoblasts in a case of reactive lymphoid hyperplasia (H & E × HP).

Cytology

Fine needle aspiration cytology usually yields high cellularity in RLH. The smears show abundant discrete polymorphic population of lymphoid cells consisting of large number of mature lymphocytes, follicular center cells (centrocytes and centroblasts), immunoblasts, plasma cell, polymorphs, eosinophils, and tingible body macrophages (Box 28.4). The tingible body macrophages are large histiocytes with phagocytosed nuclear debris. These represent the cell turnover in the smear. Background of the smear shows LG. The presence of LG body indicates only the presence of lymphoid tissue. It has no other significance. RLH shows aggregates of lymphoid cells and histiocytes known as lymphohistiocytic tangles. The lymphohistiocytic aggregates are the hallmark of RLH. Frequent mitotic activities are also seen as the lymphoid cells always get mitogenic stimulation and undergo proliferation. It should always be remembered that abundant cellularity and mitosis are not the criteria of malignancy in the FNAC of lymph node.

The cytopathologist often faces difficulty to differentiate RLH and low-grade NHL. Small lymphocytic lymphoma or mantle cell lymphoma (MCL) shows small monomorphic population of lymphoid cells and at times is difficult to differentiate from RLH. The characteristic cytological features such as polymorphic population of cells, tingible body macrophages, and lymphohistiocytic tangles along with clinical details of the patients are helpful in distinguishing reactive changes versus NHL. Occasional cases may need demonstration of light chain restriction or aberrant T-cell markers expression to confirm the diagnosis of NHL.

Box 28.4: Reactive lymphoid hyperplasia.

- Polymorphic population
- Lymphocytes
- Centrocytes
- Centroblasts
- Immunoblasts
- Plasma cells
- Occasional neutrophils, eosinophils, mast cells, etc.
- Tingible body macrophages
- Lymphohistiocytic tangles
- Lymphoglandular bodies.

Abundant population of reactive lymphoid cells and the presence of occasional Reed-Sternberg (RS) cell in HL are often confused with RLH particularly in early evolving HL and lymphocyte predominant cases.

Viral infections particularly infectious mononucleosis infection may show large atypical cells with abundant basophilic cytoplasm and eccentric nuclei. These cases may be misdiagnosed as malignancy. However, a good clinical history is helpful to avoid any false positive diagnosis.

At times, FNAC smears of RLH may show abundant number of immunoblasts and this may mislead the cytologist to the wrong diagnosis of lymphoma or nasopharyngeal carcinoma.

Rarely FNAC of small quiescent lymph nodes may show small monomorphic population of lymphoid cells mimicking small lymphocytic lymphoma. One should be careful about not to misinterpret such cases.

Differential Diagnosis

- Non-Hodgkin lymphoma
- Hodgkin lymphoma
- *Benign lymphadenopathy*: Castleman's disease, dermatopathic lymphadenitis, and HIV-associated lymphadenopathies.

Acute Lymphadenitis

Clinically the patients of acute lymphadenitis present with tender enlarged lymph node. The nodes are inflamed, red, and hot. The patients may have fever. Acute lymphadenitis is usually noted in the drainage area of acute abscess and predominantly is caused by bacterial infection.

Cytology

Fine needle aspiration cytology smears show abundance of neutrophils and other inflammatory cells along with background necrosis. Later on aspirate of the node yields purulent material.

Granulomatous Lymphadenitis[9]

Granulomatous lymphadenitis occurs in a variety of infective conditions, foreign body reactions, and sarcoidosis. The detailed causes of granulomatous inflammation have been discussed in Chapter 3 (Box 3.7). In the Indian subcontinent tuberculosis is the most common cause of granulomatous lymphadenitis.

Tuberculosis

Tuberculosis is most commonly caused by mycobacterium tubercle infection. The other two mycobacteria causing tuberculosis are *Mycobacterium bovis* and *M. africanum*. Due to pasteurization of milk, *M. bovis* infection is almost rare in human. Nontuberculous mycobacteria (NTM) infection is now on the rise in both developed and developing countries. *M. scrofulaceum*, *M. avium-intracellulare* complex, and *M. kansaii* are three common NTM. Out of these, *M. avium-intracellulare* is the most common causative agent of nontuberculous adenitis.

Tuberculosis usually indicates pulmonary tuberculosis. The isolated involvement of other body sites by tuberculosis is known as extrapulmonary tuberculosis. Tuberculous lymphadenitis is the most common site of extrapulmonary tuberculosis and represents 35% all extrapulmonary tuberculosis.[10] The tuberculous lymphadenitis may occur in any age group. The patients typically complaints of painless enlarged lymph node. In addition, various systemic symptoms, e.g. evening rise of temperature, malaise, and loss of body weight may also be present.

The tuberculous infection of the lymph node most likely occurs due to spread of the bacilli through lymphatic from the lung parenchyma. Chavollo et al. hypothesize that the other routes such as the tonsils and adenoids, may be responsible to spread the infection to the lymph node.[11]

Cytology (Figs. 28.9 to 28.12): FNAC smears of tuberculous lymphadenitis show multiple epithelioid cell granulomas, multinucleated Langhan's type of giant cell, and reactive

Fig. 28.9: Multiple epithelioid cell granulomas in a background of reactive lymphoid cells in tuberculous lymph node (MGG × MP).

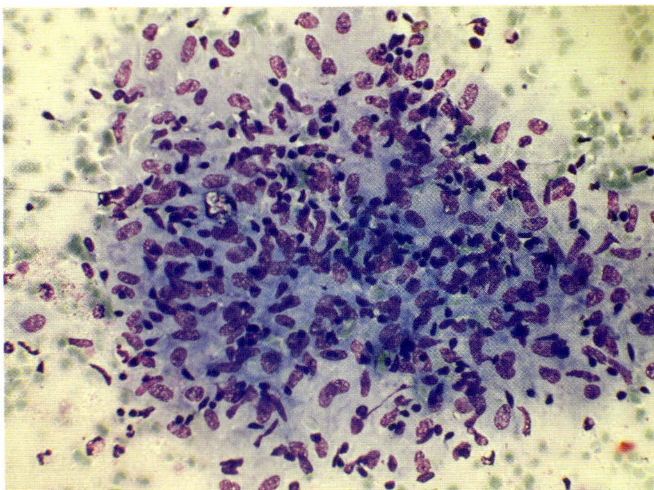

Fig. 28.10: Higher magnification showing the epithelioid cell granuloma in tuberculous lymph node. Note the close admixture of lymphocytes with the epithelioid cells in this granuloma (MGG × OI).

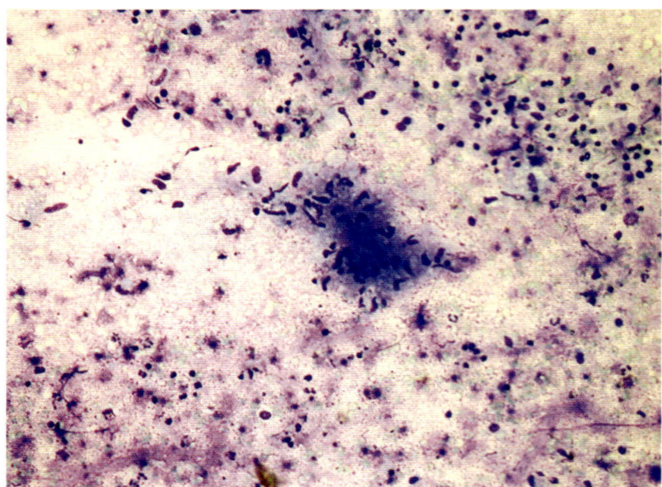

Fig. 28.11: Epithelioid cell granuloma in the background of necrosis in tuberculous lymph node (MGG × HP).

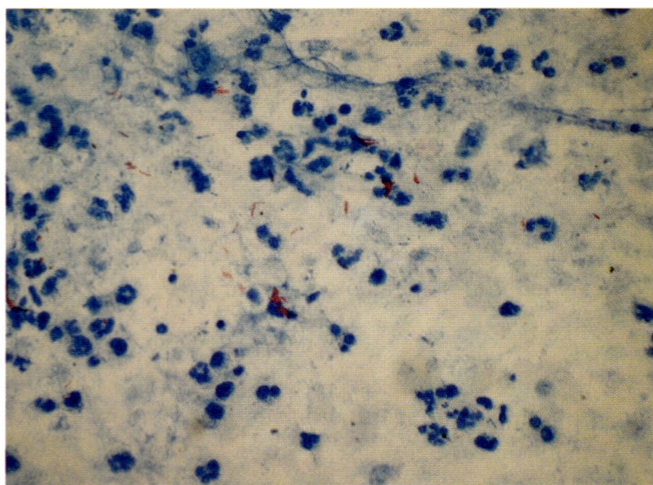

Fig. 28.12: Many acid fast bacilli in the necrotic background (Ziehl-Neelsen stain × oil immersion).

Box 28.5: Granulomatous lymphadenitis.

- Multiple epithelioid cell granulomas
- Multinucleated Langhan's type giant cells
- Necrosis
- Reactive lymphoid cells.

Box 28.6: Epithelioid cell granulomas noted in malignancies.

- Hodgkin lymphomas
- T-cell rich B cell lymphomas
- Seminoma
- Metastatic squamous cell carcinomas.

lymphoid cells in a necrotic background (Box 28.5). The epithelioid cell granuloma consists of well-circumscribed aggregation of epithelioid cells and lymphocytes. The individual epithelioid cells show moderate amount of pale distinct cytoplasm along with spindle-shaped nuclei with blunt ends. The multinucleated Langhan's giant cells contain abundant cytoplasm with multiple nuclei that are arranged in horseshoe-shaped manner. The total number of nuclei is 15–30. The shape of nuclei may be round to spindle shaped. The reactive lymphoid population shows follicular center cells, mature lymphocytes, plasma cells, eosinophils, and immunoblasts. FNAC of tuberculous lymphadenitis may present as following patterns of smears:

- *Predominantly reactive lymphoid cells and occasional epithelioid cell granulomas*: In this type the abundant reactive lymphoid cells may mislead the pathologists and diagnosis may be missed unless a thorough search is made.
- *Epithelioid cell granulomas and multinucleated giant cells in a necrotic background*: This type of smear is readily identifiable for tuberculous infection.
- *Only necrosis*: The smear shows only necrotic cells. There may not be any evidence of tuberculosis other than the demonstration of acid fast bacilli in Ziehl-Neelsen (Z-N) stain.
- *Only reactive lymphoid cells*: This is the most uncommon type of smear pattern and may be noted in HIV-infected patients due to lack of any immunological response.

Hodgkin lymphoma often shows multiple epithelioid cell granulomas. Demonstration of typical RS cell is helpful in confirmation of HL. The epithelioid cell granulomas in HLs are usually ill formed. Certain lymphomas such as T-cell rich B-cell lymphomas show epithelioid cell granulomas. Background immature lymphoid cells are helpful diagnostic clue in these cases. Epithelioid cell granulomas are also seen in seminoma and metastatic squamous cell carcinomas (Box 28.6).

Demonstration of acid-fast bacilli (AFB): In each suspected case of tuberculous lymphadenitis, Z-N stains should always be done to demonstrate mycobacterium. The sensitivity of Z-N stain for the detection of mycobacteria is 33–59% and specificity is 100%.[9] Usually smears with necrosis and epithelioid cell granulomas have the highest chance of AFB positivity. The overall rate of isolation of mycobacteria on culture is 35–49%.[12] The combined use of Z-N stain of the direct smear and mycobacterial culture of aspirated material increases the sensitivity of detection of mycobacteria.[9] Nowadays many newer culture techniques of mycobacteria are available such as the BACTEC 460 radiometric system, BACTEC MGIT 960 system, MB/BacT system, ESP II culture system, and microcolony detection on solid media. These techniques improve mycobacterial isolation rate and substantially reduce detection time as compared to culture in Löwenstein-Jensen (L-J) medium, these techniques have significantly improved the isolation of bacteria and also have reduced the reporting time.[13]

Polymerase chain reaction (PCR) on the aspirated material increases the sensitivity of the detection of mycobacteria. The sensitivity and specificity of PCR in FNAC material of tuberculous lymphadenitis are 84% and 75%, respectively. It has been noted that the combined use of FNAC smear and PCR increases the sensitivity and specificity to 84% and 100%, respectively.[14]

Differential Diagnosis

- Hodgkin lymphoma
- Non-Hodgkin lymphoma
- Fibroblasts.

Sarcoidosis

Sarcoidosis is a systemic disease of unknown etiology. The disease may occur in any age group but it is commonly noted in third to fourth decade. The disease invariably involves lung and thoracic group of lymph nodes and occasionally peripheral lymph nodes in head and neck region.[15] The diagnosis of the sarcoidosis depends on the clinical, radiological, and histopathological features. Non-caseating epithelioid cell granuloma in the absence of any organism is suggestive of sarcoidosis.

Cytology: FNAC smear of sarcoidosis shows multiple non-caseating epithelioid cell granulomas, multinucleated giant cells, and lymphoid cells (Box 28.7). The giant cells may rarely contain calcium oxalate crystals and asteroid bodies. The epithelioid cell granuloma of sarcoidosis is indistinguishable from the granulomas of other diseases. However, the cytology smear in sarcoidosis does not show any organisms or necrosis.

Differential Diagnosis

- Other granulomatous disease.

Lepromatous Lymphadenitis

Fine needle aspiration cytology is rarely done in lepromatous lymphadenitis cases. The cytology smears show many foamy histiocytes arranged discretely or in loose clusters (Box 28.8). The individual cells have abundant multivacuolated soap bubble type of cytoplasm (Figs. 28.13 and 28.14). The nuclei are centrally placed with fine chromatin

Box 28.7: Sarcoidosis.

- Multiple epithelioid cell granulomas
- Multinucleated giant cells
- No necrosis
- Reactive lymphoid cells
- Negative for acid-fast bacilli or fungi.

Box 28.8: Leprosy lymphadenitis.

- Foamy multivacuolated cells
- Multinucleated giant cells
- Epithelioid cell granuloma
- Modified Ziehl-Neelsen stain: bundles of intracytoplasmic lepra bacilli.

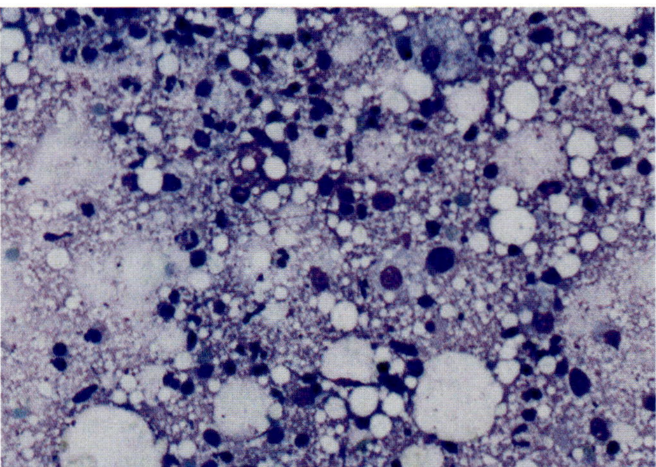

Fig. 28.13: Lepromatous lymphadenitis—large number of foamy cells (MGG × HP).

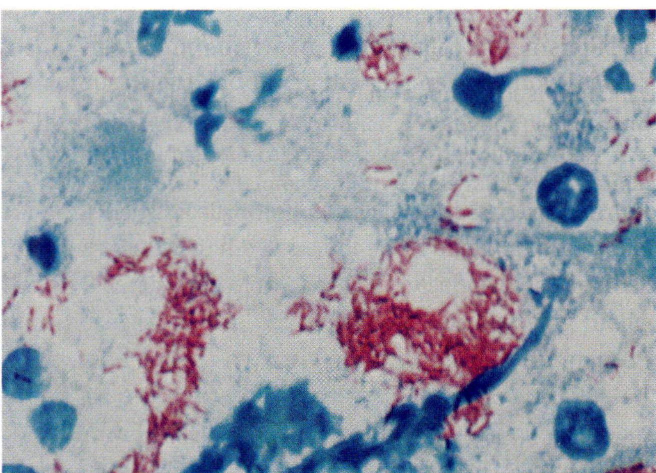

Fig. 28.14: Lepra stain—strongly positive leprae bacilli.

and prominent nucleoli. Intracytoplasmic unstained areas may also be noted. In addition, the cytology smears show multinucleated giant cells and epithelioid cell granulomas. The number or abundance of epithelioid cell granulomas depends on the type of the disease. Tuberculoid leprosy will have more number of epithelioid cell granulomas than lepromatous leprosy.[16] Modified Z-N staining of the smear shows bundles of leprae bacilli within the histiocytes.

Leishmania Lymphadenitis

Leishmaniasis is caused by protozoa of the genus *Leishmania*. Visceral leishmaniasis is caused by Leishmania donovani infection. The sandfly inoculates promastigote form of leishmania into the skin. These promastigote forms of leishmania are phagocytosed by the macrophages. The promastigotes are transformed into amastigotes within the histiocytes. The amastigotes come out from the histiocytes by rupturing the cells. These amastigotes multiply in the reticuloendothelial cells of the body. Lymph nodal involvement of leishmania is rare.

Cytology[17]

Cytology smear of leishmania lymphadenitis shows mixed population of cells consisting of lymphocytes, plasma cells, histiocytes, etc. The smears may also show occasional multinucleated giant cells and epithelioid cell granulomas. Histiocytes contain large number of amastigotes (Fig. 28.15). These amastigotes are also known as Leishman-Donovan bodies. They are tiny 1–3 μm diameter membrane bound oval structures with a relatively large nucleus. Many parasites may remain free in the background of air-dried smear.

Filarial Lymphadenitis

Wuchereria bancrofti may cause lymphadenopathy in tropical countries (Fig. 28.16). The microfilaria parasites may occasionally be noted in the FNAC of the lymph node. The smears show the extracellular long sheathed parasite with a pointed tail that is free of nuclei. In addition, the smear may show eosinophils, reactive lymphoid cells, and epithelioid cell granulomas.[18]

Toxoplasma Lymphadenitis

Toxoplasmosis is a zoonotic infection. Feline such as cat is the definitive host and man is intermediate host. In human it is caused by an intracellular parasite, *Toxoplasma gondii*. FNAC of toxoplasma lymphadenitis shows necrosis, reactive lymphoid cells, and large histiocytes with finely granular cytoplasm. Within the necrotic exudate numerous small, elongated, and crescent-shaped organism may be seen. This is best visualized by MGG stain. *T. gondii* may also be present within the histiocytes.

Rosai-Dorfman Disease[19]

Rosai-Dorfman disease is also known as sinus histiocytosis with massive lymphadenopathy (SHML). SHML is commonly seen in the first and second decade of life. However, it

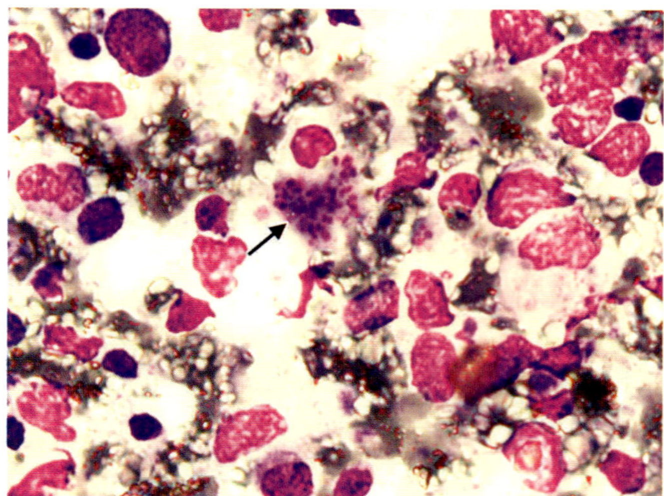

Fig. 28.15: Leishmania lymphadenitis—amastigote form of leishmania (*see* arrow) (MGG × OI).

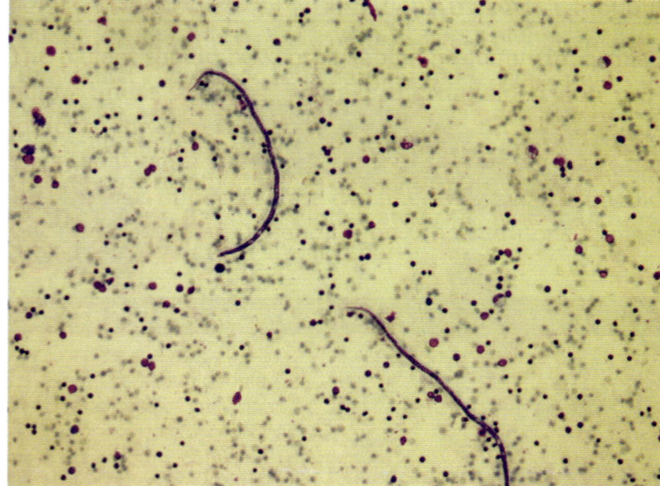

Fig. 28.16: Microfilaria in a background of reactive lymphoid cells (MGG × LP).

may affect the patient in any age group. The patient of SHML presents with painless massive bilateral cervical lymphadenopathy, fever, joint pain, loss of weight, leukocytosis, elevated erythrocyte sedimentation rate (ESR), and polyclonal hypergammaglobulinemia. Clinically the symptoms and signs of the patient may often mimic lymphoma. In 25% of cases there may be extranodal involvement of SHML and include salivary glands, ocular adnexa, bone and skin regions. Extranodal involvement of SHML is usually associated with massive enlargement of the lymph node. SHML is a self-limiting condition and regress spontaneously.

Cytology

Cytology smears of SHML exhibit polymorphic population of cells consisting of many dissociated large histiocytes, plasma cells, and reactive lymphoid cells (Box 28.9). The histiocyte contains abundant pale cytoplasm and centrally placed nuclei with prominent nucleoli. Nuclear enlargement and pleomorphism is also noted. The histiocyte characteristically contains phagocytosed lymphocytes and plasma cells. This phenomenon is known as emperipolesis.[18] Even polymorphs may be phagocytosed by this histiocyte. There remains a clear halo around the phagocytosed blood cells (Figs. 28.17A and B).

Box 28.9: Rosai-Dorfman disease.

- Reactive lymphoid cells
- Discrete large histiocytes with abundant pale cytoplasm
- Central round, pleomorphic nuclei
- Phagocytosed lymphocytes and plasma cells (emperipolesis).

Due to the presence of abundant reactive lymphoid cells, SHML may simulate as reactive lymph nodal hyperplasia. However, the characteristic emperipolesis is a clue to diagnosis along with clinical features of massive lymph nodal enlargement.

Nuclear enlargement and mild pleomorphism of the histiocytes in SHML may simulate malignant histiocytosis particularly in the extranodal sites. However, the nuclear atypia is more marked in case of malignant histiocytosis. The presences of abundant histiocytes in SHML may mimic Langerhans cell histiocytes. The prominent nuclear grooves in the histiocytes, large number of eosinophils, and absence of emperipolesis are important differentiating cytological features of Langerhans cell histiocytosis from SHML.

The hemophagocytosis syndrome may also present with lymph nodal enlargement and FNAC smear shows phagocytosis of red blood cells and platelets whereas, SHML shows phagocytosis of lymphocytes and plasma cells.

Immunocytochemistry

The histiocytes are positive for CD 68 and S 100, CD 11c, CD 14, CD 33 immunostaining and negative for CD 1a.

Differential Diagnosis

- Reactive lymphoid hyperplasia
- Malignant histiocytosis
- Langerhans cell histiocytosis
- Hemophagocytosis syndrome
- Lymphoma.

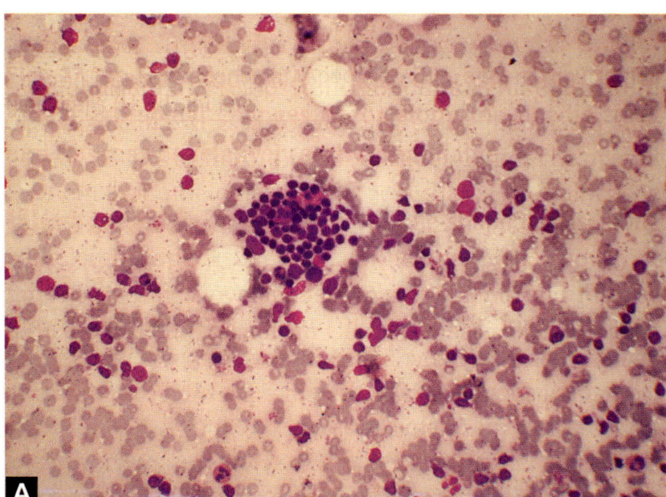

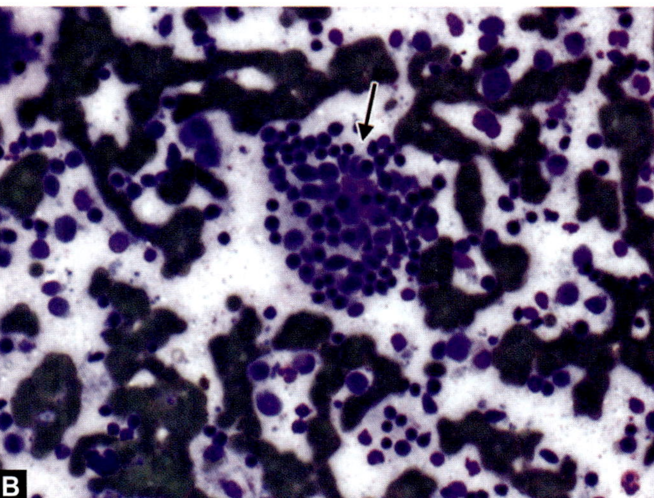

Figs. 28.17A and B: Rosai-Dorfman disease (A) phagocytosed lymphocytes (MGG × MP); (B) histiocyte with phagocytosed lymphocytes (*see* arrow) (H & E × HP).

Box 28.10: Kimura's disease.

- Polymorphic population
- Lymphocytes, histiocytes
- Numerous eosinophils-forming abscess.

Box 28.11: Kikuchi's lymphadenitis.

- Necrotic debris
- Histiocytes with angulated crescent-shaped eccentric nuclei
- Almost complete absence of polymorphs and plasma cells.

Kimura's Disease[20]

This is an inflammatory condition of the lymph node with unknown etiology. The patient presents with involvement of lymph nodes in the head and neck region, salivary gland enlargement, and subcutaneous manifestation. This is an uncommon entity in Indian subcontinent.

Cytology

Histology section of Kimura's lymph node shows reactive follicular hyperplasia with well-vascularized GCs containing polykaryocytes and eosinophilic abscess (Box 28.10). Cytology smear shows abundant eosinophils, reactive lymphoid cells, endothelial cells, and occasional multinucleated giant cells known as Warthin-Finkeldey giant cells. These findings are nonspecific; however, the presence of excessive eosinophils in a clinical setting is suggestive of Kimura's disease.

Polymorphic population of cells along with background of abundant eosinophils may pose diagnostic difficulty with HL. However, classical RS cell is the diagnostic feature of HL and usually these cells are readily identifiable on cytology smear. The numerous eosinophils in Kimura's disease may simulate a parasitic infection and thorough search for parasites should be done.

Differential Diagnosis

- Parasitic infection
- Hodgkin lymphoma.

Kikuchi's Disease[21]

Kikuchi's disease is commonly noted in Japan and other Asian countries. However, it may also occur in USA and Europe. The patient is usually young woman and presents with fever and painless cervical lymphadenopathy. This is a self-limited disease.

Cytology

On histology, the section of the lymph node shows well-defined paracortical necrotizing lesions. Characteristically the lesion is devoid of any neutrophil and plasma cells.

The cytology smear shows abundant karyorrhectic debris and histiocytes (Box 28.11). There is remarkable absence of polymorphs and plasma cells. The histiocytes show angulated crescent-shaped eccentric nuclei that are peripherally pushed. In a proper clinical setting, the diagnosis of Kikuchi's lymphadenitis may be possible on cytology smear.

Marked necrosis in granulomatous inflammation may mimic Kikuchi's disease. However, the absence of polymorphs and the crescent-shaped nuclei of the histiocytes are helpful diagnostic features of Kikuchi's disease. Epithelioid histiocytes in granulomatous reaction have plump-shaped nuclei with smooth outer margin.

Differential Diagnosis

- Necrotizing granulomatous lymphadenitis
- Reactive lymphoid hyperplasia with abundant tingible body macrophages.

HIV Lymphadenopathy

Lymphadenopathy is one of the earliest manifestations of HIV infections. The predominant type of lymph nodal lesions in HIV are:[22]

- Reactive lymphoid hyperplasia
- Various opportunistic infections
- Kaposi sarcoma
- Non-Hodgkin lymphoma
- Hodgkin lymphoma.

Out of all these type of lesions, the most common lesion is florid RLH.

Cytology[23]

There is persistent generalized lymphadenopathy (PGL) and the cytology smears show predominantly florid reactive lymphoid cells consisting of follicular center cells, immunoblasts, and monocytoid B cells having relatively abundant, clear cytoplasm. It is not possible to differentiate HIV-induced PGL from a simple RLH on FNAC sample.

Later on, in the "burn out" phase, there are numerous plasma cells along with scanty tingible body macrophages,

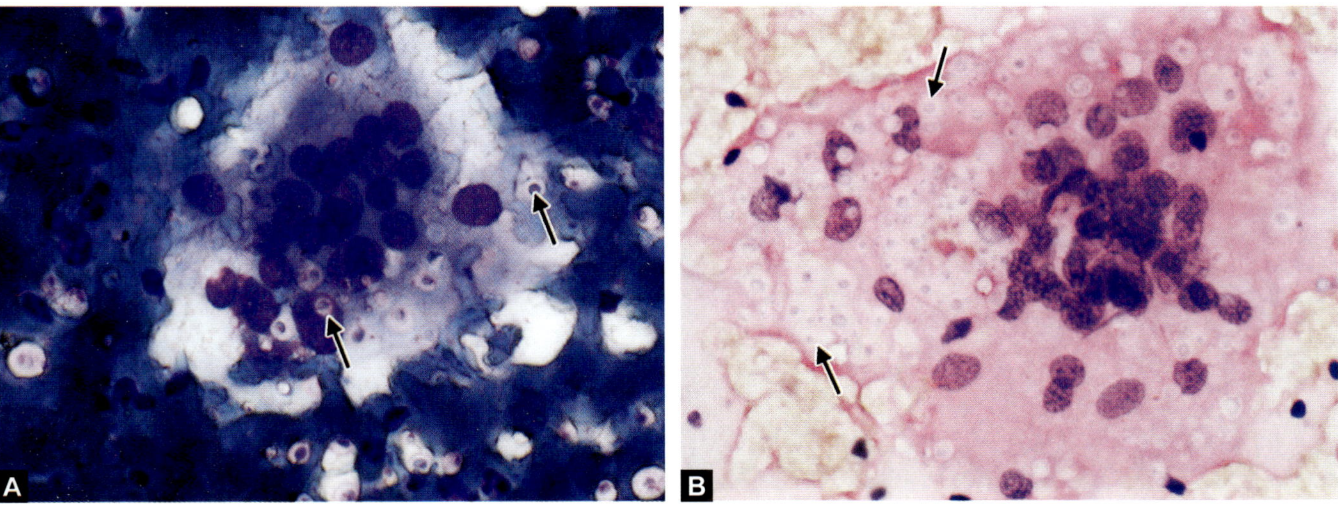

Figs. 28.18A and B: (A) Round encapsulated cryptococci in HIV lymphadenopathy case (*see* arrows) (MGG × OI). (B) Multiple cryptococci within the multinucleated giant cells in HIV lymphadenopathy case (*see* arrows) (H & E × OI).

Box 28.12: Langerhans cell histiocytosis.

- Abundant histiocytes
- Mono and multinuclear
- Oval to bean-shaped nuclei, with characteristic linear folds or grooves in the nuclear membrane
- Many eosinophils.

Immunocytochemistry: S 100 and CD 1a positive. CD 68 negative
Electron microscopy: Birbeck granules present.

and follicular center cells. In all such cases a thorough search is needed to find out any fungi (Figs. 28.18A and B). Z-N stain should always be done to exclude the possibility of tuberculosis even in the background of RLH.

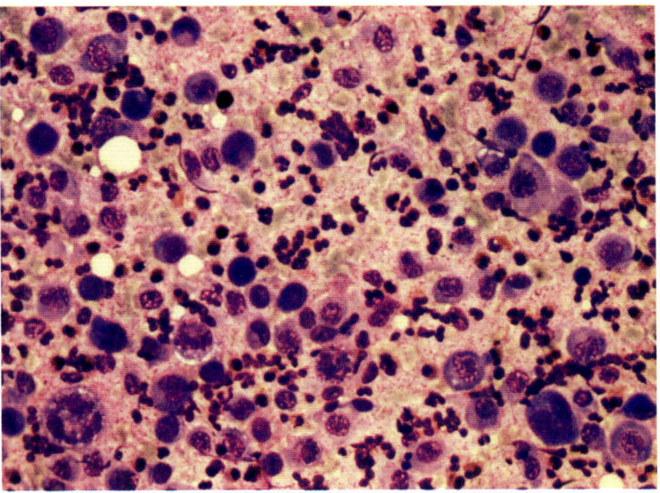

Fig. 28.19: Abundant mononuclear and multinuclear histiocytes along with background eosinophils in Langerhans cell histiocytosis of lymph node (MGG × MP).

Langerhans Cell Histiocytosis[24]

Langerhans cell histiocytosis is a systemic disorder and commonly involves bone, skin, lymph nodes, bone marrow, lungs, hypothalamic pituitary axis, spleen, and liver. The disease is characterized by the clonal proliferation of Langerhans cell, a distinct type of immune "accessory" cells. The patients are usually children; however, no age group is exempted from this lesion.

Cytology

The cytology smears show many mononuclear and multinucleated histiocytes, reactive lymphoid cells and abundant eosinophils (Box 28.12). The histiocytes contain abundant cytoplasm with centrally placed nuclei. The nuclei are characteristically bean-shaped with deep longitudinal nuclear grove. The cytoplasm of the histiocytes is usually free from any phagocytosed material. In addition, the smear shows abundant eosinophils. Large number of eosinophils may cause diagnostic difficulty with parasitic or fungal infections. The presence of deep nuclear grooves in the histiocytes is characteristic of Langerhans cell histiocytosis (Figs. 28.19 and 28.20).

Immunocytochemistry

Langerhans cells are positive for S 100 and CD 1a.

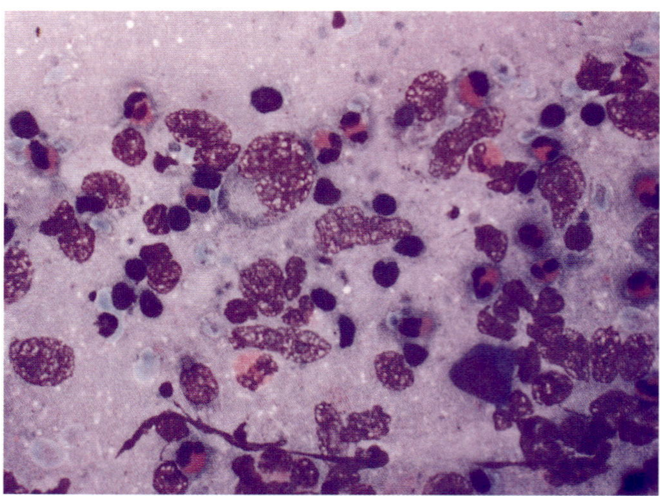
Fig. 28.20: Higher magnification showing deep nuclear convolution of the histiocytes in Langerhans cell histiocytosis of lymph node (MGG × OI).

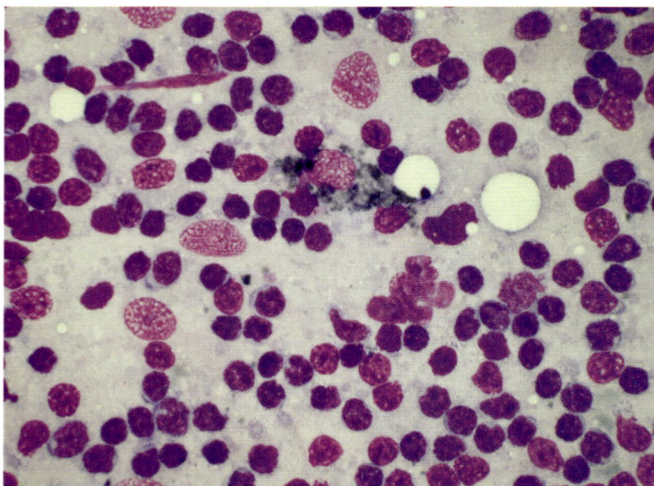
Fig. 28.21: Histiocyte containing melanin pigment in dermatopathic lymphadenitis (MGG × HP).

Electron Microscopy

Positive for Birbeck granules.

Differential Diagnosis

- Parasitic or fungal infection.

Dermatopathic Lymphadenitis

This is commonly seen in the drainage area of any dermatitis lesion.

Cytology

The cytology smear shows a reactive lymphoid cell population consisting of follicular center cells, lymphocytes, plasma cells, and immunoblasts along with many histiocytes containing dark brown melanin pigments. The dermatopathic lymphadenitis should be differentiated from metastatic melanoma because of melanin-containing cells in both the lesions. However, the nuclei of the melanin-containing cells are benign in look in case of dermatopathic lymphadenitis (Fig. 28.21).

Differential Diagnosis

- Metastatic melanoma.

Castleman's Disease

Castleman's disease is also known as angiofollicular lymph node hyperplasia. This is a type of lymph nodal hyperplasia with unknown etiology. Castleman's disease commonly occurs in adults; however, rarely children may be affected. The patient presents with localized or generalized lymphadenopathy. Mediastinal lymph nodes are commonly enlarged. There are two histological types of Castleman's disease: hyaline vascular type and plasma cell type. Hyaline vascular type is more common and represents 90% cases, whereas, the plasma-cell variant is much less common and is associated with multifocal lymphadenopathy and systemic symptoms.

Cytology

Cytology smears of Castleman's lymph node show abundant discrete polymorphic population of lymphoid cells admixed with follicular dendritic cells and tingible body macrophages. Eosinophilic granular material and hyalinized capillaries are seen within the follicular center cells. Follicular dendritic cells are large with abundant pale cytoplasm having ill-defined outlines. The nuclei are variable sized and often convoluted giving a coffee bean appearance. Nuclear chromatin is fine with small chromocenter. Occasionally the nuclei show coarse chromatin with an appearance of a wrinkled tissue paper. Most of the time the nuclei of such cells are monomorphic, however, occasionally large atypical nuclei may be seen. The cytologists should be careful not to mistake these cells as RS cells of Hodgkin disease.[25]

The recognition of Castleman's disease on FNAC smear is difficult because the characteristic hyaline vascular appearance can only be seen in histopathology section. However, in appropriate clinical setting, the certain cytomorphological features may be helpful in recognition of Castleman's disease.

Differential Diagnosis

- Reactive lymphoid hyperplasia
- Hodgkin lymphoma.

METASTATIC MALIGNANCY[26-28]

Majority of the malignant tumors spread through the lymphatic and, therefore, the lymph nodes are frequently involved by metastasis. The different types of carcinomas, malignant melanomas, germ cell tumors, and certain sarcomas metastasize in the lymph node. The detailed clinical history is necessary for the accurate typing and detecting the primary site of the malignancy. The following data helps in this aspect:

- Chief complaints of the patient
- Past and present history about any malignancy
- Histopathology report of the primary, if available
- Complete physical examination.

The detailed information of laboratory investigations may also indicate the possible origin of the primary site. Chest radiographs and CT scan of thorax and abdomen may show space-occupying lesion. In addition, simple blood test, urine analysis, and biochemical investigations are also important.

Cytology

Fine needle aspiration cytology of the various metastatic malignancy usually show a polymorphic population of cells consisting of reactive lymphoid cells and discrete or clusters of foreign cells. Monotonous population of malignant cells is seen in case of complete effacement of the lymph node by malignancies.

Squamous Cell Carcinoma

Fine needle aspiration cytology of the metastatic squamous cell carcinoma in lymph node often shows cystic degeneration and the aspirate yield turbid fluid. The cyst should always be reaspirated to have more cells. The smears show polyhedral squamoid cells with moderate cytoplasm and enlarged hyperchromatic, pleomorphic nuclei. Papanicolaou's stained smear shows orangeophilic cytoplasm indicating intracellular keratin. Many tadpole and fiber cells are also seen. At times, there may be only mature-looking squamous cells in the smear and therefore a definite diagnosis of metastatic squamous cell carcinoma may be difficult. Histopathology should be done in such cases (Fig. 28.22).

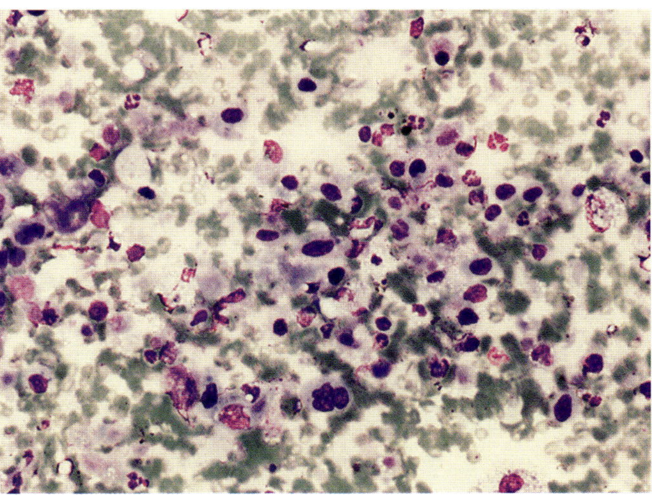

Fig. 28.22: Many discrete malignant squamous cells along with polymorphs in a metastatic squamous cell carcinoma (MGG × MP).

Adenocarcinoma

Fine needle aspiration cytology smears of adenocarcinoma show loose clusters and discrete cells along with glandular arrangement of malignant cells. The individual cells show moderate amount of vacuolated cytoplasm and central to eccentric nuclei with prominent nucleoli. In addition, the background of the smear may show mucinous material. In case of gastric carcinoma characteristic signet ring cells are noted (Fig. 28.23).

Small Cell Carcinoma

The smears show predominantly discrete cells and occasional small loosely cohesive cells. The cells are small with scanty cytoplasm having round minimally pleomorphic hyperchromatic nuclei along with characteristic nuclear molding (Fig. 28.24).

Germ Cell Tumor

Testicular or ovarian germ cell tumor often metastasizes in the paraaortic or mediastinal lymph node. The smear shows foamy vacuolated background and tigroid appearance. The cells are predominantly discrete round having central large nuclei. Nuclear chromatin is fine with

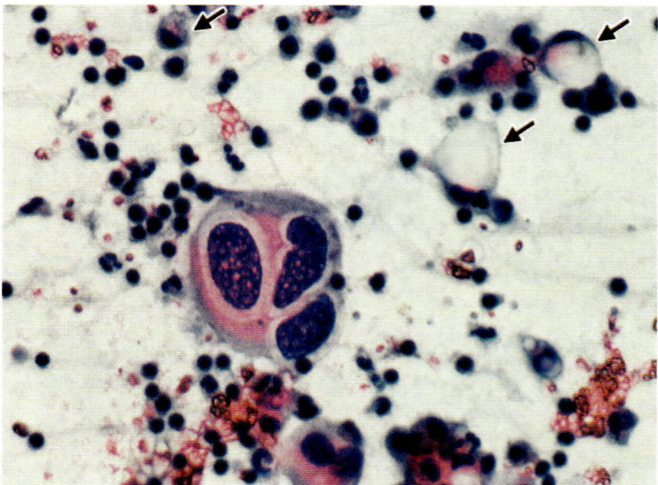

Fig. 28.23: Metastatic adenocarcinoma in supraclavicular lymph node in a gastric carcinoma (MGG × HP). The arrows indicate signet ring cells.

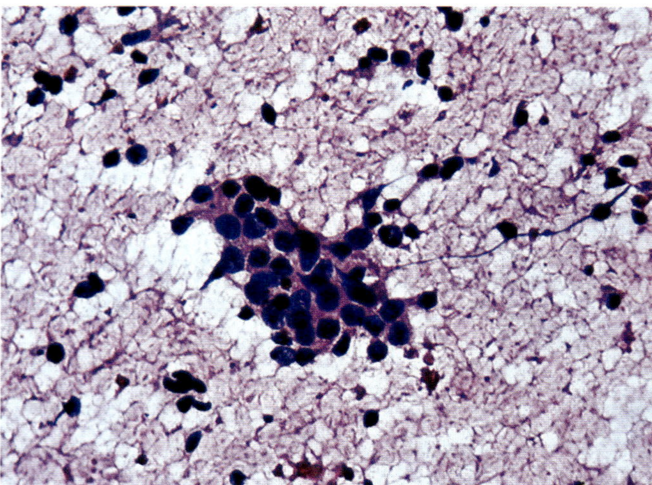

Fig. 28.24: Metastatic small cell carcinoma from lung in supraclavicular lymph node (H & E × HP).

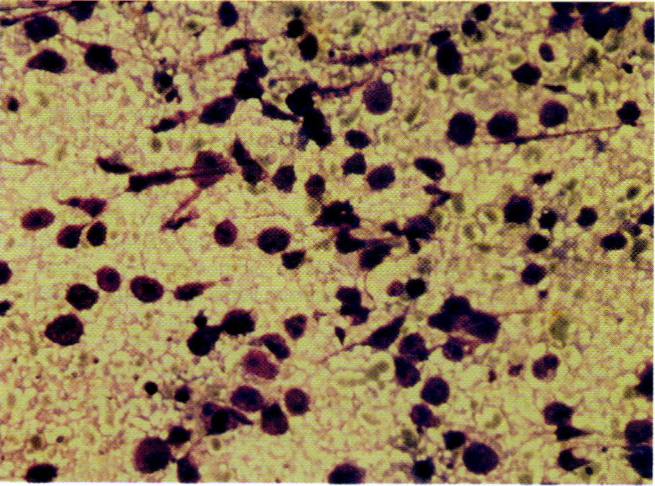

Fig. 28.25: Metastatic seminoma in a paraaortic lymph node. Note the typical tigroid background (MGG × MP).

single prominent nucleoli. Individual cell morphology along with typical background indicates the possibility of metastatic dysgerminoma or seminoma. Cell of endodermal sinus tumor are severely pleomorphic with large prominent nucleoli (Fig. 28.25).

Sarcoma

Sarcomas may also metastasize in the lymph node and 2–5% of patients with soft-tissue sarcomas may have nodal metastases.[29]

The common sarcomas that may be seen in the lymph node aspirates are:[28]

- Embryonal rhabdomyosarcoma
- Synovial sarcoma
- Leiomyosarcoma
- Fibrosarcoma
- Malignant fibrous histiocytoma.

The cytomorphology of the metastatic sarcoma depends on the morphology of the primary malignancy. Without the proper clinical history, the diagnosis of metastatic rhabdomyosarcoma is difficult only on the basis of cytomorphology. The differential diagnosis includes NHL, undifferentiated carcinoma, or neuroblastoma. Immunohistochemistry particularly desmin and myogenin are helpful in the diagnosis of metastatic rhabdomyosarcoma.

Metastatic spindle cell sarcoma is relatively easy to diagnose. However, the exact subtyping may be difficult or impossible in FNAC. The differential diagnosis includes spindle cell carcinoma and melanoma.

Others

Various other malignancies such as melanoma, carcinoid, renal cell carcinoma, etc. may also metastasize in the lymph node (Fig. 28.26). Cytological features and thorough clinical history are helpful in diagnosis. In difficult situation immunocytochemistry may also help.

Immunocytochemistry: Immunocytochemistry is of great help in identifying various types of malignancy particularly poorly differentiated occult malignancies (Table 28.1).

Squamous cell carcinoma strongly expresses the CK5, CK14, and CK17 as well as CK6 and CK16. It is important to remember that the demonstration of CK5 and CK6

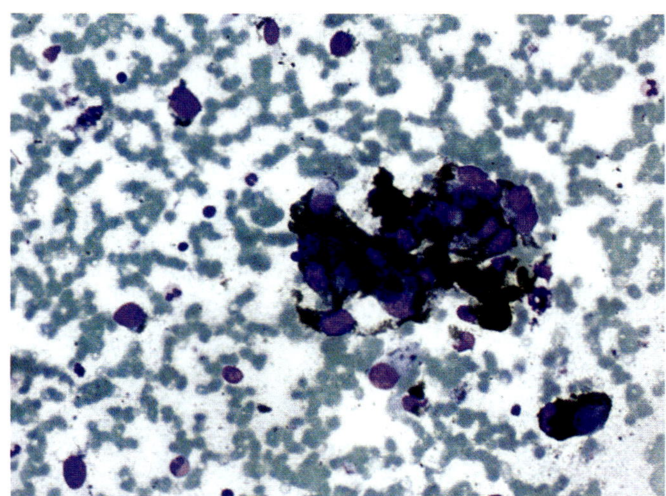

Fig. 28.26: Metastatic malignant melanoma in lymph node showing dark black melanin pigment within the malignant cells (MGG × MP).

expression is particularly helpful to distinguish a poorly differentiated squamous cell carcinoma from a poorly differentiated adenocarcinoma.[30]

The detection of primary location of adenocarcinoma is possible by dual use of CK7 and CK20 on FNAC sample (Table 28.2). Colorectal adenocarcinomas exhibit a CK7–/CK20+ expression in majority of the cases. Ovary and endometrial carcinomas are always positive for CK7 and negative for CK20. In addition, they are also positive for CK8, CK18, and CK19. Both ductal and lobular carcinomas of breast are positive for CK7, CK8, CK18, and CK19 and negative for CK20, CK5/6, and CK14. Therefore, CK7+ and CK20– along with ER, PR positivity are helpful markers to differentiate metastatic breast carcinoma from other adenocarcinomas.[30]

In addition to cytokeratin different other antibodies may also be helpful in identifying the primary malignancy of the metastatic malignancy such as prostate specific antigen for metastatic prostatic carcinoma, placental alkaline phosphatase (PLAP) for metastatic seminoma, alpha fetoprotein for endodermal sinus tumor, etc.

Table 28.1: Immunocytochemistry of different categories of malignancies.

Immunocytochemistry (antibody)	*Tumor type*
Keratin and EMA	Epithelial tumors
Vimentin	Mesenchymal tumor
Desmin	Myogenic tumor
CD 45 (leukocyte common antigen)	NHL
Mic-2	PNET
NB 40	Neuroblastoma
HMB 45	Malignant melanoma

(EMA: Epithelial membrane antigen; NHL: Non-Hodgkin lymphoma; PNET: Primitive neuroectodermal tumor).

Table 28.2: Cytokeratin expression in different malignancies.

	Cytokeratin expression			
Malignancy	*CK7*	*CK20*	*CK5*	*CK19*
Colorectal carcinoma	–	+	–	+
Adenocarcinoma stomach	+	Focal+	–	+
Ovarian adenocarcinoma (non-mucinous)	+	–	–	+
Transitional cell carcinoma	+	Focal +	–	+
Adenocarcinoma of lung	+	–	–	+
Squamous cell carcinoma of lung	–	–	+	Occasional +
Small cell carcinoma of lung	–	–	–	Focal +
Invasive carcinoma of breast	+	–	+ in basal type	+
Renal cell carcinoma, clear cell	–	–	–	Focal +

LYMPHOMAS

Lymphomas are the neoplasm of lymphoid origin. At the time of developmental stages of B or T cells, NHL may originate at any point. The malignant lymphoid cells usually carry the various diagnostic immunological markers of their parental origin. FNAC is one of the most popular and the first-line investigations in the diagnosis of lymphomas. The cytopathologist may help in

- Establishing the primary diagnosis of lymphomas
- Differentiating NHL from HL
- Subclassification of NHL
- Staging of lymphomas
- Diagnosis of recurrent lymphomas.

Lymphoma Classification

In the year 1994, Revised European American Lymphoma (REAL) classification was recommended by the International Lymphoma Study Group.[31] Within a couple of years, this was modified by the WHO group.[32] This WHO classification of lymphoma is mainly based on the cell lineage of the lymphoid cells and the stage of maturation of the presumed normal counterparts (Table 28.3). In the year 2016, WHO revised classification of lymphoid neoplasm was published.[33]

Table 28.3: World Health Organization's classification[33] of non-Hodgkin lymphoma in brief.

B-cell non-Hodgkin lymphoma	*T-cell non-Hodgkin lymphoma*
Precursor B-cell neoplasm • Lymphoblastic leukemia/lymphoma Peripheral B-cell neoplasm • B-cell CLL/SLL • B-cell prolymphocytic leukemia • Lymphoplasmacytic lymphoma • Extranodal marginal zone lymphoma of mucosa-associated lymphoid tissue (MALT lymphoma) • Nodal marginal zone B-cell lymphoma • Mantle cell lymphoma • Follicular lymphoma • Diffuse large B-cell lymphoma • Burkitt lymphoma • Mediastinal large B-cell lymphoma • Plasma cell myeloma • Plasmacytoma	Precursor T-cell neoplasm • Lymphoblastic leukemia/lymphoma Peripheral T-cell neoplasm • T-cell prolymphocytic leukemia • T-cell LGL leukemia • NK cell leukemia • Adult T-cell leukemia/lymphoma • Angioimmunoblastic T-cell lymphoma • Anaplastic large cell lymphoma, T/null-cell • Mycosis fungoides • Sezary syndrome • Hepatosplenic T-cell lymphoma

(CLL: Chronic lymphocytic leukemia; SLL: Small lymphocytic lymphoma; LGL: Large granular lymphocytic; NK: Natural killer).

Modifications of WHO Classification in 2016[33]

The several newer entities have been included in WHO 2016 lymphoma classification and some of them are highlighted here (Table 28.4).

WHO classification is relatively easily applicable on the FNAC smear. For the implementation of WHO lymphoma classification one should have the following information:

- Detailed cytomorphology of the lymphoid cells
- Immunophenotype of the cells
- Molecular genetic markers and cell proliferation markers (preferable).

The different types of NHL have their unique cytomorphology and immunophenotype expression.[34-37]

B-cell Small Lymphocytic Lymphoma

B-cell small lymphocytic lymphoma (SLL) or chronic lymphocytic leukemia (CLL) is the neoplasm of mature B cells and represents 6% of NHL. This is an indolent, less aggressive, and incurable tumor. The patients are in elderly age groups and the median age of the patient is 65 year. Clinically the patients are mostly asymptomatic. Occasionally they may have weakness, hemolytic anemia, lymphadenopathy, and hepatosplenomegaly. SLL patients also show leukemia like picture at the time of presentation.

Table 28.4: Newer entities included in WHO 2016 lymphoma classification.

Mature B-cell type	*Peripheral T-cell neoplasm*

• In situ follicular neoplasia
• Duodenal-type follicular lymphoma
• Pediatric-type follicular lymphoma
• Large B-cell lymphoma with IRF4 rearrangement
• In situ mantle cell neoplasia
• DLBCL, NOS
  - Germinal center B-cell type
  - Activated B-cell type
• Burkitt-like lymphoma with 11q aberration
• High-grade B-cell lymphoma, with MYC and BCL 2 and/or BCL 6 rearrangements
• High-grade B-cell lymphoma, NOS
	• Systemic EBV1 T-cell lymphoma of childhood
	• Hydroa vacciniforme–like lymphoproliferative disorder
	• Monomorphic epitheliotropic intestinal T-cell lymphoma
	• Indolent T-cell lymphoproliferative disorder of the GI tract
	• Primary cutaneous acral CD 81 T-cell lymphoma
	• Primary cutaneous CD 41 small/medium T-cell lymphoproliferative disorder
	• Follicular T-cell lymphoma
	• Anaplastic large cell lymphoma, ALK2
	• Breast implant-associated anaplastic large cell lymphoma

(DLBCL: Diffuse large B-cell lymphoma; EBV1: Epstein-Barr virus 1; IRF4: Interferon regulatory factor 4; GI: Gastrointestinal).

Box 28.13: Small lymphocytic lymphoma or chronic lymphocytic leukemia.

- Small lymphocytes
- Small round regular nucleus
- Regular nuclear membrane
- Coarsely clumped chromatin
- No nucleoli

Immunophenotype:

- Positive for: CD 5, CD 23, CD 19, CD 20
- Coexpression of CD 5 and CD 23
- Negative for: CD 10.

Cytomorphological and phenotypic picture of SLL and CLL are indistinguishable (Box 28.13).

Cytomorphology

Cytology smear of SLL shows a monomorphic population of small round cells, slightly larger than mature lymphocytes. The individual cells have scanty barely visible thin rim of cytoplasm. Nuclei of the cells are round with minimal pleomorphism and almost regular nuclear margin. Nuclear chromatin is coarsely clumped with absent to inconspicuous nucleoli. Mitotic activity is very low. Scanty-to-moderate number of prolymphocytes and paraimmunoblasts are also seen in FNAC smear. The prolymphocytes are medium-sized cells, larger than the small lymphocytes, with fine chromatin and small nucleoli. The paraimmunoblasts are medium to large with scanty basophilic cytoplasm and vesicular nuclei having central prominent nucleoli. These cells are present in clusters in the proliferation center and may not be easily distinguishable from each other. The presence of more than 10% prolymphocytes indicates more aggressive course of the disease. About 3.5% cases of SLL may undergo transformation to high-grade NHL in course of time. The most common type of transformation is diffuse large B-cell lymphoma (DLBCL). The aspirates of these cases show more than 50% large lymphoma cells that have scanty-to-moderate amounts of cytoplasm with one or two prominent nucleoli. In addition the smears show increased mitotic figures and apoptotic bodies with dirty necrotic background. Ki-67 index more than 30% is another helpful indicator of transformation to high-grade NHL (Figs. 28.27 to 28.29).[38]

Immunophenotype

Positive for CD 5+, CD 23+, CD 19+, and CD 20+ (weak) and negative for CD 10 and FMC-7. The cells show coexpression of CD 5 and CD 23.

Genetics

Trisomy 12 or 13q present in some cases.

Mantle Cell Lymphoma

Mantle cell lymphoma is an aggressive B-cell tumor and represents 3–10% of NHL. The disease occurs in elderly patient above 60 years of age with a higher male predominance. The patients of MCL usually present in higher stage with generalized lymphadenopathy and hepatosplenomegaly. The peripheral blood may show involvement in one fourth of the case at the time of presentation. MCL commonly involves lymph node and spleen. The most common extranodal site of involvement of MCL is gastrointestinal tract. It is an aggressive disease with multiple relapses and the most of the patients are not cured. The median survival of this NHL is only 3–5 years. Morphologically MCL is indistinguishable from SLL (Box 28.14).

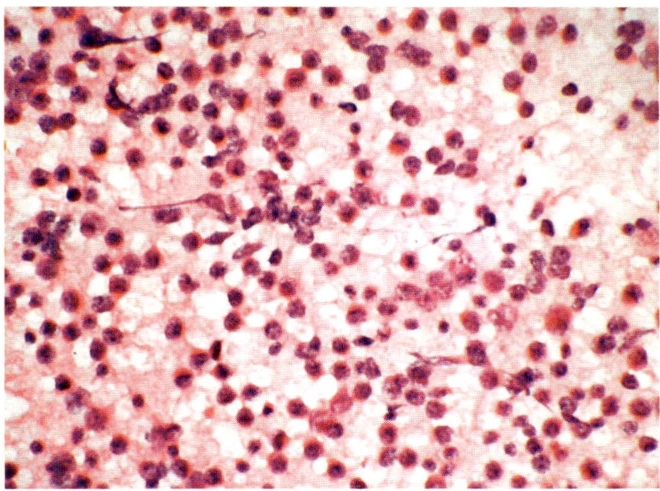

Fig. 28.27: Discrete round monomorphic cells in B-cell small lymphocytic lymphoma (H & E × LP).

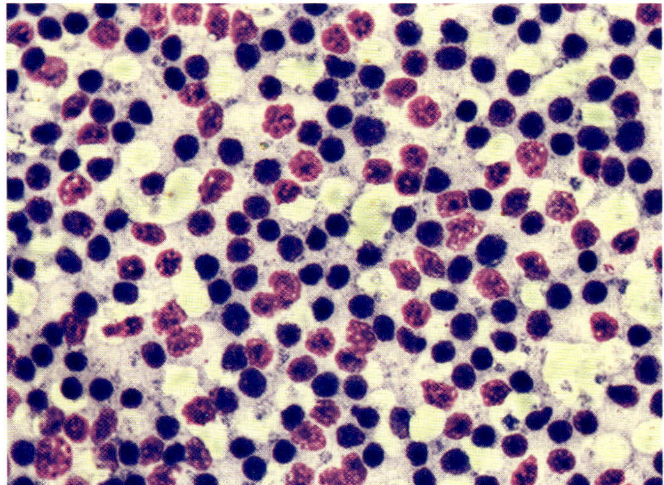

Fig. 28.28: Fine needle aspiration cytology smear of B-cell small lymphocytic lymphoma showing round cells with scanty cytoplasm. Nuclei show condensed clumped chromatin (MGG × HP).

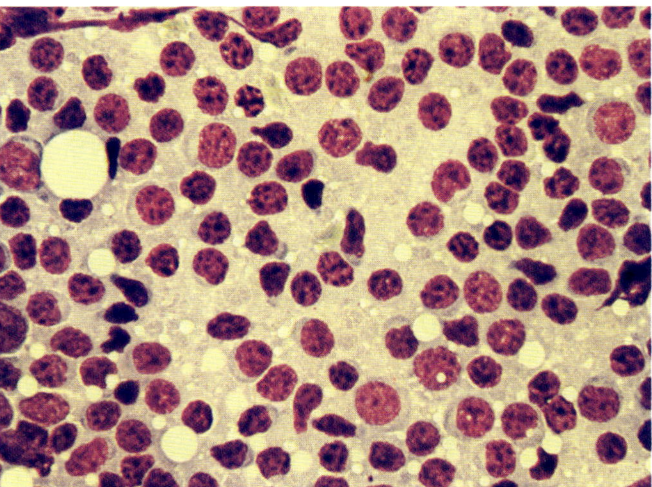

Fig. 28.29: Higher magnification showing typical clumped chromatin in nuclei of B-cell small lymphocytic lymphoma case (MGG × OI).

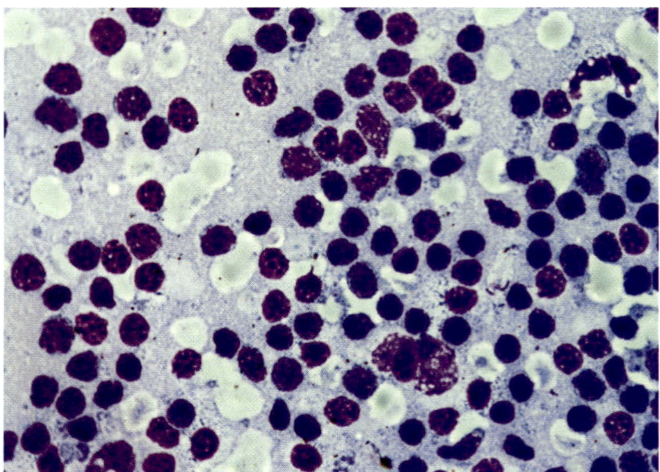

Fig. 28.30: Fine needle aspiration cytology smear of mantle cell lymphoma showing small lymphoid cells with scanty thin rim of cytoplasm and monomorphic nuclei with dispersed fine chromatin and inconspicuous nucleoli (MGG × OI).

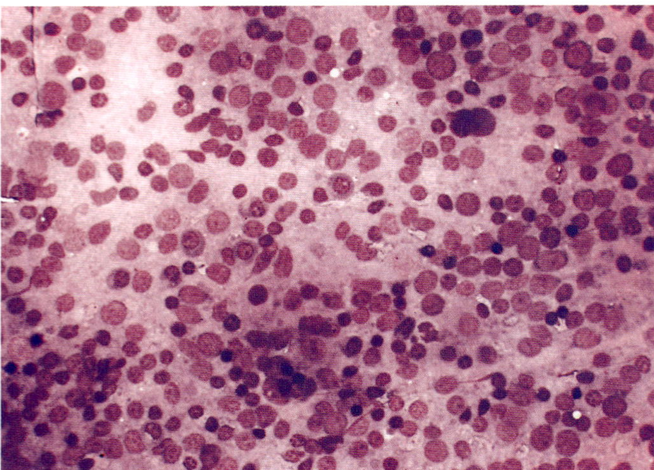

Fig. 28.31: Follicular lymphoma—mixed small and large lymphoid cells in follicular lymphoma (MGG × HP).

Box 28.14: Mantle cell lymphoma.

- Small to medium sized cells
- Irregular nuclear contour
- Fine nuclear chromatin
- Inconspicuous nucleoli

Immunophenotype: CD 5+, CD 10−, CD 19+, CD 20+, CD 23−, cyclin D1 positive.

Cytomorphology

Cytology smears show small lymphoid cells with scanty thin rim of cytoplasm. Nucleus is monomorphic with irregular margin, dispersed fine chromatin, and inconspicuous nucleoli. There is absence of prolymphocytes or paraimmunoblasts. The lymphoid cells may be in aggregation in about one third of cases. In the blastic variant of MCL, the cells are intermediate-to-large having irregular nuclear margin with fine, evenly distributed chromatin. Mitotic activity is high in blastic variant of MCL. This type of MCL has poorer prognosis (Fig. 28.30).[39]

Immunophenotype

- *Positive*: CD 20, CD 5, FMC 7, cyclin D1
- *Negative*: CD 23

Genetics

t(11:14); BCL 1 gene rearrangement.

Follicular Lymphoma

Follicular lymphoma (FL) is a neoplasm of follicular center B cells. It is the most common variety of NHL and represents 20–35% NHL. FL lymphoma usually occurs in elderly patient with a median age 59 years. The most patients present with generalized lymphadenopathy along with involvement of spleen and also bone marrow.[40] This is an indolent lymphoma and 5 years survival rate is high. However, the patients are refractory to treatment (Box 28.15).

Box 28.15: Follicular lymphoma.

- A mixture of cleaved and non-cleaved small and large cells
- Small cells with cleaved nuclei
  - Coarse chromatin
  - Absent nucleoli
- Large non-cleaved cells
  - Round regular nuclei
  - Fine nuclear chromatin and multiple nucleoli.

Immunophenotype: Surface Ig+, CD 5−, CD 10+, CD 19+, CD 20+, BCL 2+.

Cytomorphology

World Health Organization recommends three grades system of FL on histology (Fig. 28.31).

- Grade 1: Predominantly centrocytes—0–5 centroblasts or high power field
- Grade 2: Mixture of centrocytes and centroblasts—6–15 centroblasts or high power field
- Grade 3: Predominantly centroblasts—more than 15 centroblasts or high power field
  - Grade 3a: Centrocytes present
  - Grade 3b: Solid sheets of centroblasts only.

The cells are morphologically neoplastic equivalent of the normal germinal cell. FNAC smears show a monomorphic population of cell consisting of centrocytes and mixed with cleaved and non-cleaved centroblasts like cells. The small cleaved cells are small in size with cleaved nuclei having coarse chromatin and absent nucleoli. They resemble centrocytes. The centroblast like cells have large regular nuclei having fine nuclear chromatin and multiple nucleoli. The number of these large cells is between 20% and 50%. In addition the smear may also show aggregation of dendritic histiocytes in 33% cases.[41] On cytology smear, it is almost impossible to say about the follicular pattern of the cells. The grade of FL on cytology smear is also subjective as the count of centrocytes and centroblasts is subjective in a smear. It is almost impossible to differentiate a grade 3 FL and DLBCL in FNAC smears.

Immunophenotype

- Positive: CD 19, CD 20, CD 10, BCL 2
- Negative: CD 5.

Genetics

t(14:18) and BCL 2 gene rearrangement.

Lymphoplasmacytic Lymphoma

This is a relatively uncommon lymphoma and accounts for 1.5% of all nodal lymphoma. This is a neoplasm of the small B lymphocytes, plasma cells, and plasmacytoid cells. Lymphoplasmacytic lymphoma (LPL) is commonly seen in the elderly patients. The tumor involves lymph node, spleen, and bone marrow. The majority of the patients show immunoglobulin M (IgM) monoclonal protein in the serum. If the serum level of IgM protein exceeds 3 g/100 mL then the disease is labeled as Waldenstrom's macroglobulinemia. The patients with high IgM may have hyperviscosity syndrome. LPL has an indolent course and only a small fraction of the lymphoma may transform to DLBCL (Box 28.16).

Cytology

Smears show a mixture of lymphocytes, plasma cells, and plasmacytoid cells. In some cases intracytoplasmic PAS-positive inclusion bodies (Dutcher bodies) are seen. Immunoblasts, epithelioid histiocytes, and mast cells may be rarely present in the smear.[40] The LPL is the disease of exclusion as various other lymphomas such as FL, MCL, and SLL also simulate similar morphological features (Fig. 28.32).

Box 28.16: Lymphoplasmacytic lymphoma.

- Lymphocytes
- Plasma cells
- Plasmacytoid cells
- Occasionally immunoblasts, epithelioid histiocytes, and mast cells

Immunocytochemistry:
Positive: Cytoplasmic immunoglobulin, CD I9. CD 20, CD 22, CD 79a, CD 38 and negative for CD 5, 23, CD 10.

Immunocytochemistry

- *Positive*: Cytoplasmic immunoglobulin, CO 19, CD 20, CD 22, CD 79a, CD 38
- *Negative*: CD 5, CD 23, CD 10.

Marginal Zone Lymphoma

Marginal zone lymphoma (MZL) is relatively uncommon low-grade B-cell lymphoma. MZL may be nodal and extranodal MZL. Extranodal marginal zone lymphoma is commonly known as mucosa-associated lymphoid tissue (MALT) lymphoma and represents 7–8% of all lymphomas. The extranodal MZL occurs in various body sites such as stomach, eye, thyroid, salivary gland, lung, and skin. The stomach is the most frequently involved area of MALT lymphoma. In many cases of MALT lymphoma a strong association with autoimmune diseases is noted such as Hashimoto's thyroiditis in thyroid lymphoma, Sjogren's syndrome in the salivary gland and Helicobacter Pylori infection induced gastritis in stomach lymphomas (Box 28.17).

Cytomorphology

Cytology smear of MZL shows a heterogeneous population of cells consisting of small-to-medium-sized lymphoid cells with irregular nuclear contour, plasma cells, plasmacytoid cells, and variable numbers of monocytoid cells. The small lymphoid cells show convoluted nuclei and inconspicuous to absent nucleoli. The cells resemble

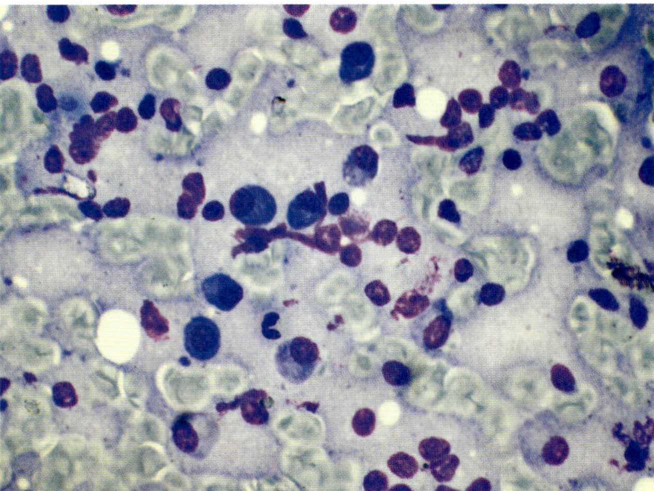

Fig. 28.32: Lymphoplasmacytoid lymphoma showing plasmacytoid cells and small mature looking lymphoid cells (MGG × HP).

centrocytes. The monocytoid cells have moderate amount of pale staining cytoplasm with centrally placed convoluted nuclei having dispersed chromatin and inconspicuous nucleoli. Many tingible body macrophages and lymphohistiocytic tangles may be present in the smear.

Immunophenotype

Surface Ig+, CD 5–, CD 10–, CD 19+, 20+, CD 23–.

Box 28.17: Marginal zone or mucosa-associated lymphoid tissue lymphoma.

- Heterogeneous population
- Small centrocyte like cells
- Plasma cells
- Plasmacytoid cells
- Monocytoid B cells with pale cytoplasm

Immunophenotype: Surface Ig+, CD 5–, CD 10–, CD 19+, CD 20+, CD 23–.

Approach to Small B-cell Lymphomas

On FNAC smears it is important to differentiate these B-cell lymphomas from RLH. The following features are suggestive of RLH:

- Polymorphic population of lymphoid cells
- Lymphohistiocytic aggregates
- Tingible body macrophages.

These features are however not applicable to distinguish NHL and all cases of RLH. In case of partially involved NHL there may be admixture of polymorphic population of lymphoid cells. Unlike other NHL, MZL may show a polymorphic population of lymphoid cells consisting of centrocytes, centroblasts, plasma cells, and plasmacytoid cells. Dendritic-lymphocytic aggregates and tingible body macrophages may be seen in FL. Therefore, to resolve the issue FCI and the demonstration of light chain restriction are necessary (Figs. 28.33A to F).[1]

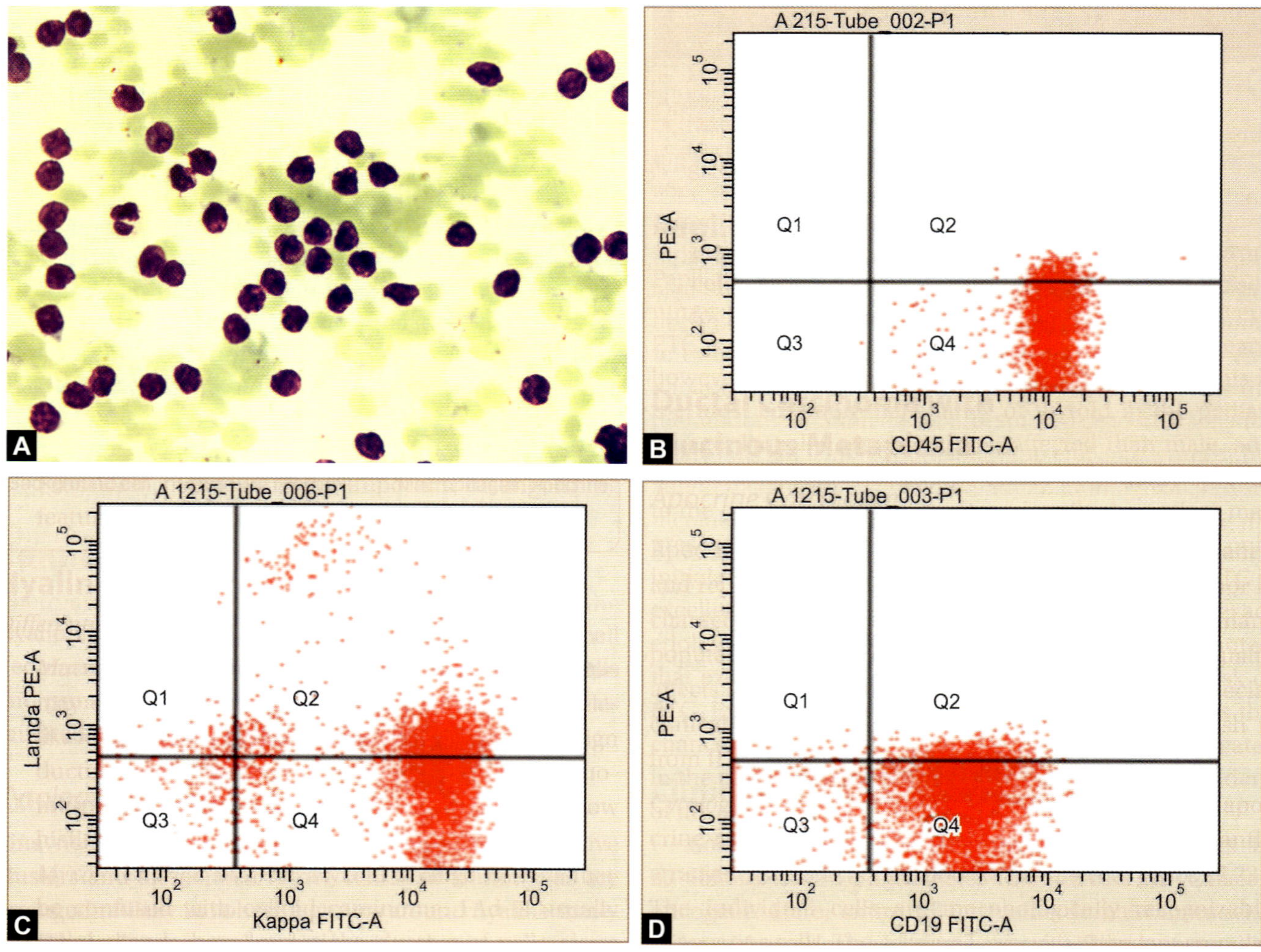

Figs. 28.33A to D

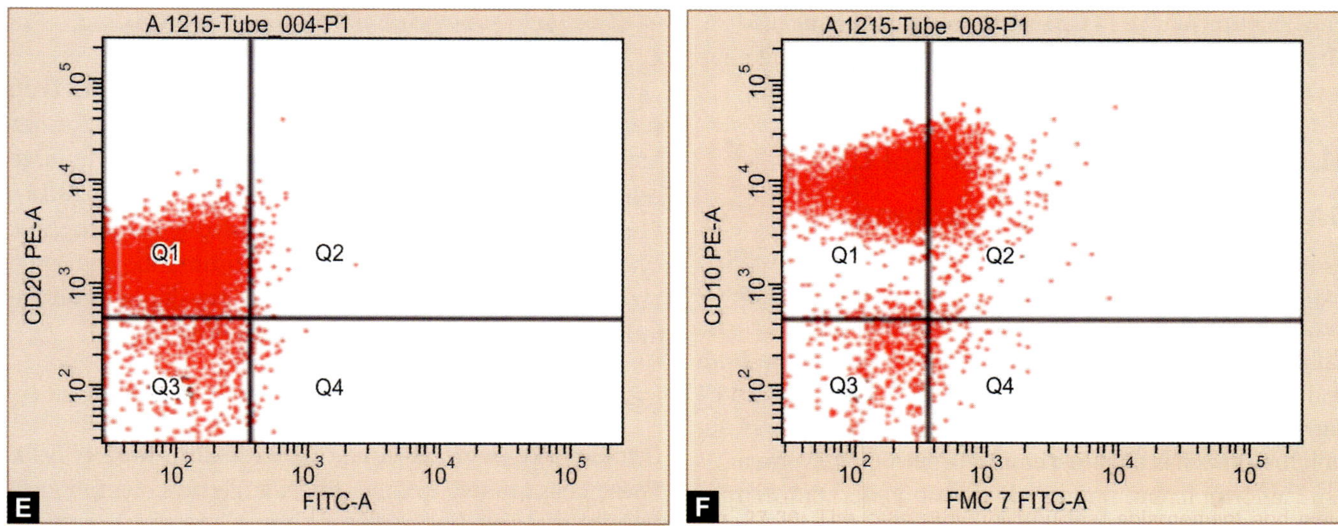

Figs. 28.33A to F: A case of follicular lymphoma in intra-abdominal lymph node showing small mature looking lymphoid cells. Flow cytometric immunophenotyping shows CD 45, CD 19, CD 20, and CD 10 positivity. The cells also show light chain restriction (predominant kappa chain expression).

Table 28.5: Immunophenotype of small mature B-cell lymphomas.

	Antigen					
Lymphomas	*CD 10*	*CD 5*	*CD 23*	*Cyclin D1*	*CD 20*	*CD 38*
SLL	Negative	Positive	Positive	Negative	Weak positive	–
MCL	Negative	Positive	Negative	Positive	Positive	–
FCC	Positive	Negative	Variable positivity	Negative	Positive	–
LPL	–	–	–	–	+	+
MZL	–	–	–	–	+	–

(FCC: Follicular center cell; LPL: Lymphoplasmacytic lymphoma; MCL: Mantle cell lymphoma; MZL: Marginal zone lymphoma; SLL: Small lymphocytic lymphoma).

The non-lymphoid malignancies, particularly small cell carcinoma may also simulate NHL in FNAC. The frequent nuclear molding, paranuclear blue bodies, and background crushing artifact are helpful features in the diagnosis of small cell carcinoma. In addition, positive synaptophysin and chromogranin further confirm the later diagnosis.

The five common types of mature B-cell NHL often poses diagnostic difficulties. Table 28.5 shows detailed immunophenotyping features to distinguish these lymphomas.

Small lymphocytic lymphoma and MCL both are positive for CD 5. However, SLL cases show dual expression of CD 5 and CD 23, whereas MCL shows only CD 5 positivity. FL, LPL, and MZL all are negative for CD 5. Among these three entities, CD 10 positivity is noted only in FL. Cyclin D1 expression is quite specific for MCL (Flowchart 28.1).

Flowchart 28.1: Mature small B-cell lymphoma.

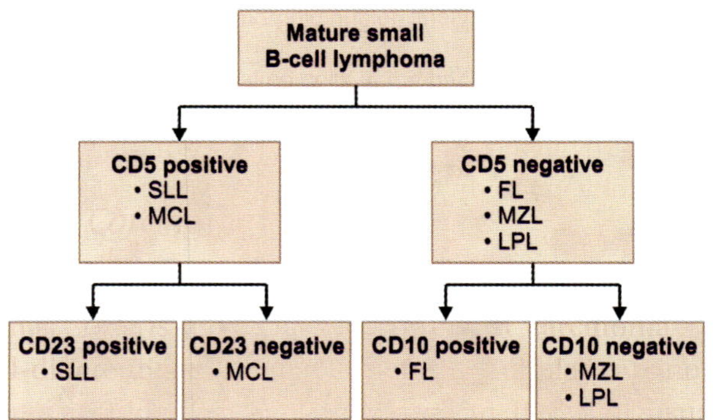

(FL: Follicular lymphoma; LPL: Lymphoplasmacytic lymphoma; MCL: Mantle cell lymphoma; MZL: Marginal zone lymphoma; SLL: Small lymphocytic lymphoma).

In addition, molecular genetics study is also helpful in difficult cases where aberrant expression of FCI happens. SLL cases often show trisomy 12 or 13q (Box 28.18). The translocation of t(11;14) (q13;q32) is characteristic of MCL. FL shows t(14:18) (q32;q21) translocation and BCL 2 gene rearrangement in majority of the cases.[1]

LYMPHOMAS OF LARGE CELLS

Diffuse Large B-cell Lymphoma

Diffuse large B-cell lymphoma is a commonly encountered NHL and represents 30–40% of adult NHL. The elderly patients are usually commonly affected; however, the children are not exempted from DLBCL. There are both nodal and extranodal involvement of DLBCL and about 40% patients of DLBCL show extranodal involvement and out which, stomach is the most common site of involvement.[40]

This lymphoma commonly develops de novo or may represent the transformation or progression of other less aggressive lymphomas such as SLL, FL, and MALT/MZL lymphomas and nodular lymphocytic predominant Hodgkin lymphoma (NLPHL).

Cytomorphology

On histology section, DLBCL shows discrete large lymphoid cells with different morphologic variants (Figs. 28.34A and B):

- Centroblastic
- Immunoblastic
- T-cell or histiocyte rich
- Anaplastic large B cell.

The recognition of these morphologic variants is to some extent subjective and may not have any further prognostic value.[31] FNAC smears show monomorphic large cells two to three times of mature lymphocytes (Box 28.19). The individual cells have scanty thin rim of basophilic cytoplasm, round nuclei with fine chromatin, and large prominent nucleoli. The cytomorphology depends on the individual morphologic variants of DLBCL.

Centroblastic

Cytology smears of this variant show medium-to-large cells. These cells are two to three times larger than lymphocyte and have scanty basophilic cytoplasm. Nuclei are round vesicular with fine chromatin. Each nucleus has two to three prominent membrane bound nucleoli. The cells may be admixed with multilobated cells and immunoblasts.

Immunoblastic

In immunoblastic variant predominant population of cells are immunoblast (90%). The cells are large with

Box 28.18: Molecular genetics of mature small B-cell non-Hodgkin lymphoma.

Small lymphocytic lymphoma: Trisomy 12 or 13q
Mantle cell lymphoma: Translocation of t(11;14) (q13;q32)
Follicular lymphoma: t(14:18) (q32;q21) translocation.

Box 28.19: Diffuse large B-cell lymphoma.

- Monomorphic large cells two to three times of mature lymphocytes
- Prominent nucleoli and basophilic cytoplasm
- Variable mitotic figures
- Ki-67 index less than 90%.

Immunophenotype: Surface Ig+/−, CD 5−, CD 10+/−, CD 19+, 20+.

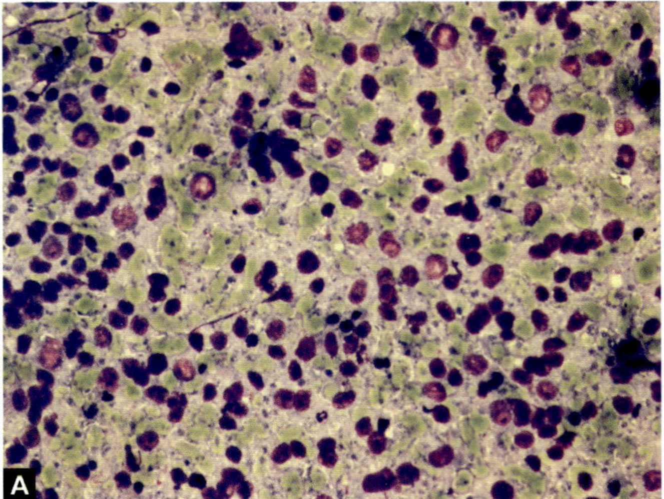

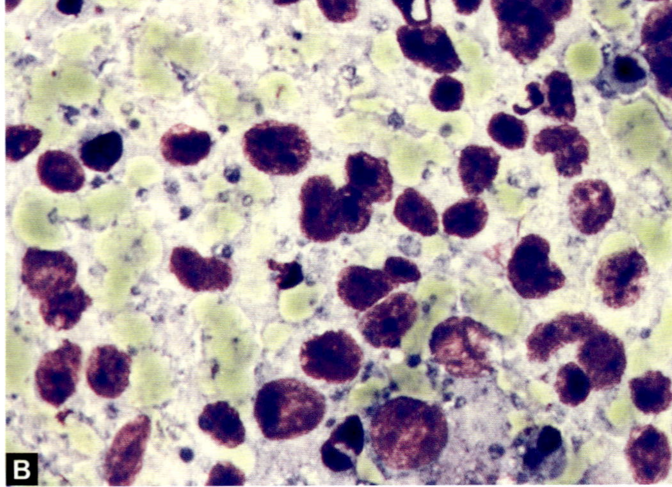

Figs. 28.34A and B: (A) Discrete immature lymphoid cells in diffuse large B-cell lymphoma (MGG × MP). (B) Higher magnification showing large cells with scanty cytoplasm and occasional prominent nucleoli (MGG × OI).

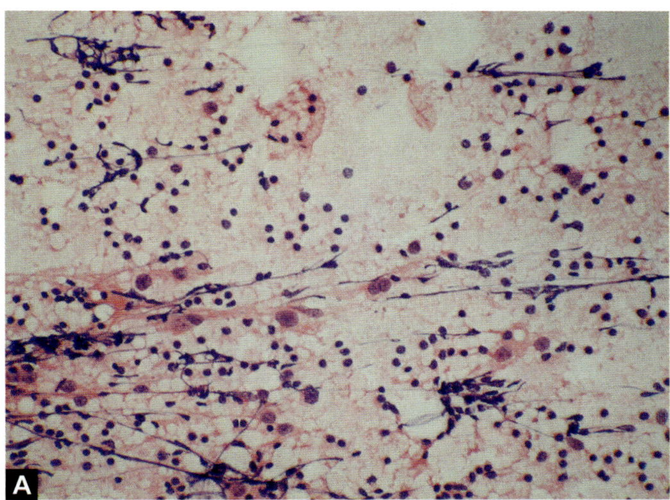

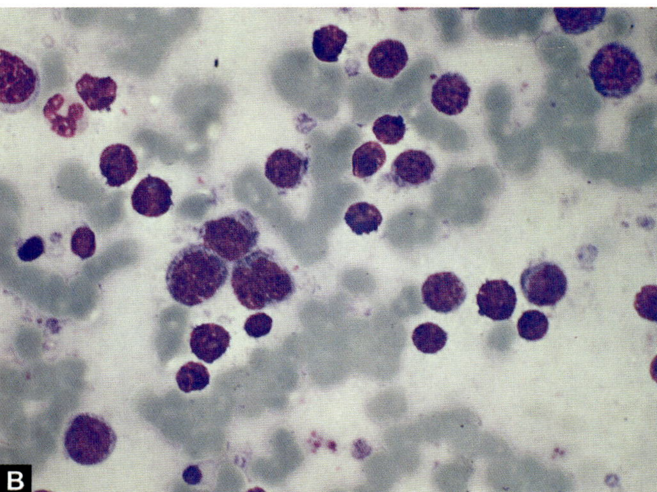

Figs. 28.35A and B: (A) Discrete occasional atypical lymphoid cells in the reactive lymphoid cell background in T-cell rich B-cell lymphoma (MGG × MP). (B) Higher magnification showing better morphology of the neoplastic lymphoid cells (MGG × OI).

Box 28.20: Lymphoblastic lymphoma.

- Small-to-medium-sized cells
- Scanty basophilic cytoplasm
- Condensed nuclear chromatin and small inconspicuous nucleoli
- Nuclear contour irregularity may or may not be present.

Immunophenotype: Tdt+, CD 10+, CD 19+.

scanty-to-moderate amount of basophilic cytoplasm. Nuclei show central large nucleoli with peripheral clearing of chromatin. The smear shows less than 10% centroblasts. Occasionally there may be plasmacytoid differentiation of the immunoblasts and may pose difficulty to distinguishing with plasmablastic multiple myeloma.

T Cell or Histiocytes Rich

The smear is composed of more than 90% reactive T cells and less than 10% neoplastic large B cells that resemble immunoblasts, centroblasts, or RS cell. In addition, there may be variable numbers of non-neoplastic histiocytes. These histiocytes often give epithelioid cell like appearance and may simulate epithelioid cell granuloma. This NHL may be mistakenly diagnosed as granulomatous reaction in FNAC (Figs. 28.35A and B).

Anaplastic

In this variant the smear is composed of large round to oval cells with bizarre pleomorphic nuclei.

- This variant has no relation with anaplastic large-cell lymphoma.

Immunophenotype

- *Positive*: CD 19, CD 20, and CD 79a, surface and cytoplasmic Ig. DLBCL variably expresses CD 10
- *Negative*: CD 5.

The FCI of DLBCL is often difficult as the cells are fragile besides that the large cells may not come into the usual lymphoid-gated population.

Genetics

t(14:18) in 30% cases.

B Lymphoblastic Lymphoma

Precursor lymphoblastic lymphoma (LBL) is also called as acute lymphoblastic leukemia. LBL is commonly seen in children and young adults

Cytomorphology

The tumor shows small-to-medium-sized immature lymphoid cells with scanty basophilic cytoplasm and round nuclei (Box 28.20). Nuclear chromatin is condensed with inconspicuous nucleoli. Occasional cells may have moderate amount of vacuolated cytoplasm and prominent nucleoli (Figs. 28.36 and 28.37).

Immunophenotype

Lymphoblastic lymphoma is characteristically positive for terminal deoxynucleotidyl transferase (Tdt). The cells are positive for CD 10 and CD 19.

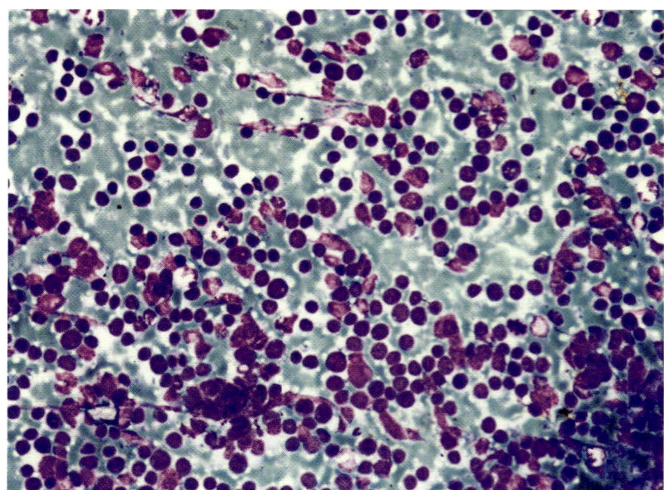

Fig. 28.36: Fine needle aspiration cytology smear of lymphoblastic lymphoma showing discrete immature lymphoid cells (MGG × MP).

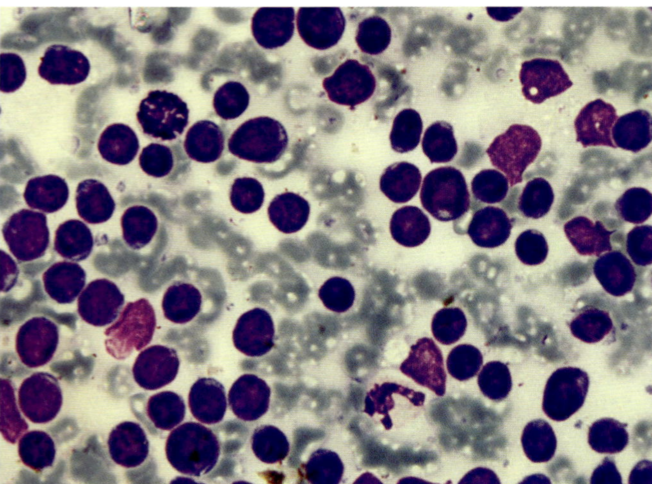

Fig. 28.37: Higher magnification of lymphoblastic lymphoma showing detailed nuclear morphology. The cells have scanty cytoplasm, round nuclei with homogenous condensed chromatin and inconspicuous nucleoli (MGG × OI).

Box 28.21: Burkitt lymphoma.

- Medium-sized cells
- Moderate amount of deep basophilic vacuolated cytoplasm
- Coarse nuclear chromatin with multiple prominent nucleoli
- Starry sky appearance
- High mitotic rate
- High apoptotic rate.

Immunophenotype: Surface Ig+, CD 5−, CD 23−, CD 10+, CD 19+, 20+, Ki-67 index is more than 85%.

Genetics: t(8:14), t(8:22). Rearrangement of c-MYC gene.

Burkitt Lymphoma

Burkitt lymphoma is an aggressive B-cell NHL with frequent extranodal involvement and is characterized by chromosomal translocation resulting in rearrangement of c-MYC oncogene. There are three clinical variants of BL (Box 28.21).

Endemic

It is commonly noted in Africa and also to a lesser extent in New Guinea and South America. This is the most common malignancy in childhood in this zone. The endemic type of BL usually presents with jaw swelling and abdominal mass.

Sporadic

It occurs throughout the world. The children and young adults are commonly affected by sporadic variant of BL. It is often associated with Epstein-Barr virus (EBV) infection and poor socioeconomic condition. The sporadic variant represents 30–50% of all childhood lymphomas.

Immunodeficiency-related Burkitt Lymphoma

It is associated with HIV infection with the initial manifestation of AIDS.

Cytomorphology

Cytology smear of BL shows a dimorphic population of cells, the dark-colored lymphoid cells and pale scattered tingible body macrophages. This gives a starry sky appearance of the smear (Figs. 28.38 and 28.39).[42]

The lymphoid cells are medium-sized with moderate amount of deep basophilic vacuolated cytoplasm. The nucleus is round with coarse chromatin having two to three variable-sized prominent nucleoli. Frequent mitotic activity is also seen. Background of the smear contains many tingible body macrophages.

Immunophenotype

- *Positive*: Surface Ig, CD 10, CD 19, CD 20
- *Negative*: CD 5, CD 23
- *Cell proliferation markers*: Ki-67 index is more than 85%
- Endemic form of BL harbors latent EBV genome.

Genetics

t(8:14), t(8:22) and rearrangement of c-MYC gene.

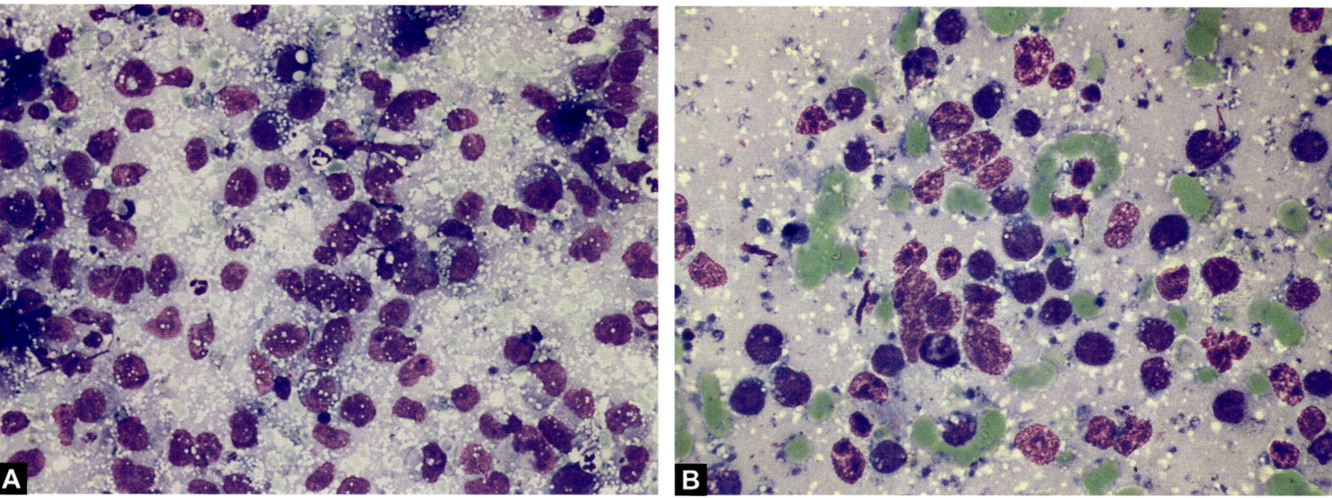

Figs. 28.38A and B: Burkitt's lymphoma (A) discrete lymphoid cells with vacuolated cytoplasm (MGG × MP); (B) lymphoid cells with vacuolated cytoplasm and relatively large nuclei with multiple prominent nucleoli (MGG × HP).

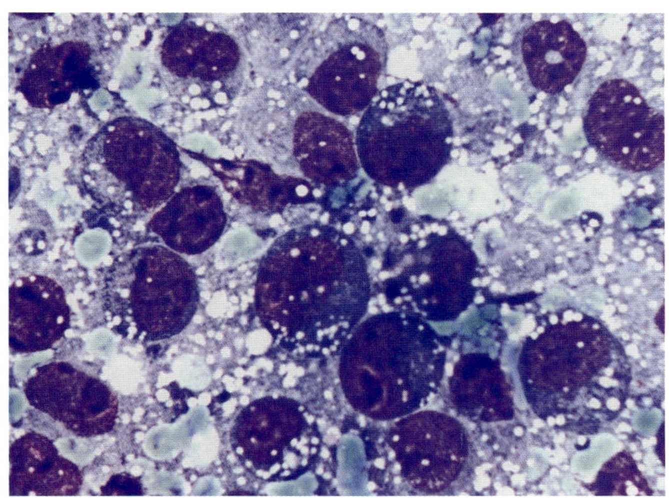

Fig. 28.39: Burkitt's lymphoma—individual cell morphology is better seen in higher magnification. Enlarged cells with large nuclei having prominent nucleoli (MGG × OI).

T-cell Lymphoma

T-cell NHL represents 10% of all NHL. It usually occurs in adults. WHO classified this NHL as precursor T lymphoblastic lymphomas and mature T-cell lymphomas.

T Lymphoblastic Lymphoma

It is highly aggressive and usually occurs in young adults. Most of the patients present with palpable neck node along with mediastinal lymphadenopathy that often compresses the superior venal cava causing superior venal caval obstruction. FNAC diagnosis of this lymph node and rapid therapy gives a great relief to the patient.

Cytomorphology: FNAC smears show similar morphology as that of B-LBL.

Immunophenotype: Tdt+, CD 3+, CD 7+, CD 4+/–, CD 8+.

Box 28.22: Anaplastic Large cell lymphoma.

- Large cells
- Multilobated nuclei
- "Hallmark" cells with abundant cytoplasm, large horse-shoe-shaped convoluted nuclei and single to multiple prominent nucleoli
- Doughnut cells
- Multinucleated giant cells with abundant cytoplasm and multiple nuclei in a wreath-like pattern
- Plasmacytoid cell with clumped chromatin and prominent nucleoli.

Immunophenotype: CD 30 (Ki-1)+, EMA+, ALK+.

Anaplastic Large-cell Lymphoma

Anaplastic large-cell lymphoma is a T-cell neoplasm and accounts for 3% of all adult NHL and 30% of pediatric NHL. The majority of the patients present with higher stage and extranodal involvement at the time of first presentation. Systemic symptoms especially fever is also noted.

The diagnostic cytological features are mentioned in Box 28.22.

Cytomorphology[43] *(Figs. 28.40 to 28.42)*: FNAC smears show many large cells and medium-sized cells with bilobated and multilobated bizarre nuclei, clumped chromatin, and

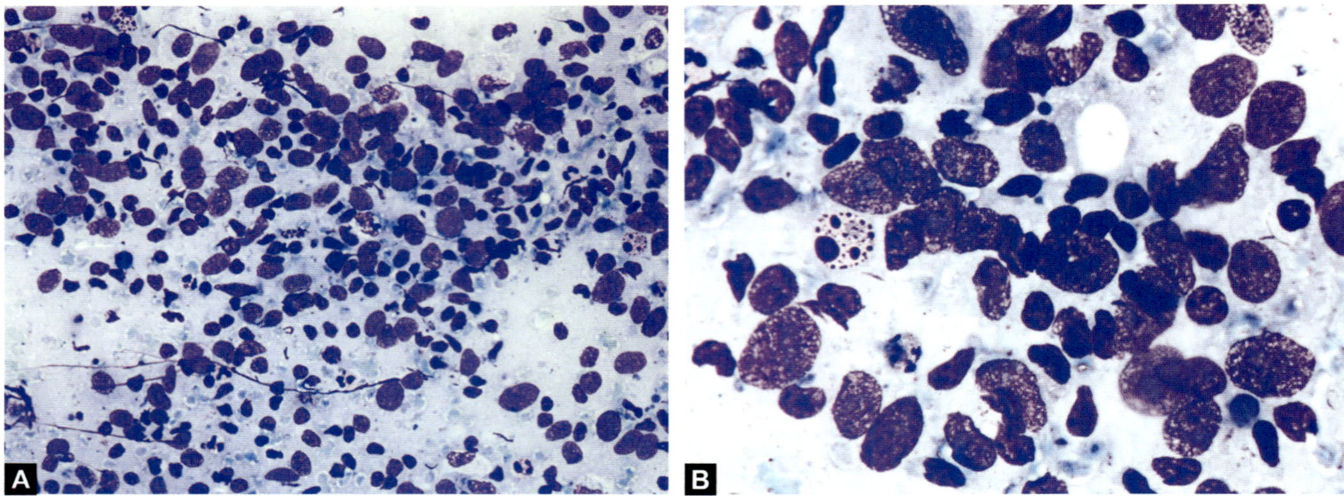

Figs. 28.40A and B: Anaplastic large cell lymphoma. (A) Discrete cells with mild-to-moderately pleomorphic nuclei (MGG × HP). (B) Higher magnification showing better morphology of the cells. Individual cells are large with fine chromatin and prominent nucleoli (MGG × OI).

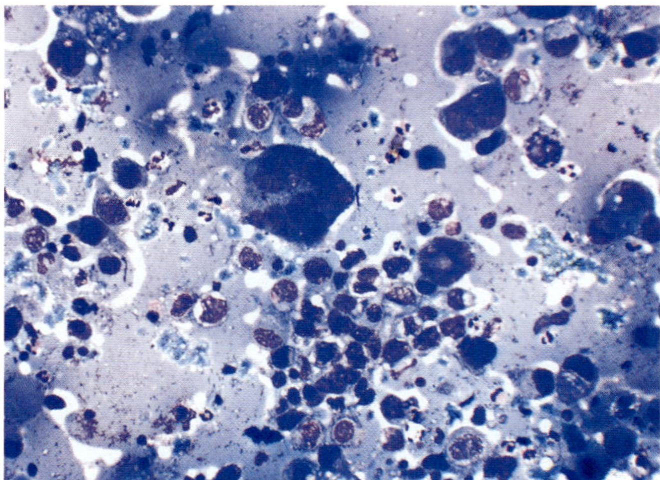

Fig. 28.41: Large doughnut-shaped nuclei in anaplastic large cell lymphoma (MGG × OI).

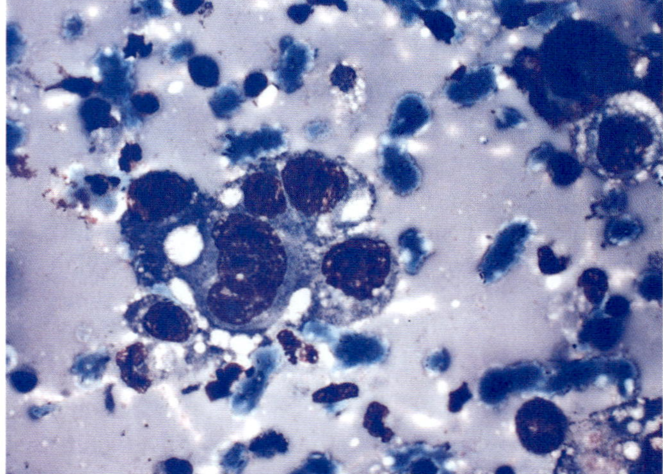

Fig. 28.42: Fine needle aspiration cytology smear of anaplastic large cell lymphoma showing large cells with moderate amount of cytoplasm. Nuclei have irregular margin, fine chromatin, and multiple prominent nucleoli (MGG × OI).

prominent nucleoli (Box 28.22). The smears show variable numbers of the characteristic "Hallmark" cells. These cells contain abundant amphophilic cytoplasm with central to eccentric large horseshoe-shaped convoluted nuclei having single to multiple prominent nucleoli. Occasionally such kidney-shaped nuclei show a smooth convex surface. This gives the nuclei a jellyfish-like appearance. In addition the smear may show "doughnut" cells that contain a large pseudonuclear cytoplasmic inclusion due to the deep cytoplasmic invaginations into the nuclei. In addition, there may be multinucleated giant cells with abundant cytoplasm and multiple nuclei in a wreath-like pattern with variable-sized single to multiple nucleoli. These cells resemble RS cells.

The tumor often shows cells with moderate cytoplasm and eccentric nuclei giving a "plasmacytoid" appearance.

Immunophenotype: Only two-thirds cases of ALCL are positive for CD 45. As the tumor cells are T cells, so they are positive for CD 3 marker. The tumor cells of ALCL are positive for CD 30 (Ki-1) and epithelial membrane antigen (EMA). Majority of ALCL cases (80%) show membranous or cytoplasmic positivity of anaplastic lymphoma kinase (ALK) which is a useful diagnostic and prognostic marker.

Genetics: t(2:5), causing fusion of ALK and NPM genes in majority of the cases.

Peripheral T-cell Lymphoma (Unspecified)

Peripheral T-cell lymphoma (PTCL) is a mature T-cell neoplasm and presents with generalized lymphadenopathy along with organ involvement. Most of the PTCL patients are adults.

Cytology

Fine needle aspiration cytology smears show discrete medium-sized to large cells with pleomorphic nuclei and prominent nucleoli. The nucleus of the cell shows marked irregularity of the membrane with deep notching and convolution. The nuclear chromatin is coarsely clumped with parachromatin clearing.

Immunophenotyping

Positive for CD 3, CD 7, and CD 4/CD 8 or coexpression of both.

HODGKIN'S LYMPHOMA

Hodgkin lymphoma was first time described by Thomas Hodgkin in 1832 and further recognized as a specific entity by Samuel Wilks.[44,45] HL is almost always lymph nodal in origin. Patient of any age group may have HL. There is a bimodal distribution of HL: one peak of incidence in 15–30 years of age another in older age. The patient may have fever, weight loss, and other systemic symptoms. The consistency of the lymph node is soft to hard depending on the fibrosis of the node. HL is of B cell in origin. WHO classification of HL is mentioned in Box 28.23.[40]

Classic subtype of HL represents near about 95% of HL. There is no special clinical significance of recognition of the variants of HL.[46]

Box 28.23: World Health Organization's classification of non-Hodgkin lymphoma.

Classical Hodgkin lymphoma
- Nodular sclerosis Hodgkin lymphoma
- Lymphocyte-rich Hodgkin lymphoma
- Mixed cellularity Hodgkin lymphoma
- Lymphocyte-depleted Hodgkin lymphoma

Nodular lymphocyte predominant Hodgkin lymphoma.

Cytomorphology[46]

Classical Hodgkin Lymphoma

Smear of classical HL shows polymorphic population of cells consisting of mature lymphocytes, eosinophils, plasma cells, and immunoblasts (Box 28.24). Excess eosinophils in the FNAC smear immediately draw attention. The presence of classical RS cells is characteristic of HL. RS cells are large cells of 20–50 μm diameter with abundant amphophilic cytoplasm and bilobed or polylobed nuclei. The nuclei may truly be binucleated or multinucleated. The nuclei are vesicular with coarse clumped chromatin. Each lobe of nuclei shows very large round-shaped acidophilic central nucleoli. In a classical RS cell the two nuclear lobes face each other containing the prominent nucleoli resulting in the mirror image with each other. This is also known as owl-eyed appearance. In case of mononuclear variants of RS cell, the cell contains single nucleus with all the above features as described. The RS cell may be very large with large pleomorphic nuclei simulating the cells of anaplastic carcinoma or pleomorphic sarcoma. Many other cells may simulate RS cell (Box 28.25). Lymphocyte

Box 28.24: Hodgkin's lymphoma.

- Polymorphic population
- Mature lymphocytes, eosinophils, plasma cells, and immunoblasts
- Classical Reed-Sternberg cells: Large binucleated cell with prominent nucleoli
- Many mononuclear large atypical Hodgkin's cells
- Lymphocyte and histiocyte (L&H) cell or popcorn cell in lymphocyte predominance type
- Ill-formed epithelioid cell granulomas
- Scattered elongated cells in nodular sclerosing variety.

Box 28.25: Reed-Sternberg cells (RS cell).

- RS cell is essential for primary diagnosis of Hodgkin lymphoma (HL).

Morphology
- Large cell
- Abundant cytoplasm
- Bilobed nuclei or double nuclei
- Peripheral coarsely clumped chromatin
- Single macronucleoli, basophilic in May-Grünwald Giemsa (MGG).
- Mirror image nuclei

Variants: Suggestive but not diagnostic of HL
- Mononuclear variants of RS cell
- Multilobated anaplastic type
- Mummified
- Popcorn type

Immunocytochemistry
- CD 15+, CD 30+, CD 45−

Differential diagnosis
- Immunoblasts, infectious mononucleosis, malignant melanoma.

(CLL: Chronic lymphocytic leukemia; MCL: Mantle cell lymphoma; SLL: Small lymphocytic lymphoma).

and histiocyte (L & H) cell or popcorn cell is noted in lymphocyte predominance type of HL. In addition, there may be ill-formed epithelioid granulomas in FNAC smear. It may be difficult to get adequate material in nodular sclerosing variety of HL. The smear of nodular sclerotic variety shows scanty cellularity. The smears may have increased amount of fibroblasts and collagenous material and lacunar type of RS cells. The classical RS cells are also infrequent in this variety of HL. The various other cells may simulate RS cells such as immunoblasts, cells of infectious mononucleosis and malignant melanoma. The immunoblasts have irregular nuclear contour, peripheral or marginated basophilic colored nucleoli (Figs. 28.43 to 28.48).

The presence of epithelioid cell granulomas may create diagnostic difficulties with granulomatous inflammation and HL. A careful search for RS cells may be helpful in this aspect. The presence of binucleated large cells simulating RS cell may be a serious diagnostic problem to differentiate ALCL and HL. HL shows a polymorphic population of cells with excess eosinophils. However, it may not be possible to differentiate these two entities based on cytology alone and detailed immunophenotyping is necessary, particularly in cell block.

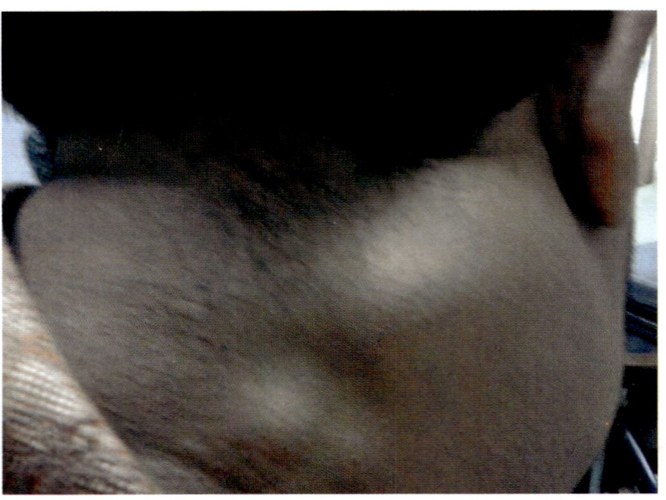

Fig. 28.43: Massive enlargement of neck node in a case of Hodgkin lymphoma.

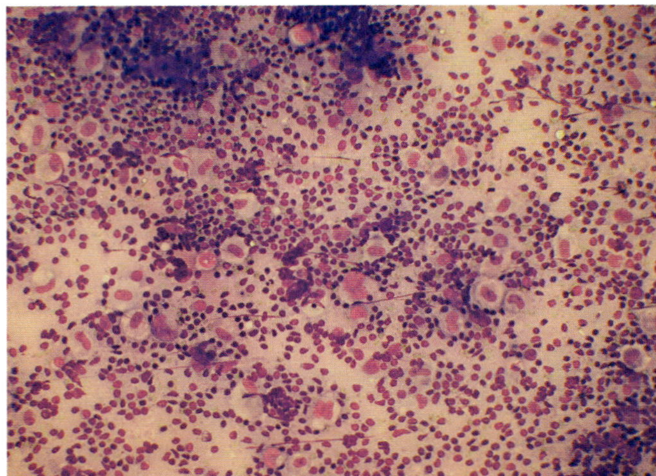

Fig. 28.44: Fine needle aspiration cytology smear of Hodgkin lymphoma showing polymorphic population of reactive lymphoid cells along with Reed-Sternberg cell and mononuclear Hodgkin cells (MGG × MP).

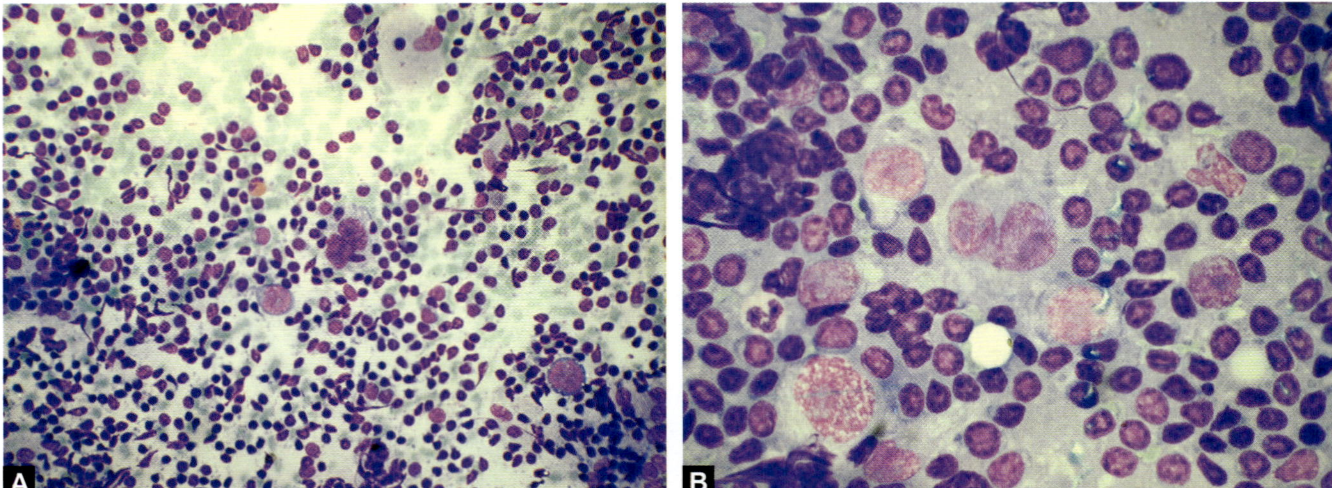

Figs. 28.45A and B: (A) Classical Reed-Sternberg cell along with mixed population of reactive lymphoid cells in Hodgkin lymphoma (MGG × HP). (B) Higher magnification showing classical Reed-Sternberg cell. Note the binucleated cell with moderate amount of cytoplasm and nucleus shows large prominent nucleoli (MGG × OI).

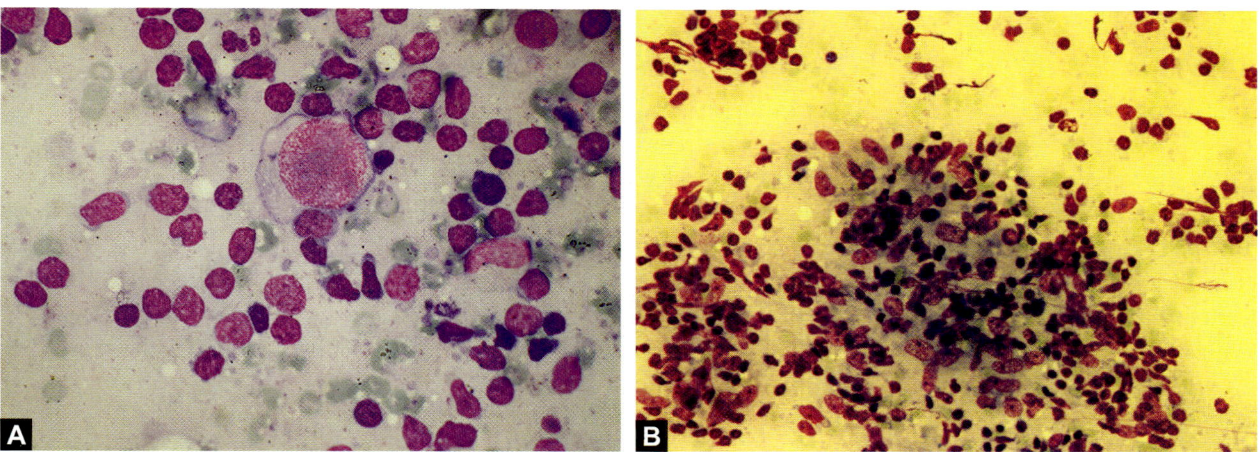

Figs. 28.46A and B: (A) Higher magnification of large mononuclear Hodgkin cell in Hodgkin lymphoma (MGG × OI). (B) Hodgkin lymphoma—ill-formed epithelioid cell granuloma (MGG × HP).

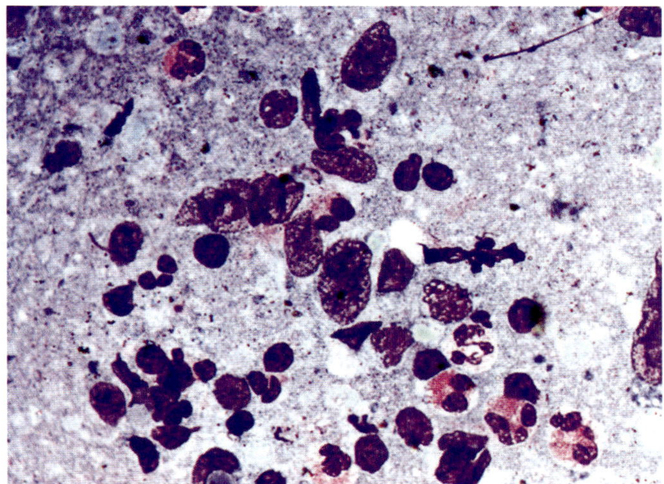

Fig. 28.47: Hodgkin lymphoma—many mononuclear Hodgkin cell in lymphocytic depletion type (MGG × OI).

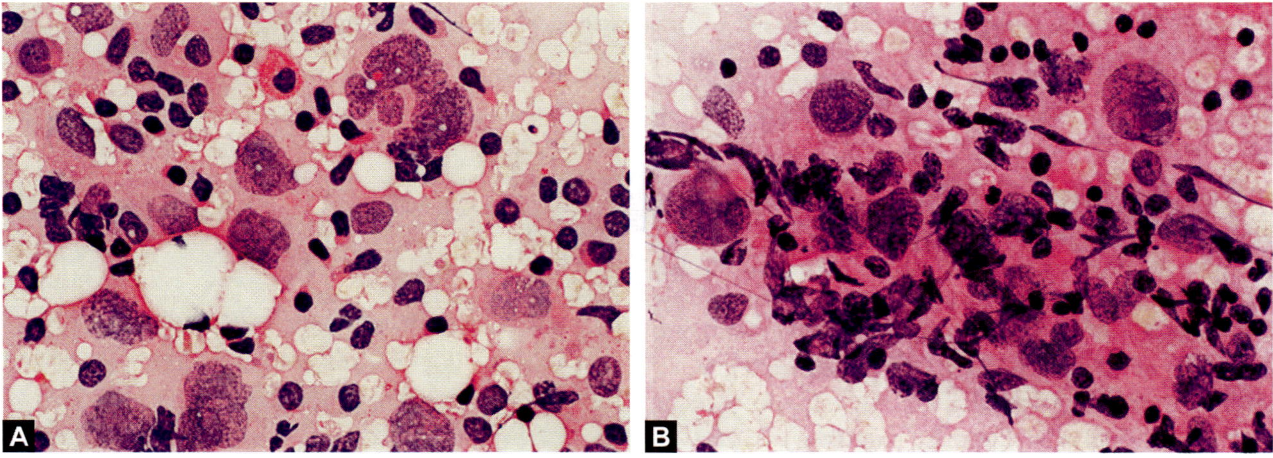

Figs. 28.48A and B: Nodular Sclerosis Classical Hodgkin lymphoma (A) discrete large pleomorphic cells (H & E × HP); (B) syncytial group of cells (H & E × HP).

Nodular Lymphocytic Predominant Hodgkin Lymphoma[47,48]

It is a less common type of HL and most of the patients present with localized lymphadenopathy. Cytology smear of NLPHL shows abundant small lymphoid cells along with occasional L & H cells. These cells are large with scanty amount of cytoplasm and multilobated extremely folded popcorn-like nucleus with thin nuclear membrane. The nuclear chromatin is vesicular with multiple small nucleoli.

Lymphocyte and histiocyte cells are positive for CD 20 and CD 45, in contrast to classical RS cells that are negative for CD 20 and CD 45. L & H cells are also negative for CD 15 and occasionally positive for CD 30 (Table 28.6).

At times, it may be difficult to differentiate RLH from NLPHL because dense population of lymphocytes may hide L & H cells. A careful search of L & H cell may be helpful.

Differential Diagnosis

- Granulomatous inflammation
- Anaplastic large-cell lymphoma
- Reactive lymphoid hyperplasia
- Nasopharyngeal carcinoma
- T-cell rich B-cell lymphoma
- Infectious mononucleosis.

Table 28.6: Distinguishing immunological markers between Reed-Sternberg cell and lymphocytic and/or histiocytic cells.

Immunostain	Lymphocytic and/or histiocytic cells	Reed-Sternberg cell
CD 20	Positive	Negative
CD 45	Positive	Negative
CD 15	Negative	Positive
CD 30	Occasional positive	Positive
Epithelial membrane antigen (EMA)	Often positive	Negative

APPROACH TO DIAGNOSIS OF LYMPH NODE LESIONS

Flowcharts 28.2 and 28.3 show the overall cytological and immunocytochemical approach to diagnosis of lymph node lesions.

The following ancillary investigations are necessary for the exact diagnosis and subtyping of lymphoproliferative disorders:

- Flow cytometric immunophenotyping
- Immunocytochemistry on cell block (supplementary to FCI)
- Proliferative or S-phase cell fraction
- Molecular cytogenetics.

Flow Cytometry

Detailed description and utility of FCI has been already discussed in Chapter 20. Overall this is now almost mandatory for diagnosis and subtyping of lymphomas. However, its main disadvantage is loss of cytomorphology. FCI may not be helpful in ALCL and HL.

After initial assessment of cytomorphology of the cell, a panel of antibodies should be used for FCI (Box 28.26). In case of NHL with large-cell morphology it is advisable to proceed for immunocytochemistry because of fragile nature of the cell and high false positive result.

Immunocytochemistry

Immunocytochemistry can be done on cell block section or cytospin preparation. The morphology of the cell is well

Flowchart 28.2: Diagram showing overall approach in the diagnosis of Fine needle aspiration cytology of lymph node.

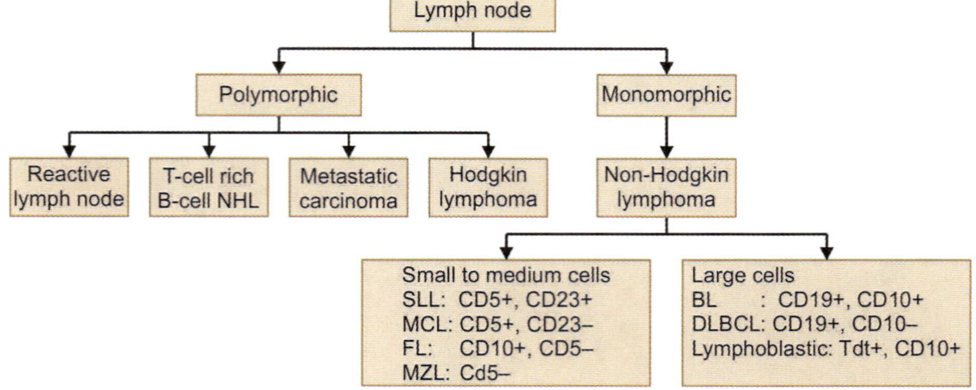

(BL: Burkitt lymphoma; DLBCL: Diffuse large B-cell lymphoma; FL: Follicular lymphoma; MCL: Mantle cell lymphoma; MZL: Marginal zone lymphoma; NHL: Non-Hodgkin lymphoma; SLL: Small lymphocytic lymphoma).

Flowchart 28.3: Diagram showing overall approach of immunocytochemistry application in the diagnosis of metastatic tumor in the lymph node aspirate.

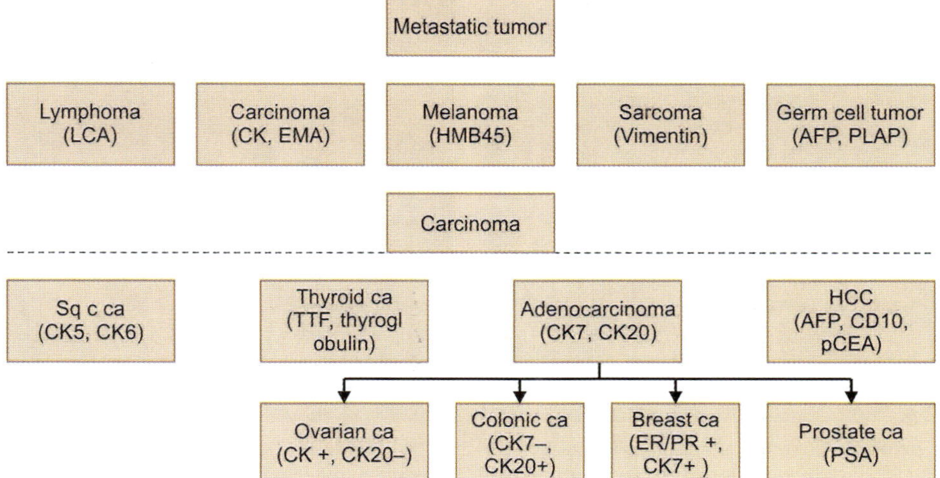

(Sq c ca: Squamous cell carcinoma; ca: Carcinoma; HCC: Hepatocellular carcinoma).

Box 28.26: Basic panel of markers for lymphoma subtyping.

Panel for small cell morphology
- Light chain: Kappa and lambda for B-cell clonality.
- CD 45: Majority of the lymphoid cells
- CD 19: B cell
- CD 20: B cell
- CD 3: T cell
- CD 10:
- CD 5: T cell, CLL, MCL
- CD 23: SLL/CLL

Panel for medium to large cell (additional)
- CD 10
- Tdt
- CD 15
- CD 30.

(CLL: Chronic lymphocytic leukemia; MCL: Mantle cell lymphoma; SLL: Small lymphocytic lymphoma).

Box 28.27: Chromosomal alterations in lymphomas.

Diagnosis
- MCL: t (11;14)
- MALT lymphoma: t(11: 18)
- SLL/CLL: Trisomy 12
- FCC lymphoma: t(14:18)
- DLBCL: t(3:14)
- BL: t(8:14)
- ALCL: t(2:5)

Prognosis
- MALT lymphoma: The t(1;14) and t(11,18) translocations have bad prognosis
- ALCL: t(2;5) translocation and overexpression of ALK have better prognosis
- DLBCL: BCL 10 and CD 10 expressions have better prognosis.

(ALCL: Anaplastic large cell lymphoma; CLL: Chronic lymphocytic leukemia; DLBCL: Diffuse large B-cell lymphoma; MALT: Mucosa-associated lymphoid tissue; MCL: Mantle cell lymphoma; SLL: Small lymphocytic lymphoma).

preserved in case of immunocytochemistry. However, immunocytochemistry technique is time consuming and laborious in comparison to flow cytometry (FCM).

Molecular Diagnostic Tests

Molecular diagnostic tests can be performed from FNAC material.[1] The following molecular tests may be necessary:

- Fluorescent in situ hybridization (FISH)
- Polymerase chain reaction (PCR)
- Microarray to see gene expression profile.

Molecular genetics have assisted in the diagnosis of many lymphomas (Box 28.27). Translocation of t(14;18) and BCL 2 expression are useful in distinguishing RLH from FL. In case of MZL translocation of t(11;14) is diagnostic. Similarly translocation of t(8:14) is the diagnostic hallmark of BL. ALCL, also shows the specific t(2;5) translocation. Molecular genetics also has definite role in assessing prognosis of NHL. It has been noted that t(2;5) translocation and overexpression of ALK in ALCL bears a good prognosis. In case of gastric MALT lymphoma the t(1;14) and t(11,18) translocations and overexpression of BCL 10 has an adverse prognosis.[49]

A subset of DLBCL with BCL 10 and CD 10 expression conveys better prognosis.[50]

LEUKEMIC INFILTRATION[51]

All types of leukemia may involve the lymph nodes. A prior history of leukemia or at least peripheral blood smear should be present at the time of interpretation of the FNAC.

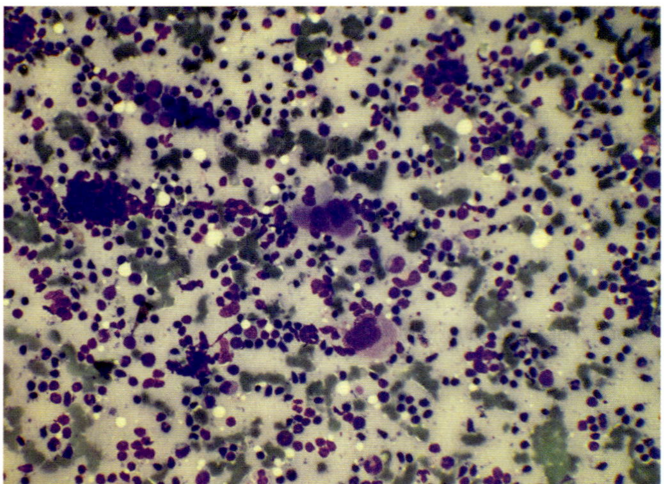

Fig. 28.49: Chronic myeloid leukemia infiltration in the lymph node showing myelocytes, metamyelocytes, and megakaryocytes (MGG × MP).

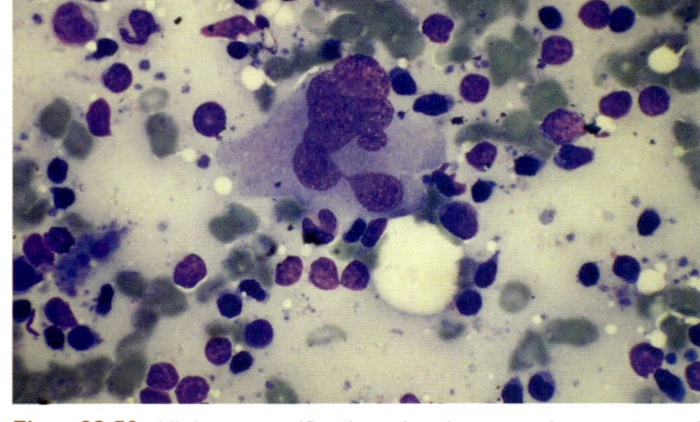

Figs. 28.50: Higher magnification showing megakaryocyte and immature myeloid cells (MGG × HP).

Acute Lymphoblastic Leukemia

The FNAC smear shows discrete blasts which are often admixed with mature lymphocytes. The blasts are round cell with scanty deep blue cytoplasm having fine nuclear chromatin and inconspicuous nucleoli. At present, there is no clinical relevance to separate lymphoblastic lymphoma from a leukemic infiltration in the lymph node.

Acute Myeloid Leukemia

Infiltration by acute myeloid leukemia shows large number of blasts along with variable number of nucleated red blood cells (RBCs), myelocytes, metamyelocytes and promyelocytes. The presence of Auer rods within the cytoplasm confirms the presence of myeloblasts; however, they may not be noted in every case. In case of promyelocytic leukemia, large numbers of promyelocytes are seen in the smear. Cytochemistry or immunophenotyping in the bone marrow aspirate is needed for the primary diagnosis of leukemia.

Chronic Myeloid Leukemia

In chronic myeloid leukemia (CML), the cytology smear shows variable population of cells of myeloid series along with nucleated RBC, basophil, and megakaryocytes. In case of CML with blast crisis, a large number of blasts are seen in the FNAC smear (Figs. 28.49 and 28.50).

There is no clinical relevance to distinguish infiltration by chronic lymphocytic leukemia in the lymph node from small lymphocytic lymphoma.

REFERENCES

1. Dey P. Role of ancillary techniques in diagnosing and subclassifying non-Hodgkin lymphomas on fine needle aspiration cytology. Cytopathology. 2006;17(5):275-87.
2. Schwickert TA, Lindquist RL, Shakhar G, et al. In vivo imaging of germinal centres reveals a dynamic open structure. Nature. 2007;446(7131):83-7.
3. Prasad RR, Narasimkan R, Sankarou U, et al. Fine needle aspiration cytology in the diagnosis of superficial lymphadenopathy: and analysis of 2418 cases. Diagn Cytopathol. 1996;15(5):382-6.
4. Steel B, Schwartz MR, Ramzy I. Fine needle aspiration biopsy in the diagnosis of lymphadenopathy in 1,103 patients. Role, limitations and analysis of diagnostic pitfalls. Acta Cytol. 1995; 39(1):76-81.
5. Dey P, Amir T, Al Jassar A, et al. Combined applications of fine needle aspiration cytology and Flow cytometric immunphenotyping for diagnosis and classification of non Hodgkin Lymphoma. Cytojournal. 2006;3:24.
6. Hehn ST, Grogan TM, Miller TP. Utility of Fine needle aspiration as a diagnostic technique in lymphoma. J Clin Oncol. 2004;22(15):3046-52.
7. Lioe TF Elliott H, Allen DC, et al. The role of fine needle aspiration cytology (FNAC) in the investigation of superficial lymphadenopathy; uses and limitations of the technique. Cytopathology. 1999;10(5):291-7.
8. Kocjan G. The role of FNAC in diagnosis of lymph node enlargements. Cytopathology. 1997;8(Suppl):2-3.
9. Radhika S, Gupta SK, Chakrabarti A, et al. Role of culture for mycobacteria in Fine needle aspiration diagnosis of tuberculous lymphadenitis. Diagn Cytopathol. 1989;5(3):260-2.
10. Sharma SK, Mohan A. Extrapulmonary tuberculosis. Indian J Med Res. 2004;120(4):316-53.
11. Chavollo R, Dolci GF, Hernández JF, et al. Primary tuberculosis of the tonsil. Int J Pediatr Otolaryngol Extra. 2006;1:150-3.
12. Gupta SK, Chugh TD, Sheikh ZA, et al. Cytodiagnosis of tuberculous lymphadenitis. A correlative study with microbiologic examination. Acta Cytol. 1993;37(3):329-32.

13. Aggarwal P, Singal A, Bhattacharya SN, et al. Comparison of the radiometric BACTEC 460 TB culture system and Löwenstein-Jensen medium for the isolation of mycobacteria in cutaneous tuberculosis and their drug susceptibility pattern. Int J Dermatol. 2008;47(7):681-7.
14. Manitchotpisit B, Kunachak S, Kulapraditharom B, et al. Combined use of fine needle aspiration cytology and polymerase chain reaction in the diagnosis of cervical tuberculous lymphadenitis. J Med Assoc Thai. 1999;82(4):363-8.
15. Frable MA, Frable WJ. Fine needle aspiration biopsy in the diagnosis of sarcoid of the head and neck. Acta Cytol. 1984;28(2):175-7.
16. Bhake AS, Desikan KV, Jajoo UN. Cytodiagnosis of histoid leprosy. Lepr Rev. 2001;72(1):78-82.
17. Dey P, Radhika S, Rajwanshi A, et al. Fine needle aspiration cytology of leishmania lymphadenitis. Diagn Cytopathol. 1992;8(5):551-2.
18. Dey P, Radhika S, Jain A. Microfilariae of Wuchereria bancrofti in a lymph node aspirate. A case report. Acta Cytol. 1993;37(5):745-6.
19. Kumar B, Karki S, Paudyal P. Diagnosis of sinus histiocytosis with massive lymphadenopathy (Rosai-Dorfman disease) by fine needle aspiration cytology. Diagn Cytopathol. 2008; 36(10):691-5.
20. Jayaram G, Peh KB. Fine needle aspiration cytology in Kimura's disease. Diagn Cytopathol. 1995;13(4):295-9.
21. Tsang WY, Chan JK. Fine needle aspiration cytologic diagnosis of Kikuchi's lymphadenitis. A report of 27 cases. Am J Clin Pathol. 1994;102(4):454-8.
22. Said JW. AIDS-related lymphadenopathies. Semin Diagn Pathol. 1988;5(4):365-75.
23. Saikia UN, Dey P, Jindal B, et al. Fine needle aspiration cytology in lymphadenopathy of HIV-positive cases. Acta Cytol. 2001;45(4):589-92.
24. Ramadas PT, Kattoor J, Mathews A, et al. Fine needle aspiration cytology of Langerhans cell thyroid histiocytosis and its draining lymph nodes. Acta Cytol. 2008;52(3):396-8.
25. Nanda A, Handa U, Punia RS, et al. Fine needle aspiration in retroperitoneal Castleman's disease: a case report. Acta Cytol. 2009;53(3):316-8.
26. Mohanty SK, Dey P, Ghoshal S, et al. Cytologic features of metastatic nasopharyngeal carcinoma. Diagn Cytopathol. 2002;27(6):340-2.
27. Dey P, Amir T, Jogai S, et al. Fine needle aspiration cytology of metastatic transitional cell carcinoma. Diagn Cytopathol. 2005;32(4):226-8.
28. Khirwadkar N, Dey P, Das A, et al. Fine needle aspiration biopsy of metastatic soft tissue sarcomas to lymph nodes. Diagn Cytopathol. 2001;24(4):229-32.
29. Weingrad DW, Rosenberg SA. Early lymphatic spread of osteogenic and soft-tissue sarcomas. Surgery. 1978;84(2):231-40.
30. Dey P, Togra J, Mitra S. Intermediate filament: structure, function, and applications in cytology. Diagn Cytopathol. 2014;42(7):628-35.
31. Chan JK, Banks PM, Cleary ML, et al. A proposal for classification of lymphoid neoplasms (by the International Lymphoma Study Group). Histopathology. 1994;25(6):517-36.
32. Harris NL, Jaffe ES, Diebold J, et al. The World Health Organization classification of neoplasms of the hematopoietic and lymphoid tissues: report of the clinical advisory committee meeting—Airlie House, Virginia, November, 1997. Hematol J. 2000;1(1):53-66.
33. Swerdlow SH, Campo E, Pileri SA, et al. The 2016 revision of the World Health Organization classification of lymphoid neoplasms. Blood. 2016;127(20):2375-90.
34. Das DK, Gupta SK, Datta BN, et al. FNA cytodiagnosis of non-Hodgkin's lymphoma and its subtyping under working formulation of 175 cases. Diagn Cytopathol. 1991;7(5):487-98.
35. Das DK. Value and limitations of Fine needle aspiration cytology in diagnosis and classification of lymphomas: a review. Diagn Cytopathol. 1999;21(4):240-9.
36. Zeppa P, Vigliar E, Cozzolino I, et al. Fine needle aspiration cytology and flow cytometry immunophenotyping of non-Hodgkin lymphoma: can we do better? Cytopathology. 2010; 21(5):300-10.
37. Kocjan G. Best Practice No 185. Cytological and molecular diagnosis of lymphoma. J Clin Pathol. 2005;58(6):561-7.
38. Shin HJ, Caraway NP, Katz RL. Cytomorphologic spectrum of small lymphocytic lymphoma in patients with an accelerated clinical course. Cancer. 2003;99(5):293-300.
39. Rassidakis GZ, Tani E, Svedmyr E, et al. Diagnosis and subclassification of follicle center and mantle cell lymphomas on Fine needle aspirates. A cytology and immunocytochemical approach based on the revised European-American lymphoma (REAL) classification. Cancer. 1999; 87(4):216-23.
40. Jaffe ES, Harris NL, Stein M, et al. (Eds). World Health Organization Classification of Tumours. Pathology and Genetics of Tumours and Haematopoietic and Lymphoid Tissues. Lyon, France: IARC Press; 2001.
41. Gascoyne RD. Establishing the diagnosis of lymphoma: From initial biopsy to clinical staging. Oncology. 1998;12(10 Suppl 8): 11-6.
42. Das DK, Gupta SK, Pathak IC, et al. Burkitt-type lymphoma. Diagnosis by fine needle aspiration cytology. Acta Cytol. 1987;31(1):1-7.
43. Ng WK, Ip P, Choy C, et al. Cytologic and immunocytochemical findings of anaplastic large cell lymphoma: analysis of ten Fine needle aspiration specimens over a 9-year period. Cancer. 2003;99(1):33-43.
44. Bonadonna G. Historical review of Hodgkin's disease. Br J Haematol. 2000;110(3):504-11.
45. Kass AM, Kass EH. Perfecting the world: the life and times of Dr Thomas Hodgkin 1798–1866. Boston, Harcourt Brace Jovanovich. 1988;1:642.
46. Jogai S, Al-Jassar A, Dey P, et al. Fine needle aspiration cytology of Hodgkin's lymphoma: A cytohistologic correlation study from a cancer center in Kuwait. Acta Cytol. 2006;50(6):656-62.
47. Jogai S, Dey P, Al-Jassar A, et al. The role of fine needle aspiration cytology in nodular sclerosis variant of Hodgkin's lymphoma. Acta Cytol. 2006;50(5):507-12.
48. Sharma S, Dey P, Mitra S, et al. Nodular sclerosis classical Hodgkin lymphoma grade 2: A diagnostic challenge to the cytopathologists. Cancer. 2017;125(2):104-13.
49. Isaacson PG, Du MQ. MALT lymphoma: from morphology to molecules. Nat Rev Cancer. 2004;4(8):644-53.
50. Iqbal J, Sanger WG, Horsman DE, et al. BCL2 translocation defines a unique tumor subset within the germinal center B-cell-like diffuse large B-cell lymphoma. Am J Pathol. 2004;165(1):159-66.
51. Dey P, Varma S, Varma N. Fine needle aspiration cytology of extramedullary leukaemia. Acta Cytol. 1996;40(2):252-6.

Review Questions

1. **A 28-year female presented with a swelling in the upper cervical lymph node for 4 months. Fine needle aspiration cytology of the swelling yielded 1 mL clear fluid.**
   a. **What is your diagnosis from the microphotograph of the smears (Figs. 28.51A to D)?**
      a. Metastatic adenocarcinoma
      b. Metastatic papillary carcinoma of thyroid
      c. Branchial cyst
      d. Metastatic squamous cell carcinoma
   b. **What do you suggest for further investigation in this patient?**
2. **A 19-year-old boy presented with 5 cm diameter firm swelling in the left mid-cervical region. He had history of malaise and fever. Fine needle aspiration cytology of the swelling yielded particulate material.**
   a. **What is your diagnosis from the microphotograph of the smear (Figs. 28.52A to D)?**
      a. Reactive lymphoid hyperplasia
      b. Metastatic carcinoma
      c. Hodgkin's lymphoma
      d. Non-Hodgkin lymphoma
   b. **What special stains are helpful in this case?**
3. **A 12-year-boy presented with bilateral multiple 2–4 cm diameter lymph nodes for 3 months. He also had loss of weight. Fine needle aspiration cytology was done from the lymph node.**
   a. **What is your provisional diagnosis from the microphotographs (Figs. 28.53A and B)?**
      a. Burkitt's lymphoma
      b. Hodgkin's lymphoma
      c. Reactive lymphoid hyperplasia
      d. Acute leukemic infiltration
   b. **What will be the possible immunophenotype and genetic markers of this case?**
4. **A 15-year-girl presented with 5 cm diameter enlarged bilateral cervical lymph nodes for 6 months. Figures 28.54A and B show the representative microphotographs of the Fine needle aspiration cytology of the lymph node. What is your diagnosis?**
   a. Reactive lymphoid hyperplasia
   b. Cryptococci
   c. Rosai-Dorfman disease
   d. Lepromatous lymphadenitis

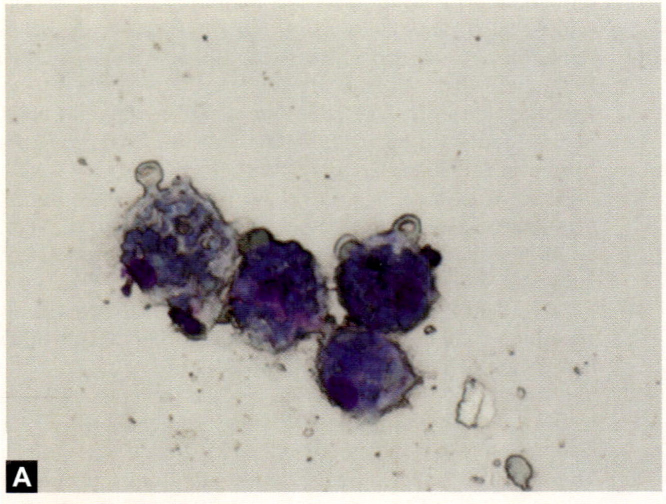

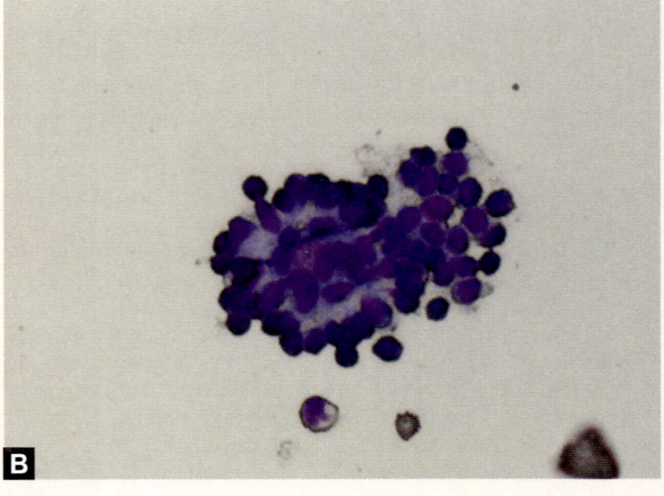

Figs. 28.51A and B

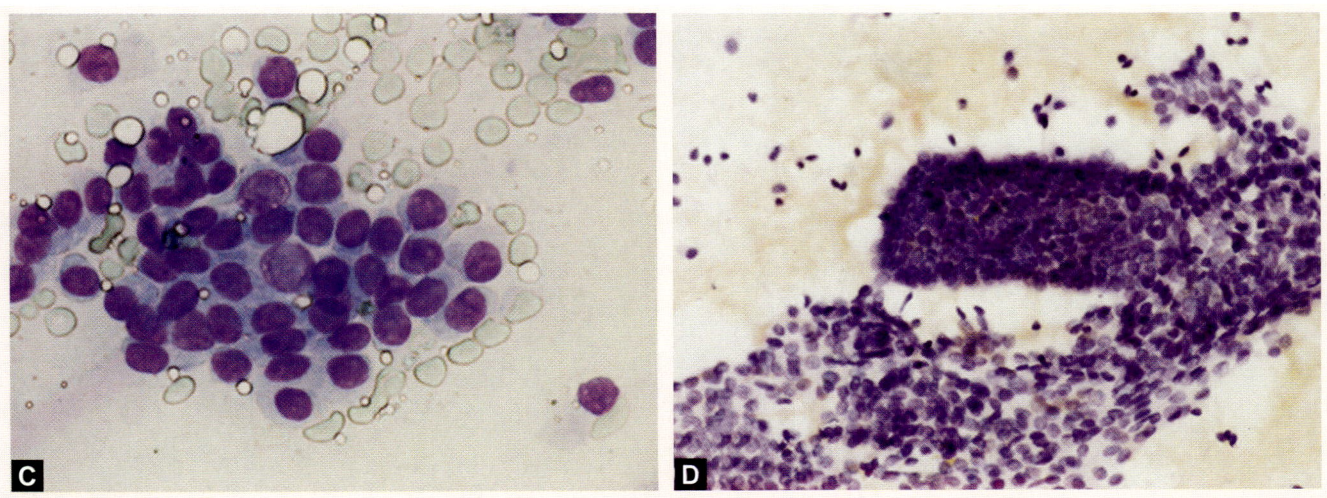

Figs. 28.51A to D: Fine needle aspiration cytology smear of question 1.

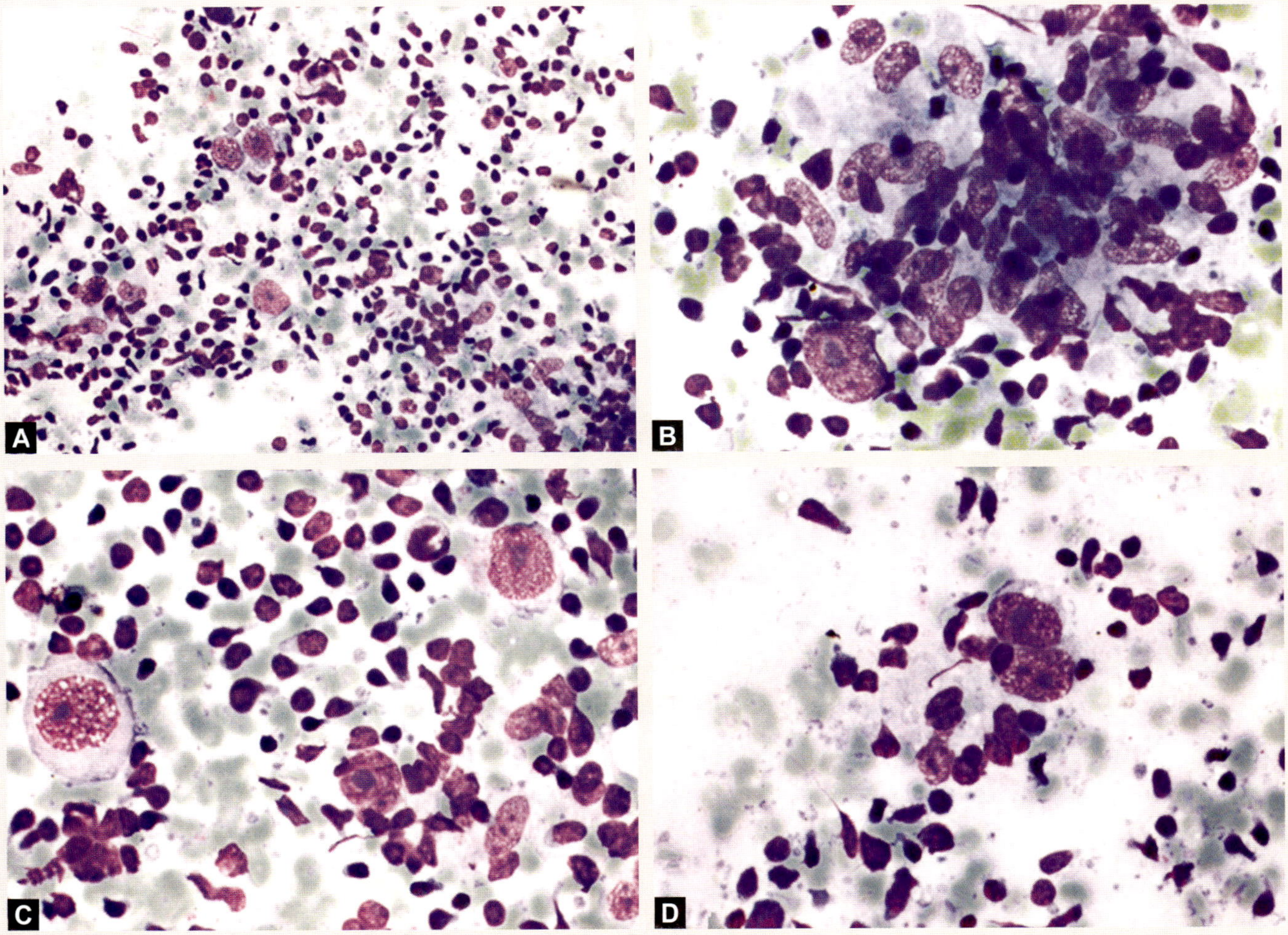

Figs. 28.52A to D: Fine needle aspiration cytology smear of case of question 2.

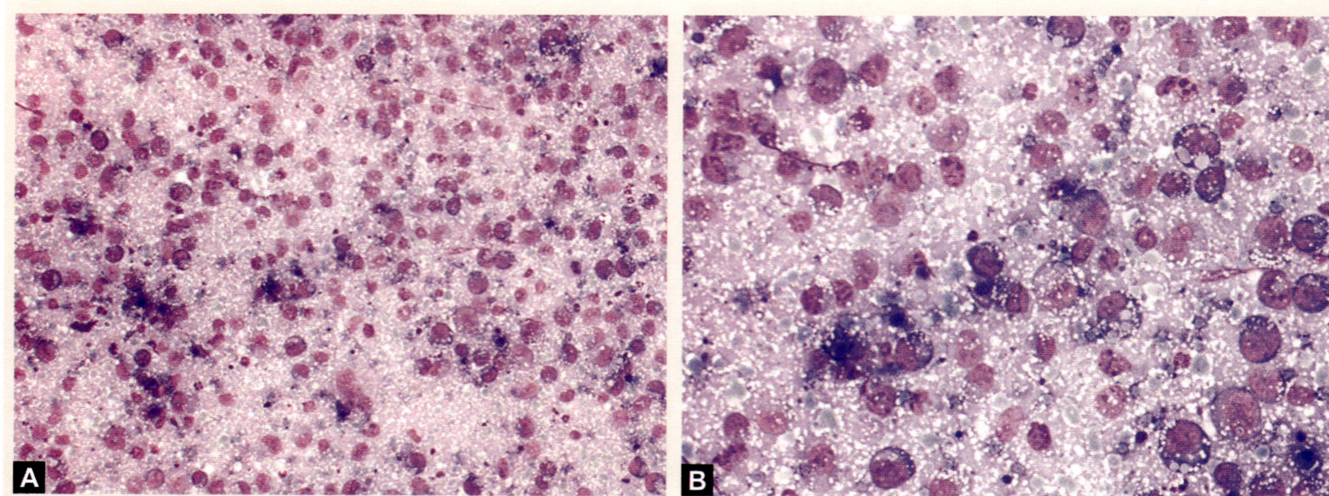

Figs. 28.53A and B: Fine needle aspiration cytology smear of case of question 3.

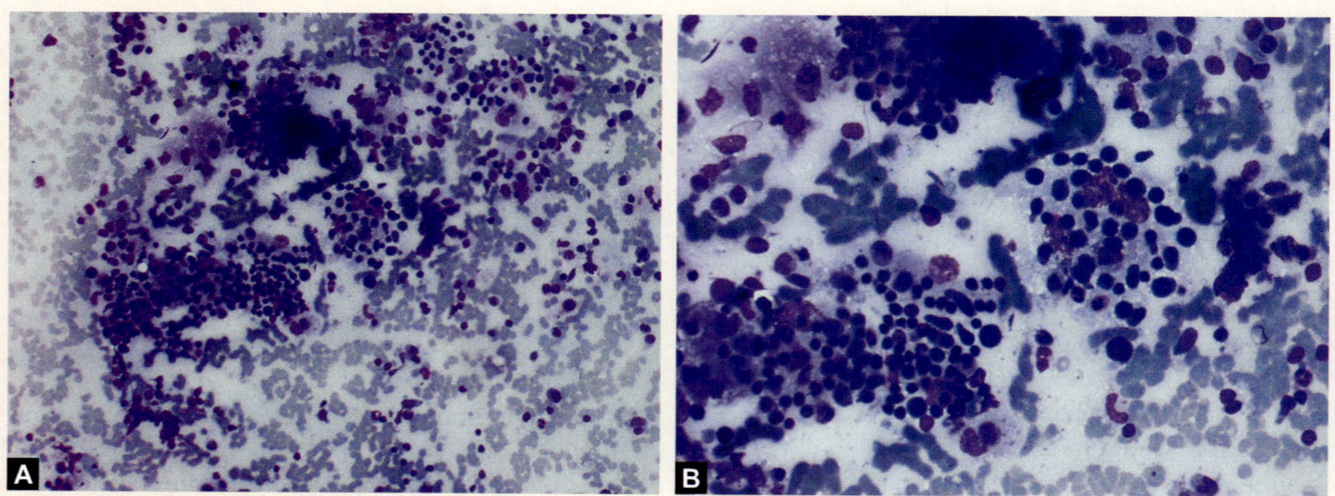

Figs. 28.54A and B: Fine needle aspiration cytology smear of case of question 4.

Answers

1. a. Answer is (b) Metastatic papillary carcinoma of thyroid
   b. The following investigations are necessary in this case:
   - USG of thyroid
   - Thyroid scan
   - FNAC of thyroid swelling if any

   Note: The presence of fragmented papillary structures and intranuclear pseudoinclusions in this case suggest the diagnosis of a metastatic papillary carcinoma of thyroid. The complete examination of the thyroid gland is necessary to find out the primary tumor.
2. a. Answer is (c) Hodgkin's lymphoma
   b. Immunocytochemistry:

- CD 15: Positive
- CD 30: Positive
- CD 45: The large atypical cells are negative.

Note: The microphotograph shows a polymorphic population of cells, epithelioid granulomas along with large mononuclear cells and classical Reed-Sternberg cells. All these features suggest the diagnosis of a Hodgkin's lymphoma.

3. a. Answer is (a) Burkitt's lymphoma

   b. Immunological markers of Burkitt's lymphoma

   - CD 19 and CD 20: Positive
   - CD 10: Positive
   - CD 5: Negative
   - CD 23: Negative
   - Genetics: t(8: 14). Rearrangement of c-myc gene

   Note: The smears show discrete large lymphoid cells with deep blue vacuolated cytoplasm. The nuclei show fine chromatin and occasional prominent nucleoli.

4. c. Rosai-Dorfman disease

   Note: The reactive lymphoid cells along with prominent emperipolesis in this case favor the diagnosis of Rosai-Dorfman disease.

CHAPTER

29 Mediastinum

ANATOMY OF THE MEDIASTINUM AND GENERAL CONSIDERATIONS

The mediastinum is the anatomical space bounded laterally by the pleura of right and left lungs, anteriorly by the sternum and posteriorly by the thoracic vertebra, superiorly by thoracic inlet and inferiorly by the diaphragm. The mediastinum is arbitrarily divided into four parts: (1) anterior, (2) posterior, (3) superior, and (4) middle mediastinum. The mediastinum contains heart, great vessels, and nerves. The topography of mediastinal lesions is important because certain tumors have predilection in particular part of the mediastinum. Thymoma, thymic carcinoids and thymic lymphomas are more frequently seen in superior mediastinum. Certain tumors such as thymoma, lymphoma and germ cell tumors are common in the anterior mediastinum. Lymphomas and metastatic tumors are more frequent in the middle mediastinum. Tumors of neurogenic origin are more frequent in the posterior mediastinum (Fig. 29.1).

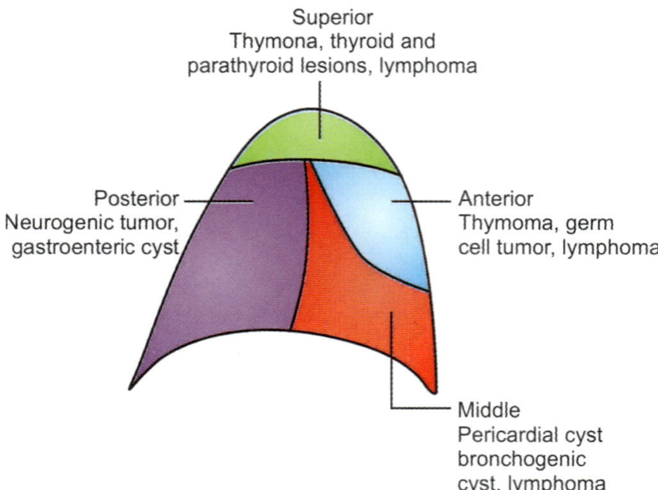

Fig. 29.1: Schematic diagram showing relative preponderance of different tumors in different parts of mediastinum.

The mediastinum contains several different types of tumors with variable cytomorphology and often creates diagnostic dilemmas.[1-8] The cytological diagnosis of the mediastinal lesions should always be correlated with a combination of clinical, radiological and biochemical findings.

CLINICAL HISTORY

Majority of the mediastinal lesions are asymptomatic and detected in routine screening or during screening for some other purposes. The common complaints of the patients are cough, chest pain, dyspnea, hemoptysis, and superior vena cava syndrome due to the pressure effect on the great vessels. Younger patients are commonly affected by the germ cell tumors and thymoma. Thymoma is often associated with clinical history of the myasthenia gravis. Patients may often give the history of primary malignancy in the lung, breast, kidney, ovary, and testis. The patients with generalized lymphadenopathy and/or hepatosplenomegaly on physical examination may indicate lymphoma or leukemic involvement in the mediastinal lymph nodes.

TECHNIQUES

The mediastinal fine needle aspiration cytology (FNAC) should be done as a team approach of cytologists, radiologists, surgeons and general physicians. The radiologists should localize the lesion and put the needle accordingly. FNAC is done with the help of computed tomography (CT), ultrasonography (USG) or fluoroscopic guidance. CT-guided FNAC provides excellent resolution and it is helpful to aspirate from the small lesions. It also helps to avoid the puncture of great vessels. In comparison, USG-guided FNAC provides real-time monitoring and it is free of radiation exposure. Transbronchial FNAC of the mediastinal swelling can also be done in case of

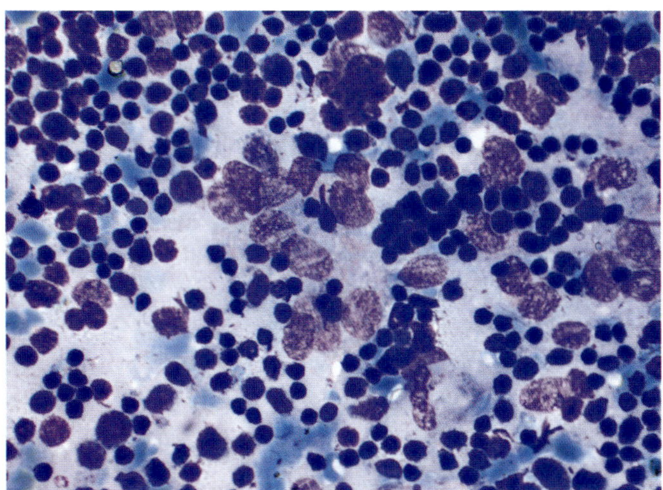

Fig. 29.2: Abundant reactive lymphoid cells along with scattered epithelial cells in thymoma (MGG × HP).

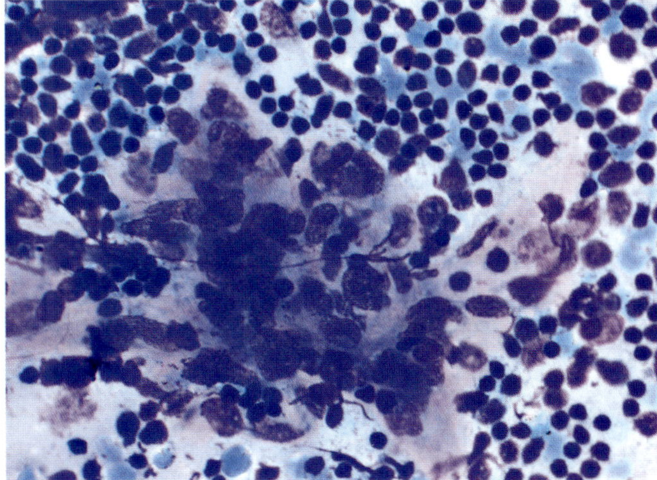

Fig. 29.3: Cluster of oval to elongated epithelial cells with moderate amount of cytoplasm in thymoma (MGG × HP).

central lesions around the bronchus. This technique also gives real-time imaging and assessment of the lesion during the time of the procedure. It has an added advantage to get material from the small lesions of the mediastinum.

There are no absolute contraindications of mediastinal FNAC. However, it should better be avoided in case of bleeding disorders. FNAC of the mediastinum is usually free of any serious complication. However, hemoptysis, localized bleeding and minor pneumothorax are common complications of FNAC. The pneumothorax can be managed conservatively.

LESIONS

Thymoma[9-11]

Thymoma is the neoplasm that develops from common thymic epithelial stem cell of endodermal origin. This is one of the unique tumors in the mediastinum. It commonly occurs in adults. The thymoma is most common in the anterior and superior mediastinum. The patients of thymoma usually complain of local pressure symptoms of the mass, such as pain, tachycardia, superior vena cava syndrome and respiratory distress. Thymoma is often associated with myasthenia gravis. In addition, thymomas are also associated with large number of autoimmune disorders, such as autoimmune hemolytic anemia, autoimmune hepatitis, myositis, myocarditis, dermatomyositis, systemic lupus erythematosus, rheumatoid arthritis, scleroderma, Addison's disease, Graves' disease, etc.

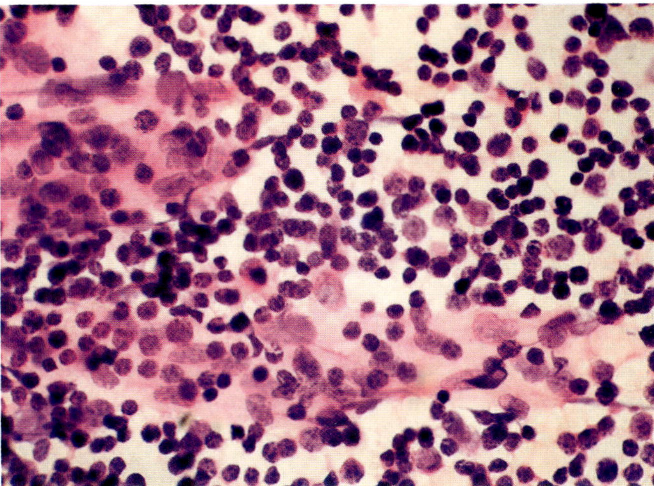

Fig. 29.4: Better morphology of epithelial cells in hematoxylin and eosin-stained smear (H & E × HP).

Cytology (Figs. 29.2 to 29.4)

According to recent World Health Organization (WHO) classification, thymoma is classified as[12] (Box 29.1):

A: Predominant spindle-shaped neoplastic epithelial cells and

B: Predominant round or polygonal epithelial cells.

The B cell component is further subdivided into B1, B2 and B3, depending on the degree of atypia and lymphocytic infiltrate. Now depending on the admixture of the A and B components, the thymoma is classified as A, B or AB. It is generally seen that thymomas with a predominantly spindly epithelial component behaved as benign tumor,

Box 29.1: Thymoma classification.

- *Type A*: Predominant spindle cells
- *Type B*: Predominant round or polygonal cells
- *Type AB*: Mixed foci of types A and B
- *B1*: Richest in lymphocytes
- *B2*: In between B1 and B3
- *B3*: Richest in epithelial cells
- Type B3 (epithelial, atypical, squamoid, well-differentiated thymic carcinoma).

Box 29.3: Thymoma.

- Clusters of oval to polyhedral epithelial cells
  - Moderate cytoplasm with indistinct cell margins
  - Nuclei are vesicular with pale homogenous chromatin
  - Absent nucleoli
- Elongated spindle cells in small fascicles
- Background lymphoid cells
- *Immunocytochemistry*: Epithelial cells of thymomas are positive for cytokeratin, epithelial membrane antigen (EMA), and carcinoembryonic antigen (CEA).

whereas thymomas that contain polygonal epithelial cells behave in an aggressive manner.

The term malignant thymoma is used in the cases of advanced thymomas that are locally invasive or show metastasis. Thymic epithelial tumors with marked nuclear atypia are also designated as malignant thymoma, irrespective of stage (Box 29.2).

Thymic carcinoma shows marked nuclear atypia and features of malignancy.

Fine needle aspiration cytology of thymoma depends on the type of thymoma.[10] Cytology smear shows dual population of multiple clusters of epithelial cells in the background of lymphoid cells. It is easy to diagnose the cases that contain mixed population of lymphocytes and epithelial cells.

The epithelial cells in thymoma are arranged singly or as large clusters. The clusters are large and irregular in shape and size (Box 29.3). Occasional clusters may show cyst-like spaces within them. The clusters of these cells surrounded by arborizing capillary networks are also noted.

The individual epithelial cells are three to four times larger than lymphocytes. The epithelial cells are widely variable in size and shape. They are oval to spindle-shaped depending on the type of thymoma. The cells have moderate cytoplasm with indistinct cell margins. The nuclei are vesicular with pale homogenous chromatin and single prominent nucleoli. The background of the smear shows single naked cells with stripped of cytoplasm.

Box 29.2: Malignant thymoma: Many features.

- Locally invasive
- Pleural or pericardial implants
- Distant metastasis
- Marked nuclear atypia.

Abundant monomorphic populations of small, mature lymphocytes along with lymphoglandular bodies and tingible body macrophages are also noted. The nuclear chromatin of lymphocytes is condensed with inconspicuous nucleoli. Occasional large transformed lymphocytes are also seen. Lymphocytes in thymoma are T-cell in origin. Hassall's corpuscle is uncommonly seen in thymomas, however, its presence is characteristic of this lesion.

Spindle cell variant of thymoma shows oval to elongated spindle cells in small clusters. The cells are arranged in small fascicles that are better appreciated in cell block preparation. Variable amount of mature lymphocytes are seen in the background.

Lymphocyte-rich thymoma in FNAC shows predominantly lymphocytes and scanty epithelial cells. The presence of large number of lymphoid cells in the thymoma often gives rise the diagnostic possibility of non-Hodgkin's lymphoma (NHL). The cells in NHL are immature lymphoid cells. Cystic thymoma yields drops of clear or yellowish fluid with sparse cellularity.

Immunocytochemistry

Epithelial cells of thymomas are positive for cytokeratin (CK), epithelial membrane antigen (EMA), and carcinoembryonic antigen (CEA). Thymic tumor cells are strongly positive for AE1-defined acidic CKs and negative for AE3-defined basic CKs. The epithelial cells also show focal positivity for CD20, and the B-cell marker.

Differential Diagnosis

- Non-Hodgkin's lymphoma
- Hodgkin's lymphoma
- *Metastatic carcinoma*: The cells in metastatic carcinoma show significant nuclear enlargement and pleomorphism. The clinical history of primary malignancy is also an important clue.
- *Neurogenic tumors*: Spindle cell variant of thymoma may simulate the peripheral nerve sheath tumors. Neural sheath tumors are seen in posterior mediastinum. In addition, the cells of nerve sheath tumor have long slender nuclei with pointed ends along with characteristic nuclear kinking.

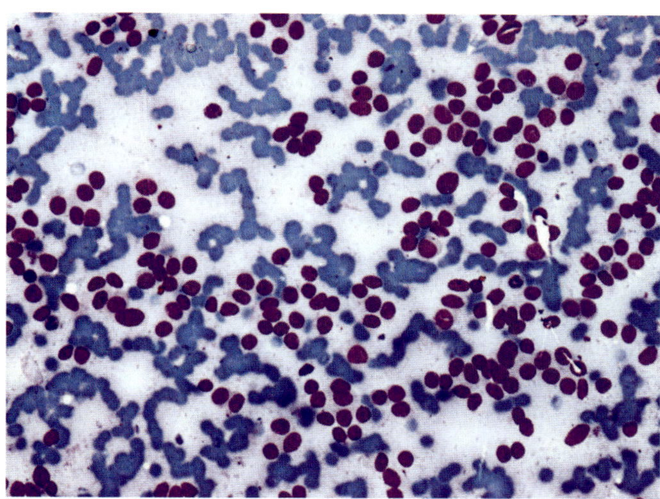

Fig. 29.5: Monomorphic round to oval discrete cells in thymic carcinoid (MGG × MP).

Malignant Thymoma[13-15]

Malignant thymoma may be invasive thymoma or thymic carcinomas.

Invasive thymoma: This tumor is aggressive and shows cytological evidences of malignancy, invasion or metastasis.

Cytology: On FNAC smear it is almost impossible to detect an invasive thymoma.

Cytology smears show epithelial cells with bland nuclei and background lymphoid cells. Occasionally the cells may show large nuclei and prominent nucleoli.

Thymic carcinoma: It is a relatively rare malignancy of thymus and predominantly involves the adults. The unique features of thymic carcinomas are:

- No association with myasthenia gravis
- Rarely associated with autoimmune diseases
- Positive for CD5, CD70 and CD117
- Almost always invasive, and
- Mostly unresectable tumor.

The epithelial element of thymus undergoes malignant changes. The various morphologic types of thymic carcinomas are squamous cell carcinoma, anaplastic carcinoma, small-cell carcinoma, lymphoepithelial carcinoma, etc.

Cytology: Fine needle aspiration cytology smears of thymic carcinoma usually show abundant epithelial cells with moderate nuclear enlargement and pleomorphism. Nuclei show marked hyperchromasia with prominent nucleoli. Frequent mitotic activities and necrosis may also be seen. Immunocytochemistry shows positivity for CD5, CD70 and CD117.

Box 29.4: Thymic carcinoid.

- Dissociated cells
- Round cells with moderate amount of reddish granular cytoplasm
- Round nuclei, minimal pleomorphism
- Salt and pepper chromatin and inconspicuous nucleoli
- Spindle cells.

Differential diagnosis:

Metastatic carcinoma: It is impossible to differentiate primary thymic carcinoma from metastatic carcinoma on the basis of cytomorphology. Clinical history of primary carcinoma is helpful in this aspect.

Thymic Carcinoid

Thymic carcinoid develops from the primitive cells with neuroendocrine differentiation. These are rare tumors and represent only 2–5% of all thymic tumors.[12] Thymic carcinoids are classified as:

- Well-differentiated neuroendocrine carcinoma:
  - Typical carcinoids
  - Atypical carcinoids
- Poorly differentiated neuroendocrine carcinoma.

The patient often presents with various endocrine manifestations.

Cytology (Fig. 29.5)

Cytologic appearance of thymic carcinoid is similar as seen in other sites. The smear shows round to oval discrete cells with occasional rosettes-like arrangement (Box 29.4). The individual cells show moderate amount of reddish granular cytoplasm. Nuclei are round and regular with typical salt and pepper chromatin with inconspicuous to absent nucleoli. Variable amount of spindle cells are also noted. Occasional pseudonuclear cytoplasmic inclusions may also be seen.

Atypical Carcinoid

Cytomorphology of the atypical carcinoid shows abundant dissociated round cells with moderate nuclear enlargement and pleomorphism. Occasional cells may show nuclear molding. In addition, the smears show high mitotic activity and necrosis.

Neuroendocrine carcinoma (NEC) of thymus is positive for the neuroendocrine markers such as chromogranin, and synaptophysin. The cells are also positive for CK.

Differential diagnosis:

- *Small-cell carcinoma*: Rosette-like arrangement, cells with moderate amount of cytoplasm and salt and pepper-like appearance of nuclear chromatin indicate the diagnosis of carcinoid.
- *Non-Hodgkin's lymphoma*: Immature lymphoid cells of NHL may simulate carcinoid. Individual cell morphology and immunocytochemistry are helpful in diagnosis.

GERM CELL TUMORS[16,17]

Mediastinum is the most frequent site of the origin of the extragonadal germ cell tumors. The germ cell tumor is commonly seen in the anterior mediastinum. It is worthwhile to mention that metastatic germ cell tumor is more common than the primary germ cell tumor. Therefore, one should be careful to search the presence of the primary tumor in the gonads first in case of mediastinal germ cell tumors.

Mature Cystic Teratoma

Mature cystic teratoma is the most common germ cell tumor in the mediastinum. It represents 7–9% of all mediastinal germ cell tumors. It predominantly occurs in young adults and the mean age of the adult is 28 years. Teratoma may be solid or cystic. The patients are usually asymptomatic. The chief complaints of the patients are chest pain, fever or cough.

Cytology

Fine needle aspiration cytology smear of mature cystic teratoma usually yields pultaceous cheesy material. The smear shows anucleated squames and mature squamous cells (Box 29.5). There may be the other elements of skin, neural structure, respiratory lining cells, glandular elements, etc. The smears also show multinucleated giant cells and epithelioid cell granulomas.

Differential Diagnosis

Squamous cell carcinoma: The presence of mature squamous cells and anucleated squames may often mislead to the false diagnosis of metastatic squamous cell carcinoma.

Box 29.5: Mature cystic teratoma.

- Mature squamous cells
- Anucleated squames
- Keratin flakes, skin adnexal cells
- Glandular cells
- Neural elements.

Immature Teratoma

It is a rare tumor in the mediastinum. The presence of immature neuroectodermal elements such as rosettes and tubules indicate the presence of immature teratoma.

Seminomas

Seminomas are rare germ cell tumors in the mediastinum. They represent only 8% of all extranodal germ cell tumors. Seminoma of the mediastinum is commonly seen in young male and most of the cases occur in the 3rd and 4th decades of life. Seminoma commonly occurs in the anterior mediastinum.

Cytology (Figs. 29.6 and 29.7)

Fine needle aspiration cytology smear of the seminoma shows abundant dispersed round cells. Background of the smear shows typical tigroid or stripped appearance (Box 29.6). Necrosis and cells with naked nuclei are also noted. The individual tumor cells have abundant vacuolated cytoplasm containing glycogen. The nuclei are large round and moderately pleomorphic. The nuclear chromatin is fine with single to multiple prominent nucleoli. These cells are admixed with many lymphocytes and plasma cell. This characteristic appearance of germinoma is due to rupture of the cytoplasmic content into the background. Mitosis and apoptosis are common. Occasional scattered large "syncytiotrophoblast-like" cells are seen. The smears also show ill-formed epithelioid granulomas.

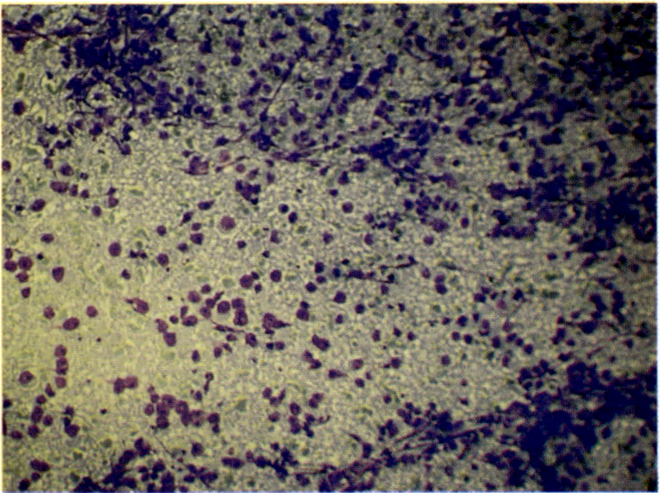

Fig. 29.6: Fine needle aspiration cytology (FNAC) smear of a germinoma in mediastinum showing scattered round cells in a tigroid background (MGG × MP).

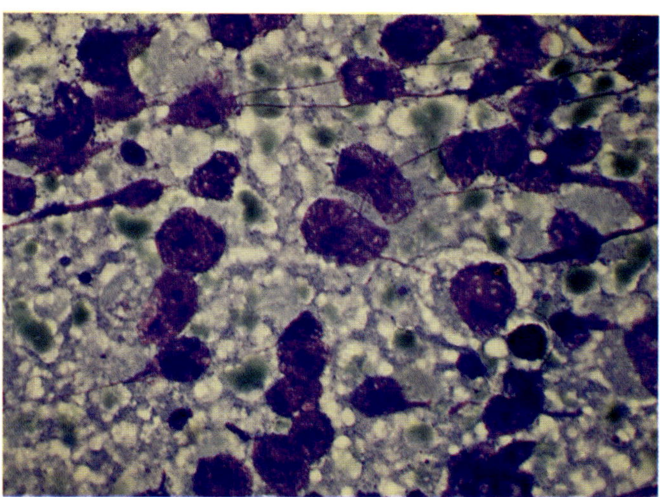

Fig. 29.7: Higher magnification showing individual cell morphology. The cells are round, moderately pleomorphic with fine chromatin and prominent nucleoli (MGG × HP).

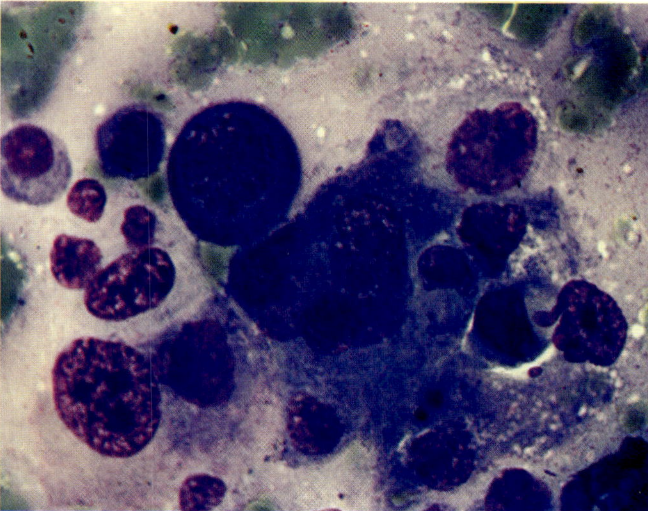

Fig. 29.8: Mediastinal embryonal carcinoma showing markedly pleomorphic cells with multiple prominent nucleoli (MGG × OI).

Box 29.6: Seminomas.

- Discrete cells
- Tigroid background
- Round cells
- Abundant vacuolated cytoplasm
- Moderately pleomorphic nuclei
- Fine chromatin
- Single to multiple nucleoli
- High mitotic activity
- Lymphocytes
- Ill-formed epithelioid cell granulomas.

Immunohistochemistry

Majority of the mediastinal seminomas are positive for placental leukocyte alkaline phosphatase (PLAP). Large numbers of cases are also positive for vimentin and CD117. Focal weak positivity for pancytokeratin is also seen.

Differential diagnosis

- Non-Hodgkin's lymphoma
- Poorly differentiated carcinoma
- Other germ cell tumor such as embryonal carcinoma (EC).

Embryonal Carcinoma

Embryonal carcinoma represents about 12% of all germ cell tumors of the mediastinum. It commonly occurs in the young males and the mean age of the tumor is 27 years. Cytology smear of EC is similar to that of the gonad.

Box 29.7: Embryonal carcinoma.

- Cohesive clusters of cells
- Large cells with granular to vacuolated cytoplasm
- Moderate to marked pleomorphic nuclei
- Single to multiple nucleoli
- Macronucleoli.

Cytology (Fig. 29.8)

Fine needle aspiration cytology smears show multiple small cohesive clusters and discrete malignant cells (Box 29.7). The individual cells have scanty to moderate amount of vacuolated cytoplasm with ill-defined cell border. The nuclei of the cells are enlarged and moderately pleomorphic. The nuclei show vesicular chromatin with single to multiple large nucleoli.

Immunocytochemistry

The majority of ECs are positive for CD30. The cells are also positive for CK.

Diagnostic difficulty

- Seminoma
- Poorly differentiated carcinoma.

Endodermal Sinus Tumor

This is a rare tumor in the mediastinum and occurs predominantly in infant and young child. Cytology smear shows small clusters, papillae and discrete malignant cells. The cells are round with vacuolated cytoplasm

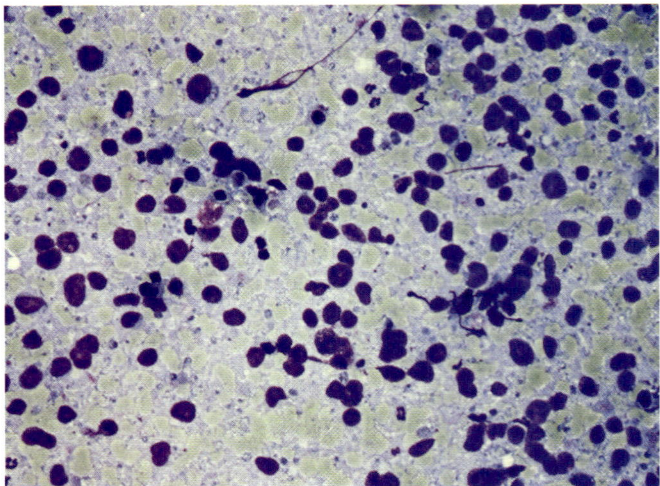

Fig. 29.9: Discrete large round cells in diffuse large B-cell lymphoma (DLBCL) (MGG × MP).

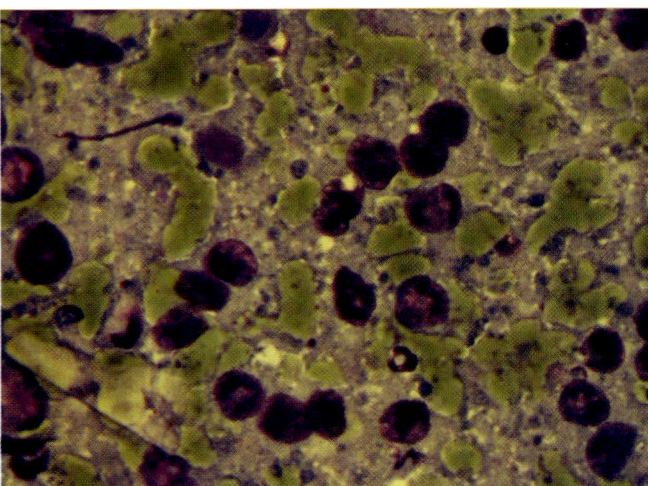

Fig. 29.10: Higher magnification showing enlarged cells, fine chromatin and large prominent nucleoli (MGG × OI).

and mild-to-moderate pleomorphic nuclei. Nucleoli are relatively small in size. Occasional intracytoplasmic and extracytoplasmic small round pink globules are also seen. Schiller-Duval bodies are rarely present in endodermal sinus tumor (EST).

Immunocytochemistry

The cells show low-molecular weight CK. The cells are also positive for alpha-fetoprotein.

LYMPHOMAS[18-20]

Non-Hodgkin's Lymphoma

Non-Hodgkin's lymphoma in the mediastinum develops from the mediastinal lymph node or from the thymic lymphocytes. Precursor T-lymphoblastic lymphoma (T-cell) and diffuse sclerosing large B-cell lymphomas are the common types of mediastinal lymphomas.

Diffuse Large Cell Non-Hodgkin's Lymphoma

Primary mediastinal large B-cell lymphoma (PMLBCL) is type of diffuse large B-cell NHL that undergoes sclerosis. Primary B-cell lymphomas represent for 2–3% of all NHLs. Unlike diffuse large B-cell lymphoma (DLBCL), this tumor commonly occurs in young adults. Due to marked sclerosis of the lymph node, the cellular yield may be poor. PMLBCL is seen in the anterosuperior mediastinum. This lymphoma develops from the thymic lymphoid cells and secondarily involves the adjacent lymph nodes of the thymus. Superficial lymphadenopathy and hepatosplenomegaly are not seen in PMLBCL.

Box 29.8: Large cell non-Hodgkin's lymphoma (NHL).

- Discrete large cells, three times larger than lymphocytes
- Variable amount of cytoplasm, minimal to moderate in amount
- Round to convoluted nuclear margin
- Vesicular chromatin, prominent nucleoli
- Lymphoglandular bodies.

Cytology (Figs. 29.9 and 29.10): Fine needle aspiration cytology smear shows dispersed population of large lymphoid cells in the background of lymphoglandular bodies (Box 29.8). Occasional small clusters of cells are also seen. The size of the lymphoid cell is three times more than the mature lymphocyte. The cells are round with variable amount of cytoplasm. The nuclei are round, moderately pleomorphic having irregular margin and convolution. Nuclear chromatin is fine with one or more prominent nucleoli located in the peripheral membrane of the nuclei. The tumor shows increased mitotic activity. Occasional spindle cells may be seen. In addition, there may be large cells with abundant cytoplasm and moderately pleomorphic nuclei. These cells may resemble Reed-Sternberg (RS) cells of Hodgkin's lymphoma.[3]

Immunocytochemistry: Primary mediastinal large B-cell lymphoma expresses B-cell markers, such as CD19, CD20 and CD22. Focal weak positivity of CD30 is also demonstrated.

Diagnostic difficulty:

- Seminoma
- Hodgkin's lymphoma

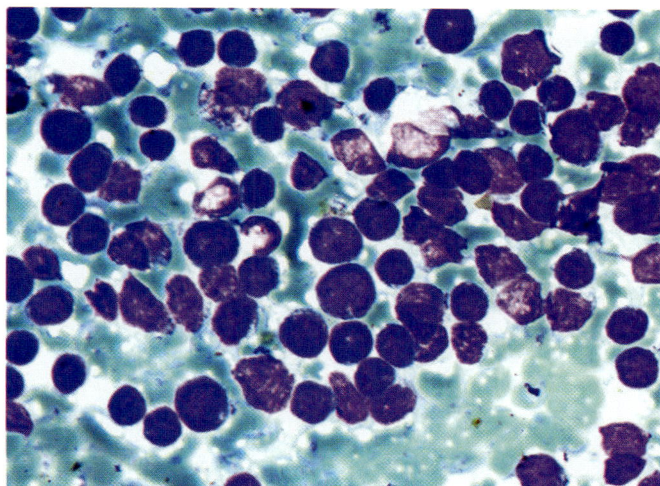

Fig. 29.11: Lymphoblastic lymphoma showing cells with scanty thin rim of deep blue cytoplasm and round relatively monomorphic nuclei with inconspicuous nucleoli (MGG × HP).

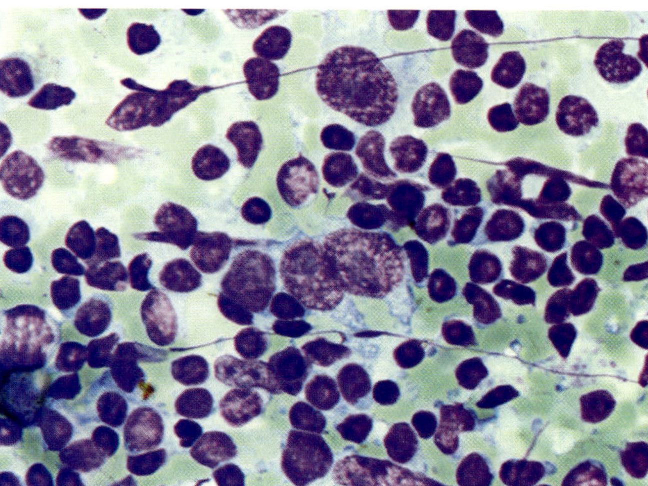

Fig. 29.12: Polymorphic population of cells along with classical Reed-Sternberg cells in Hodgkin's lymphoma (MGG × HP).

- *Spindle cell tumor*: Due to sclerosis in this lymphoma, the lymphoid cells often show spindle-shaped distortion and may give rise to the mistaken diagnosis of soft tissue sarcomas, spindle cell variant of thymoma and malignant melanoma.
- *Metastatic carcinoma*: Occasional small clusters of the lymphoid cells may give rise to the wrong diagnosis of poorly differentiated carcinoma.

Lymphoblastic Lymphoma

Precursor T-lymphoblastic lymphoma develops from T-cell. This is common in children and young adults. It is a high-grade aggressive lymphoma that typically involves the thymus and mediastinal lymph nodes.

Cytology (Fig. 29.11): Precursor T-lymphoblastic lymphoma shows dispersed monotonous population of small to medium-sized lymphoid cells (Box 29.9). The cells are 1.5 to 2 times larger than the mature lymphocytes. The individual cells have a scanty thin rim of deep blue cytoplasm with round relatively monomorphic nuclei. The nuclear margin may be irregular. Chromatin is fine reticulated with inconspicuous nucleoli. Increased mitotic figures and many tingible body macrophages are seen in the background.

Immunocytochemistry: The cells are positive for TdT along with T-cell markers such as CD3 and CD5.

Differential diagnosis:

- Various small round blue cell tumors, such as neuroblastoma, rhabdomyosarcoma, etc. comes in the differential diagnosis of precursor T-lymphoblastic lymphoma.

Box 29.9: Lymphoblastic lymphoma.

- Medium-sized cell, twice the size of mature lymphocyte
- Scanty rim of cytoplasm
- Irregular nuclear margin
- Fine reticular chromatin, inconspicuous nucleoli.

Anaplastic Large Cell Lymphomas

Anaplastic large cell lymphoma (ALCL) is uncommon in the mediastinum. It usually occurs in children and young adults. FNAC of ALCL has already been described in lymphoma section. The cytology smear shows typical "hallmark" cells characterized by large cells with abundant cytoplasm and kidney-shaped or embryo-shaped nuclei. Flow cytometry (FCM) is needed to confirm the diagnosis of ALCL. The tumor cells are positive for T-cell markers, such as CD3, and CD45RO. The cells are also positive for EMA, CD30 and anaplastic lymphoma kinase (ALK).

Hodgkin's Lymphoma

Among the different types of Hodgkin's lymphoma, nodular sclerosing Hodgkin's lymphoma is the most common primary lymphoma in the mediastinum. It affects young adult, particularly young female.

Cytology (Fig. 29.12)

Fine needle aspiration cytology of Hodgkin's lymphoma shows similar cytological features as that noted in other superficial lymph nodes. The yield of the cell may be

Box 29.10: Hodgkin's lymphoma.

- Polymorphic population of lymphoid cells
- Classical Reed-Sternberg cells
- Mononuclear Hodgkin's cells.

Box 29.11: Neuroblastoma.

- Dissociated and small cluster
- Pseudorosettes
- Small round cell
- Scanty cytoplasm
- Round monomorphic nuclei
- Hyperchromatic nuclei
- Small nucleoli
- Neurofibrillary material.

poor in these cases due to sclerosis. The smear shows a polymorphic population of reactive lymphoid cells consisting of mature lymphocytes, follicular center cells, eosinophils, plasma cells and characteristic typical RS cells (Box 29.10).

NEUROGENIC TUMOR[21,22]

The neurogenic tumors are commonly located in the posterior mediastinum. Neuroblastoma is the most common tumor of neurogenic origin in children. In adult, the peripheral nerve sheath tumors are common.

Neuroblastoma

This is a small blue round cell tumor. The salient cytological features of neuroblastomas are highlighted in Box 29.11.

Cytology (Fig. 29.13)

Neuroblastoma shows monomorphic small round cells arranged in loose cluster and discretely. Pseudorosettes are also seen. The cells show scanty deep blue cytoplasm with hyperchromatic round monomorphic nuclei having small nucleoli. Neural filamentous material may be seen in the background.

Ganglioneuroblastoma

The cells with ganglionic differentiation are seen in ganglioneuroblastoma. The ganglion cells are polygonal in shape with abundant cytoplasm having centrally placed nuclei. The nuclear chromatin is vesicular with prominent nucleoli.

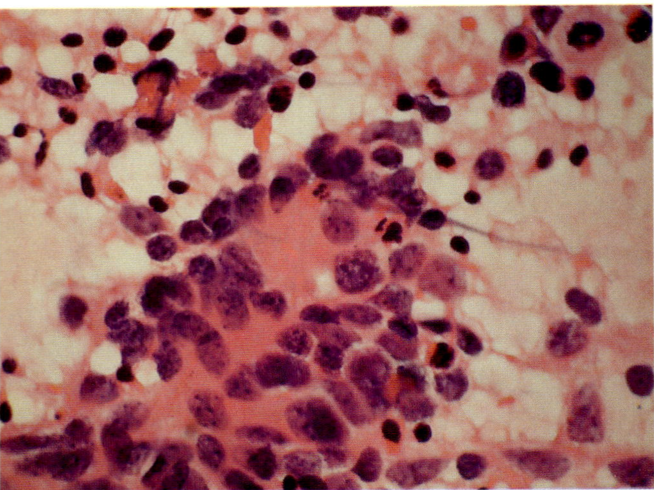

Fig. 29.13: Mediastinal neuroblastoma showing rosette formation (H & E × OI).

Box 29.12: Neurofibroma and schwannoma.

- Small fascicles of cells
- Oval-to-spindle-shaped cells
- Scanty cytoplasm
- Long and slender nuclei
- Thin-pointed ends
- Nuclear waving and kinking.

PERIPHERAL NERVE SHEATH TUMOR

Neurofibroma and Schwannoma

Schwannoma is the most common neurogenic tumor in the posterior mediastinum. Neurofibromas are also seen in the posterior mediastinum mostly in association with von Recklinghausen's disease.

Cytology

Fine needle aspiration cytology smear of the peripheral nerve sheath tumor shows small fascicles and dissociated cells. The cells are long slender with elongated wavy nuclei having thin-pointed ends (Box 29.12). Characteristic nuclear kinking is also seen. Nuclear chromatin is fine with prominent nucleoli. The background of the smear shows eosinophilic fibrillar material.

MALIGNANT PERIPHERAL NERVE SHEATH TUMORS (FIG. 29.14)

The cytomorphology of malignant peripheral nerve sheath tumor (MPNST) has been described in soft tissue tumor section. FNAC smear shows oval-to-spindle-shaped cells in small clusters. The cells show whorling appearance. The tumor cells are spindle-shaped with elongated moderate-to-marked pleomorphic nuclei. Mitotic activity is high. Background necrosis is frequently seen.

Diagnostic Difficulties

- Spindle cell type of thymoma
- Large cell sclerosing lymphoma
- Other soft tissue tumors
- Malignant melanoma.

Paraganglioma

Paraganglioma arises from the sympathetic chain of the posterior mediastinum. The detailed cytomorphology has been described in head and neck section.

METASTATIC CARCINOMA

Different types of metastatic tumors may involve the mediastinal lymph nodes. The most common primary sites of the malignancies are lung, breast, head neck region, gastrointestinal tract and kidney. Clinical history along with detailed cytomorphology is helpful in diagnosis and subtyping of malignancies. In certain situations, detailed immunocytochemistry on cell block section is helpful.

APPROACH TO THE DIAGNOSIS OF MEDIASTINAL TUMORS

As mentioned before, the following data is helpful in the diagnosis of mediastinal lesions:

- Relevant clinical history
- Radiological localization
- Cytomorphology database, and
- Ancillary investigations.

Relevant clinical history and radiological localization help to make a shortlist of diagnostic possibilities. In addition, the basic cytomorphology also helps in the provisional diagnosis of most of the lesions, such as:[23]

- *Round cell morphology*:
    - *Cohesive cells*: Thymoma, metastatic carcinoma
    - *Discohesive cells*: Non-Hodgkin's lymphoma, seminoma, Hodgkin's lymphoma
- *Spindle cell morphology*: Spindle cell thymoma, spindle cell melanoma, neurofibroma/schwannoma, MPNST
- *Pleomorphic cells*: Metastatic carcinoma, ALCL, embryonal carcinoma.

Once provisional diagnosis is made, then further ancillary tests may be done to confirm the diagnosis. The common ancillary investigations are:

- *Special stains*: Ziehl-Neelsen (ZN) stain, mucicarmine, etc.
- *Culture*: Bacterial and fungal culture
- Flow cytometry
- Immunocytochemistry (Table 29.1)
- *Others*: Polymerase chain reaction (PCR), biochemical markers, etc.

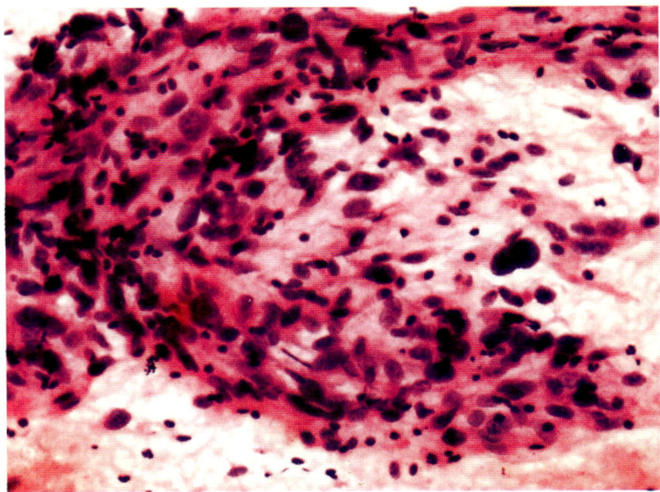

Fig. 29.14: Malignant peripheral nerve sheath tumor of posterior mediastinum showing loose cluster and discrete oval-to-elongated spindle cells with moderate nuclear pleomorphism (H & E × MP).

Table 29.1: Immunocytochemistry of different mediastinal tumors.

	Immunocytochemistry				
Lesions	*CK*	*LCA*	*Chromogranin*	*PLAP*	*NB45*
Thymoma	+	–	–	–	
NHL	–	+	–	–	
Seminoma	+ (occasional)	–	–	+	
Neuroblastoma	–	–	–	–	+
Small cell carcinoma	–	–	+	–	–

(CK: Cytokeratin; LCA: Leukocyte common antigen; NB: Neuroblastoma; NHL: Non-Hodgkin's lymphoma; PLAP: Placental leukocyte alkaline phosphatase).

REFERENCES

1. Singh HK, Silverman JF, Powers CN, et al. Diagnostic pitfalls in fine needle aspiration biopsy of the mediastinum. Diagn Cytopathol. 1997;17(2):121-6.
2. Linder J, Olsen GA, Johnston WW. Fine needle aspiration biopsy of the mediastinum. Am J Med. 1986;81(6):1005-8.
3. Shabb NS, Fahl M, Shabb B, et al. Fine needle aspiration of the mediastinum: a clinical, radiologic, cytologic, and histologic study of 42 cases. Diagn Cytopathol. 1998;19(6):428-36.
4. Wakely PE. Cytopathology-histopathology of the mediastinum: epithelial, lymphoproliferative, and germ cell neoplasms. Ann Diagn Pathol. 2002;6(1):30-43.
5. Geisinger KR. Differential diagnostic considerations and potential pitfalls in fine needle aspiration biopsies of the mediastinum. Diagn Cytopathol. 1995;13(5):436-42.
6. Assaad MW, Pantanowitz L, Otis CN. Diagnostic accuracy of image-guided percutaneous fine needle aspiration biopsy of the mediastinum. Diagn Cytopathol. 2007;35(11):705-9.
7. Desai F, Shah M, Patel S, et al. Fine needle aspiration cytology of anterior mediastinal masses. Indian J Pathol Microbiol. 2008;51(1):88-90.
8. Goel D, Prayaga AK, Sundaram C, et al. Utility of fine needle aspiration cytology in mediastinal lesions: a clinicopathologic study of 1617 cases from a single institution. Acta Cytol. 2008;52(4):404-11.
9. Ali SZ, Erozan YS. Thymoma. Cytopathologic features and differential diagnosis on fine needle aspiration. Acta Cytol. 1998;42(4):845-54.
10. Chhieng DC, Rose D, Ludwig ME, et al. Cytology of thymomas: emphasis on morphology and correlation with histologic subtypes. Cancer. 2000;90(1):24-32.
11. Wakely PE. Cytopathology of thymic epithelial neoplasms. Semin Diagn Pathol. 2005;22(3):213-22.
12. Travis WD, Brambilla E, Müller-Hermelink HK, et al. World Health Organization Classification of Tumours: Pathology and Genetics of Tumours of the Lung, Pleura, Thymus and Heart. Lyon: IARC Press; 2004.
13. Kuo TT, Chan JK. Thymic carcinoma arising in thymoma is associated with alterations in immunohistochemical profile. Am J Surg Pathol. 1998;22(12):1474-81.
14. Riazmontazer N, Bedyat C, Izadi B. Epithelial cytologic atypia in a fine needle aspirate of an invasive thymoma. A case report. Acta Cytol. 1992;36(3):387-90.
15. Shin HJ, Katz RL. Thymic neoplasia as represented by fine needle aspiration biopsy of anterior mediastinal masses. A practical approach to the differential diagnosis. Acta Cytol. 1998;42(4):855-64.
16. Dehner LP. Germ cell tumors of the mediastinum. Semin Diagn Pathol. 1990;7(4):266-84.
17. Collins KA, Giesinger KR, Wakely PE, et al. Extragonadal germ cell tumors: a fine needle aspiration biopsy study. Diagn Cytopathol. 1995;12(3):223-9.
18. trickler JG, Kurtin PJ. Mediastinal lymphoma. Semin Diagn Pathol. 1991;8(1):2-13.
19. Hughes JH, Katz RL, Fonseca GA, et al. Fine needle aspiration cytology of mediastinal non-Hodgkin's nonlymphoblastic lymphoma. Cancer. 1998;84(1):26-35.
20. Silverman JF. Raab SS, Park HK. Fine needle aspiration cytology of primary large-cell lymphoma of the mediastinum: cytomorphologic findings with potential pitfalls in diagnosis. Diagn Cytopathol. 1993;9(2):209-14.
21. Reeder LB. Neurogenic tumors of the mediastinum. Semin Thorac Cardiovasc Surg. 2000;12(4):261-7.
22. Slagel DD, Powers CN, Melaragno MJ, et al. Spindle-cell lesions of the mediastinum: diagnosis by fine needle aspiration biopsy. Diagn Cytopathol. 1997;17(3):167-76.
23. Dey P. Diagnostic dilemma: diagnostic algorithm in fine needle aspiration cytology of mediastinal tumors. Ind J Pathol Microbiol. 2010;53(3):395-402.

Review Questions

1. A 25-year-old female presented with cough and dyspnea for 3 months. Her chest radiograph showed 6-cm diameter superior mediastinal tumor. Fine needle aspiration cytology of the mass yielded particulate material. Figures 29.15A to D represent the microphotograph of the cytology smear.

a. What is your possible diagnosis?

a. Metastatic squamous cell carcinoma
b. Thymoma
c. Granulomatous inflammation
d. Metastatic sarcoma

b. What do you expect will be the immunocytochemistry in this case?

2. A 64-year-old male had history of cough and hemoptysis. His chest radiograph showed a 5-cm diameter anterior mediastinal lesion. Ultrasonography-guided fine needle aspiration cytology of the mass was done. Figures 29.16A and B are the representative of the cytology smears.

a. What is your diagnosis?

b. What do you expect will be the immunocytochemistry in this case?

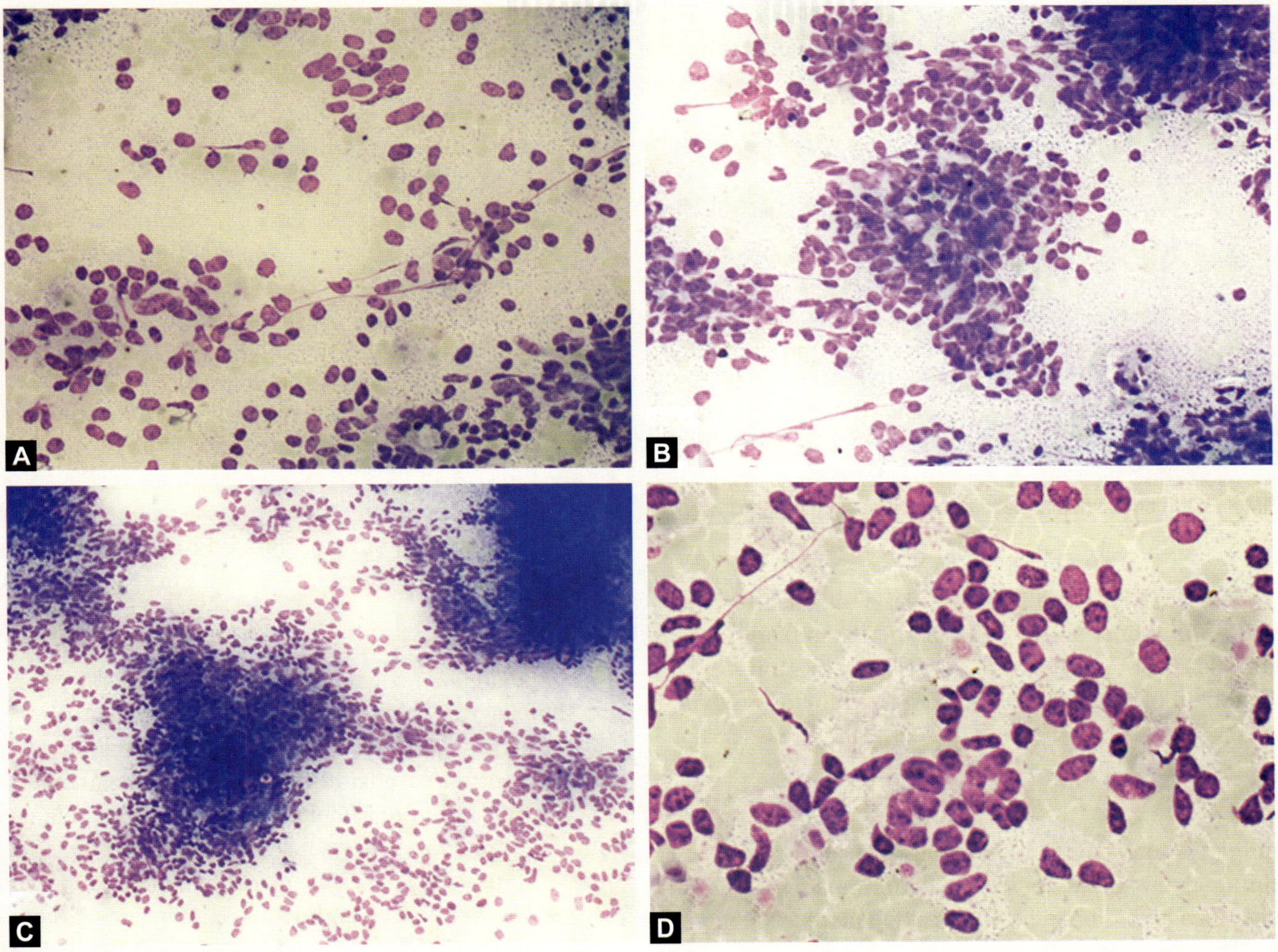

Figs. 29.15A to D: Cytology smears of case of question 1.

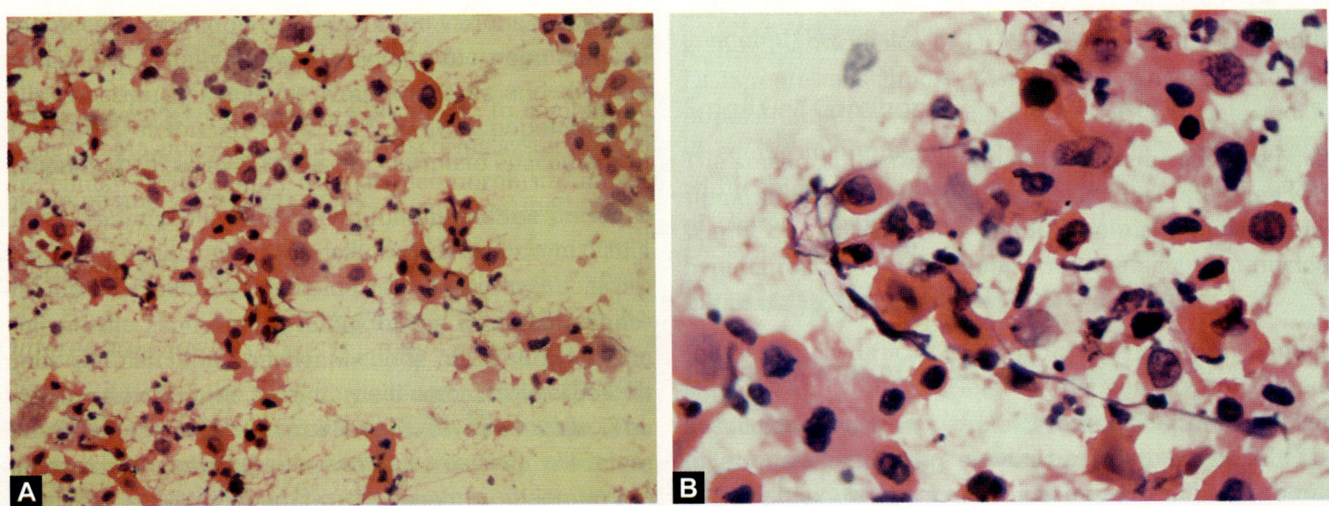

Figs. 29.16A and B: The fine needle aspiration cytology smear of the case of question 2.

Answers

1. a. Answer is (b) Thymoma
   b. Immunocytochemistry:
   - Epithelial cells of thymomas are positive for cytokeratin, epithelial membrane antigen (EMA), and carcinoembryonic antigen (CEA).

   Note: The presence of round cells and spindle looking discrete and clusters of cells with bland chromatin favour the diagnosis of thymoma.
2. a. Metastatic squamous cell carcinoma
   b. Immunocytochemistry:
   p 63 = positive
   p40 = positive
   CK5/6 = positive
   TTF = negative
   CK7 = negative

   Note: The discrete large polyhedral cells with hyperchromatic enlarged nuclei indicate the diagnosis of squamous cell carcinoma.

CHAPTER

30

Liver and Spleen

LIVER

INTRODUCTION

Fine needle aspiration cytology (FNAC) of the liver is mainly useful for the diagnosis of neoplastic lesion particularly to distinguish a primary liver tumor from a metastatic one and also to identify the type of metastatic or primary malignancy. FNAC is done under the guidance of ultrasonography (USG), computed tomography (CT) scan, or via endoscopy. The diagnostic accuracy of liver FNAC is near about 100%. The sensitivity and specificity of FNAC of liver in the diagnosis of malignancy are about 95% and 100%, respectively. FNAC is of little help in the diffuse parenchymal lesions of the liver such as cirrhosis, hepatitis, etc. except in certain conditions such as amyloidosis and hemochromatosis. Occasionally, metastatic malignancy may be diffusely infiltrative such as breast carcinoma and lymphoma. FNAC may be helpful in such conditions.[1-3]

Ultrasonography guidance FNAC of liver can be done from multiple sites in a single setting and the adequate material can be obtained from a lesion as small as 1-cm diameter. A space occupying lesion in the liver may be hepatocellular carcinoma (HCC), metastatic carcinoma, hydatid cyst, amoebic, or pyogenic abscess. FNAC diagnosis in these lesions guides the surgeons or physician to manage the case accordingly.

There is almost no complication of the FNAC of the liver lesion. However, rarely focal hemorrhage, biliary peritonitis, and anaphylactic shock (in hydatid cyst) may occur. Bleeding diathesis is the contraindication of liver FNAC and therefore prothrombin time or prothrombin index should be done before this procedure. The diameter of the needle preferably should be small and 22–25-gauge needle reduces the risk of any complication. It is better to avoid FNAC from a hydatid cyst, as there is a chance of spillage of cyst fluid and development of allergic reaction.

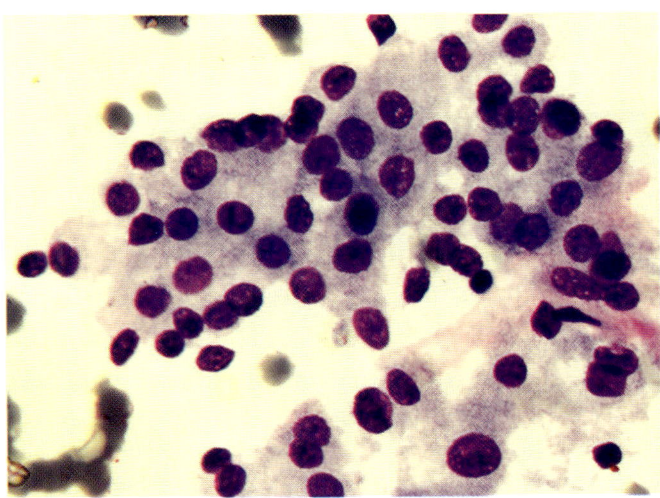

Fig. 30.1: Benign hepatocytes in cluster. Polygonal cells with abundant cytoplasm having monomorphic nuclei (MGG × HP).

NORMAL CELLS

Normal cellular contents of FNAC of the liver are as follows.

Hepatocytes (Fig. 30.1)

Hepatocytes are present in small clusters or discretely. The cells are large polygonal with abundant cytoplasm containing golden-brown bile pigment. The nuclei are centrally placed round monomorphic with fine granular chromatin and prominent nucleoli (Box 30.1). Pseudoinclusions are also noted. Mild degree of nuclear pleomorphism may be seen in the benign hepatocyte.

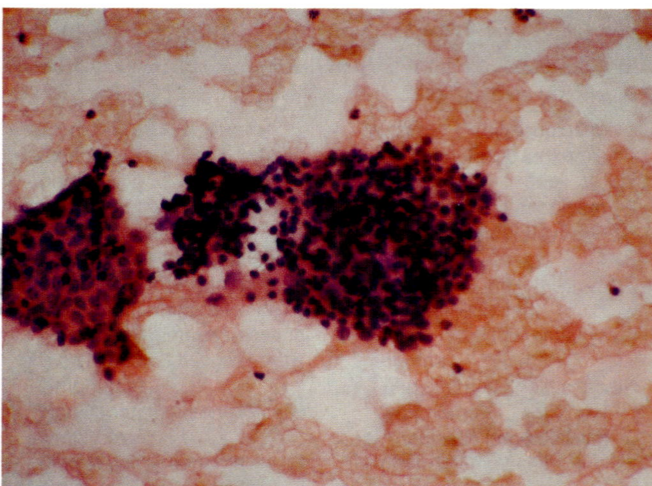

Fig. 30.2: Bile ductular cells in small clusters. The cells are round monomorphic having scanty cytoplasm (H and E × MP).

Box 30.2: Bile ductular cells.
- Small clusters or honeycomb sheet
- Small round cells
- Scanty cytoplasm

Bile Ductules (Fig. 30.2)

The bile ductular cells are present usually in small cohesive clusters. The cells are well spaced and give a honeycomb-like appearance (Box 30.2). The individual cells are small with scanty cytoplasm and small round monomorphic nuclei.

Kupffer Cells

The Kupffer cells are usually present in between the hepatocytes. These cells are of histiocytic in origin. The Kupffer cells have scanty cytoplasm, bean-shaped nuclei with inconspicuous nucleoli. Phagocytosed materials are often noted within the Kupffer cell.

Endothelial Cells

These cells surround the cluster of hepatocytes. Individual cells have spindle-shaped elongated nuclei with prominent nucleoli and scanty delicate cytoplasm.

LIVER LESIONS

The common space-occupying lesions in the liver encountered by FNAC are listed in Table 30.1.

Box 30.1: Hepatocytes.
- Polygonal cells
- Abundant cytoplasm
- Central round nuclei
- Prominent nucleoli
- Nuclear pseudoinclusion
- Bile pigments in cytoplasm

Table 30.1: Common space-occupying lesions in liver.

Non-neoplastic:	*Neoplastic*:
• Hepatic abscess • Hydatid cyst • Granulomas • Focal nodular hyperplasia	*Benign*: • Liver adenoma • Cavernous hemangioma *Malignant* *Primary*: • Hepatocellular carcinoma • Hepatoblastoma • Cholangiocarcinoma *Secondary*: • Metastatic carcinoma • Metastatic sarcoma

Non-neoplastic Lesions

Cysts

Congenital cysts: These are usually unilocular. The wall of the cyst is lined by cuboidal to columnar epithelium. FNAC of the congenital cyst yields clear fluid and the smear is usually hypocellular that shows predominantly macrophages and cuboidal to columnar epithelial cells.

The ciliated foregut cyst is also solitary and remains beneath the falciform ligament. These cysts are lined by ciliated columnar epithelium. FNAC smears of the cyst show mucus cells and ciliated columnar cells. At times, the cilia may be lost and the cells may be mistaken as malignant cells.

Hydatid cysts: Hydatid cyst is caused by Echinococcus granulosus, a tape worm. Infection of this parasite invades multiple organs in the human body. Liver is the most common site of hydatid cyst. The cyst in the liver is usually solitary and on imaging the cyst is covered by a membrane and filled with fluid. The membrane is acellular. From the germinal layer, many multiple daughter cysts may grow. The daughter cysts contain many scolices with hooklets.

Cytology (Fig. 30.3): FNAC from the hydatid cyst is not recommended because of the risk of anaphylactic shock. However, it may be done accidentally from the hydatid cyst. FNAC yields clear fluid. The smear shows polymorphs, laminated membrane like structure, occasional multinucleated giant cells, and many scoleces with hooklets (Box 30.3). The presence of hooklets is diagnostic of hydatid cyst.

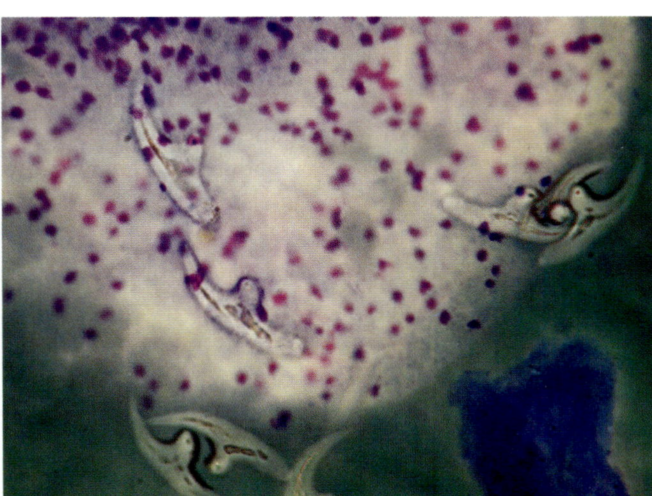

Fig. 30.3: Multiple hooklets of hydatid cyst in an aspirate from liver (MGG × HP).

Box 30.4: Pyogenic abscess.

- Polymorphs
- Necrotic debris
- Degenerated hepatocytes
- Reactive atypia of hepatocytes

Pyogenic abscess: This is usually caused by bacterial infection due to sepsis or ascending cholangitis. The common organisms are *Streptococci* and *Staphylococci*. Cytology smear shows numerous polymorphs, necrotic debris, and degenerated hepatocytes. The hepatocytes in the wall of the cyst may show significant reactive atypia (Box 30.4).

Amoebic abscess: This is due to infection of amoeba. FNAC smear shows both polymorphs and lymphocytes along with the amoebic trophozoites. *Entamoeba histolytica* have small vesicular nuclei and vacuolated cytoplasm with phagocytosed red blood cell (RBC).

Benign Neoplastic Lesion

World Health Organization has classified the neoplastic lesions of liver as:[4]

Epithelial Tumors

- *Benign*:
  - Hepatocellular adenoma (liver cell adenoma)
  - Focal nodular hyperplasia (FNH)
  - Intrahepatic bile duct adenoma
  - Intrahepatic bile duct cystadenoma
  - Biliary papillomatosis

Box 30.3: Hydatid cyst.

- Laminated membrane
- Scolices
- Hooklets
- Multinucleated giant cells

Box 30.5: Focal nodular hyperplasia.

- Benign hepatocytes
- Many fibroblasts
- Bile ductular cells

- *Malignant*:
  - Hepatocellular carcinoma (liver cell carcinoma)
  - Intrahepatic cholangiocarcinoma
  - Peripheral bile duct carcinoma
  - Bile duct cystadenocarcinoma
  - Combined hepatocellular and cholangiocarcinoma
  - Hepatoblastoma
  - Undifferentiated carcinoma.

Focal nodular hyperplasia: More than 90% FNH is seen in females of reproductive age group. Occasionally, it may occur in pediatric age group.[5] FNH possibly results due to hyperplastic response to arterial malformation. CT scan of the liver shows a mass with central stellate scar. The scar enhances in the arterial phase and disappears in the portal venous phase. FNAC of FNH yields a chunk of liver tissue that is difficult to spread on the slide. The smear shows abundant discrete benign hepatocytes along with many fibroblasts in the background (Box 30.5). The hepatocytes look completely benign and a diagnosis of FNH is not possible in the cytology smear.

Liver cell adenomas: Liver cell adenomas predominantly occur in females under 30-year of age who take oral contraceptive for more than 5 years.[6] The liver cell adenoma may present with pain abdomen due to rupture of the adenoma into the surrounding tissue. CT scan of liver shows an encapsulated, well circumscribed, low-density mass with marked centripetal pattern of enhancement on arterial phase.

Histology of the liver cell adenoma shows only benign hepatocytes without any portal triads.

Cytology (Figs. 30.4 and 30.5): FNAC smear of the liver cell adenoma shows abundant three-dimensional clusters and also dissociated cells. The hepatocytes are normal polygonal in shape with often vacuolated cytoplasm (Box 30.6). Nuclei are round and monomorphic appearances. The background of the smear does not show any

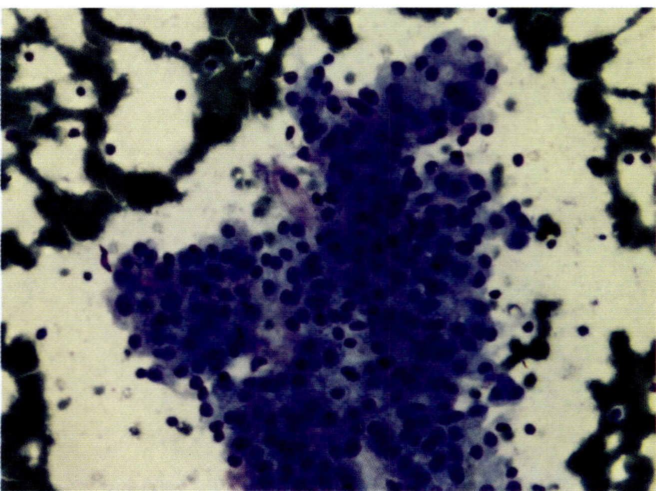

Fig. 30.4: Large cluster of benign looking hepatocytes in fine needle aspiration cytology smear of liver cell adenoma (MGG × MP).

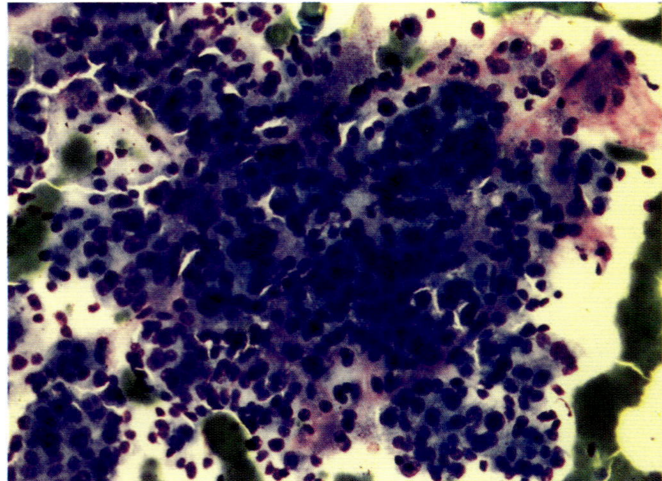

Fig. 30.5: Fine needle aspiration cytology smear of liver cell adenoma showing benign looking hepatocytes (MGG × HP).

Box 30.6: Liver cell adenoma.

- Three-dimensional clusters of hepatocytes
- Normal looking hepatocytes
- Mild atypia
- Absence of bile duct epithelial cells
- *CT scan*: well encapsulated, low-density mass with centripetal enhancement on arterial phase

(CT: Computed tomography).

bile duct epithelium. The cytological features of liver cell adenoma are nonspecific and the diagnosis is impossible on FNAC smear alone. Clinical history, CT scan findings along with cytology may be helpful in diagnosis of liver cell adenoma.

Differential Diagnosis

- Hepatocellular carcinoma
- *Reactive hepatocytes*: The cells in reactive hepatocytes show more nuclear pleomorphism than liver cell adenoma. The absence of bile duct epithelial cells favors liver cell adenoma
- *Cirrhotic nodule*: Lack of atypia and absent bile ductules favor liver cell adenoma.

Malignant Tumor

Hepatocellular Carcinoma[7-15]

Hepatocellular carcinoma is the malignant tumor that develops from the hepatocytes. It is one of the most common malignant tumors in Asia and also a worldwide major public health problem. Males are more commonly affected by HCC than females. It may in any group, however, the incidence of HCC is more in 30–40 years of age.

It is also the most common primary malignant tumors of the liver. The common etiologic causes of HCC are:

- Hepatitis B (HBV) and hepatitis C virus (HCV) infection
- Alcoholic cirrhosis
- Dietary ingestion of high dose of aflatoxin
- Long-standing use of oral contraceptives
- High-dose anabolic steroid
- Iron overload.

Out of all these causes, chronic viral infections by HBV and HCV are the most common etiological factors. It has been noted that the individuals with chronic HBV infection carry 100 times more risk of HCC than the uninfected people. HBV vaccination reduces the incidence of HCC.

Cirrhosis of liver is another important risk factor of HCC and almost 90% of HCC develops from cirrhosis. In 60% of HCC cases, alpha-fetoprotein (AFP) level is high. This is one of the important diagnostic markers of HCC. A significantly raised level of AFP level or continuous rising level of the same suggests the possibility of HCC.

The patient of HCC usually presents with generalized weakness, malaise, and pain abdomen. Physical examination of the patients shows hepatomegaly, jaundice, and ascites.

Biochemical features: The patients of HCC may show rise of liver enzymes such as aspartate aminotransferase, alanine aminotransferase, alkaline phosphatase, gamma-glutamyl transpeptidase, and bilirubin. These raised enzymes depend on the underlying liver disease and damage. They are nonspecific for HCC. AFP level is also raised in HCC. Serum AFP level more than 500 ng/mL is highly suggestive of HCC. Des-gamma carboxyprothrombin (DCP), an abnormal prothrombin is produced from the tumor cells in HCC. Serum level of DCP is a useful marker of HCC and is well correlated with tumor size and inversely correlated with grade of HCC. A combination of AFP and DCP is more effective as diagnostic serological markers rather than single marker.

Imaging study: Various radiological imaging studies are helpful for the detection of HCC such as USG, CT scan, magnetic resonance imaging, and color Doppler USG.

Cytology (Figs. 30.6 to 30.12): FNAC smear of the liver should be thoroughly studied in low-power magnification of the microscope (Box 30.7). The smears should be studied for:

- Pattern of the spread of cells
- Individual tumor cells
- Background hepatocytes or other evidences.

Smears with hypercellularity and regularly arranged cells usually indicate the possibility of HCC.

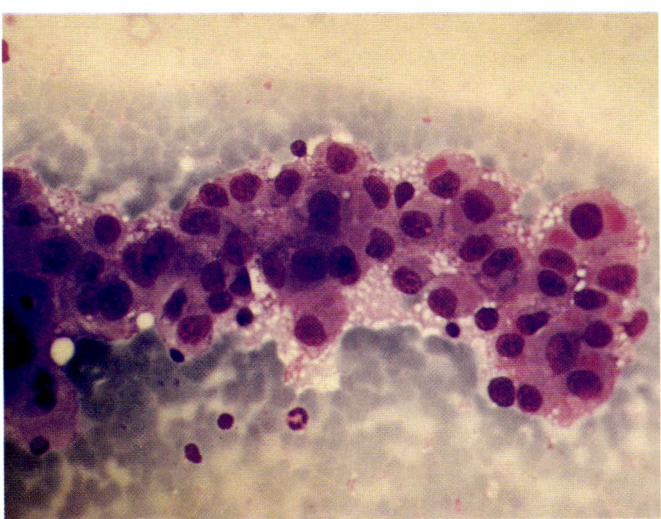

Fig. 30.6: Hepatocellular carcinoma. The cells are arranged in long cord (MGG × HP).

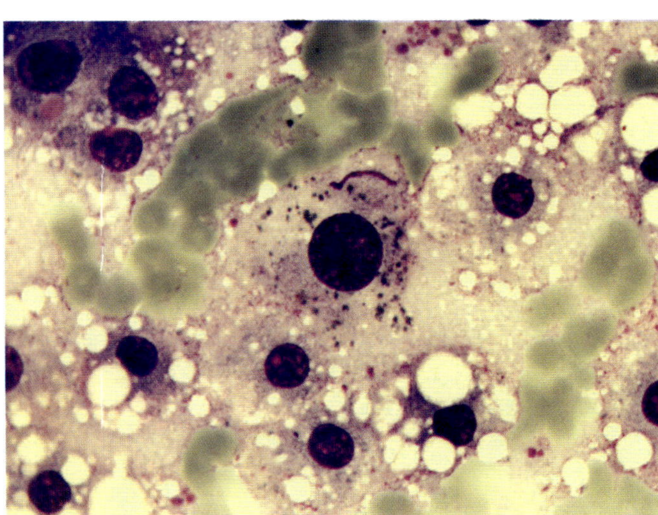

Fig. 30.7: Hepatocellular carcinoma: Bile within the malignant hepatocytes (MGG × HP).

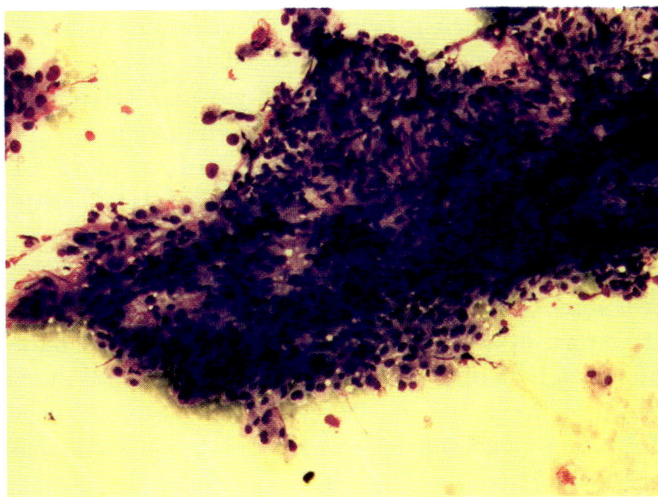

Fig. 30.8: Hepatocellular carcinoma: Transgressing capillaries within the hepatocytes (MGG × MP).

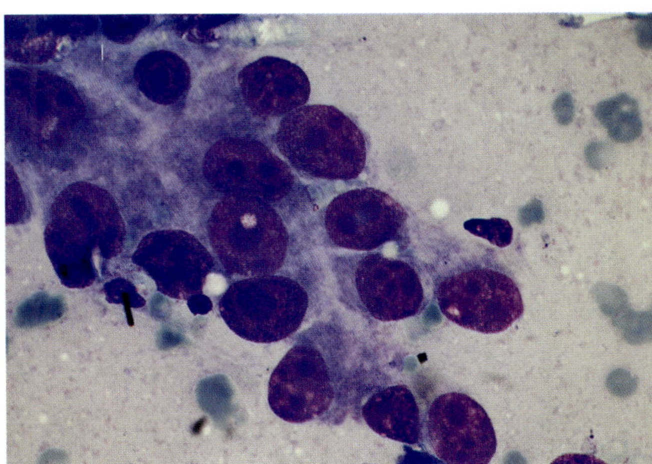

Fig. 30.9: Hepatocellular carcinoma: Higher magnification showing large cells resembling hepatocytes. The nuclei are large, pleomorphic, and show multiple prominent nucleoli (MGG × OI).

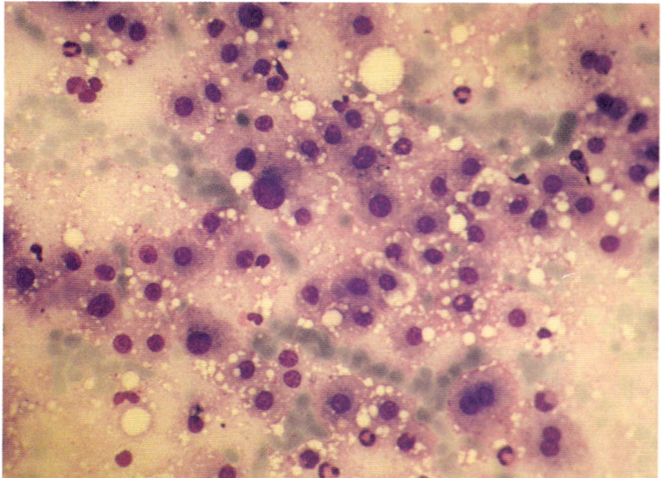

Fig. 30.10: Hepatocellular carcinoma: Well-differentiated hepatocellular carcinoma resembles normal hepatocytes (MGG × MP).

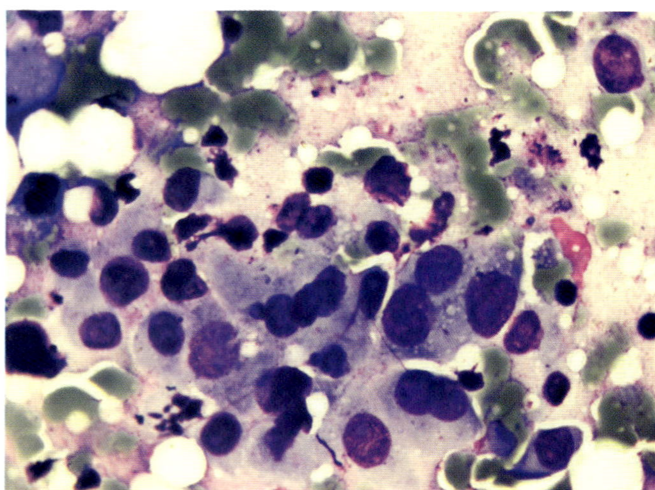

Fig. 30.11: Poorly differentiated hepatocellular carcinoma: Large moderately pleomorphic cells (MGG × HP).

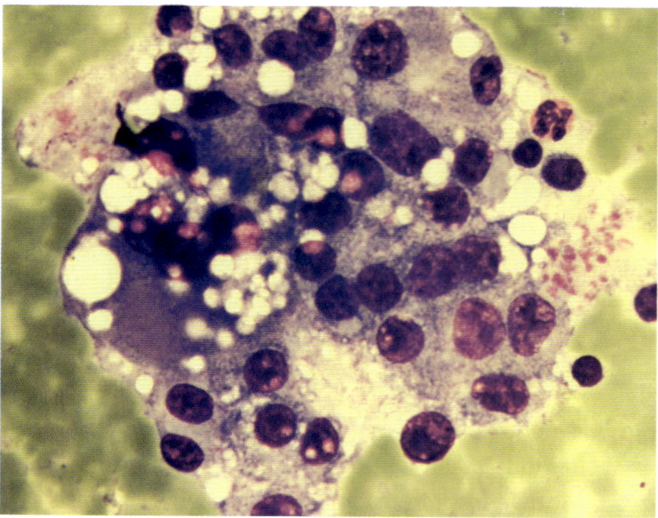

Fig. 30.12: Clear cell type hepatocellular carcinoma: Cells with marked clear vacuolated cytoplasm (MGG × HP).

The tumor cells are arranged in following pattern:

- *Trabecular*: Trabecular pattern is characterized by column of three to four cells and surrounded by endothelial cells
- *Acinar or glandular*: The acinar pattern shows a central lumen surrounded by five to eight cells
- *Thin cords*: One to two cells thick rows of cells.

The single most important feature of HCC is that the tumor cells resemble hepatocytes. The individual tumor cells are large polygonal with well-defined cytoplasmic border. The nuclei show mild-to-severe degree of pleomorphism with large prominent macronucleoli. The nuclear membrane is well defined, irregular, and often shows folds and deep indentations. The nuclear chromatin is fine granular. Intranuclear cytoplasmic inclusions may also be seen in HCC and they are not specific.

Box 30.7: Hepatocellular carcinoma.

- Hypercellular
- Trabecular, acinar, cord of cells
- Polygonal malignant cell resembling hepatocytes
- Well-defined cell margin
- Atypical bare nuclei
- Transgressing capillaries within clusters
- Enlarged pleomorphic nuclei
- Macronucleoli
- Intracytoplasmic bile pigments
- Intracytoplasmic eosinophilic globules

Immunocytochemistry: Positive for alpha-fetoprotein, Hep Par-1, glypican-3, polyclonal carcinoembryonic antigen (p-CEA) and CD10

Intracytoplasmic pale hyaline globules resembling Mallory hyaline bodies and vacuoles containing fat, and glycogen may also be noted. The presence of intracytoplasmic bile pigments is found in almost one-third of HCC cases and this is specific for the diagnosis of HCC.

Transgressing thin capillaries lined by the endothelial cells within the large clusters of tumor cells are also noted. Uncommonly, pseudoacini are seen with central dark-brown blobs of bile. The cytology smears also show many atypical stripped bare nuclei that are similar to the nuclei present in intact hepatocytes. Isolated tumor giant cells may also be noted.

Reactive or regenerative hepatocytes may often show nuclear enlargement and pleomorphism. Bi- and

Table 30.2: Differentiating points between hepatocellular carcinoma and metastatic adenocarcinoma.

Features	*Hepatocellular carcinoma*	*Metastatic adenocarcinoma*
Pattern of cells	Trabecular, acinar, small cluster	Glandular
Transgressing capillaries	Present	Absent
Associated benign hepatocytes	Usually absent	Present
Bare nuclei	Present	Absent
Cell shape	Polygonal	Columnar
Cytoplasm	Eosinophilic granular	Vacuolated
Macronucleoli	Present	Usually absent
Intracytoplasmic bile pigment	Present	Absent
HbsAg	Positive	Negative
Alpha-fetoprotein level in serum	Raised	Mostly normal
Immunocytochemistry: Hep Par-1, glypican-3, p-CEA, and CD10	Positive	Negative

(HbsAg: Hepatitis B surface antigen; Hep Par-1: Hepatocyte antibody; p-CEA: Polyclonal carcinoembryonic antigen).

multinucleated hepatocytes are also seen. The differentiating cytological features of HCC from reactive hepatocytes are abundant cellularity, trabecular pattern of cells, moderate to marked nuclear atypia, stripped atypical nuclei, and macronucleoli.

On FNAC, it is difficult to differentiate a metastatic adenocarcinoma from the HCC. However, certain cytological features such as polygonal cells resembling hepatocytes, trabecular pattern of cells, background stripped nuclei, eosinophilic granular cytoplasm, and intracellular bile pigments favor a diagnosis of HCC rather than metastatic adenocarcinoma (Table 30.2).

At times, it is difficult to differentiate liver cell adenoma from HCC. Both the conditions may show abundant cellularity and nuclear atypia. However, clinical history of cirrhosis raised AFP level, absence of history of steroid intake along with the cytological features of trabecular arrangement of cell surrounded by endothelial lining, stripped atypical cell, and significant nuclear atypia favor a diagnosis of HCC.

Box 30.8: Fibrolamellar variant of hepatocellular carcinoma.

- It is commonly noted in 2nd and 3rd decade of life
- Surgically resectable
- Dyscohesive large polygonal liver cells
- Dense granular eosinophilic oncocytic cytoplasm
- Cytoplasmic pale bodies
- Nuclei are round, monomorphic with coarse chromatin
- Many benign spindle-shaped fibroblasts and fragments of collagen

Variants of Hepatocellular Carcinoma

1. *Fibrolamellar variant of HCC*: It is a distinct clinical pathological entity. Fibrolamellar variant of HCC is a rare variant of HCC and is commonly noted in 2nd and 3rd decade of life. This tumor presents as single nodule and therefore it is surgically resectable. On histology section, the tumor cells are arranged in sheets or small trabeculae. The cells are separated by hyalinized collagen bundles with a characteristic lamellar pattern.

   Cytology (Box 30.8): Aspiration cytology smears show dyscohesive large polygonal liver cells with abundant dense granular eosinophilic oncocytic cytoplasm. The nuclei are round and monomorphic with coarse chromatin. Cytoplasmic pale bodies are also characteristic of this tumor. Many benign spindle-shaped fibroblasts and fragments of collagen are seen in the background.
2. *Clear cell variant*: The clear cell variant comprises of almost 10% cases of HCC. Here, the cells show abundant clear vacuolated cytoplasm due to accumulation of glycogen. Focal clear cell change may also be seen in classical HCC. This case may be difficult to distinguish from metastatic renal cell carcinoma.
3. *Giant cell variant of HCC*: Pure giant cell HCC is very uncommon. In this tumor, the FNAC smear shows multiple tumor giant cells. The cell may be large mononuclear or multinucleated.
4. *Small cell variant*: The cytology smears of this variant of HCC resemble as neuroendocrine tumor. The tumors show dyscohesive or acinar arrangement of small round to oval cells with scanty cytoplasm. Nuclear features of the cells resemble neuroendocrine tumor. Trabecular pattern is absent in this variant.
5. *Spindle cell variant*: The pure form of spindle cell variant is uncommon. The cytology smear shows spindle-shaped hepatocytes in small clusters along with many giant hepatocytes. The individual cells show spindle-shaped nuclei with moderate nuclear pleomorphism.

Box 30.9: Immunocytochemical markers of hepatocellular carcinoma.

Alpha-fetoprotein:
- Cytoplasmic positivity
- Neoplastic hepatocytes
- Low sensitivity, good specificity
- Confirmation of HCC

Hepatocyte Paraffin 1 (Hep Par-1):
- A hepatocyte mitochondrial epitope
- Cytoplasmic granular positivity
- High sensitivity (100%) in well-differentiated HCC
- 90% specific for HCC
- Distinguishes HCC from cholangiocarcinoma and metastatic adenocarcinoma

Glypican-3:
- Sulfate proteoglycan on cell membrane
- Very high sensitivity and specificity
- Only malignant hepatocytes are positive

p-CEA:
- Stains bile canaliculi and bile duct epithelium
- Low sensitivity and high specificity
- Distinguishes HCC from metastatic adenocarcinoma

(HCC: Hepatocellular carcinoma).

If the smear contains predominantly spindle cells then it may be difficult to differentiate this tumor from a metastatic spindle cell sarcoma such as fibrosarcoma or leiomyosarcoma.

6. *HCC with fatty change*: In this variant, the smears show malignant hepatocytes with remarkable fatty changes. This variant of HCC may be mistaken for fatty change in the liver. Poorly differentiate HCC with fatty change may be mistaken for metastatic liposarcoma.

Immunocytochemistry and serological markers of HCC (Box 30.9): Immunocytochemistry or serological markers are helpful for confirmation of the primary malignancy in liver or the histogenetic origin of the tumor.

- *Alpha-fetoprotein*: This is one of the commonly used markers for the diagnosis of HCC. This protein is secreted by the neoplastic liver cells and the normal hepatocytes do not express AFP. The sensitivity of this marker is near about 50%.[16] The specificity of AFP is relatively high. However, the raised AFP level may be noted in malignancies other than HCC such as gastric adenocarcinoma and large cell neuroendocrine carcinoma.[17] There is a growing tendency to drop this marker from the diagnostic panel of HCC
- *Hepatocyte Paraffin 1 (Hep Par-1)*: Hep Par-1 recognizes a hepatocyte mitochondrial epitope. It shows cytoplasmic granular positivity. Hep Par-1 is relatively sensitive, specific, and very helpful in detecting HCC, especially the well-differentiated HCC.[18,19] Unfortunately, its sensitivity drops remarkably in poorly differentiated HCC. Hep Par-1 staining may also be seen in tumors other than HCC such as gastric, pulmonary, colon, breast, and pancreatic adenocarcinoma[20]
- *Polyclonal carcinoembryonic antigen (p-CEA)*: The presence of intercellular canaliculi is one of the important diagnostic features of HCC. p-CEA stains bile canaliculi and duct but not the hepatocytes. In well-differentiated HCC, this can be demonstrated as long linear pattern, whereas in poorly differentiated HCC, it is thick and short
- *CD 10*: This is expressed in normal and neoplastic liver cells and therefore helps in differentiation of HCC from metastatic carcinoma. It shows similar canalicular pattern to p-CEA
- *Glypican-3*: This is a member of the sulfate proteoglycans family. The glypican-3 gene is located on xq26.1. Glyciphan 3 is expressed in the cell membrane and plays an important role in cell growth, migration, and differentiation. Immunocytochemistry displays cytoplasmic reaction with membranous accentuation. It is a highly sensitive and specific marker of HCC and is more useful than Hep Par-1 in detecting poorly differentiated HCC. Glypican-3 is especially useful in detecting mass lesions of HCC from other benign and premalignant liver nodules such as liver cell adenoma, dysplastic nodules, and FNH nodules
  - *Differential diagnosis*:
    - Reactive hepatocytes
    - Adenocarcinoma
    - Liver cell adenoma.

Cholangiocarcinoma

This is far less common than HCC. The tumor arises from the bile duct epithelium, intrahepatic bile ducts, or extrahepatic biliary tree. Cholangiocarcinoma is often associated with Clonorchis sinensis infestation, hemochromatosis, thorotrast injection and chronic ulcerative colitis.[21] The patients usually present with weakness, malaise, and obstructive jaundice.

Cytology (Figs. 30.13A and B): FNAC smear shows small clusters and microglandular arrangement of cells. The individual cells are cuboidal to columnar with scanty cytoplasm and resemble atypical bile duct epithelial cells (Box 30.10). Nuclei are mildly enlarged with prominent nucleoli. Occasional cells show vacuoles in the cytoplasm. On FNAC, smear cholangiocarcinoma cannot be distinguished from metastatic pancreatic adenocarcinoma.

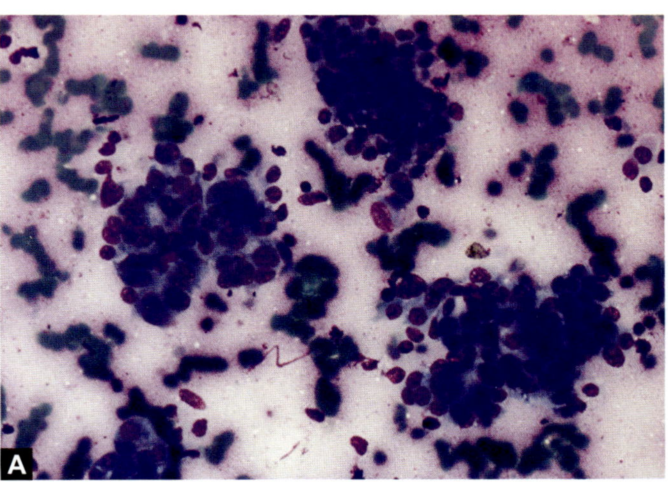

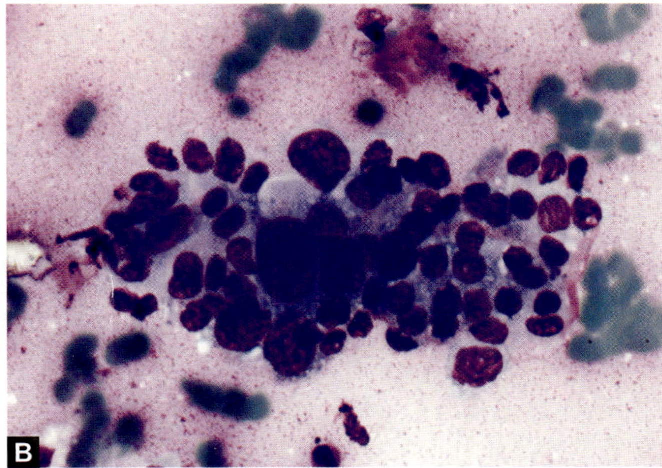

Figs. 30.13A and B: (A) Cholangiocarcinoma: Clusters of malignant cells with round nuclei and scanty cytoplasm. The cells are CK 7 and CK19 positive (MGG × MP). (B) Cholangiocarcinoma: The cells show moderate nuclear pleomorphism. Occasional cells have vacuolated cytoplasm (MGG × HP).

Box 30.10: Cholangiocarcinoma.

- Small clusters and sheets
- Small cuboidal to columnar cells
- Round hyperchromatic nuclei
- Scanty cytoplasm
- Normal alpha-fetoprotein level

Immunocytochemistry: Positive for CK7, CK17, CK19, EMA, and diffusely positive for p-CEA

The cells of cholangiocarcinoma are positive for CK7, CK17, CK19, EMA, and diffusely positive for p-CEA. In contrast, HCC cells are positive for CK8 and CK18.[22] Cholangiocarcinoma is characteristically positive for both CK7 and CK20.

Differential diagnosis:

- Metastatic adenocarcinoma
- *HCC*: Small ovoid cells with clean background in cholangiocarcinoma distinguish it from HCC that shows polygonal cells with many bare nuclei. HCC cells are CK8 and CK18 positive and negative for CK7, CK17, and CK19.

Hepatoblastoma[23-26]

Hepatoblastoma is the tumor of the children and young adults and 90% of this tumor occurs before 5 years of age. This is a relatively rare tumor. However, hepatoblastoma is the most common malignant tumor of liver in children. The tumor is usually solitary space-occupying lesion in liver. The children with hepatoblastoma are presented with a large bulging abdominal mass, hepatomegaly with abdominal swelling, and fever.

Cytology (Figs. 30.14 to 30.17): Hepatoblastoma may be of three types (Box 30.11):

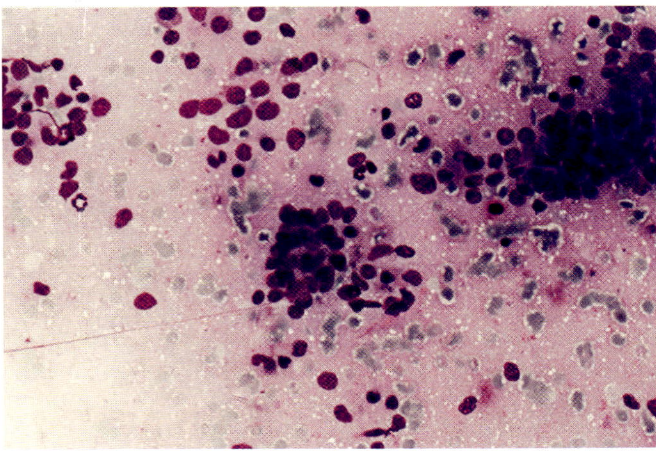

Fig. 30.14: Hepatoblastoma: Round to oval cells in cluster and ill-defined acini (MGG × MP).

- *Anaplastic*: The anaplastic type of hepatoblastoma shows small round cells with scanty cytoplasm and round nucleus. Anaplastic type of hepatoblastoma may cause diagnostic difficulties with other small round cell tumors such as neuroblastoma and rhabdomyosarcomas
- *Embryonal*: The cells of embryonal type are arranged in sheets, clusters, and rosette like structures. The individual cells are larger than the small round cells of anaplastic type. They are immature with high N/C ratio, irregular hyperchromatic nuclei. Nuclear chromatin is dense with single to multiple nucleoli. The cytoplasm is scanty to moderate in amount. The cells lack the differentiation of hepatocytes

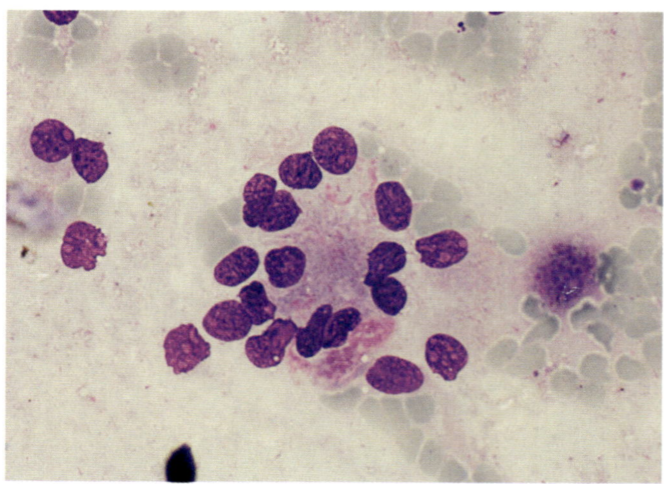

Fig. 30.15: Hepatoblastoma: Acinar arrangement (MGG × HP).

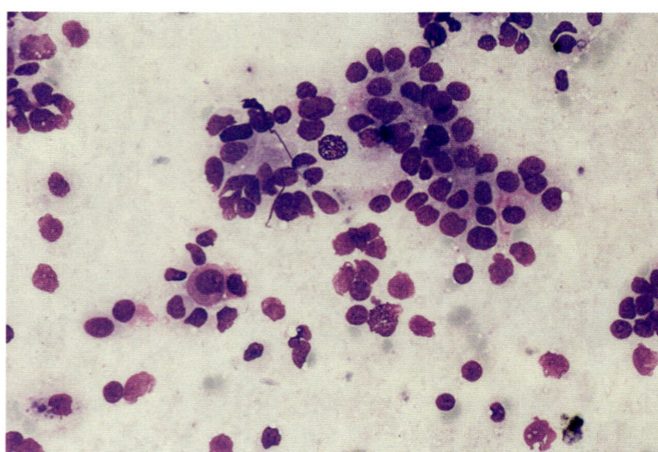

Fig. 30.16: Hepatoblastoma: Round to oval cells with relatively monomorphic nuclei (MGG × MP).

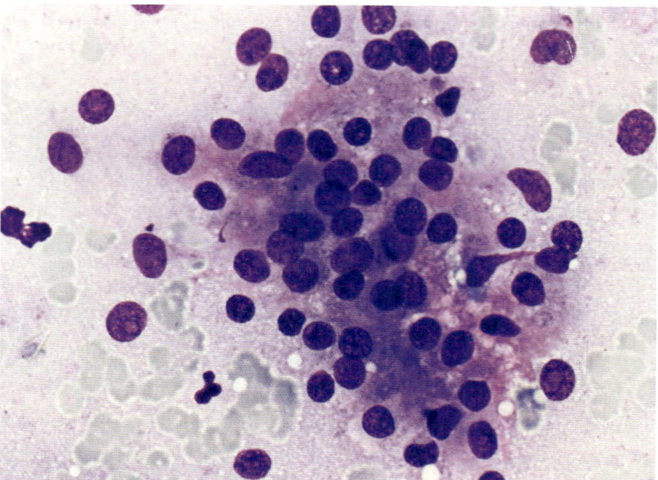

Fig. 30.17: Hepatoblastoma: Higher magnification of the cells showing moderate cytoplasm and fine nuclear chromatin (MGG × HP).

- *Fetal*: Fetal cells resemble fetal hepatocytes and form well-formed acini. These cells are larger than the embryonal cells. The cells are round to polygonal with well-defined cytoplasmic border and high N/C ratio. Nuclei are round with minimal nuclear pleomorphism and finely granular chromatin. These cells may contain bile pigment. Many traversing capillaries may be seen with perivascular arrangement of tumor cells resembling sinusoids. Mesenchymal components are seen in the form of clusters of spindle cells with elongated nuclei. Osteoid material or skeletal muscle differentiation may also be seen. Extramedullary hematopoiesis in the form of nucleated RBC, megakaryocytes and myeloid series of cells are frequently noted. Fetal type of hepatoblastoma may be confused with HCC. The presence of metaplastic elements and extramedullary hematopoiesis favor a diagnosis of hepatoblastoma.

Differential diagnosis:
- Hepatocellular carcinoma
- Other small round cell tumor.

Primary Sarcomas

Angiosarcoma

This is the most common sarcoma of liver. However, angiosarcoma is a rare tumor. The tumor occurs in 6th–7th decade. The exact etiological cause of this tumor is unknown in majority of the cases. However, this tumor is often associated with prior administration of Thorotrast (a radiographic dye), exposure to vinyl chloride monomer and use of androgenic-anabolic steroids.

Cytology (Figs. 30.18 and 30.19): The cytology smear shows discrete and tight cohesive clusters of malignant spindle cells (Box 30.12). The nuclei are oval to elongate with blunt ends having moderate pleomorphism. The cytoplasm shows fine vacuolations and intracytoplasmic lumen.

The cells of angiosarcoma are positive for CD31 and CD34 immunostaining.

Epithelioid hemangioendothelioma: This is also a rare tumor in the liver arising from vascular endothelial cells. This is less aggressive tumor than angiosarcoma.

Cytology: FNAC smears are usually paucicellular. There are loose clusters and discrete large cells with abundant lacy cytoplasm (Box 30.13). Many of the tumor cells have

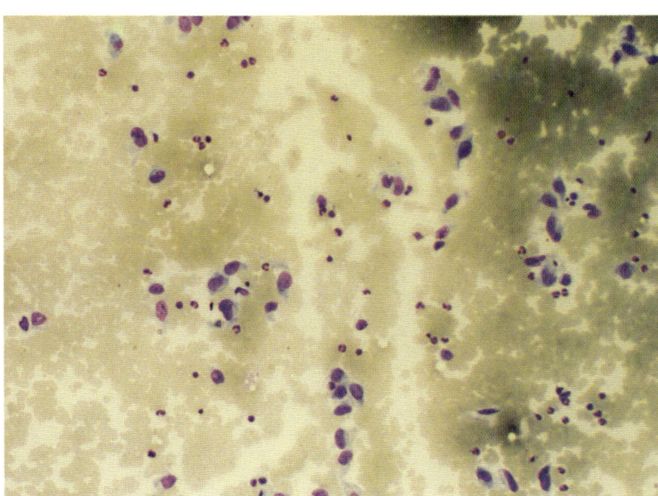

Fig. 30.18: Angiosarcoma: Discrete oval to spindle cells (MGG × MP).

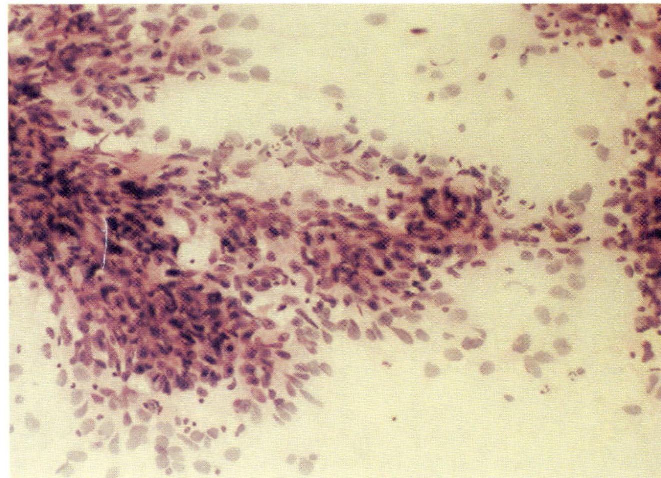

Fig. 30.19: Angiosarcoma: Perivascular arrangement of oval to spindle-shaped tumor cells (H & E × HP).

Box 30.11: Hepatoblastoma.

Anaplastic:
- Small round cells

Embryonal:
- Sheets, clusters, and rosettes
- Larger than anaplastic type
- Immature cells with high N/C ratio, irregular hyperchromatic nuclei

Fetal:
- Larger than the embryonal cells
- Round to polygonal with well-defined cytoplasmic border
- Round nuclei
- Minimal nuclear pleomorphism
- Finely granular chromatin
- *Mesenchymal components*: Osteoid material or skeletal muscle
- Extramedullary hematopoiesis

Box 30.12: Angiosarcoma.

- Cohesive clusters and discrete cells
- Oval to spindle-shaped nuclei
- Moderate nuclear pleomorphism
- Tumor giant cells
- Cytoplasmic vacuolations

Immunostain: CD31, CD34

Box 30.13: Epithelioid hemangioendothelioma.

- Hypocellular
- Large pleomorphic cells
- Tadpole like cells
- Abundant lacey cytoplasm
- Pleomorphic nuclei with folding
- Intranuclear cytoplasmic inclusions
- Bi- and multinucleated giant cells

Immunostain: CD31, CD34

tail like elongated cytoplasm. The nuclei are moderately pleomorphic with prominent nuclear folding and distinct nucleoli. Intranuclear cytoplasmic inclusions are also seen. In addition, there may be many bi- and multinucleated giant cells.[27]

Metastatic Malignancies

Liver is a highly vascular organ and therefore commonly harbors metastatic tumors. In our institution, more than 90% of FNAC of liver mass are diagnosed as metastatic carcinoma. The common sources of metastasis are from gastrointestinal tract, breast, lung, kidney, gall bladder, and pancreas. Malignant tumors from the adjacent organs such as gall bladder, pancreas, and stomach may directly invade to the liver parenchyma. Sarcomas, melanomas, and lymphomas may also infiltrate in the liver. At times, the metastatic tumors may simulate HCC and pose diagnostic problems.

Cytology (Figs. 30.20 to 30.24): Cytology features of metastatic malignancies depend on the morphology of the primary tumor (Box 30.14). Therefore, a thorough look of the smear by low-power magnification is essential. The study of cell arrangement, overall cell morphology, and background material are helpful.

Adenocarcinoma: FNAC smear of metastatic carcinoma shows clusters and glandular arrangement of cuboidal to columnar epithelial cells. The recognition of such foreign cells is very important to distinguish them from the cells of HCC.

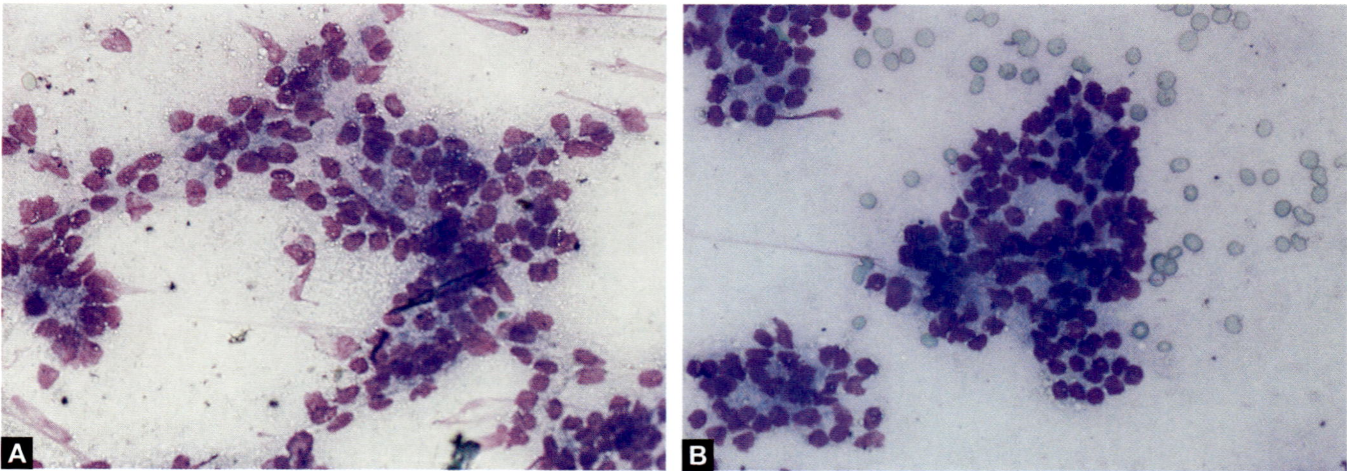

Figs. 30.20A and B: (A) Metastatic adenocarcinoma from prostate: Cluster of malignant cells with gland like structure (MGG × MP). (B) Metastatic adenocarcinoma from prostate: Gland like structure (MGG × MP).

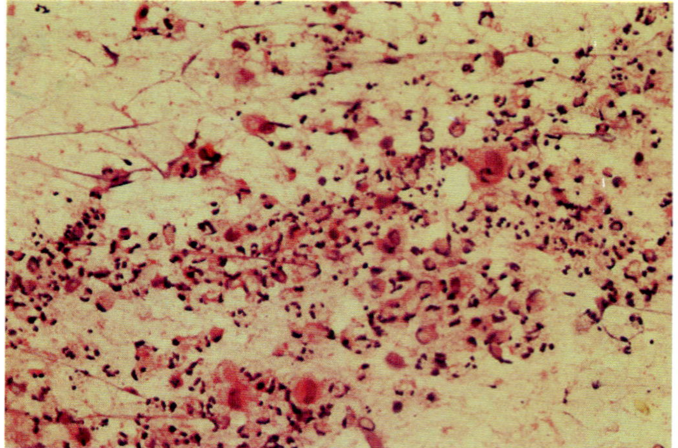

Fig. 30.21: Metastatic signet ring cell carcinoma: Discrete signet ring cells with abundant vacuolated cytoplasm and eccentric signet ring like nuclei. The primary tumor was in stomach (H & E × MP).

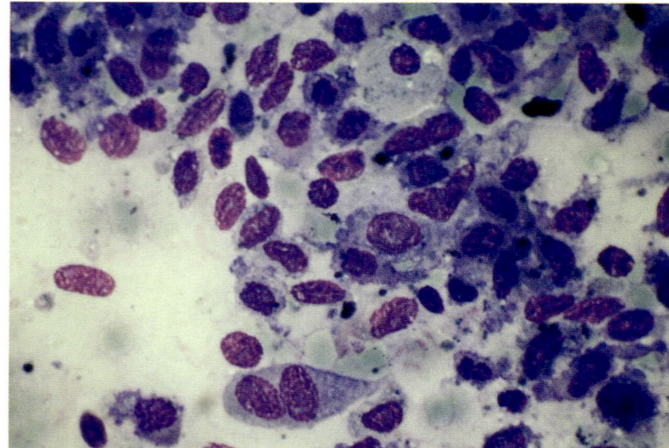

Fig. 30.22: Metastatic malignant melanoma: Discrete melanoma cells with dark-black melanin pigment within the cytoplasm (MGG × OI).

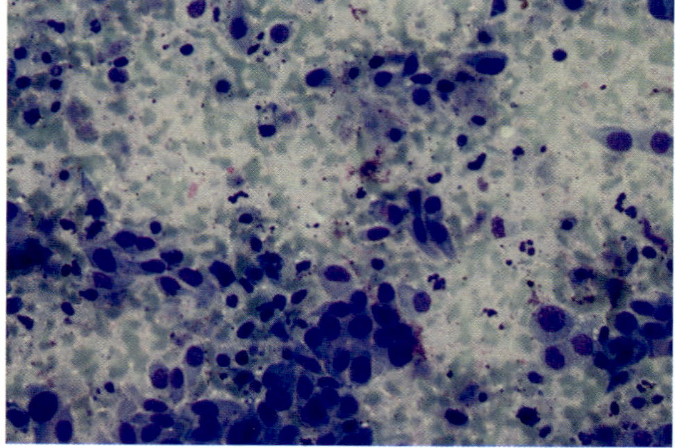

Fig. 30.23: Metastatic transitional cell carcinoma: Discrete cells with elongated cytoplasm and basally placed nuclei (MGG × HP).

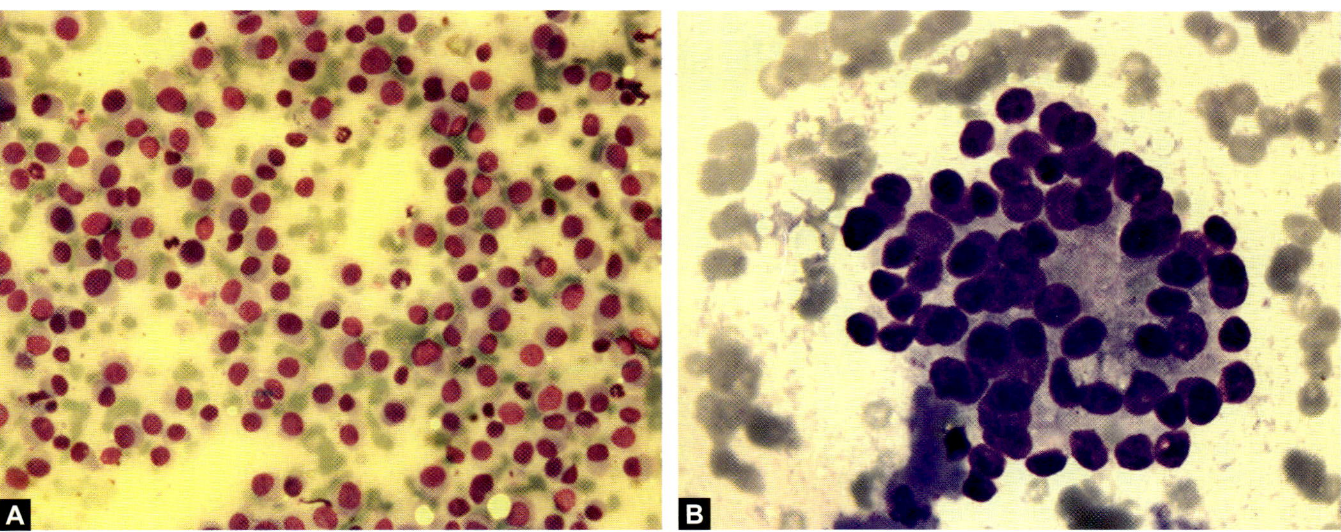

Figs. 30.24A and B: (A) Metastatic neuroendocrine tumor: Loose clusters of round monomorphic cells (MGG × MP). (B) Metastatic neuroendocrine tumor: High-powered view shows rosette-like structure (MGG × HP).

Box 30.14: Metastatic malignancies in liver.

- Cells look foreign to liver
- Glandular arrangement
- Cuboidal to columnar cells
- Benign hepatocytes
- Round moderately pleomorphic nuclei with prominent nucleoli
- Normal alpha-fetoprotein level

The cytological features depend on the type of the metastatic lesions. In case of metastatic adenocarcinoma, the individual cells have scanty to moderately vacuolated cytoplasm. Nuclei are round, moderately pleomorphic having prominent nucleoli. Benign hepatocytes may be admixed with the malignant cells.

Squamous cell carcinoma: FNAC of metastatic squamous cell carcinoma shows oval to polyhedral cells with enlarged hyperchromatic nuclei. Cytoplasmic orangeophilia in Papanicolaou's staining is characteristic of squamous cells. The smears also show fiber cells and tadpole like cells.

Small cell carcinoma: Cytology smears of small cell carcinoma show abundant discrete and loose clusters of small cells slightly larger than lymphocytes. The cells show nuclear molding. Individual cells have scanty cytoplasm and round hyperchromatic nuclei with inconspicuous to absent nucleoli. Crushing artifact may also be seen in the background.

Malignant melanoma: FNAC smears of melanoma may present with variable morphology. The cells are usually round to oval. However, spindle cells may also be seen. The individual cells show moderate to marked nuclear enlargement and pleomorphism. Nucleoli are large and variable sized. Cytoplasmic dark-black melanin pigment indicates the diagnosis of melanoma.

Metastatic neuroendocrine tumors: Neuroendocrine tumors from pancreas or other part of the gastrointestinal tract often metastasize in the liver. The malignant cells are usually monomorphic with round regular nuclei and scanty cytoplasm. Pseudorosettes are also seen.

Differential diagnosis:

- Hepatocellular carcinoma.

Malignant Lymphoma

Primary lymphoma of the liver is rare and it is defined as an extranodal lymphoma where the main bulk of the tumor is localized in the liver. However, the secondary lymphoma is not an uncommon entity and 50–60% cases of non-Hodgkin's lymphoma (NHL) involve liver in advanced stage. The primary lymphomas of liver include diffuse large B-cell lymphoma (DLBCL) and Burkitt's lymphoma. Occasionally, mucosa-associated lymphoid tissue (MALT) lymphomas of liver is also described. As the liver involvement is patchy and diffuse in MALT lymphoma, so FNAC may miss such lesion.

SPLEEN

INTRODUCTION

Fine needle aspiration cytology of the spleen is mainly indicated in diagnosis of metastatic carcinoma and lymphomas that cause space-occupying lesion. Occasionally, FNAC of spleen is done in diffuse-infiltrative process such as storage disorder or infective process such as leishmaniasis. Spleen is an extremely vascular organ and therefore FNAC of this organ is not free from complications. The major complication of FNAC is hemorrhage followed by shock. If small-bore needle is used (22-gauge) and the procedure is rapidly done under USG guidance then no serious complications are encountered. In our institution, we routinely perform FNAC of the spleen and fortunately we did not face any serious complication.

NON-NEOPLASTIC PROCESS

Granulomatous Infection

Tuberculosis is one of the most common causes of granulomatous inflammation of spleen. Multiple epithelioid cell granulomas, multinucleated giant cells, and necrosis are common findings.

Sarcoidosis of spleen shows noncaseating granulomatous inflammation and on FNAC smear, it is not possible to diagnose sarcoidosis.

Large variety of fungi may be present in splenic aspirate (Fig. 30.25). The fungal infections may show granulomatous inflammation. The smears show typical fungal profile along with epithelioid cell granuloma, eosinophils, and multinucleated giant cells.

Storage Disorders

Fine needle aspiration cytology smears of Gaucher's disease show classical large histiocytes with abundant foamy cytoplasm. Biochemical analysis is needed for the confirmation of Niemann-Pick disease.

Neoplasm

Lymphoma

The cytomorphology and the diagnostic criteria of NHL and Hodgkin's lymphoma of the spleen are essentially same as that of noted in lymph nodes (Fig. 30.26). At times, low-grade lymphoma or follicular lymphomas is difficult to diagnose on the FNAC of spleen.

Sarcomas

Rarely, angiosarcoma may occur in spleen. Cytomorphology of this tumor is essentially same as has been described before in connection with liver.

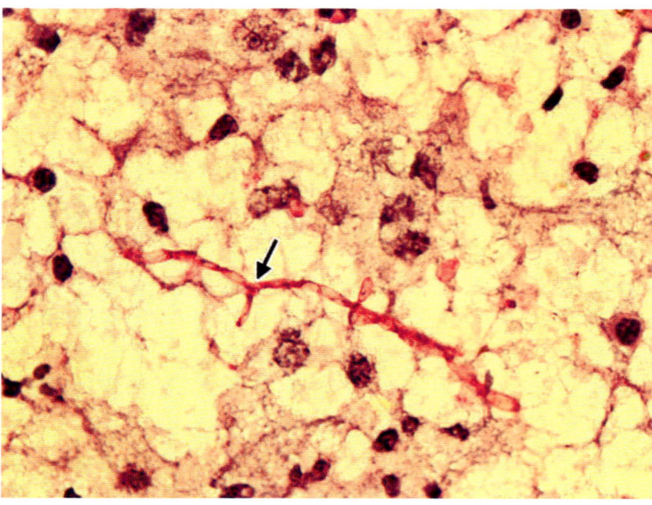

Fig. 30.25: Aspergillus in spleen fine needle aspiration cytology (MGG × HP). Arrow indicates acute angle branching of aspergillus.

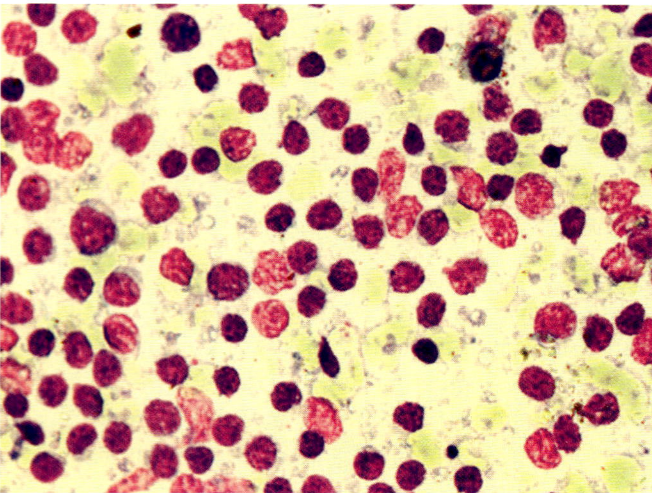

Fig. 30.26: Non-Hodgkin's lymphoma of spleen: Discrete immature lymphoid cells in spleen (MGG × HP).

REFERENCES

1. Dusenbery D, Ferris JV, Thaete FL, et al. Percutaneous ultrasound-guided needle biopsy of hepatic mass lesions using a cytohistologic approach: comparison of two needle types. Am J Clin Pathol. 1995;104:583-7.
2. Edoute Y, Tibon-Fisher O, Ben Haim S, et al. Ultrasonically guided fine needle aspiration of liver lesions. Am J Gastroenterol. 1992;87:1138-41.
3. Sheikh M, Sawhney S, Dey P, et al. Deep-seated thoracic and abdominal masses: Usefulness of ultrasound and computed tomography guidance in fine needle aspiration cytology diagnosis. Australas Radiol. 2000;44:155-60.
4. Hamilton SR, Aaltonen LA. World Health Organization Classification of Tumours. Pathology and Genetics of Tumours of the Digestive System. IARC Press Lyon; 2000.
5. Nguyen BN, Flejou JF, Terris B, et al. Focal nodular hyperplasia of the liver: a comprehensive pathologic study of 305 lesions and recognition of new histologic forms. Am J Surg Pathol. 1999;23:1441-54.
6. Klatskin G. Hepatic tumors: possible relationship to use of oral contraceptive. Gastroenterology. 1977;73:386-94.
7. Kuo FY, Chen WJ, Lu SN, et al. Fine needle aspiration cytodiagnosis of liver tumors. Acta Cytol. 2004;48:142-8.
8. Yang GC, Yang GY, Tao LC. Cytologic features and histologic correlations of microacinar and microtrabecular types of well-differentiated hepatocellular carcinoma in fine needle aspiration biopsy. Cancer. 2004;102:27-33.
9. Das DK. Cytodiagnosis of hepatocellular carcinoma in fine needle aspirates of the liver: its differentiation from reactive hepatocytes and metastatic adenocarcinoma. Diagn Cytopathol. 1999;21:370-7.
10. Yang GC, Yang GY, Tao LC. Distinguishing well-differentiated hepatocellular carcinoma from benign liver by the physical features of fine needle aspirates. Mod Pathol. 2004;17:798-802.
11. Soyuer I, Ekinci C, Kaya M, et al. Diagnosis of hepatocellular carcinoma by fine needle aspiration cytology. Cellular features. Acta Cytol. 2003;47:581-9.
12. Lau SK, Prakash S, Geller SA, et al. Comparative immunohistochemical profile of hepatocellular carcinoma, cholangiocarcinoma, and metastatic adenocarcinoma. Hum Pathol 2002;33:1175-81.
13. Saleh HA, Aulicino M, Zaidi SY, et al. Discriminating hepatocellular carcinoma from metastatic carcinoma on fine-needle aspiration biopsy of the liver: the utility of immunocytochemical panel. Diagn Cytopathol. 2009;37:184-90.
14. Wang L, Vuolo M, Suhrland MJ, et al. HepPar1, MOC-31, pCEA, mCEA and CD10 for distinguishing hepatocellular carcinoma vs. metastatic adenocarcinoma in liver fine needle aspirates. Acta Cytol. 2006;50:257-62.
15. Saad RS, Luckasevic TM, Noga CM, et al. Diagnostic value of HepPar1, pCEA, CD10, and CD34 expression in separating hepatocellular carcinoma from metastatic carcinoma in fine needle aspiration cytology. Diagn Cytopathol. 2004; 30:1-6.
16. Gokden M, Shinde A. Recent immunohistochemical markers in the differential diagnosis of primary and metastatic carcinomas of the liver. Diagn Cytopathol. 2005;33: 166-72.
17. Wee A, Thamboo TP, Thomas A. Alpha-fetoprotein-producing liver carcinomas of primary extrahepatic origin. Acta Cytol. 2003;47:799-808.
18. Siddiqui MT, Saboorian MH, Gokaslan ST, et al. Diagnostic utility of the HepPar1 antibody to differentiate hepatocellular carcinoma from metastatic carcinoma in fine needle aspiration samples. Cancer Cytopathol. 2001;96:49-52.
19. Massoll NA, Brown HM. The use of HepPar-1 in distinguishing common and uncommon metastatic liver lesions from hepatocellular carcinoma in fine needle aspiration. Mod Pathol. 2002;15:80A.
20. Gokden M, Shinde A. Recent immunohistochemical markers in the differential diagnosis of primary and metastatic carcinomas of the liver. Diagn Cytopathol. 2005;33:166-72.
21. Weinberg CD, Ranchod M. Thorotrast induced hepatic cholangiocarcinoma and angiosarcoma. Hum Pathol. 1979; 10:108-12.
22. Stroescu C, Herlea V, Dragnea A, et al. The diagnostic value of cytokeratins and carcinoembryonic antigen immunostaining in differentiating hepatocellular carcinomas from intrahepatic cholangiocarcinomas. J Gastrointestin Liver Dis. 2006;15:9-14.
23. Jain R, Jain M. Mixed hepatoblastoma diagnosed by fine needle aspiration biopsy cytology: a case report. Diagn Cytopathol. 1998;19:306-8.
24. Dekmezian R, Sneige N, Popok S, et al. Fine needle aspiration cytology of pediatric patients with primary hepatic tumors: a comparative study of two hepatoblastomas and a liver-cell carcinoma. Diagn Cytopathol. 1988; 4:162-8.
25. Jain BL, Mathur DR, Vyas MC, et al. Cytologic diagnosis of hepatoblastoma by fine needle aspiration biopsy cytology. Acta Cytol. 1997;41:1858-60.
26. Iyer VK, Kapila K, Agarwala S, et al. Fine needle aspiration cytology of hepatoblastoma. Recognition of subtypes on cytomorphology. Acta Cytol. 2005;49:355-64.
27. Cho NH, Lee KG, Jeong MG. Cytologic evaluation of primary malignant vascular tumors of the liver. One case each of angiosarcoma and epithelioid hemangioendothelioma. Acta Cytol. 1997;41:1468-76.

Review Questions

1. A 35-year-old male presented with loss of weight and malaise for 25-day's duration. USG detected single 4 cm space occupying lesion in right lobe of liver. Figures 30.27A to D show the FNAC smear of the mass.

a. What is your possible diagnosis?
   a. Metastatic adenocarcinoma
   b. Metastatic neuroendocrine tumor
   c. Cirrhosis of liver
   d. Hepatocellular carcinoma

b. What markers in the blood may be helpful in this case?

2. A 48-year-old male presented with pain upper abdomen. USG showed multiple 3-cm diameter space occupying lesions in the right lobe of liver. Figures 30.28A to D show the FNAC smear of the mass.

a. What is your possible diagnosis?
   a. Hepatocellular carcinoma
   b. Angiosarcoma
   c. Cirrhosis of liver
   d. Metastatic carcinoma

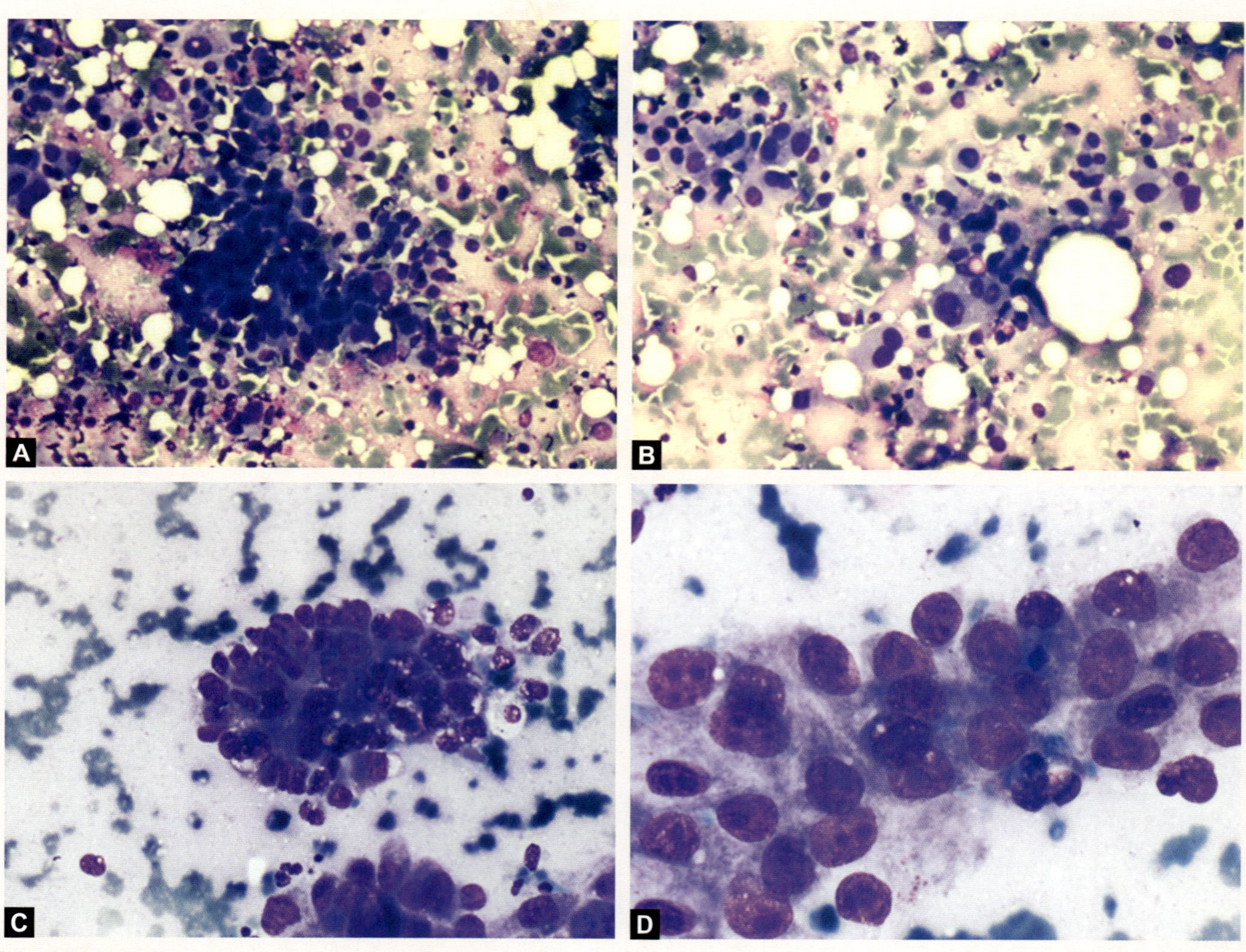

Figs. 30.27A to D: Cytology smear of the case of question 1.

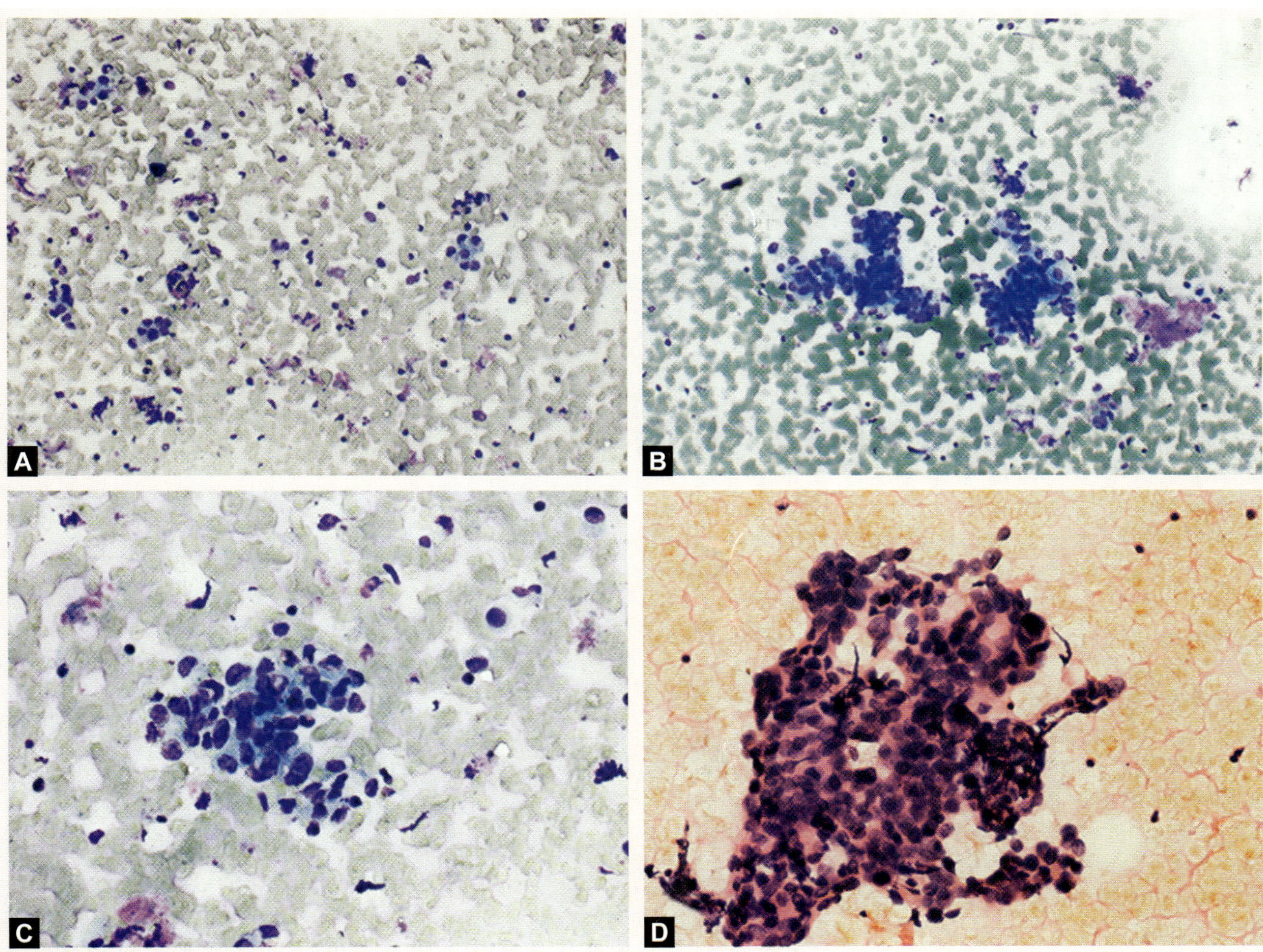

Figs. 30.28A to D: Cytology smear of the case of question 2.

Answers

1. a. Answer is (d) Hepatocellular carcinoma
   b. Markers:
      - Alpha feto protein level in serum
      - HbsAg positivity
      - High Des-gamma-carboxy prothrombin (DCP)

   Note: The presence of discrete and loos clusters of malignant cells, trabecular and acinar pattern along with polyhedral shape and moderately pleomorphic nuclei, favour the diagnosis of hepatocellular carcinoma.

2. d. Metastatic carcinoma

   Note: The smear shows discrete round cells with glandular arrangement (Fig. 30.28C). The cells are round with scanty cytoplasm and enlarged pleomorphic nuclei. The cytological features indicate metastatic carcinoma.

CHAPTER 31 Pancreas

INTRODUCTION

This is the retroperitoneal organs with both endocrine and exocrine glands. Most of the space occupying lesions in the pancreas are malignant in nature. In addition, various imaging technologies such as computed tomography (CT) scan, ultrasonography (USG) and magnetic resonance imaging (MRI) provide important information on the location, extent and nature of the lesion. However, many times a chronic inflammatory reaction in the pancreas is difficult to differentiate from a malignant tumor, even after open surgical exploration. Fine needle aspiration cytology (FNAC) is very helpful in confirming or excluding a malignant tumor of pancreas. FNAC, in fact, has little contribution in the early diagnosis of pancreatic carcinoma. It just helps to confirm the malignant nature of the lesion and prevents unnecessary surgical exploration. Rarely, FNAC diagnosis of a benign lesion may help the patient immensely. In case of pancreatic pseudocyst FNAC is both a diagnostic and therapeutic procedure. Occasionally during endoscopic-guided FNAC of the pancreas the stent can be inserted in the stenotic duct in the same sitting after FNAC of the tumor.

Fine needle aspiration cytology of pancreas can be done by: (1) USG guidance, (2) CT scan guidance, and (3) Endoscopic ultrasound-guided-FNAC (EUS-FNAC) guidance. The material from the lesion can also be procured during endoscopic retrograde cholangiopancreatography (ERCP) or brushing the biliary tract.[1-3]

Transabdominal USG guidance FNAC is easy to perform and a rapid technique. The tip of the needle is also visible in real time. The major disadvantage is the reduction of visibility in case of fatty patient and by the abdominal bowel gas. In contrast CT-guided FNAC provides better visualization than USG.

Endoscopic ultrasound-guided-fine needle aspiration cytology is a relative newer technique that can be performed endoscopically by inserting high frequency ultrasound probe and needle within the gastrointestinal tract.[4] EUS-FNAC is a reliable diagnostic test for the diagnosis and grading of malignant tumor. EUS-FNAC is a cheap and less risky, technique of getting material from the small pancreatic lesion.

Echoendoscope has a transducer attached in anterior to the optic lens. A *radial scanning* echoendoscope gives a 360° view and a *liner array* echoendoscope produces an oblique 100° range real-time view. The later one is preferable for FNAC. Tumor as less as 5 mm diameter can be detected by echoendoscopy and FNAC can be done by this technique.

Overall sensitivity and specificity of pancreatic FNAC are as high as 90% and 100%, respectively.[5-9] The false-negative cytology is due to sampling error. This may happen in very small lesion, fibrotic lesion or sampling from the necrotic area of the tumor. Interpretation error giving rise to false-negative cytology mainly occurs in well-differentiated pancreatic carcinoma. False-positive cytology rarely happens in pancreatic FNAC.

The complications of FNAC are rare if thin needle of 21- or 22-gauge is used. Minor complications such as pain, small hemorrhage and vasovagal attack are known. The major complications of pancreatic FNAC include massive hemorrhage and pancreatitis. We routine use FNAC of pancreas in our institution and have never faced severe pancreatitis after FNAC.

NORMAL ANATOMY AND HISTOLOGY

Pancreas is situated in upper part of the abdomen behind the peritoneum. It has four parts: (1) uncinate process, (2) head, (3) body, and (4) tail part. Pancreas is composed of both exocrine and endocrine glands. The exocrine part of the pancreas consists of lobules that are made of bunches of acini. The acini are connected to the small ducts and these ducts communicate with each other to form larger ducts. The acini are lined by cells with abundant granular

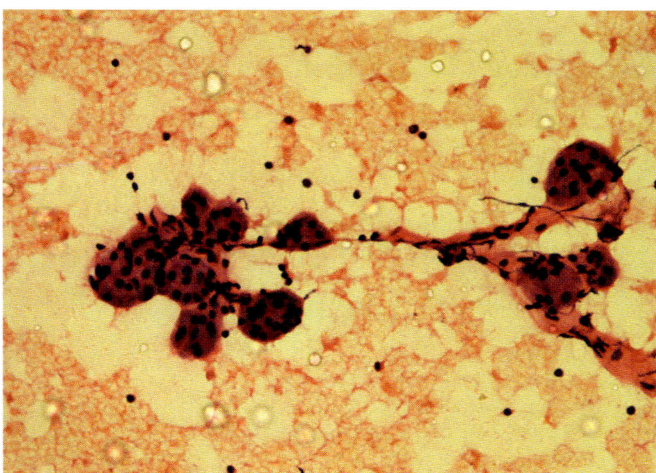

Fig. 31.1: Pancreatic acinar cells: Multiple clusters of cells with abundant cytoplasm and round central nuclei (H & E × MP).

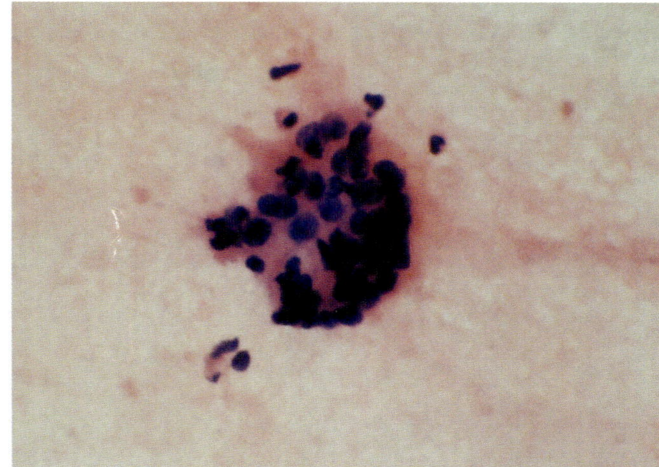

Fig. 31.2: Pancreatic ductular cells: Tight clusters of cells with scanty cytoplasm and round nuclei (H & E × MP).

Box 31.1: Pancreatic acinar cells.

- Acinar arrangement
- Ill-defined border
- Abundant granular cytoplasm
- Small round bland nucleus.

cytoplasm and small monomorphic round nuclei. The ducts are lined by flattened to cuboidal epithelium depending on the size of the ducts. The acini secrete many digestive enzymes that include pancreatic amylase, pancreatic lipase, trypsinogen, chymotrypsinogen, procarboxypeptidase, elastase, etc. The endocrine pancreas is composed of spherical aggregates of endocrine cells that are commonly known as Islets of Langerhans. These are small polyhedral cell arranged in small nests. The endocrine cells are dispersed throughout the entire pancreas, however, they are more concentrated in body and tail region of the pancreas. There are several types of islet cells based on the hormone production: (1) alpha cells: secretes glucagon, (2) beta cells: insulin, (3) delta cells: somatostatin, (4) G cell: gastrin, (5) enterochromaffin cells: 5-hydroxytryptamine, and (6) pancreatic polypeptide cells: pancreatic polypeptide.

NORMAL CELLS

Pancreatic Acinar Cells

Pancreatic acinar cells are commonly present in small acinar-like structures or in loose cohesion (Fig. 31.1). The cells are large with indistinct cell border having abundant and granular cytoplasm (Box 31.1). The nuclei are round and monomorphic with granular chromatin and inconspicuous nucleoli.

Ductular Cells (Fig. 31.2)

The pancreatic ductular cells are present in small clusters and in monolayered sheets. The cells are round with scanty cytoplasm having monomorphic small round nuclei with fine granular chromatin and small nucleoli.

CYSTS OF PANCREAS

Pancreatic cysts may be: acquired or congenital. The acquired cysts may be benign or malignant.

Congenital Cyst

These are benign cysts and rarely found in the pancreas. Benign cysts are commonly associated with inherited polycystic disease. FNAC yields clear fluid and smears are usually paucicellular. Occasional clusters of benign columnar cells are seen.

Acquired Cysts

Pancreatic Pseudocyst

Pseudocyst of the pancreas is a benign acquired cyst. This occurs after an acute bout of pancreatitis or reflux of bile from the biliary tree to pancreatic duct. This causes leakage of bile from the pancreatic duct and accumulation of secretion resulting in cyst formation. The patient presents with pain abdomen, nausea, vomiting and jaundice.

Box 31.2: Pseudocyst: cytology.

- Foamy histiocytes
- Polymorphs and lymphocytes
- Fibroblasts
- Reactive mesothelial cells
- Absent epithelial cells.

Box 31.4: Pancreatic serous cystadenoma.

- Clear, watery fluid
- Bland looking round to polygonal cells
- Scanty to moderate cytoplasm
- Bland, round monomorphic nuclei.

Cytology: Fine needle aspiration cytology of pseudocyst has therapeutic value because the evacuation of the cyst gives immediate symptomatic relief to the patient. FNAC from the cyst yields clear fluid (Box 31.2). The smear shows foamy macrophages, mixed inflammatory cells and spindle-shaped fibroblasts. Characteristically epithelial cells are absent in the smear. The presence of epithelial cells excludes the possibility of pseudocyst. The histiocytes often show multinucleation. In addition the smear may also show mesothelial cells. At times these cells show reactive atypia.

NEOPLASTIC LESION OF PANCREAS

World Health Organization (WHO) classified pancreatic neoplasm as epithelial, nonepithelial and metastatic tumors.[10] The simplified version of the classification is shown in Box 31.3.

Box 31.3: World Health Organization (WHO) classification of pancreatic tumors.[10]

- Benign:
  - Serous cystadenoma
  - Mucinous cystadenoma
  - Intraductal papillary mucinous adenoma
- Borderline:
  - Mucinous cystic neoplasm with moderate dysplasia
  - Intraductal papillary mucinous neoplasm with moderate dysplasia
  - Solid pseudopapillary neoplasm
- Malignant:
  - Ductal adenocarcinoma
  - Serous cystadenocarcinoma
  - Mucinous cystadenocarcinoma
  - Intraductal papillary mucinous carcinoma
  - Acinar cell carcinoma
  - Acinar cell cystadenocarcinoma
  - Mixed acinar-endocrine carcinoma
  - Pancreatoblastoma
  - Solid pseudopapillary carcinoma
- Nonepithelial tumors
- Metastatic tumors.

Serous Cystadenoma

Serous cystadenomas are rare tumor and represents only 1% of the pancreatic exocrine tumors. The tumor predominantly occurs in female with a mean age of 66 years. Serous cystadenomas commonly presents as large cystic mass in the body and tail of the pancreas.

Cytology

Fine needle aspiration cytology of the cyst yields clear thin fluid. The smear shows small clusters and monolayered flat sheets of cells. The cells have scanty to moderate cytoplasm with monomorphic round nuclei (Box 31.4). The nuclei show fine chromatin and inconspicuous nucleoli.[11]

Mucinous Cystic Neoplasia[12,13]

Mucinous cystic neoplasia (MCN) is a very rare lesion in the pancreas and accounts for 2–3% of exocrine pancreatic tumors. This is usually seen in young to middle-aged patients. The tumor may present as small 2–3 cm D cyst to large more than 8 cm cyst. The vast majority of the tumors occur in the body and tail of the pancreas. CT scan of the tumors shows thick-walled multiloculated cystic mass.

Cytology (Figs. 31.3 and 31.4)

Fine needle aspiration cytology of MCN yields thick mucinous material. The smears show abundant mucin along with cohesive cells arranged in monolayered sheets, small tight clusters and papillae-like fashion. Small loosely cohesive cells may be present as freely floating on the mucinous background (Box 31.5). The epithelial cells have moderate to abundant vacuolated cytoplasm resembling benign endocervical cells. The nuclei are eccentrically placed with varying degree of atypia. In case of borderline MCN the nuclei are enlarged and show mild to moderate pleomorphism. Free floating goblet cells may also be seen.

CARCINOMA

Ductal Adenocarcinoma[7,8,14-16]

Ductal adenocarcinoma accounts for 85–90% of all pancreatic neoplasm. This tumor exclusively occurs in elderly patient and rarely seen under the age of 40 years. Majority of the carcinomas (60–70%) are present in the head of the pancreas. Pancreatic ductal adenocarcinoma

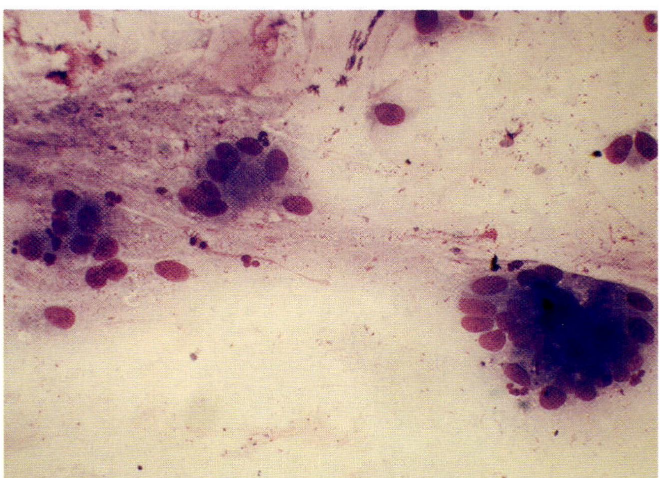

Fig. 31.3: Mucinous cystic neoplasm: Small tight clusters of cells embedded in thick mucinous material (MGG × HP).

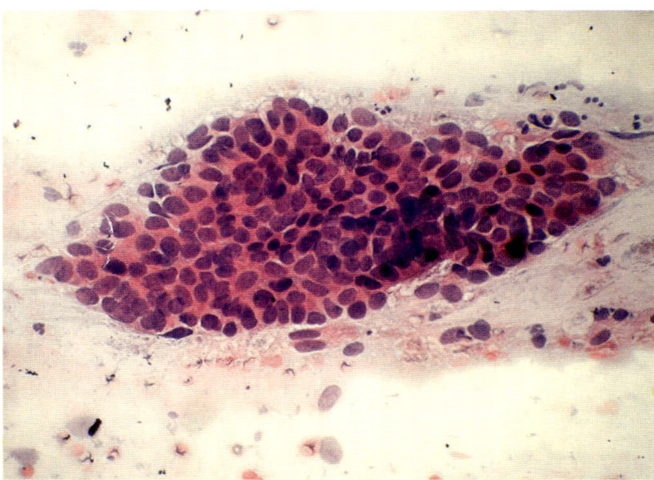

Fig. 31.4: Mucinous cystic neoplasm: Cells with moderate amount of cytoplasm and mildly pleomorphic nuclei (H & E × HP).

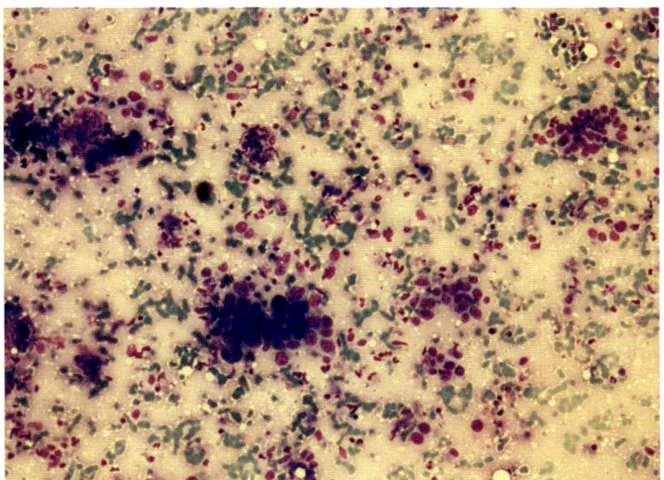

Fig. 31.5: Ductal adenocarcinoma: Multiple loose clusters and discrete malignant cells (MGG × MP).

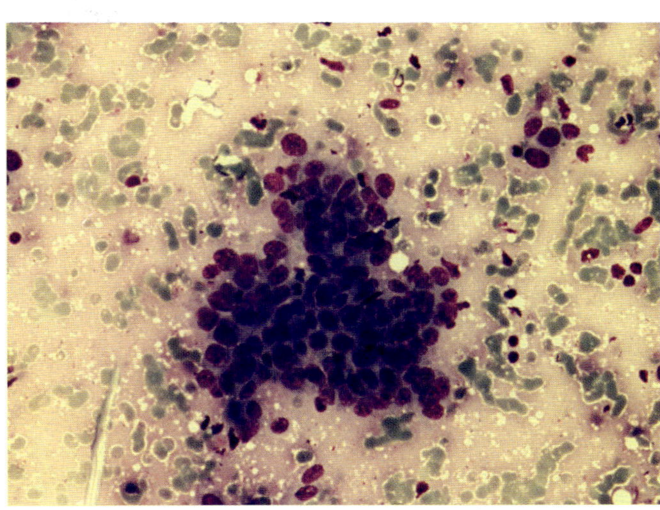

Fig. 31.6: Ductal adenocarcinoma: Cells with nuclear overlapping (MGG × HP).

Box 31.5: Mucinous cystic neoplasia.

- Thick mucinous material
- Cells arranged in monolayered sheets, small tight clusters and papillae
- Cell with moderate cytoplasm
- Cytoplasmic vacuolations
- Monomorphic nuclei in benign mucinous cystic neoplasia (MCN).

is strongly related with cigarette smoking. There is also association of ductal adenocarcinoma of pancreas and intake of diet low in fiber and high in meat. The patient presents with the classical triad of symptoms: jaundice, pain and weight loss.

Cytology (Figs. 31.5 to 31.8)

Fine needle aspiration cytology smears show multiple cohesive clusters, monolayer flat sheets and microglandular pattern of tumor cells. The smears also show many dissociated single cells (Box 31.6). The clusters of cells show nuclear overlapping and crowding. Nuclear crowding indicates loss of polarity and this is one of the important diagnostic features of pancreatic adenocarcinoma. The malignant cells show scanty cytoplasm in nonsecretary carcinomas and moderately vacuolated cytoplasm in secretary (mucinous) carcinoma. The nuclei show moderate pleomorphism with irregular nuclear contour. Nucleoli are prominent. Multivariate logistic-regression analysis of

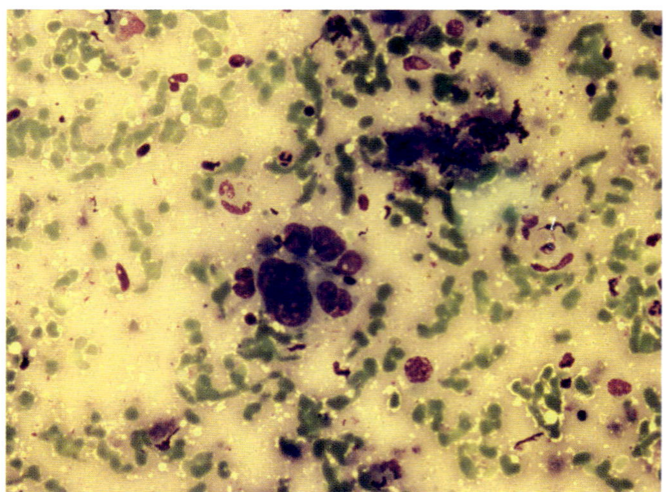

Fig. 31.7: Ductal adenocarcinoma: Nuclear margin irregularity (MGG × HP).

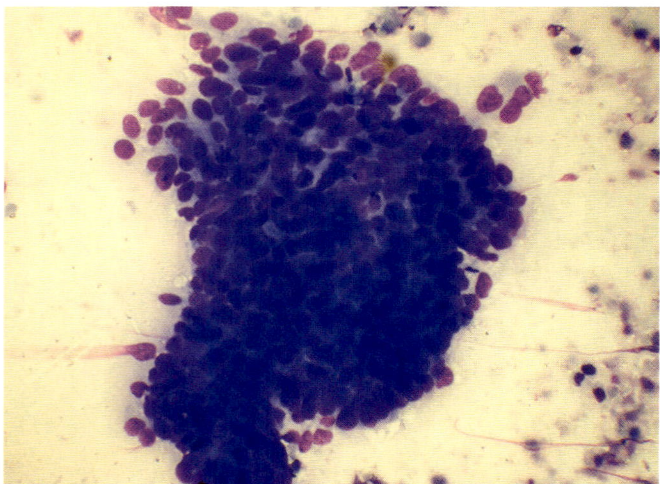

Fig. 31.8: Ductal adenocarcinoma: Large three-dimensional clusters (MGG × HP).

Box 31.6: Adenocarcinoma of pancreas.

- Three-dimensional clusters of cells
- Nuclear overcrowding
- Single discrete cells
- Microacini
- Absence of normal acinar and ductal cells
- Round to oval cells, scanty to moderate cytoplasm
- Anisonucleosis
- Nuclear contour irregularity
- Prominent nucleoli.

FNAC of pancreatic carcinoma shows:[17]

- *Three major criteria*:
  - Three-dimensional clusters with loss of polarity of the cells
  - Irregular chromatin distribution
  - Nuclear margin irregularity.
- *Four minor criteria*:
  - Nuclear enlargement
  - Single epithelial cells
  - Necrosis, and
  - Mitoses.

Definitive Diagnosis

- Two major and one minor or
- One major and two minor criteria.

Fine needle aspiration cytology diagnosis of moderate and poorly differentiated adenocarcinoma is usually straightforward. It is difficult to diagnose a well-differentiated adenocarcinoma of pancreas. Lin and Staerkel. noted that features such as anisonucleosis, nuclear membrane irregularity, nuclear crowding/overlapping/three-dimensional clusters, and nuclear enlargement are the most important criteria to diagnose well-differentiated pancreatic adenocarcinoma.[14]

Table 31.1: Chronic pancreatitis versus adenocarcinoma of pancreas.

Features	*Adenocarcinoma*	*Chronic pancreatitis*
Nuclear crowding and polarity	Nuclear overlapping and loss of polarity	Usually maintained polarity
Microacini	Many	Occasional to absent
Discrete cells	Many	Scanty to absent
Nuclear pleomorphism	Moderate to marked	Mild
Nuclear margin	Irregular	Regular
Nucleoli	Prominent, often large	Inconspicuous

Differential Diagnosis

- *Chronic pancreatitis*: Cells of chronic pancreatitis may often show nuclear atypia. The cytological features such as nuclear crowding, anisonucleosis, nuclear margin irregularities and altered nucleocytoplasmic ratio favor the diagnosis of adenocarcinoma (Table 31.1).
- *Well-differentiated adenocarcinoma*: It is often difficult to distinguish well-differentiated adenocarcinoma from normal pancreatic aspirate. However, nuclear crowding, nuclear margin irregularity, chromatin abnormality and nucleolar prominence favor the diagnosis of well-differentiated adenocarcinoma.

Variants of Ductal Carcinoma

Osteoclastic Giant Cell Carcinoma

The tumor shows multiple multinucleated osteoclast-like giant cells with bland looking nuclei.

Anaplastic Carcinoma (Fig. 31.9)

Anaplastic carcinoma is also known as giant cell carcinoma or sarcomatoid carcinoma. This tumor represents 2.7% of ductal carcinomas. The prognosis of this tumor is bad. The aspirates show many large bizarre multinucleated giant cells, large pleomorphic epithelial cells and spindle cells. The cells are present in loose clusters or discretely. The background of the smear shows blood, necrosis and inflammatory cells. Small foci of glandular differentiation may also be noted.[18]

Differential diagnosis: Malignant melanoma, pleomorphic sarcoma.

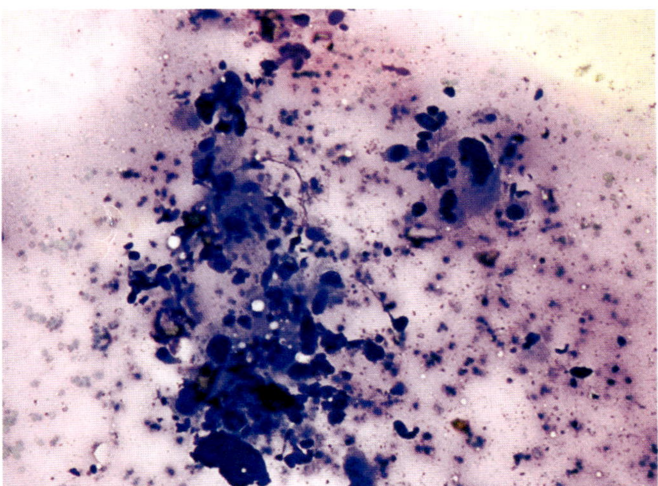

Fig. 31.9: Anaplastic carcinoma: Loose clusters of pleomorphic cells (MGG × HP).

Small Cell Carcinoma

This is an extremely rare carcinoma of pancreas and represents less than 1% of pancreatic malignancies. On cytomorphology this tumor simulates small cell carcinoma of lung. FNAC smear shows discrete small cells with scanty cytoplasm, small hyperchromatic nuclei and nuclear molding. In fact, before diagnosis of such tumor in pancreas, metastatic small cell carcinoma should be excluded.

Adenosquamous Carcinoma

Adenosquamous carcinoma is a rare neoplasm and represents only 3–4% of exocrine pancreatic malignancies.[19] The tumor contains both the glandular elements and squamous components. The cell with glandular differentiation shows abundant intracellular mucin with vacuolated cytoplasm and eccentric nuclei. The squamous cells are oval to polyhedral with hyperchromatic nuclei. Tadpole cells are also seen. Intracellular keratinization may be seen in Papanicolaou's staining. The dual differentiation may be focal and may be overlooked in FNAC smears. In the absence of any squamoid cells the tumor may be diagnosed as poorly differentiated carcinoma.[20]

Signet Ring Carcinoma

This is an extremely uncommon carcinoma of pancreas. Cytology smears show freely floating cells in the pool of mucus. The individual cells have abundant vacuolated cytoplasm with eccentric nuclei. Metastatic signet ring carcinoma from the stomach should be excluded before the diagnosis primary signet ring cell carcinoma of pancreas.

Pancreatic Acinar Carcinoma[21]

Acinar cell carcinoma of the pancreas is a rare tumor and comprises less than 2% of the exocrine pancreatic neoplasm. This tumor exhibits phenotypic and immunohistochemical evidence of acinar cell differentiation. It is usually seen in adult male. The neoplasm bears a poor prognosis, and 5 year survival rate is less than 10%.[22]

Cytology (Figs. 31.10 and 31.11): Fine needle aspiration cytology smears are richly cellular and the cells show a combination of loose clusters and single cells. Acinar formation is characteristically present and the tumor cells resemble normal pancreatic acinar cells. The cells are large and polygonal with granular cytoplasm (Box 31.7). Cytoplasmic granularity is one of the important characteristic features of this tumor. The nuclei are centrally placed mildly pleomorphic round nuclei with smooth nuclear contour. Chromatin is clumped and prominent nucleoli are present.[23]

Differential diagnosis:

- Islet cell tumor
- Solid pseudopapillary tumors.

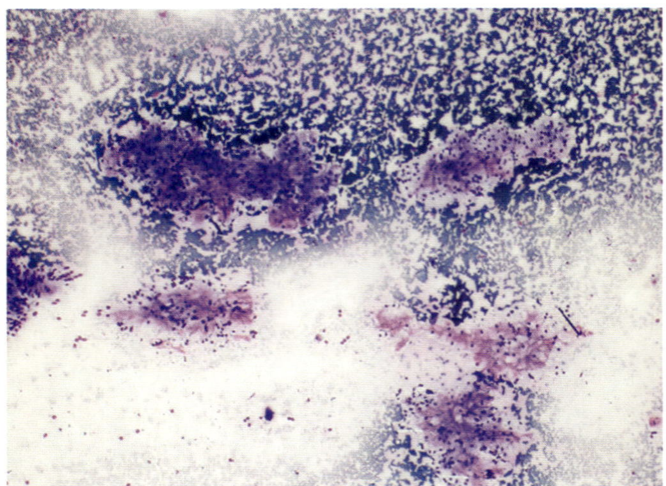

Fig. 31.10: Pancreatic acinar carcinoma: Loose clusters of cells resembling pancreatic acinar cells (H & E × MP).

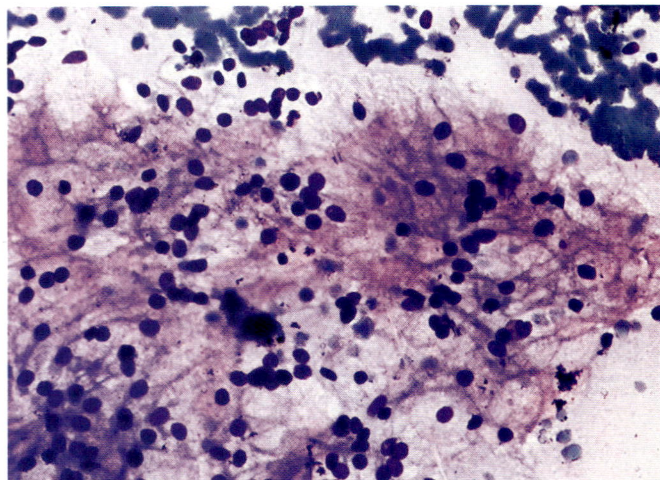

Fig. 31.11: Pancreatic acinar carcinoma: Large polygonal cells with granular cytoplasm having enlarged nuclei (MGG × HP).

Box 31.7: Acinar cell carcinoma.

- Loose clusters and discrete cells
- Polygonal cells
- Abundant granular cytoplasm
- Monomorphic round nuclei
- Smooth nuclear contour
- Prominent nucleoli.

NEUROENDOCRINE TUMOR

Pancreatic Endocrine Tumor (Islet Cell Tumor of Pancreas)[24-26]

The terminology of "islet cell tumor" has been replaced by pancreatic endocrine tumor (PET).[27] The endocrine tumors of pancreas probably develop from the endocrine cells of the diffuse endocrine system. There are about 15 cell types that produce hormonal peptides or biogenic amines in the pancreas. The recognition of specific tumor cell type needs hormone immunohistochemistry. PET is a relatively uncommon tumor and represents less than 5% of all pancreatic tumors. The tumors typically occur in adults, however, the children may also be affected by this tumor. PET arises more commonly in body and tail of the pancreas.

The hormonally active or functional PET may secrete various hormones depending on the tumor of the particular type of endocrine cells. The patient may present with severe hypoglycemia in case of insulinoma, peptic ulcer in case of gastrinoma, watery diarrhea in case of vasoactive intestinal polypeptide-producing tumor. Nonfunctioning tumors are asymptomatic and are detected incidentally.

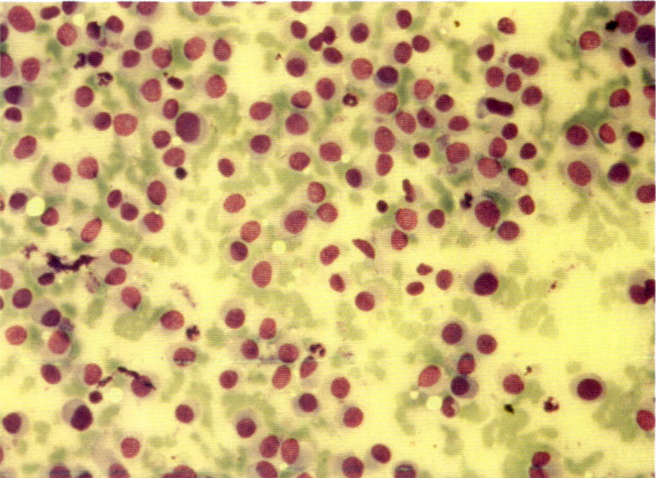

Fig. 31.12: Pancreatic endocrine tumor: Dissociated and loose cohesive clusters of cells with monomorphic nuclei (MGG × MP).

The resection of the tumor cures the low stage tumors and therefore accurate FNAC diagnosis of PET is helpful for the patient.

Cytology (Figs. 31.12 to 31.15)

Fine needle aspiration cytology smear shows predominantly dissociated and loose cohesive cells along with trabecular and acinar pattern (Box 31.8). The cells are also arranged along the thin-walled capillaries. The individual cells are small to medium sized with scanty to moderate amount of cytoplasm. The cytoplasmic reddish granularity in May-Grünwald Giemsa (MGG) stained smear is one of the important characteristic features of PET.[28] The nuclei

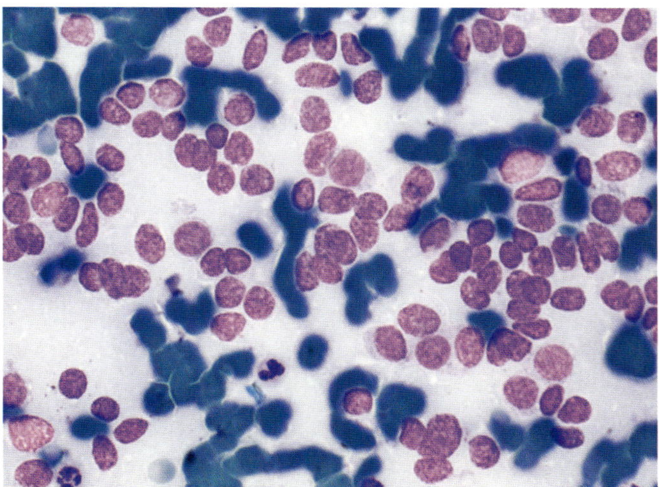

Fig. 31.13: Pancreatic endocrine tumor: Discrete monomorphic cells with salt and pepper chromatin (MGG × HP).

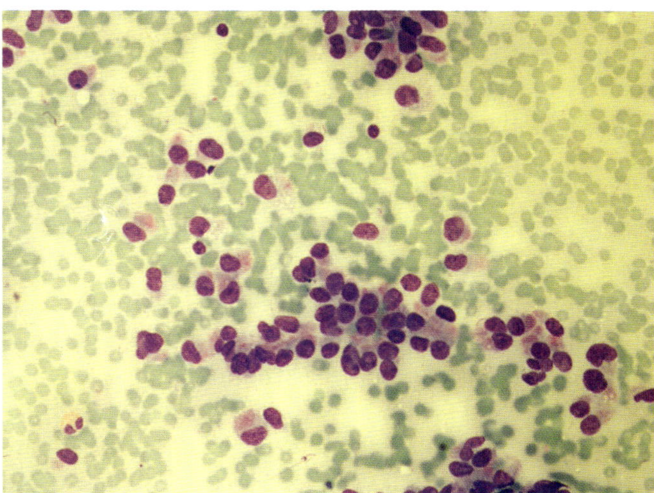

Fig. 31.14: Pancreatic endocrine tumor metastasized in liver: Discrete cells with mild pleomorphism having abundant reddish cytoplasm. No characteristic feature of malignancy is seen (MGG × MP).

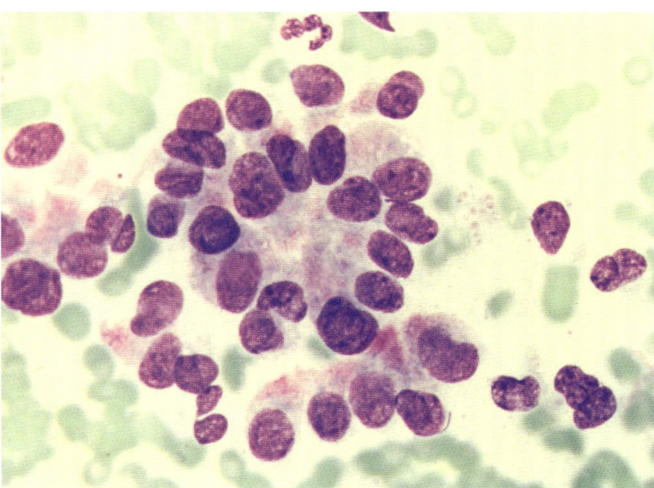

Fig. 31.15: Pancreatic endocrine tumor metastasized in liver: Higher magnification showing better morphology of the cells. Rosette-like structure is also seen (MGG × MP).

are central to eccentric in position, round monomorphic and often show binucleation. The nuclear chromatin shows characteristic salt and pepper appearance. The nucleoli are usually inconspicuous. However, occasional prominent nucleoli may be seen. Nuclear pleomorphism and mitotic activity may also be noted and these features are present both in benign and malignant PET. On cytology smear, it is not possible to differentiate benign from malignant PET.

Immunocytochemistry

The tumors are positive for neuron-specific enolase (NSE), chromogranin A and synaptophysin.

Box 31.8: Pancreatic endocrine tumor.

- Dissociated cells
- Loose clusters and acinar arrangement
- Round cells with moderate fine reddish granular cytoplasm
- Central to eccentric, monomorphic nuclei
- Salt and pepper chromatin.

Differential Diagnosis

- *Solid and cystic papillary neoplasm*: Cytology smears of solid and cystic papillary neoplasm (SCPN) often simulate PET as both the tumors show monomorphic round cells. However, the typical young female, radiological appearance of solid and cystic components and the presence of papillae and macrophages favor the diagnosis of SCPN of pancreas.
- *Well-differentiated adenocarcinoma*: Cells in PET are usually discrete and have reddish granular cytoplasm. In contrast, well-differentiated pancreatic adenocarcinoma shows cluster of cells with scanty nongranular cytoplasm. Nuclear chromatin of these cells is fine with prominent nucleoli (Table 31.2).

Solid and Cystic Papillary Neoplasm of Pancreas[29-31]

This is a relatively uncommon tumor and represents only 1–2% pancreatic tumors. The other name of this tumor is solid pseudopapillary tumor. This tumor characteristically occurs in young female. USG and CT scan of SCPN shows a multilocular cystic mass having both solid and fluid-filled cystic components. The radiologic features are quite suggestive of SCPN in a proper clinical setting.[32] The tumor has low malignant potentiality and most of the patients have a prolonged survival after adequate local surgery.[33]

Cytology (Figs. 31.16 to 31.20)

The cytology smears of SCPN show papillae-like structures, pseudopapillae, and discrete cells (Box 31.9). The branching papillary fronds or pseudopapillae are made of central thin fibrovascular stalks lined by one to more layers of cuboidal tumor cells. The tumor cells are also arranged around the blood vessels. Occasional cases may show acinar or rosettes formation. The discrete cells are monotonous with scanty to moderate cytoplasm and eccentrically placed round nuclei. The cytoplasm is pale or acidophilic and may show vacuolations. The nuclei are monomorphic with fine chromatin having occasional small nucleoli. Nuclear pleomorphism, and grooves of the nuclear membrane have been occasionally described.[34] Degenerative changes such as hyaline droplets or pink cytoplasmic inclusions in MGG stain have also been described. Many foamy macrophages are also noted in the background.

Table 31.2: Pancreatic endocrine tumor versus well-differentiated adenocarcinoma.

Pancreatic endocrine tumor	*Pancreatic well-differentiated adenocarcinoma*
Discrete cells	Clusters and glandular
Moderate amount of reddish granular cytoplasm	Scanty amount of vacuolated cytoplasm
Regular, monomorphic nuclei with salt and pepper chromatin	Irregular and hyperchromatic nuclei with prominent nucleoli
Positive for chromogranin and synaptophysin	Negative for chromogranin and synaptophysin

Immunohistochemistry

Solid and cystic papillary neoplasm shows keratin, vimentin, desmoplakin, trypsin, chymotrypsin, amylase, galectin-3, CD10, and CD56 positivity. The cells also show positivity for NSE and other neuroendocrine markers.

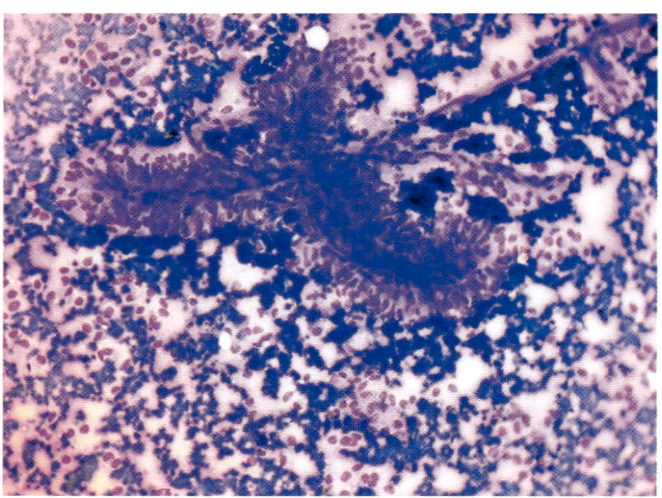

Fig. 31.16: Solid and cystic papillary neoplasm of pancreas: Papillary structure and discrete cells (MGG × MP).

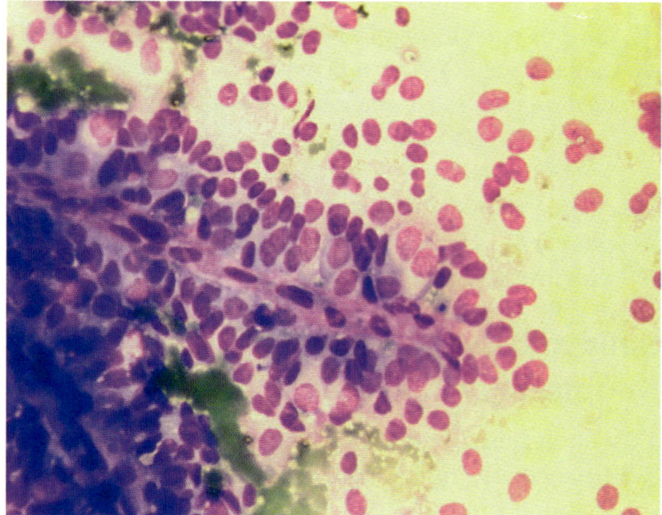

Fig. 31.17: Solid and cystic papillary neoplasm of pancreas: Higher magnification of the papillary structure (MGG × HP).

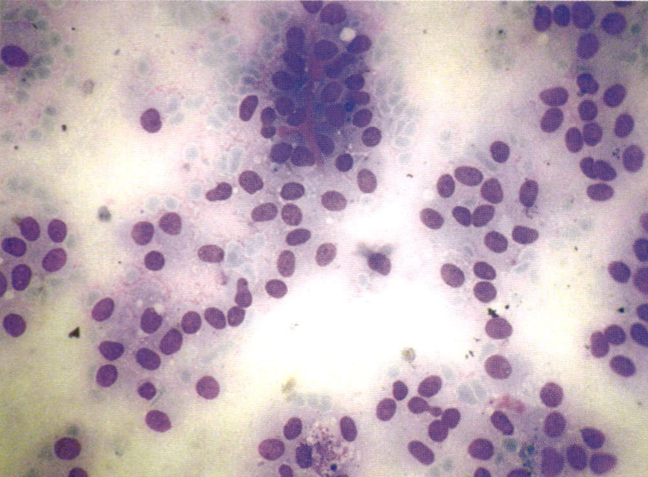

Fig. 31.18: Solid and cystic papillary neoplasm of pancreas: Discrete round monomorphic cells with reddish moderate amount of cytoplasm (MGG × HP).

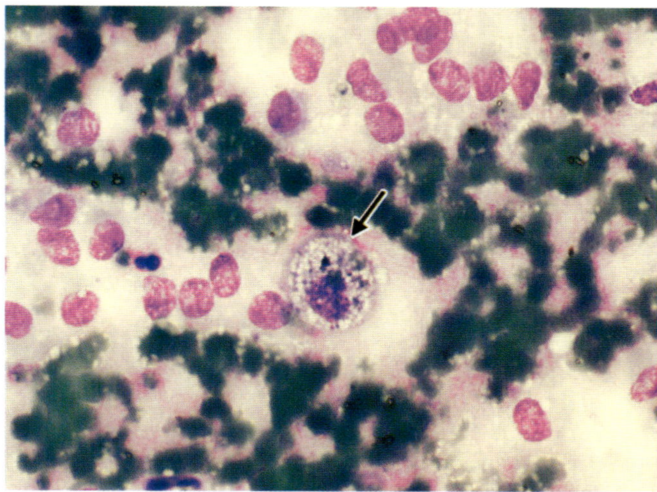

Fig. 31.19: Solid and cystic papillary neoplasm of pancreas: The arrow indicates foamy macrophage in the background (MGG × MP).

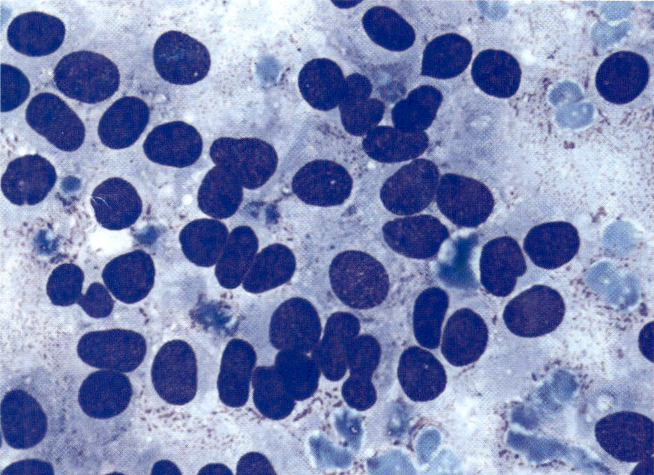

Fig. 31.20: Solid and cystic papillary neoplasm of pancreas: Higher magnification showing better morphology of the cells. Cell shows round nuclei with stippled chromatin and inconspicuous nucleoli (MGG × OI).

Box 31.9: Solid and cystic papillary neoplasm.

- Papillae with fibrovascular core
- Small round cells
- Scanty to moderate cytoplasm
- Eccentric nucleus
- Fine chromatin
- Nuclear grooves
- Foamy macrophages
- Positive for CD10, NSE and CK.

(CK: Cytokeratin; NSE: Neuron-specific enolase).

Differential Diagnosis

- *Islet cell tumors*: See earlier
- *Papillary carcinoma*: The presence of multiple papillary structures may be confused with that of papillary ductal carcinoma of pancreas. The discrete monomorphic cell component is helpful distinguishing feature.

REFERENCES

1. Palazzo L, Roseau G, Gayet B, et al. Endoscopic ultrasonography in the diagnosis and staging of pancreatic adenocarcinoma. Results of a prospective study with comparison to ultrasonography and CT scan. Endoscopy. 1993;25(2):143-50.
2. Brugge WR. Advances in the endoscopic management of patients with pancreatic and biliary malignancies. South Med J. 2006;99(12):1358-66.
3. Volmar KE, Vollmer RT, Jowell PS, et al. Pancreatic FNA in 1000 cases: a comparison of imaging modalities. Gastrointest Endosc. 2005;61(7):854-61.
4. Bardales RH, Stelow EB, Mallery S, et al. Review of endoscopic ultrasound-guided fine needle aspiration cytology. Diagn Cytopathol. 2006;34(2):140-75.
5. Afify AM, al-Khafaji BM, Kim B, et al. Endoscopic ultrasound-guided fine needle aspiration of the pancreas. Diagnostic utility and accuracy. Acta Cytol. 2003;47(3): 341-8.
6. Di Stasi M, Lencioni R, Solmi L, et al. Ultrasound-guided fine needle biopsy of pancreatic masses: results of a multicenter study. Am J Gastroenterol. 1998;93(8): 1329-33.
7. Lerma E, Musulen E, Cuatrecasas M, et al. Fine needle aspiration cytology in pancreatic pathology. Acta Cytol. 1996; 40(4):683-6.
8. Dey P, Radhika S, Rajwanshi A, et al. Fine needle aspiration biopsy of pancreas. Indian J Pathol Microbiol. 1994; 37(3):269-74.
9. Bret PM, Nicolet V, Labadie M. Percutaneous fine needle aspiration biopsy of the pancreas. Diagn Cytopathol. 1986; 2(3):221-7.
10. Hamilton SR, Aaltonen LA. World Health Organization Classification of Tumours. In: Pathology and Genetics of Tumours of the Digestive System. Lyon: IARC Press; 2000.
11. Nguyen GK, Vogelsang PJ. Microcystic adenoma of the pancreas. A report of two cases with fine needle aspiration cytology and differential diagnosis. Acta Cytol. 1993; 37(6):908-12.
12. Gupta RK, Scally J, Stewart RJ. Mucinous cystadenocarcinoma of the pancreas: diagnosis by fine needle aspiration cytology. Diagn Cytopathol. 1989;5(4):408-11.
13. Dodd LG, Farrell TA, Layfield LJ. Mucinous cystic tumor of the pancreas: an analysis of FNA characteristics with an emphasis on the spectrum of malignancy associated features. Diagn Cytopathol. 1995;12(2):113-9.

14. Lin F, Staerkel G. Cytologic criteria for well differentiated adenocarcinoma of the pancreas in fine needle aspiration biopsy specimens. Cancer. 2003;99(1):44-50.
15. Cohen MB, Egerter DP, Holly EA, et al. Pancreatic adenocarcinoma: regression analysis to identify improved cytologic criteria. Diagn Cytopathol. 1991;7(4):341-5.
16. Mitchell ML, Carney CN. Cytologic criteria for the diagnosis of pancreatic carcinoma. Am J Clin Pathol. 1985;83(2):171-6.
17. Robins DB, Katz RL, Evans DB, et al. Fine needle aspiration of the pancreas. In quest of accuracy. Acta Cytol. 1995; 39(1):1-10.
18. Silverman JF, Dabbs DJ, Finley JL, et al. Fine needle aspiration biopsy of pleomorphic (giant cell) carcinoma of the pancreas. Cytologic, immunocytochemical, and ultrastructural findings. Am J Clin Pathol. 1988;89(6):714-20.
19. Chen J, Baithun SI. Morphological study of 391 cases of exocrine pancreatic tumours with special reference to the classification of exocrine pancreatic carcinoma. J Pathol. 1985;146(1):17-29.
20. Rahemtullah A, Misdraji J, Pitman MB. Adenosquamous carcinoma of the pancreas: cytologic features in 14 cases. Cancer. 2003;99(6):372-8.
21. Villanueva RR, Nguyen-Ho P, Nguyen GK. Needle aspiration cytology of acinar-cell carcinoma of the pancreas: report of a case with diagnostic pitfalls and unusual ultrastructural findings. Diagn Cytopathol. 1994;10(4):362-4.
22. Klimstra DS, Heffess CS, Oertel JE, et al. Acinar cell carcinoma of the pancreas. A clinicopathologic study of 28 cases. Am J Surg Pathol. 1992;16(9):815-37.
23. Samuel LH, Frierson HF. Fine needle aspiration cytology of acinar cell carcinoma of the pancreas: a report of two cases. Acta Cytol. 1996;40(3):585-91.
24. Gu M, Ghafari S, Lin F, et al. Cytological diagnosis of endocrine tumors of the pancreas by endoscopic ultrasound-guided fine needle aspiration biopsy. Diagn Cytopathol. 2005;32(4):204-10.
25. Collins BT, Cramer HM. Fine needle aspiration cytology of islet cell tumors. Diagn Cytopathol. 1996;15(1): 37-45.
26. Jiménez-Heffernan JA, Vicandi B, López-Ferrer P, et al. Fine needle aspiration cytology of endocrine neoplasms of the pancreas. Morphologic and immunocytochemical findings in 20 cases. Acta Cytol. 2004;48(3):295-301.
27. Capella C, Heitz PU, Höfler H, et al. Revised classification of neuroendocrine tumors of the lung, pancreas and gut. Virchows Arch. 1995;425:547-60.
28. Leiman G, Mair S. Aspiration cytology of neuroendocrine tumors below the diaphragm. Diagn Cytopathol. 1989;5(3): 263-8.
29. Buchino JJ. Fine needle aspiration of solid and papillary cystic tumor of the pancreas. Pediatr Pathol Lab Med. 1996; 16(2):235-42.
30. Pelosi G, Iannucci A, Zamboni G, et al. Solid and cystic papillary neoplasm of the pancreas: a clinico-cytopathologic and immunocytochemical study of five new cases diagnosed by fine needle aspiration cytology and a review of the literature. Diagn Cytopathol. 1995;13(3): 233-46.
31. Stachura J, Popiela T, Pietro M, et al. Cytology of solid and papillary epithelial neoplasms of the pancreas: a case report. Diagn Cytopathol. 1988;4(4):339-41.
32. Buetow PC, Buck JL, Pantongrag-Brown L, et al. Solid and papillary epithelial neoplasm of the pancreas: imaging-pathologic correlation on 56 cases. Radiology. 1996;199(3): 707-11.
33. Kaufman SL, Reddick RL, Stiegel M, et al. Papillary cystic neoplasm of the pancreas: a curable pancreatic tumor. World J Surg. 1986;10(5):851-9.
34. Pettinato G, Di Vizio D, Manivel JC, et al. Solid-pseudopapillary tumor of the pancreas: a neoplasm with distinct and highly characteristic cytological features. Diagn Cytopathol. 2002;27(6):325-34.

Review Questions

1. **A 35-year-female presented with diarrhea and vague pain in the upper abdomen. Ultrasonography (USG) of her abdomen revealed 4 cm space occupying lesion in the head of the pancreas. Fine needle aspiration cytology (FNAC) of the mass was done under USG guidance. Figures 31.21A to D represent the cytology smear along with immunocytochemistry such as chromogranin (C) and neuron-specific enolase (NSE) (D). What is your diagnosis?**
   a. Solid and cystic papillary neoplasm of the pancreas
   b. Well differentiated adenocarcinoma
   c. Pancreatic neuroendocrine tumor
   d. Small cell carcinoma
2. **A 32-year-female presented with vague pain in the upper abdomen. The ultrasonography (USG) shows a predominantly solid and also cystic space occupying lesion in the pancreas. Figures 31.22A to D show the microphotographs of fine needle aspiration cytology (FNAC) of the lesion. What is your diagnosis?**
   a. Acinic cell carcinoma
   b. Solid and cystic papillary neoplasm of the pancreas
   c. Adenocarcinoma
   d. Pancreatic neuroendocrine tumor

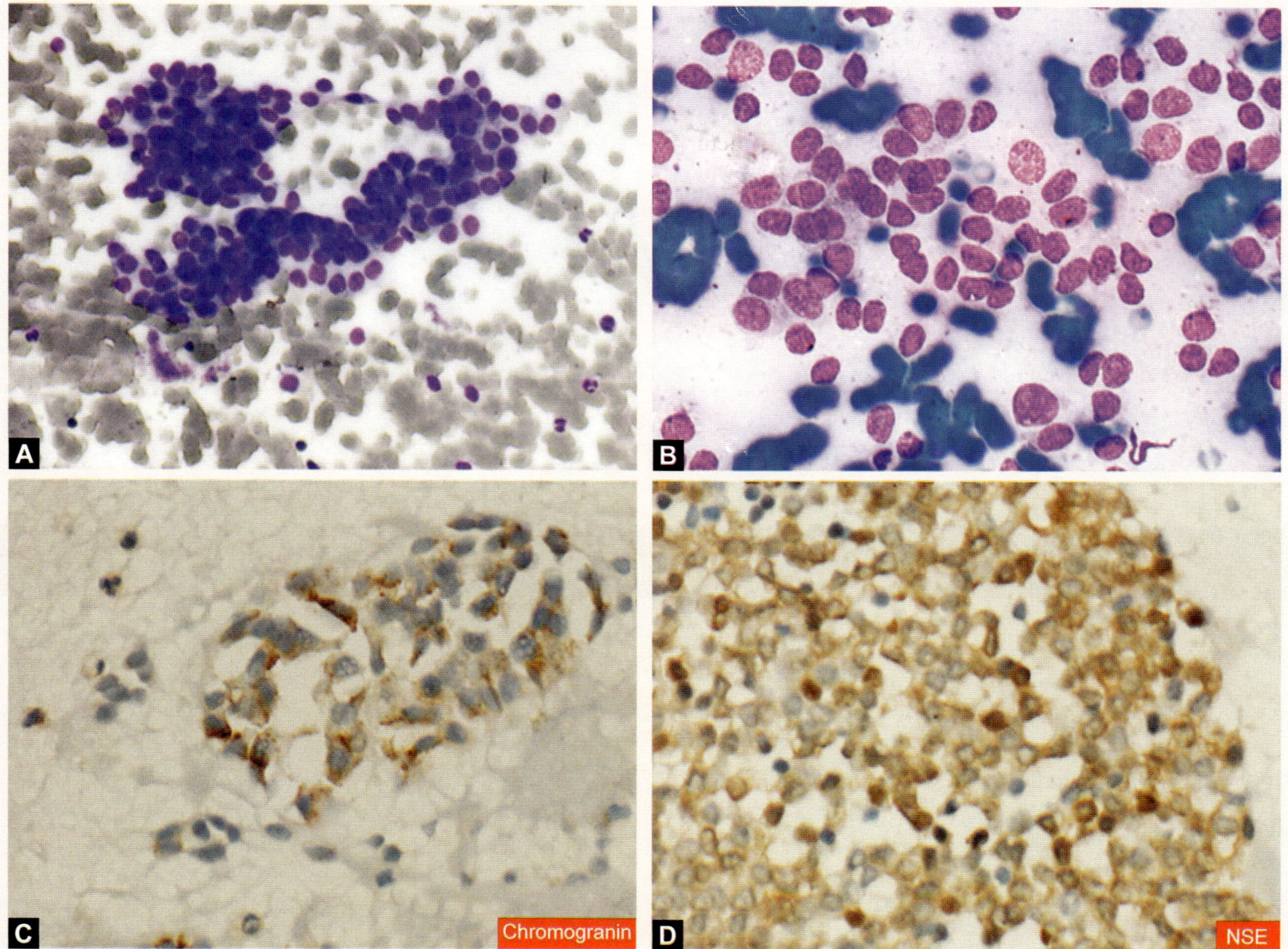

Figs. 31.21A to D: Cytology smear of the case of question 1 along with immunocytochemistry.

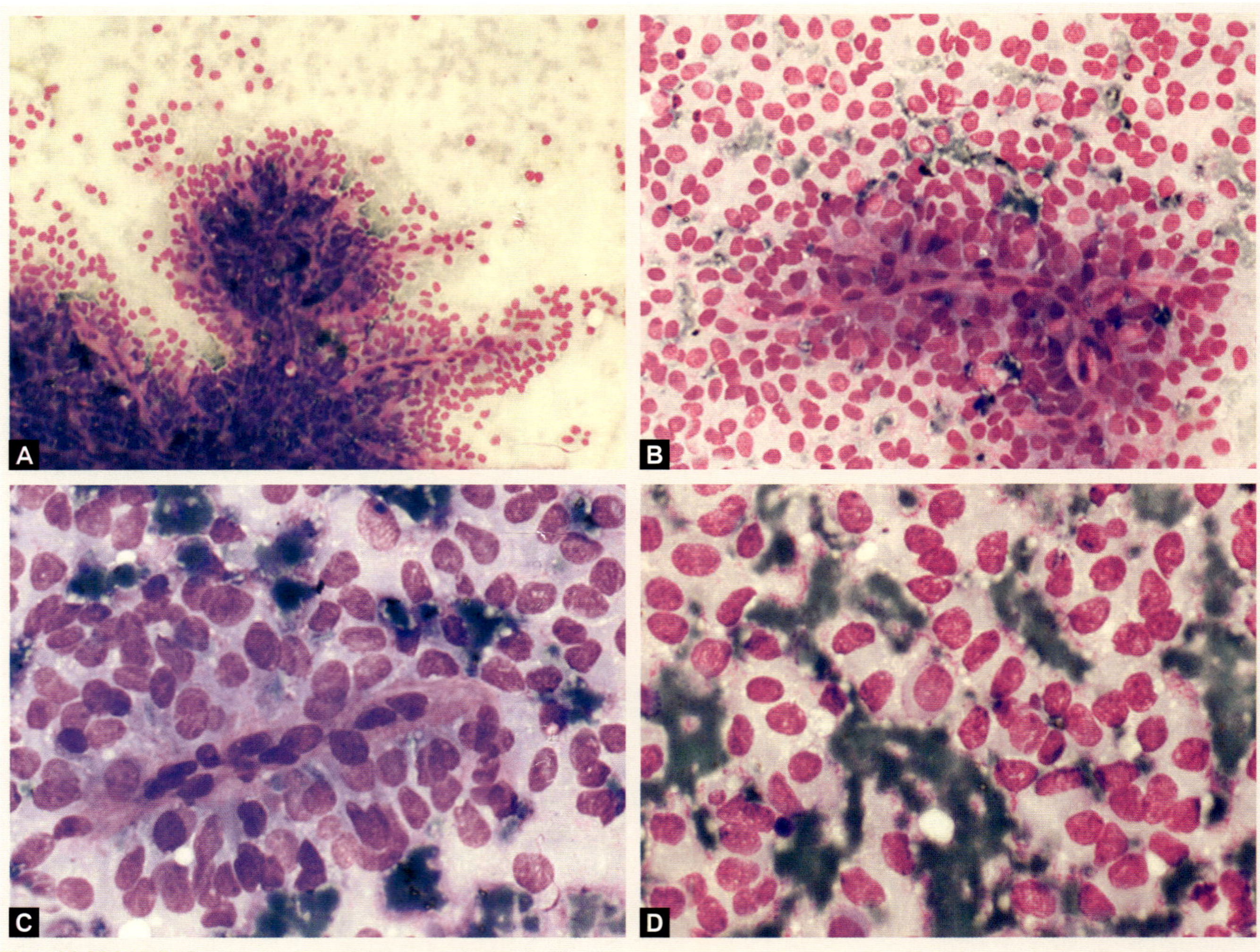

Figs. 31.22A to D: Cytology smear of the case of question 2.

Answers

1. c. Pancreatic neuroendocrine tumor

   Note: Round relatively monomorphic cells with strongly positive chromogranin and NSE favor the diagnosis of neuroendocrine tumor of pancreas.

2. b. Solid and cystic papillary neoplasm of the pancreas

   Note: The clinical history of a young female with solid–cystic pancreatic space occupying lesion along with the cytological features of multiple papillae and round cells with reddish granulated cytoplasm and relatively monomorphic nuclei indicate the diagnosis of solid and cystic pancreatic neoplasm.

CHAPTER

32 Kidney and Adrenal

INTRODUCTION

There are many diagnostic modalities of the space occupying lesions of the kidney such as ultrasonography (USG), computed tomography (CT) scan, and magnetic resonance imaging (MRI). The diagnostic accuracy of these imaging technologies is quite high. These investigative procedures have considerably reduced the need of fine needle aspiration cytology (FNAC). However, FNAC is still indicated:

- To confirm the diagnosis of kidney lesions particularly where radiological diagnosis is equivocal
- In advanced cases of renal cell carcinoma (RCC) where radical surgery is not needed
- To confirm metastasis from the other lesions
- Radical nephrectomy is contraindicated due to medical reason
- Small kidney lesions in young patient who needs partial nephrectomy
- Therapeutic application of cyst fluid evacuation, and
- Suspected cases of pyelonephritis where the patient can be treated medically.

Fine needle aspiration cytology of the kidney lesion is usually done by USG, CT, or MRI guidance. USG-guided FNAC is easy, cheap, and flexible, whereas CT scan can localize small lesion with better resolution. FNAC is done with a 22 gauze needle and stylet. The patient is kept in prone position and local anesthesia is applied at the site of FNAC. Both air-dried and alcohol-fixed smears are made. It is always preferable to take sample for cell block for immunostaining. Complications of FNAC of the kidney are rare. Local hemorrhage, pain, hematuria, and pneumothorax are occasionally encountered. Needle tract seeding due to FNAC is extremely rare and does not occur if thin bore needle is used.[1] The diagnostic sensitivity of FNAC is more than 80% with a high specificity rate of near about 98%.[2-5] False negative cases are mainly due to sampling error. Well-differentiated RCC may be mistaken as benign cells. False positive reports are rare. This may occur particularly in cases of angiomyolipoma (AML) and xanthogranulomatous pyelonephritis.

NORMAL CELLS

Fine needle aspiration cytology of normal kidney elements are predominantly tubular cells, which are derived from the distal convoluted tubules, proximal convoluted tubules, and the loop of Henle.

Tubular cells (Fig. 32.1): Tubular cells are usually present as small clusters and discretely. They have abundant granular cytoplasm with indistinct border. The nuclei are monomorphic round and central in position. Chromatin of the nuclei are fine granular with inconspicuous nucleoli. The cells often contain coarse dark lipofuscin pigments.

Endothelial cells: Oval- to spindle-shaped endothelial cells may also be noted in the background.

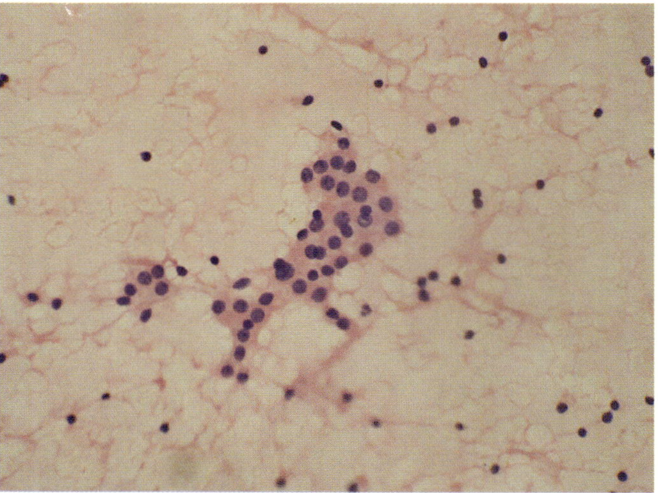

Fig. 32.1: Renal tubular cells: Small clusters and discrete cells with abundant indistinct cytoplasm and monomorphic round nuclei (H & E × MP).

Glomerular fragments: Uncommonly fragments of glomerulus may be aspirated. These are cohesive clusters of small round cells with scanty cytoplasm. These cells are surrounded by the thin capillaries.

RENAL LESIONS

Renal Cyst[6]

Renal cysts are very common and represent near about 70–80% of all renal lesions.[7] Most of these cysts are benign lesion and rarely may represent cystic RCC. The majority of the benign renal cysts are accidentally detected in the course of investigation of other diseases. The cysts are diagnosed accurately by USG and rarely needs cytological examination. However in selected conditions, the cyst should be distinguished from the cystic renal tumor. Bosniak MA has classified renal cyst in four categories based on radiological imaging.[8,9]

Category I: Clearly simple cysts.

Category II: The cysts are a bit more complicated and contain thin smooth septa, minimal wall thickening, and minimal calcification. These cysts are clearly not worrisome.

Category III: These cysts are more complicated with irregular thick septa or wall. They may be the feature of both benign and malignant lesions.

Category IV: These are clearly malignant lesions and show enhanced soft tissue areas adjacent to the wall.

The cysts of category I are all benign and do not need any FNAC. Whereas the cysts of category IV type need surgical intervention.

Cytology

Evacuation of the large simple cyst is therapeutically helpful. FNAC of the benign renal cyst usually yields thin clear fluid (Box 32.1). The aspirate shows scanty cellularity. There may be scattered foamy macrophages along with bland looking renal epithelial cells. In occasional cases the tubular epithelial cells may show mild degree of nuclear atypia. Atypia in the category II and III renal cyst should be considered as significant.

Differential Diagnosis

- *Renal cell carcinoma*: Occasionally RCC may show considerable cystic changes and may be difficult to distinguish from a simple cystic lesion. Nuclear atypia in RCC may be helpful in this aspect.

Xanthogranulomatous Inflammation

Xanthogranulomatous inflammation is a chronic inflammatory condition characterized by recurrent urinary tract infection, flank pain, and solid space occupying lesion in kidney. The lesion may mimic RCC on radiology.

Cytology (Figs. 32.2 and 32.3)

The cytology smear shows large clusters of foamy histiocytes around the capillaries. Multinucleated giant cells

Box 32.1: Renal cyst.

- Clear fluid
- Foamy macrophages
- Degenerated epithelial cells.

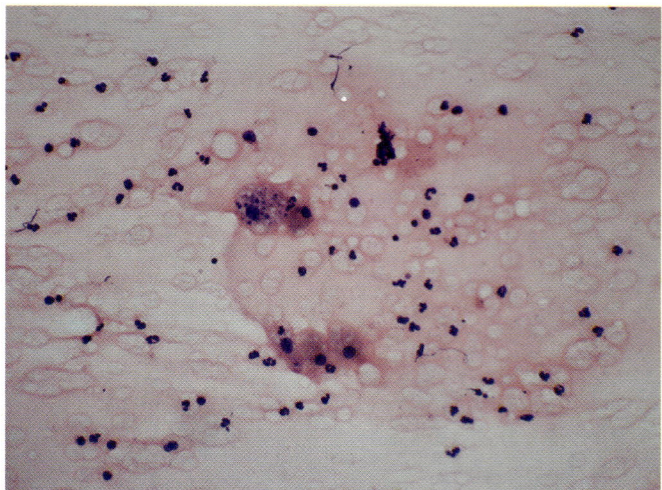

Fig. 32.2: Xanthogranulomatous inflammation: Discrete foamy histiocytes and lymphocytes (H & E × MP).

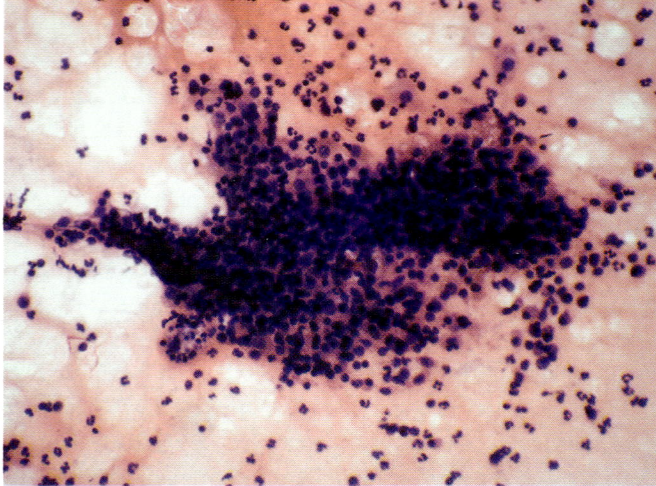

Fig. 32.3: Xanthogranulomatous inflammation: Renal tubular cells admixed with foamy histiocytes and lymphocytes (H & E × MP).

may also be seen. The individual cells have abundant vacuolated cytoplasm with central round bland nuclei. Unlike RCC, the nuclei of the histiocytes do not show any atypia. Necrosis and lymphocytes may be seen in the background.

Differential Diagnosis

- Renal cell carcinoma.

RENAL NEOPLASMS

World Health Organization (WHO) has classified renal cell neoplasms[13] as mentioned in Table 32.1.

Angiomyolipoma[8,9]

Angiomyolipoma (AML) is an uncommon benign renal tumor that shows intimate admixture of adipose tissue, smooth muscle, and blood vessels. It represents about 1% of all surgically resected renal mass. Almost 50% of AML occurs with tuberous sclerosis, an autosomal inherited disorder.[10] An USG examination and angiography may suggest a diagnosis of AML particularly due to high fat content. However, FNAC is indicated when the lesion contains low amount of fat and cannot be distinguished from RCC. The patients without tuberous sclerosis presents with flank pain, hematuria, and solid renal mass. However, the patients with tuberous sclerosis are asymptomatic. The correct preoperative diagnosis of AML is necessary for the conservative surgery and therefore FNAC has a definitive role in such cases. The salient diagnostic features of AML are mentioned in Box 32.2.

Table 32.1: Tumors of kidney.

- Renal cell tumors
  - Clear cell renal cell carcinoma
  - Multilocular clear cell renal cell carcinoma
  - Papillary renal cell carcinoma
  - Chromophobe renal cell carcinoma
  - Carcinoma of the collecting ducts of Bellini
  - Renal medullary carcinoma
  - Xp11 translocation carcinomas
  - Carcinoma associated with neuroblastoma
  - Mucinous tubular and spindle cell carcinoma
  - Renal cell carcinoma, unclassified
  - Papillary adenoma
  - Oncocytoma
  - Papillary adenoma
- Metanephric tumors
  - Metanephric adenoma
  - Metanephric adenofibroma
  - Metanephric stromal tumor
- Nephroblastic tumor
  - Nephroblastoma
  - Cystic partially differentiated nephroblastoma
- Mesenchymal tumor
  - Clear cell sarcoma
  - Rhabdoid tumor
  - Leiomyosarcoma
  - Angiosarcoma
  - Angiomyolipoma
- Neuroendocrine tumor
  - Carcinoid
  - Neuroblastoma
  - Pheochromocytoma
- Germ cell tumor, hematopoietic tumor, etc.
- Metastatic tumor.

Cytology (Figs. 32.4 and 32.5)

Smear shows abundant clusters of mature fat cells. There are multiple fragments of thick-walled blood vessel fragments. The vessels are lined by endothelial cells. The leiomyomatous cells are present in small clusters or in dissociation. These cells are round- to spindle-shaped with moderate amount of vacuolated cytoplasm.[11] The nuclei are oval- to spindle-shaped with blunt ends giving rise to cigar-shaped appearance. The nuclear chromatin is fine granular with single prominent nucleoli. Occasionally, these smooth muscle cells with spindle-shaped nuclei show marked nuclear pleomorphism and these cells should be carefully interpreted to avoid false positive diagnosis of sarcomatoid RCC.

Immunocytochemistry

The cells are positive for HMB-45 and Melan A. These are useful markers to differentiate AML from RCC.

Differential Diagnosis

- *Renal cell carcinoma*: The presence of atypical mesenchymal cells with bizarre nuclei may mislead the cytologist to the diagnosis of RCC. However, the nuclear chromatin of the cells of AML is bland and the nucleoli are inconspicuous. The presence of adipose tissue usually favors AML. CT scan features are usually characteristic of this tumor.

Box 32.2: Angiomyolipoma.

- Mature fat cells
- Thick-walled blood vessels
- Round- to spindle-shaped mesenchymal cells
- Vacuolated cytoplasm
- Epithelioid cells with nuclear atypia
- CT scan characteristics.

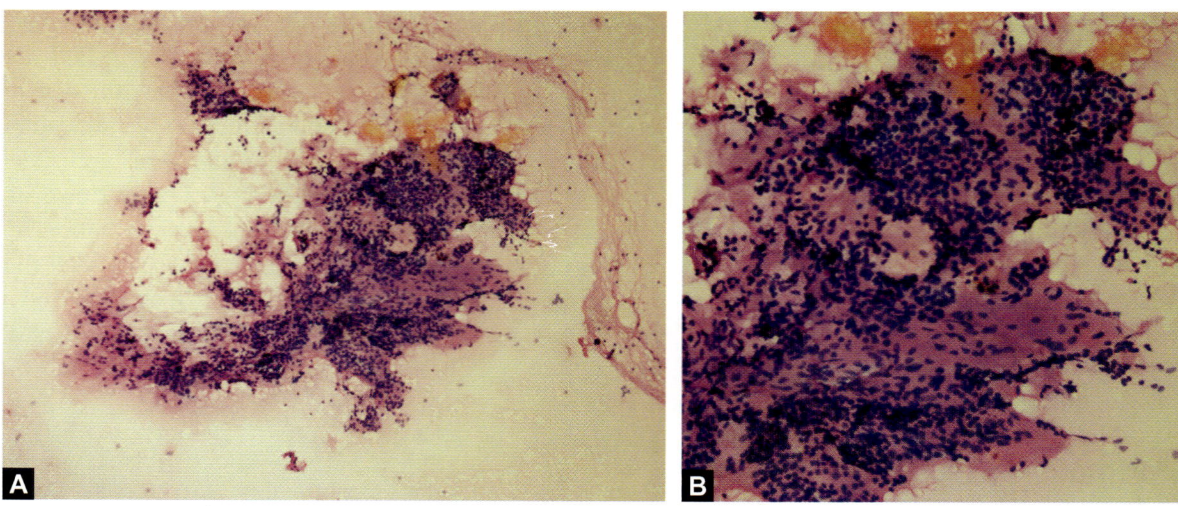

Figs. 32.4A and B: (A) Angiomyolipoma: Clusters and discrete oval to spindle cells along with renal tubular cells (H & E × LP). (B) Angiomyolipoma: Spindle cells embedded in the stroma (H & E × HP).

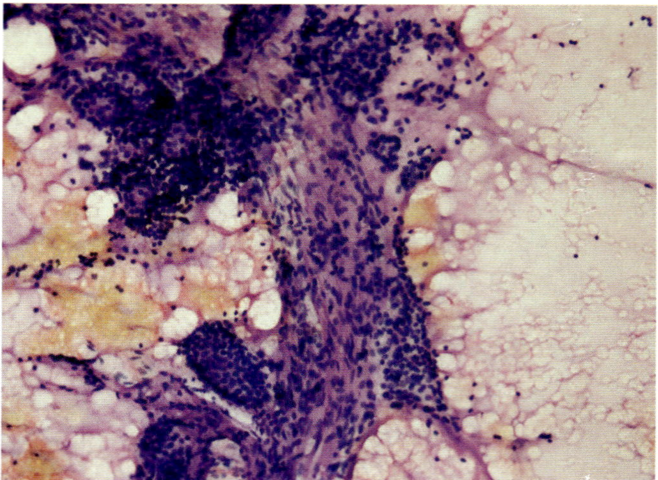

Fig. 32.5: Angiomyolipoma: Spindle cells are arranged in long bundles (H & E × HP).

Renal Cell Carcinoma[2,4,5,12-14]

Renal cell carcinoma develops from the renal tubules and is the most common primary malignant tumor in the kidney. RCC represents about 90% of the malignant tumors of the kidney. It generally occurs in the adults of late fifties, and males are commonly affected than female. The children may also develop RCC. Tobacco smoking, obesity, and exposure to carcinogenic arsenic compounds are the common risk factors of RCC. A small proportion (4%) of RCC occurs as hereditary cancer.[15] von Hippel-Lindau tumor suppressor gene is located on chromosome 3p25. Inactivation of this tumor suppressor gene plays an important role in hereditary and sporadic clear cell renal carcinoma. Based on molecular cytogenetics and histogenetic study of RCC, it is strongly recommended that these tumors are histogenetically heterogeneous group of tumors with significantly different prognostic outcome.

The patients of RCC usually present with the classical triad of hematuria, flank pain, and abdominal mass. However, 40% patients of RCC may present with loss of weight loss, abdominal pain, anorexia, and fever.

Cytology (Figs. 32.6 to 32.8)

Clear cell type of renal cell carcinoma: Near about 75% of RCC is clear cell carcinoma. The FNAC smear of clear cell carcinoma is usually highly cellular (Box 32.3). The cells are arranged in large cohesive clusters and singly. Transgressing blood vessels within the clusters of cells are also noted. The individual cells have abundant cytoplasm with distinct cytoplasmic outline. Nucleocytoplasmic ratio of the cell is low. The nuclei are round and variably enlarged. The nuclear position is central to eccentric. Depending on the grade of the tumor, the cells show nuclear enlargement and nucleolar prominence. The higher grade tumors have moderate to markedly enlarged nuclei with irregular nuclear contour. There is frequent binucleation. Nuclear chromatin is fine to coarse depending on the grading of the tumor. Nucleoli may be indistinct to large and prominent. It is important to differentiate the benign tubular cells and low-grade RCC as they may often simulate each other (Table 32.2).

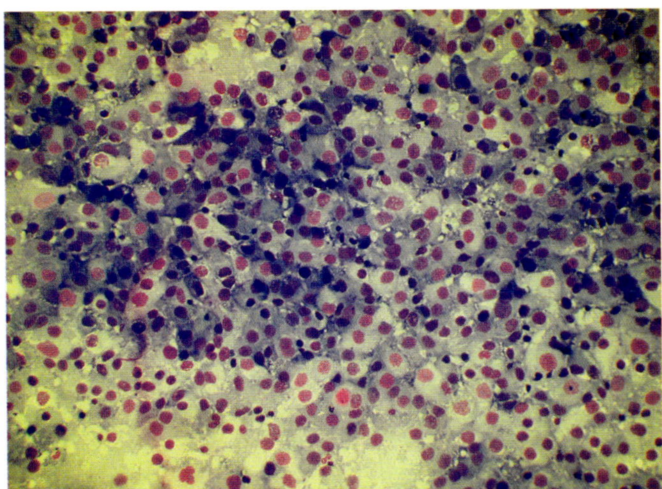

Fig. 32.6: Renal cell carcinoma: Abundant discrete cells with clear cytoplasm and mildly enlarged nuclei in a well-differentiated renal cell carcinoma (MGG × MP).

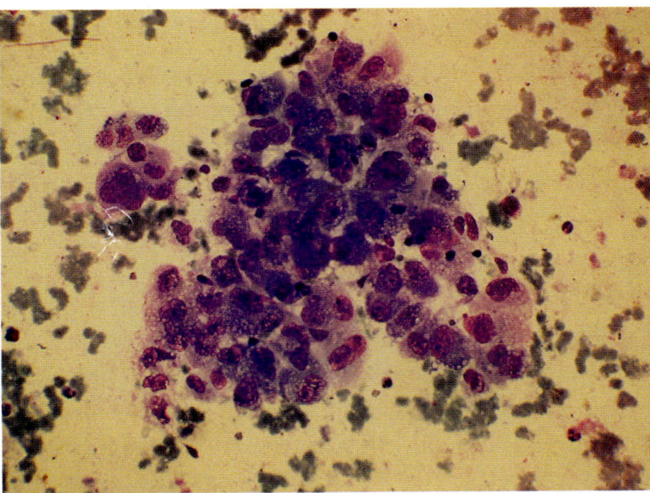

Fig. 32.7: Renal cell carcinoma: Loosely cohesive clusters of cells with moderate amount of vacuolated cytoplasm. Nuclei are moderately enlarged and pleomorphic (MGG × HP).

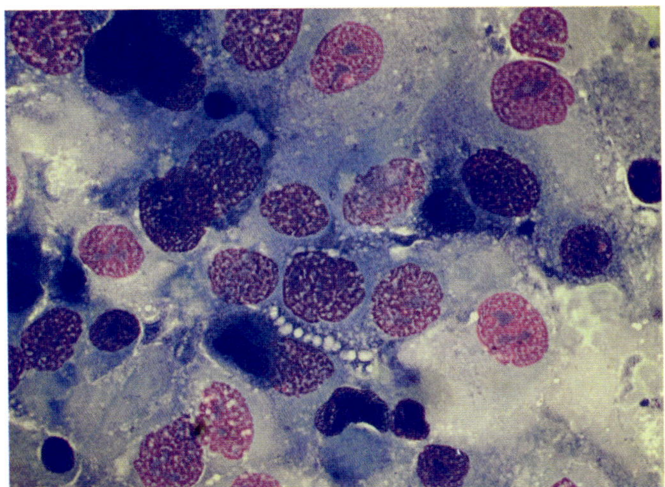

Fig. 32.8: Renal cell carcinoma: Higher magnification showing better morphology of the cells. The cells have abundant cytoplasm. Nuclei show fine chromatin and prominent nucleoli (MGG × OI).

Box 32.3: Renal cell carcinoma.

- Multiple clusters, papillary fragments, and discrete cells.
- Cell with well-defined cytoplasmic outline.
- Abundant granular or finely vacuolated pale cytoplasm.
- Central round nuclei with variable pleomorphism.
- Fine to coarse nuclear chromatin depending on grade.
- Frequent binucleation.
- Inconspicuous to large prominent nucleoli.

Immunocytochemistry: Positive for cytokeratin, vimentin, and CD10.

Table 32.2: Differentiating features between clear cell carcinoma and benign tubular cells.

Features	*Renal cell carcinoma cells*	*Benign tubular cells*
Cells	Large cohesive clusters	Discrete
Cytoplasm	Vacuolated	No vacuolations
Nuclei	Enlarged: mild to moderate	No enlargement
Nucleoli	Prominent	Inconspicuous to absent

Papillary Carcinoma

The papillary renal carcinoma is defined as a malignant tumor of the kidney composed of more than 50% papillae. Smears show multiple papillae and cohesive three-dimensional (3D) clusters of cells (Box 32.4). On cell block, the papillae may show fibrovascular core. The individual cells show dense cytoplasm and small round relatively monomorphic bland nuclei. The nucleoli are inconspicuous to absent. The nuclei often show deep nuclear grooves and intranuclear pseudoinclusion. Occasional cases show intracytoplasmic hemosiderin pigments. In minority of the cases psammoma bodies are also seen. High-grade papillary carcinoma shows cells with abundant granular cytoplasm having enlarged nuclei and large nucleoli. High-grade papillary carcinoma is difficult to differentiate from the clear cell carcinoma.

Box 32.4: Papillary carcinoma of kidney.

- Multiple papillae and cohesive clusters of cells
- Small round cells
- Monomorphic bland nuclei
- Deep nuclear groove
- Intranuclear pseudoinclusion
- Intracytoplasmic hemosiderin pigments
- Psammoma bodies.

Differential Diagnosis

Clear cell renal cell carcinoma: The presence of occasional papillae in the ordinary RCC may be confused with papillary carcinoma. The relatively bland nuclei, nuclear grooving, intracellular hemosiderin, and the presence of psammoma bodies favor the diagnosis of papillary carcinoma.

Chromophobe Type

Chromophobe RCC comprises 5% of all RCCs. The cytology smears are relatively cellular and consist of small groups and isolated cells. The individual cells show abundant floppy, granular cytoplasm with well-defined cytoplasmic margins (Box 32.5). In May-Grünwald Giemsa (MGG)-stained smears, the cytoplasm shows perinuclear reticulated zone instead of typical clear vacuolated area. Cytoplasmic vacuolations are usually not seen. The nuclei are round moderately pleomorphic and show frequent binucleation. Nuclear margin may be irregular and intranuclear pseudoinclusion may be seen.[18] Chromophobe cell carcinoma may often simulate as oncocytoma as both the tumor show cells with abundant granular cytoplasm and frequent binucleation. However, nuclear pleomorphism is more severe in chromophobe RCC. Chromophobe RCC may also mimic clear cell RCC on cytology. The cells of chromophobe RCC are dispersed. And more pleomorphic than clear cell RCC.

Immunocytochemistry

Chromophobe RCC is positive for CK7 and c-Kit. The cells are negative for vimentin.

Sarcomatoid Type

This tumor comprises only 1% of RCC. It is relatively aggressive in behavior. The tumors usually have the admixture of sarcomatoid and epithelial components. FNAC smears show predominantly clusters and dissociated spindle cells in a necrotic or clean background. The cells have moderate to marked pleomorphic spindle-shaped nuclei with irregular nuclear margin and large prominent nucleoli. These cells are admixed with high-grade epithelial component with abundant clear or granular cytoplasm. Osteoid, cartilaginous fragments, and multinucleated giant cells may also be seen. In case of lack of epithelial component cytokeratin positivity is required to confirm the diagnosis.

Box 32.5: Chromophobe renal cell carcinoma.

- Abundant floppy, granular cytoplasm
- Well-defined cytoplasmic margins
- Perinuclear reticulated zone
- Intranuclear pseudoinclusion
- Round moderately pleomorphic nuclei
- Frequent binucleation
- Intranuclear pseudoinclusion.

Differential Diagnosis

Angiomyolipoma: The presence of only spindle cells and complete lack of epithelial component may simulate AML. However, the spindle cells are less pleomorphic and there may be other components such as fat in the smear of AML.

Collecting Duct Type

This is a very rare type of RCC. The tumor probably originates from the collecting ducts. The FNAC smear shows single and clusters of cells. Occasional papillary arrangements of cells are also noted. The cells are relatively small with scanty to moderate cytoplasm and round hyperchromatic nuclei. Psammoma bodies are also noted.[19] The tumor may often be mistaken as metastatic carcinoma.

Nuclear Grading of Renal Cell Carcinoma

Nuclear grading[12,13] of RCC has been highlighted in Table 32.3.

Table 32.4 highlights the cytological features of different types of RCC.

Differential Diagnosis of Renal Cell Carcinoma

- Benign renal tubular cells.
- *Hepatocytes*: Hepatocytes with reactive atypia may be mistaken as low-grade RCC. The hepatocytes are polygonal in shape with centrally placed nuclei having very low nucleocytoplasmic ratio. The cytoplasm of the hepatocyte often contains bile pigments.
- Angiomyolipoma.
- *Xanthogranulomatous pyelonephritis*: Discussed in xanthogranulomatous pyelonephritis section.
- Benign cysts.

Table 32.3: Nuclear grading of renal cell carcinoma.

Grade	*Nuclear size*	*Nucleoli*
Grade 1	Small, round regular	Inconspicuous to absent
Grade 2	Mildly enlarged, irregular	Small conspicuous
Grade 3	Moderately enlarged, irregular	Prominent
Grade 4	Severely pleomorphic enlarged	Macronucleoli

Table 32.4: Salient cytological features of different types of renal cell carcinoma.

Type	*Cell pattern*	*Cytoplasm*	*Nucleus*	*Additional features*	*Immunocytochemistry*
Clear	Clusters	Abundant, clear vacuolated	Round, low N/C ratio, monomorphic		Negative for CK7, C-Kit and positive for EMA and CD10
Papillary	Papillae	Moderate dense	Round, low N/C ratio, monomorphic	Necrosis present, intranuclear inclusions, psammoma bodies	Positive for CK7, EMA, vimentin, and CD10
Sarcomatoid	Dissociated	Mild to moderate	Spindle-shaped, high N/C ratio, pleomorphic	Necrosis present, malignant epithelial component	Positive for CK and vimentin
Chromophobe	Dissociated	Abundant floppy, granular	Round, low N/C ratio, monomorphic		Positive for C-Kit

(N/C ratio: Nuclear-cytoplasmic ratio, EMA: Epithelial membrane antigen; CK: Cytokeratin).

Table 32.5: The clinical, cytological, immunocytochemistry, and electron microscopy to distinguish adrenocortical carcinoma from renal cell carcinoma.

	Renal cell carcinoma	*Adrenocortical carcinoma*
Cushing's syndrome	Absent	May be present
Cell arrangement	Papillary and tubular	Discrete and clusters
Cytoplasmic glycogen	Present	Usually absent
Immunocytochemistry		
Keratin AE1 and AE3	Positive	Negative
EMA	Positive	Negative
Vimentin	Positive	Positive
Melan A	Negative	Positive
Inhibin alpha	Negative	Positive
Calretinin	Negative	Positive
Electron microscopy	Microvillus present	Mitochondria with tubular or vesicular cristae

- *Adrenal tumor*: At times it is very difficult to differentiate a clear cell RCC located in the upper pole of kidney from an adrenocortical carcinoma. Table 32.5 highlights the possible differentiating points to distinguish adrenocortical carcinoma from RCC.

Oncocytoma

Oncocytoma is a benign renal epithelial neoplasm and represents less than 3% of all renal tumors. The majority of the patients are asymptomatic (Box 32.6).

Box 32.6: Oncocytoma.

- Dissociated cells
- Abundant granular eosinophilic cytoplasm
- Small bland nuclei.

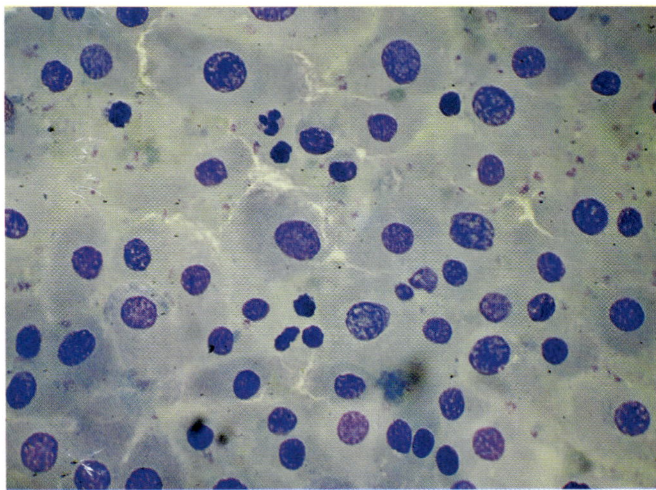

Fig. 32.9: Renal oncocytoma: Discrete cells with abundant cytoplasm and monomorphic round nuclei (MGG × HP).

Cytology (Fig. 32.9)

The FNAC smear shows predominantly dissociated cells. The cells are rarely arranged in clusters (Fig. 32.9). The individual cells have abundant eosinophilic granular cytoplasm with well-defined cell border. Cytoplasm of the cells does not show any vacuolations. The nuclei are bland, round, and monomorphic with inconspicuous nucleoli. Oncocytoma cells are negative for Hale's colloidal iron staining.

Diagnostic Difficulties

- *Chromophobe type of renal cell carcinoma*: Oncocytoma can be confused with chromophobe type of RCC. These cells are positive for Hale's colloidal iron staining.
- *Hepatocytes*: Normal hepatocytes have also abundant granular cytoplasm and these cells may be aspirated in case of FNAC of right kidney. Hepatocytes may rarely be mistaken as oncocytes.

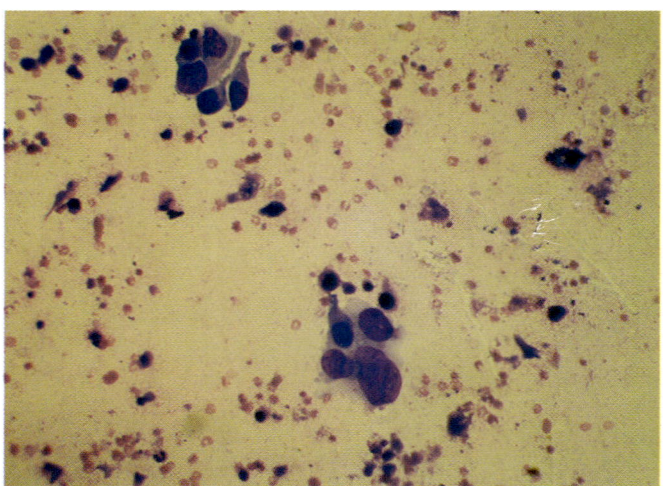

Fig. 32.10: Urothelial carcinoma: Oval to elongated cells with basally placed nuclei (MGG × HP).

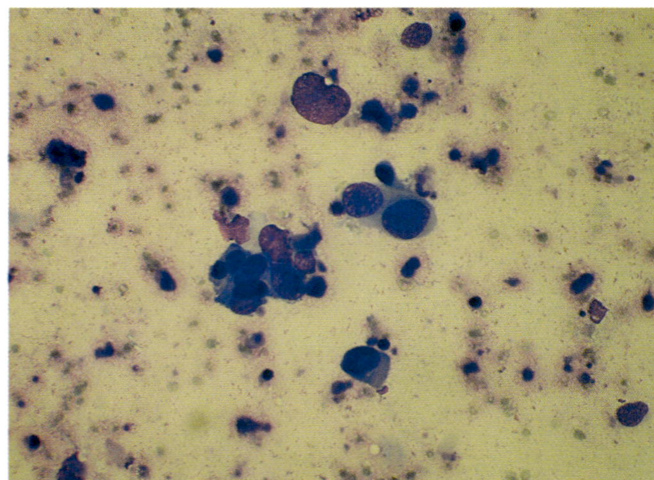

Fig. 32.11: Urothelial carcinoma: Columnar looking cells with moderately pleomorphic nuclei (MGG × HP).

Box 32.7: Urothelial carcinoma.

- Clusters and papillae
- Elongated cells
- Medium to low nucleocytoplasmic ratio
- Glassy homogeneous cytoplasm
- Cercariform cells.

Urothelial Carcinoma

Urothelial carcinoma (UC) was previously known as transitional cell carcinoma. It represents about 7% of all primary carcinomas of kidney. The tumor is often multifocal in origin. The common risk factors of the UC are cigarette smoking, analgesic abuse, renal papillary necrosis, and renal stone. The patient usually presents with painless, hematuria, flank pain, and palpable mass.

Cytology (Figs. 32.10 and 32.11)

Smear shows usually small clusters, papillae, and single cells. The tumor cells are spindle shaped with glassy homogeneous cytoplasm (Box 32.7). The nucleocytoplasmic ratio is low to medium. Depending of the grade of the tumor, the nuclei show mild to moderate pleomorphism. In many cases, elongated cells with thin long tail of cytoplasm, known as cercariform cells, are seen. These cells have wide cytoplasm in the ends and thin in the middle.[20]

Differential Diagnosis

- *Papillary renal cell carcinoma*: The papillary RCC shows histiocytes and occasionally psammoma bodies.
- *Reactive transitional cells*: Abundant reactive transitional cells are seen in renal stone and a false positive diagnosis of papillary TCC may be given. Nuclear morphology is helpful in differentiating TCC from reactive transitional cells.

METASTATIC TUMORS OF KIDNEY

Metastasis in kidney represents only 7% of renal tumor. Metastatic kidney rarely presents any symptomatic manifestation. Lung is the most common primary site followed by breast, colon, and pancreas. It is very difficult to recognize the metastatic tumor on FNAC smear. However, if the tumor affects bilateral kidneys with a history of primary tumor and the smear shows large pleomorphic cells or small undifferentiated cells then a possibility of metastatic tumor should be considered.

PEDIATRIC RENAL TUMORS

Nephroblastoma (Wilms' Tumor)[21,22]

Nephroblastoma is also known as Wilms' tumor (WT). It is primarily a neoplasm of the infants that develops from the nephrogenic blastemal cells. The tumor occurs in both sexes with equal frequencies and 98% of the tumor occurs before 10 years of age. WT is the most common renal tumor in the pediatric patients. The tumor is usually detected as an abdominal mass by the parents of the children.

Cytology (Figs. 32.12 to 32.14)

Fine needle aspiration cytology smear of the WT shows three major components of cells: (1) blastemal cells, (2) epithelial cells, and (3) stromal cells (Box 32.8).

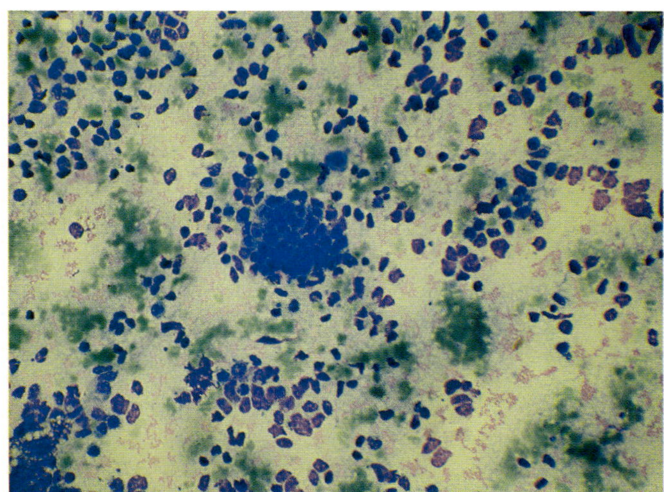

Fig. 32.12: Wilms' tumor: Discrete blastemal cells and tight glomeruloid-like body (MGG × MP).

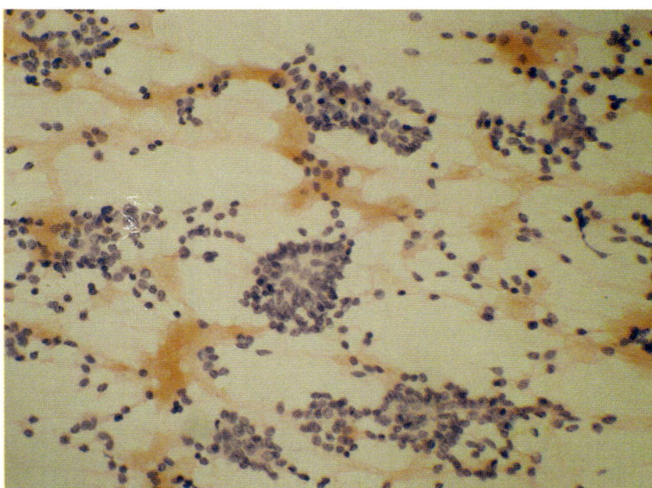

Fig. 32.13: Wilms' tumor: Tubular structures and blastemal cells (H & E × MP).

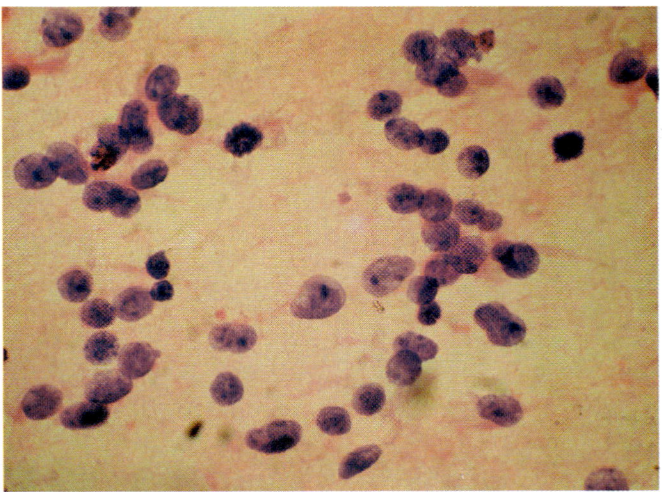

Fig. 32.14: Wilms' tumor: Scanty thin rim of cytoplasm and round nuclei with finely dispersed chromatin (H & E × OI).

1. *Blastemal cells*: These cells are predominantly discrete cells and occasionally in loose cluster. The cells are round and twice the size of the lymphocytes. The cytoplasm is scanty and deep blue forming a thin rim around the nucleus. The nuclei are round with finely chromatin and small single to multiple nucleoli.
2. *Epithelial cells*: These cells are present in cohesive clusters, small tubules, or rosette-like arrangement. These so called rosettes are possibly nothing but the transversely cut tubules. The epithelial cells are larger than the blastemal cells and have moderate amount of cytoplasm. The tight 3D clusters of cell resembling glomeruloid bodies are also noted.

Box 32.8: Wilms' tumor.

- Small round dissociated blastemal cells
- Blastemal cells have scanty deep blue cytoplasm, round hyperchromatic nuclei
- Tubular epithelial cells
- Round well circumscribed glomeruloid-like bodies
- Spindle-shaped mesenchymal component.

3. *Mesenchymal cells*: These cells are oval- to spindle-shaped with bland nuclei. In between the cells, deep pink collagenous material is also seen. Cells with smooth muscle or rhabdoid differentiation may be present.

Occasional cases of Wilms' tumor may show large markedly pleomorphic nuclei that usually indicate bad prognosis.

Immunocytochemistry

The blastemal cells are positive for vimentin and also show focal expression of desmin, cytokeratin, and NSE.

Differential Diagnosis

Fineneedle aspiration cytology of WT may resemble the cytomorphology of small blue round cell tumor.

- *Neuroblastoma*: The blastemal cell morphology and Rosette's in neuroblastoma may simulate the tubules of WT. However, the rosettes of neuroblastoma contain neurofibrillary material and the surrounding cells are multilayered. The presence of typical mesenchymal cells may be helpful in diagnosis of WT.

- *Rhabdomyosarcoma*: Round cells with frequent bi- and multinucleation and strap cells with cross striation are often seen in rhabdomyosarcoma. On immunocytochemistry, the cells are positive for desmin.
- *Primitive neuroectodermal tumor*: FNAC smears of primitive neuroectodermal tumor (PNET) show relatively more vacuolated cytoplasm in comparison to WT. True rosettes with central neurophilic material are seen in PNET. On immunocytochemistry, the cells are positive for synaptophysin and Mic 2 and negative for WT1.

Mesoblastic Nephroma[23]

It is a low-grade fibrosarcoma of the infant kidney. This is a congenital neoplasm and is usually detected before the age of 6 months. The infant presents with an abdominal mass.

Cytology (Box 32.9)

The FNAC smears show abundant clusters and dissociated oval to elongated spindle cells (Figs. 32.15A to C). The tumor cells show scanty cytoplasm with elongated spindle-shaped bland nuclei. The nuclear chromatin is fine and nucleoli are inconspicuous. The cellular mesoblastic nephroma may show considerable nuclear pleomorphism, coarse chromatin, and occasionally necrosis.[24] These cases may be mistaken as sarcoma. The cells of mesoblastic nephroma are positive for CD34 immunostaining.[25]

Box 32.9: Mesoblastic nephroma.

- Clusters and dissociated spindle cells
- Spindle-shaped nuclei with blunt ends
- Fine chromatin
- Inconspicuous nucleoli
- Positive for CD34 immunostaining.

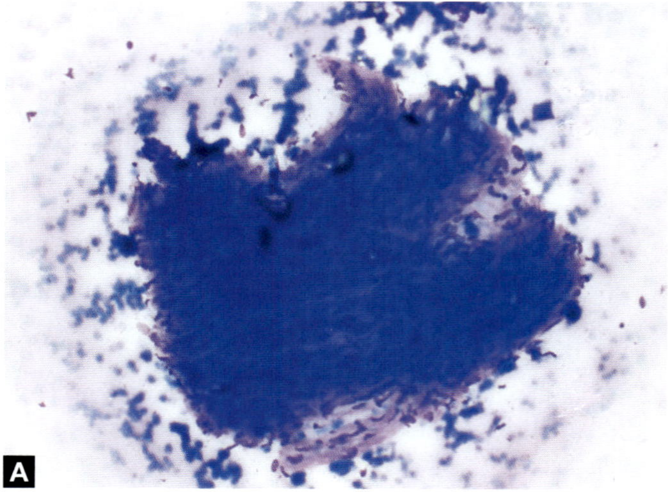

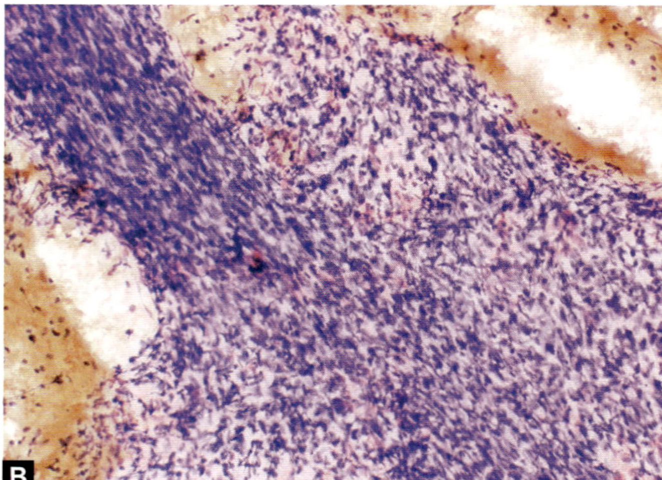

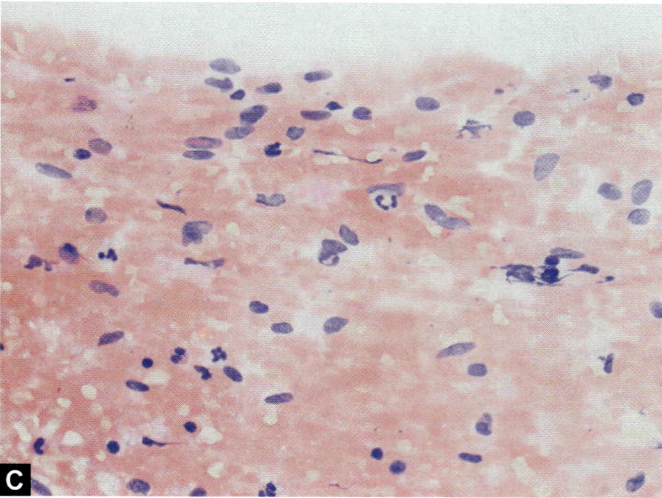

Figs. 32.15A to C: (A) Mesoblastic nephroma: Tight cluster of spindle cells (MGG × MP), (B) Mesoblastic nephroma: Cluster of cells with long slender nuclei (H & E × MP), (C) Mesoblastic nephroma: Discrete spindle cells (H & E × MP).

Differential Diagnosis

Congenital fibrosarcoma: The cells of congenital fibrosarcoma show moderate nuclear pleomorphism. Nuclear chromatin is fine and often shows prominent nucleoli.

Rhabdoid Tumor

Rhabdoid tumor of kidney (RTK) is a highly invasive aggressive tumor. It represents 2% of all pediatric kidney tumors and 80% of the tumor occurs before the age of 2 year. The mean age of the patient is 1 year. RTKs are often associated with midline posterior fossa tumor such as medulloblastoma and hence accurate cytological recognition is important. The patient usually presents with hematuria.

Cytology

The FNAC smear shows predominantly dispersed population and cluster of small cells.[26] Stripped bare nuclei are also seen in the background (Box 32.10). The individual cells are round with moderate amount of cytoplasm. The nuclei are large with irregular margin and show large prominent nucleoli. The cytoplasm shows round, dense, pinkish (MGG stain), and variably sized inclusions. This cytoplasmic inclusion is considered as one of the characteristic features of RTK.

Box 32.10: Rhabdoid tumor.

- Discrete and small clusters
- Small cell with moderate cytoplasm
- Rhabdoid cell shows
  - Abundant cytoplasm
  - Macronucleoli
  - Round, dense, variable sized intracytoplasmic inclusions.

Immunocytochemistry

The cells show strong positivity for vimentin and focal EMA (epithelial membrane antigen) positivity.

Differential Diagnosis

Rhabdoid differentiation of WT: Rhabdoid tumor should be differentiated from the rhabdoid differentiation of WT. The rhabdomyosites of WT are large cells with abundant cytoplasm and focal cross striations.

Clear Cell Sarcoma[27]

Clear cell sarcoma of kidney (CCSK) is a rare childhood sarcoma of kidney and constitutes only 4% of all pediatric kidney tumors. It is also known as bone-metastasizing tumor as it has a propensity to metastasize in the bone. CCSK is three times more common in male child. The mean age of the patient is 3 years.

Cytology (Fig. 32.16 and 32.17)

Cytology smear shows cord cells, septal cells, arborizing vasculature, and mucopolysaccharide substance (Box 32.11).

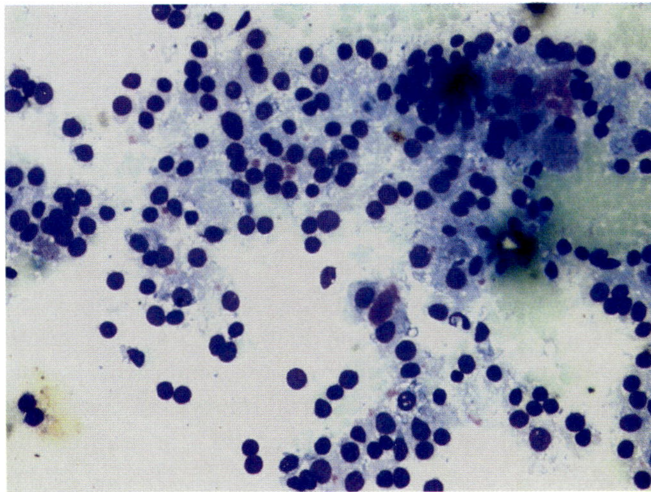

Fig. 32.16: Clear cell sarcoma of kidney: Abundant discrete cells with moderate to abundant vacuolated cytoplasm (MGG × MP).

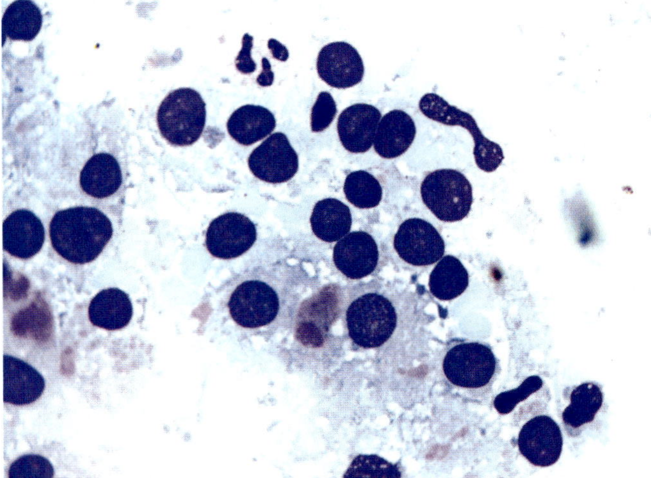

Fig. 32.17: Clear cell sarcoma of kidney: Higher magnification showing cells with abundant vacuolated cytoplasm and mildly enlarged nuclei having fine chromatin (MGG × OI).

Box 32.11: Clear cell sarcoma of kidney.

- Clusters and discrete cells
- Polygonal cells with wispy clear cytoplasm
- Eccentrically placed grooved nuclei
- Background magenta-colored mucopolysaccharide material
- Prominent arborizing vessels with spindle-shaped septal cells adjacent to endothelium.

The cord cells are polygonal with wispy clear cytoplasm. The nuclei are central to eccentric with deep grooves. Nuclear chromatin is fine with prominent nucleoli. Magenta-colored mucopolysaccharide ground substances are often seen in the background. One important clue to diagnosis of this tumor is the arborizing blood vessels with the septal spindle-shaped cells adjacent to endothelium. The pyknotic apoptotic cells may also be noted. Occasionally FNAC smears show normal tubular cells that may simulate the epithelial component of WT.

ADRENAL

Adrenal glands are vascular retroperitoneal organ that secrets various hormones. Adrenal gland behaves as a fertile land for various tumors, both primary and secondary. Majority of these masses are asymptomatic and individuals usually present with incidental masses or are being investigated for other primary complaints. Moreover, differentiating primary adrenal cortical carcinomas, from metastatic lesions, on imaging alone, can pose a diagnostic difficulty at times. Advances in the current radiological techniques have aided in rapid diagnosis by enabling fine needle aspiration even from deep abdominal masses. The main indications of adrenal FNAC is to identify the metastatic lesions (Box 32.12). The primary adrenal lesions are also recognizable by FNAC. In addition, various infective organism particularly tuberculosis and fungal infections may also produce a space occupying lesions and can be confirmed by FNAC.

Fine Needle Aspiration Cytology Technique

Fine needle aspiration cytology of adrenal is usually done from the back side and patient should lie in prone position. The procedure is performed usually with the help of CT scan using 20–22 gauge needle. Both air-dried and wet-fixed smears are prepared. It is preferable to have a cell block preparation. Sample can also be collected for bacterial or fungal culture.

Fine needle aspiration cytology is usually free of major complications except minor hematuria and hypotension.

Box 32.12: Indications of FNAC of adrenal.

- Recognition of metastatic tumor
- Identification of primary tumor
- Infective cases.

However, major complications such as surgical emphysema and shock have been reported. Severe fatal hypertensive crisis may occur particularly during FNAC of pheochromocytoma due to sudden release of catecholamines.[28] The sensitivity and specificity of FNAC of adrenal varies from 85% to 90%, respectively.[15-18] The false positive result of FNAC is rare.

Anatomy and Histology

Both the adrenal glands are located in the upper pole of kidney and each weighs about 8–10 gm. The gland has a outer cortex and inner medulla. The cortex is divided in three zones as (1) zona glomerulosa, (2) zona fasciculata, and (3) zona reticularis. The parenchymal cells of zona glomerulosa, zona fasciculata, and zona reticularis synthesize and release aldosterone, cortisol, and dehydroepiandrosterone, respectively. The medullary part of adrenal gland liberates catecholamine.

The cells of the zonal glomerulosa are large with foamy cytoplasm and small round nuclei having one or two prominent nucleoli. The zona fasciculata occupies 80% of the adrenal cortex and is composed of cords of large polygonal cells with abundant vacuolated cytoplasm. The innermost layer zona reticularis constitutes only 7% of the cortex and is composed of anastomosing cords of small round cells with scanty cytoplasm.

Adrenocortical Neoplasm[28-31]

Adrenal neoplasm is divided into adenoma and carcinoma. It is a relatively rare tumor and commonly occurs in the middle-aged person. However, the children are rarely affected by this neoplasm. The children with adrenocortical neoplasm is frequently (50% cases) associated with Li-Fraumeni syndrome.[32] The adrenal neoplasms are unilateral compared to adrenal hyperplasia which are bilateral. The majority of adrenal adenomas (85%) patients are nonfunctional, whereas most of the adrenocortical carcinomas (ACC) are functional. The tumors may be found during routine radiological investigations or they may be detected due to hormonal activities such as primary aldosteronism, Cushing's syndrome, or virilization. The size of the tumor is an important criterion of malignancy and most of the ACC is larger than 6 cm diameter on radiology.

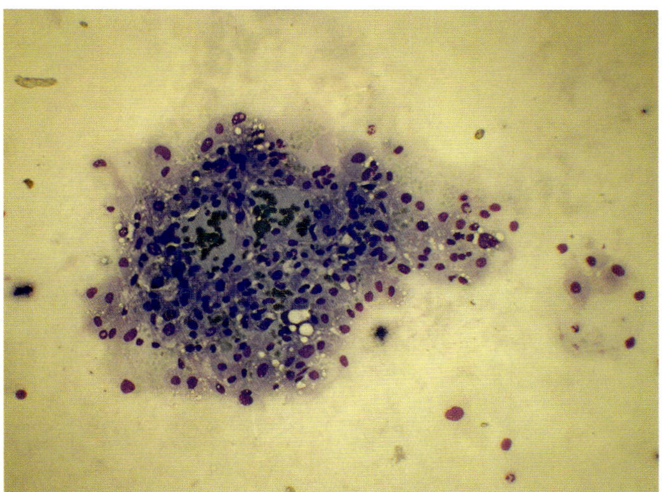

Fig. 32.18: Adrenal adenoma: Cohesive cluster of cells with abundant vacuolated cytoplasm and mildly pleomorphic nuclei (MGG × MP).

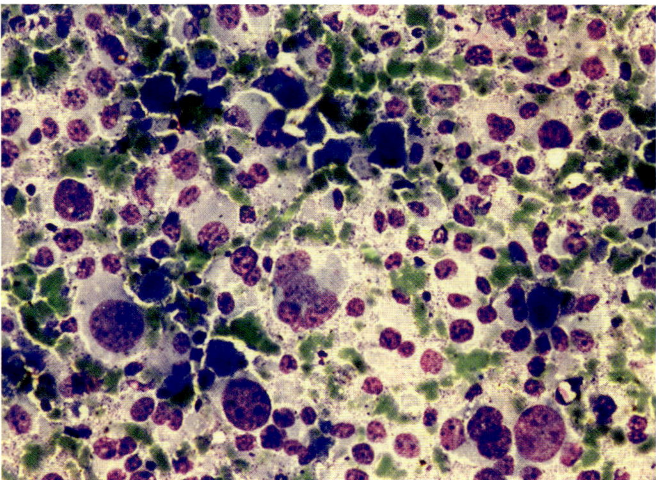

Fig. 32.19: Adrenocortical carcinoma: Abundant dissociated cells in bubbly vacuolated cytoplasm (MGG × MP).

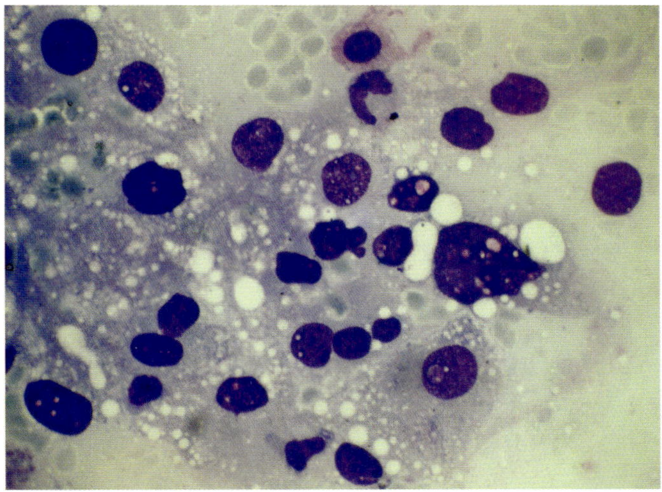

Fig. 32.20: Adrenocortical carcinoma: Large cells with moderate amount of vacuolated cytoplasm and centrally placed moderately pleomorphic nuclei (MGG × HP).

Cytology (Fig. 32.18)

On histology section, it is difficult to differentiate adrenal adenoma from carcinoma. The certain characteristic gross features of adrenal adenoma are: (1) usually less than 5 cm in diameter, (2) rarely more than 50 g in weight, (3) homogeneous gross appearance without any necrosis, and (4) well encapsulated (Box 32.13). Morphologically necrosis, high mitosis, and capsular invasion are the characteristic features of ACC. However, these features are not easy to assess in FNAC smears particularly capsular invasion is not possible to assess cytologically. Therefore, at times, it is difficult to distinguish adrenal adenoma from carcinoma.

Box 32.13: Adrenal adenoma.

- Bubbly lipid-filled background
- Abundant round bare nuclei
- Large cohesive clusters of cells
- Vacuolated cytoplasm
- Mildly enlarged monomorphic nuclei.

Box 32.14: Adrenocortical carcinoma.

- Dissociated and small cohesive clusters
- Numerous bare nuclei
- Bubbly background
- Round cells with vacuolated cytoplasm
- Centrally placed nuclei showing variable degree of pleomorphism
- Necrosis and bizarre cells.

Fine needle aspiration cytology smears of adrenal adenoma are usually paucicellular. The smears show three important characteristic features.

1. *Large cohesive clusters of cells*: These cells have abundant vacuolated cytoplasm and mildly enlarged monomorphic nuclei. The cells are admixed with sinusoidal endothelial cells,
2. Bubbly vacuolated lipid background, and
3. Abundant round bare nuclei.[33]

Fine needle aspiration cytology smears of ACC shows high cellularity (Figs. 32.19 to 32.21). The cells are predominantly arranged discretely and occasional loose cohesive groups (Box 32.14). The individual cells are large with moderate amount of vacuolated cytoplasm and centrally placed nuclei. The nuclei are hyperchromatic with coarsely granular chromatin. Depending on the grade of ACC the nuclei show variable degree of pleomorphism.

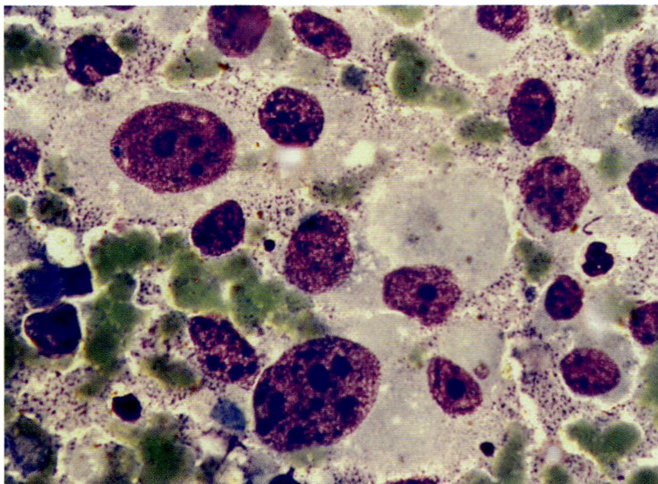

Fig. 32.21: Adrenocortical carcinoma: Higher magnification showing individual cells morphology. Markedly enlarged cells with moderately pleomorphic nuclei having multiple prominent nucleoli (MGG × OI).

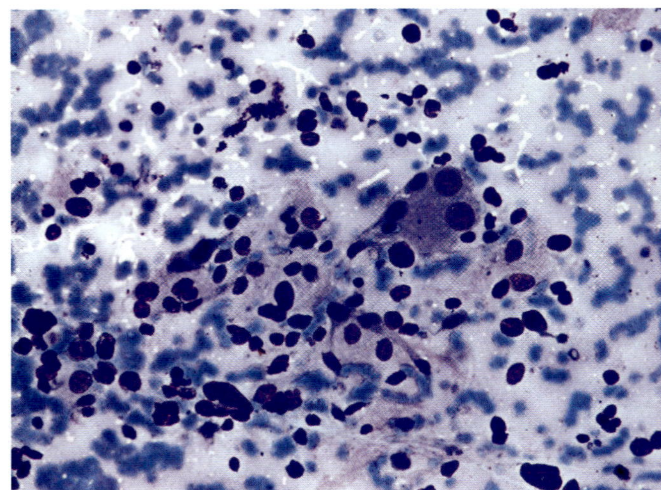

Fig. 32.22: Pheochromocytoma: Discrete oval to polygonal cells and spindle cells (MGG × MP).

Table 32.6: Immunocytochemistry of renal cell carcinoma and adrenocortical carcinoma.

Immunocytochemistry	*Renal cell carcinoma*	*Adrenocortical carcinoma*
• Keratin AE1 and AE3	• Positive	• Negative
• EMA	• Positive	• Negative
• Vimentin	• Positive	• Positive
• Melan A	• Negative	• Positive
• Inhibin alpha	• Negative	• Positive
• Calretinin	• Negative	• Positive

Moderately differentiated ACC may show flocculent aggregates of lipid material in the cytoplasm. Background necrosis and increased mitotic figures are noted in poorly differentiated ACC.

Immunocytochemistry

The tumor cells are positive for Melan A, calretinin, inhibin-alpha, and synaptophysin. In addition, the cells are also variably positive for cytokeratin (Table 32.6).

Differential Diagnosis

Renal cell carcinoma: Cytomorphologically it is difficult to differentiate RCC from adrenocortical carcinoma. Radiological localization also may not help in renal upper pole lesions. Immunocytochemically, RCC is positive for CK and EMA (Table 32.6).

Pheochromocytoma[34]

This is the tumor of the chromaffin cells of the medulla of adrenal gland and is also known as paraganglioma of the adrenal gland. Pheochromocytoma is also famous as 10% tumor. About 10% of pheochromocytomas are bilateral, 10% are extra-adrenal, and 10% malignant in nature. It may occur in all age group. The clinical symptom of pheochromocytoma is due to liberation of catecholamines. Patients often present with triad of paroxysmal hypertension, sweating, and tachycardia that are virtually diagnostic of this disease.

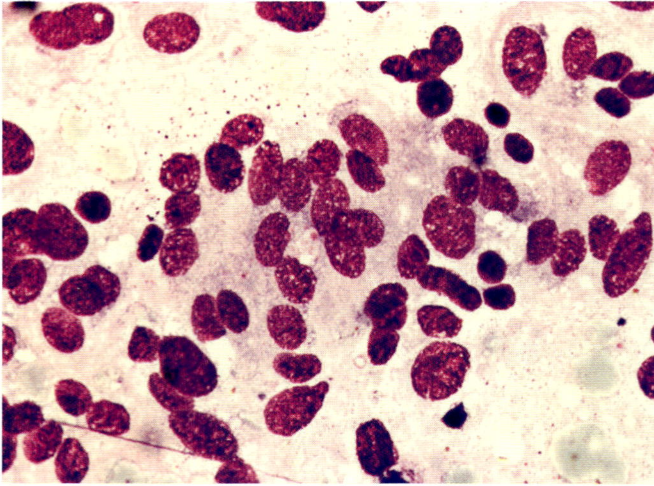

Fig. 32.23: Pheochromocytoma: Oval to elongated cells with moderate pleomorphism and fine nuclear chromatin (MGG × HP).

Cytology (Figs. 32.22 to 32.24)

Cytology smear of pheochromocytoma shows predominantly three types of cells (Box 32.15).

1. *The Epithelial Cell*: These cells are medium-sized polygonal cells with moderate amount of reddish granular cytoplasm. Cytoplasm often contains pinkish globular bodies. The nuclei are central, round, and monomorphic. The cells usually show low nucleocytoplasmic ratio. However, there may be cells with moderate nuclear enlargement and pleomorphism. Nuclear chromatin is fine with prominent nucleoli. Sudden anisonucleosis may be present.
2. *Spindle Cells*: The cells have elongated nuclei, coarse chromatin, and abundant cytoplasm.
3. *Ganglionic Cells*: These cells show abundant pale cytoplasm and eccentrically placed large nuclei with prominent nucleoli.

Nuclear enlargement and pleomorphism have no relation with the behavior of pheochromocytoma.

Differential Diagnosis

- *Adrenocortical carcinoma*: Poorly differentiated ACC often shows moderate nuclear pleomorphism and is often difficult to distinguish from pheochromocytoma. The presence of reddish globular material in the cytoplasm favors pheochromocytoma. Pheochromocytoma is positive for S-100 and chromogranin.
- *Metastatic carcinoma*: Clinical history of known primary along with immunocytochemistry may be helpful to confirm the cases of metastatic carcinoma. The cells of pheochromocytoma are CK and EMA negative and positive for chromogranin.

Box 32.15: Pheochromocytoma.

- Discrete and loose clusters
- Small- to moderate-sized polygonal cells
- Fine reddish granular cytoplasm
- Relatively monomorphic round nuclei with low nucleocytoplasmic ratio
- Spindle cells
- Occasional ganglion cell
- Sudden anisonucleosis.

Metastatic Tumors[35]

Metastasis in the adrenal gland is frequent and about one-fifth of cancer shows metastasis in cancer.[36] The common primary sites of malignancies are from lung, kidney, and breast (Figs. 32.25A and B). Metastatic carcinoma in the

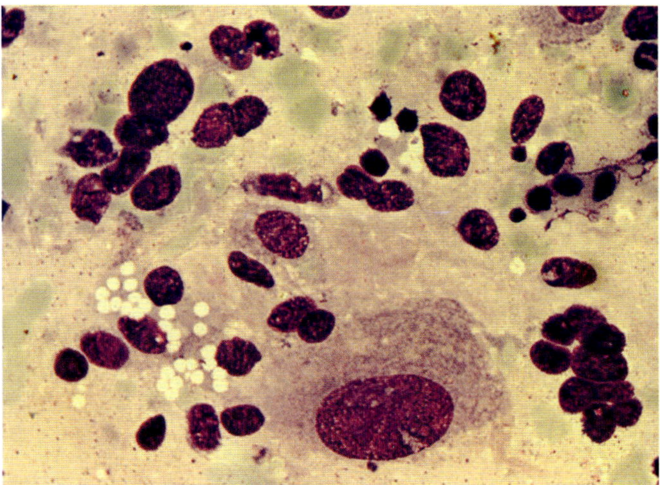

Fig. 32.24: Pheochromocytoma: Sudden nuclear pleomorphism (MGG × OI).

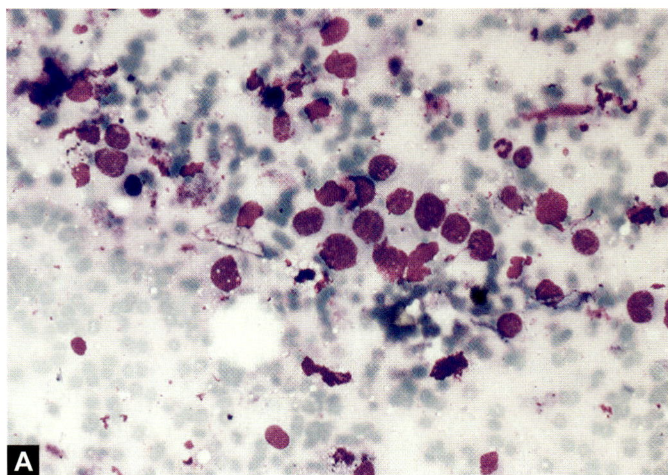

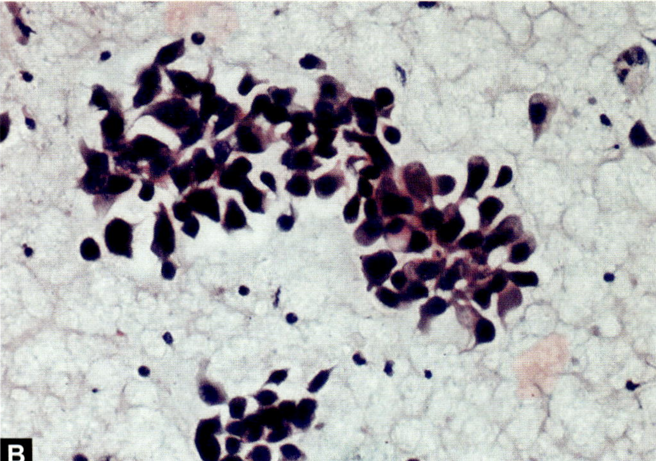

Figs. 32.25A and B: (A) Metastatic adenocarcinoma: Gland formation seen (MGG × MP), (B) Metastatic adenocarcinoma: Higher magnification shows tall columnar looking cells (PAP × MP).

Table 32.7: Characteristic features of metastasis.

Primary tumors	*Cytology*	*Immunocytochemistry*
Renal cell carcinoma	Cells with abundant clear cytoplasm	EMA, CK, and vimentin
Lung carcinoma: Small cell	Small cells, scanty cytoplasm, hyperchromatic nucleus, nuclear molding	NSE, chromogranin, CK
Prostatic adenocarcinoma	Glandular differentiation	PSA
Melanoma	Large pleomorphic cells, spindle cells, cytoplasmic melanin pigment	HMB-45
Colorectal adenocarcinoma	Glandular differentiation	CK20 positive and CK7 negative
Breast carcinoma	Malignant ductular cells	CK7 positive, CK20 negative. ER, PR, and GCDPF 15 positive

(EMA: Epithelial membrane antigen; CK: Cytokeratin; NSE: Neuron-specific enolase; PSA: Prostate-specific antigen).

adrenal may mimic poorly differentiated adrenocortical carcinoma or pheochromocytoma. Cytomorphologically it is very difficult to distinguish adrenocortical carcinoma from metastatic adenocarcinoma and immunocytochemistry may be helpful in this aspect (Table 32.7). Cells in ACC are positive for Melan A, inhibin, calretinin and negative for cytokeratin.

REFERENCES

1. Kiser GC, Totonchy M, Barry JM. Needle tract seeding after percutaneous renal adenocarcinoma aspiration. J Urol. 1986;136:1292-3.
2. Renshaw AA, Granter SR, Cibas ES. Fine needle aspiration of the adult kidney. Cancer Cytopathol. 1997;81:71-88.
3. Kelley CM, Cohen MB, Raab SS. Utility of fine needle aspiration biopsy in solid renal masses. Diagn Cytopathol. 1996;14:14-9.
4. Zardawi IM. Renal fine needle aspiration cytology. Acta Cytol. 1999;43(2):184-90.
5. Truong LD, Todd TD, Dhurandhar B, et al. Fine needle aspiration of renal masses in adults: analysis of results and diagnostic problems in 108 cases. Diagn Cytopathol. 1999;20:339-49.
6. Todd TD, Dhurandhar B, Mody D, et al. Fine needle aspiration of cystic lesions of the kidney. Morphologic spectrum and diagnostic problems in 41 cases. Am J Clin Pathol. 1999;111(3):317-28.
7. Lang EK. Renal cyst puncture studies. Urol Clin N Am.1987;14:91-102.
8. Bosniak MA. The Bosniak renal cyst classification: 25 years later. Radiology. 2012;262(3):781-5.
9. Bosniak MA. The current radiological approach to renal cysts. Radiology. 1986;158:1-10.
10. Kennelly MJ, Grossman HB, Cho KJ. Outcome analysis of 42 cases of renal angiomyolipoma. J Urol. 1994;152:1988-91.
11. Glentoj A, Partoft S. Ultrasound-guided percutaneous aspiration of renal angiomyolipoma. Report of two cases diagnosed by cytology. Acta Cytol. 1984;28:265-8.
12. Helpap B, Knüpffer J, Essmann S. Nucleolar grading of renal cancer: correlation of frequency and localization of nucleoli to histologic and cytologic grading and stage of renal cell carcinomas. Mod Pathol. 1990;3:671-8.
13. Furhman SA, Lasky LC, Limas C. Prognostic significance of morphologic parameters in renal cell carcinoma. Am J Surg Pathol. 1982;6:655-63.
14. Cajulis R, Katz R, Dekmezian R, et al. Fine needle aspiration biopsy of renal cell carcinoma. Cytologic parameters, its concordance with histology and flow cytometric (FCM) data. Lab Invest. 1993;37(3):367-72.
15. Kaelin WG Jr. The von Hippel–Lindau tumor suppressor protein and clear cell renal carcinoma. Clin Cancer Res. 2007;13(2 Pt 2):680s-4s.
16. van den Berg E, van der Hout AH, Oosterhuis JW, et al. Cytogenetic analysis of epithelial renal-cell tumors: relationship with a new histopathological classification. Int J Cancer. 1993;55:223-7.
17. Storkel S, Eble JN, Adlakha K, et al. Classification of renal cell carcinoma: Workgroup No 1. Union Internationale Contre le Cancer (UICC) and the American Joint Committee on Cancer (AJCC). Cancer. 1997;80:987-9.
18. Salamanca J, Alberti N, Lopez-Rios F, et al. Fine needle aspiration of chromophobe renal cell carcinoma. Acta Cytol. 2007;51(1):9-15.
19. Layfield LJ. Fine needle aspiration biopsy of renal collecting duct carcinoma. Diagn Cytopathol. 1994;11:74-8.
20. Powers CN, Elbadawi A. "Cercariform" cells: a clue to the cytodiagnosis of transitional cell origin in metastatic neoplasms? Diagn Cytopathol. 1995;13:15-21.
21. Shet T, Viswanathan S. The cytological diagnosis of paediatric renal tumours. J Clin Pathol. 2009;62(11):961-9.
22. Dey P, Radhika S, Rajwanshi A, et al. Aspiration cytology of Wilms' tumour. Acta Cytol. 1993:37(4):477-82.
23. Dey P, Radhika S, Nijhawan R, et al. Fine needle aspiration cytology of mesoblastic nephroma. Acta Cytol. 1992;36: 404-6.
24. Portugal R, Barroca H. Clear cell sarcoma, cellular mesoblastic nephroma and metanephric adenoma: cytological features and differential diagnosis with Wilms tumour. Cytopathology. 2008;19:80-5.
25. Schmidt D, Beckwith JB. Histopthology of childhood renal tumors. Hematol Oncol Clin North Am. 1995;9:1179-2000.
26. Drut R. Malignant rhabdoid tumor of the kidney diagnosed by fine needle aspiration cytology. Diagn Cytopathol. 1990;6(2):124-6.
27. Radhika S, Dey P, Das A. Fine needle aspiration cytology of clear cell sarcoma and its distinction with Wilms' tumor. Acta Cytol. 1997;41:950-1.
28. McCorkell SJ, Niles NL. Fine needle aspiration of catecholamine-producing adrenal masses: a possibly fatal mistake. AJR. 1985;145(1):113-4.

29. Saboorian MH, Katz RL, Charnsangavej C. Fine needle aspiration cytology of primary and metastatic lesions of the adrenal gland. A series of 188 biopsies with radiologic correlation. Acta Cytol. 1995;39:843-51.
30. Fassina AS, Borsato S, Fedeli U. Fine needle aspiration cytology (FNAC) of adrenal masses. Cytopathology. 2000;11:302-11.
31. Sharma S, Singh R, Verma K. Cytomorphology of adreno-cortical carcinoma and comparison with renal cell carcinoma. Acta Cytol. 1997;41(2):385-92.
32. Gonzalez KD, Noltner KA, Buzin CH, et al. Beyond Li Fraumeni syndrome: clinical characteristics of families with p53 germline mutations. J Clin Oncol. 2009;27: 1250-6.
33. Wu HH, Cramer HM, Kho J. Fine needle aspiration cytology of benign adrenal cortical nodules. A comparison of cytologic findings with those of primary and metastatic adrenal malignancies. Acta Cytol. 1998;42(6):1352-8.
34. Shidham VB, Galindo LM. Phaeochromocytoma. Cytologic findings on intraoperative scrape smears in five cases. Acta Cytol. 1999;43(2):207-13.
35. Lee JE, Evans DB, Hickey RC, et al. Unknown primary cancer presenting as an adrenal mass: frequency and implications for diagnostic evaluation of adrenal incidentalomas. Surgery. 1998;124:1115-22.
36. Page DL, DeLellis RA, Hough AJ. Tumors of the Adrenal. In Atlas of Tumor Pathology, second series, fascicle 23. Washington, DC: Armed Forces Institute of Pathology; 1995.

Review Questions

1. **A 55-year-old male presented with hematuria. Ultrasonography (USG) revealed a 3.5 cm diameter space occupying lesion in the middle of the kidney near the pelvic region. USG-guided fine needle aspiration cytology (FNAC) of the mass was done. Figures 32.26A to F represent the cytology and immunocytochemistry such as vimentin (D), CK 7 (E) and CK 20 (F). What is your diagnosis?**
   a. Renal cell carcinoma
   b. Renal transitional cell carcinoma
   c. Metastatic adenocarcinoma
   d. Renal oncocytoma

2. **A 65-year-old male presented with dysphagia. Ultrasonography (USG) revealed a 1.5 cm diameter space occupying lesion in the adrenal gland. Figures 32.27A to C represent the fine needle aspiration cytology (FNAC) smear of the adrenal lesion. What is your possible diagnosis?**
   a. Metastatic adenocarcinoma
   b. Adrenocotical carcinoma
   c. Pheochromocytoma
   d. Neuroblastoma

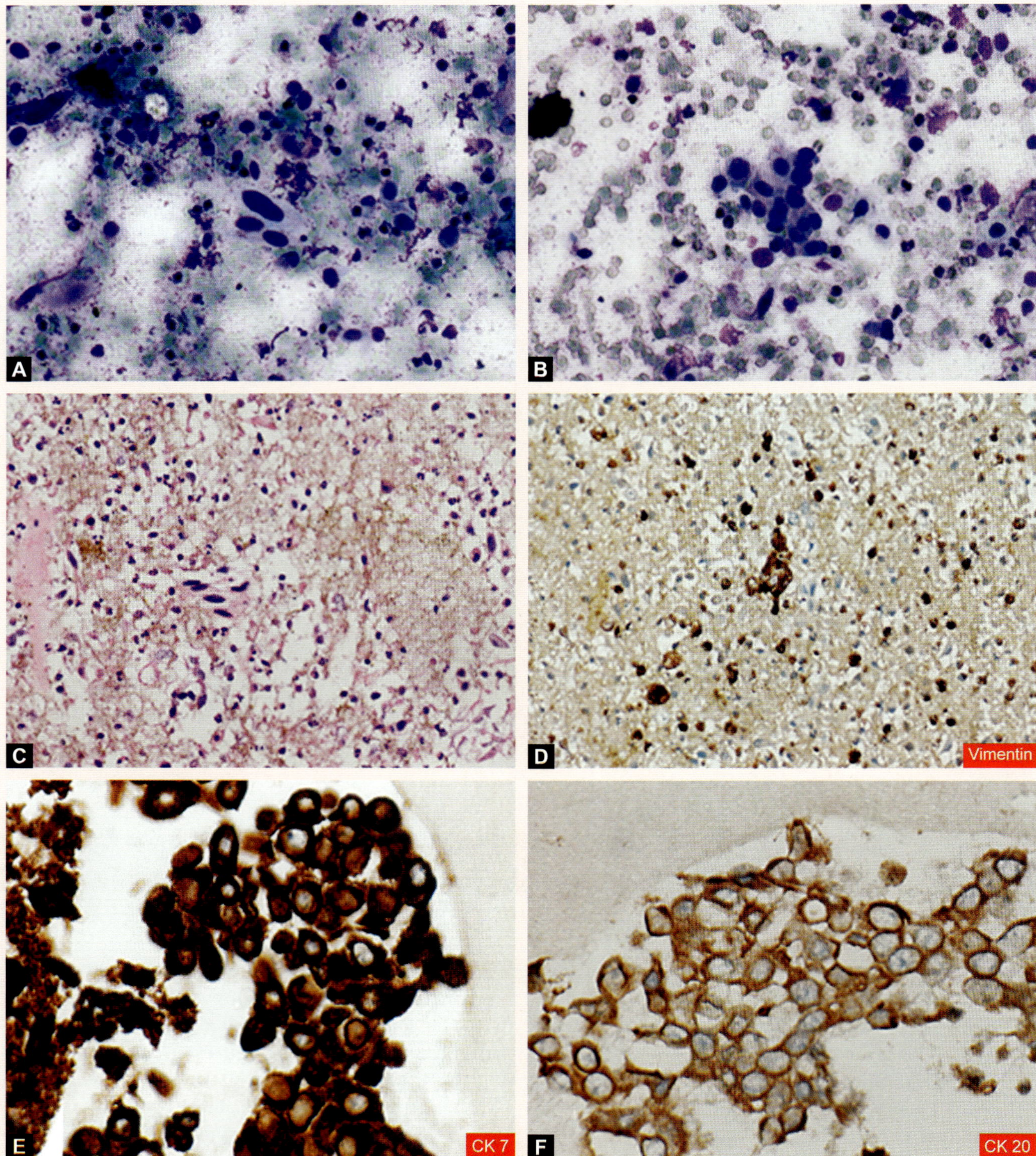

Figs. 32.26A to F: Fine needle aspiration cytology smear and immunocytochemistry of the kidney of question 1.

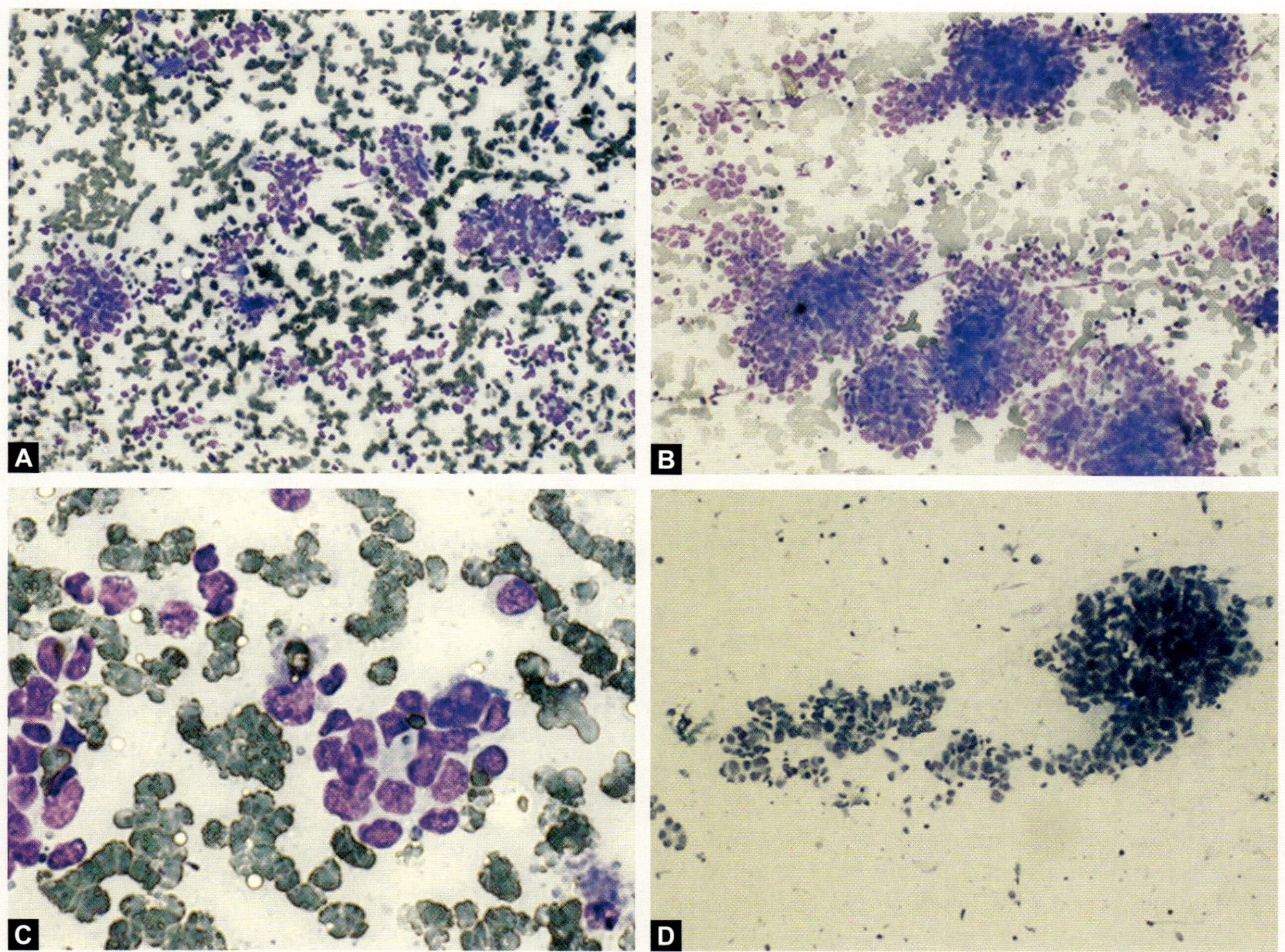

Figs. 32.27A to D: Fine needle aspiration cytology smear of the adrenal gland of question 2.

Answers

1. b. Renal transitional cell carcinoma

   Note: The cytology smear shows discrete and loose clusters of malignant cells. Occasional cells show elongated nuclei. These cells are positive for vimentin, CK 7 and CK 20. Overall features indicate the diagnosis of transitional cell carcinoma.

2. a. Metastatic adenocarcinoma

   Note: The presence of clusters and glandular arrangement of cells with round moderately pleomorphic nuclei favor a metastatic lesion. This patient had adenocarcinoma of esophagus.

CHAPTER

33 Gonads and Prostrate

TESTIS

Introduction

Testis is the male gonad situated within the scrotal sac. Fine needle aspiration cytology (FNAC) of the testis is now a well-established technique. It is mainly done to investigate the nature of the swelling and also to investigate the cases of male infertility. There is an unproven risk of dissemination of malignancy by FNAC through the needle tract. Therefore, many people doubt the necessity of testicular FNAC. In our experience in PGIMER, Chandigarh, we did not encounter any case of dissemination of malignancy through needle tract during testicular FNAC. We have not faced any case of local recurrence or inguinal metastasis due to FNAC of testis. FNAC of the testis is a rapid, economic, and reliable procedure and provides the important information about the nature of the lesion. FNAC of the testicular masses helps in accurate preoperative diagnosis for the management of the patient. FNAC of the scrotal swelling is, however, less controversial and it can be used to diagnose the various cysts and inflammatory lesions.

ANATOMY AND HISTOLOGY OF TESTIS

Each testis is approximately 4 cm long and 2–3 cm wide. Testis develops in the abdominal cavity and then descends in the scrotal sac dragging a part of peritoneum known as tunica vaginalis.

Testis is composed of numerous seminiferous tubules that are surrounded by richly vascular loose connective tissue. In the connective tissue, there are small conglomerations of endocrine cells present which are known as the interstitial cells (of Leydig). Within the seminiferous tubule the germ cells undergo maturation through various stages: spermatocytes to spermatids to spermatozoa. The mature spermatozoa travels from seminiferous tubules to rete testis to ductus efferens and finally stores in epididymis.

NORMAL CELLS OF TESTIS FINE NEEDLE ASPIRATION CYTOLOGY (FIG. 33.1)

Sertoli Cells

These are relatively large cells with fragile cytoplasm and indistinct cell border. The cytoplasm may show fine vacuolations and spermatozoa. The nuclei are round to oval, with granular chromatin having a prominent nucleolus.

Spermatocytes

The primary spermatocytes show scanty deeply basophilic cytoplasm and round nuclei with fine chromatin. Nucleoli are indistinct. Secondary spermatocytes are not identified.

Spermatids

These cells are often present in small groups. The cytoplasm of the cell is scanty and vacuolated. The nuclei are round with clumped chromatin and indistinct nucleoli.

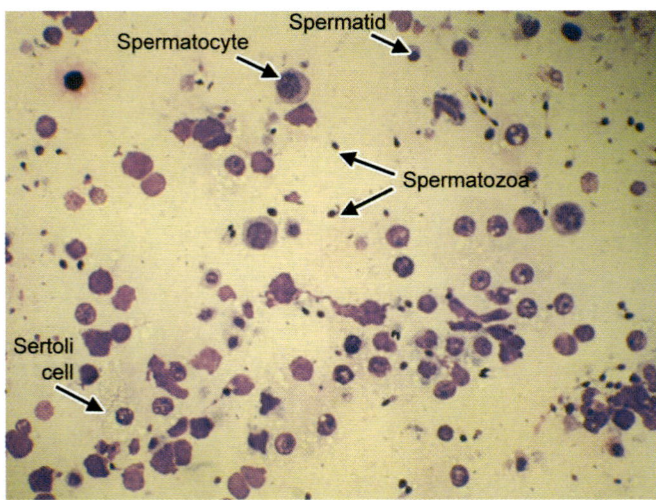

Fig. 33.1: Normal testicular tissue: Sertoli cells, spermatocytes, spermatids, and spermatozoa (MGG × HP).

Spermatozoa

These are triangular-shaped cells with eccentric nuclei. Chromatin of the nuclei is condensed. The tip of the spermatozoa shows a clear cytoplasmic outline. Sperm shows a long tail.

Leydig Cells

These are large cells with abundant granular cytoplasm.

The nuclei are centrally in position with fine granular chromatin and prominent nucleoli. Crystalloids of Reinke are occasionally seen as unstained areas in May-Grünwald Giemsa (MGG)-stained smears.

PERITESTICULAR LESIONS

Hydrocele

Hydrocele is the accumulation of fluid in the tunica vaginalis. Hydrocele may be congenital or acquired. The acquired hydrocele is often associated with inflammation of the tunica vaginalis. Aspirates of hydrocele yields clear straw colored fluid and smears show many sheets of benign tunica lining mesothelial cells.

Spermatocele (Fig. 33.2)

Spermatocele is the cystic dilatation of the efferent ducts. The cyst is filled with spermatozoa. This is usually associated with a history of local operation such as vasectomy etc. FNAC smears show many spermatozoa and foamy macrophages with ingested sperms.

INFLAMMATION

Tuberculous Epididymitis

Tuberculosis of the epididymitis is common in the Indian subcontinent. The aspirate usually yields thick cheesy material. The FNAC smear shows multiple epithelioid cell granulomas, multinucleated giant cells, and lymphocytes on a necrotic background. Ziehl-Neelsen stain for AFB is positive in half of such cases.

Other Causes of Granulomatous Epididymitis

There are other causes of granulomatous inflammation in epididymitis such as fungal infection, granulomatous ischemic lesion, and idiopathic granulomatous epididymitis.

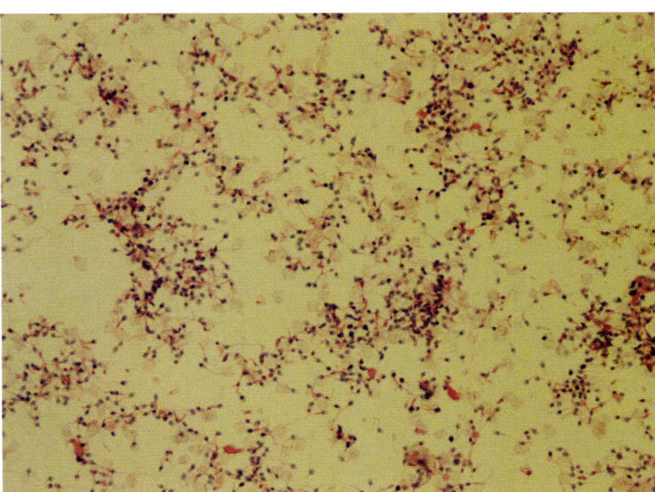

Fig. 33.2: Spermatocele: Abundant spermatozoa in the centrifuged fluid of the spermatocele (H & E × MP).

Filarial Inflammation

Microfilarial infestation in the epididymis often provokes chronic inflammation. Cytology smear shows microfilaria along with variable amount of multinucleated giant cells and granulomas. It is preferable to screen the smear in lower magnification to detect such parasites.

Adenomatoid Tumor[1]

This is the most common tumor of the epididymis and occurs in third and fourth decade of life. The cytology smear shows multiple clusters and sheets of monotonous population of round to oval cells monomorphic nuclei (Fig. 33.3). The nuclei shows fine chromatin and small inconspicuous nucleoli. Discrete spindle cells are also seen.

The tumor cells show strong reactivity for CK (cytokeratin), EMA (epithelial membrane antigen), calretinin, and WT1 (Wilms' tumor 1). The cells are negative for carcinoembryonic antigen (CEA) and factor VIII (FVIII)-related antigen.[2]

Spermatocytic Granuloma[1] (Figs. 33.4 and 33.5)

Spermatocytic granuloma presents as a nodule in the head of the epididymitis. FNAC smears show mixed inflammatory cells consisting of lymphocytes, macrophages, and occasional ill-formed epithelioid cell granulomas. The background of the smear usually contains many

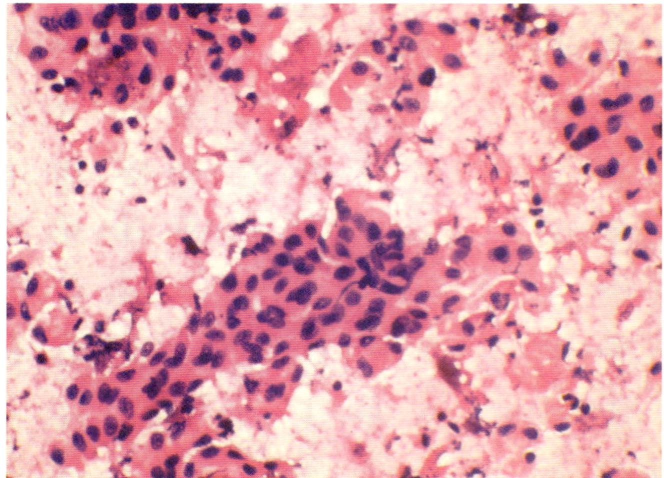

Fig. 33.3: Adenomatoid tumor: Multiple clusters and discrete monomorphic epithelial cells (H & E × HP).

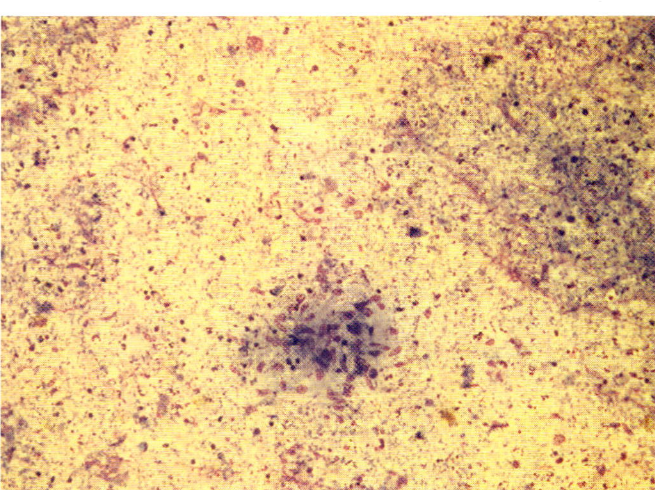

Fig. 33.4: Spermatocytic granuloma: Epithelioid cell granulomas along with many spermatozoa in a dirty necrotic background (MGG × MP).

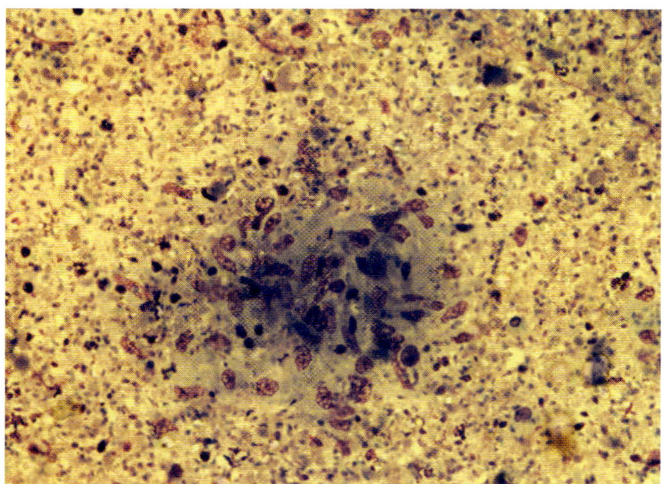

Fig. 33.5: Spermatocytic granuloma: Higher magnification of the epithelioid cell granuloma (MGG × HP).

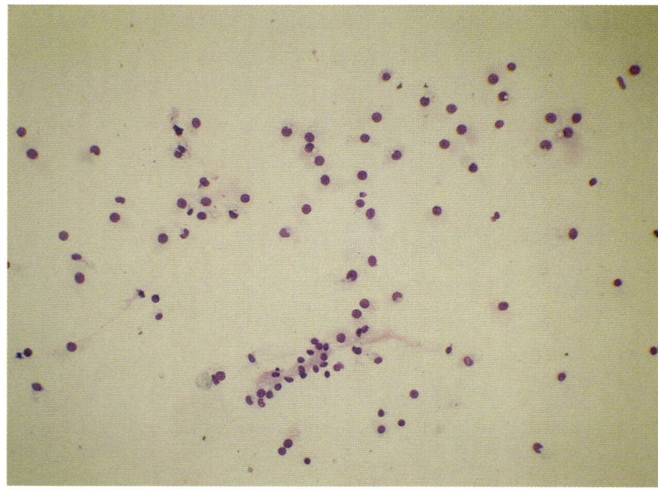

Fig. 33.6: Sertoli cell only syndrome: Only Sertoli cells present (MGG × MP).

spermatozoa or sperm heads. Macrophages with ingested sperm heads are frequently seen. Z-N stain for AFB is always negative in this granulomatous inflammation.

EVALUATION OF MALE INFERTILITY[3-7]

In 1965, Obrant and Persson described FNAC for getting material for cytological evaluation of spermatogenesis.[7] The testicular FNAC for evaluation of male infertility was not popular for long time as many clinicians were afraid of trauma and hemorrhage. However, FNAC of the testis is almost free of complications. FNAC is a relatively easy and quick procedure to assess any obstruction in the efferent duct system and the status of spermatogenesis. The various cells in maturation are easily identified in FNAC smears. FNAC of testis has almost 100% diagnostic accuracy in the evaluation of male azoospermic patient.[6]

Sertoli Cell Only Syndrome (Fig. 33.6)

The smears show large number of Sertoli cells. No other cells are seen. Smear may also show variable number of mast cells.

Early Maturation Arrest

Fine needle aspiration cytology smears show spermatocytes and Sertoli cells in early maturation arrest. No spermatids or sperm are seen.

Late Maturation Arrest

The smears show Sertoli cells, spermatocytes, and spermatids; however, no sperm is seen.

In case of normal spermatogenesis all types of cells are seen. The presence of normal maturation up to the level of spermatozoa in FNAC smear in an azoospermic male indicates the possibility of obstruction in the pathway of semen.

NEOPLASM OF TESTIS

Testicular tumor is classified by WHO[8] as described in Box 33.1.

Seminoma[9-13]

This is the most common germ cell tumor of testis and represents about one third of all testicular tumors. The incidence of this tumor increases sharply after puberty. It commonly occurs between 30 years and 40 years of age. The patient usually presents as painless enlargement of testis.

Cytology (Figs. 33.7 and 33.8)

Here are two histological types of seminoma: (1) classical and (2) spermatocytic. The classical seminoma shows discrete malignant cells in a typical lace like vacuolated background known as tigroid background (Box 33.2). This is due to the cytoplasmic contents of the fragile cells. The individual cells are round to oval in shape and three to four times larger than the mature lymphocytes. The cells show

Box 33.1: Testicular tumor classification (modified WHO).[8]

Germ cell tumors
- Intratubular germ cell neoplasia, unclassified
- Other types

Tumors of one histological type (pure forms)
- Seminoma
- Spermatocytic seminoma
- Embryonal carcinoma
- Yolk sac tumor
- Trophoblastic tumors
  - Choriocarcinoma
  - Trophoblastic neoplasms other than choriocarcinoma
    - Monophasic choriocarcinoma
    - Placental site trophoblastic tumor

Teratoma
- Dermoid cyst
- Monodermal teratoma
- Teratoma with somatic type malignancies

Tumors of more than one histological type (mixed forms)

Sex cord or gonadal stromal tumors
- Leydig cell tumor
- Malignant Leydig cell tumor
- Sertoli cell tumor
- Malignant Sertoli cell tumor
- Granulosa cell tumor

Tumors of the thecoma or fibroma group
- Thecoma
- Fibroma
- Sex cord or gonadal stromal tumor
- Others

Miscellaneous tumors of the testis: Carcinoid, paraganglioma, etc.

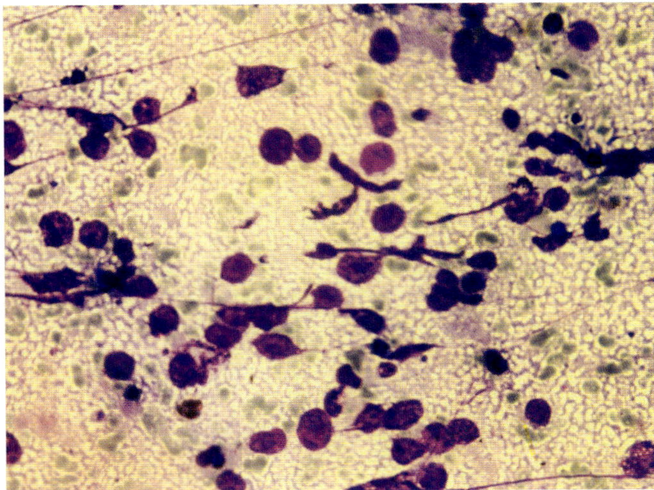

Fig. 33.7: Seminoma: Discrete round cells in a tigroid background (MGG × MP).

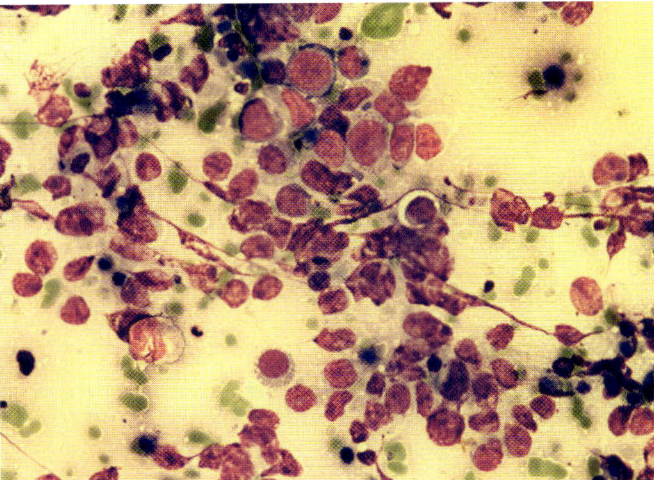

Fig. 33.8: Seminoma: Round cells with vacuolated cytoplasm. Nuclei are enlarged with fine chromatin and prominent nucleoli (MGG × OI).

scanty to moderate amount of vacuolated cytoplasm. Nuclei are round, mildly pleomorphic with fine granular chromatin and prominent nucleoli. The fragile nucleus often gives rise to thin long chromatin threads. Cytoplasmic fragments of the cells resembling lymphoglandular bodies are also noted. In addition, the mature lymphocytes are also seen in the background. Epithelioid cell granulomas are occasionally noted in case of seminoma of testis. Seminoma is positive for placental alkaline phosphatase (PLAP) and CD117. The cells are negative for high molecular weight keratin, epithelial membrane antigen (EMA), and CD30.

Spermatocytic seminoma represents only 4% of all seminoma. They show variable population of cells consisting of small, medium, and large cells. The medium sized cells usually are the dominant population. These cells show scanty to moderate cytoplasm and large central nuclei with coarse nuclear chromatin and prominent nucleoli. Small cells show scanty deep blue cytoplasm with irregular nuclei having dense chromatin. The large cells have abundant cytoplasm and moderately pleomorphic large nuclei. The cells often are binucleated with multiple prominent nucleoli.

Unlike classical seminoma, the spermatocytic seminoma shows a clean background that is free of any lymphocytes. Tigroid lacy vacuolated background is absent in such tumor.

Differential Diagnosis

- *Nonseminomatous germ cell tumor*: The other germ cell tumors may simulate seminoma. The typical tigroid background, lymphocytes and individual cell morphology may be helpful. Frequent admixture of different germ cell tumors may pose significant problem in diagnosis.
- *Non-Hodgkin lymphoma*: NHL shows lack of tigroid background. Lymphoglandular bodies are always present in NHL. NHLs are positive for CD45 and negative for placental alkaline phosphatase.
- *Metastatic carcinoma*: Metastatic carcinoma shows cohesive clusters of malignant cells with moderate nuclear enlargement and pleomorphism. The cells are positive for CK and negative for LCA and placental alkaline phosphatase.

Box 33.2: Seminoma.

- Discrete cells
- Tigroid lacy vacuolated background
- Scanty vacuolated cytoplasm
- Round mildly pleomorphic nuclei, fine chromatin, prominent nucleoli
- Background lymphocytes
- Epithelioid cell granulomas

Immunocytochemistry: Positive for placental alkaline phosphatase (PLAP) and CD117 (C-Kit).

Box 33.3: Embryonal carcinoma.

- Cohesive three-dimensional clusters
- Small acinar, tubular, and papillary pattern
- Large cells, moderately pale vacuolated cytoplasm
- Large moderate to marked pleomorphic nuclei
- Single to multiple prominent nucleoli, often macronucleoli.

Embryonal Carcinoma

The cytological features of embryonal carcinomas are mentioned in Box 33.3.

Cytology (Figs. 33.9 and 33.10)

The aspirates of embryonal carcinoma show predominantly cohesive clusters of cells along with acinar, tubular, and papillary arrangement. The tumor cells show large highly pleomorphic nuclei with irregular nuclear margin. The nuclei contain multiple prominent nucleoli. Background of the smear may show necrosis. The tumor cells are positive for AFP, high molecular weight keratin, CD30 and negative for CD117.

Yolk Sac Tumor

Yolk sac tumor is also called as endodermal sinus tumor. The tumor may occur in pure form or as a component of mixed germ cell tumor. The smear shows multiple cohesive clusters of cells in a mucoid background. The tumor cells

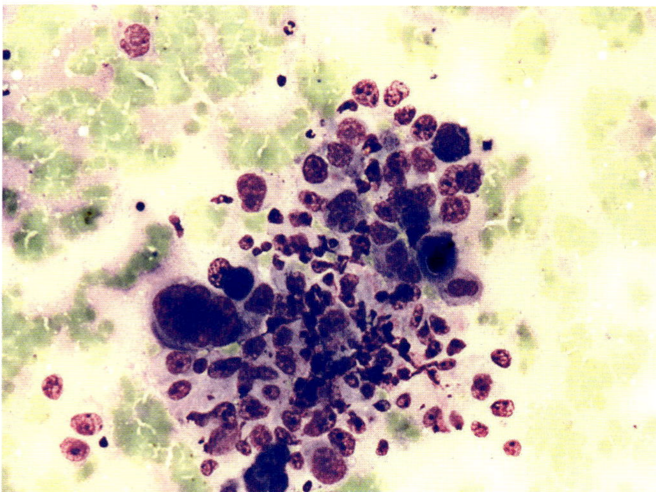

Fig. 33.9: Embryonal carcinoma: Loose cluster of cells with markedly pleomorphic cells (MGG × HP).

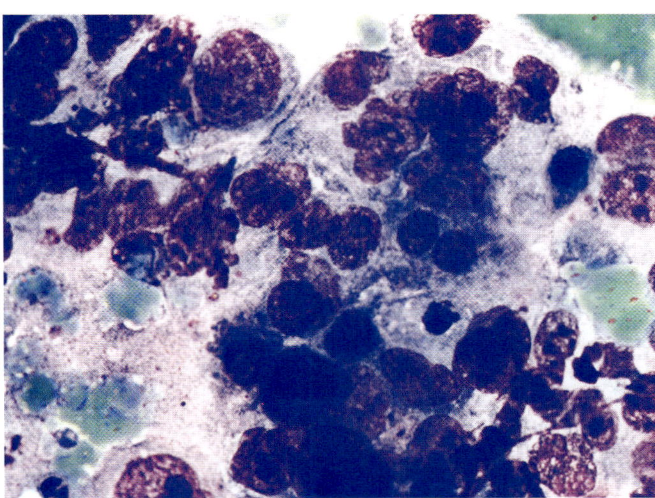

Fig. 33.10: Embryonal carcinoma: Large cells with enlarged nuclei having multiple prominent nucleoli (MGG × OI).

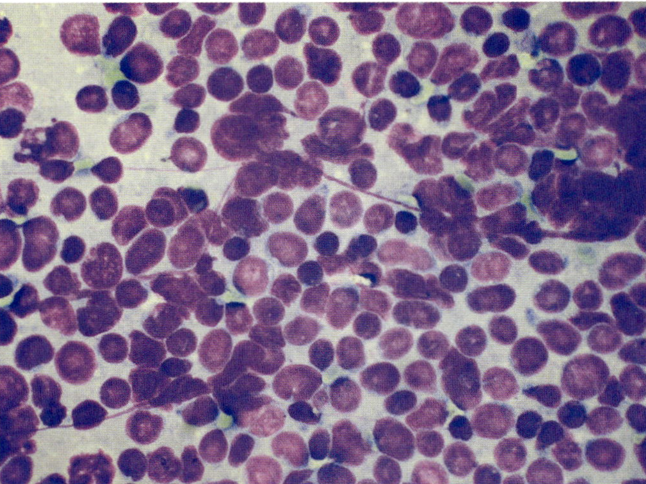

Fig. 33.11: Non-Hodgkin limphoma (NHL) testis: Lymphoblastic lymphoma secondarily involved in testis (MGG × OI).

are moderately pleomorphic with vacuolated cytoplasm. Nuclei show multiple prominent nucleoli. Intracytoplasmic and extracellular pink globules may also be noted. These globules are PAS positive and diastase resistant. The cells of endodermal sinus tumor are positive for PLAP and AFP.

Choriocarcinoma

Choriocarcinoma represents 5% of all testicular tumors. The tumor is usually small in size and there may not be any enlargement of testis. The cytology smear shows syncytio and cytotrophoblast. The syncytiotrophoblasts are relatively large cells with abundant cytoplasm and large severely pleomorphic nuclei with multiple prominent nucleoli. The cytotrophoblastic cells are small sized with scanty vacuolated cytoplasm having round mildly pleomorphic nuclei and indistinct nucleoli. Background of the smear usually shows large amount of necrosis. The cells are consistently positive for hCG and keratin.

Other Tumors of Testis

Non-Hodgkin lymphoma of the testis represents only 2% of all the testicular tumors. NHL of testis usually affects the elderly patient. Most of the testicular lymphomas are diffuse large B-cell lymphoma. The cytomorphology of NHL is similar as that of other areas (Fig. 33.11).

Female Genital System

Many clinicians do not recommend FNAC of frankly malignant operable ovarian tumor because of possible rupture and spillage of cyst material to the peritoneal cavity. Moreover, the preoperative diagnosis of malignant ovarian tumor may not be needed because the surgical excision may be the treatment of choice. FNAC of ovarian tumor is indicated in:

- Confirmation of recurrence of the malignant tumor
- To diagnose advanced un-resectable ovarian tumor
- Confirmation of benign incidental ovarian tumor
  - Presently the preoperative FNAC diagnosis is needed before neoadjuvant chemotherapy

Fine needle aspiration cytology of ovarian tumor is done under USG or CT scan guidance. The benign cyst in USG is usually thin walled, simple cyst without any septation. No solid areas are seen. FNAC from the ovary is almost free of any complications. In our institution, we have never seen any needle tract seeding after FNAC of ovarian malignancy. Due to heterogeneity of the ovarian histology in various parts of the ovarian mass it is not always possible to have proper sampling from the representative area and malignancy may be underdiagnosed. The sensitivity of ovarian tumor is as high as 90%. The false negative FNAC report is particularly seen in case of borderline tumors.

NON-NEOPLASTIC CYST

Follicular Cyst

Follicular cyst of ovary may be of variable sized and unilateral. USG shows unilocular thin-walled fluid-filled cyst. The majority of them spontaneously regressed within a few months.

Fine needle aspiration cytology of the cyst yields clear fluid. The smear of the fluid is usually paucicellular. However, occasionally the smears may be hypercellular. The cells are discrete granulosa cells with scanty to moderate amount of vacuolated cytoplasm and round monomorphic nuclei. The nuclei show granular chromatin and 1–2 prominent nucleoli. Nuclear grooves may be seen in occasional cells.

Corpus Luteal Cyst

This is due to persistent presence of corpus luteal cyst. The cyst is usually unilocular and lined by corpus luteal cell.

Cytology smear of the corpus luteal cyst shows discrete corpus luteal cells (Box 33.4). The cells are large with abundant finely vacuolated cytoplasm. Nuclei are central and pyknotic. In addition, the smear may show golden brown hemosiderin-laden histiocytes.

Endometriotic Cyst

Fine needle aspiration cytology smears of the endometriotic cyst show hemosiderin-laden histiocytes and occasional degenerated endometrial glandular cells and endometrial stromal fragments (Box 33.5). The endometrial cells are arranged in small clusters. The cells are small with scanty cytoplasm. The nuclei are monomorphic hyperchromatic with inconspicuous nucleoli. The endometrial stromal cells are round with moderate cytoplasm and oval nuclei.

OVARIAN TUMOR[14-18]

Serous and Mucinous Adenocarcinoma (Figs. 33.12 to 33.14)

The cytology smears of serous adenocarcinoma show multiple cohesive clusters and discrete cells. Smears may also show multiple glands or papillary arrangement of cells. The malignant cells are round to oval with moderate amount of vacuolated cytoplasm (Box 33.6). The nuclei show moderate pleomorphism with vesicular chromatin having prominent nucleoli. In addition, psammoma bodies are also seen. Tumor necrosis and increased mitotic activities are the indicators of malignancy. At times, it is very difficult to distinguish a borderline serous cystadenoma from the serous cystadenocarcinoma. In difficult case histopathology is needed.

Box 33.4: Corpus luteal cyst.

- Large cells
- Abundant finely vacuolated cytoplasm
- Central pyknotic nuclei
- Hemosiderin-laden histiocytes.

Box 33.5: Endometriotic cyst.

- Hemosiderin-laden histiocytes
- Endometrial cells
- *Stromal cells*: Round with moderate cytoplasm.

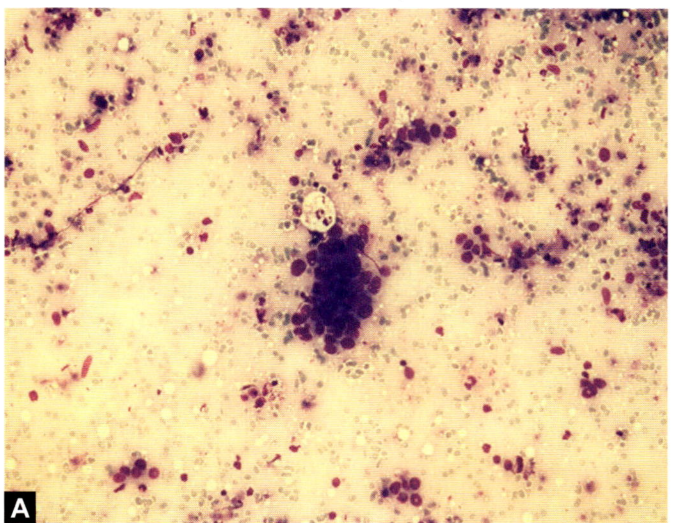

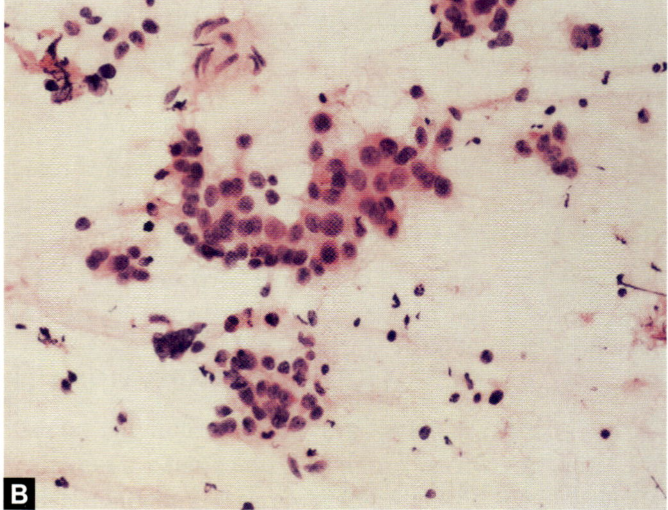

Figs. 33.12A and B: (A) Serous cystadenocarcinoma: Cohesive cluster and discrete malignant cells (MGG × MP). (B) Serous cystadenocarcinoma: Loose clusters of round cells with moderately pleomorphic enlarged nuclei (H & E × MP).

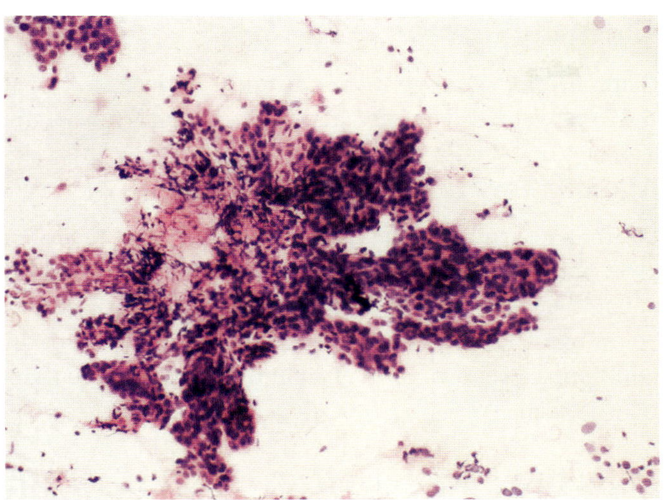

Fig. 33.13: Serous cystadenocarcinoma: Papillary clusters of malignant epithelial cells (H & E × MP).

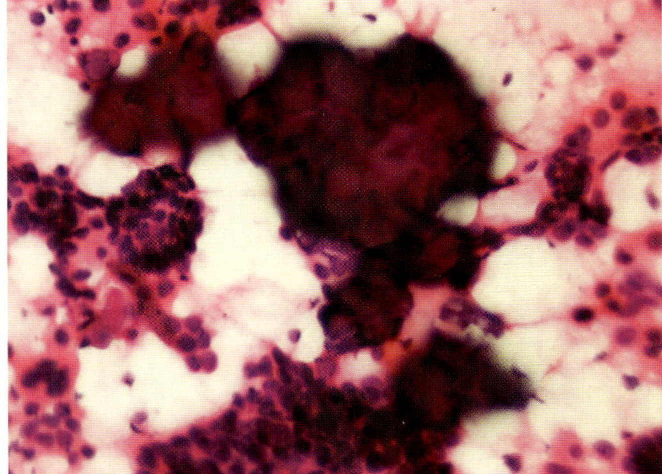

Fig. 33.14: Serous cystadenocarcinoma: Concentric laminated psammoma body (H & E × HP).

Box 33.6: Serous cystadenocarcinoma.

- Cohesive clusters, single cells, and glandular arrangement
- Large round cells
- Pleomorphic nuclei
- Prominent nucleoli
- Psammoma bodies

Box 33.7: Mucinous cystadenocarcinoma.

- Mucinous material
- Columnar cells
- Intracellular mucin
- Pleomorphic nuclei
- Prominent nucleoli.

Mucinous Cystadenocarcinoma

Fine needle aspiration cytology smears of mucinous adenocarcinoma show multiple three-dimensional (3D) cohesive clusters of malignant cells in the background of mucinous material (Box 33.7). The individual cells are columnar in shape with central to eccentric basally placed nuclei. The cytoplasm of the cell is moderately vacuolated. The nuclei are large with mild to moderate pleomorphism and prominent nucleoli.

Differential Diagnosis

- *Metastatic carcinoma*: Metastatic carcinoma particularly metastatic colonic carcinoma is difficult to differentiate from the primary ovarian carcinoma.
- *Borderline malignancy*: It is impossible to differentiate a borderline ovarian malignancy from a frank malignancy in FNAC.

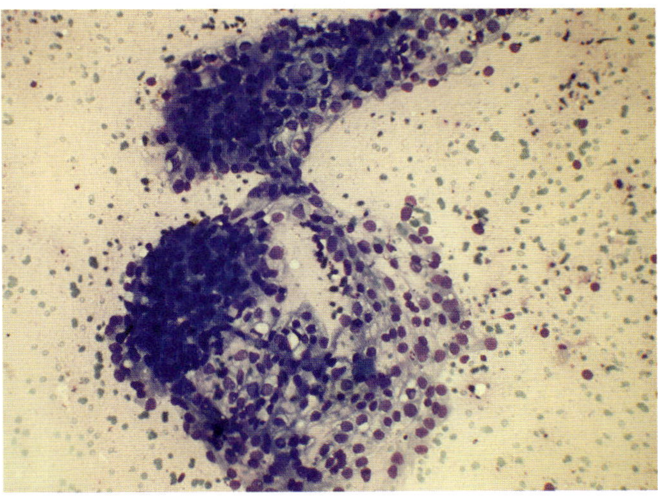

Fig. 33.15: Clear cell carcinoma: Cluster of cell with clear vacuolated cytoplasm (MGG × MP).

Endometrioid Carcinoma

On FNAC smear it is difficult to distinguish endometrioid carcinoma from serous adenocarcinoma. The smears show discrete cells and small clusters or fragments of cells. The cells are columnar in look with moderately pleomorphic nuclei. Background may show hemorrhage, necrosis, and hemosiderin-laden macrophages.

Clear Cell Carcinoma (Figs. 33.15 and 33.16)

Fine needle aspiration cytology smear shows clusters and discrete tumor cells. These cells have abundant clear pale vacuolated cytoplasm with centrally placed moderately pleomorphic nuclei (Box 33.8). The nuclei show frequent binucleation and prominent nucleoli.[19] Extracellular hyaline material may also be noted.

Differential Diagnosis

- *Metastatic renal cell carcinoma*: The cells of clear cell carcinoma of ovary may simulate metastatic renal cell carcinoma.

Box 33.8: Clear cell carcinoma.

- Clear vacuolated cytoplasm
- Central nucleus
- Moderate nuclear pleomorphism.

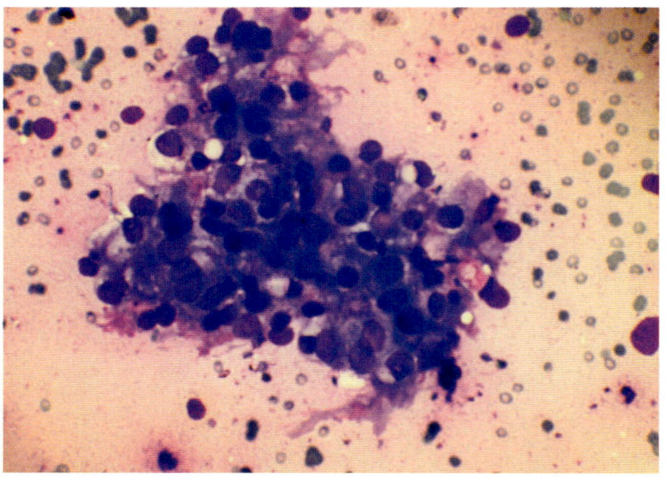

Fig. 33.16: Clear cell carcinoma: Higher magnification showing round to oval cells with moderate amount of vacuolated cytoplasm and enlarged nuclei (MGG × HP).

Germ Cell Tumor

Cytomorphology of germ cell tumor is similar to that of testicular germ cell tumor. This is already described before.

Mature Teratoma

Fine needle aspiration cytology smears of mature teratoma yield pultaceous material. Smears show many anucleated squamous cells, hair follicles, sebaceous cells, ciliated columnar epithelial cells, and intestinal epithelial cells. In addition, mesenchymal and mature neural components may be seen.

Immature Teratoma (Figs. 33.17 to 33.20)

Immature teratoma is an intermediate type of malignancy and graded in histopathology according to the presence of immature neural elements. In addition to mature components, the FNAC smears show immature neural components such as rosette-like structures and round cells simulating cells of neuroblastoma. These cells show scanty cytoplasm, round nuclei, and fine chromatin. Occasionally the tumor shows other germ cell tumors particularly yolk sac tumors. The presence of hyaline globules and large cells with severely pleomorphic nuclei having multiple prominent nucleoli suggest the possibility of yolk sac tumors. Serum AFP is elevated in such cases.

Dysgerminoma

Cytomorphological features of dysgerminoma are similar to that of seminoma of the testis. The tumor cells are

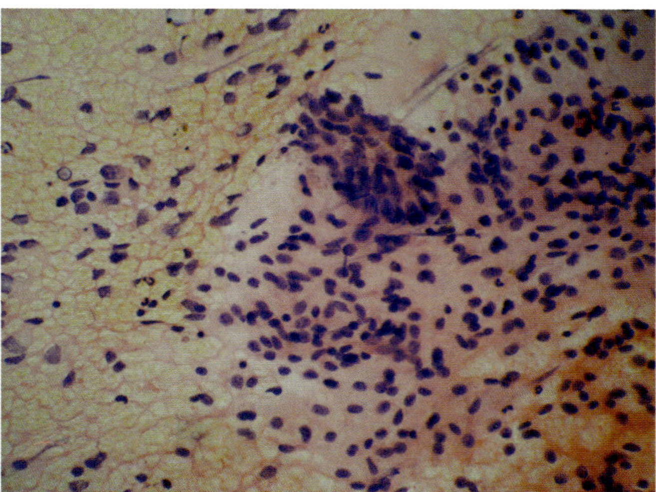

Fig. 33.17: Immature teratoma: Discrete round to oval cells and loose cluster of spindle cells embedded in connective tissue (H & E × MP).

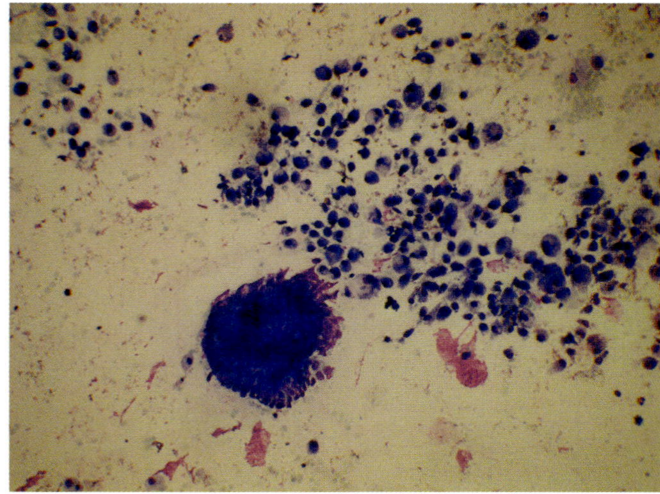

Fig. 33.18: Immature teratoma: Discrete columnar cells and cluster of round cells (MGG × MP).

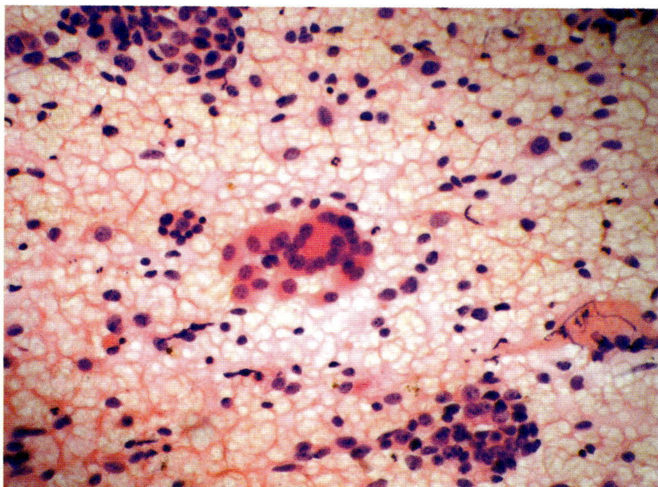

Fig. 33.19: Immature teratoma: Round discrete cells and tubules (H & E × MP).

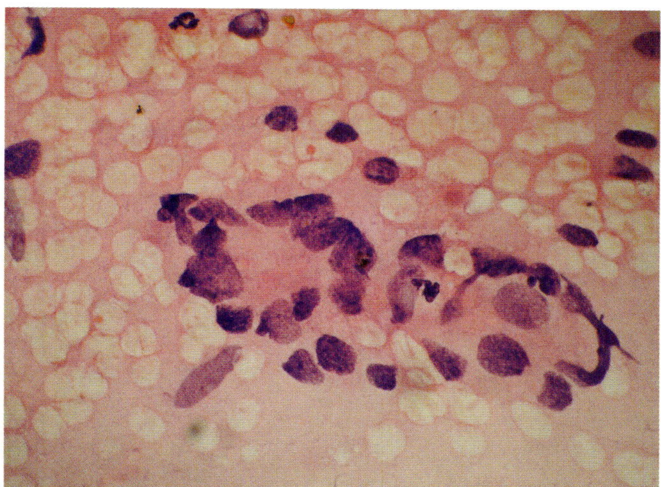

Fig. 33.20: Immature teratoma: Vague rosette like structure (H & E × HP).

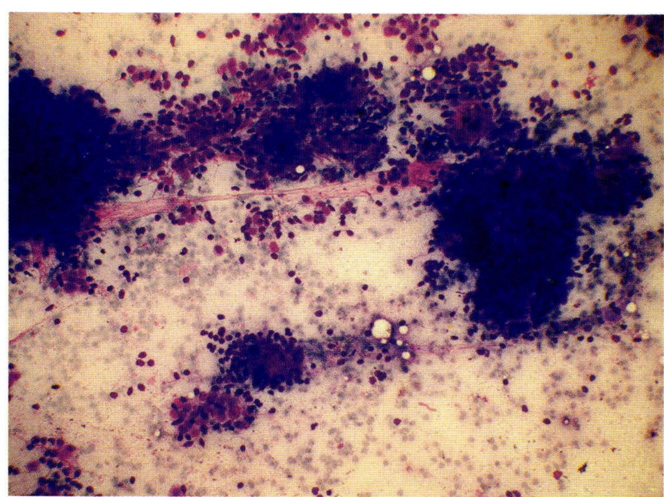

Fig. 33.21: Granulosa cell tumor: Monomorphic round cells in clusters and arranged around reddish globules (MGG × MP).

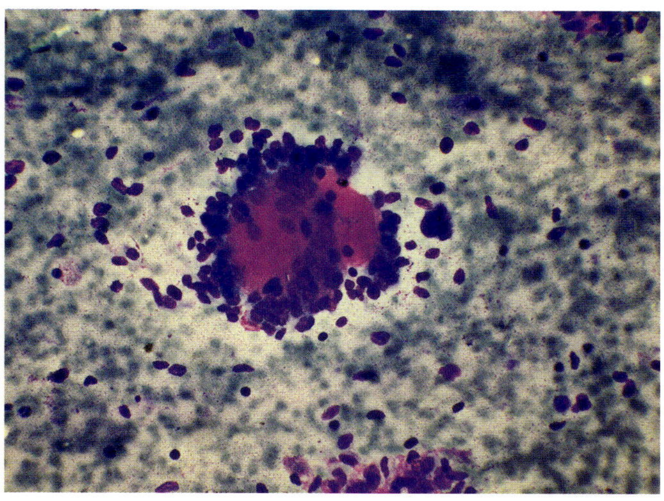

Fig. 33.22: Granulosa cell tumor: Cells are arranged around pinkish material (MGG × HP).

predominantly discrete in a tigroid background. The cells are large round with scanty vacuolated cytoplasm and mildly pleomorphic nuclei with prominent nucleoli. Mature lymphocytes are admixed with the tumor cells.

Granulosa Cell Tumor (Figs. 33.21 and 33.22)

This tumor develops from the granulosa cells of ovary and represents 1% of all ovarian tumors. The tumor occurs in all age group. The functional granulosa cell tumor may show hyperestrogenic symptoms such as irregular bleeding in postmenopausal woman, menstrual disorders in reproductive age group and pseudoprecocious puberty in prepubertal girl.

Cytology

The FNAC smears of the granulosa cell tumor show both discrete and small cohesive clusters of cells (Box 33.9). Occasionally the cells are arranged around deep pink PAS positive material. The cells are round with scanty to moderate amount of pale cytoplasm having indistinct borders. Unlike adenocarcinoma, the nuclei of the cells are monomorphic, round and often have characteristic coffee bean-like groove.

Sertoli Cell Tumor

Cytological diagnosis of Sertoli cell tumor is difficult. The smear shows discrete monomorphic round to oval cells (Figs. 33.23 and 33.24). Occasional tubules are also noted. The background may be fatty vacuolated.

Prostate[20,21]

The major indication of FNAC of prostrate is to differentiate from benign prostatic enlargement from malignancy. Prostate-specific antigen (PSA) is a useful serum biomarker for screening of prostate carcinoma. Core needle biopsy of the prostate along with serum PSA level estimation has greatly replaced FNAC of the prostrate. However, FNAC has the added advantage of multiple sampling from the different area of the prostrate. The detailed description of prostrate FNAC has been described in previous chapter. FNAC of prostate is almost free of any complications except minor hematuria, pyrexia, and hematospermia. Diagnostic accuracy of prostate FNAC is well established.

Box 33.9: Granulosa cell tumor.

- Discrete cells
- Cells arranged around pink material
- Monomorphic nuclei
- Longitudinal coffee bean-like nuclear groove

Normal Cells in Prostrate Fine Needle Aspiration Cytology

Prostrate epithelial cells: The normal prostate epithelial cells are usually present in small monolayered sheets. The cells are arranged as honeycomb-like pattern. The individual cells are round, with scanty cytoplasm and round monomorphic nuclei having indistinct nucleoli.

Seminal vesicle cells: These cells are quite large with hyperchromatic enlarge nuclei. Seminal vesicle cells may be mistaken as malignant cells. However, these cells are readily identifiable because of yellow lipochrome pigment in the cytoplasm and accompanying spermatozoa.

Spermatozoa: Occasionally spermatozoa are seen in prostate FNAC.

Rectal epithelial cells: Benign columnar epithelial cells from the rectum are also seen in FNAC smears of the prostrate. The cells are columnar in shape with round monomorphic nuclei and vacuolated cytoplasm.

Urothelial cells: The lining epithelial cells of the bladder may be seen if the needle passes through the bladder wall to the superficial mucosa.

BENIGN PROSTATIC HYPERPLASIA

Cytology (Fig. 33.25)

The cytology smear of the benign prostatic hyperplasia shows multiple clusters of monolayered sheets and

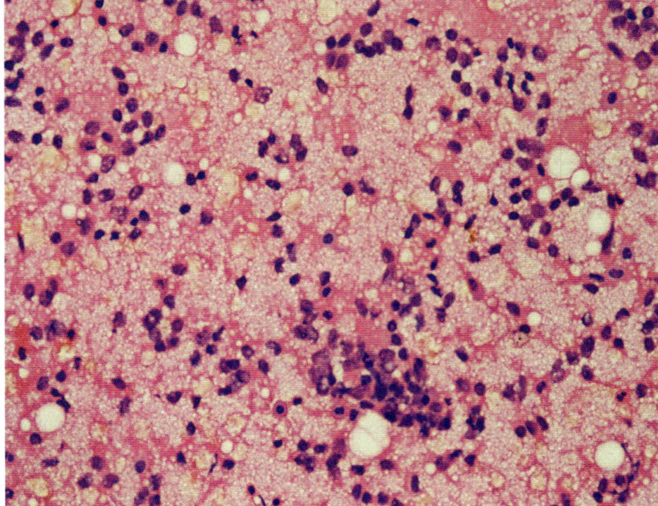

Fig. 33.23: Sertoli cell tumor: Monomorphic round to oval cells in vacuolated background (H & E × MP).

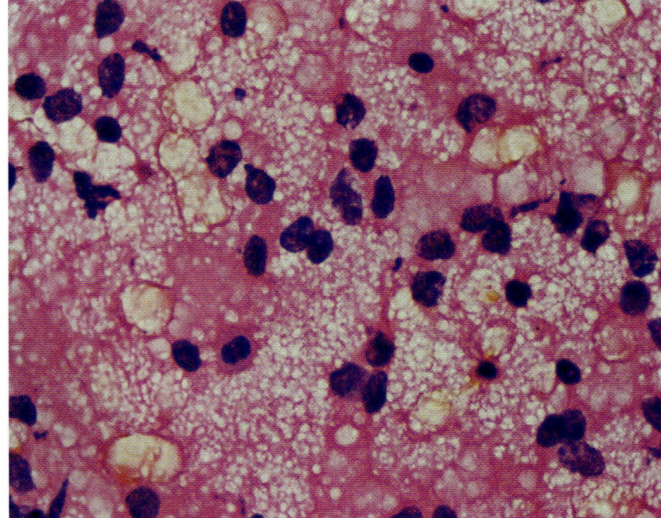

Fig. 33.24: Sertoli cell tumor: Higher magnification showing better morphology. Round cells with blunt nuclear chromatin (H & E × HP).

occasionally gland-like arrangement (Box 33.10). The cells are round with scanty cytoplasm and remarkably monomorphic nuclei with regular nuclear membrane. Nuclear chromatin is finely granular with indistinct nucleoli.

CARCINOMA

Cytology (Figs. 33.26 and 33.27)

The FNAC smear of the prostrate shows 3D tight clusters of cells, multiple microacinar arrangement, and dyscohesive cells (Box 33.11). There are abundant microacinar structures present in adenocarcinoma. Considerable amount of dissociated cells are also present. Nuclei of the cells are enlarged, pleomorphic with high N/C ratio. Nuclear margin is irregular with large prominent nucleoli. The most important characteristics of adenocarcinoma include:

- Three-dimensional clusters
- Microacini
- Dissociated cells
- Pleomorphic cells with high N/C ratio
- Prominent macronucleoli.

Box 33.10: Benign prostatic hyperplasia.

- Monolayered sheets
- Round, monomorphic nuclei
- Granular chromatin
- No nuclear enlargement.

Box 33.11: Adenocarcinoma of prostate.

- Three-dimensional clusters, dissociated cells, and multiple microacinar structures
- Nuclear enlargement and high nucleocytoplasmic ratio
- Prominent nucleoli
- Irregular nuclear membrane

Prostate-specific antigen (PSA) is high (more than 4 ng/mL).

Differential Diagnosis

- Seminal vesicle cells
- *Rectal mucosal cell*: Rectal mucosal cells may be misinterpreted as malignant cells. However, individual cells do not show any features of malignancy.

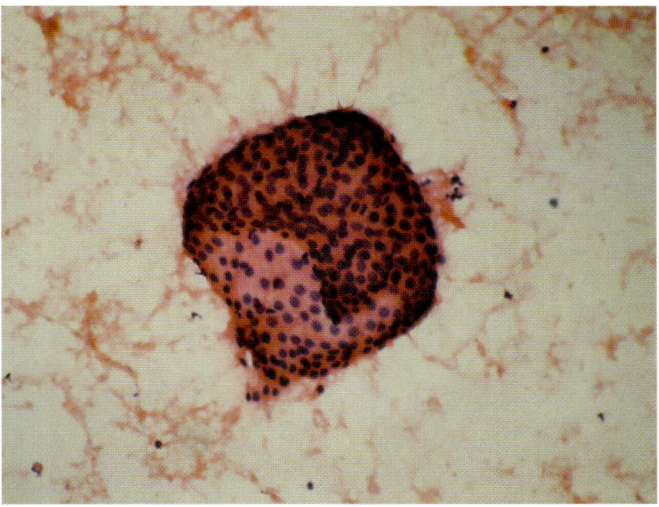

Fig. 33.25: Prostrate epithelial cells: Monolayer sheet of benign prostatic epithelial cells (H & E × MP).

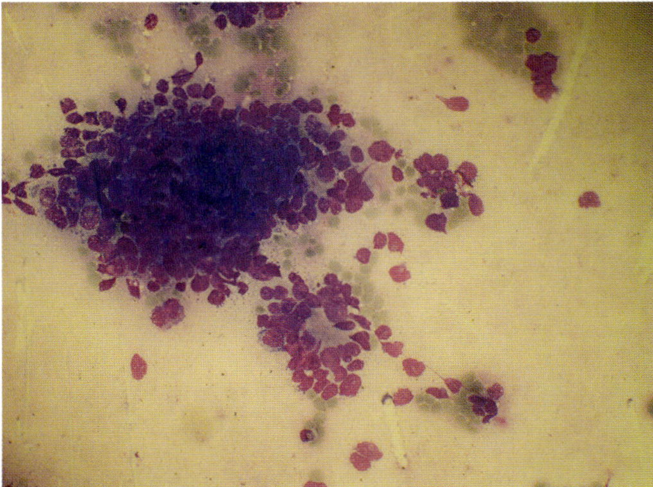

Fig. 33.26: Adenocarcinoma of prostate: Cluster and glandular arrangement of cells (MGG × MP).

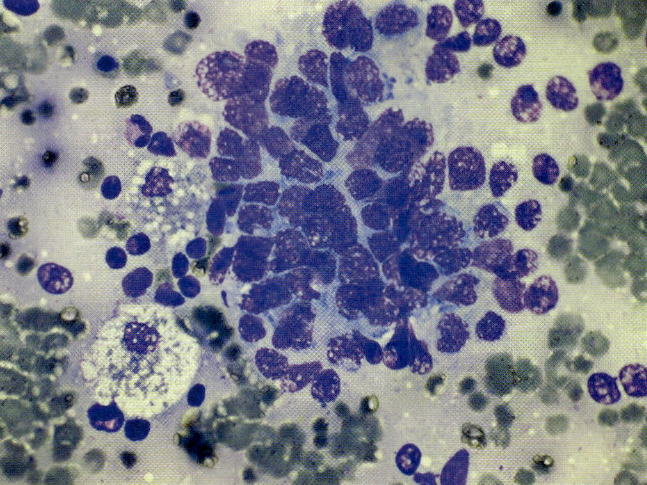

Fig. 33.27: Adenocarcinoma of prostate: Three-dimensional cluster of malignant cells with moderately pleomorphic nuclei (MGG × HP).

- *Well-differentiated carcinoma versus benign lesion*: It is often difficult to differentiate well-differentiated carcinoma from the benign prostatic hyperplasia.

Other tumors: Tumors from the adjacent area such as rectum or bladder may also involve prostrate.

Rarely sarcoma may develop from the native prostratic stroma and muscle. Leiomyosarcomas are most frequently seen among all other sarcomas. The tumor cells are usually arranged in small tight clusters and fascicles. The cells are elongated with spindle-shaped blunt ended nuclei. The cells of leiomyosarcoma are positive for desmin and smooth muscle actin.

REFERENCES

1. Gupta N, Rajwanshi A, Srinivasan R, et al. Fine needle aspiration of epididymal nodules in Chandigarh, north India: an audit of 228 cases. Cytopathology. 2006;17(4):195-8.
2. Sangoi AR, McKenney JK, Schwartz EJ, et al. Adenomatoid tumors of the female and male genital tracts: a clinicopathological and immunohistochemical study of 44 cases. Mod Pathol. 2009;22:1228-35.
3. Jain M, Kumari N, Rawat A, et al. Usefulness of testicular fine needle aspiration cytology in cases of infertility. Indian J Pathol Microbiol. 2007;50(4):851-4.
4. Srivastava A, Raghavendran M, Jain M, et al. Fine needle aspiration cytology of the testis: can it be a single diagnostic modality in azoospermia? Urol Int. 2004;73(1):23-7.
5. Arora VK, Singh N, Bhatia A, et al. Testicular fine needle aspiration cytology for the diagnosis of azoospermia and oligospermia. Acta Cytol. 2000;44(3):349-56.
6. Rajwanshi A, Indudhara R, Goswami AK, et al. Fine needle aspiration cytology in azoospermic males. Diagn Cytopathol. 1991;7(1):3-6.
7. Obrant KO, Persson PS. Zytologis Che untersuchung des Hodens durch. Aspiration biopsie, Zur Beuteilung der. Fertil Urol Int. 1965;20:176-89.
8. Eble JN, Sauter G, Epstein JI, et al. World Health Organization Classification of Tumours. Pathology and Genetics of Tumours of the Urinary System and Male Genital Organs. IARC Press. Lyon; 2004.
9. Caraway NP, Fanning CV, Amato RJ, et al. Fine needle aspiration cytology of seminoma: a review of 16 cases. Diagn Cytopathol. 1995;12(4):327-33.
10. Assi A, Patetta R, Fava C, et al. Fine needle aspiration of testicular lesions: report of 17 cases. Diagn Cytopathol. 2000;23(6):388-92.
11. García-Solano J, Sánchez-Sánchez C, Montalbán-Romero S, et al. Fine needle aspiration (FNA) of testicular germ cell tumours; a 10-year experience in a community hospital. Cytopathology. 1998;9(4):248-62.
12. Saran RK, Banerjee AK, Gupta SK, et al. Spermatocytic seminoma: a cytology and histology case report with review of the literature. Diagn Cytopathol. 1999;20(4):233-6.
13. Fleury-Feith J, Bellot-Besnard J. Criteria for aspiration cytology for the diagnosis of seminoma. Diagn Cytopathol. 1989;5(4):392-5.
14. Dey P, Saha SC, Dhar KK. Fine needle aspiration biopsy of ovarian neoplasm. Indian J Pathol Microbiol. 2001;44(2): 103-6.
15. Andersen WA, Nichols GE, Avery SR, et al. Cytologic diagnosis of ovarian tumors: factors influencing accuracy in previously undiagnosed cases. Am J Obstet Gynecol. 1995;173(2):457-63.
16. Uguz A, Ersoz C, Bolat F, et al. Fine needle aspiration cytology of ovarian lesions. Acta Cytol. 2005;49(2):144-8.
17. Ganjei P. Fine needle aspiration cytology of the ovary. Clin Lab Med. 1995;15(3):705-26.
18. Sood T, Handa U, Mohan H, et al. Evaluation of aspiration cytology of ovarian masses with histopathological correlation. Cytopathology. 2010;21(3):176-85.
19. Atahan S, Ekinci C, Icli F, et al. Cytology of clear cell carcinoma of the female genital tract in fine needle aspirates and ascites. Acta Cytol. 2000;44(6):1005-9.
20. Maksem JA, Berner A, Bedrossian C. Fine needle aspiration biopsy of the prostate gland. Diagn Cytopathol. 2007;35:778-5.
21. Pérez-Guillermo M, Acosta-Ortega J, García-Solano J. Pitfalls and infrequent findings in fine needle aspiration of the prostate gland. Diagn Cytopathol. 2005;33(2):126-37.

Review Questions

1. A 12-year-old boy presented with scrotal mass 4 cm diameter for 2 months. On examination the swelling appears to be adjacent to testis. Clinical diagnosis was non-Hodgkin's lymphoma or seminoma. Figures 33.28A to F show the fine needle aspiration cytology smear (a, b), cell block section (c), CD 45 (d), desmin (e), and myogenin (f) stain.

What is your diagnosis?

2. A 49-year-old female presented with a pelvic mass. USG of pelvis shows a 20 cm diameter solid-cystic swelling in the right adnexal region. Figures 33.29A to D show the fine needle aspiration cytology smears of the mass. What is your diagnosis?

a. Mucinous carcinoma
b. Endometriosis
c. Granulosa cell tumor
d. Clear cell carcinoma

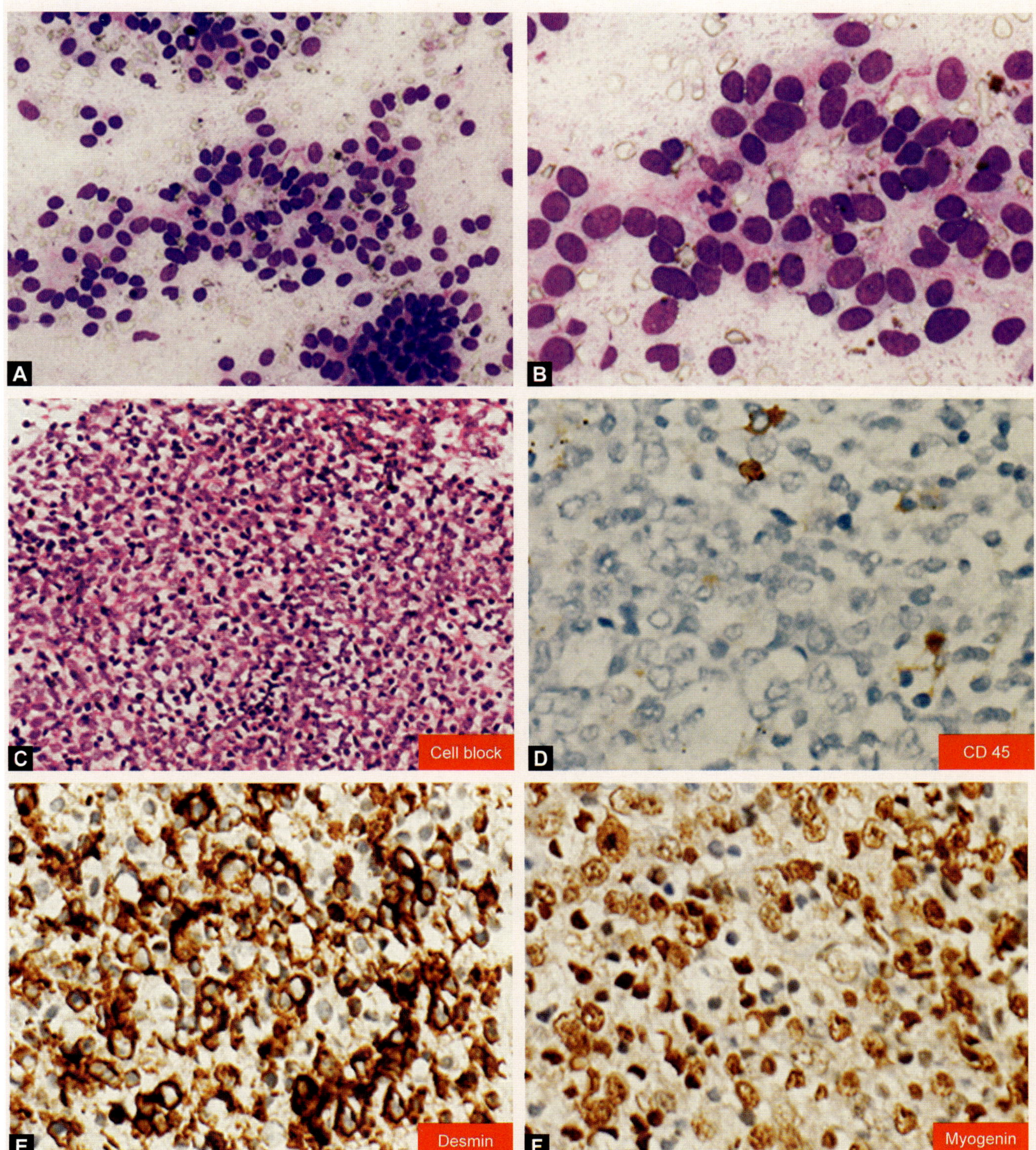

Figs. 33.28A to F: Fine needle aspiration cytology smears and immunocytochemistry on cell block in question 1.

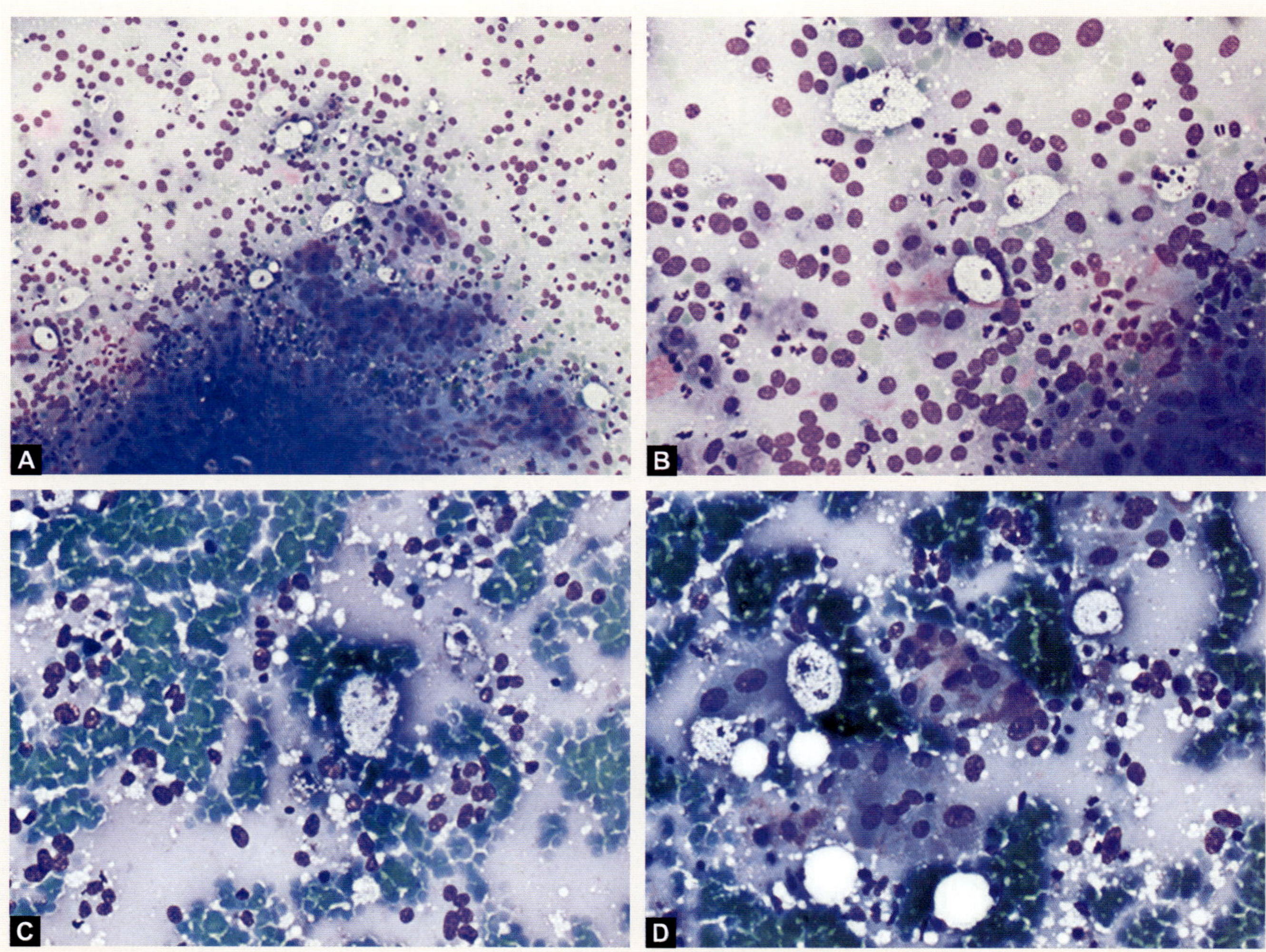

Figs. 33.29A to D: Fine needle aspiration cytology smears of the right adnexal mass in question 2.

Answers

1. Rhabdomyosarcoma

   Note: This is a case of malignant round cell tumor. The strongly positive desmin and myogenin indicate the diagnosis of rhabdomyosarcoma. Negative CD 45 eliminates the possibility of NHL.

2. d. Clear cell carcinoma

   Note: Many discrete cells with abundant vacuolated cytoplasm and moderately pleomorphic nuclei indicate the carcinoma and most likely clear cell carcinoma.

CHAPTER

34 Soft Tissue Lesions

INTRODUCTION

Soft tissue tumor comprises of wide variety of lesions with different architectural pattern. It is often difficult to assess the exact histological type of soft tissue lesions on fine needle aspiration cytology (FNAC). The primary diagnosis of soft tissue tumor with the help of FNAC is not well accepted and it is still a controversial issue. In fact, there is a negative attitude of surgeons, oncologist, and even histopathologists regarding FNAC diagnosis of soft tissue lesions.[1] However, FNAC is useful in recurrent soft tissue sarcomas (STSs), metastatic sarcomas, and also to confirm various benign lesions (Box 34.1). It also provides necessary information about the nature of the soft tissue lesion. Ancillary investigations can be done from the FNAC material to reach a conclusive diagnosis in certain situations.[2]

Compared to open biopsy or core needle biopsy, FNAC of soft tissue can be done in outpatient department and the procedure is well tolerated, rapid, and cost effective. If needed, repeat samples can be taken for ancillary investigations such as immunohistochemistry, electron microscopy (EM), DNA ploidy analysis, and molecular genetics (Box 34.2).

The FNAC of soft tissue lesion is almost free of any complication. Needle tract seeding is a myth and has no practical importance.

Box 34.1: Indications of fine needle aspiration cytology fine needle aspiration cytology of soft tissue lesions.

- Initial confirmation of nature of the lesion for further management
- Recurrent sarcoma.
- Metastatic sarcoma
- To exclude a metastatic tumors in the soft tissue.

Box 34.2: Advantages of fine needle aspiration cytology of soft tissue lesions.

- Well tolerated
- Rapid
- Cost effective
- Multiple sampling
- Ancillary investigation possible.

DIAGNOSTIC ACCURACY

The overall diagnostic sensitivity and specificity of soft tissue tumors are more than 90%.[3-5] The false negative rate of soft tissue tumor is as high as 15%. The main causes of false negative diagnosis are inadequate sampling, nonrepresentative sampling, and misinterpretation of the smear (Box 34.3). Inadequate or suboptimal sampling may be due to FNAC of richly vascular tissue such as hemangioma or angiosarcoma. The tumor may be hyalinized or collagenous and FNAC may yield poor amount of cells. Nonrepresentative sampling may be due to entry of the needle to the adjacent reactive tissue. The rate of false negative report can be reduced if multiple sampling is done from the different areas of the tumor and immediate assessment of the material is done. False positive diagnosis of FNAC is about 5%. In case of any doubt, histopathological examination of the tumor should be recommended. Mutilating surgery should not be done on the basis of primary FNAC diagnosis.

Box 34.3: False negative diagnosis.

Inadequate sampling
- Less number of needle passes
- Hyalinized tissue
- Collagenous tissue
- Necrosis
- Richly vascular
- Deep seated lesion may be missed.

Nonrepresentative sample
- Sampling from adjacent reactive tissue

Interpretation error

FINE NEEDLE ASPIRATION CYTOLOGY TECHNIQUE AND PREREQUISITES FOR INTERPRETATION OF SMEAR

The FNAC of soft tissue lesion is done as usual with a syringe, pistol handle, and needle (Box 34.4). The diameter of the needle should not be more than 0.7 mm (22 gauge). FNAC should be done from multiple sites to avoid the problem of tumor heterogeneity and also to get adequate representative tissue. Immediate rapid Giemsa staining may provide necessary information about the adequacy of the material and also about the need for ancillary studies. Both alcohol-fixed and air-dried smears should be kept for Papanicolaou's stain and May-Grünwald Giemsa (MGG) stain, respectively. One part of the aspirate should be collected in 10% buffered formalin for cell block to do further immunostaining. If necessary a repeat FNAC could be done for flow cytometry (FCM) and molecular genetics study.

For accurate diagnosis of soft tissue tumor, following information are needed:

- *Age*: Many soft tissue tumors are age specific. Rhabdomyosarcoma and soft tissue Ewing's tumor usually occur in young patients.
- *Chief complaints*: Rapidly growing tumor within a short duration is likely to be malignant.
- *Size*: Tumor with more than 5 cm diameter should be carefully interpreted as the chance of malignancy is more in large sized mass.
- *Computed tomography (CT) scan or magnetic resonance imaging (MRI)*: Deeper tissue or bone infiltration by the tumor indicates its malignant behavior.

In addition, a past history of sarcoma or other malignancy is helpful in accurate interpretation of the FNAC smear. One can diagnose a soft tissue tumor as benign, sarcoma, other malignancy, and inadequate. In case of difficulty you can give a thorough description of the smear along with possible differential diagnosis.[3]

Many authors recommend the use of cytomorphological subtypes of the soft tissue lesions based on predominant cell morphology such as.[6,7]

- *Spindle cell types*: Fibrosarcoma, leiomyosarcoma, malignant peripheral nerve sheath tumor, synovial sarcoma (SS) (monophasic), dermatofibrosarcoma protuberans.
- *Round cell type*: Embryonal and alveolar rhabdomyosarcoma, soft tissue Ewing's tumor, and round cell liposarcoma (LPS).
- *Pleomorphic cell type*: Malignant fibrous histiocytoma, pleomorphic LPS, and pleomorphic rhabdomyosarcoma.
- *Biphasic tumors*: Synovial sarcoma.

However, there may be overlapping of the cell morphology and it may be difficult to put the lesion in one such category.

Exact histological subclassification of soft tissue tumor may not be always feasible. Grading of STS probably is more important than histological subtyping regarding management and prognosis. Currently, National Cancer Institute (NCI) grading system proposed by Costa et al. and the French grading system proposed by Guillou et al. from the Fédération Nationale des Centers de Lutte Contré le Cancer (FNCLCC) are commonly used in grading STS.[8,9] NCI system graded STS in three grades: grade 1, 2, and 3. This system uses grading of STS based on histological type, cellularity, pleomorphism, mitotic rate, and necrosis. Depending on the amount of necrosis the grade 2 (less than 15% necrosis) and grade 3 (more than 15% necrosis) STSs are assigned. FNCLCC system of grading gives importance more on tumor differentiation, mitotic rate, and amount of tumor necrosis. A score is given to each factor and a combined score is used for grading of STS. We have successfully used NCI grading system to grade STS.[10] However, a two-tier grading system is also proposed on cytology smear for better reproducibility (Table 34.1).[11]

World Health Organization (WHO) classified soft tissue tumor according to histological type and behavior of the tumor (Box 34.5).[12]

ANCILLARY TECHNIQUES

Ancillary techniques are often needed for the exact typing of STS. The important techniques in this respect are:

Box 34.4: Fine needle aspiration cytology techniques.

- *Needle*: 22 gauge
- Multiple area should be sampled
- Air-dried and alcohol-fixed smear
- MGG and Papanicolaou (or H & E) staining
- On site assessment of material
- *Material for cell block*: Immunocytochemistry
- *Material for other ancillary studies*: Flow cytometry, molecular genetics.

Table 34.1: Two tiered grade of sarcoma.

Features	*Low-grade sarcoma*	*High-grade sarcoma*
Cellularity	Low	High
Nuclear atypia	Minimal	Moderate to severe
Nuclear overlap	Minimal	Moderate to marked
Necrosis	Absent	Present
Mitosis	Absent	Present

Box 34.5: WHO Classification of soft tissue tumor (modified).

Tumors of adipocytes
- Benign
  - Lipoma and it variants such as myolipoma, angiolipoma, spindle cell, pleomorphic lipoma
- Intermediate (locally aggressive)
  - Atypical lipomatous tumor or well-differentiated liposarcoma
- Malignant
  - Dedifferentiated liposarcoma, myxoid liposarcoma, round cell liposarcoma, pleomorphic liposarcoma, mixed-type liposarcoma, liposarcoma, not otherwise specified

Fibroblastic or myofibroblastic tumors
- Benign
  - Nodular fasciitis, proliferative fasciitis, proliferative myositis, myositis ossificans
- Intermediate (locally aggressive)
  - Superficial fibromatoses, desmoid-type fibromatoses, lipofibromatosis
- Intermediate (rarely metastasizing)
  - Solitary fibrous tumor, hemangiopericytoma, infantile fibrosarcoma
- Malignant
  - Adult fibrosarcoma, myxofibrosarcoma, low-grade fibromyxoid sarcoma

Fibrohistiocytic tumors
- Benign
  - Giant cell tumor of tendon sheath, diffuse-type giant cell tumor
- Intermediate (rarely metastasizing)
  - Plexiform fibrohistiocytic tumor, giant cell tumor of soft tissues
- Malignant
  - Pleomorphic MFH, giant cell MFH, inflammatory MFH

Smooth muscle tumors
- Leiomyoma
- Leiomyosarcoma

Pericytic (perivascular) tumors
- Glomus tumor, malignant glomus tumor

Skeletal muscle tumors
- Benign
  - Rhabdomyoma
- Malignant
  - Embryonal rhabdomyosarcoma, alveolar rhabdomyosarcoma, pleomorphic rhabdomyosarcoma

Vascular tumors
- Benign
  - Hemangiomas, epithelioid hemangioma, lymphangioma
- Intermediate (locally aggressive)
  - Kaposiform hemangioendothelioma
- Intermediate (rarely metastasizing)
  - Retiform hemangioendothelioma, papillary intralymphatic angioendothelioma, kaposi sarcoma
- Malignant
  - Epithelioid hemangioendothelioma, angiosarcoma of soft tissue

Chondro-osseous tumors
- Soft tissue chondroma, mesenchymal chondrosarcoma, extraskeletal osteosarcoma

Tumors of uncertain differentiation
- Benign
  - Myxoma
- Intermediate (rarely metastasizing)
  - Mixed tumor, myoepithelioma
- Malignant
  - Synovial sarcoma, epithelioid sarcoma, alveolar soft part sarcoma, clear cell sarcoma of soft tissue, PNET or extraskel etal Ewing tumor, desmoplastic small round cell tumor, neoplasms with perivascular epithelioid cell differentiation (PEComa).

(MFH: Malignant Fibrous Histiocytoma).

Box 34.6: Immunocytochemistry of sarcoma.

- *Leiomyosarcoma*: Smooth muscle actin
- *Rhabdomyosarcoma*: Desmin, myogenin
- *Synovial sarcoma*: CK, EMA
- *Desmoplastic small round cell tumor*: CK, EMA, vimentin, desmin
- *Angiosarcoma*: CD31, CD34.

Table 34.2: Cytogenetic of soft tissue tumor.

Tumor	*Chromosomal abnormalities*	*Gene involved*
Alveolar soft part sarcoma	der(X)t(X;17)(p11;q25)	ASPL-TFE3
Clear cell sarcoma	t(12;22)(q13;q12)	AFT1-EWS
Desmoplastic small round cell tumor	t(11;22)(p13;q12)	WTI-EWS
Epithelioid sarcoma	t(8;22)(q22;q11); +2	
Ewing's tumor	t(11;22)(q24;q12)	FLII-EWS
Inflammatory myofibroblastic tumor	2p23 rearrangement	ALK
Liposarcoma, myxoid	t(12;16)(q13;p11)	EWSR1/FUS-DDIT3
Rhabdomyosarcoma, alveolar	t(2;13)(q37;q14); del(13)(q14)	PAX3-FKHR
Rhabdomyosarcoma, embryonal	t(8;11)(q12;q21); +11 (trisomy); del(11)	
Synovial sarcoma	t(X;18)(p11;q11)	SSX1-SYT

- *Cell block for immunocytochemistry*: Cell block is needed to do immunocytochemistry. This is mainly helpful in spindle cell and round cell tumor (Box 34.6).
- *FISH and reverse transcription polymerase chain reaction (RT-PCR) for molecular genetics*: Specific chromosomal abnormalities indicate certain sarcomas such as t(11;22)(q24;q12) is specific for Ewing's tumor, and t(X;18)(p11;q11) is unique in SS (Table 34.2).
- *Electron microscopy*: EM is helpful in diagnosis of certain SFS. Demonstration of melanosomes is specific for clear cell sarcoma. Similarly cross striations can be shown in rhabdomyosarcoma. Weibel-Palade bodies are specifically seen in vascular tumors.

INDIVIDUAL SOFT TISSUE TUMORS

Lipoma and Its Variants

This is the most common soft tissue tumor and accounts for 50% of all soft tissue tumors. The tumor is common in elderly obese person. Lipoma may occur in any anatomic locations. It may be seen in superficial subcutaneous tissue or deep soft tissue.

Cytology (Fig. 34.1)

The FNAC smears show multiple clusters of mature adipocytes (Box 34.7). The fat cells show abundant vacuolated cytoplasm with centrally placed monomorphic round nuclei. The cytoplasm is thin and peripherally pushed. Smears may also show fat-filled histiocytes and thin capillaries.

Spindle Cell Lipoma or Pleomorphic Lipoma (Fig. 34.2)

They probably represent a single entity with overlapping clinical, morphologic, and cytogenetic features. Spindle cell lipoma or pleomorphic lipoma commonly occurs in posterior part of neck, upper back, and shoulder area as well-circumscribed, painless, and slow growing mass.

Cytology: The FNAC smear shows a mixed population of spindle cells, adipocytes, and collagen bundles (Box 34.8). The spindle cells are arranged in short fascicles in between the adipocytes. The spindle cells are usually bland; however, they may show mild nuclear pleomorphism. In addition, the smears may also show hyaline, ropy collagen fibers, and mast cells.[13]

Box 34.7: Lipoma.

- Mature adipocytes
- Abundant vacuolated cytoplasm
- Central monomorphic bland nuclei.

Box 34.8: Spindle cell lipoma.

- Adipocytes
- Spindle cells
  - Bland looking nuclei
  - Small fascicles
- Collagen bundles
- Mast cells
- No lipoblasts.

Pleomorphic Lipoma

The FNAC smear shows fat cells with enlarged moderately pleomorphic, hyperchromatic nuclei, and floret cells. Floret-like cells may also be noted.

The floret cells show large round cells with abundant cytoplasm and multiple nuclei arranged in a circle or semicircle manner (Box 34.9). No lipoblasts are seen.

Differential diagnosis

- *Liposarcoma*: Pleomorphic lipoma and atypical lipoma may be mistaken for LPS.

Hibernoma

This is a rare benign lipomatous tumor composed of brown fat cells. It commonly occurs in young adults and the mean age of the tumor is 38 years. The common sites of hibernoma are thigh, trunk, upper extremity, and neck region.

Box 34.9: Pleomorphic lipoma.

- Adipocytes with enlarged hyperchromatic nuclei
- Floret cells
  - Multiple nuclei arranged in semicircular manner
- No lipoblasts.

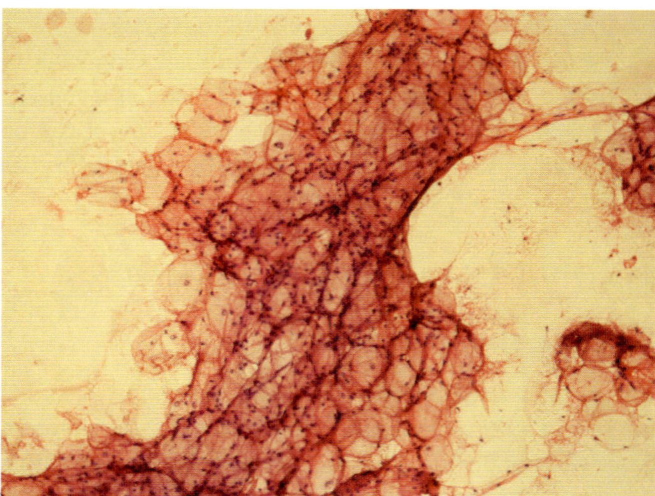

Fig. 34.1: Lipoma: Lobules of mature fat (H & E × MP).

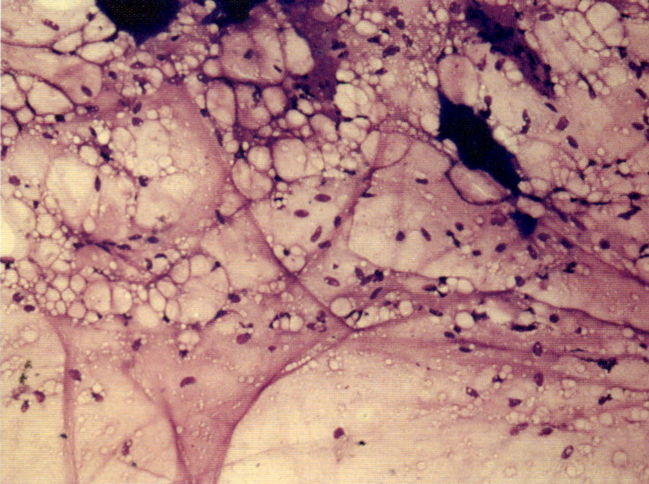

Fig. 34.2: Spindle cell lipoma: Predominantly spindle cells (MGG × MP).

Cytology: The FNAC smears show three populations of cells: (1) mature adipocytes, (2) hibernoma cells, and (3) lipoblast-like cells. Hibernoma cells are large with pale multiple small uniformly vacuolated cytoplasm. Nuclei are round centrally placed. The lipoblast-like cells are large with larger fat vacuoles. In addition, the smear also shows delicate thin capillaries.[14]

Liposarcomas[15,16]

Atypical Lipomatous Tumor or Well-differentiated Liposarcoma (Figs. 34.3 to 34.5)

The atypical lipomatous tumor (ALT) is considered as an intermediate grade of malignant tumor and is synonymous with well-differentiated LPS. ALT represents 40–45% of all LPSs and commonly occurs in the sixth decade of life. The common sites of the tumor are deep soft tissue of the extremities, retroperitoneum, the paratesticular area, and the mediastinum.

Cytology: The FNAC smears show fat cell with enlarge pleomorphic nuclei. The nuclei may be multilobated. There may be admixture of lipoblasts. The presence of lipoblasts in a sarcoma usually indicates LPS. The important characteristics of lipoblast are:

- Multivacuolated round cells
- Scalloping vacuoles around nucleus
- Occasionally compressed nuclei may give signet ring-like appearance.

It is often difficult to distinguish such lesion from lipoma. It is therefore always advisable to have histopathological examination in any deep lipomatous lesion.[15]

Myxoid Liposarcoma

Myxoid liposarcoma (MLS) is the second most common type of LPS and accounts for 10% of all adult STSs. MLS is commonly seen in deep soft tissue of thigh. The tumor commonly occurs in the fourth and fifth decade of life. The patient presents commonly complaints of a large painless swelling in the deep soft tissue.

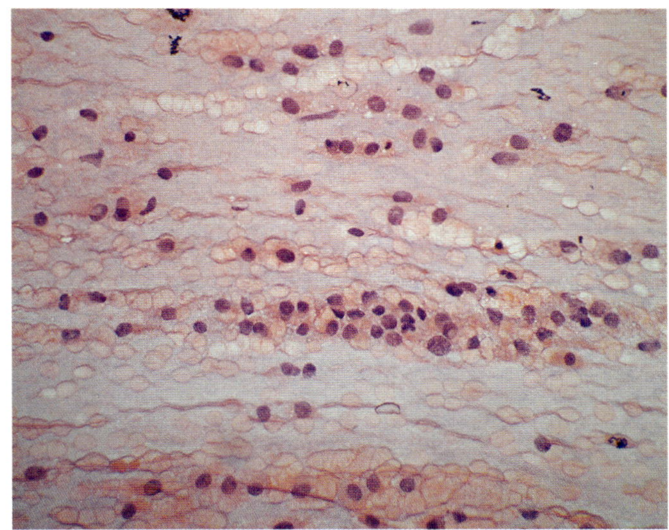

Fig. 34.3: Well-differentiated liposarcoma: Monomorphic round cells with moderate amount of vacuolated cytoplasm (H & E × MP).

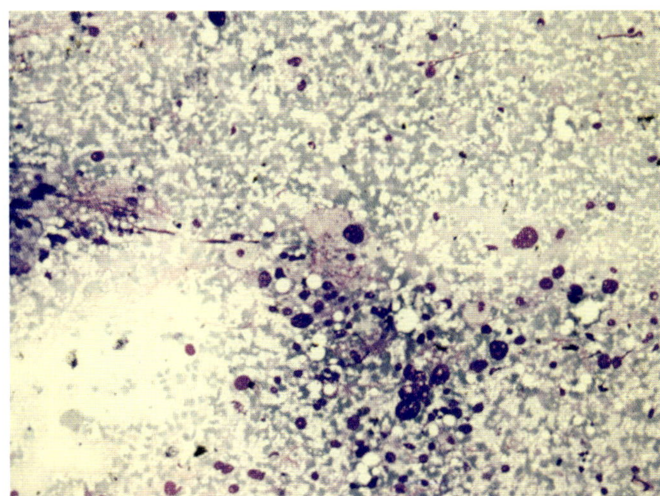

Fig. 34.4: Well-differentiated liposarcoma: Scattered large atypical cells with abundant vacuolated cytoplasm (MGG × MP).

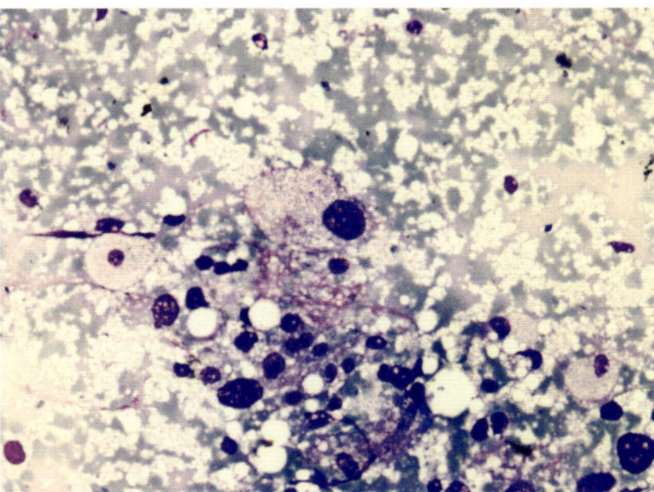

Fig. 34.5: Well-differentiated liposarcoma: Scattered cells with enlarged and pleomorphic nuclei (MGG × HP).

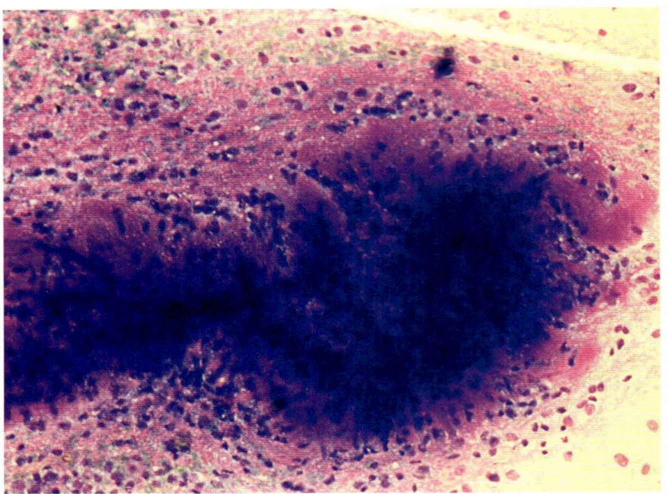

Fig. 34.6: Myxoid liposarcoma: Thin arborizing capillaries in myxoid stroma (MGG × MP).

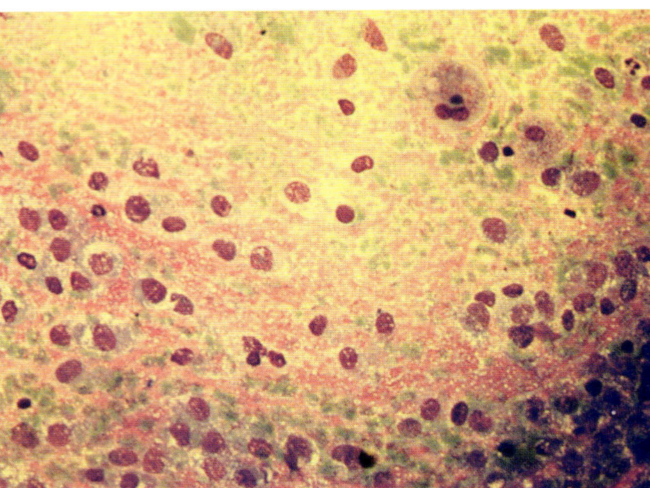

Fig. 34.7: Myxoid liposarcoma: Scattered round cells with vacuolated cytoplasm in the myxoid material (MGG × MP).

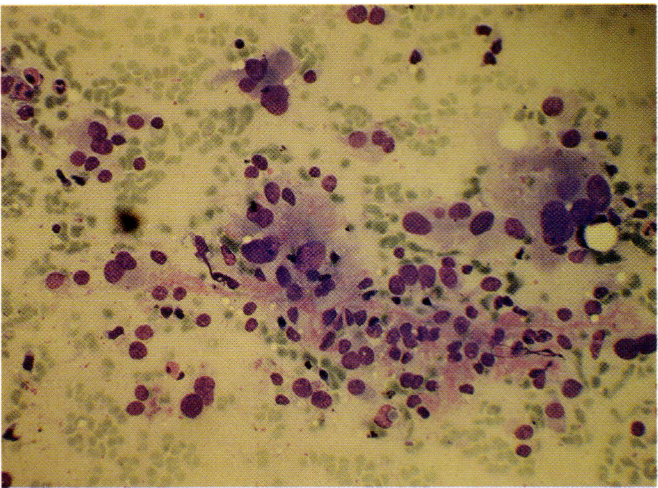

Fig. 34.8: Pleomorphic liposarcoma: Large cells with markedly pleomorphic nuclei having moderate to abundant cytoplasm (MGG × MP).

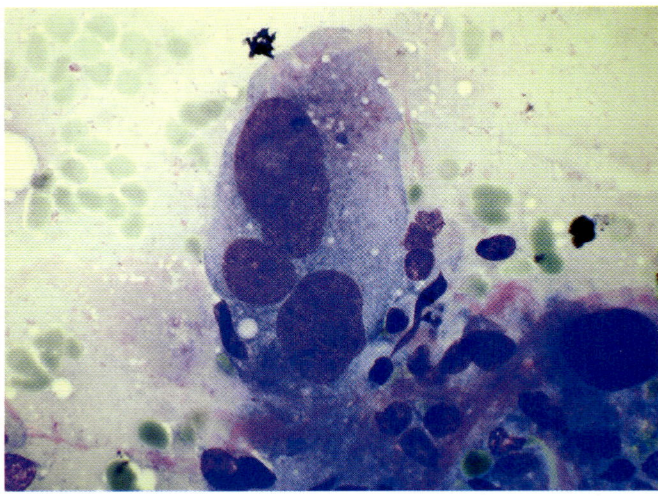

Fig. 34.9: Pleomorphic liposarcoma: Higher magnification of the large bizarre cells (MGG × OI).

Box 34.10: Myxoid liposarcoma.

- Abundant granular myxoid material
- Thin-walled arborizing capillaries
- Uni- or multivacuolated lipoblasts
- Round cells with high N/C ratio
- Spindle-shaped cells with cytoplasmic vacuoles.

Cytology[17] *(Figs. 34.6 and 34.7)*: FNAC smear shows tumor cells entrapped in the abundant granular myxoid material. There are many arborizing thin-walled capillaries (Box 34.10). The tumor cells show oval-shaped bland nuclei with high nuclear-cytoplasmic (N/C) ratio. The presence of uni- or multivacuolated lipoblasts with scalloped nuclear margin is essential for diagnosis of myxoid LPS. This tumor lacks nuclear pleomorphism, bizarre tumor giant cells, or any mitotic activity.

Pleomorphic Liposarcoma

Pleomorphic LPS is a high-grade sarcoma and accounts for 5% of all LPS. This tumor occurs in elderly patient and has no sex predilection. The most common location of this tumor is in the deep tissue of thigh. The patient usually presents as firm rapidly enlarging mass in the extremity.

Cytology (Figs. 34.8 and 34.9): FNAC smears are usually rich in cells. The tumor cells are in dissociation and small loose clusters. The cells show moderate amount of vacuolated cytoplasm. The nuclei are markedly pleomorphic with coarse chromatin and prominent nucleoli. Many multinucleated giant cells and bizarre mononuclear cells are also noted (Box 34.11). The smears also show variable number of atypical lipoblasts. The identification of lipoblasts is an important feature of pleomorphic LPS.[18]

Differential diagnosis

- *Myxoid tumor versus myxoid liposarcoma*: Myxoid LPS may pose diagnostic difficulty with other soft tissue tumor with myxoid change such as intramascular myxoma or myxoid variant of malignant fibrous histiocytoma. Intramuscular myxoma (IM) shows lack of branching capillaries and typical lipoblast. Myxoid variant of malignant fibrous histiocytoma shows significant nuclear pleomorphism.
- *Other pleomorphic sarcomas versus pleomorphic liposarcoma*: Other pleomorphic sarcomas such as malignant fibrous histiocytoma or rhabdomyosarcoma also come in the differential diagnosis of pleomorphic LPS.

Fibroblastic or Myofibroblastic Lesion

Fibromatosis

Fibromatosis is a locally aggressive infiltrative tumor of fibroblasts that never metastasize. The exact etiology of this tumor is unknown. These tumors are composed of fibrous tissue and are broadly divided into two groups: (1) superficial and (2) deep. The superficial fibromatosis involves palmer, planter, and penile region. The deeper fibromatosis includes the abdominal and extra-abdominal region.

Box 34.11: Pleomorphic liposarcoma.

- Large cells with vacuolated cytoplasm
- Markedly pleomorphic nuclei
- Coarse chromatin
- Prominent nucleoli
- Atypical lipoblasts
- Mitotic activities
- Necrosis.

Box 34.12: Fibromatosis.

- Variable amount of cells
- Oval to spindle cell
- Spindle-shaped nuclei
- Bland chromatin
- Collagenous stroma
- No mitotic activity.

Cytology (Fig. 34.10): Cytology smear shows scanty to moderate cellularity. The cells are in clusters and embedded in collagenous stroma (Box 34.12). The individual cells are oval to spindle shaped with elongated nuclei and pointed ends. The nuclei are hyperchromatic with minimal atypia. The mitotic activity is absent. The background of the smear is clean and shows fragments of dense collagenous stroma.

Differential diagnosis

- *Fibrosarcoma*: Fibrosarcoma may be difficult to differentiate from fibromatosis. Absence of nuclear pleomorphism and mitotic activity favor a diagnosis of fibromatosis.

Nodular Fasciitis

Nodular fasciitis is the fibrous proliferation resulting mass-like lesion. It occurs in all age groups, but more commonly occurs in younger patient. Nodular fasciitis may affect any part of the body but it commonly involves the upper extremity, trunk, and head. It grows rapidly and may simulate malignancy.

Cytology: Cytology smear shows cohesive clusters and dissociated cells in a myxoid background. The cells are arranged around thin capillaries. The individual cells have plump spindly nucleus with blunt ends. Nuclear chromatin is open with small nucleoli. Mitotic activity may be high; however, no atypical mitosis is seen.

Differential diagnosis

- *Sarcoma*: Increased cellularity and high mitotic activity may mislead the diagnosis of sarcoma.

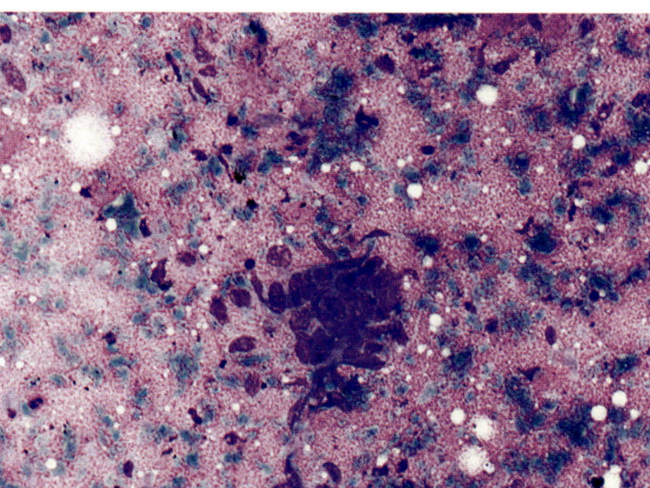

Fig. 34.10: Fibromatosis: Cluster and dissociated spindle cells (MGG × MP).

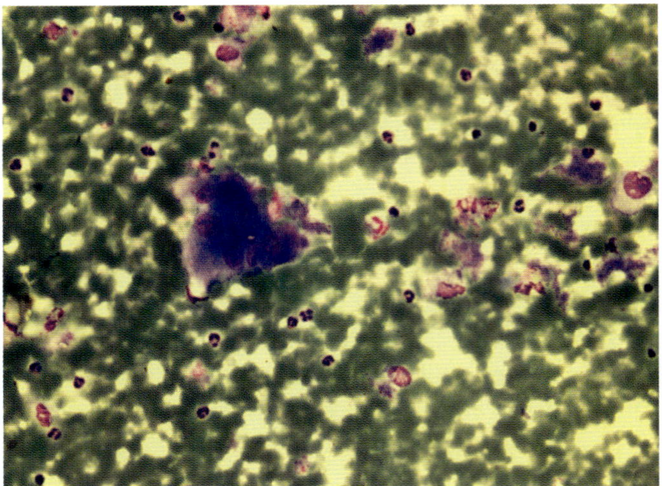

Fig. 34.11: Myositis ossificans: Osteoclastic giant cells and occasional osteoblasts (MGG × MP).

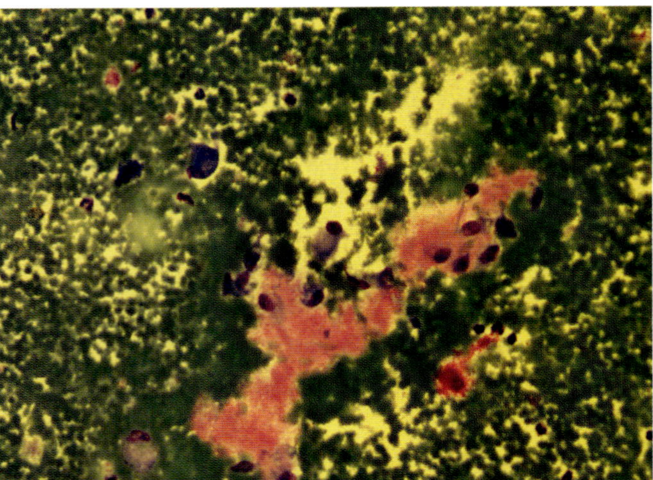

Fig. 34.12: Myositis ossificans: Many osteoblasts and fragments of osteoid material (MGG × MP).

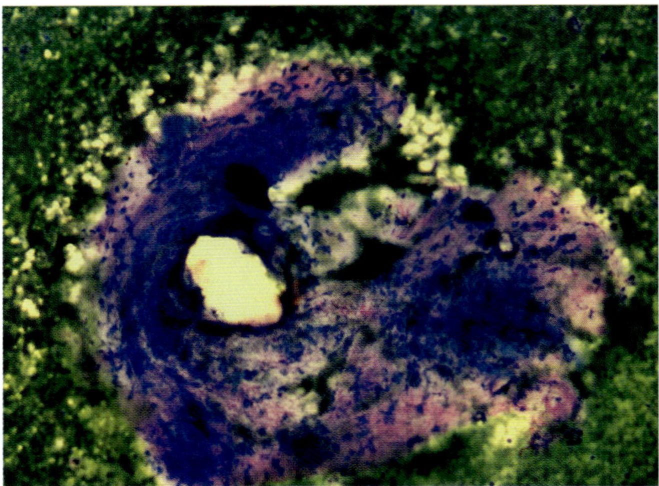

Fig. 34.13: Myositis ossificans: Bundle of oval- to spindle-shaped muscle cells and calcified material (MGG × MP).

Myositis Ossificans[19]

Myositis ossificans (MO) is a self-limiting reparative lesion. It characteristically occurs in a young male who may or may not recall the history of trauma. The swelling commonly occurs in extremities, trunk, head, and neck. The swelling shows the characteristic radiological appearance in its osteoid-producing phase and may mislead the clinical diagnosis of periosteal osteosarcoma.

Cytology (Figs. 34.11 to 34.13): FNAC of MO yield low cellularity. The aspiration may be hindered due to ossified material. The smear often contains fragment of muscles and that may raise the doubt about adequacy of the sample (Box 34.13).

Box 34.13: Myositis ossificans.

- Granular matrix material
- Myofibroblast
  - Oval to polygonal cells
  - Feathery cytoplasm
  - Eccentrically placed round nuclei
- Osteoblast
- Osteoclast.

The cells are dispersed in dirty granular or metachromatic stromal material. Cytology smears of MO show many multinucleated osteoclastic giant cells, osteoblasts, proliferating fibroblasts, and myofibroblasts embedded at places in pink stroma. The myofibroblasts are large ovoid or polygonal cells with abundant feathery cytoplasm and eccentrically placed round nuclei. The osteoblasts are round to oval with eccentric nuclei. The nuclei may show mild reactive atypia. The atypical osteoblasts are the potential source of misdiagnosis of this lesion as osteosarcoma.

Differential diagnosis

- *Osteosarcoma*: MO may be misdiagnosed as osteosarcoma due to the presence of atypical osteoblasts, large atypical myofibroblasts, and clinical history of rapid growth. A careful observation of the nuclear character of osteoblasts and identification of myofibroblasts may help in the accurate diagnosis of MO.

Solitary Fibrous Tumor

Solitary fibrous tumor (SOFT) is the fibroblastic neoplasm. It commonly occurs as deep seated mass near the pleural cavity in peritoneum, pericardium, mediastinum, orbit, etc.

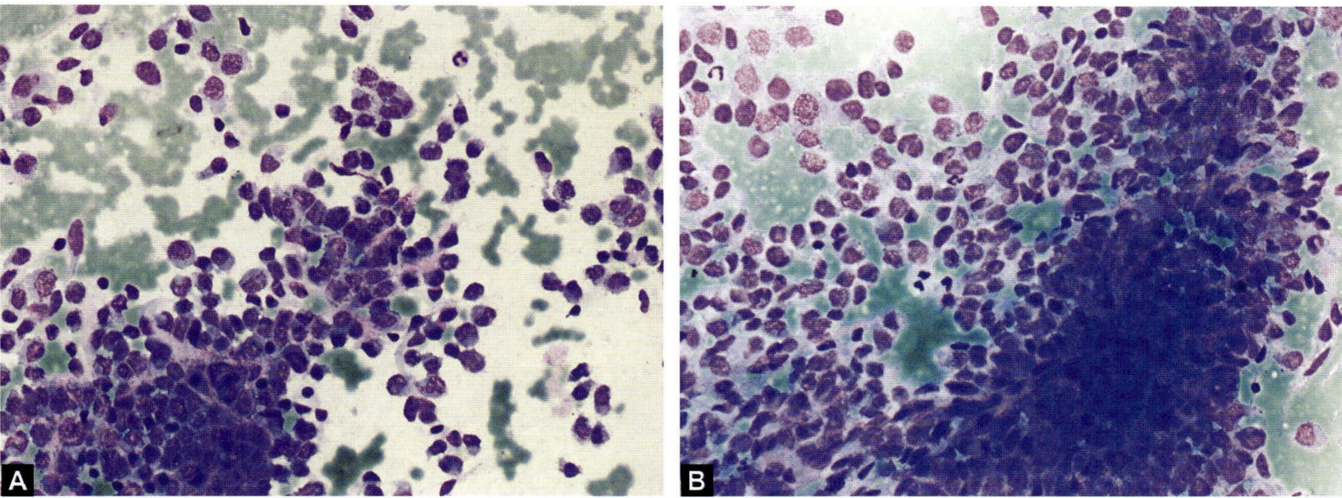

Figs. 34.14A and B: (A) Solitary fibrous tumor: Cluster of spindle cells with mild nuclear pleomorphism (MGG × MP). (B) Solitary fibrous tumor: Abundant oval to spindle cells (MGG × MP).

Box 34.14: Solitary fibrous tumor.

- Fascicles, cohesive clusters, and dispersed cells
- Thick collagenous material
- Naked nuclei
  - Oval to spindle cells with spindle-shaped blunt ended nuclei and scanty friable cytoplasm
  - Fine chromatin with inconspicuous nucleoli

Immunocytochemistry: Positive for CD34 and negative for smooth muscle actin.

Majority (90%) of the SOFTs are benign and only 10% cases may behave as malignant tumor. The exact cell of origin is debatable; however, it is most likely developed from the mesenchymal tissue.[20]

Cytology[21,22] *(Figs. 34.14A and B)*: FNAC smear shows small fascicles and discrete oval to spindle cells admixed with thick collagenous matrix material (Box 34.14). Many naked nuclei are also seen. Necrosis or mitosis is absent in benign tumors. The individual cells show spindle to polygonal nuclei with thin and frayed cytoplasm. Malignant SOFT shows abundant clusters of cells with moderate nuclear atypia, frequent mitosis, and absent of collagenous material SOFT.[22]

Immunocytochemistry: The tumors are characteristically positive for CD34 and negative for smooth muscle actin (SMA).

Interpretation and diagnostic problems: SOFT may come in the differential diagnosis of other soft tissue tumors with spindle cell morphology [malignant peripheral nerve sheath tumor (MPNST), SS (monophasic), fibromatosis, and leiomyosarcoma].

Fibrosarcoma

Fibrosarcoma is a malignant tumor of fibroblastic in origin. The exact incidence of fibrosarcoma is difficult to assess as it is a tumor of exclusion. Possibly, fibrosarcoma represents 1–3% of all adult sarcomas.[23] It commonly occurs between 35 years and 55 years of age. It commonly affects the extremities, trunk, head, and neck region. A distinct variant is the infantile fibrosarcoma that affects children.

Cytology[23] *(Figs. 34.15A and B)*: FNAC smears show abundant cellularity. The cells are arranged in small clusters, bundles, and dissociated spindle cells (Box 34.15). The cells are in interwoven pattern. Typical herringbone pattern may not be evident in case of cytology smear of fibrosarcoma. The tumor cells show elongated spindle-shaped nuclei with pointed ends and irregular nuclear membrane. The nuclear chromatin is finely granular with absent nucleoli. The cells show variable nuclear pleomorphism depending on the grade of the tumor. Nuclear pleomorphism is less in well-differentiated fibrosarcoma than in poorly differentiated fibrosarcoma. The amount of stromal matrix material varies and it is generally indirectly proportional to the cellularity of the smear. There may be blood and necrotic material in FNAC smear and the cells may be obscured. The diagnosis of fibrosarcoma depends in the elimination of other spindle cell sarcomas and the tumor is often missed in cytology smear.

Differential diagnosis

- *Other spindle cell sarcomas*: The differential diagnosis of fibrosarcoma comes along with other sarcomas of spindle cell morphology such as leiomyosarcoma, SS, malignant peripheral nerve sheath tumor, etc.

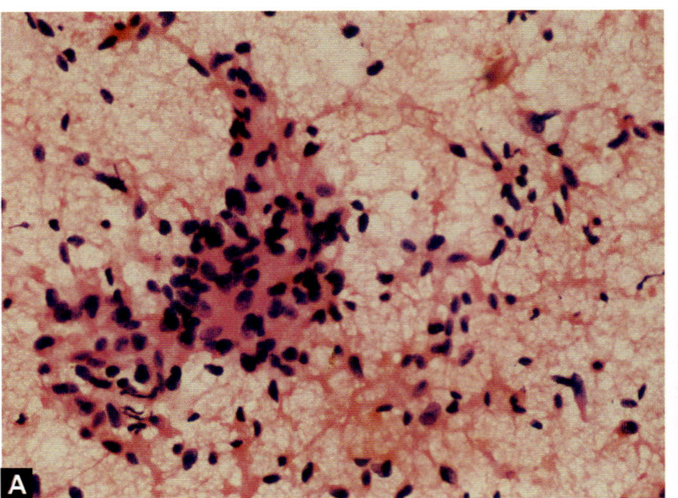
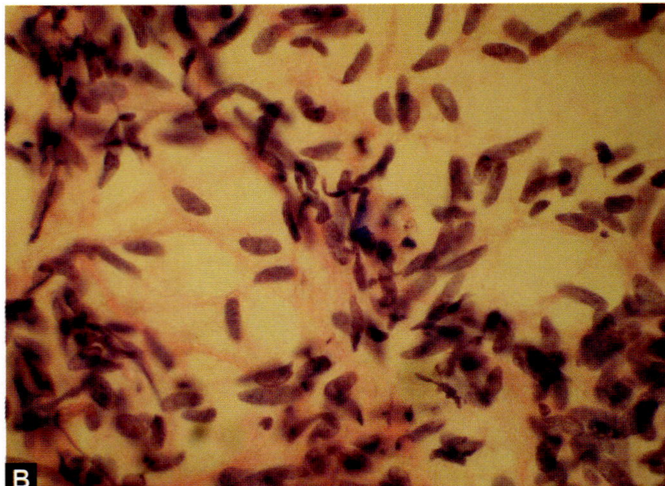

Figs. 34.15A and B: (A) Fibrosarcoma: Discrete oval to spindle cells (H & E × MP). (B) Fibrosarcoma: Higher magnification showing b□

Box 34.15: Fibrosarcoma.

- Small fascicles of cells
- Herring bone pattern
- Spindle cells
- Pointed nuclei
- Irregular nuclear membrane
- Finely granular chromatin
- Variable nuclear pleomorphism
- Blood and necrosis.

So Called "Fibrohistiocytic Tumors"

Giant Cell Tumor of Tendon Sheath[24,25]

Giant cell tumor of tendon sheath (GCTTS) is a benign lesion that occurs due to proliferation of synovial like cells of the joints, bursae, and tendon sheath. The tumor is also known as tenosynovitis. GCTTS may occur in any age group; however, it is commonly seen in 30–50 years of age. It is commonly seen as a soft tissue nodule in relation to the tendon sheath of the fingers, wrist, ankle, and knee. Radiological examination of the swelling always reveals a soft tissue mass free from the underlying bone.

Cytology (Figs. 34.16A and B): FNAC smear shows moderate to abundant cellularity. There are homogenous admixture of large number of multinucleated giant cells and mononuclear stromal cells (Box 34.16). The giant cells are morphologically identical with osteoclastic giant cells. The giant cells are large with widely variable in size. They have average 20 nuclei. The nuclei often show grooves and indentation. Nuclear chromatin is stippled. Occasional prominent nucleoli are also seen. Nuclear character of these giant cells is same as that of stromal cells.

The stromal cells are oval to polygonal with abundant cytoplasm and centrally placed variable shaped nuclei. Nuclear chromatin is finely granular. Nuclear grooves and occasional intranuclear inclusions are also seen. These cells show minimal nuclear pleomorphism and anisocytosis. Occasional mitotic figures may also be seen; however, no atypical mitosis is noted. The background of the smear often shows many hemosiderin-laden macrophages.

Immunocytochemistry: Mononuclear stromal cells are positive for CD68 and SMA. Multinucleated giant cells are positive for CD68 and CD45. These cells also show tartrate resistant acid phosphatase.

Differential diagnosis

- *Giant cell tumor of bone*: FNAC smears of giant cell tumor of bone and GCTTS show almost similar cytological features. Giant cell tumor of bone shows characteristic bone involvement.

Malignant Fibrous Histiocytoma

This category of tumor is almost nonexistent. In fact, the concept of fibrohistiocytic differentiation has been challenged. The various histopathological types of malignant fibrous histiocytoma (MFH) are nothing but the features of other sarcomas.[26] Therefore, the term "malignant fibrous histiocytoma (MFH)" is used only in a small subset of tumor that lacks definite differentiation.

Pleomorphic malignant fibrous histiocytoma: This is a group of undifferentiated pleomorphic sarcoma. Originally, it was considered as the most common sarcoma. However, now it is demonstrated that wide variety of

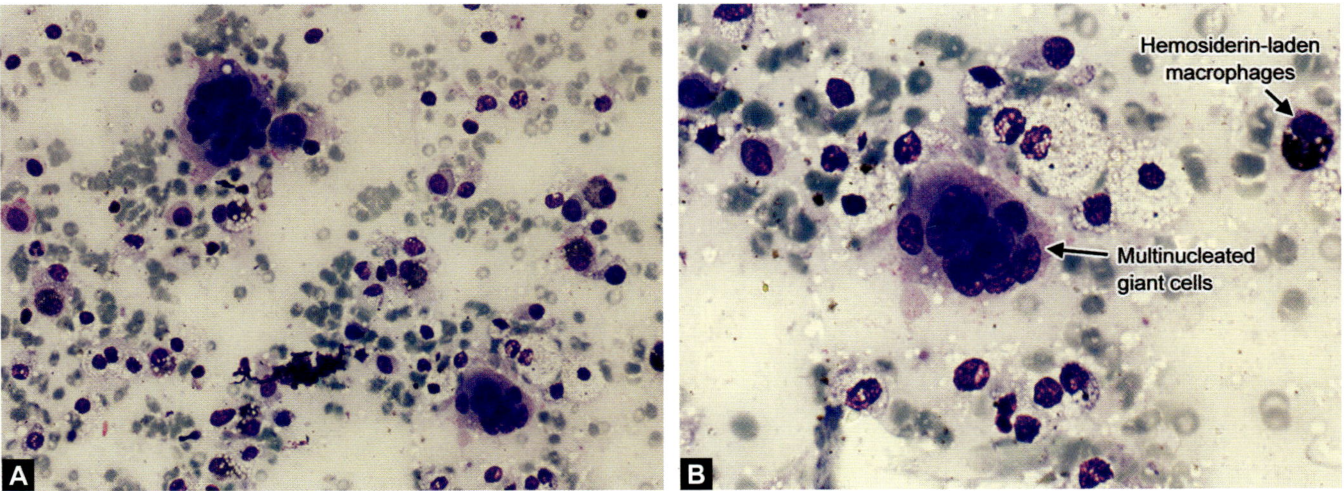

Figs. 34.16A and B: (A) Giant cell tumor of tendon sheath: Many multinucleated osteoclast-like giant cells and foamy histiocytes (MGG × MP). (B) Giant cell tumor of tendon sheath: Multinucleated osteoclast-like giant cells and pigment laden foamy histiocytes (MGG × HP).

Box 34.16: Giant cell tumor of tendon sheath.

- Many multinucleated osteoclast-like giant cells
- Mononuclear stromal cells
- Oval to polygonal
- Abundant cytoplasm
- Round nuclei
- Nuclear grooves
- Intranuclear inclusions
- No atypical mitosis
- Hemosiderin-laden macrophages.

poorly differentiated malignant neoplasm may demonstrate similar morphological features.[26]

Cytology: FNAC smear shows multiple clusters and dissociated spindle cells. The cells are often arranged in small fascicles. The tumor cells have moderate amount of pale blue vacuolated cytoplasm. The nuclei are plump to spindle shaped with irregular coarse chromatin and prominent nucleoli. The smears also show many large pleomorphic bizarre tumor cells and giant cells.

Diagnostic difficulties

- *Other pleomorphic sarcomas*: All the other pleomorphic sarcomas such as pleomorphic LPS and rhabdomyosarcoma should be excluded before diagnosis of this tumor.
- *Anaplastic carcinoma*: Any poorly differentiated carcinoma may simulate pleomorphic MFH.
- *Anaplastic large cell lymphoma*: ALCL lacks connective tissue matrix material and the cells of ALCL are more discrete. The cells of ALCL are positive for CD30 and ALK1.

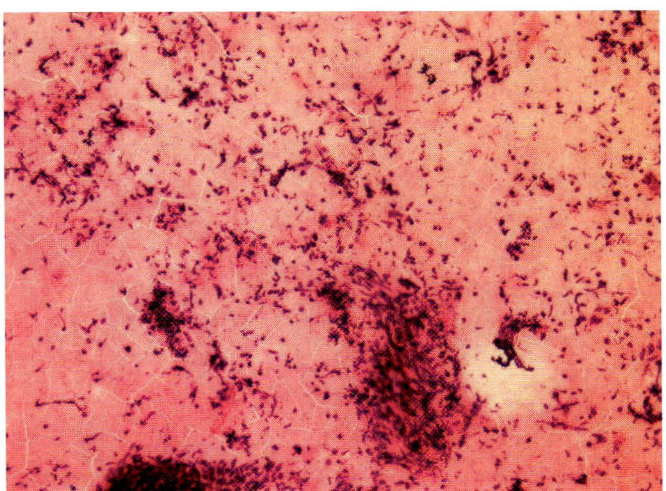

Fig. 34.17: Peripheral nerve sheath tumor: Small clusters and discrete oval to spindle cells (H & E × MP).

Tumors of Nerve Sheath

Benign Peripheral Nerve Sheath Tumor[27]

Schwannoma: Schwannoma arises from the Schwann cells of the nerve sheath. This tumor commonly affects the adults and usually involves flexor surface of the extremities, neck, mediastinum, retroperitoneum, and cerebellopontine angle. Most of the tumors occur sporadically and occasional cases occur with neurofibromatosis type 2.

Cytology (Figs. 34.17 and 34.18): Aspiration of schwannomas is often painful. FNAC smears show many clusters and discrete spindle cells. The cells are often embedded

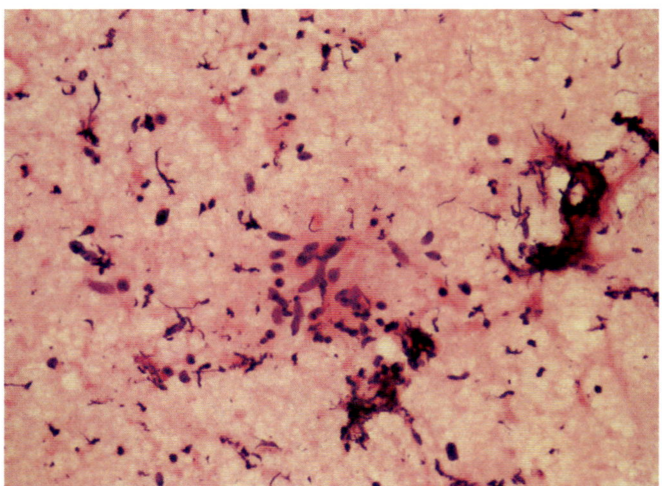

Fig. 34.18: Peripheral nerve sheath tumor: Elongated spindle cells with pointed ends (H & E × HP).

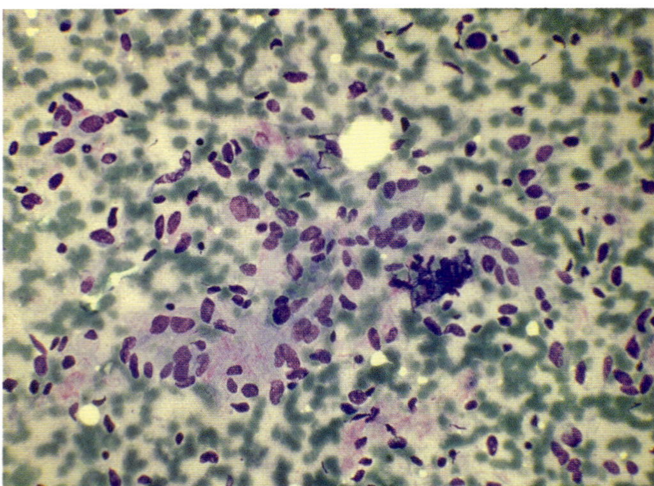

Fig. 34.19: Malignant peripheral nerve sheath tumor: Discrete and loose cluster of spindle cells (MGG × MP).

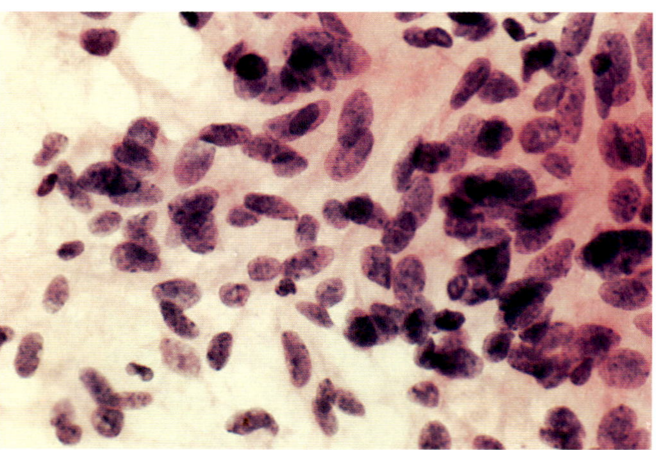

Fig. 34.20: Malignant peripheral nerve sheath tumor: Spindle cells showing moderate to marked nuclear pleomorphism (H & E × HP).

Box 34.17: Schwannoma.

- Clusters and dissociated cells
- Palisading arrangement of cells
- Spindle cells
- Long slender nuclei
- Wavy nuclear margin with kinking
- Pointed nuclear ends.

in pinkish fibrillary matrix material (Box 34.17). The tumor cells are spindle shaped with long slender nuclei having pointed ends. The nuclei often show wavy margin and frequent kinking. Nuclear palisading like arrangement is also seen. At times the ancient schwannomas may show significant nuclear pleomorphism. These large pleomorphic cells may be falsely recognized as malignant cells. Mitotic

Box 34.18: Malignant peripheral nerve sheath tumor.

- Small fascicles
- Discrete cells
- Spindle-shaped cells
- Fibrillar cytoplasm
- Wavy kinked nuclei
- Pointed ends
- Fibrillar collagenous matrix.

activity is rarely seen in schwannomas. FNAC of ganglioneuroma shows admixture of ganglion cells along with many clusters of elongated spindle cells

Differential diagnosis

- *Sarcoma*: Ancient schwannoma may deceive as sarcoma because of nuclear pleomorphism.

Malignant Peripheral Nerve Sheath Tumor[28]

Malignant peripheral nerve sheath tumor (MPNST) is also known as neurofibrosarcoma. Half of the tumor arises as de novo and the other half arises from neurofibromatosis. The tumor develops from the large peripheral nerve or preexisting neurofibroma. This tumor commonly affects the proximal part of the extremities, pelvis, and retroperitoneum. It is commonly seen in the third and fourth decades of life.

Cytology (Figs. 34.19 and 34.20): FNAC smear shows abundant cellularity. The cells are arranged in small bundles and discretely. The tumor cells are embedded in pale violet fibrillary matrix (Box 34.18). The cells are elongated with delicate indistinct fibrillar cytoplasm. The nuclei are spindle shaped with indentation and kinking and

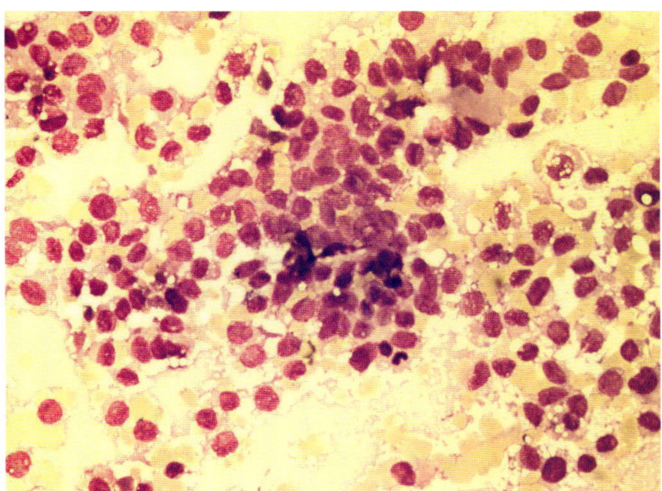

Fig. 34.21: Rhabdomyosarcoma: Discrete round to oval cells with scanty cytoplasm (MGG × MP).

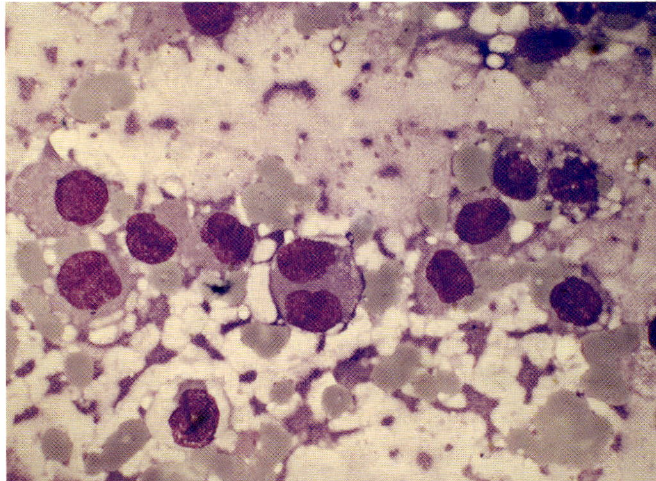

Fig. 34.22: Rhabdomyosarcoma: Discrete cells with binucleation (MGG × OI).

pointed ends. The nuclei show moderate pleomorphism with nuclear hyperchromasia and prominent nucleoli. N/C ratio is high. Mitotic activities are frequent with background necrosis.

Differential diagnosis

- *Other spindle cell sarcoma*: Various spindle cell sarcomas such as fibrosarcoma, leiomyosarcomas, and SS should be distinguished from MPNST.

Tumors of Muscle Origin

Rhabdomyoma

This benign tumor shows skeletal muscle differentiation. This tumor may occur both in adults and in children and 90% of rhabdomyoma is seen in the head and neck region.

Cytology: FNAC smears show large regenerating muscle fibers. The cells show abundant dense cytoplasm. Cytoplasmic cross striations are also evident. Nuclei are central and round shaped. Intranuclear cytoplasmic inclusions are often seen.

Rhabdomyosarcoma[29] (Figs. 34.21 and 34.22)

Rhabdomyosarcoma (RMS) commonly occurs in children. It usually involves the head and neck region. RMS also occurs in the pelvic region particularly in bladder. This is the most common bladder tumor in children.

There are three types of rhabdomyosarcoma: (1) pleomorphic, (2) embryonal, and (3) alveolar. Out of these varieties, pleomorphic RMS is the rarest. Rhabdomyoblasts are seen in all these three types in varying amount.

Table 34.3: Distinguishing features of different types of rhabdomyoblasts.

Features	*Early rhabdomyoblast*	*Intermediate rhabdomyoblast*	*Late rhabdomyoblast*
Size	Small	Large	Same as intermediate
Shape	Round	Oval to polygonal	Oval to polygonal
Cytoplasm	Scanty deep blue	Abundant vacuolated	Abundant opaque
Nucleus	Large irregular single nuclei	Single to bi-nucleation, prominent nucleoli	Pleomorphic nuclei

Rhabdomyoblasts may be divided into early, intermediate, and late rhabdomyoblasts depending on the differentiation (Table 34.3).

Embryonal rhabdomyosarcoma: This is a primitive STS that simulates embryonic skeletal muscle. This is the most common type of RMS and most occurs in children below 10 years of age. The common sites of involvement are head and neck region, genitourinary system (urinary bladder, prostrate, paratesticular soft tissue), and extremities.

Cytology: FNAC smear of embryonal rhabdomyosarcoma shows predominantly two main cell types. One of these two types shows small round cells with scanty deep blue vacuolated cytoplasm. Nuclei are round, mildly pleomorphic having opened up fine chromatin and prominent nucleoli. These cells represent early rhabdomyoblasts. The second cell type is large with abundant cytoplasm. These cells display great variation in shape such as round, tadpole, or ribbon shaped. These cells represent intermediate to late rhabdomyoblasts. Frequent bi- and multinucleation are noted. The nuclei of these cells are round with fine chromatin and prominent nucleoli. Multinucleated giant cells and strap cells are also seen in embryonal RMS. Tigroid-like background has also been described in RMS.

Pleomorphic rhabdomyosarcoma: This is a relatively uncommon and highly malignant tumor. It predominantly occurs in the thigh region and is exclusively seen in adult patient.

Cytology: FNAC smear shows discrete and loosely cohesive large tumor cells. These cells show moderate amount of cytoplasm and severely pleomorphic large nuclei having multiple prominent nucleoli. Many multinucleated tumor giant cells are also seen. The smears also show increased mitotic activities.

Alveolar rhabdomyosarcoma: Alveolar rhabdomyosarcoma is seen in all ages and does not show any predilection for children. It commonly occurs in extremities followed by paraspinal and perineal region.

Cytology: Cytology smear contains large number of early and small number of intermediate rhabdomyoblasts. Smear shows predominantly discrete small round cells with deep blue cytoplasm. Cytoplasm of the cells often shows small uniform vacuolations. Nuclei are round and mild to moderately pleomorphic with fine nuclear chromatin and prominent nucleoli. Cytoplasmic cross striations are usually absent. Alveolar RMS often shows large tumor giant cells with multiple nuclei. These nuclei are arranged in semicircular manner around the periphery of the cytoplasm.

Alveolar RMS shows a characteristic molecular cytogenetics t(2; 13) (q35; q14) in majority of the cases and a small subset shows translocation t(1; 13)(p36; q14).

Immunocytochemistry: The cells of RMS are positive for vimentin, desmin, and myo D1.

Differential diagnosis

- *Other small blue round cell tumor*: Small blue round cell tumor such as neuroblastoma, soft tissue Ewing's and lymphomas come in the differential diagnosis of embryonal and alveolar RMS. The presence of strap cells is helpful in the identification of RMS.

Leiomyosarcomas[30]

Leiomyosarcomas (LS) usually occurs in adult. It is commonly seen in retroperitoneum and mesentery. It may also occur in deep tissue of the extremities.

Cytology (Figs. 34.23 and 34.24): Aspirate of leiomyosarcoma shows cohesive clusters and small fascicles of cells. The discrete cells are also present (Box 34.19). The individual cells have moderate to abundant finely granular cytoplasm with elongated nuclei. The nuclei are cigar shaped with blunt ends. Smears may also show many atypical cells with nuclear pleomorphism and multinucleated giant cells. The mitotic activity on cytology smear may not be reliable enough to distinguish leiomyosarcoma from a leiomyoma. However, dissociated cell population, increased number of mitosis, and nuclear pleomorphic are suggestive of leiomyosarcoma.

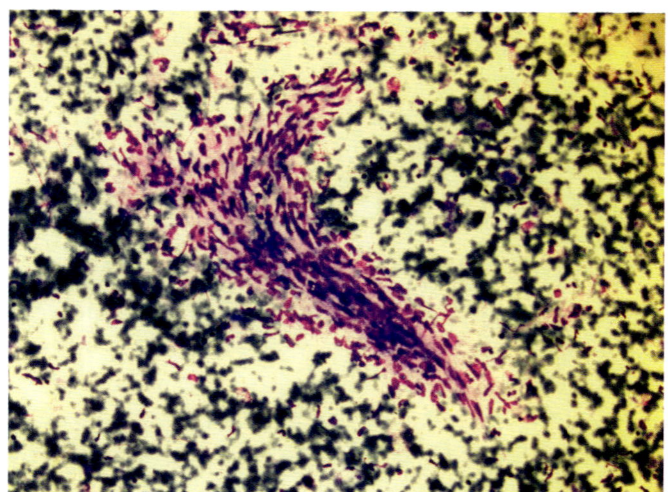

Fig. 34.23: Leiomyosarcoma: Small fascicle of oval to spindle cells (MGG × LP).

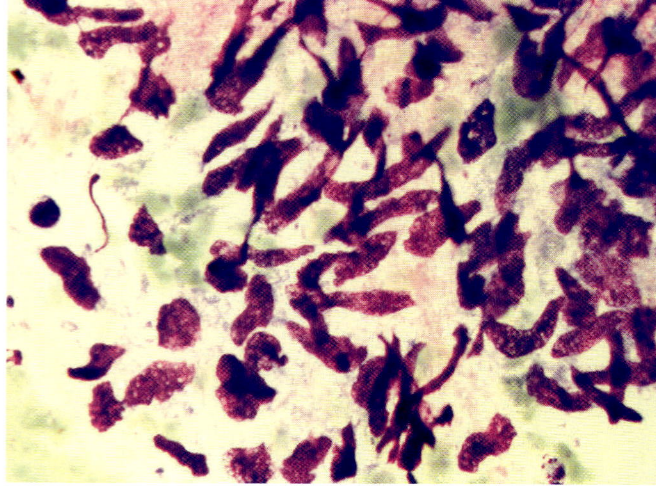

Fig. 34.24: Leiomyosarcoma: Higher magnification showing cigar-shaped nuclei (MGG × OI).

Box 34.19: Leiomyosarcomas.

- Bundles and small fascicles
- Dissociated cells
- Necrosis
- Spindle-shaped cells
- Abundant finely granular cytoplasm
- Cigar-shaped nuclei with blunt ends
- Nuclear atypia
- Multinucleated giant cells
- Increased mitotic activity.

Box 34.21: Glomus tumor.

- Discrete round cells
- Myxoid fibrillary background
- Abundant ill defined cytoplasm
- Round bland nuclei
- Nucleoli are inconspicuous.

Immunocytochemistry: Positive for SMA muscle specific actin, desmin, and caldesmon.

Differential diagnosis

- *Other spindle cell tumor*: Leiomyosarcoma should be distinguished from the other spindle cell tumors such as MPNST, fibrosarcoma, schwannoma, etc.

Tumor of Vascular Origin

Hemangiopericytoma

Hemangiopericytoma is a well-circumscribed tumor of the pericyte. This is also called as solitary fibrous tumor. This tumor usually occurs in the fourth to fifth decade and preferentially distributes in the extremities, intra-abdominal region, mediastinum, and orbit.

Cytology: FNAC smear are usually bloody with scanty to moderate cellularity (Box 34.20). The smear shows oval to elongated spindle cells that are arranged in short fascicles and also discretely. The tumor cells have scanty cytoplasm and elongated spindle-shaped nuclei with pointed ends. The nuclear chromatin is reticular. Mitotic count is variable. Background of the smear shows many naked nuclei and ropy collagenous material.

Immunocytochemistry: Positive for CD34 and negative for desmin, CD99, and S-100 immunostaining.

Glomus Tumor

These are rare tumors and represents less than 2% of all soft tissue tumors. The most common site is the distal extremities, particularly the subungual region of the fingers, the wrist, and foot. However, it may occur in any part of the body. The tumor usually occurs in young and middle aged persons. Characteristically the patient presents with a small red-blue painful nodule along with cold intolerance.

Box 34.20: Hemangiopericytoma.

- Discrete and small fascicles
- Oval to elongated spindle cells
- Spindle-shaped nuclei with pointed ends
- Reticular nuclear chromatin
- Ropy collagenous material
- Naked nuclei.

Box 34.22: Hemangioma.

- Bloody smear
- Elongated spindle-shaped nuclei
- Capillary fragments
- Occasional histiocytes.

Cytology: FNAC is rarely performed in glomus tumor. The smear shows discrete round cells embedded in myxoid fibrillary background. The individual cells have abundant ill-defined cytoplasm with round bland nuclei. Nucleoli are inconspicuous (Box 34.21).

Immunocytochemistry: The tumor cells are positive for CD31, CD34, and SMA.

Hemangioma

This is a benign vascular neoplasm. However, evidences suggest that these are hamartomatous malformations rather than tumor. Hemangioma commonly occurs in children and majority of the tumors are seen in the head and neck region and also in the extremities.

Cytology: FNAC of hemangioma is usually not indicated. In majority of the cases, clinical and radiological examinations are helpful in the diagnosis of hemangioma. FNAC yields blood from the lesion (Box 34.22). Smears are usually paucicellular. The cells are dissociated with oval to elongated spindle-shaped nuclei and pointed ends. The smears may also show variable number of histiocytes and fragments of capillaries.

Angiosarcoma

This is a rare malignant tumor of endothelial cells that commonly occurs in the elderly patient. Angiosarcoma commonly affects the deeper tissue of the lower extremities, arm, trunk and head, and neck region.

Cytology: FNAC usually yields blood. Smears are paucicellular. There are scatted and occasional clusters of oval to elongated spindle cells (Box 34.23). The nuclei are spindle-shaped, moderately pleomorphic, and hyperchromatic. Nuclear chromatin is fine. Smears also show signet ring-like cells with intracytoplasmic red blood cell.

Immunocytochemistry: The tumor cells are positive for CD34 and CD31.

Box 34.23: Angiosarcoma.

- Predominantly blood
- Scanty cellularity
- Spindle cells
- Moderate pleomorphism
- Hyperchromatic nuclei
- Signet ring cells with intracytoplasmic red blood cell.

Tumor of Uncertain Histogenesis

Synovial Sarcoma[5,31]

The SS represents about 5% of all STSs. This tumor has no relation with synovium. SS commonly occurs in 20–40 years. The vast majority of the tumor is seen in the deep soft tissue of the extremity around the knee joints. However, SS may occur at any sites. SS shows characteristic chromosomal alteration t(x;18) (p11;q11).

Cytology (Figs. 34.25 to 34.28)

Biphasic (Box 34.24): The biphasic SS shows admixture of two types of cells: (1) spindle cells and (2) epithelial-like

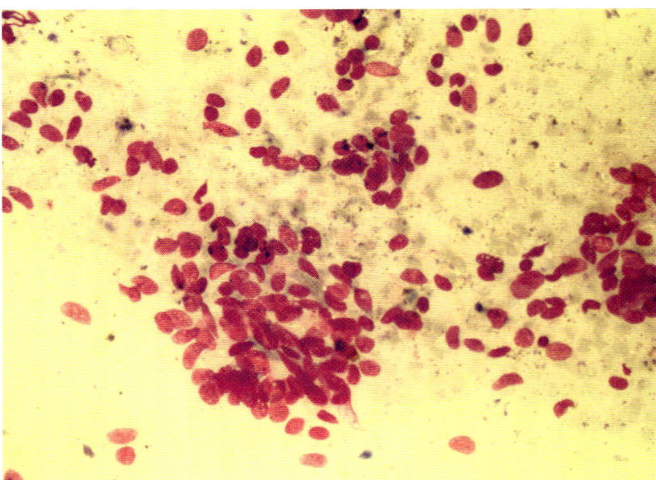

Fig. 34.25: Synovial sarcoma: Clusters and discrete round and spindle cells with occasional tubular arrangement (MGG × MP).

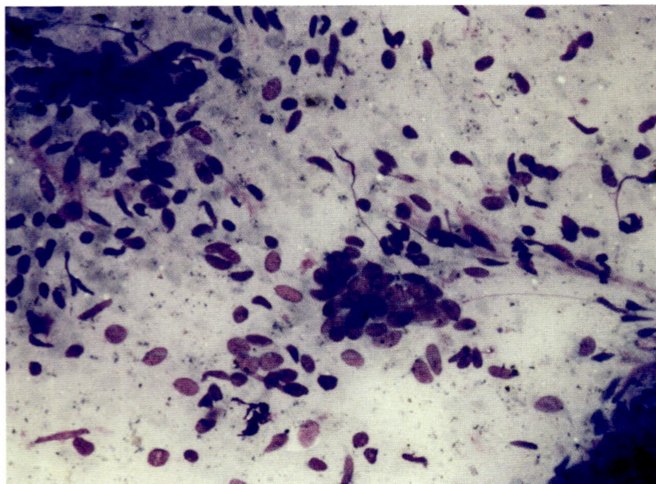

Fig. 34.26: Synovial sarcoma: Round to oval epithelial cells and scattered spindle cells (MGG × HP).

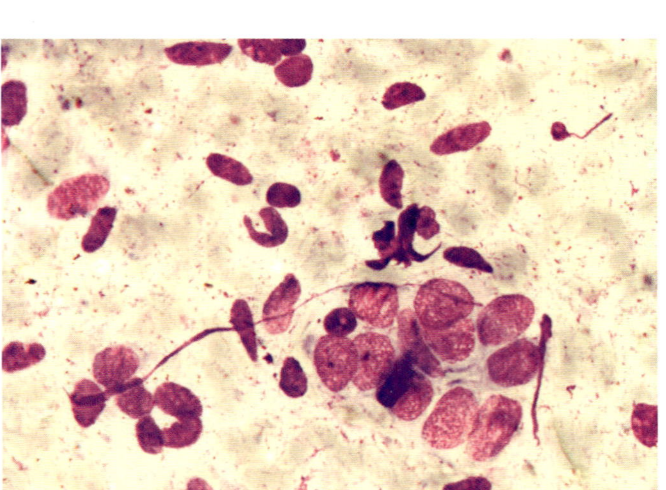

Fig. 34.27: Synovial sarcoma: Higher magnification showing spindle cells and round cells (MGG × OI).

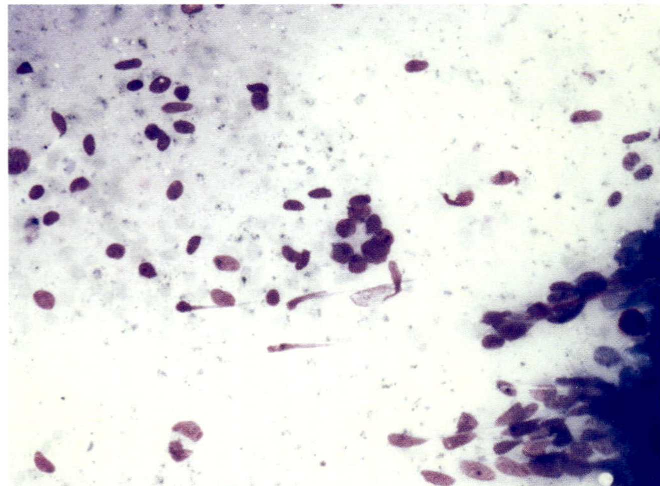

Fig. 34.28: Synovial sarcoma: Tubular arrangement of the epithelial cells (MGG × HP).

Box 34.24: Synovial sarcoma.

- Dual population of cells in biphasic synovial sarcoma (SS)
- Predominant spindle cell component in monophasic SS
- *Spindle cells*:
  - Small fascicles and discretely arranged cells
  - Spindle-shaped nuclei
  - Hyperchromatic, irregular nuclear margin, and prominent nucleoli.
- *Epithelial cells*:
  - Tubular or glandular arrangement
  - Round cells, monomorphic nuclei, prominent nucleoli.

Immunocytochemistry: Positive for CK, vimentin, EMA, S-100 protein.
Molecular genetics: Characteristic chromosomal alteration t(x;18)(p11;q11).

cells. The epithelial cells are arranged as glands-, tubules-, and papillae-like structures. These cells are round to oval shaped with moderate to abundant cytoplasm and round relatively monomorphic nuclei. The nuclear chromatin is fine with occasional prominent nucleoli.

The spindle cells are arranged in clusters with fascicles or whorled pattern. They are oval to elongated cells with scanty, delicate cytoplasm. The nuclei are sspindle shaped and monomorphic with irregular margin. Nuclei are hyperchromatic and often show single to multiple prominent.

Monophasic Synovial Cell Sarcoma

The monophasic SS shows absence of any epithelial cells. The cells are predominantly arranged in small bundles and discretely. The individual cells have elongated spindle-shaped nuclei. Background of the smear may show fibrosis and calcified materials. FNAC smears of SS may show increased mitosis, mast cells, and occasionally necrosis.

Diagnostic difficulties

- *Fibrosarcoma and other spindle cell sarcomas*: Predominant population of spindle cells may pose diagnostic difficulty with fibrosarcoma, leiomyosarcoma, and other spindle cell sarcomas.

Clear Cell Sarcoma[32]

Clear cell sarcoma (CCS) is also known as malignant melanoma of the soft part. This is a STS with melanocytic differentiation. The tumor typically involves the tendon and aponeuroses of the lower extremities followed by the hand and wrist. CCS is slow growing malignant tumor and commonly affects the young adults.

Cytology: The smear shows predominantly discrete and loosely cohesive cells. The tumor cells are round to polygonal and spindle shaped with abundant vacuolated

Box 34.25: Clear cell sarcoma.

- Predominantly discrete and loosely cohesive cells
- Round to polygonal and spindle-shaped cells
- Abundant vacuolated cytoplasm
- Round, moderately pleomorphic, and eccentrically placed nuclei
- Prominent nucleoli
- Intranuclear pseudoinclusions
- Multinucleated tumor giant cells
- Cytoplasmic pigmentation.

cytoplasm (Box 34.25). Occasional cells show cytoplasmic pigmentation. The nuclei of the cells are round, moderately pleomorphic, and eccentrically placed with prominent nucleoli. Intranuclear pseudoinclusions are also noted. Multinucleated tumor giant cells and binucleated cells are also present. Clear cell sarcomas are positive for HMB-45 and S-100 protein.

Differential diagnosis

- *Epithelioid sarcoma*: Epithelioid sarcoma are strongly positivity for keratin and negative for HMB-45 and S-100 protein.
- *Synovial sarcoma*: Monophasic SS may simulate clear cell sarcoma. However, the nuclei of the cells of SS show fine chromatin and indistinct nucleoli.
- *Metastatic carcinoma*: Metastatic carcinoma may also look like clear cell sarcomas. Metastatic carcinomas are positive for CK and negative for HMB-45.

Epithelioid Sarcoma[33]

Epithelioid sarcoma (ES) is a sarcoma of unknown etiology. ES usually occurs in the second to fourth decade of life and affects finger, hand, wrist, and forearm.

Cytology (Figs. 34.29 and 34.30): FNAC smears show both single and loose clusters of cells. The individual cells are round to polyhedral cells with dense eosinophilic cytoplasm (Box 34.26). Small intercellular spaces are also seen. The nuclei of the cells are large round and eccentric in position giving a plasmacytoid appearance. Nuclei show fine chromatin and prominent macronucleoli. Frequent binucleation is also seen. Smears may also show ill formed granuloma-like structures and inflammatory cells.

Differential diagnosis

- Clear cell sarcoma
- Poorly differentiated metastatic carcinoma.

Alveolar Soft Part Sarcoma[34]

Alveolar soft part sarcoma is an uncommon tumor and represents only 0.5% of all STS. This tumor occurs mainly

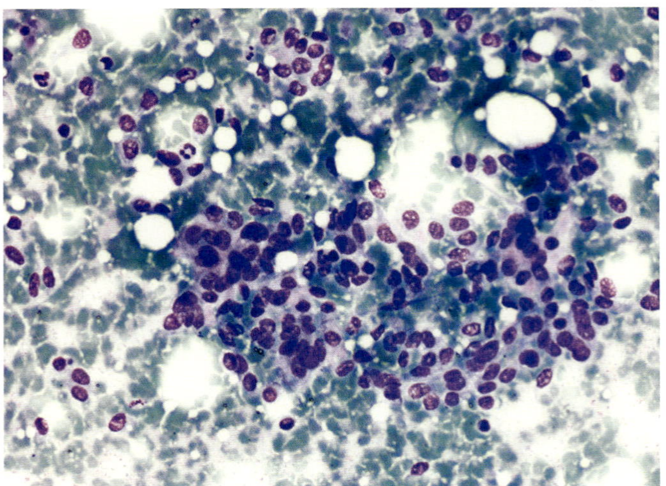

Fig. 34.29: Epithelioid sarcoma: Loose clusters and discrete round to oval cells (MGG × MP).

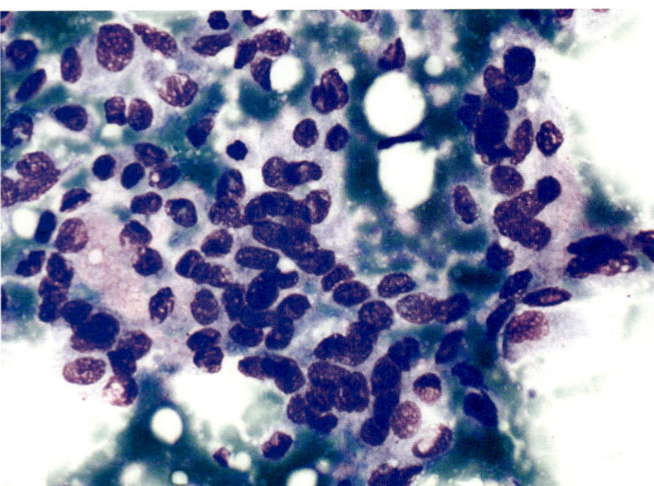

Fig. 34.30: Epithelioid sarcoma: Discrete cells with mild to moderate amount of cytoplasm and central to eccentric nuclei (MGG × HP).

Box 34.26: Epithelioid sarcoma.

- Round to polyhedral cells
- Dense eosinophilic cytoplasm
- Large round and eccentrically located nuclei
- Prominent macronucleoli
- Epithelioid granuloma-like structures
- Inflammatory cells.

Box 34.27: Alveolar soft part sarcoma.

- Single and loose clusters of cells
- round to polygonal with well-defined cell border
- Abundant granular cytoplasm
- Nuclei are enlarged, round, central to eccentric in position
- Chromatin is stippled with large prominent nucleoli
- Occasional intranuclear inclusions.

in adolescents and young adults between 15 years and 35 years of age. The tumor commonly affects the lower extremities preferentially deep tissue of thigh and buttock. It usually presents as painless slowly growing mass. However, early metastasis to lung is common.

Cytology: The FNAC smear shows both clusters and discrete cells. The individual cells are round to polygonal with well-defined cell border (Box 34.27). The cytoplasm of the cell is abundant granular. Due to fragile cytoplasm, many bare nuclei are also noted in the background. Nuclei are enlarged, round, central to eccentric in position. Nuclear chromatin is stippled with large prominent nucleoli. Occasional intranuclear inclusions are also seen. Many cells show bi- and multinucleation.

Immunostaining: The tumor cells are consistently positive to the antibody against carboxy terminal portion of TFE3. The tumor cells are often positive for MyoD1 and desmin.

REFERENCES

1. Kilpatrick SE, Ward WG, Cappellari JO, et al. Fine needle aspiration biopsy of soft tissue sarcomas. A cytomorphologic analysis with emphasis on histologic subtyping, grading and therapeutic significance. Am J Clin Pathol. 1999;112:179-88.
2. Sapi Z, Antal I, Pápai Z, et al. Diagnosis of soft tissue tumors by fine needle aspiration with combined cytopathology and ancillary techniques. Diagn Cytopathol. 2002;26:232-42.
3. Dey P, Mallik MK, Gupta SK, et al. Role of fine needle aspiration cytology in the diagnosis of soft tissue tumors and tumor like lesions. Cytopathology. 2004;15(1):32-7.
4. Nagira K, Yamamoto T, Akisue T, et al. Reliability of fine needle aspiration biopsy in the initial diagnosis of soft-tissue lesions. Diagn Cytopathol. 2002;27(6):354-61.
5. Bezabih M. Cytological diagnosis of soft tissue tumours. Cytopathology. 2001;12(3):177-83.
6. Singh HK, Kilpatrick SE, Silverman JF. Fine needle aspiration biopsy of soft tissue sarcomas: utility and diagnostic challenges. Adv Anat Pathol. 2004;11(1):24-37.
7. Kilpatrick SE. Histologic prognostication in soft tissue sarcomas: grading versus subtyping or both? A comprehensive review of the literature with proposed practical guidelines. Ann Diagn Pathol. 1999;3(1):48-61.
8. Guillou L, Coindre JM, Bonichon F, et al. Comparative study of the National Cancer Institute and French Federation of Cancer Centers Sarcoma Group grading systems in a population of 410 adult patients with soft tissue sarcoma. J Clin Oncol. 1997;15(1):350-62.

9. Costa J. The grading and staging of soft tissue sarcomas. In: Fletcher CDM, McKee Ph(Eds). Pathology of soft tissue tumors. Edingburgh, UK: Churchill Livingstone; 1990. pp. 221-38.
10. Mallik MM, Dey P, Gupta SK, et al. Grading of soft tissue sarcomas on fine needle aspiration cytology smear. Diagn Cytopathol. 2010;38(2):109-12.
11. Palmer HE, Mukunyadzi P, Culbreth W, et al. Subgrouping and grading of soft-tissue sarcomas by fine needle aspiration cytology: a histopathologic correlation study. Diagn Cytopathol. 2001;24(5):307-16.
12. Fletcher CDM, Unni KK, Mertens F. Pathology and Genetics of Tumours of Soft Tissue and Bone. World Health Organization Classification of Tumours. Lyon: IARC Press; 2002.
13. Guo Z, Voytovich M, Kurtycz DF, et al. Fine needle aspiration diagnosis of spindle-cell lipoma: a case report and review of the literature. Diagn Cytopathol 2000;23(5):362-5.
14. Lemos MM, Kindblom LG, MeisKindblom JM, et al. Fine needle aspiration characteristics of hibernoma. Cancer. 2001;93(3):206-21.
15. Dey P. Fine needle aspiration cyology of well differentiated liposarcoma. Acta Cytol. 2000;44:459-62.
16. Nemanqani D, Mourad WA. Cytomorphologic features of fine needle aspiration of liposarcoma. Diagn Cytopathol. 1999;20(2):67-9.
17. Szadowska A, Lasota J. Fine needle aspiration cytology of myxoid liposarcoma; a study of 18 tumours. Cytopathology. 1993;4(2):99-106.
18. Klijanienko J, Caillaud JM, Lagacé R. Fine needle aspiration in liposarcoma: cytohistologic correlative study including well-differentiated, myxoid, and pleomorphic variants. Diagn Cytopathol. 2004;30(5):307-12.
19. Barwad A, Banik T, Gorsi U, et al. Fine needle aspiration cytology of Myositis ossificans. Diagn Cytopathol. 2011; 39(6):432-4.
20. Suster S, Nascimento AG, Miettinen M, et al. Solitary fibrous tumors of soft tissue. A clinicopathologic and immunohistochemical study of 12 cases. Am J Surg Pathol. 1995;19(11):1257-66.
21. Cho EY, Han JJ, Han J, et al. Fine needle aspiration cytology of solitary fibrous tumours of the pleura. Cytopathology. 2007;18(1):20-7.
22. Khairwa A, Dey P, Nada R. Fine needle aspiration cytology of malignant solitary fibrous tumour. Cytopathology. 2015; 26(6):391-3
23. Mathur S, Kapila K, Verma K. Accuracy of cytological grading of spindle-cell sarcomas. Diagn Cytopathol. 2003; 29(2):79-83.
24. Gupta K, Dey P, Goldsmith R, et al. Comparison of cytologic features of giant-cell tumor and giant-cell tumor of tendon sheath. Diagn Cytopathol. 2004;30(1):14-8.
25. Batra VV, Jain S, Singh DK, et al. Cytomorphologic spectrum of giant cell tumor of tendon sheath. Acta Cytol. 2008;52(2): 152-8.
26. Fletcher CD. Pleomorphic malignant fibrous histiocytoma: fact or fiction? A critical reappraisal based on 159 tumors diagnosed as pleomorphic sarcoma. Am J Surg Pathol. 1992;16:213-28.
27. Domanski HA, Akerman M, Engellau J, et al. Fine needle aspiration of neurilemoma (schwannoma). A clinicocytopathologic study of 116 patients. Diagn Cytopathol. 2006; 34(6):403-12.
28. Gupta K, Dey P, Vashisht R. Fine needle aspiration cytology of malignant peripheral nerve sheath tumors. Diagn Cytopathol. 2004;31(1):1-4.
29. Akhtar M, Ali MA, Bakry M, et al. Fine needle aspiration biopsy diagnosis of rhabdomyosarcoma: cytologic, histologic and ultrastructural correlations. Diagn Cytopathol. 1992;5:465-74.
30. Domanski HA, Akerman M, Rissler P, et al. Fine needle aspiration of soft tissue leiomyosarcoma: an analysis of the most common cytologic findings and the value of ancillary techniques. Diagn Cytopathol. 2006;34(9):597-604.
31. Klijanienko J, Caillaud JM, Lagace R, et al. Cytohistologic correlations in 56 synovial sarcomas in 36 patients: The Institut Curie Experience. Diagn Cytopathol. 2002;27(2): 96-102.
32. Rau AR, Kini H, Verghese R. Tigroid background in fine needle aspiration cytology of clear cell sarcoma. Diagn Cytopathol. 2006;34(5):355-7.
33. Barwad A, Dey P, Das A. Fine needle aspiration cytology of epithelioid sarcoma. Diagn Cytopathol. 2011;39(7):517-20.
34. Shabb N, Sneige N, Fanning CV, et al. Fine needle aspiration cytology of alveolar soft-part sarcoma. Diagn Cytopathol. 1991;7(3):293-8.

Review Questions

1. **A 27-year-old male presented with 6 cm diameter swelling near the right joint region for 19 days. Figures 34.31A to D represent the fine needle aspiration cytology smears of the swelling.**

a. **What is your diagnosis?**
   a. Synovial sarcoma
   b. Malignant peripheral nerve sheath tumor
   c. Rhabdomyosarcoma
   d. Liposarcoma

b. **What immunostains and cytogenetics can be done to further confirm your diagnosis?**

2. **A 25-year-old male presented with a soft 3 cm swelling over the right ankle for 6 months. Radiograph of his ankle is free of any bony lesion. Figures 34.32A to D represent the fine needle aspiration cytology smears of the swelling.**
   What is your diagnosis?
   a. Synovial sarcoma
   b. Giant cell tumor of tendon sheath
   c. Osteosarcoma
   d. Ewing's sarcoma

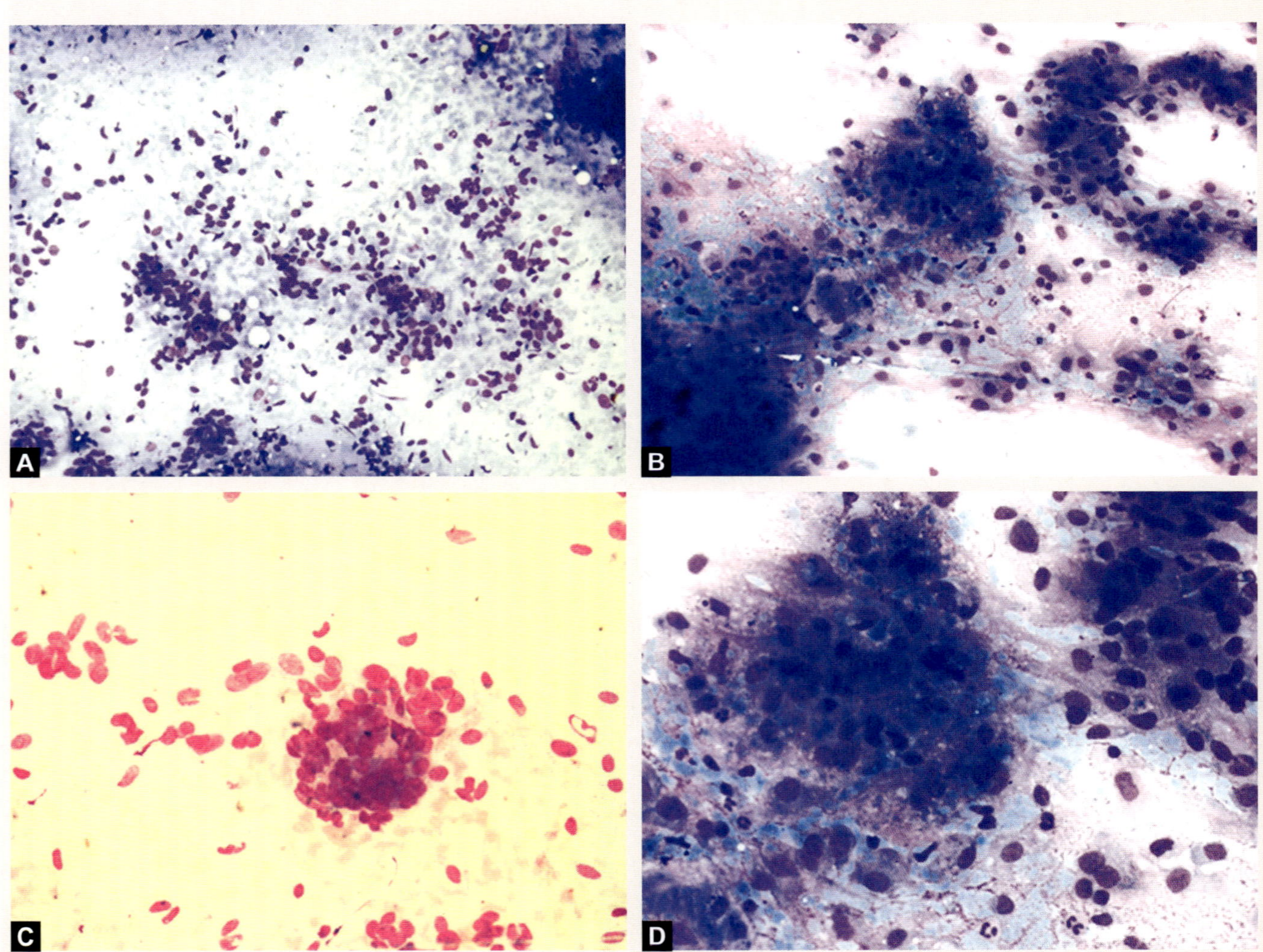

Figs. 34.31A to D: Cytology smear of the case of question 1.

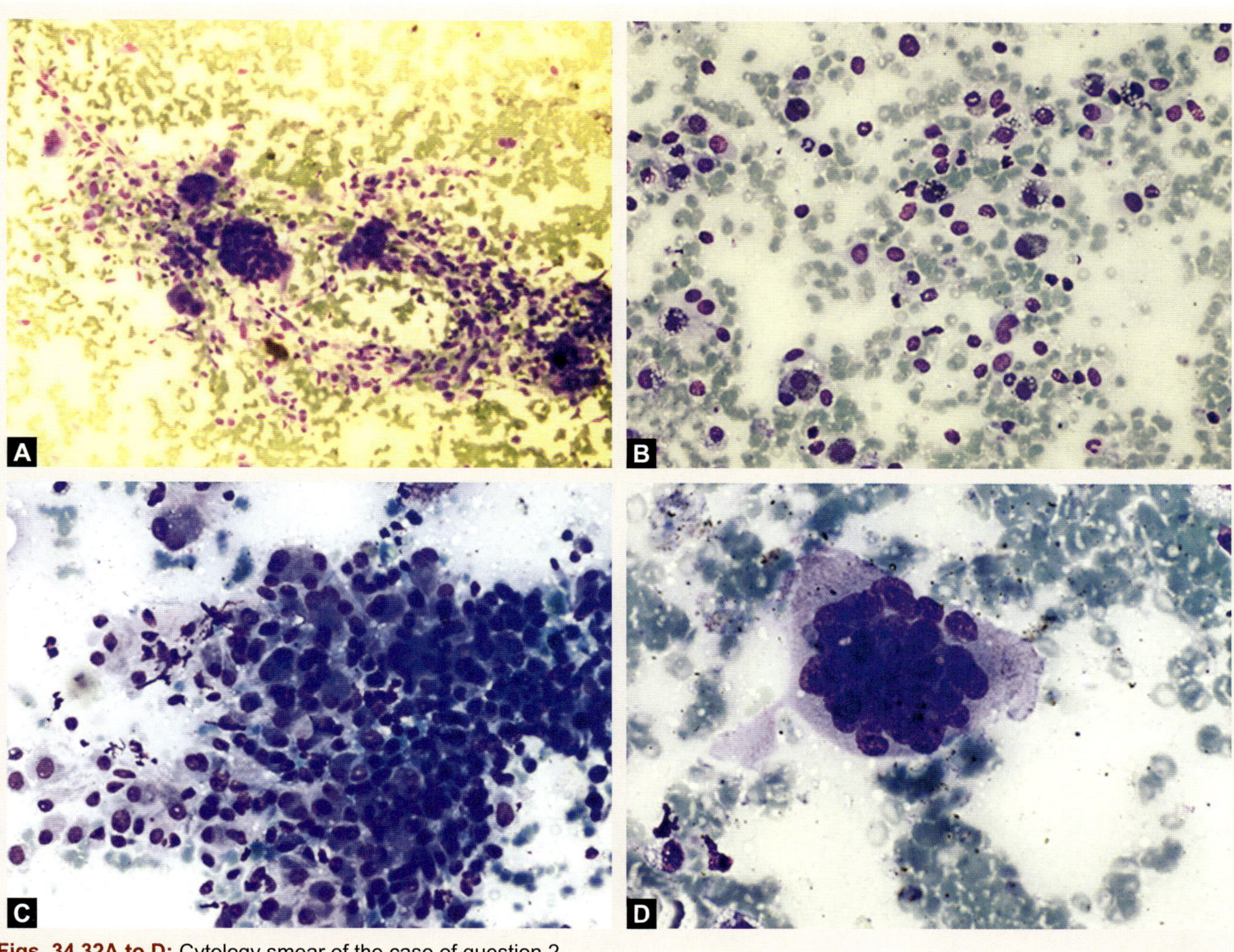

Figs. 34.32A to D: Cytology smear of the case of question 2.

Answers

1. a. Answer is (a) Synovial sarcoma
   b. Immunostains:
   - CK= positive
   - EMA= positive
   - Vimentin= positive

   Cytogenetics:
   - t(X;18)(p11;q11)

   Note: The tumor shows a biphasic pattern having both round and spindle cells. Occasional gland like pattern is present. The individual cells show nuclear enlargement and pleomorphism. All these features suggest the diagnosis of synovial sarcoma.
2. b. Giant cell tumor of tendon sheath

   Note: The presence of many multinucleated giant cells along with round to oval monomorphic stromal cells in this case favour the diagnosis of giant cell tumor of tendon sheath. The close differential diagnosis is giant cell tumor of bone which is eliminated as the bone is free of any lesion.

CHAPTER 35

Skin

INTRODUCTION

The various skin lesions are easily accessible and a punch biopsy provides the diagnosis. Therefore, fine needle aspiration cytology (FNAC) of skin lesions is not much popular. However, like all other sites, FNAC can provide rapid and reliable diagnosis, particularly in differentiating inflammatory lesion from a tumor. It is also helpful in diagnosis of various metastatic lesions in skin (Box 35.1). FNAC material from the neoplastic lesions in skin can be processed for various ancillary investigations, such as cell block for immunocytochemistry in case of Merkel-cell carcinoma or flow cytometry in case of non-Hodgkin's lymphoma (NHL) of skin. A thorough knowledge of cytology of skin tumors may help to avoid false-positive diagnosis.[1-5]

Scrapping from the ulcer can be taken in small-ulcerated lesions of skin. Larger lesions can be sampled by FNAC.

NON-NEOPLASTIC LESIONS

Inflammation

Viral Infection

Viral infection can best be diagnosed by simple scrapping from the base of the ulcer. The smears from molluscum contagiosum show classical 'molluscum bodies' within the cytoplasm of the squamous cells replacing the nucleus to the periphery of the cell. The cytology smears from the herpes simplex infection show similar picture as described in cervical cytology section of this book. The smears show characteristic multinucleated cells with nuclear molding along with intranuclear large ground glass-like inclusion.

Box 35.1: Advantages of fine needle aspiration cytology of skin.

- Rapid
- Cost effective
- Reliably differentiates neoplastic lesion from inflammation
- Helps in identification of metastatic tumor in skin
- Ancillary investigation can be performed such as FCM and immunocytochemistry

(FCM: Flow cytometry).

Fungal Infection

Scrapping from the ulcer base of the skin lesion may show fungal lesions. Individual morphology of the fungi studied by methylene blue stain is helpful to identify the type of fungus.

Bacterial Infection

Bacterial infection gives rise to nonspecific inflammation. FNAC or scrapping of the lesion usually yields large number of inflammatory cells. In case of skin tuberculosis, FNAC smears may show epithelioid cell granulomas, multinucleated giant cells, and lymphocytes. Z-N stain should be done to show the presence of acid-fast bacilli.

Parasitic Infection

Leishmania donovani in dermal leishmaniasis is often identified in cytology smears. FNAC of the cysticercus infection yields clear fluid and the smears show tegument layer of the parasite (Fig. 35.1). Background of the smear may show collection of histiocytes, lymphocytes, and giant cell.

Rare Benign Diseases of Skin

Rarely calcinosis cutis, rheumatoid arthritis, or sarcoidosis may present as a nodular skin lesion.[6]

Fine needle aspiration cytology of calcinosis cutis shows abundant granular calcified material along with occasional histiocytes (Fig. 35.2).

Aspirates from the rheumatoid arthritis and sarcoidosis show granulomatous inflammation and smear contains

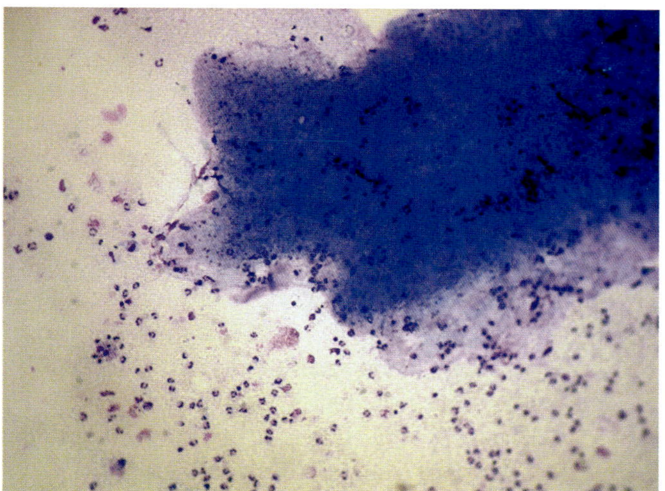

Fig. 35.1: Cysticercus infection: Tegument layer of cysticercus along with many polymorphs and eosinophils in the background (MGG × MP).

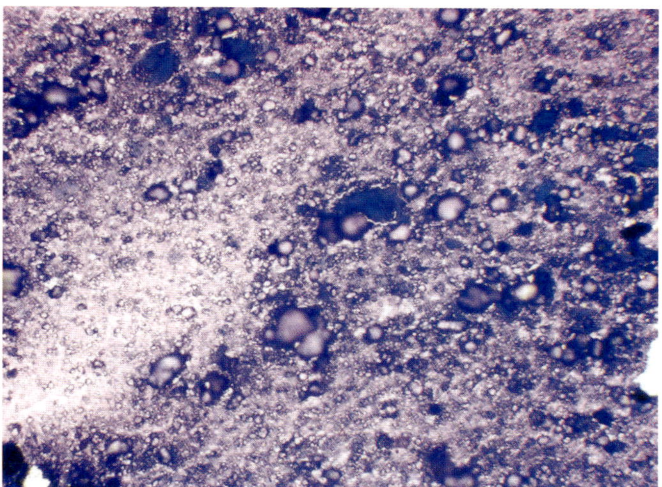

Fig. 35.2: Calcinosis cutis: Granular calcified material (MGG × MP).

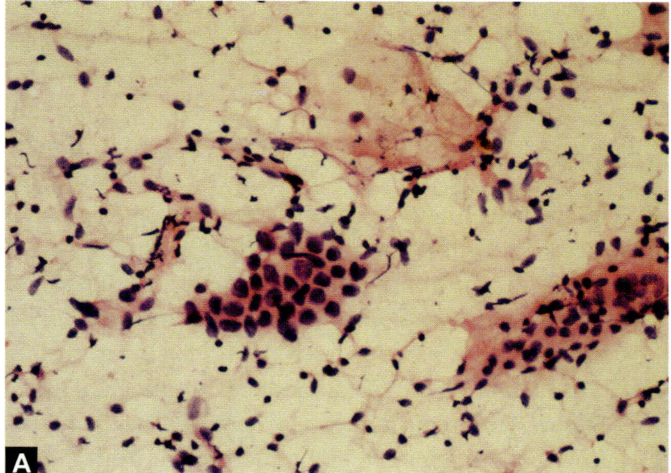

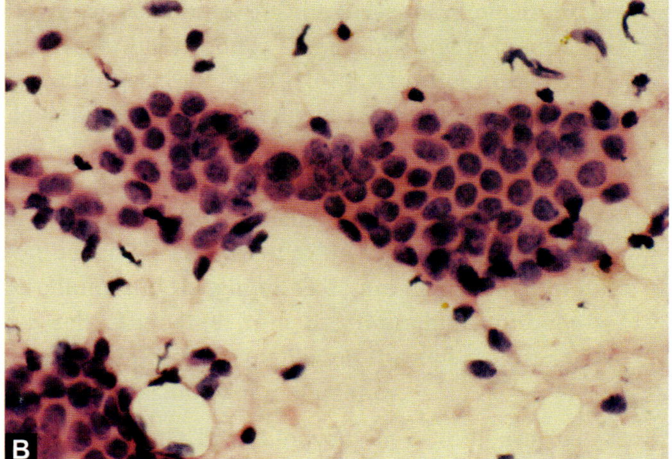

Figs. 35.3A and B: (A) Endometriosis: Glandular epithelium and stromal fragment (H & E × MP). (B) Endometriosis: Endometrial glandular epithelium (H & E × HP).

multiple epithelioid cell granulomas, multinucleated giant cells, and inflammatory cells. The granulomas of sarcoidosis are noncaseating.

Endometriosis (Figs. 35.3A and B)

Endometriosis may present as nodular lesions in skin. Cytology smears show glandular epithelial cells, oval to spindle-shaped endometrial stroma, and hemosiderin-laden histiocytes. The characteristic clinical history of painful enlargement of the swelling during menstruation and bland nuclear morphology of the glandular epithelial cells are helpful in diagnosis of endometriosis.

Other Non-neoplastic Lesions

Epidermal Inclusion Cyst (Fig. 35.4)

Epidermal inclusion cyst is frequently aspirated. FNAC of epidermal inclusion cyst yields thick whitish material. The smear shows abundant anucleated squamous cells. Occasionally, the cells may show reactive atypia and it may be difficult to distinguish well-differentiated squamous cell carcinoma from epidermal inclusion cyst. However, careful search may show malignant cells in FNAC smear of squamous cell carcinoma. A good clinical history of primary malignancy may also be helpful. The smears also show many multinucleated giant cells.

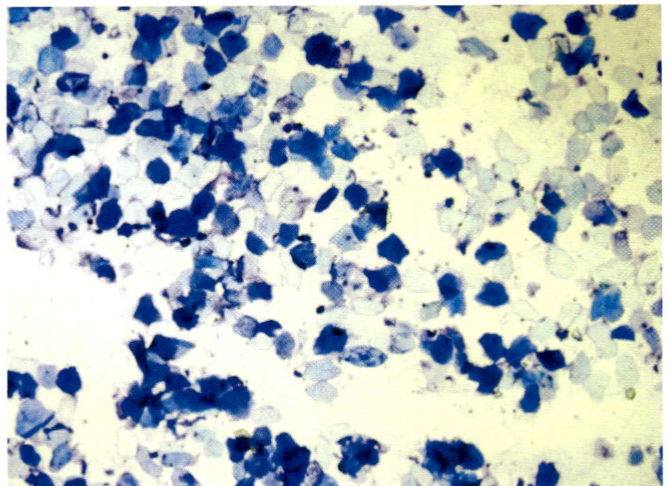

Fig. 35.4: Epidermal inclusion cyst: Anucleated squamous cells (MGG × HP).

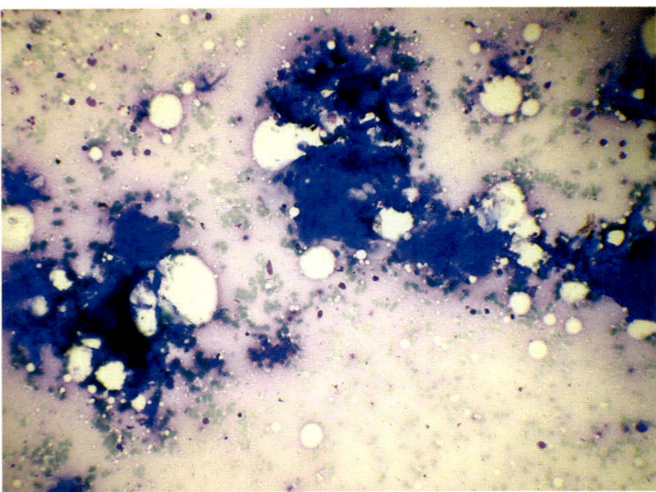

Fig. 35.5: Pilomatrixoma: Ghost of squamous cells, multinucleated giant cells, and calcified material (MGG × MP).

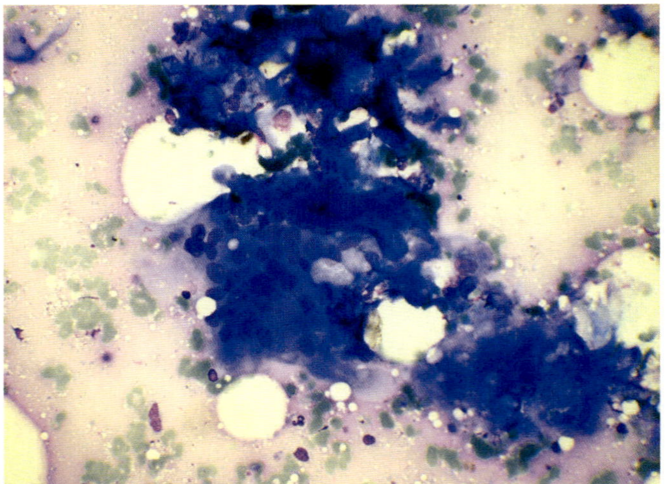

Fig. 35.6: Pilomatrixoma: Higher magnification of the previous smear showing giant cells and calcified material (MGG × HP).

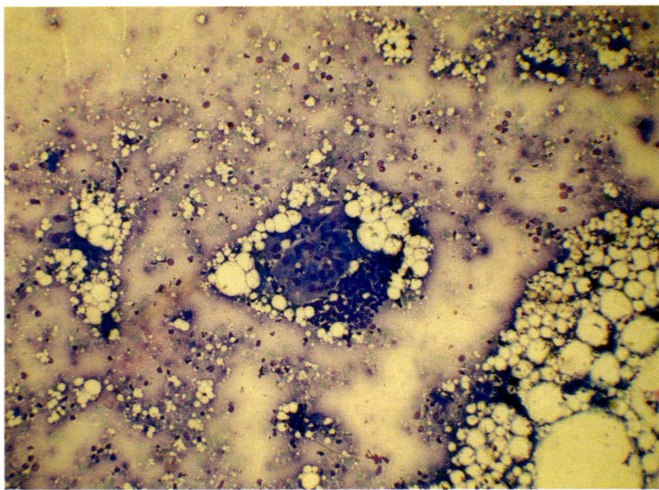

Fig. 35.7: Pilomatrixoma: Cluster and discrete round monomorphic basal cells along with multinucleated giant cells.

Differential diagnosis:

- Well-differentiated squamous cell carcinoma.

NEOPLASTIC LESIONS OF SKIN

Benign Tumor of Skin Adnexa

Pilomatrixoma[4,7]

This is a benign adnexal tumor of the hair follicle and represents 0.2% of all routine dermatological samples. The tumor predominantly occurs in the young individuals and the common sites of involvement are head and neck region and upper extremities. The patient commonly presents as skin colored 1–3-cm diameter firm nodule.

Cytology (Figs. 35.5 to 35.7): The cytology smears show a mixed population of basaloid cells, ghost cells, and multinucleated giant cells in a background of calcified material (Box 35.2). The basaloid cells have scanty bluish cytoplasm. The cell margin is usually ill defined. The nuclei are round with high N/C ratio and monomorphic. Nuclear chromatin is fine with single prominent nucleoli. The smear also shows many discrete anucleated squamous cells, known as ghost cells. They may often be present as small clumps. Many multinucleated giant cells are also seen. Background of the smear shows dark bluish, calcified material, and myxoid material.

Differential diagnosis:

- Metastatic squamous cell carcinoma
- Epidermal inclusion cyst
- Foreign body reaction.

Chondroid Syringoma

This is a benign skin adnexal tumor analogous to mixed tumor of the salivary gland. It commonly occurs in adults. Head and neck regions are commonly affected by chondroid syringoma.

Cytology: Fine needle aspiration cytology of chondroid syringoma shows discrete and small clusters of round to oval epithelial cells embedded in purple fibrillary chondromyxoid material (Box 35.3). The cells have moderate amount of dense cytoplasm with central to eccentric round nuclei. Nuclear chromatin is fine with single prominent nucleoli.[8]

Box 35.2: Pilomatrixoma.

- Anucleated squamous cells: ghost cells
- Monomorphic round basaloid cells:
  - Round
  - Scanty ill-defined cytoplasm
  - Monomorphic nuclei
  - Fine chromatin
- Multinucleated giant cells
- Calcified material

Differential diagnosis:

- Basal cell carcinoma (BCC).

Cylindroma (Box 35.4)

Cylindroma usually occurs in the scalp. Aspiration cytology smears simulate adenoid cystic carcinoma of the salivary gland. FNAC smear shows multiple homogenous purple-colored hyaline globules [May-Grünwald Giemsa (MGG) stain] surrounded by round to oval epithelial cells (Figs. 35.8A and B). These cells have scanty cytoplasm and round monomorphic hyperchromatic nuclei.

Eccrine Spiradenoma

This is a benign skin adnexal tumor. FNAC smear of eccrine spiradenoma simulates adenoid cystic carcinoma. The

Box 35.3: Chondroid syringoma.

- Discrete and small clusters of round to oval epithelial cells
- Round cells
- Well-defined cytoplasmic margin
- Round nuclei with fine chromatin
- Prominent nucleoli
- Fibrillary chondromyxoid material

Box 35.4: Cylindroma.

- Homogenous purple-colored globules
- Basaloid cells:
  - Round cells
  - Scanty cytoplasm
  - Monomorphic round nuclei
  - Hyperchromatic nuclei

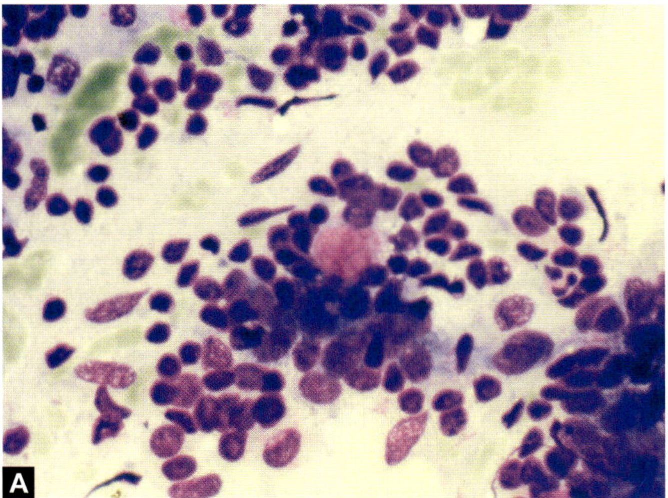

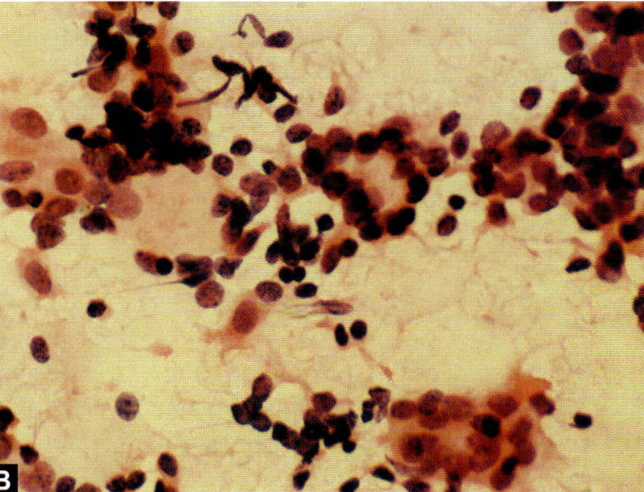

Figs. 35.8A and B: (A) Cylindroma: Multiple homogenous purple-colored hyaline globules surrounded by round to oval epithelial cells (MGG × MP). (B) Cylindroma: Cells are round with scanty cytoplasm (H & E × HP).

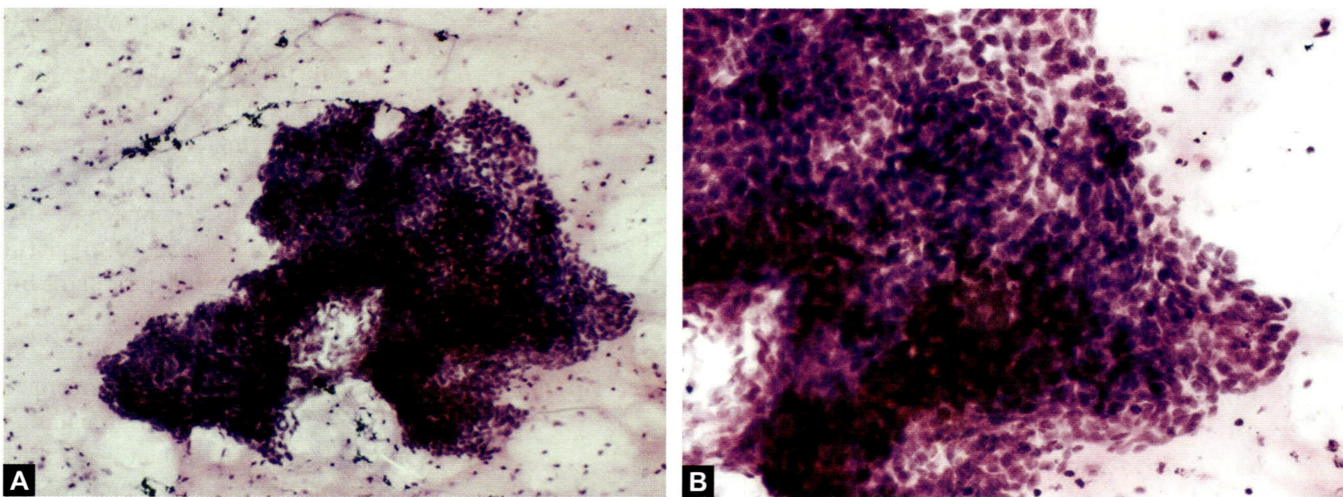

Figs. 35.9A and B: (A) Hidradenoma: Cohesive papillary like cluster of cells (H & E × MP). (B) Hidradenoma: Cells with scanty cytoplasm and monomorphic nuclei (H & E × HP).

Box 35.5: Eccrine spiradenoma.

- Stromal matrix material surrounded by epithelial cells
- Cuboidal epithelial cells:
  - Scanty cytoplasm
  - Round nuclei and inconspicuous nucleoli
- Myoepithelial cells
- Lymphocytes

Box 35.6: Hidradenoma.

- Cohesive clusters and tubules
- Cuboidal to polyhedral in cells
- Scanty cytoplasm
- Monomorphic round nuclei
- Bland chromatin
- Dense round metachromatic-staining globules

cytology smear shows stromal matrix material surrounded by epithelial cells giving a rosette-like arrangement (Box 35.5). The epithelial cells are also arranged as cell balls. The epithelial cells are cuboidal cells with scanty cytoplasm having round nuclei and inconspicuous nucleoli. In addition, the smears also show discrete myoepithelial cells and scattered lymphocytes.

Hidradenoma

This is a benign skin adnexal tumor of eccrine sweat gland. This is also known as clear cell hidradenoma. This tumor commonly occurs in adult. Hidradenomas commonly involves the scalp, trunk, and proximal extremities.

Cytology:[9,10] FNAC smear shows cohesive clusters and tubule-like structures of cells. Occasional scattered cells with naked nuclei are also seen (Box 35.6). The cells are cuboidal to polyhedral in shape with scanty cytoplasm. The nuclei are monomorphic round with bland chromatin and inconspicuous nucleoli (Figs. 35.9A and B). Background of the smear shows scattered-dense round metachromatic-staining globules.

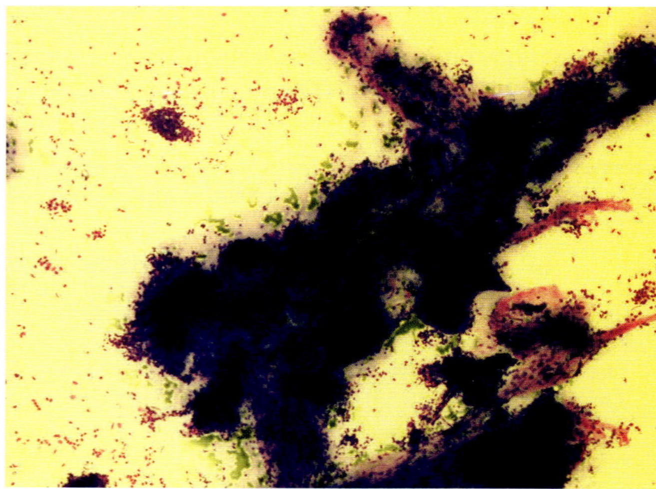

Fig. 35.10: Syringocystadenoma papilliferum: Multiple papillary structures (MGG × LP).

Syringocystadenoma Papilliferum (Figs. 35.10 to 35.14)

Syringocystadenoma papilliferum is a rare cutaneous adnexal neoplasm. The average age at the time of presentation is 28 years. The tumor commonly occurs in the trunk and scalp region. FNAC smears show multiple

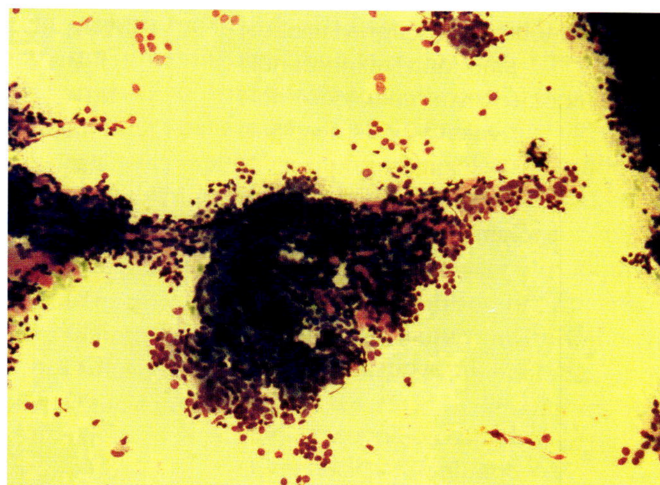

Fig. 35.11: Syringocystadenoma papilliferum: Papillary cluster along with round to oval epithelial cells and elongated spindle cells (MGG × MP).

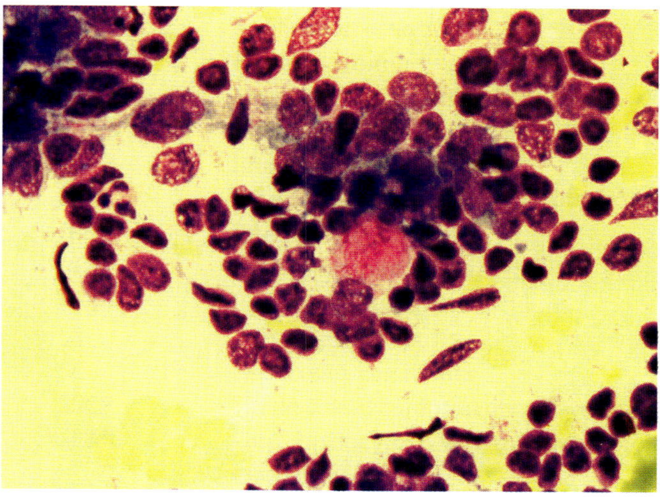

Fig. 35.12: Syringocystadenoma papilliferum: Higher magnification showing better morphology of the cells. The cells are round with scanty cytoplasm having monomorphic bland nuclei. Cells occasionally arranged around pinkish globules (MGG × OI).

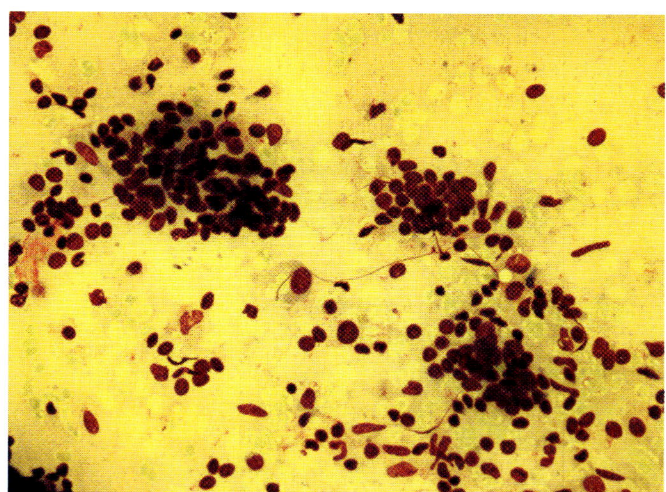

Fig. 35.13: Syringocystadenoma papilliferum: Discrete round and spindle-shaped cells along with few inflammatory cells (MGG × HP).

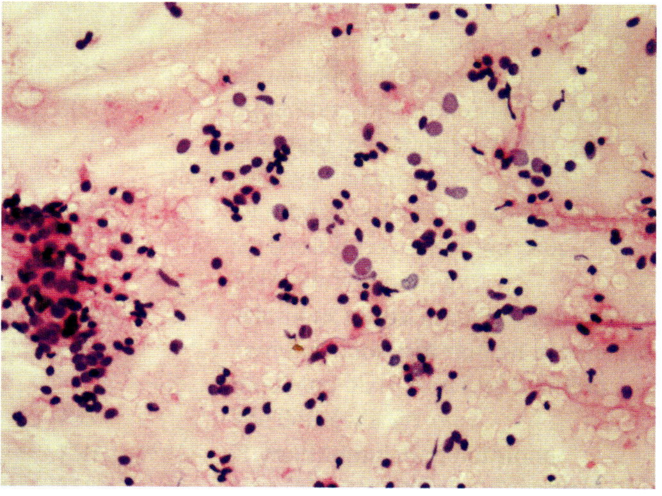

Fig. 35.14: Syringocystadenoma papilliferum: Nuclear morphology is better seen in hematoxylin and eosin-stained smear (H & E × HP).

papillae-like structures along with discrete monomorphic epithelial cells and occasional spindle cells. Smears may also show chronic inflammatory cells.

Malignant Tumors of Skin

Basal Cell Carcinoma[11-13]

Basal cell carcinoma is also known as trichoblastic carcinoma. This is the most frequent primary skin cancer. It predominantly affects the sun-exposed skin area. BCC is commonly seen in adults and usually affects in the head and neck region as slow-growing ulcerated nodule or papule.

Cytology (Fig. 35.15): FNAC smears show small tight cluster of cells (Box 35.7). The cells are often arranged as palisading manner around the periphery of the clusters. The tumor cells contain scanty cytoplasm with very high N/C ratio. The nuclei of the cells are round, monomorphic, and hyperchromatic. Occasional cells may show small distinct nucleoli.

Differential diagnosis:
- Small-cell carcinoma
- Merkel-cell carcinoma
- Poorly differentiated skin adnexal carcinoma.

Sebaceous Carcinoma[14-16]

Sebaceous carcinoma (SC) is commonly seen in the lacrimal gland of eye. It usually occurs in elderly adults and commonly presents as painless mass in the eyelid. It may be mistaken clinically as chalazion blepharitis or conjunctivitis.

Cytology (Figs. 35.16A and B): FNAC smears show predominantly discrete cells and tight three-dimensional clusters. Occasional glandular arrangements are also seen. Background of the smear shows fatty material and keratin debris (Box 35.8). The individual cells are large with moderate to abundant amount of finely vacuolated cytoplasm and well-defined cytoplasmic margin. Cytoplasmic vacuoles are positive for oil red O. Nuclei are central in position and round to oval with moderate pleomorphism. Occasional nuclei may be notched or indented. Smears may show individual cell necrosis and background necrosis. Occasional multinucleated giant cells may also be seen.

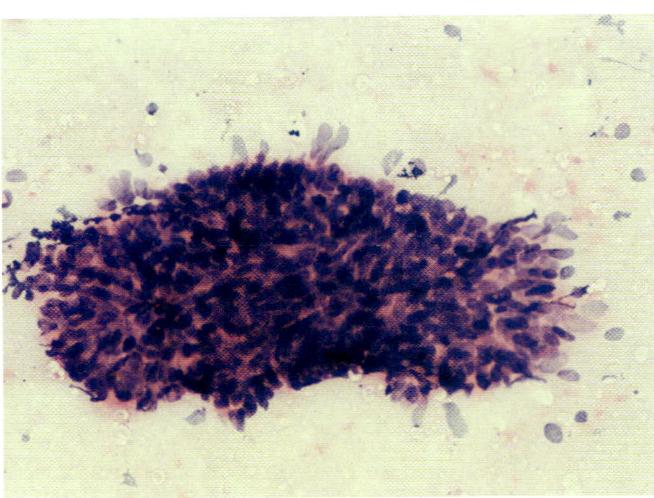

Fig. 35.15: Basal cell carcinoma: Round cells with hyperchromatic nuclei arranged as palisading manner (H & E × HP).

Box 35.7: Basal cell carcinoma.
- Tight clusters of round cells
- Peripheral palisade-like arrangement
- Round cells
- Scanty cytoplasm
- Very high N/C ratio
- Hyperchromatic round nuclei
- Occasional prominent nucleoli

Box 35.8: Sebaceous carcinoma.
- Discrete cells and tight three-dimensional clusters
- Large cells with well-defined borders
- Abundant amount of finely vacuolated cytoplasm
- Nuclei are central
- Round to oval with moderate pleomorphism
- Individual cell necrosis and background necrosis
- Multinucleated giant cells

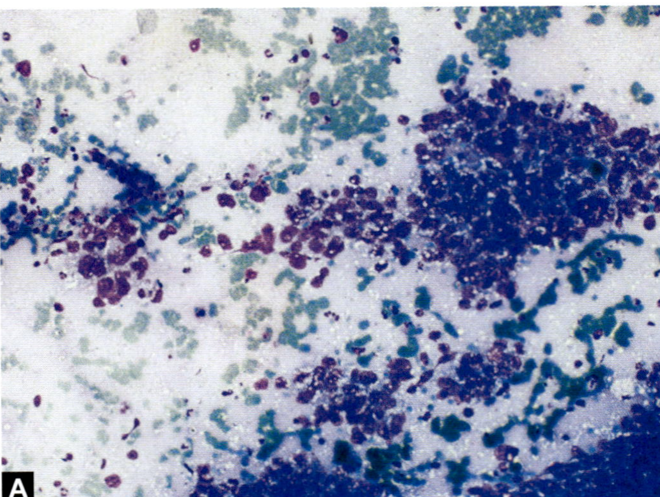

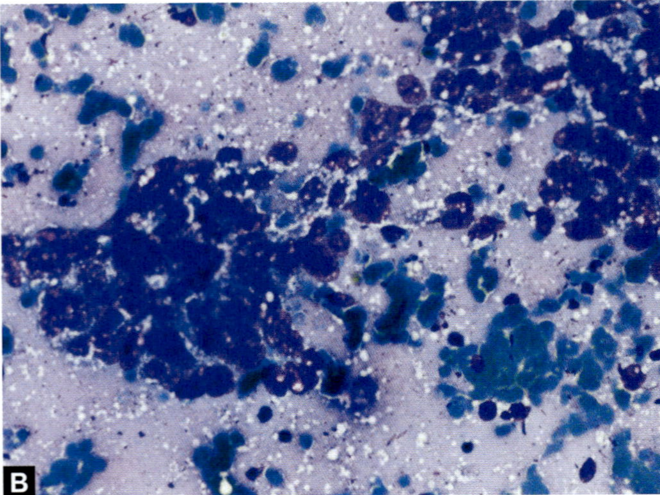

Figs. 35.16A and B: (A) Sebaceous carcinoma: Clusters of cells with vacuolated cytoplasm and round pleomorphic nuclei (MGG × MP). (B) Sebaceous carcinoma: Higher magnification of the same (MGG × HP).

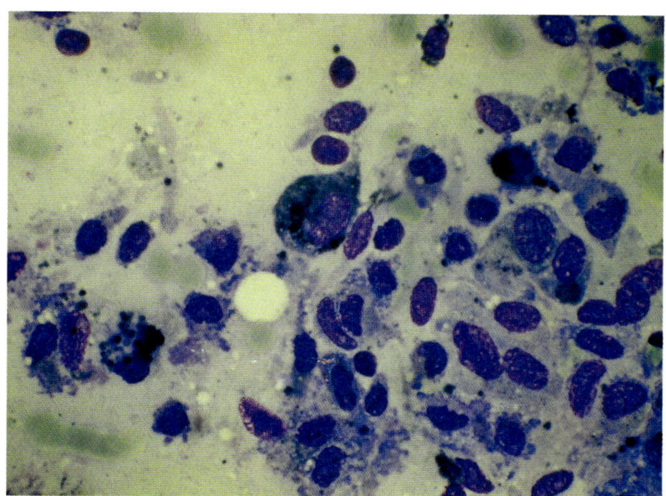

Fig. 35.17: Malignant melanoma: Discrete moderately pleomorphic cells with melanin in the cytoplasm (MGG × MP).

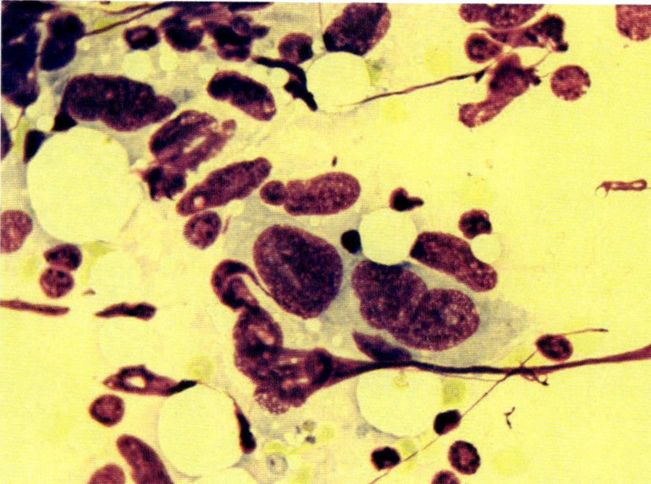

Fig. 35.18: Malignant melanoma: Cells with markedly pleomorphic nuclei having prominent nucleoli (MGG × HP).

Differential diagnosis:

- Pagetoid malignant melanoma
- Paget's disease.

Malignant Melanoma[4,17,18]

Malignant melanomas develop from the melanocytes of the skin and are the aggressive cancers. They are commonly noted in the sun-exposed area such as head and neck region and lower extremities. The tumor usually occurs in adults but may also develop before puberty. Malignant melanoma usually develops spontaneously or occasionally from the pigmented nevi.

Cytology (Figs. 35.17 and 35.18): FNAC of primary melanoma is not common. Most of the cases are aspirated from the metastatic sites. The smears show predominantly dyscohesive cells (Box 35.9). The individual cells have abundant cytoplasm with central to eccentric large round moderately pleomorphic nuclei. The nuclei often show single-to-multiple prominent nucleoli. Macronucleoli are often seen. Intranuclear cytoplasmic inclusions are also noted. Dark-brown melanin pigment in the cell is characteristic for the diagnosis of melanoma. Occasionally, malignant melanoma shows predominant spindle-cell morphology. The spindle cells are arranged in interlacing fascicles and whorls and also discretely. The individual cells contain variable amount of cytoplasm with bipolar-elongated cytoplasmic process. The cytoplasm of these cells often shows dark-brown melanin pigment. Nuclei are moderately pleomorphic oval to elongated having finely granular chromatin. Binucleation and multinucleation are also noted. In the absence of melanin, malignant melanoma with spindle cells is difficult to diagnose only on cytology smear.

Box 35.9: Malignant melanoma.

- Discrete round cells
- Moderate cytoplasm with dark-brown pigment
- Moderately pleomorphic nuclei
- Many bi- and multinucleated cells
- Macronucleoli
- Intranuclear inclusions
- Spindle cells
- HMB-45 and S-100 positive

Immunocytochemistry: Melanoma cells are positive for HMB-45, melan-A, and S-100 protein. HMB-45 is more specific than S-100 protein immunostaining. Melan-A, a melanocytic differentiation antigen, is present in 80% of malignant melanoma cases.

Diagnostic difficulties:

- Carcinoma
- Non-Hodgkin's lymphoma
- Sarcoma.

Squamous Cell Carcinoma

It is the malignant tumor of the keratinocytes of the epidermis with squamous differentiation. The tumor usually involves the exposed area of the body such as forehead, face, and hand. The patient usually presents as shallow ulcer with indurated margin.

Cytology: Smear shows discrete tumor cells. The tumor cells are polyhedral with moderate amount of cytoplasm.

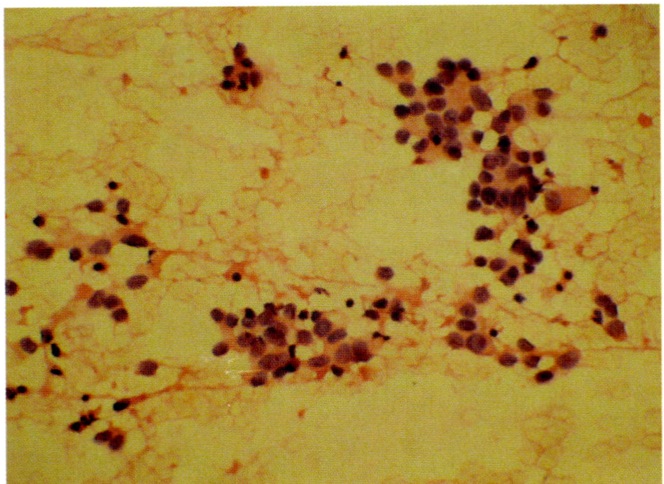

Fig. 35.19: Merkel cell carcinoma of skin: Discrete and occasional rosette-like arrangement of small round cells with scanty cytoplasm having round monomorphic nuclei (H & E × MP).

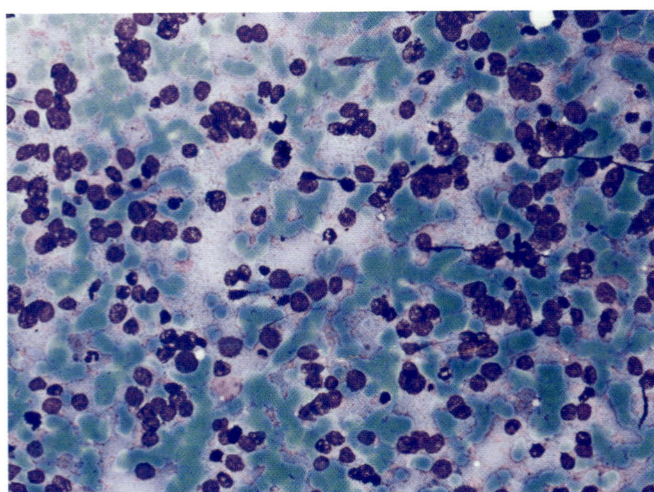

Fig. 35.20: Merkel cell carcinoma of skin: Discrete small round cells (MGG × MP).

Box 35.10: Squamous cell carcinoma.

- Polyhedral cells
- Abundant cytoplasm
- Orangeophilia in Papanicolaou's stain
- High N/C ratio
- Moderate nuclear pleomorphism
- Anucleated squamous cells
- Fiber and tadpole cells

Cytoplasmic orangeophilia are seen in Papanicolaou's staining (Box 35.10). Nuclei are enlarged with high N/C ratio and moderately pleomorphic. Nuclear chromatin is condensed with inconspicuous nucleoli. Occasional fiber cells and tadpole-like cells may also be seen. In addition, mature looking anucleated cells may also be seen.

Malignant Sweat Gland Tumor[19,20]

Cytology smear of malignant sweat gland tumor shows abundant cells. The cells are discrete and also with tubular arrangement. The tumor cells show abundant pale cytoplasm with central mildly pleomorphic nuclei. Cytological diagnosis of malignant sweat gland tumor is often difficult. Detailed clinical history may be helpful in diagnosis of malignant sweat gland tumor.

Merkel Cell Carcinoma[21,22]

Merkel cell tumor is a relatively rare primary malignant tumor of the skin. Most of the tumor arises on the sun-exposed skin area and head and neck regions are commonly affected.

Box 35.11: Merkel cell tumor.

- Discrete cells
- Occasional pseudorosette
- Scanty deep-blue cytoplasm
- Round nuclei, fine chromatin, occasional molding

Cytology (Figs. 35.19 and 35.20): FNAC smear of Merkel cell carcinoma shows predominant discrete small round cells and occasional pseudorosette-like arrangement (Box 35.11). The tumor cells are small round with scanty deep-blue cytoplasm. The nuclei are small round with fine chromatin and multiple small nucleoli. Occasional cell shows nuclear molding. Mitosis is usually frequent. Many histiocytes may also be noted in the background.

Immunocytochemistry: Merkel cell carcinomas are positive for CK20, neuron-specific enolase (NSE), epithelial membrane antigen (EMA), and S-100. The cells are also positive for CD117. In contrast, small-cell carcinomas are negative for CK20 and positive for thyroid transcription factor-1 (TTF-1).

Differential diagnosis:

- Small-cell carcinoma
- NHL.

Metastasis[23,24]

Skin often shows metastasis from various sources. The common sources of metastasis are from lung, breast, large intestine, melanoma, and kidney. Metastatic soft-tissue tumor is also not rare (Fig. 35.21). Occasionally, solitary metastatic

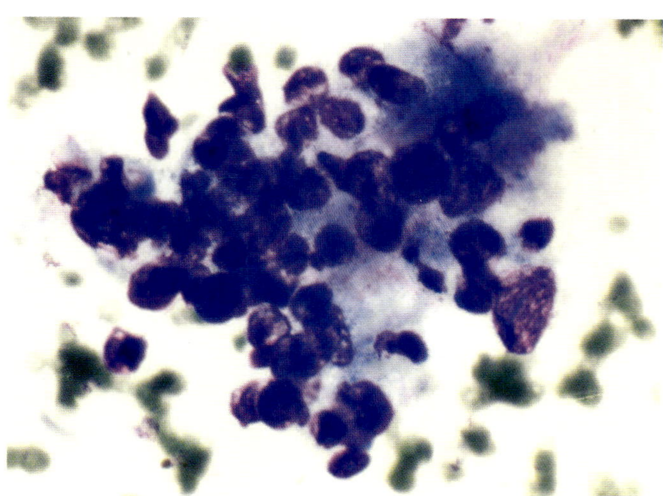

Fig. 35.21: Metastatic adenocarcinoma: Moderately pleomorphic cells from an ovarian carcinoma to skin (MGG × HP).

skin lesion may simulate a primary skin tumor on clinical examination. Cytomorphology of metastatic carcinoma of skin depends on the type of primary malignancy. Some of the metastatic tumors are readily identifiable from the cytomorphology such, as signet ring carcinoma of the stomach and clear cell carcinoma of kidney.

Differential diagnosis:

- Endometriosis
- Primary skin tumor.

Hematopoietic Malignancy

Certain lymphomas often involve the skin such as anaplastic large-cell lymphomas in pediatric population and mycosis fungoides in adult population. The cytomorphology of these lymphomas is same as that of lymph node. Leukemia also involves the subcutaneous tissue of skin. Cytology smear shows myeloid series of cells and blasts.

REFERENCES

1. Kapila K, Chopra P, Verma K. Fine needle aspiration cytology of alveolar soft-part sarcoma. A case report. Acta Cytol. 1985;29:559-61.
2. Rege J, Shet T. Aspiration cytology in the diagnosis of primary tumors of skin adnexa. Acta Cytol. 2001;45:715-22.
3. Daskalopoulou D, Galanopoulou A, Statiropoulou P, et al. Cytologically interesting cases of primary skin tumors and tumor-like conditions identified by fine needle aspiration biopsy. Diagn Cytopathol. 1998;19:17-28.
4. Dey P, Das A, Radhika S, et al. Cytology of primary skin tumors. Acta Cytol. 1996;40:708-13.
5. Layfield LJ, Glasgow BJ. Aspiration biopsy cytology of primary cutaneous tumors. Acta Cytol. 1993;37:679-88.
6. Agrawal P, Banik T, Dey P. Calcinosis cutis: diagnosis by fine needle aspiration cytology—a rare case report. Diagn Cytopathol. 2011;39:917-8.
7. Dubb M, Michelow P. Fine needle aspiration cytology of pilomatrixoma and differential diagnoses. Acta Cytol. 2009;53:683-8.
8. Srinivasan R, Rajwanshi A, Padmanabhan V, et al. Fine needle aspiration cytology of chondroid syringoma and syringocystadenoma papilliferum. A report of two cases. Acta Cytol. 1993;37:535-8.
9. Gottschalk-Sabag S, Glick T. Fine needle aspiration of nodular hidradenoma: A case report. Diagn Cytopathol. 1996;15:395-7.
10. Rollins SD. Fine needle aspiration diagnosis of a vulvar papillary hidradenoma: A case report. Diagn Cytopathol. 1994;10:60-1.
11. Fang X, Ma B. Fine needle aspiration cytology of basal cell carcinoma of the skin: a clinical and cytopathological appraisal. J Dermatol. 1999;26:640-6.
12. Malberger E, Tillinger R, Lichtig C. Diagnosis of basal-cell carcinoma with aspiration cytology. Acta Cytol. 1984;28:301-4.
13. Vega-Memije E, De Larios NM, Waxtein LM, et al. Cytodiagnosis of cutaneous basal and squamous cell carcinoma. Int J Dermatol. 2000;39:116-20.
14. Garbyal RS, Gupta P, Kumar M, et al. A cytologic perspective on meibomian gland carcinoma. Acta Cytol. 2007;51:171-7.
15. Das DK, Das J, Natarajan R, et al. Meibomian gland carcinoma initially identified by cytology. Diagn Cytopathol. 1986;2:154-6.
16. Jain P, Nanda A, Handa U. FNA Diagnosis of Recurrent Sebaceous Carcinoma. Diagn. Cytopathol. 2006;34:124-6.
17. Murali R, Doubrovsky A, Watson GF, et al. Diagnosis of metastatic melanoma by fine needle biopsy: analysis of 2,204 cases. Am J Clin Pathol. 2007;127:385-97.
18. Doubrovsky A, Scolyer RA, Murali R, et al. Diagnostic accuracy of fine needle biopsy for metastatic melanoma and its implications for patient management. Ann Surg Oncol. 2008;15:323-32.
19. Gangane N, Joshi D, Sharma SM. Cytomorphological diagnosis of malignant eccrine tumors: report of two cases. Diagn Cytopathol. 2008;36:801-4.
20. Agrawal V, Gupta RL, Kumar S, et al. Malignant chondroid syringoma. J Dermatol. 1998;25:547-9.
21. Dey P, Jogai S, Amir T, et al. Fine needle aspiration cytology of Merkel cell carcinoma. Diagn Cytopathol. 2004;31:364-5.
22. Al-Kaisi NK. Fine needle aspiration cytology of a metastatic Merkel-cell carcinoma. Diagn Cytopathol. 1991;7:184-8.
23. Sharma S, Kotru M, Yadav A, et al. Role of fine needle aspiration cytology in evaluation of cutaneous metastases. Diagn Cytopathol. 2009;37:876-80.
24. Srinivasan R, Ray R, Nijhawan R. Metastatic cutaneous and subcutaneous deposits from internal carcinoma. An analysis of cases diagnosed by fine needle aspiration. Acta Cytol. 1993;37:894-8.

Review Questions

1. **A 27-year-old male presented with a 2.5-cm diameter swelling in the scalp for 7 months. Figures 35.22A to D represent the cytology smears from the FNAC of the scalp swelling. What is your possible diagnosis?**
   a. Skin adnexal tumor possibly hidradenoma
   b. Metastatic carcinoma
   c. Pilomatrixoma
   d. Markel cell tumor
2. **A 37-year-old female presented with a left multiple small 0.5-cm diameter subcutaneous nodule in the left chest wall. She had polyuria and hypercalcemia and was operated for parathyroidectomy in thoracic route in the same site about 3-year-back. Figures 35.23A and B highlight the FNAC smear of the skin nodule.**
   The most likely diagnosis is:
   a. Parathyromatosis
   b. Fibroadenosis of breast
   c. Skin adnexal tumor
   d. Leprosy

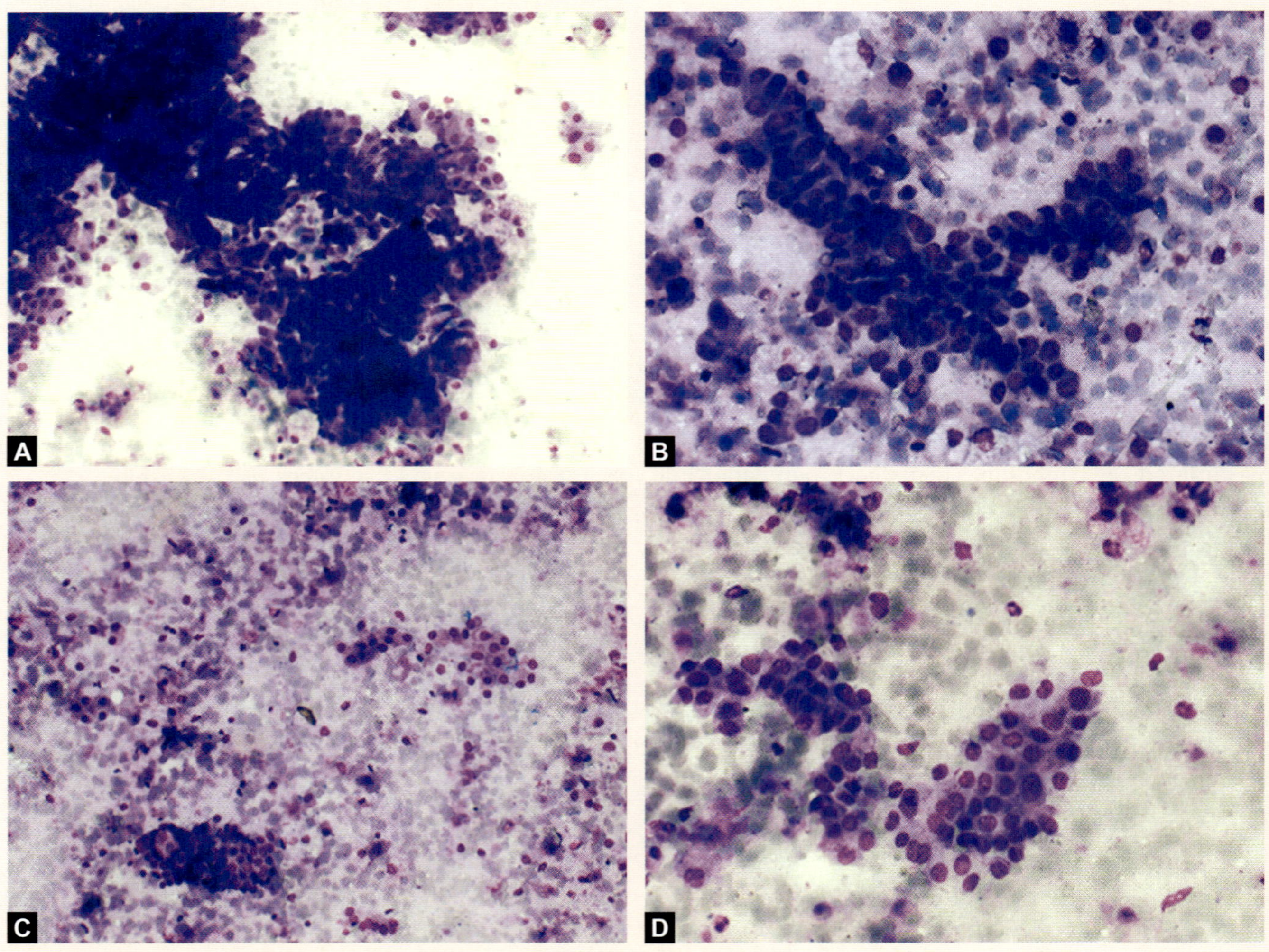

Figs. 35.22A to D: Fine needle aspiration cytology smears of the case of question 1.

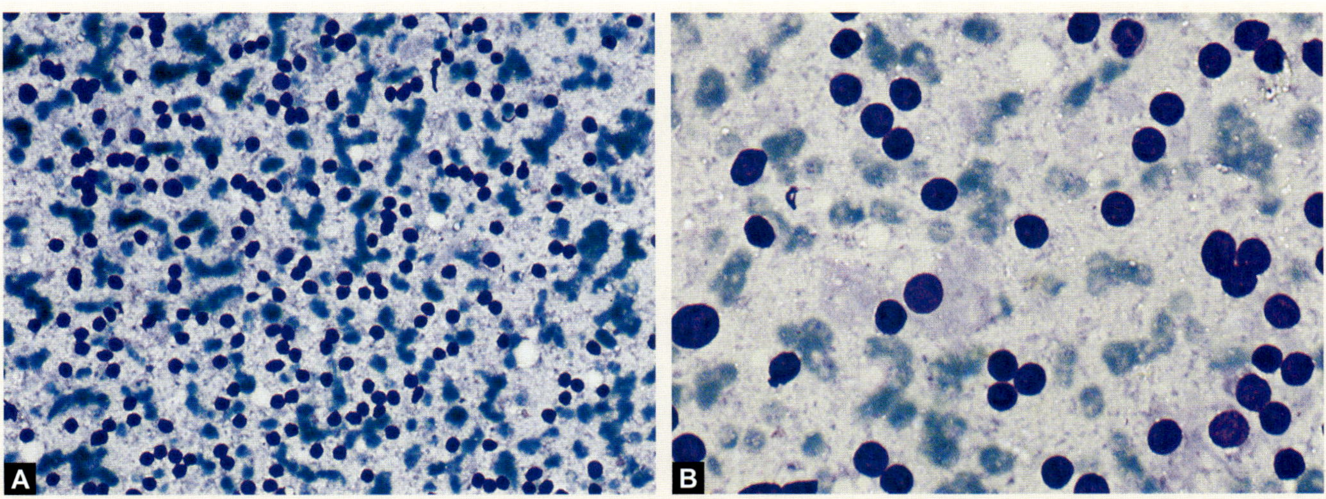

Figs. 35.23A and B: Fine needle aspiration cytology smears of the case of question 2.

Answers

1. a. Skin adnexal tumor possibly hidradenoma
   Note: The cytology smear shows many papillary structures along with discrete cell. The cells have moderate cytoplasm with round monomorphic bland nuclei. The features are that of a skin adnexal tumor consistent with hidradenoma.

2. a. Parathyromatosis
   Note: The abundant discrete cell population with monomorphic nuclei having moderate cytoplasm and indistinct cell margin indicate the possibility of parathyroid implant during the operative procedure.

CHAPTER

36 Bone

INTRODUCTION

Fine needle aspiration cytology (FNAC) is still not well popularized for the primary diagnostic technique in bone tumors and there are many concerns regarding its use.[1-5] The cytologists are not aware of the detailed morphology of many primary benign lesions of bone and at times it may be difficult to provide the exact histological type of the bone tumor. Ancillary investigations, particularly immunocytochemistry and molecular genetics, are not always possible from FNAC material. Moreover, FNAC may not yield adequate diagnostic material particularly in benign bony lesions. However, in case of malignant bone lesion the needle can easily pierce the bone and adequate material can be aspirated. The insufficiency rate of FNAC of bone lesions varies from 8% to 31%.[6-8] The adequacy of FNAC material depends on the type of the lesion and radiological appearance. Overall low yield of material is seen predominantly in cystic lesion with thick intact bone cortex, e.g. aneurysmal bone cyst (ABC) and simple bone (Box 36.1). Severely sclerotic bony lesions (osteoid osteoma and osteoblastoma) may also yield insufficient material for diagnosis. Similarly, bony lesions, which are predominantly calcified, cartilaginous or necrotic, may also yield nonrepresentative material. Careful selection of the patient for FNAC helps to reduce the insufficiency rate. The diagnostic accuracy of FNAC of bone varies from 80% to 93%.[1-5,9,10] The accuracy rate depends on the experience of the cytologist and careful correlation of radiological pictures and FNAC findings.

Box 36.1: Poor diagnostic yield of bone fine needle aspiration cytology.

- Predominant cystic lesion
- Thick intact cortex
- Densely sclerotic lesion
- Predominant cartilaginous lesion or necrotic lesion.

To increase the diagnostic accuracy of FNAC of bone, the cytologists require (1) the detailed clinical history, (2) anatomic locations of the tumor, and (3) the radiological findings.

NORMAL CELLS

Osteoblasts

Osteoblasts are round cells having abundant reddish granular cytoplasm. The nuclei are eccentric in position and give an appearance of coming out from the cell. The nuclear chromatin is fine with small nucleoli (Fig. 36.1).

Osteoclast

Osteoclasts are large cells, giant cells with abundant cytoplasm that contain about 30–50 nuclei (Fig. 36.2).

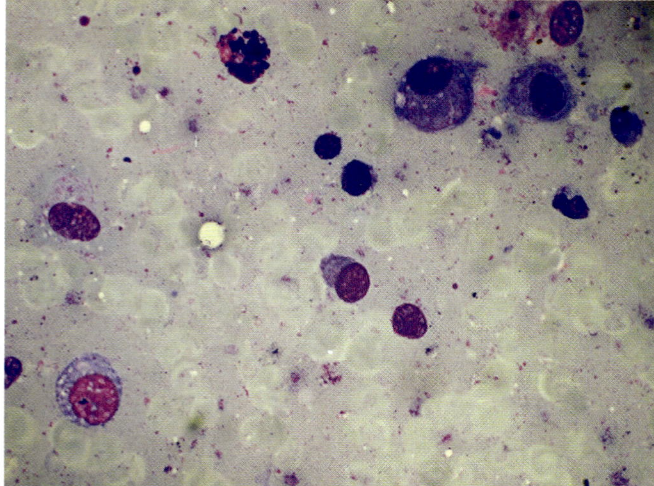

Fig. 36.1: Osteoblasts—round cell with abundant cytoplasm and peripherally placed nuclei (MGG × HP).

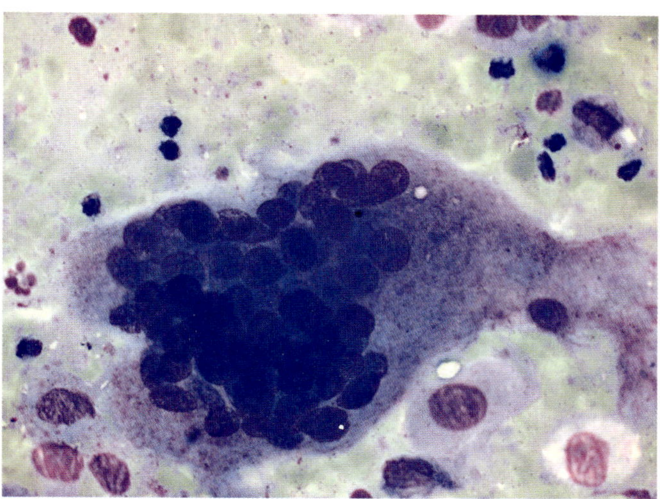

Fig. 36.2: Osteoclasts—large cell with at least 30 nuclei (MGG × HP).

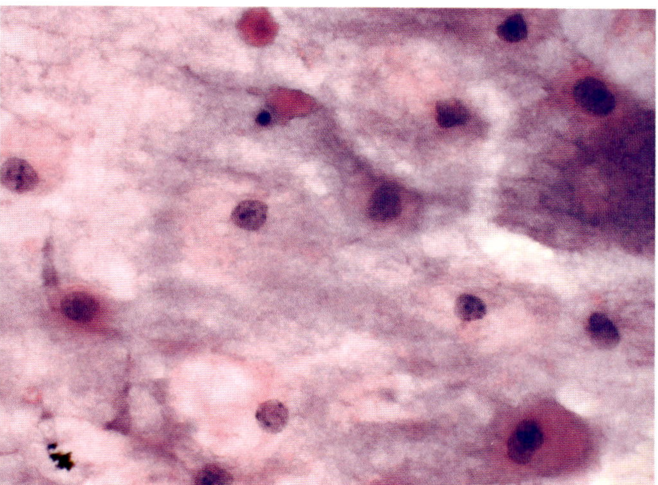

Fig. 36.3: Chondrocytes—chondroid cells in the background of chondroid material (H & E × HP).

Chondrocytes

Chondrocytes are always present in cluster and are embedded in the bright red to magenta colored chondroid material. The cells have small round pale nuclei with clear halo around the nuclei (Fig. 36.3).

World Health Organization classified bone tumors as mentioned in Box 36.2.[11]

BONE FORMING TUMOR

Osteoblastoma

This rare benign tumor represents only 1% of bone tumors. The tumor commonly affects young male and the age range varies from 10 years to 30 years. The common sites of osteoblastoma are posterior part of the spine, sacrum, femur, and proximal part of tibia. Radiography of the tumor shows well-circumscribed lytic defect surrounded by the periosteal shell.

Cytology

Fine needle aspiration cytology smears of osteoblastoma show clusters and discrete osteoblasts and osteoclastic giant cells with background pinkish osteoid material (Box 36.3). The small fascicles of monomorphic spindle cells embedded in pinkish stromal material are also present.[12,13]

Osteosarcoma[14-16]

Osteosarcoma is an aggressive malignant tumor of the bone and is commonly seen in 10–25 years of age. Osteosarcoma commonly arises from the metaphyseal area of the long

Box 36.2: World Health Organization classification of neoplasms of bone.[11]

- Neoplastic
- Osteogenic tumor
- Benign
  - Osteoid osteoma
  - Osteoblastoma
- Malignant
- Osteosarcoma
  - Conventional
  - Chondroblastic
  - Fibroblastic
  - Osteoblastic
  - Telangiectatic
  - Small cell
  - Low grade central
  - Secondary
  - Parosteal
  - Periosteal
- Cartilage forming
- Benign
  - Chondroma
  - Chondromyxoid fibroma
  - Chondroblastoma
- Malignant
- Chondrosarcoma
  - Central, primary, and secondary
  - Peripheral
  - Dedifferentiated
  - Mesenchymal
  - Clear cell
- Giant cell tumor
- Notochordal tumor: Chordoma
- Vascular tumor: Hemangioma, angiosarcoma
- Smooth muscle tumor: Leiomyoma, Leiomyosarcoma
- Fibrogenic tumor: Desmoplastic fibroma, fibrosarcoma
- Marrow tumor
  - Plasma cell tumor
  - Lymphoma
- Ewing's tumor or peripheral neuroectodermal tumor
- Miscellaneous: Aneurysmal bone cyst, Langerhans's cell histiocytosis

bone such as lower end of femur and upper end of tibia and fibula. A small percentage of osteosarcoma occurs in diaphyseal area of bone. The common sites of non-long bone involvement of osteosarcoma are jaw bones, pelvic bones, and skull.

The patients present with nonspecific pain along with bony swelling and physical examination reveals a painful tender mass. Radiological examination shows osteolytic, osteoblastic or mixed lesion that breaks the cortical bone and infiltrates into the surrounding soft tissue. The salient cytological features of osteosarcoma are mentioned in Box 36.4.

Cytology

Cytology smear of conventional osteosarcoma shows abundant cells. The cells are predominantly oval to polygonal with eccentric nuclei. The amount of cytoplasm varies from scanty to moderate in amount. The cytoplasm often shows reddish granularity and small vacuolations in May-Grünwald Giemsa (MGG) stain. The nuclei are markedly pleomorphic with coarse chromatin and inconspicuous to prominent nucleoli. Many binucleated and multinucleated tumor cells are seen. Background of the smear shows numerous mitotic activities and necrotic tissue. The smears of osteosarcoma cases show pinkish granular osteoid material. Compared to chondroid material, osteoid material is dense small aggregates. The presence of osteoid is essential for the diagnosis of osteosarcoma. In addition, the smear also shows discrete pleomorphic oval to spindle cells (Figs. 36.4 to 36.7).

Box 36.3: Osteoblastoma.

- Osteoid material
- Osteoblasts
- Osteoclasts
- Spindle cells in small fascicles.

Box 36.4: Osteosarcoma.

- Discrete and clusters of cells
- Round cells with abundant reddish granular cytoplasm resembling osteoblast
- Moderate to marked nuclear enlargement and pleomorphism with coarse chromatin
- Multinucleated tumor giant cells
- Spindle cells
- Pinkish osteoid material.

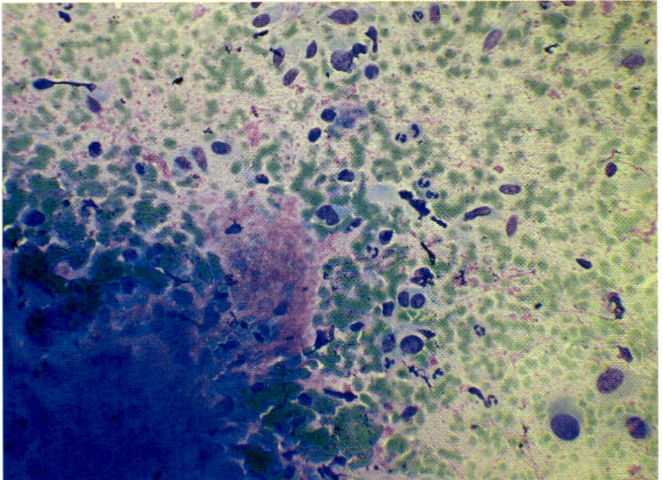

Fig. 36.4: Osteosarcoma—discrete round and spindle-shaped malignant cells along with pinkish osteoid material (MGG × HP).

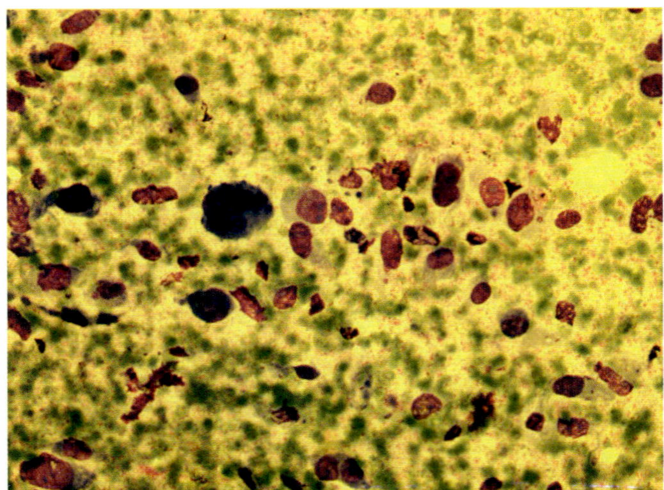

Fig. 36.5: Osteosarcoma—mononuclear, binuclear, and multinuclear malignant cells showing moderate pleomorphism (MGG × MP).

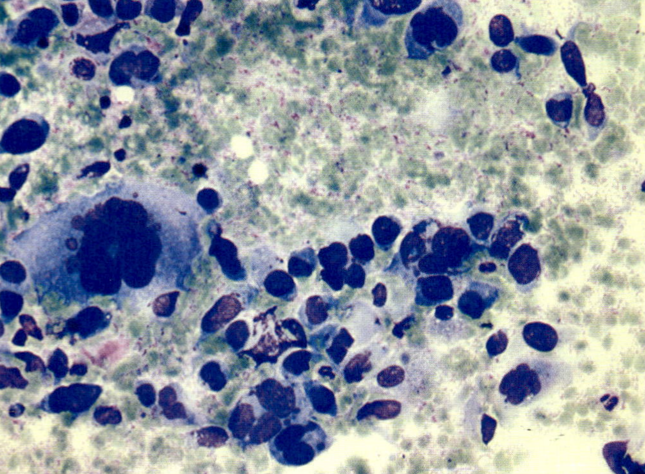

Fig. 36.6: Osteosarcoma—markedly pleomorphic bizarre cells and round pleomorphic cells in a reddish granular background (MGG × HP).

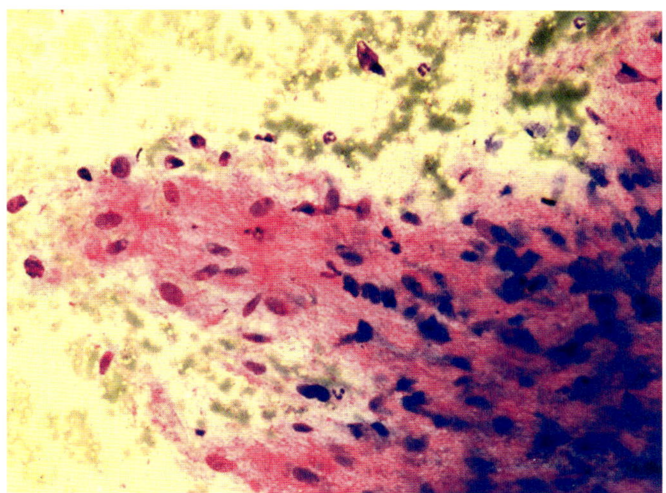

Fig. 36.7: Osteosarcoma—oval to elongated cells embedded in osteoid material (MGG × HP).

Conventional osteosarcomas are also divided into three types depending on the predominant matrix material, such as

1. *Osteoblastic*: In this type, osteoid matrix material is predominant component of the tumor stroma.
2. *Chondroblastic*: In chondroblastic osteosarcoma, there is predominant chondroid material in the FNAC smear. Hyaline type of cartilage is intimately admixed with the tumor cells.
3. *Fibroblastic osteosarcoma*: In fibroblastic variant of osteosarcoma, the osteoid material is minimal in amount and the spindle cells are the predominant population in the smear. This tumor may simulate like fibrosarcoma or malignant fibrous histiocytoma (MFH).

Small Cell Osteosarcoma

It represents only 1.5% of osteosarcomas. The smear shows small round cells with scanty cytoplasm having fine granular chromatin. The tumor cells are four times larger than lymphocytes. Small cell osteosarcoma simulates Ewing's sarcoma (EWS) of the bone.[17]

Telangiectatic Osteosarcoma

This rare subtype of osteosarcoma comprises less than 4% of all types of osteosarcoma. Telangiectatic osteosarcoma commonly arises in the distal femur and proximal tibia. The tumors are usually cystic filled with blood. FNAC yields hypocellular material. Smears show many multinucleated giant cells, atypical spindle cells, and oval mononuclear malignant cells with marked nuclear pleomorphism. In addition, the smear may also show small epithelioid-like cells.[18]

Central Low-grade Osteosarcoma

This tumor represents less than 1% of all primary bone tumors and is seen in the long bone. They are difficult to diagnose on FNAC smear because of relatively low yield of material and low nuclear grade. Radiographic picture of low-grade central osteosarcomas shows heavy mineralization and cortical bone destruction. This may simulate a fracture callus. FNAC smear shows oval-to-spindle-shaped nuclei with moderate pleomorphism along with osteoid material.

Differential Diagnosis

- *Malignant fibrous histiocytoma*: Fibroblastic type of osteosarcoma may pose diagnostic difficulty with MFH. However, the classical radiologic findings and the presence of osteoid favor osteosarcoma.
- *Ewing's sarcoma*: Small cell osteosarcoma may simulate EWS. The cells are more cohesive and nuclei show much more pleomorphism in osteosarcoma.

CARTILAGE FORMING TUMOR

Chondroma (Enchondroma)

Enchondroma is a relative common benign tumor of bone and represents about one fourth of all benign bone neoplasm. It may occur in any age group; however, it is commonly seen in 20–30 years of age. The common sites of enchondroma are short tubular bones of hand and foot. Long tubular bones like humerus and femur are also involved. The patients of enchondroma of long tubular bone are usually asymptomatic. Enchondroma of short tubular bone presents as swelling and pain. X-ray of enchondroma shows well-circumscribed radiolucent or heavily mineralized bony swelling.

Cytology

Fine needle aspiration cytology smears of enchondroma show predominantly very thick hyaline cartilage with background metachromatic material (Box 36.5). The individual cells are embedded in the cartilaginous material (Fig. 36.8). The nuclei are round with inconspicuous nucleoli. The cells do not show any binucleation. Mitotic activities are absent. Cytology smear of enchondroma and low-grade chondrosarcoma is difficult to differentiate.

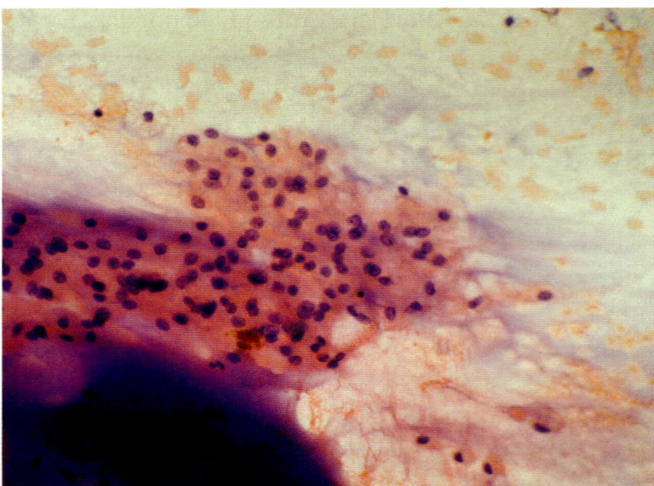

Fig. 36.8: Enchondroma—benign chondrocytes in the background of thick cartilaginous material (H & E × HP).

Box 36.5: Enchondroma.

- Hyaline cartilage
- Metachromatic material
- Round cells
- Single round bland nuclei.

Chondroblastoma

This is a benign cartilaginous neoplasm of bone and comprises less than 1% of all bone tumors. The age of the patient varies from 10 years to 25 years. The lesion typically occurs in the epiphyseal and epimetaphyseal regions of long bones particularly femur, tibia, and humerus. The patient complains of localized pain, swelling, and restricted joint movement (in case the lesion occurs near the joint). X-ray of the chondroblastoma shows a sharply demarcated lytic lesion with a sclerotic outer rim.

Cytology

The FNAC of chondroblastoma shows many chondroblasts, giant cells, and cartilaginous material (Box 36.6). The primitive chondroblasts are present as poorly cohesive or discrete round-shaped cells. The margin of the cell is well defined. The cytoplasm of the cell is dense with monomorphic round nuclei. The nuclear chromatin is fine. Nuclei of the cells show deep longitudinal groove. Occasional cells may show intranuclear inclusion. The smear shows abundant multinucleated osteoclastic giant cells.

These osteoclastic giant cells usually contain 5–20 nuclei. Occasionally large number of nuclei as many as 60 nuclei can be seen. Unlike round nuclei of the mononuclear cells, these nuclei are ovoid in appearance. The smears also show amorphous or fibrillar matrix material. This appears as purplish color in MGG smear.[19,20]

Box 36.6: Chondroblastoma.

- Chondroblasts: Polygonal to spindle cells
- Oval nuclei
- Fine chromatin
- Longitudinal nuclear groove
- Many osteoclastic giant cells
- Chondroid material.

Box 36.7: Chondrosarcoma.

- Chondroid or myxoid material
- Isolated cells
- Large cell with well-defined border
- Pale foamy cytoplasm
- Enlarged pleomorphic and hyperchromatic nuclei
- Binucleated cells.

Chondrosarcoma[21-25]

Chondrosarcoma (CHS) is a malignant cartilaginous tumor and represents 20% of all malignant bone tumors. The primary CHS commonly occurs in adults above 50 years of age. The most common sites of primary CHS are flat bones of the pelvis, proximal femur, proximal humerus, distal femur, and ribs. The patient usually presents with longstanding pain and swelling. Radiological examination of CHS shows expansile radiolucent lesion with cortical thickening. The lesion often shows cortical erosion or destruction.

Cytology

Depending on nuclear size, nuclear hyperchromasia, and cellularity the tumors are graded as grade I, grade II, and grade III. The cytological grade is well correlated with histological grade. FNAC of CHS yields gelatinous or myxoid material (Box 36.7). The smears show reddish purple cartilaginous material in MGG stain. Depending on grade of CHS the amount of the cartilaginous material varies. Low-grade CHS shows abundant cartilaginous material compared to high-grade CHS. Similarly the cellularity also increases from low-grade to high-grade CHS. Tumor cells lie predominantly singly in chondroid or myxoid material. The tumor cells are large with well-delineated cytoplasmic border. The cytoplasm is pale and vacuolated. Nuclei of the cells are central in position and round in shape. Nuclear enlargement, pleomorphism, and hyperchromasia increase with

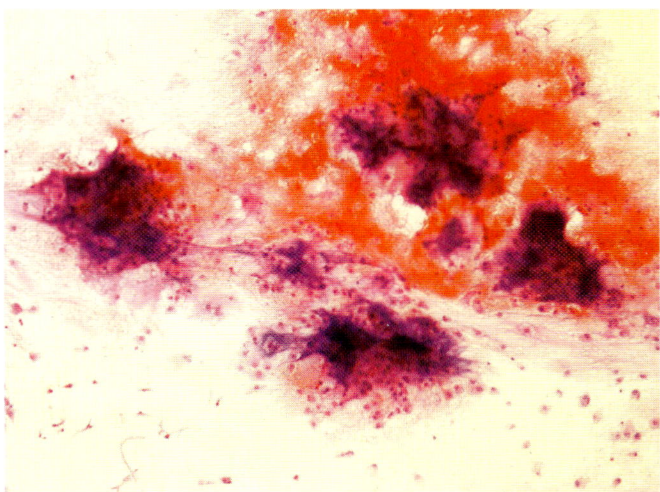

Fig. 36.9: Chondrosarcoma—abundant chondrocytes embedded in cartilaginous material (H & E × LP).

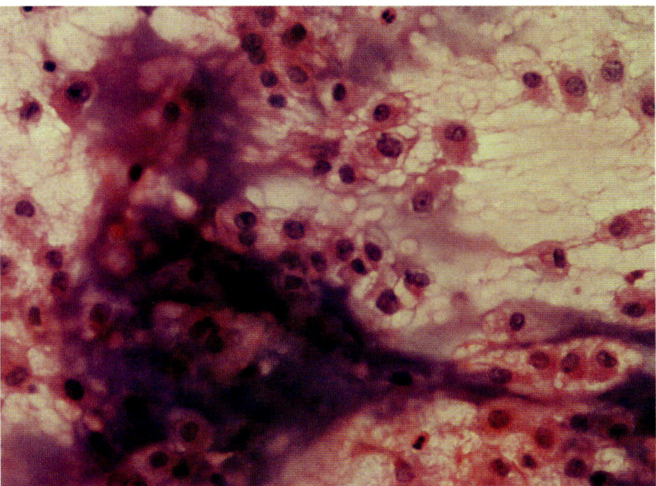

Fig. 36.10: Chondrosarcoma—chondrocytes with moderate cytoplasm and monomorphic looking nuclei. Many binucleated chondrocytes are present (H & E × MP).

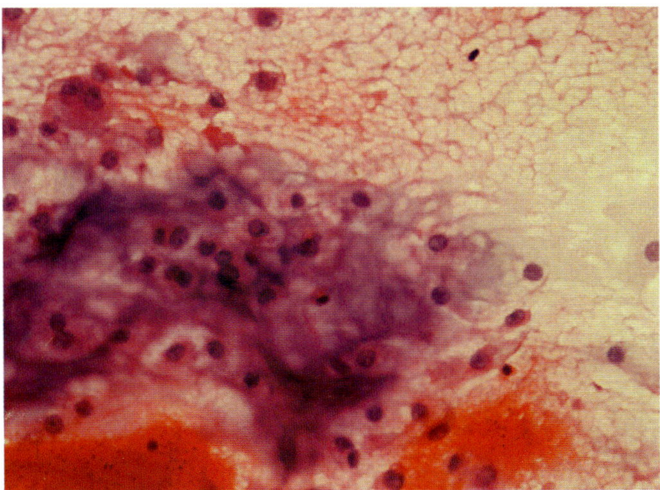

Fig. 36.11: Chondrosarcoma—higher magnification showing binucleated chondrocytes (H & E × HP).

increasing grade. The tumor cells frequently show binucleation. Mitosis is usually absent. However, necrosis is frequently present in high-grade CHS. Abundant myxoid change is more frequently seen in high-grade CHS. Fragments of thicker hyaline cartilage are seen in grade II CHS (Figs. 36.9 to 36.11).

There are various other types of chondrosarcomas such as mesenchymal CHS, clear cell variety, and dedifferentiated CHS.

Mesenchymal Chondrosarcoma

It is a rare malignant cartilaginous tumor and represents about 3% of all primary CHS. The tumor affects all age groups; however, this is more frequent in second and third decades of life. The common sites of involvement are jaw bones, ribs, pelvic bones, and vertebra. The patient usually complains of pain and swelling. Radiological examination of the tumor usually shows an osteolytic lesion with destruction of cortical bone and invasion in the neighboring soft tissue.

Box 36.8: Mesenchymal chondrosarcoma.

- Cartilaginous material
- Osteoclast like giant cells
- Small round blue cells
- High nuclear-cytoplasmic (N/C) ratio.

Cytology: The tumor is biphasic in pattern on histology with admixture of small round undifferentiated cells and hyaline cartilage. The FNAC smears are usually rich in small round cells with scanty cytoplasm. The nuclei are round with coarse chromatin having high nuclear-cytoplasmic (N/C) ratio. In addition, the smear also shows many osteoclast-like giant cells and cartilaginous material (Box 36.8). Background of the smear may show necrosis and hemorrhage.

Clear Cell Chondrosarcoma

This rare variety of tumor represents only 2% of all CHS. Clear cell CHS may occur in any age group. It commonly affects skull, spine, hands, and feet. FNAC of this tumor shows discrete large cells with clear cytoplasm and centrally placed nuclei (Box 36.9). Many multinucleated giant cells are seen. In addition, cartilaginous material is also seen.

Dedifferentiated Chondrosarcoma

This is a type of CHS that contains two types of component: (1) well-differentiated CHS and (2) high-grade noncartilaginous sarcoma. The tumor represents about 10% of all CHS. The tumor commonly affects in fifth and sixth decades of life. The common sites of dedifferentiated CHS are pelvis, femur, and humerus. Cytology smear shows chondrocytes admixed with cartilaginous material along with the cells of poorly differentiated sarcoma.

Diagnostic Difficulties

Enchondroma: Radiographic picture of cortical disruption along with high cellularity and binucleated cells in CHS help to differentiate it from enchondroma.

Giant Cell Tumor of Bone[26-28]

Giant cell tumor of bone (GCT) is a benign but locally aggressive tumor that represents 5% of all bone tumors. This is usually seen over the age of 18 years with the maximum incidence between 25 years and 45 years. GCT predominantly involves the distal femur, proximal tibia, distal radius, and proximal humerus. Radiologically the tumor represents the expanding epiphyseal osteolytic lesion. Occasionally the tumor produces a trabeculated "soap-bubble" appearance.

Box 36.9: Clear cell chondrosarcoma.

- Large cells
- Clear cytoplasm
- Central nuclei
- Multinucleated giant cells.

Box 36.10: Giant cell tumor of bone.

- Abundant multinucleated osteoclastic giant cells
- Mononuclear ovoid to spindle cells
- Giant cells are intimately attached with spindle cell clusters.

Cytology

Cytology smear shows cluster and discrete abundant multinucleated osteoclastic type of giant cells and mononuclear oval-to-spindle cells (Box 36.10). The overall arrangement of cluster and sheets of cells gives a checkerboard-like appearance. The osteoclastic giant cells are relatively large with abundant cytoplasm containing 50–100 nuclei. These cells are intimately mixed with the stromal cells. The stromal cells have moderate cytoplasm and oval-to-spindle-shaped nuclei with fine granular chromatin and distinct nucleoli. The nuclear margin is smooth. The mononuclear cells often show syncytial appearance when they are present in clusters. The nuclear character of the giant cells and that of the stromal cells are similar. It is now proved beyond doubt that the stromal cells are the neoplastic component of GCT. These cells often show increased mitotic activity; however, atypical tripolar mitosis is rarely seen and indicates the presence of sarcoma with giant cell reaction (Figs. 36.12 to 36.14).

Differential Diagnosis

Other bone lesions rich in osteoclastic giant cells: GCT of bone should be differentiated from the other bony lesions

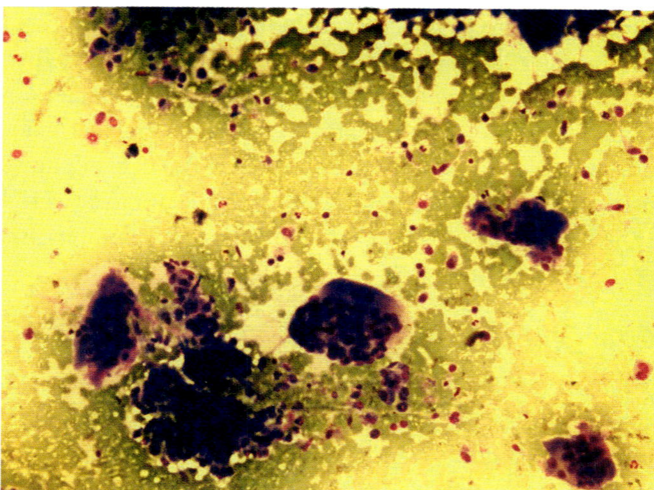

Fig. 36.12: Giant cell tumor of bone—multiple osteoclast-like giant cells along with oval to spindle-shaped stroma (MGG × MP).

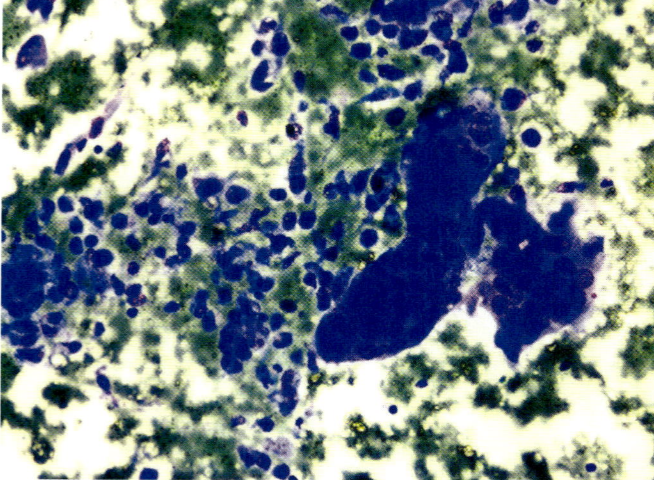

Fig. 36.13: Giant cell tumor of bone—clusters of osteoclastic giant cells along with stromal cells (MGG × MP).

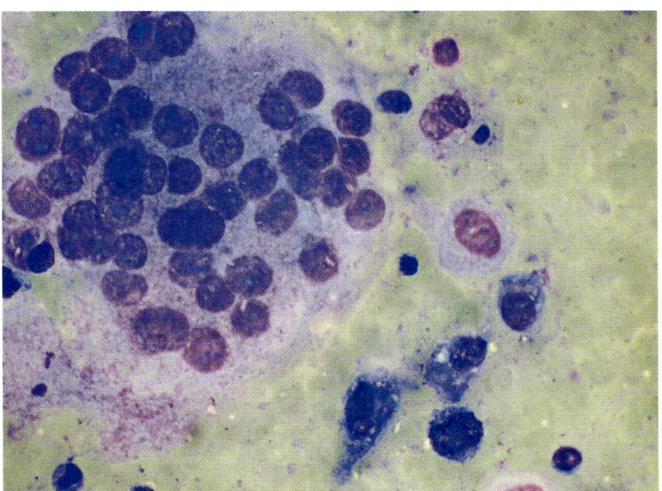

Fig. 36.14: Giant cell tumor of bone—higher magnification showing better morphology of the giant cells and stromal cells (MGG × HP).

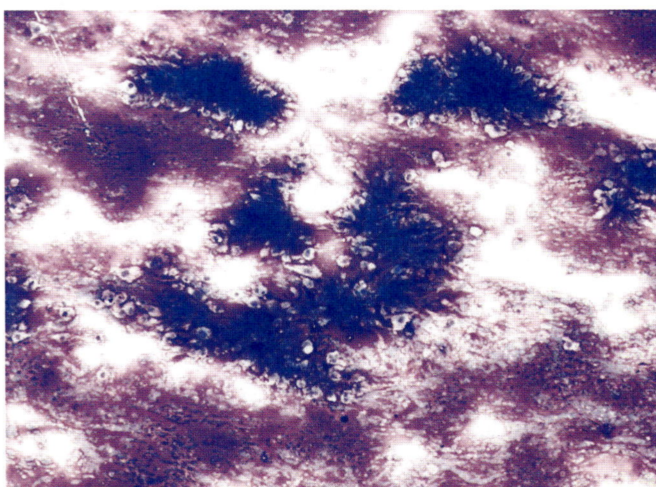

Fig. 36.15: Chordoma—multiple clusters of vacuolated cells in abundant pinkish material (MGG × MP).

Box 36.11: Chordoma.

- Abundant myxoid material
- *Physaliphorous cells*: Abundant bubbly vacuolated cytoplasm and central round nuclei
- Relatively smaller mononuclear cells with moderate amount of cytoplasm and round nuclei
- S-100 positive and negative for cytokeratin (CK).

rich in osteoclastic giant cells that include osteosarcoma, chondroblastoma, ABC, and brown tumor of hyperparathyroidism. Pleomorphic and hyperchromatic nuclei of the osteosarcoma help in differentiating it from GCT. The stromal cells of chondroblastoma are round to oval with longitudinal deep nuclear groove. ABC and brown cyst show many hemosiderin-laden macrophages.

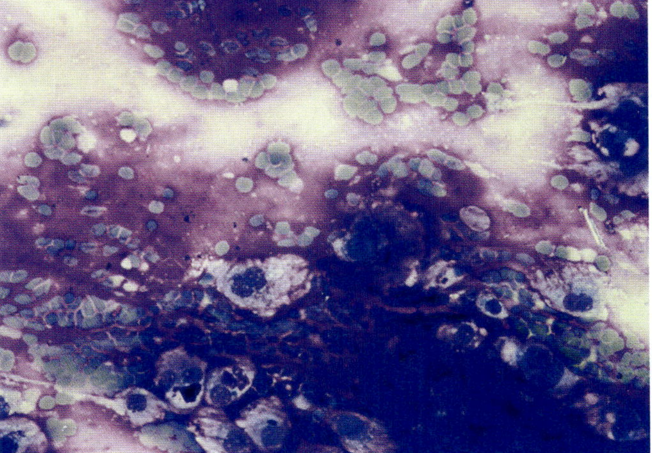

Fig. 36.16: Chordoma—physaliphorous cells showing clear multi-vacuolated cytoplasm and centrally placed nuclei (MGG × HP).

Chordoma[29-31]

Chordoma is a low-to-intermediate grade malignant tumor that develops from the remnants of notochordal rest and occurs in both ends of the neural axis. It represents 2–4% of all malignant bone tumors. Chordoma is commonly seen in middle-aged to elderly patients and rarely occurs before 30 years of age. The most common location of the tumor is sacral and spheno-occipital region.

Cytology

The FNAC of chordoma yields myxoid or mucoid material. The smear gives a reddish purple color appearance on MGG stain (Box 36.11). The bimorphic population of cell is embedded in the matrix material. There are two types of cells: large cells and relatively small mononuclear granular cells. The larger cells have abundant vacuolated bubbly cytoplasm which gives a basket-like appearance. These cells are also known as *physaliphorous* cells and are characteristic cell of chordoma. The nuclei of the cells are small round monomorphic with granular chromatin having prominent nucleoli. The most of the cells are mononuclear; however, binucleated and multinucleated cells are also seen. Mitotic activities are absent (Figs. 36.15 to 36.17).

The other cells are relatively small with moderate amount of granular cytoplasm. The nuclei are round and monomorphic with prominent nucleoli. Intranuclear cytoplasmic inclusions may also be noted.

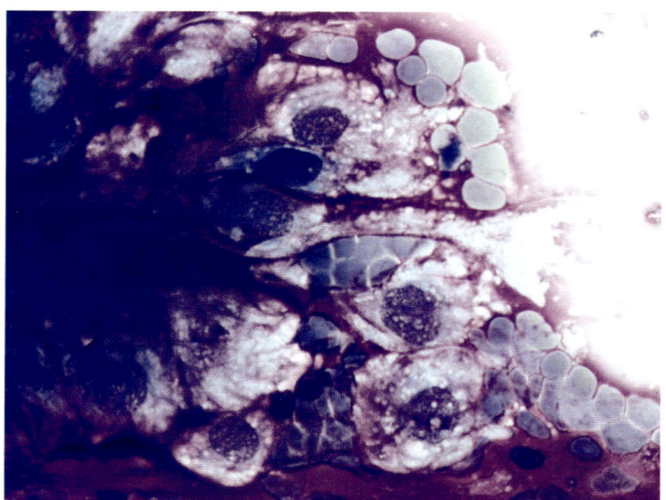

Fig. 36.17: Chordoma—higher magnification showing better morphology of the physaliphorous cells. Note the typical bubbly vacuolated cytoplasm (MGG × OI).

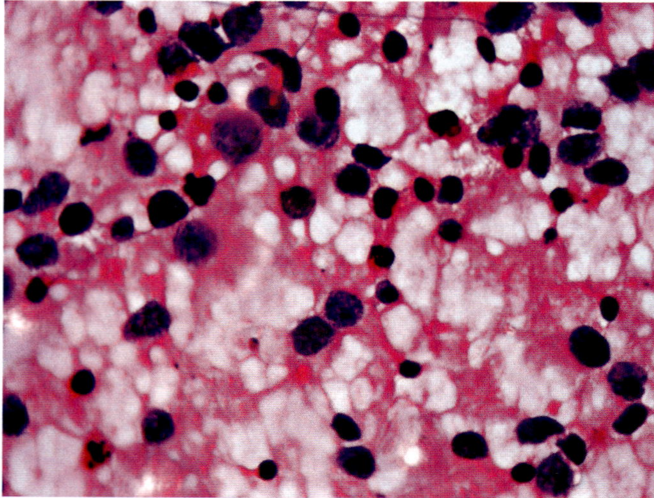

Fig. 36.18: Ewing's sarcoma—discrete small round cells with scanty cytoplasm. Nuclei are monomorphic with granular chromatin having inconspicuous nucleoli (H & E × HP).

Box 36.12: Ewing's sarcoma.

- Discrete small round cells
- *Bimodal cells*: Light and dark cells
- Dark cells show scanty deep blue cytoplasm
- Light cells show moderate vacuolated cytoplasm
- Round monomorphic nuclei
- Fine granular chromatin
- Inconspicuous to absent nucleoli
- Rosette-like structures may be seen
- CD99 (MIC2) positive. Variable positivity of vimentin, neuron-specific enolase (NSE), and cytokeratin (CK)
- t(11;22) (q24;q12) chromosomal translocation.

Immunostain

Chordomas are positive for S-100 protein, cytokeratin (CK), and epithelial membrane antigen (EMA) whereas, CHS cells are S-100 positive and negative for CK.

Differential Diagnosis

- *Chondrosarcoma*: The classical physaliphorous cells are never present in CHS. The background myxoid material encircling the individual cells is also a characteristic of chordoma.
- *Metastatic adenocarcinoma*: Renal cell carcinoma may show clear vacuolated cell and simulate chordoma. However, the nuclei of these cells are usually enlarged and pleomorphic and the smears show lack of the typical myxoid background. Adenocarcinoma cells are negative for S-100 and positive for CK.

Ewing's Sarcoma[32-34]

Ewing's sarcoma is a malignant round cell tumor with neuroectodermal differentiation and represents about 5% of all primary malignant bone tumors. It commonly occurs in the age group of 5–25 years. EWS typically shows specific t(11;22) (q24;q12) chromosomal translocation. It commonly arises from the diaphysis or metaphyseal-diaphyseal part of the long bone particularly from femur and tibia. Radiographically the tumor shows an osteolytic lesion and long bone shows onion skin like periosteal reaction. The tumor often involves the soft tissue and presents as a soft tissue mass.

Cytology

The FNAC smear of EWS shows bimodal population of light-colored and dark-colored small round cells (Box 36.12). The tumor cells are discrete round cells with scanty deep blue cytoplasm. Cytoplasmic vacuolations are often seen due to the presence of glycogen. Nuclei are round with high N/C ratio and inconspicuous nucleoli. Nuclear molding may also be seen. However, typical crushing artifact is absent. Occasional pseudorosette-like structures may be seen. The smears may also show necrosis and perivascular arrangement of cells (Figs. 36.18 and 36.19).

Immunocytochemistry

Positive for CD99 (MIC-2), vimentin, and neuron-specific enolase (NSE).

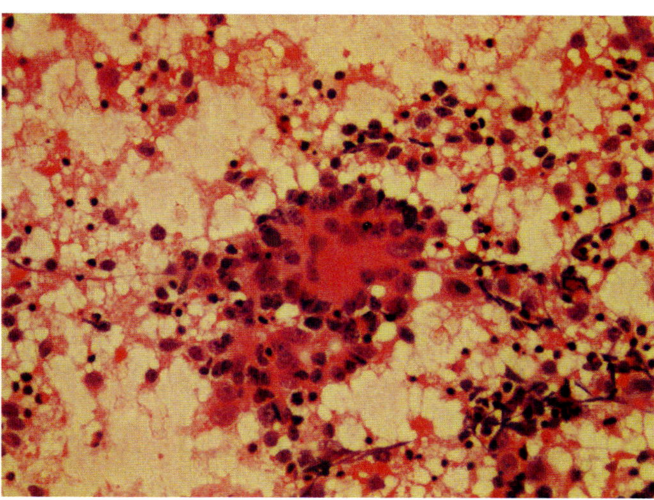

Fig. 36.19: Ewing's sarcoma—Rosette-like structure (H & E × HP).

Box 36.13: Non-Hodgkin lymphoma of bone

- Predominantly diffuse large B-cell (DLBC)
- Occasionally follicular center cell lymphoma and anaplastic large cell lymphoma
- Seven percent of all bone malignancies
- Flow cytometric immunophenotyping is needed.

Diagnostic Difficulties

Other small round cell tumor: Osteosarcoma of small cell type and non-Hodgkin lymphoma (NHL) are the differential diagnoses of EWS of the bone.

Non-Hodgkin Lymphoma

Non-Hodgkin lymphoma may involve the bone secondarily. NHL of bone represents 7% of all bone malignancies. The primary NHL of bone is rare. Lymphoma commonly affects femur followed by spine and pelvic bones. The patient commonly complains of pain or swelling of the bone. More than 90% of primary lymphoma of bone in adult is diffuse large B-cell lymphoma (DLBCL) (Box 36.13). Rarely follicular center cell lymphoma and anaplastic large cell lymphoma may occur. The patients of primary bone lymphoma present with bone pain. The patients may have (1) single site of involvement of lymphoma with or without lymph node involvement, (2) multiple skeletal sites of involvement with or without any visceral involvement, and (3) prior history of lymphoma with bone involvement in biopsy sample. The cytomorphology of NHL of bone is same as that of other body sites. Flow cytometry (FCM) may be needed for exact diagnosis and classification of NHL of bone.

Box 36.14: Plasma cell myeloma.

- Well differentiated
  - Round cells
  - Abundant cytoplasm
  - Eccentric nucleus
  - Cartwheel chromatin (peripheral clumped chromatin)
  - Perinuclear halo
- Poorly differentiated
  - Plasmablasts
  - Round cells
  - Scanty cytoplasm
  - Fine chromatin
  - Prominent nucleoli.

Plasma Cell Neoplasm[35-37]

Plasma cell myeloma (PCM) is the neoplasm of plasma cells. It is also known as multiple myeloma. This is the most common bone tumor. The tumor usually occurs in the sixth decade. PCM commonly affects vertebrae, ribs, skull, pelvis, and femur. The patient usually complains of pain and pathological fracture of bone along with symptoms of hypercalcemia and anemia. Radiographic examination of the bony lesion shows a sharply demarcated lytic area surrounded by sclerosis.

Plasma cell neoplasm may be solitary presenting as plasmacytoma or disseminated plasma cell proliferation such as multiple myeloma.

The criteria of multiple myeloma are presently changed by international myeloma groups and more emphasis has been given on the plasma cell count in the aspirate.[38]

Cytology

The FNAC smear of PCM shows abundant discrete round to oval cells of plasma cell lineage with variable cellular maturity (Box 36.14). The well-differentiated plasma cell tumors show normal looking plasma cells. The individual cells are round with moderate to abundant dense eosinophilic cytoplasm in hemotoxylin and eosin (H & E) staining. The nuclei are eccentric and show peripheral clumped chromatin giving rise to cartwheel appearance. In MGG stained smears, the cytoplasm is basophilic with a perinuclear clear halo. This is due to rough endoplasmic reticulum and prominent Golgi center. Binucleated and occasionally multinucleated plasma cells are also seen (Figs. 36.20 and 36.21).

Poorly differentiated plasma cell tumor has poor prognosis. FNAC smear shows many plasmablasts. These cells have scanty amount of cytoplasm, high N/C ratio, opened up chromatin, and prominent nucleoli. Binucleated and

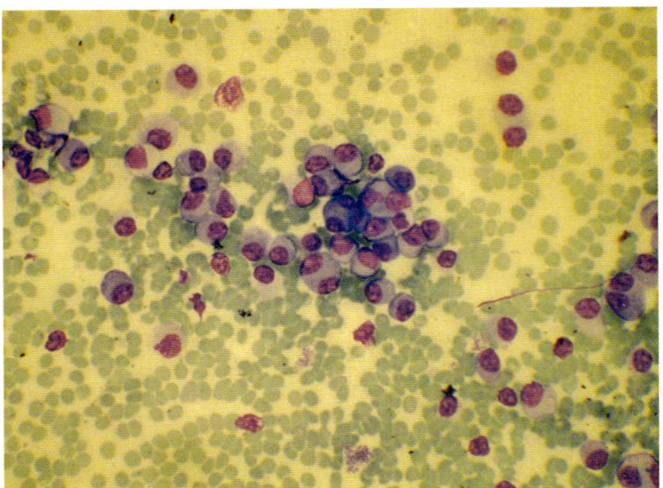

Fig. 36.20: Plasmacytoma in bone—clusters of plasma cells. Many cells are binucleated (MGG × MP).

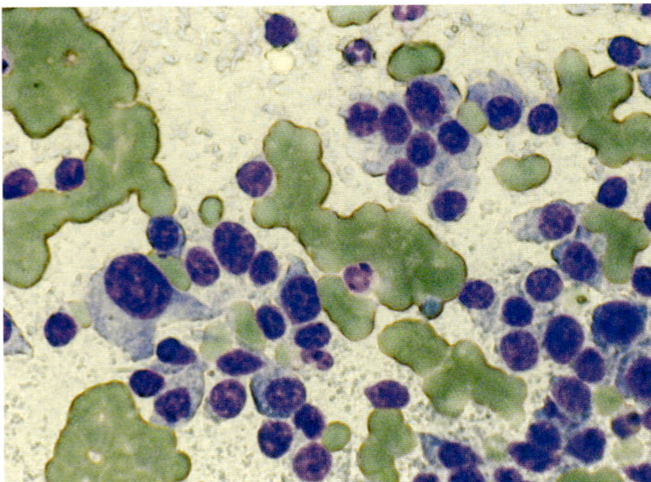

Fig. 36.21: Plasmacytoma in bone—abundant discrete plasma cells (MGG × HP).

Box 36.15: Langerhans cell histiocytosis.

- Large cells with abundant cytoplasm
- Round nuclei with longitudinal grooves
- Many binucleated and multinucleated cells
- Eosinophils
- Lymphocytes, polymorphs, and macrophages.

Immunocytochemistry: CD1a positive
Electron microscopy: Birbecks granules.

multinucleated cells are more frequent. In addition many atypical mitotic figures are also noted. A careful search always reveals typical plasma cells.

Diagnostic Difficulties

Reactive plasma cells: It is always necessary to differentiate reactive plasmacytosis from PCM. Reactive plasmacytosis may occur secondary to chronic infection, metastatic tumor in bone or due to reaction to primary bone tumor. Strict major and minor criteria of diagnosis are helpful in this occasion.

Langerhans Cell Histiocytosis[39,40]

Langerhans cell histiocytosis (LCH) is the neoplasm of Langerhans cells and represents 1% of all bone tumors. LCH commonly occurs in young patients under 10 years of age. However, it may occur in patients of any age group. LCH commonly involves the skull, pelvis, and femur. The patient usually complains of pain and swelling; however, the symptoms largely depend on the sites of involvement of bone.

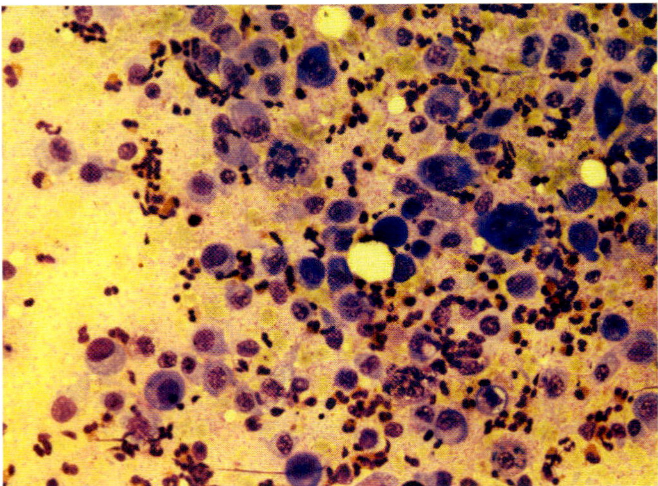

Fig. 36.22: Langerhans cell histiocytosis—many mononuclear and multinuclear histiocytes with deep nuclear groove along with abundant eosinophils (MGG × MP).

Cytology

Aspirates show discrete population of large Langerhans cells with abundant cytoplasm and distinct cell border (Box 36.15). The nuclei are large, round shaped with indented margin and characteristic longitudinal nuclear groove. Nuclear chromatin is dispersed or condensed with occasional prominent nucleoli. Background of the smear shows eosinophils, lymphocytes, polymorphs, and macrophages. In addition, large osteoclastic giant cells and histiocytes with phagocytosed materials are also noted (Fig. 36.22).

Immunocytochemistry

The cells of LCH are negative for CD45. They characteristically express CD1a and S-100 protein.

Differential Diagnosis

Fungal infections: Large number of eosinophils and histiocytes may mislead the diagnosis of fungal infection. However, the presence of Langerhans cell with deep longitudinal grooves, absence of fungal structure, and clinical features are the indicators of LCH.

Metastatic Carcinoma

Metastatic carcinomas are the most common malignant tumors of the bone. Majority of the patients are between 40 years and 60 years of age. The common sites of origin of malignancies are breast, lung, prostate, kidney, and thyroid. The metastasis commonly affects axial skeleton such as vertebra, ribs, sternum, pelvis, and skull bones. In most of the cases, the clinical history or thorough radiographic examination helps to identify the primary site of origin of carcinoma. Occasionally, solitary bone lesion from an unknown primary site may mimic as primary bone tumor.

Cytology

Cytomorphology of the individual cells depend on the type of primary malignancy. The metastatic tumor often simulates the morphology of the primary malignancies and these foreign cells are easily recognizable. Gland-like arrangement is seen in case of adenocarcinoma. Multiple follicular arrangements of cells are noted in metastatic follicular carcinoma of thyroid. Squamous cell carcinoma shows polyhedral squamoid cells with orangeophilia. Fiber and tadpole cells are also noted. Renal cell carcinoma shows large cells with clear cytoplasm and centrally placed enlarged nuclei. Metastatic spindle cell type of renal cell carcinoma may mimic sarcoma of the bone. Panel of immunocytochemistry may be helpful in difficult situation (Figs. 36.23 and 36.24).

Aneurysmal Bone Cyst

Aneurysmal bone cyst is a benign cystic lesion of bone. It commonly occurs in the second decade of life. ABC may be seen as a primary bone lesion or secondary to other benign or malignant tumors such as GCT, chondroblastoma, fibrous dysplasia, osteoblastoma, eosinophilic granulomas, and osteosarcomas.[41,42]

Aneurysmal bone cyst may occur in any bone; however, it commonly involves the metaphysis of long bones such as femur, tibia, and humerus, and the posterior part of vertebral bodies.

Cytology

The FNAC of ABC yields predominantly blood. The smears show many hemosiderin-laden histiocytes, fragments of fibroconnective tissue, and multiple osteoclastic

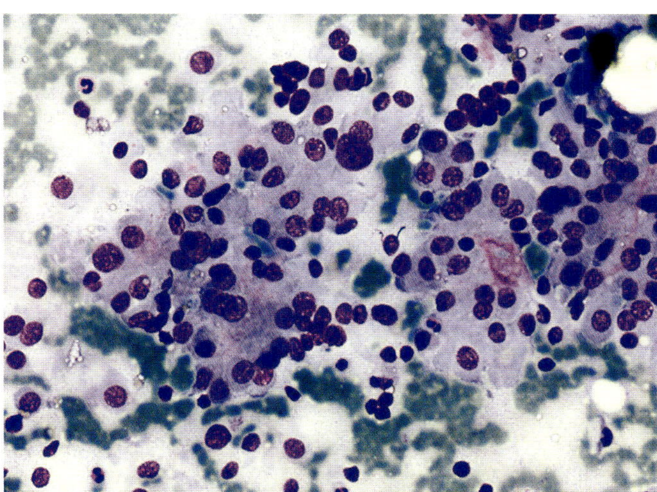

Fig. 36.23: Metastatic carcinoma—tight cluster of malignant cells in a metastatic renal cell carcinoma in bone (H & E × MP).

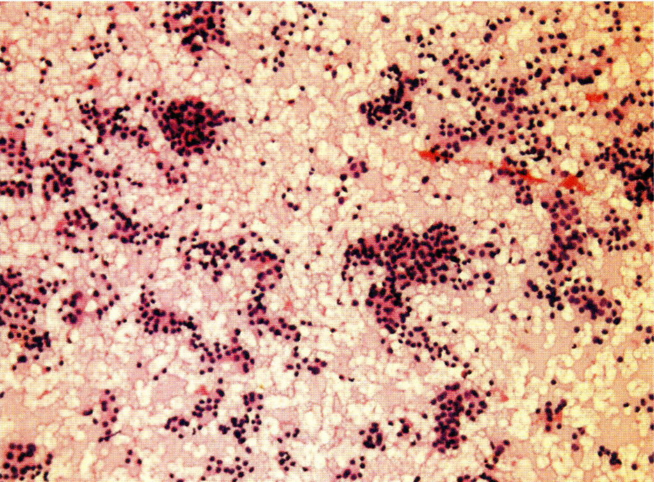

Fig. 36.24: Metastatic follicular cell carcinoma—discrete and follicular arrangement of cells in metastatic follicular carcinoma of thyroid (H & E × LP).

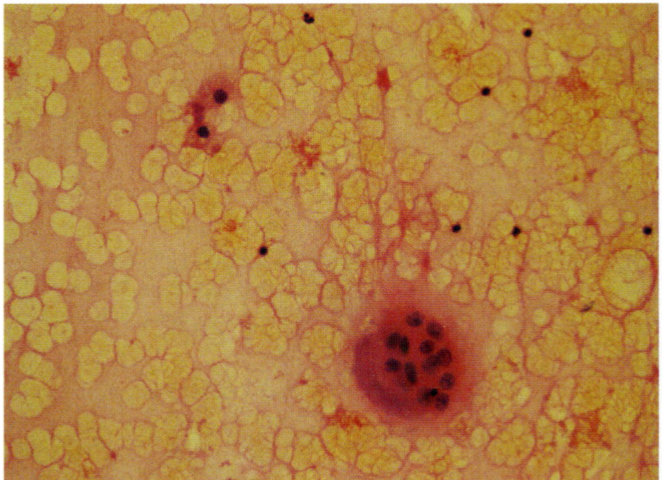

Fig. 36.25: Aneurysmal bone cyst—multinucleated giant cells and foamy histiocytes (MGG × MP).

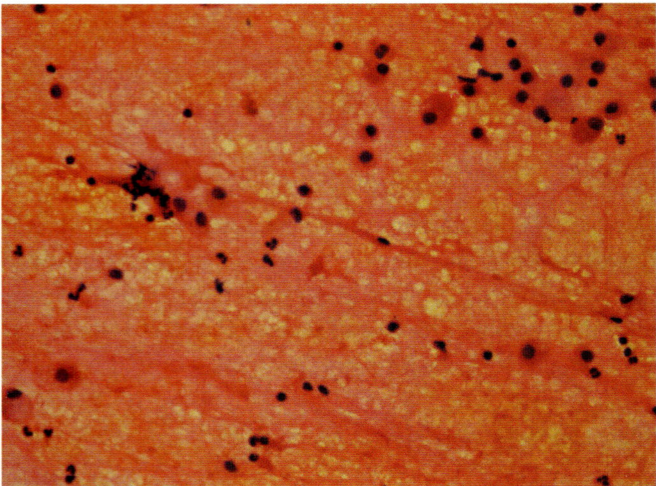

Fig. 36.26: Aneurysmal bone cyst—many foamy histiocytes are seen in the background (MGG × MP).

Box 36.16: Aneurysmal bone cyst.

- Bloody smear
- Pigment-laden histiocytes
- Osteoclastic giant cells.

giant cells (Box 36.16). Frequent mitosis may be present. Necrosis is usually absent; however, it may be seen in case of pathological fracture of bone (Figs. 36.25 and 36.26).

Adamantinoma

Adamantinoma is a rare low-grade biphasic malignant tumor of bone that represents less than 0.5 primary bone tumors. It usually occurs in young patient of 25–30 years of age. More than 90% adamantinoma occurs in the shaft of tibia. Radiograph shows a well-circumscribed, cortical, osteolytic lesion with sclerosis in the circumference.

Cytology

The FNAC of adamantinoma shows multiple clusters of malignant epithelial cells, fibroblastic stromal cells, and squamous-like cells (Box 36.17). The tumor cells are arranged in clusters with peripheral palisading arrangement. The individual cells are round to oval with monomorphic nuclei and bland chromatin.

Box 36.17: Adamantinoma.

- Malignant epithelial cells
- Palisading arrangement of cells
- Cells with high nuclear-cytoplasmic (N/C) ratio
- Monomorphic nuclei
- Squamoid cells in nest
- Scattered fibroblasts.

Differential Diagnosis

Metastatic carcinoma: Malignant epithelial cells may be mistaken as metastatic carcinoma. However, the young age, typical location of the tumor in tibial shaft, and relatively monomorphic nuclei help in the diagnosis of adamantinoma.

REFERENCES

1. Mehrotra R, Singh M, Singh PA, et al. Should fine needle aspiration biopsy be the first pathological investigation in the diagnosis of a bone lesion? An algorithmic approach with review of literature. Cytojournal. 2007;4:9.
2. Handa U, Bal A, Mohan H, et al. Fine needle aspiration cytology in the diagnosis of bone lesions. Cytopathology. 2005;16(2):59-64.
3. Yamamoto T, Nagira K, Marui T, et al. Fine needle aspiration biopsy in the initial diagnosis of bone lesions. Anticancer Res. 2003;23(1B):793-7.
4. Wedin R, Bauer HC, Skoog L, et al. Cytological diagnosis of skeletal lesions. Fine needle aspiration biopsy in 110 tumours. J Bone Joint Surg Br. 2000;82(5):673-8.
5. Bommer KK, Ramzy I, Mody D. Fine needle aspiration biopsy in the diagnosis and management of bone lesions: a study of 450 cases. Cancer. 1997;81(3):148-56.
6. Kilpatrick SE, Cappellari JO, Bos GD, et al. Is fine needle aspiration biopsy a practical alternative to open biopsy for the primary diagnosis of sarcoma? Experience with 140 patients. Am J Clin Pathol. 2001;115(1):59-68.

7. Jorda M, Rey L, Hanly A, et al. Fine needle aspiration cytology of bone: Accuracy and pitfalls of cytodiagnosis. Cancer. 2000;90(1):47-54.
8. Ruhs SA, el-Khoury GY, Chrischilles EA. A cost minimization approach to the diagnosis of skeletal neoplasms. Skeletal Radiol. 1996;25(5):449-54.
9. Layfield LJ. Cytologic diagnosis of osseous lesions: a review with emphasis on the diagnosis of primary neoplasms of bone. Diagn Cytopathol. 2009;37(4): 299-310.
10. Soderlund V. Combined radiology and cytology in the diagnosis of bone lesions–A review of 399 cases. Acta Orthop Scand Suppl. 2004;75(311):51-6.
11. Fletcher CDM, Unni K, Mertens F. World Health Organization Classification of Tumours. Pathology and Genetics of Tumours of Soft Tissue and Bone. Lyon: IARC; 2002.
12. Walaas L, Kindblom LG. Light and electron microscopic examination of fine needle aspirates in the preoperative diagnosis of osteogenic tumors: a study of 21 osteosarcomas and two osteoblastomas. Diagn Cytopathol. 1990;6(1):27-38.
13. Rhode MG, Lucas DR, Krueger CH, et al. Fine needle aspiration of spinal osteoblastoma in a patient with lymphangiomatosis. Diagn Cytopathol. 2006;34(4):295-7.
14. Nicol KK, Ward WG, Savage PD, et al. Fine needle aspiration biopsy of skeletal versus extraskeletal osteosarcoma. Cancer. 1998;84(3):176-85.
15. Kilpatrick SE, Ward WG, Bos GD, et al. The role of fine needle aspiration biopsy in the diagnosis and management of osteosarcoma. Pediatr Pathol Mol Med. 2001;20(3):175-87.
16. Domanski HA, Akerman M. Fine needle aspiration of primary osteosarcoma: a cytological-histological study. Diagn Cytopathol. 2005;32(5):269-75.
17. Park SH, Kim I. Small cell osteogenic sarcoma of the ribs: cytological, immunohistochemical, and ultrastructural study with literature review. Ultrastruct Pathol. 1999;23(2):133-40.
18. White VA, Fanning CV, Ayala AG, et al. Osteosarcoma and the role of fine needle aspiration. A study of 51 cases. Cancer. 1988;62(6):1238-46.
19. Fanning CV, Sneige NS, Carrasco CH, et al. Fine needle aspiration cytology of chondroblastoma of bone. Cancer. 1990;65(8):1847-63.
20. Jain M, Kaur M, Kapoor S, et al. Cytological features of chondroblastoma: a case report with review of the literature. Diagn Cytopathol. 2000;23(5):348-50.
21. Tunç M, Ekinci C. Chondrosarcoma diagnosed by fine needle aspiration cytology. Acta Cytol. 1996;40(2):283-8.
22. Abdul-Karim FW, Wasman JK, Pitlik D. Needle aspiration cytology of chondrosarcomas. Acta Cytol. 1993;37(5):655-60.
23. Jakowski JD, Wakely PE Jr. Cytopathology of extraskeletal myxoid chondrosarcoma: report of 8 cases. Cancer. 2007;111(5):298-305.
24. Lerma E, Tani E, Brosjö O, et al. Diagnosis and grading of chondrosarcomas on FNA biopsy material. Diagn Cytopathol. 2003;28(1):13-7.
25. Walaas L, Kindblom LG, Gunterberg B, et al. Light and electron microscopic examination of fine needle aspirates in the preoperative diagnosis of cartilaginous tumors. Diagn Cytopathol. 1990;6(6):396-408.
26. Jain M, Aiyer HM, Singh M, et al. Fine needle aspiration diagnosis of giant cell tumour of bone presenting at unusual sites. Diagn Cytopathol. 2002;27(6):375-8.
27. Gupta K, Dey P, Goldsmith R, et al. Comparison of cytologic features of giant-cell tumor and giant-cell tumor of tendon sheath. Diagn Cytopathol. 2004;30(1):14-8.
28. Vetrani A, Fulciniti F, Boschi R, et al. Fine needle aspiration biopsy diagnosis of giant-cell tumor of bone. An experience with nine cases. Acta Cytol. 1990;34(6):863-7.
29. Ramdas A, Chopra R. FNAC diagnosis of a pre-sacral chordoma: a case report. Indian J Pathol Microbiol. 2005;48(2):250-1.
30. Kay PA, Nascimento AG, Unni KK, et al. Chordoma. Cytomorphologic findings in 14 cases diagnosed by fine needle aspiration. Acta Cytol. 2003;47(2):202-8.
31. Nijhawan VS, Rajwanshi A, Das A, et al. Fine needle aspiration cytology of sacrococcygeal chordoma. Diagn Cytopathol. 1989;5(4):404-7.
32. Fröstad B, Tani E, Brosjö O, et al. Fine needle aspiration cytology in the diagnosis and management of children and adolescents with Ewing sarcoma and peripheral primitive neuroectodermal tumor. Med Pediatr Oncol. 2002;38(1): 33-40.
33. Sahu K, Pai RR, Khadilkar UN. Fine needle aspiration cytology of the Ewing's sarcoma family of tumors. Acta Cytol. 2000;44(3):332-6.
34. Mondal A, Misra DK. Ewing's sarcoma of bone—a study of 71 cases by fine needle aspiration cytology. J Indian Med Assoc. 1996;94(4):135-7, 142.
35. Söderlund V, Tani E, Skoog L, et al. Diagnosis of skeletal lymphoma and myeloma by radiology and fine needle aspiration cytology. Cytopathology. 2001;12(3):157-67.
36. Handa U, Chhabra S, Mohan H. Plasma cell tumours: cytomorphological features in a series of 12 cases diagnosed on fine needle aspiration cytology. Cytopathology. 2010; 21(3):186-90.
37. Karmakar T, Dey P. Fine needle aspiration of plasma cell disorders: special emphasis on plasma cell subtype. Diagn Cytopathol. 1994;11(2):119-23.
38. Rajkumar SV, Dimopoulos MA, Palumbo A, et al. International Myeloma Working Group updated criteria for the diagnosis of multiple myeloma. Lancet Oncol. 2014;15(12):e538-48.
39. Akhtar M, Ali MA, Bakry M, et al. Fine needle aspiration biopsy of Langerhans histiocytosis (histiocytosis-X). Diagn Cytopathol. 1993;9(5):527-33.
40. Pohar-Marinsek Z, Us-Krasovec M. Cytomorphology of Langerhans cell histiocytosis. Acta Cytol. 1996;40(6):1257-64.
41. Kransdorf MJ, Sweet DE. Aneurysmal bone cyst: concept, controversy, clinical presentation, and imaging. AJR Am J Roentgenol. 1995;164(3):573-80.
42. Martinez V, Sissons HA. Aneurysmal bone cyst. A review of 123 cases including primary lesions and those secondary to other bone pathology. Cancer. 1988;61(11):2291-304.

Review Questions

1. **A 23-year-old female presented with pain in the left wrist and hard swelling for last 4 months. Her radiographs in the left wrist showed a lytic lesion in the lower end of radius bone. Figures 36.27A to C represent the fine needle aspiration cytology smear of the lesion.**

a. What is your diagnosis?
  a. Giant cell tumor of tendon sheath
  b. Aneurysmal bone cyst
  c. Giant cell rich osteosarcoma
  d. Giant cell tumor of bone

b. What are the differential diagnoses of this lesion?

2. **A 15-year-young girl presented with pain in the right knee region after mild trauma during play. She had swelling around the right lower thigh. Radiograph of the right thigh shows a 5 cm diameter lytic lesion in lower end of the femur. Figures 36.28A to D represent the fine needle aspiration cytology smear of that lesion.**

a. What is your diagnosis?
  a. Giant cell tumor of bone
  b. Giant cell tumor of tendon sheath
  c. Osteosarcoma
  d. Chondrosarcoma

b. What may be the differential diagnosis?

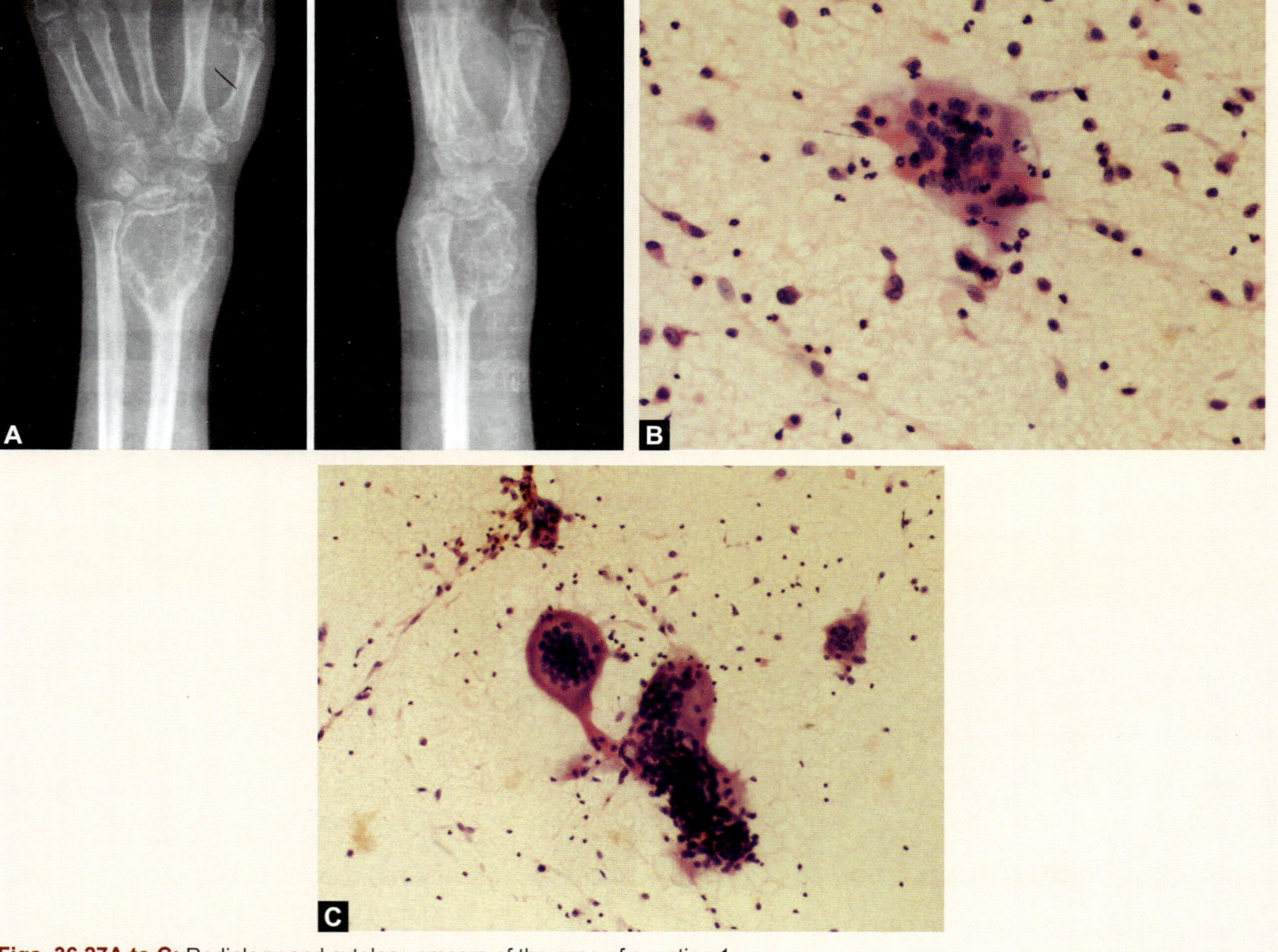

Figs. 36.27A to C: Radiology and cytology smears of the case of question 1.

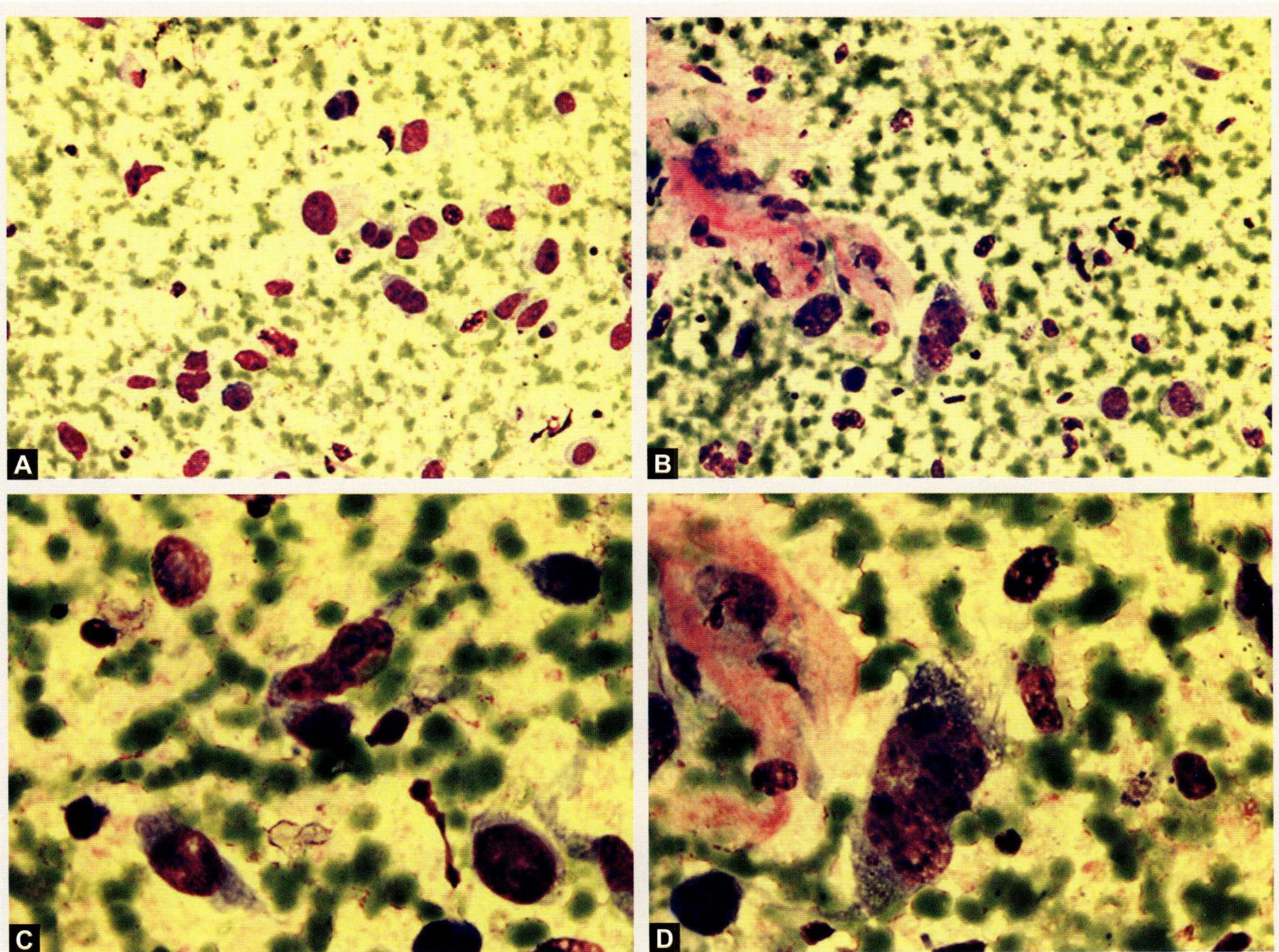

Figs. 36.28A to D: Cytology smears of the case of question 2.

Answers

1. a. Answer is (d) Giant cell tumor of bone
   b. Differential diagnosis:
   - Giant cell tumor of tendon sheath
   - Aneurysmal bone cyst
   - Giant cell rich osteosarcoma
   - Brown tumor of hyperparathyroidism

   Note: Radiograph in this young female shows typical soap bubble appearance. The cytology smear shows many multinucleated osteoclastic giant cells and round to oval monomorphic stromal cells. The overall features are that of a giant cell tumor of bone.
2. a. Answer is (c) Osteosarcoma
   b. Differential diagnosis:
   - Ewing's tumor of bone
   - Soft tissue sarcoma infiltrating in bone

   Note: The cytology smear shows many large severely pleomorphic cells along with pinkish osteoid material. Considering the age and radiological features the case should be diagnosed as osteosarcoma.

CHAPTER

37 Round Cell Tumor

INTRODUCTION

Round cell tumors are the collection of heterogeneous malignant tumors that are round in shape. These tumors only resemble in their round cell morphology otherwise they are different in origin, cytogenetic changes, and biological behavior.[1-5]

The members of these small round cell tumors (SRCT) are:

- Non-Hodgkin lymphoma (NHL)
- Neuroblastoma (NB)
- Ewing's sarcoma (EWS) or peripheral neuroectodermal tumor (PNET)
- Wilms' tumor (WT)
- Rhabdomyosarcoma (RMS)
- Desmoplastic small round cell tumor (DSRCT).

Box 37.1: Essential investigations for malignant round cell tumor.

- Clinical history
- Radiological localization
- Cytomorphology
- Immunocytochemistry
- Fluorescent in situ hybridization
- Flow cytometric immunophenotyping.

DIAGNOSTIC APPROACH

The correct diagnosis of SRCT needs a combination of history, cytological diagnosis, radiological localization, immunocytochemistry, and molecular cytogenetic (Box 37.1 and Tables 37.1 and 37.2).

It is important to remember that there may be good amount of cross-reactivity between different antigens.

CYTOMORPHOLOGY

Non-Hodgkin Lymphoma

It has been described in detail in Chapter 28.

Table 37.1: Cytomorphology of round cell tumors.

	Cytological features				
Type	*Cell dissociation*	*Arrangement*	*Background*	*Cell cytoplasm*	*Nucleus*
NHL	+++		LG body	Scanty, vacuolated	Individual cell morphology depends on type of lymphoma
NB	++	Homer Wright rosettes	Fibrillar neurophil	Scanty	Fine granular chromatin
EWS/PNET	+	Rosettes	Fibrillar	Scanty, pale blue vacuolated	Fine granular chromatin Nucleoli absent
WT	+	Tubules, glomeruloid bodies	Stromal material, spindle cells	Scanty in blastemal cells, relatively more in epithelial cell	Hyperchromatic nuclei
RMS	++	Loose clusters and discrete	Connective tissue matrix	Moderate to abundant deep blue vacuolated, deep inclusion like bodies	Fine chromatin, single to multiple nucleoli
DSRCT	++	Loose clusters and discrete	Dense connective tissue matrix	Small round cells with thin rim of deep blue cytoplasm	Fine chromatin, single to multiple nucleoli

(NHL: NonHodgkin lymphoma; NB: Neuroblastoma; EWS: Ewing's sarcoma; PNET: Peripheral neuroectodermal tumor; WT: Wilms' tumor; RMS: Rhabdomyosarcoma; DSRCT: Desmoplastic small round cell tumor; +: Occasional; ++: Many; +++: Abundant).

Table 37.2: Immunocytochemistry and cytogenetics of small round cell tumor.

	Immunocytochemistry								
	CD 45 (LCA)	*NB-84*	*Myo D1*	*CK*	*Desmin*	*CD99 (MIC-2)*	*Cytogenetics*	*Genes involved*	*Electron microscopy*
NHL	+	–	–	–	–	–	*	*	
NB	–	+	–	–	–	+	• Amplification of the proto-oncogene MYCN • Deletions of the short arm of chromosome 1p • Gain of 17q	MYCN overexpression	• Small dense core neurosecretory type granules • Abundant microtubules • Large synaptic cell junctions
EWS/ PNET	–		–	–	–	+	Translocation of • t(11;22) (q24;q12) • t(21;22) (q22;q12) • t(7;22) (p22;q12)	Chimeric gene • EWS-FLI 1 gene • EWS-ERG gene • EWS-ETV1 gene	• Cytoplasmic vacuoles • Dense core granules • Interdigitating cellular processes • Microtubules and filaments
WT	–	+	–	+	+	–	• Deletion or mutation of WT-1 and WT-2 genes • Inactivation of the WTX gene	• Zinc finger transcription factor • Tumor suppressor gene	
RMS	–		+	–	+	–	Alveolar RMS: t(2;13) (q35;q14)	Alveolar RMS: fusion genes PAX3/ FKHR and PAX7/ FKHR	• Aggregates of thick (myosin) and thin (actin) filaments • Electron dense Z filaments
DS-RCT	–	–	–	+	+	–	t(11;22) (p13;q12)	Fusion of the EWS gene on 22q12 and the Wilms' tumor gene, WT1, on 11p13	

(NHL: Non-Hodgkin lymphoma; NB: Neuroblastoma; EWS: Ewing's sarcoma; PNET: Peripheral neuroectodermal tumor; WT: Wilms' tumor; RMS: Rhabdomyosarcoma; DSRCT: Desmoplastic small round cell tumor; –: Negative; +: Positive; *: *See* Chapter 28).

Neuroblastoma

Cytology

Fine needle aspiration cytology (FNAC) smears of NB show predominantly discrete cell population. The individual cells are round with scanty cytoplasm. The nuclei of the cells are round, monomorphic with finely granular chromatin, and inconspicuous nucleoli. Spiderweb-like fibrillary neurophil material is often present. In addition, the smear may also show many rosettes (Box 37.2) (Figs. 37.1 and 37.2).

Box 37.2: Neuroblastoma.

- Cytology
  - Small clusters and discrete cells
  - Small round monomorphic nuclei
  - Fine granular chromatin
  - No nucleoli
  - Rosettes present
  - Background neurophil

Immunocytochemistry: Positive for NB 84, chromogranin
Electron microscopy: Neurosecretory granules
Cytogenetics
- Deletion or rearrangement of 1p
- Amplification of N-MYC gene.

Immunocytochemistry

Positive for

- NB 84
- Chromogranin
- Synaptophysin.

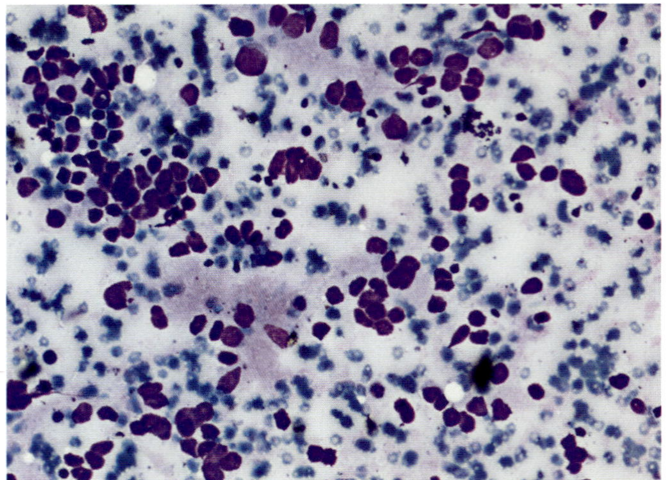

Fig. 37.1: Neuroblastoma—discrete round cells with background fibrillary material (MGG × MP).

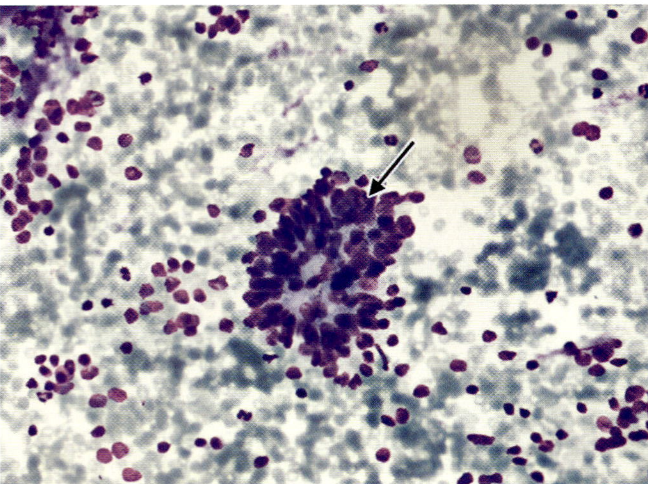

Fig. 37.2: Neuroblastoma—rosette is present (arrow) (MGG × HP).

Electron Microscopy

- Small dense core neurosecretory-type granules
- Abundant microtubules
- Large synaptic cell junctions.

Cytogenetics

- Amplification of N-MYC gene.
- Deletions of the short arm of chromosome 1p
- Gain of 17q.

Ewing's Sarcoma or Peripheral Neuroectodermal Tumor

See Chapter 36.

Wilms' Tumor

See Chapter 32.

Rhabdomyosarcoma

See Chapter 34.

Desmoplastic Small Round Cell Tumor

The DSRCT is a distinct entity. The tumor commonly occurs in young adults. The common locations of the tumor are abdomen, pelvis, scrotum, and pleura.

Box 37.3: Desmoplastic small round cell tumor.

Age: Young patient
Location: Abdomen, pelvis, scrotum and pleura
Cytology
- Small clusters and sheets of cells
- Small round with scanty cytoplasm
- Round monomorphic nuclei with granular chromatin
- No nucleoli
- Background dense connective tissue material

Immunocytochemistry: Positive for cytokeratin (CK), epithelial membrane antigen (EMA), and desmin
Cytogenetics: t(11;22) (p13;q12).

Cytology

The FNAC smear shows predominantly small clusters and sheets of round cells. The background shows desmoplastic stromal material (Box 37.3). Occasional rosette-like structures are also present. The individual cells are small round with scanty cytoplasm. The nuclei show granular chromatin with inconspicuous nucleoli and occasional molding. The desmoplastic connective tissue stromal material is an important clue to diagnosis (Figs. 37.3 and 37.4).[5]

Immunocytochemistry

Positive for cytokeratin (CK), epithelial membrane antigen (EMA), and desmin.

Cytogenetics

t(11;22) (p13;q12).

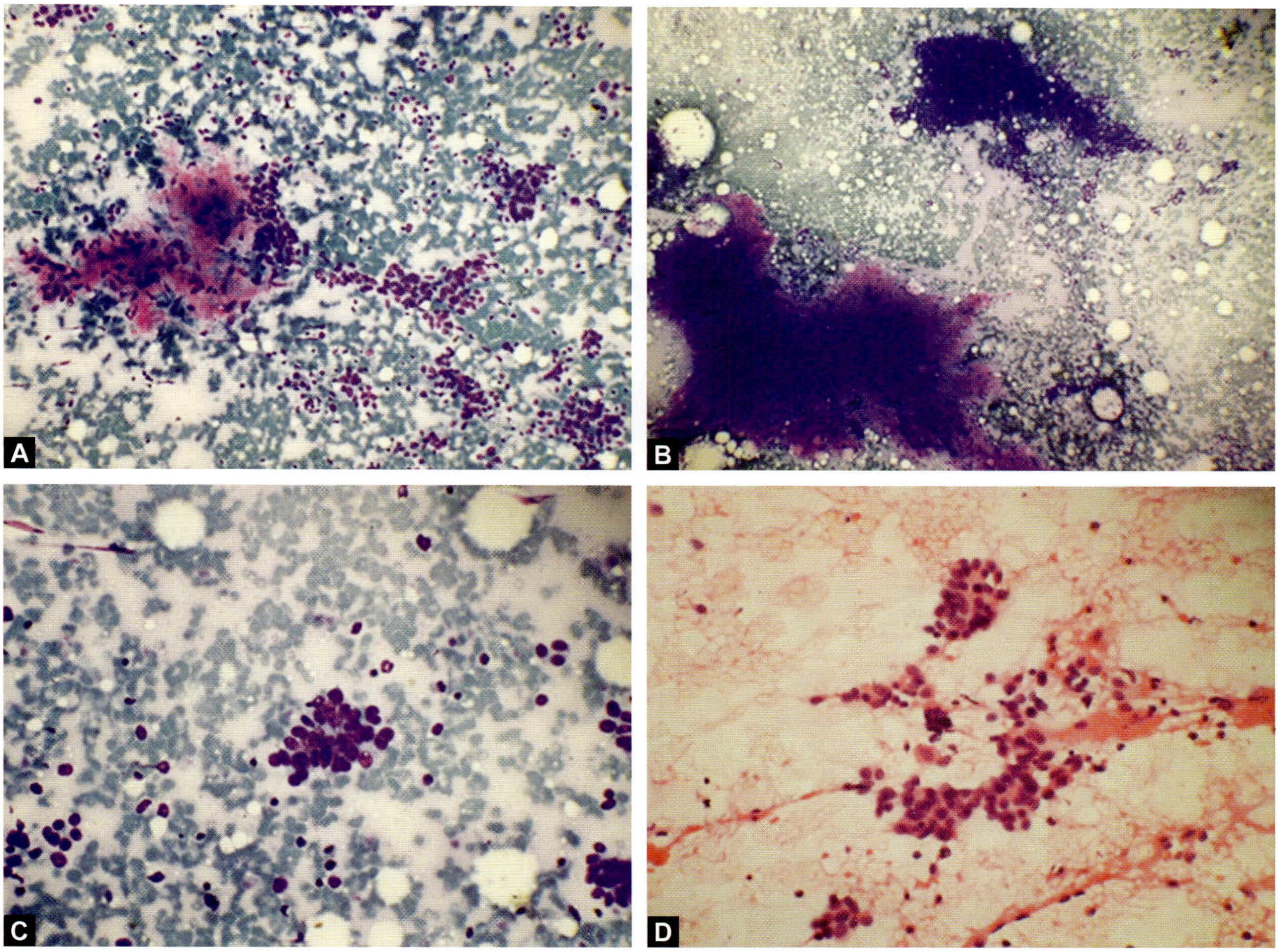

Figs. 37.3A to D: Desmoplastic small round cell tumor—Fine needle aspiration cytology smear shows (A) multiple small clusters and discrete round cells along with stromal fragment (MGG × MP); (B) large chunk of stromal fragment (MGG × MP); (C) round cells with scanty cytoplasm and predominantly monomorphic nuclei (MGG × MP); and (D) round cells with hyperchromatic nuclei. Many vague rosettes-like structures are noted (H & E × HP).

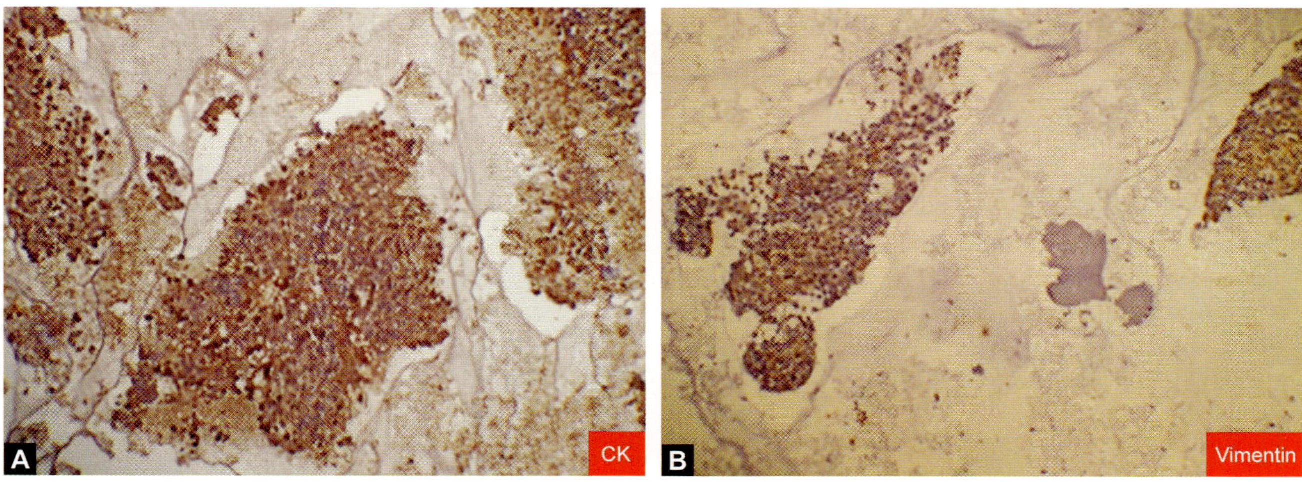

Figs. 37.4A and B

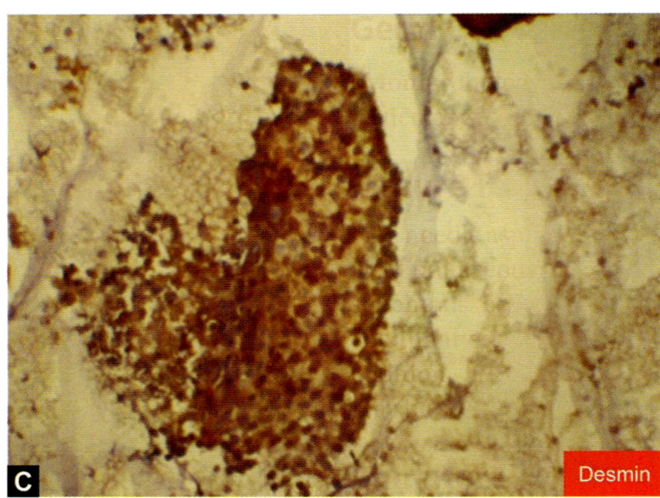

Fig. 37.4A to C: Desmoplastic small round cell tumor—immunocytochemistry from the cell block sections show (A) cytokeratin (CK), (B) vimentin. (C) Desmin positivity. Cytomorphology along with these immunostains is diagnostic of desmoplastic small round cell tumors (immunostains × MP).

REFERENCES

1. Viswanathan S, George S, Ramadwar M, et al. Evaluation of pediatric abdominal masses by fine needle aspiration cytology: a clinicoradiologic approach. Diagn Cytopathol. 2010;38(1):15-27.
2. Pohar-Marinsek Z. Difficulties in diagnosing small round cell tumours of childhood from fine needle aspiration cytology samples. Cytopathology. 2008;19(2):67-79.
3. Akhtar M, Iqbal MA, Mourad W, et al. Fine needle aspiration biopsy diagnosis of small round cell tumors of childhood: A comprehensive approach. Diagn Cytopathol. 1999;21(2):81-91.
4. Silverman JF, Joshi VV. FNA biopsy of small round cell tumors of childhood: cytomorphologic features and the role of ancillary studies. Diagn Cytopathol. 1994;10(3): 245-55.
5. Dave B, Shet T, Chinoy R. Desmoplastic round cell tumor of childhood: can cytology with immunocytochemistry serve as an alternative for tissue diagnosis? Diagn Cytopathol. 2005;32:330-5.

Review Questions

1. A 5-year-old boy presented with a palpable mass in the right upper abdomen. Ultrasonography showed a 6 cm diameter space occupying lesion in the upper pole of right kidney. Figures 37.5A to D represent the fine needle aspiration cytology smear of the mass. What is your diagnosis?

a. Rhabdomyosarcoma
b. Wilms' tumor
c. Non-Hodgkin lymphoma
d. Renal cell carcinoma

2. A 12-year male presented with an abdominal tumor. Fine needle aspiration cytology of the abdominal mass shows a malignant round cell tumor that is positive for NB 84 and chromogranin; and negative for CD 99, desmin, and CD 45. What is your diagnosis?

a. Non-Hodgkin lymphoma
b. Neuroblastoma
c. Rhabdomyosarcoma
d. Wilms' tumor

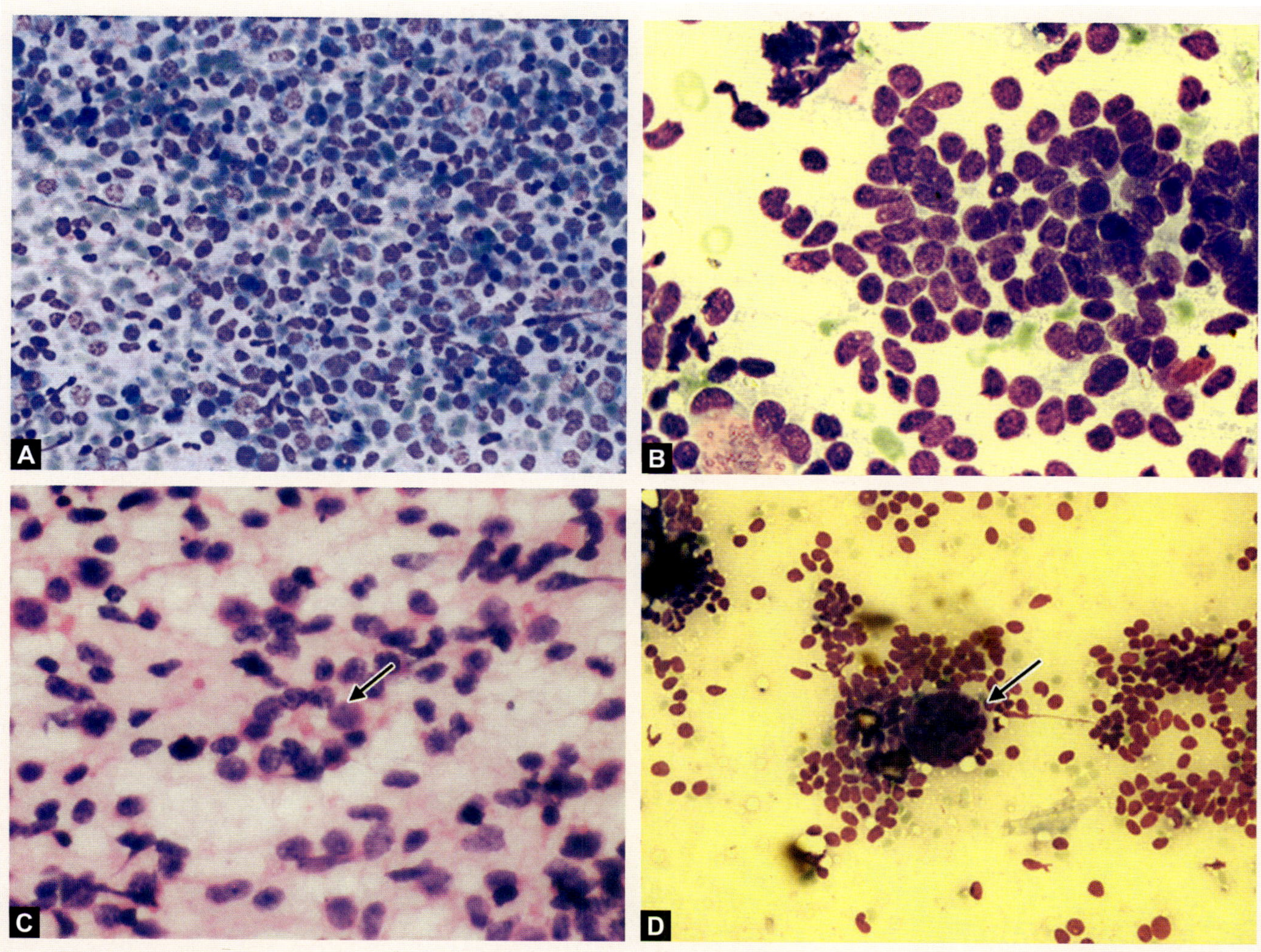

Figs. 37.5A to D: Cytology smears of the case of question 1.

Answers

1. b. Wilms' tumor
   Note: Abundant immature round cells (blastemal cells), tubules (Fig. 37.5C) and glomeruloid bodies (Fig. 37.5C) indicate the diagnosis of Wilms' tumor.
2. b. Neuroblastoma

CHAPTER

38 Infection

INTRODUCTION

Different infective organisms can infect the different organs in the body. Exfoliative cytology and fine needle aspiration cytology (FNAC) are helpful in rapid detection of most of the organisms[1,2] (Box 38.1). Morphological detection of the infective organisms is possible in routine May-Grünwald Giemsa (MGG) and hematoxylin and eosin (H & E) stains. In case of any doubt special stains on the unstained cytology smear are helpful for further confirmation. In most of the cases of infective conditions, it is advisable to have culture of the organisms at the time of FNAC. It is important to remember that the cytological technique is not a substitute of microbiological culture; it is only helpful to have rapid recognition of the organism.

COMMON SAMPLES

The common samples for the detection of infective organisms are:

- Cervical smear
- Sputum, urine, cerebrospinal fluid
- *Brush cytology*: esophageal, bronchial, etc.
- Crushed biopsy and imprint smear
- Fine needle aspiration cytology.

Both air-dried and wet-fixed samples are adequate for interpretation. Both the clinicians and cytologists may take part in the sampling procedure. However, in our laboratory, cytologists always perform FNAC procedure.

Box 38.1: Role of cytology in infectious disease.

- Rapid and easy to procure the sample
- Rapid turnaround time
- Reasonably cost effective
- Special stains combined with molecular test provide definitive diagnosis
- Additional material for culture and special stains.

STAINS AND OTHER TESTS

Routine MGG, H & E, and Papanicolaou's (PAP) stains are sufficient to raise the suspicion of infective organisms. Special stains are helpful in many conditions to further confirm the diagnosis. Special stains include:

- Acid fast stain (Ziehl Neelsen stain)
- Modified acid fast stain for leprae
- Periodic acid Schiff (PAS)
- India ink
- Gomori's methenamine silver (GMS).

In addition, the other techniques are also helpful such as:

- Immunocytochemistry
- Immunofluorescence
- In-situ hybridization
- Polymerase chain reaction (PCR).

BACTERIAL

The common bacterial infections are:

- *Mycobacterial tuberculosis*
- *Mycobacterial leprae*
- Actinomycosis
- *Helicobacter pylori*
- Nocardia species.

Mycobacterial Tuberculosis

Tuberculosis is caused by mycobacteria, tubercle bacilli. Tubercle bacilli commonly affects lung, lymph nodes, and also different organs in the body.

Cytology

The cytology smears show typical necrosis multinucleated giant cells and lymphocytic infiltration. The detailed descriptions are provided in Chapters 12 and 28.

Mycobacterium avium-intracellulare infection (MAI) is an atypical mycobacterial infection. This is a nontubercular infection and affects lung. This infection is caused by Mycobacterium avium complex. The organisms are usually in bunches and remain within the macrophages (Fig. 38.1).

Diagnosis

- Acid fast stain (Ziehl Neelsen stain) shows mycobacterial tuberculosis in 50–60% cases. The stain can be done on unstained smear or destained smear. The organisms are most often seen around granulomas or in the thin area of the smear
- *Mycobacterial culture*: Specific test
- *Polymerase chain reaction*: More sensitive but less specific. Rapid detection is possible.

Mycobacterial Leprae

Mycobacterium leprae causes leprosy. Depending on cellular immunity it may cause tuberculoid leprosy (TT), lepromatous leprosy (LL), borderline leprosy, and indeterminate leprosy (IL). The organisms mainly infect skin and peripheral nerves.

Cytology

The FNAC of lepromatous lymphadenitis shows abundant foamy histiocytes and ill-formed epithelioid granulomas. The histiocytes contain large number of mycobacterial leprae on leprae stain (Figs. 38.2A and B).

Stain

Acid fast stain for leprae.

Actinomycosis

This is a gram-positive anaerobic filamentous bacteria. This is a common saprophyte in the oral cavity and tonsillar fossa. The majority of actinomycosis infection is caused by *Actinomyces israelii* or *A. gerencseriae*. The infective organisms are often seen in cervical smear or in the cytology smears of the respiratory tract.

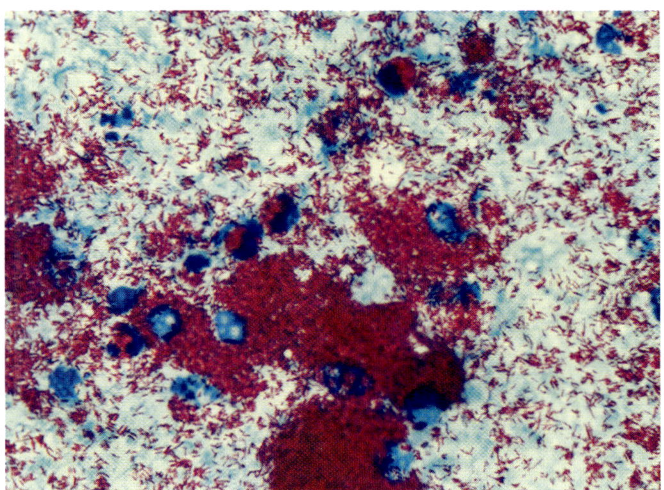

Fig. 38.1: Mycobacterium avium-intracellulare infection—abundant bacilli within the macrophages (Ziehl Neelsen stain × OI).

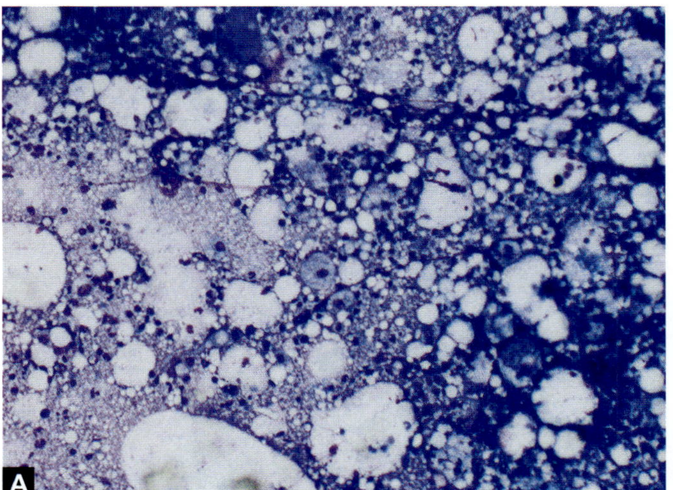

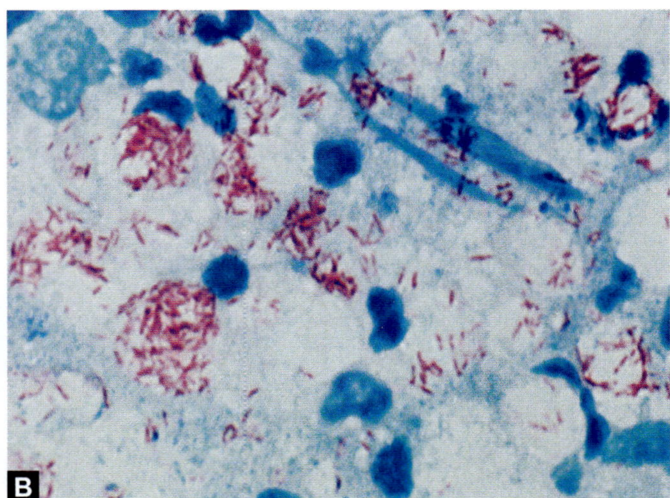

Figs. 38.2A and B: Leprosy (A) large number of foamy histiocyte in the fine needle aspiration cytology of lymph node; (B) positive leprae bacilli (modified acid fast stain for leprae bacilli × OI).

Cytology

The organisms appear as small ball like cluster with thin radiating filaments with acute angle branching. The background of the smear shows acute inflammatory cells (Fig. 38.3).

Stain

The organisms are identified by PAP, MGG, H & E, and Gram stain. GMS stain can also identify the organisms.

Helicobacter Pylori

Helicobacter pylori infection causes peptic ulcer disease and is also related with non-Hodgkin lymphoma of stomach. The gastric aspirate, brushing, and imprints are common cytological specimens that contain *H. pylori*.

Cytology

The organisms are 1–4 µm small wavy structures that are usually present in rows. *H. pylori* is commonly entangled within the mucus. In case of glandular fragments, *H. pylori* is present around the apical fragment of the glands.

Stain

Papanicolaou's stain and MGG stains.

Nocardia Species

These are opportunistic fungal infection in lung. They may occasionally present as mass-like lesion.

Cytology

Nocardia are thin (0.5 µm) and long with right angle branching (Figs. 38.4A and B). They are often mixed with acute inflammatory cells and necrosis. The cytologist needs a careful observation to identify Nocardia in such cases.

Stain

May-Grünwald Giemsa, GMS, and modified acid-fast stains (Fite's stain).

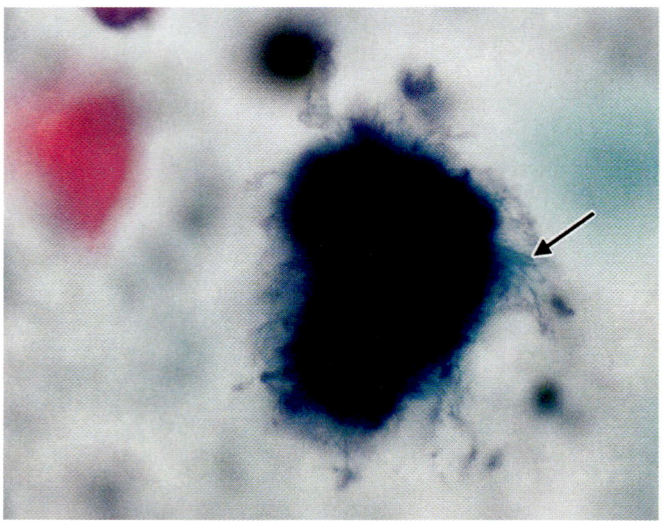

Fig. 38.3: Actinomycosis—radiating filamentous bacilli (Papanicolaou's stain × MP). Arrow indicates actinomyces.

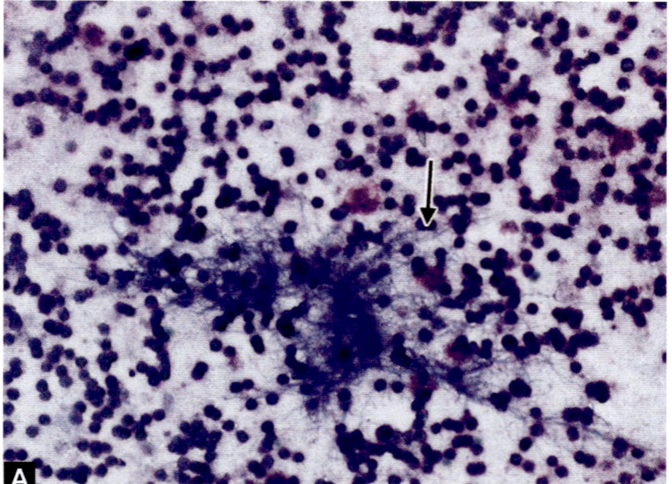

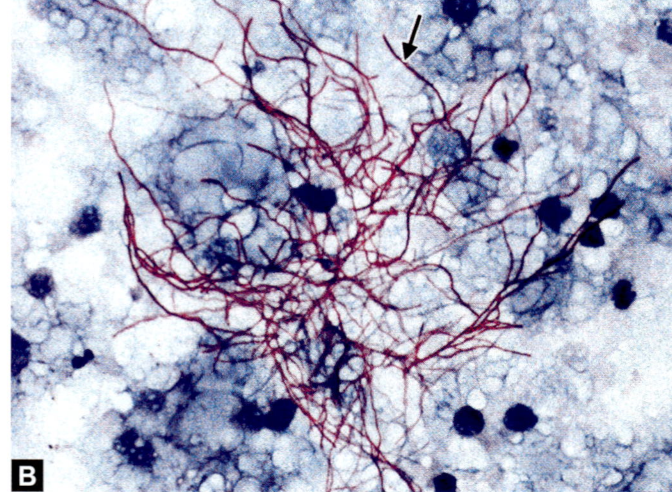

Figs. 38.4A and B: Nocardia (A) faintly visible long slender bacilli (MGG × MP); (B) thin long branching bacilli (modified acid fast stain × HP). Arrow indicates nocardia.

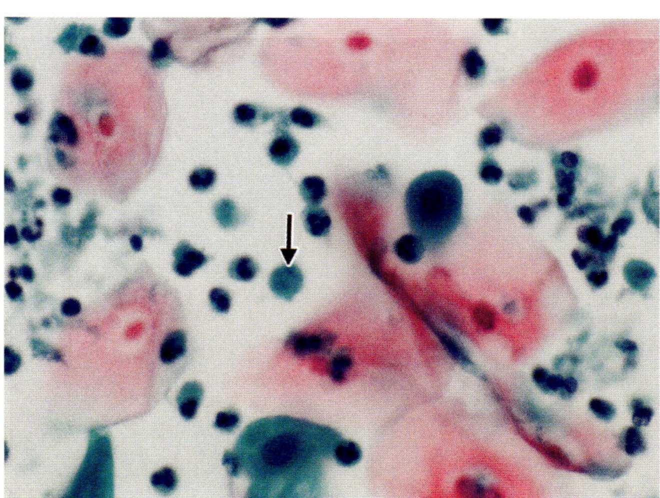

Fig. 38.5:Trichomonas vaginalis—pear-shaped organism (PAP stain × HP). Arrow indicates trichomonas vaginalis.

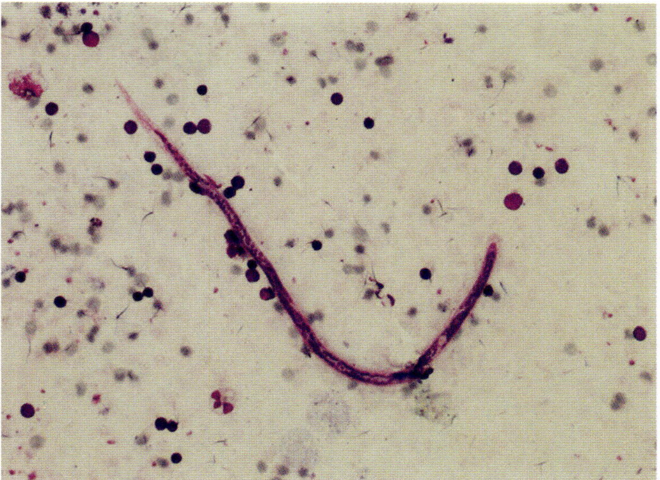

Fig. 38.6: Microfilaria—tall and straight slender parasite with tail-end free of nuclei (MGG × MP).

PARASITES

A large variety of parasites may be present in the cytology specimen. In the era of AIDS, it is essential to identify the parasitic organisms.

Trichomonas Vaginalis

Trichomonas vaginalis (TV) commonly infects the cervix of the female genital tract. The infection produces malodorous vaginal discharge.

Cytology

Trichomonas vaginalis in Papanicolaou's stained cervical smear looks like 15–30-µm diameter, round-to-oval "pear-shaped" organisms with an indistinct eccentric vesicular nucleus and red cytoplasmic granule (Fig. 38.5). Occasionally flagella are visible.

Stain

Routine Papanicolaou's.

Filariasis

Filariasis is a parasitic disease caused by nematodes. The lymphatic filariasis is commonly caused by *Wuchereria bancrofti* infection. The microfilaria of *W. bancrofti* may often present in the lymph node or various other body sites.[2]

Cytology

The parasite is visible in low power examination. Microfilaria is tall coiled to straight and is covered with hyaline sheath (Fig. 38.6). The parasite is larger than Brugia Malayi and is straight without any kinking. They contain numerous nuclei and the tail end is free of nuclei. The cytology smears may show abundant eosinophils in the background.

Echinococcus Granulosus

Echinococcus granulosus infection is also known as hydatid disease. Dog or other carnivorous animals are the definitive host of hydatid disease where the reproduction of the parasite occurs. Man is secondary host of Echinococcus granulosus and is infected by the ingestion of food contaminated with ova of the parasite. In the intestine the ova releases the oncospheres that come into the circulation and ultimately form cysts. The infection commonly occurs in liver and lung.

Cytology

The FNAC is relatively contraindicated in known case of hydatid disease. FNAC of the hydatid cyst yields fluid-like material. The smears show many hooklets and also fragments of scolices. At times the acellular homogenous material of the cyst wall may be a clue to diagnosis (Figs. 38.7A and B). The background of the smears may show inflammatory cells and multinucleated giant cells.

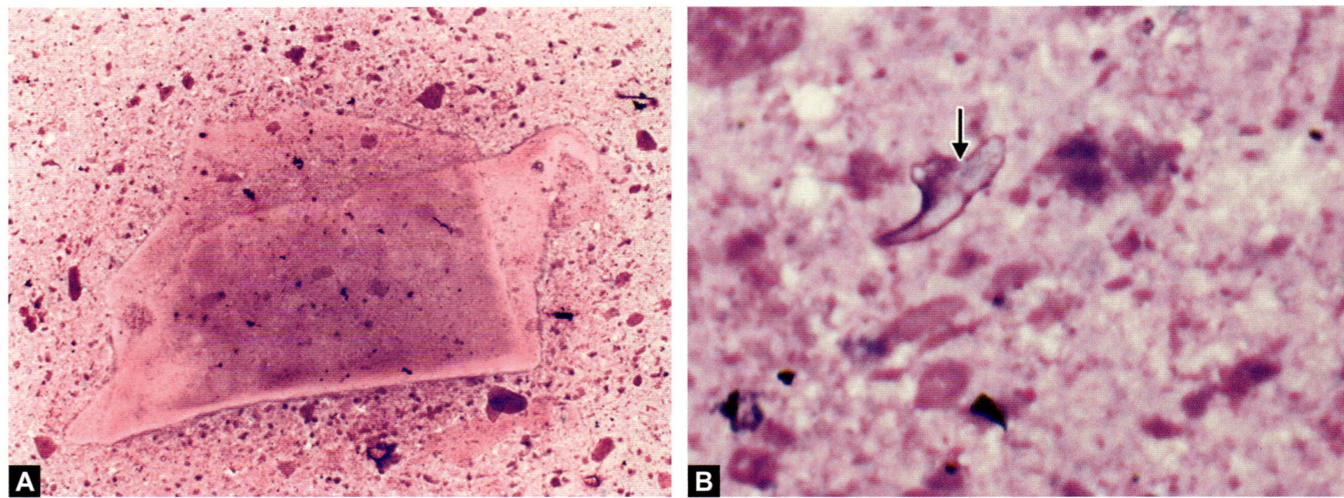

Figs. 38.7A and B: Hydatid (A) acellular membranous structure (MGG × MP); (B) characteristic spine of echinococcus (MGG × MP). Arrow indicates spine of echinococcus.

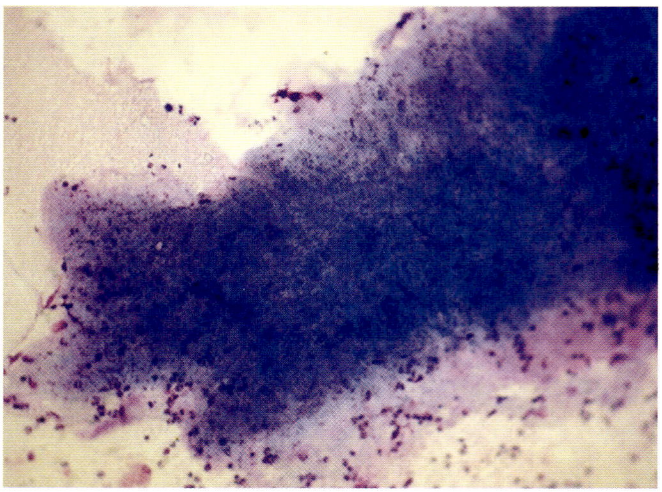

Fig. 38.8: Cysticercosis—tegument layer of cyticercous (MGG × MP).

Cysticercosis

It is caused by Taenia solium infection. It is a zoonotic parasitic disease and mainly seen in pork-eating countries. Man contains the adult worm that liberates ova. Man is the definitive host of Taenia solium and pigs are the intermediate hosts. Pigs are infected by the ingestion of food contaminated by human feces containing the ova. Man gets infection by the ingestion of undercooked pig.

Cytology

The FNAC of the cysticercus infection usually yields drops of fluid with granular material. The smears show many fragments of the tegument layer of the Taenia solium (Fig. 38.8). These are fragments of the skin with granular nuclei. The background of the smear shows inflammatory cells, giant cells, and epithelioid cell granulomas.

Leishmaniasis

Leishmaniosis is caused by the protozoa Leishmania. The disease is transmitted by the vector sandfly. There are three forms of leishmaniasis: cutaneous, mucocutaneous, and visceral. The visceral leishmaniasis presents with fever, anemia, and massive splenomegaly.

Cytology

The FNAC smears show excess plasma cells and occasional histiocytes containing Leishmania Donovani (LD) bodies (Fig. 38.9). These are 1–2 μm in size with a small kinetoplast and double dots appearance.

FUNGAL INFECTION

Majority of the fungi are visible on MGG stain and special stains only help in further confirmation of the routine cytological diagnosis.

Pneumocystis Jiroveci Pneumonia

Pneumocystis jiroveci pneumonia (PJP) is considered as fungal infection. This organism was formerly known as Pneumocystis carinii pneumonia (PCP). PJP is present in immunocompromised patient particularly in AIDS and

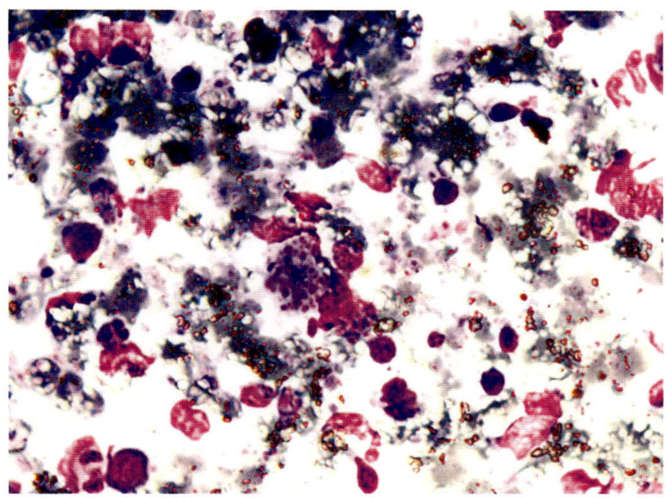

Fig. 38.9: Leishmaniasis—Leishmania Donovani (LD) bodies within the histiocyte (MGG × OI).

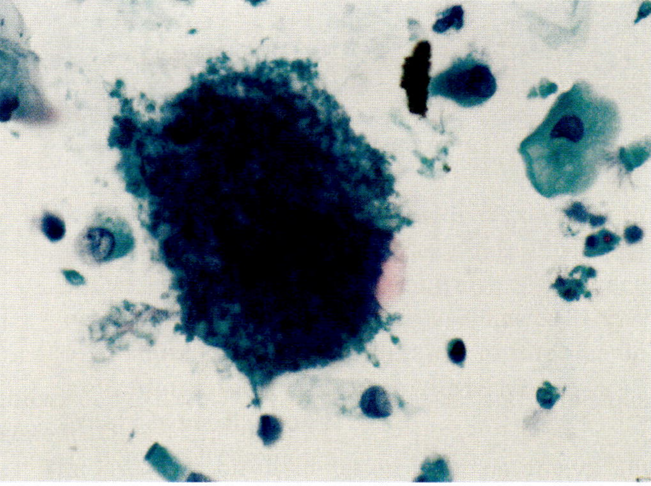

Fig. 38.10: Pneumocystis jiroveci pneumonia—frothy alveolar cast in bronchoalveolar lavage (PAP × OI).

lungs are commonly affected by PJP. Bronchoalveolar lavage (BAL) is the most common sample to diagnose PJP. However, the organisms may also be present in bronchial washing, brushing, tracheal aspirate, sputum, and FNAC material.

Morphology

The cytology smears show eosinophilic amorphous foamy proteinaceous alveolar cast. The organisms are difficult to visualize in the Papanicolaou-stained smear. Only careful observation reveals small circular objects in the frothy substance (Fig. 38.10). Pneumocystis carinii is a cup-shaped structure of 6–8 µm diameter with one surface flat and a central dark zone. The organism may vary in shape and may appear as crescent or crinkled with small dot or ring-like internal structure.[3] The smear may also show granulomatous inflammation and giant cell reaction.

Special Stain

Gomori's methenamine silver.

Aspergillosis

Aspergillosis is one of the common opportunistic infections in lung and occurs mainly in the immunocompromised patients. The causative organisms of aspergillosis are *Aspergillus fumigates*, *A. flavus*, and *A. niger*.

After the inhalation of aspergillus spore the patients may have: (1) Aspergilloma in cavitary lung disease, (2) allergic bronchopulmonary aspergillosis, (3) invasive pulmonary aspergillosis, and (4) chronic necrotizing aspergillosis. The disease pattern depends on the immune status of the patient.

Morphology

The organisms are (Fig. 38.11):

- Long septate
- Uniform
- Acute angle (45° angle) branching.

Special Stain

Periodic acid Schiff, mucicarmine, and GMS.

Mucormycosis

Mucormycosis occurs in the immunocompromised patients. It was formerly known as zygomycosis. Mucormycosis is a life-threatening opportunistic fungal infection. The infection may occur in the lung and nasal sinuses by inhalation of conidia. Normal healthy person eliminates the fungi with the help of immunity. However, in case of immunosuppressed patients the fungi invade the blood vessels resulting in thrombosis and necrosis followed by dissemination.

Morphology

The characteristic morphology of mucormycosis (Fig. 38.12):

- Broad based
- Non-septate ribbon like
- Variable in size from 6 µm to 50 µm in diameter
- Right-angled branching at irregular interval.

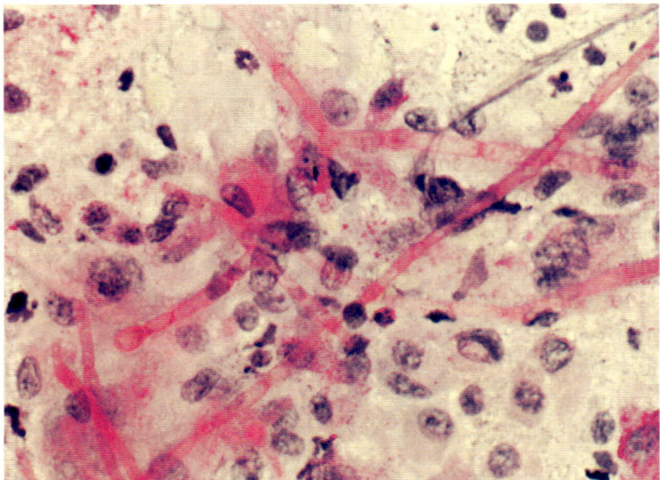

Fig. 38.11: Aspergillus—septate long with acute angle branching (PAS × OI).

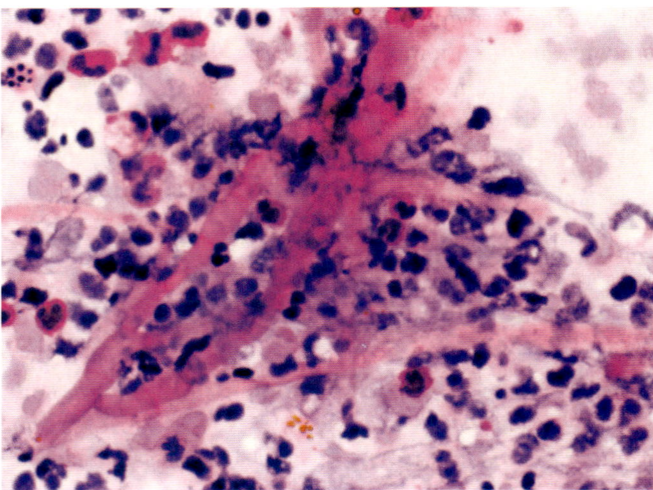

Fig. 38.12: Mucormycosis—broad hyphae branched in right angle (PAS × OI).

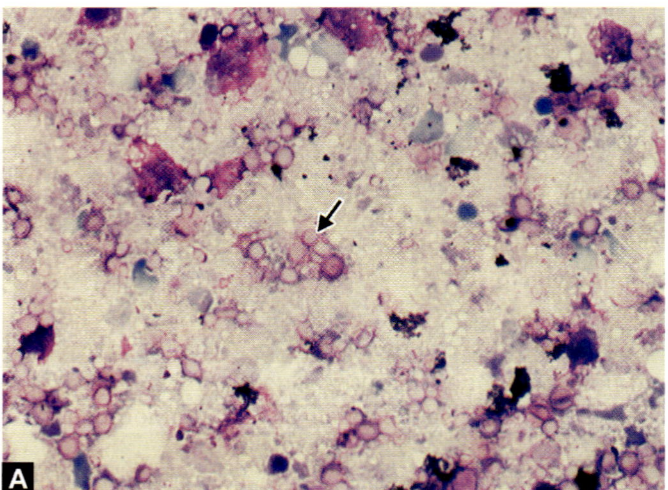

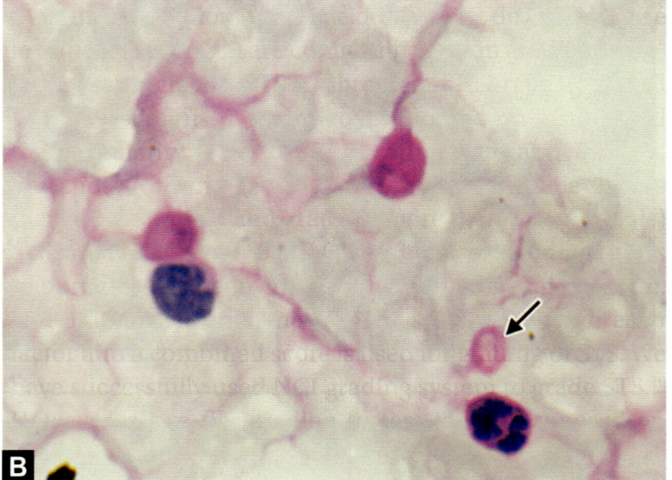

Figs. 38.13A and B: Cryptococcus (A) unstained clear halo (MGG × HP); (B) round 4–5 µm organism (PAS × OI). Arrows indicate cryptococcus.

Special Stain

Gomori's methenamine silver.

Cryptococcosis

Cryptococcosis is predominantly caused by Cryptococcus neoformans. The infection occurs in both immunocompromised and non-immunocompromised patients. It commonly affects lung and central nervous system. Lung infection occurs due to inhalation of the desiccated yeast cells or spores and the patient usually presents with cough, fever, chest pain, and blood-streaked sputum.

Morphology

The characteristic morphology of cryptococcus is (Figs. 38.13A and B):

- The organism is 5–10 µm in diameter
- Round, thick outer capsule
- Narrow based budding.

Special Stains

Periodic acid Schiff, mucicarmine, and alcian blue. The capsule of the Cryptococcus is negatively stained by India ink. The capsule is faintly stained in PAP or H & E stain.

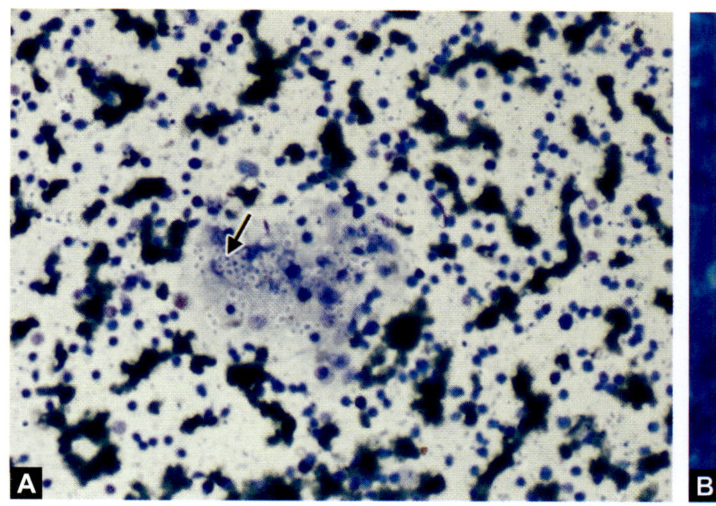
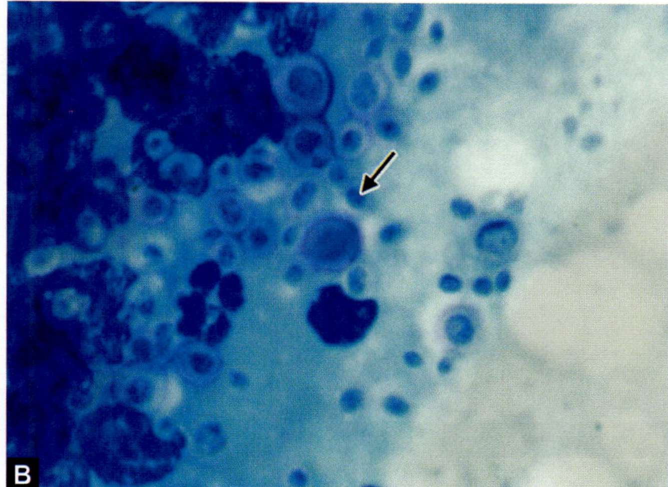

Figs. 38.14A and B: Histoplasma (A) small dot-like structure 2–3 µm in size within the histiocyte (MGG × HP); (B) clusters of organism (Ziehl Neelsen stain × OI). The arrows indicate histoplasma.

Histoplasma

Histoplasmosis is caused by Histoplasma capsulatum infection and it particularly occurs in immunocompromised and debilitated patients. The disease occurs in lung by inhalation of spore of Histoplasma capsulatum. Histoplasmosis of lung often mimics pulmonary tuberculosis.

Morphology

Histoplasma is difficult to recognize in Papanicolaou's stained smear (Figs. 38.14A and B); however, it is well visualized in MGG stain.

- Intracellular organisms and remains within the macrophages
- Small round 2–5 µm in diameter.

Special Stains

Gomori's methenamine silver.

Candidiasis

Candidiasis is predominantly caused mainly by Candida albicans. It may affect oral cavity, vagina or lung. Candidiasis is an opportunistic infection and occurs in immunocompromised patient. On cytology smear it is commonly seen as contaminants in urine or sputum. However, the presence of candidal hyphae in the FNAC of lung indicates candidiasis.

Morphology

The characteristic morphology of candidiasis (Fig. 38.15):

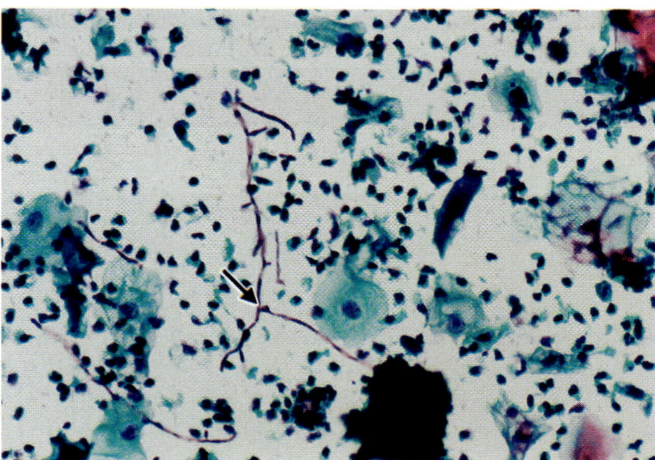

Fig. 38.15: Candida—both pseudohyphae and spore (PAP × HP). Arrow indicates candidal pseudohyphae.

- Small, oval, 2-4-µm budding yeasts
- Long thin pseudohyphae.

Special Stains

No special stain is needed. The organisms are visible in MGG and PAP stain.

VIRAL INFECTIONS

The cytological identification of the specific identification of viral infection is impossible. However, there are certain indirect evidences of viral infection in the cytology samples such as viral inclusion, nuclear changes, and koilocytosis.

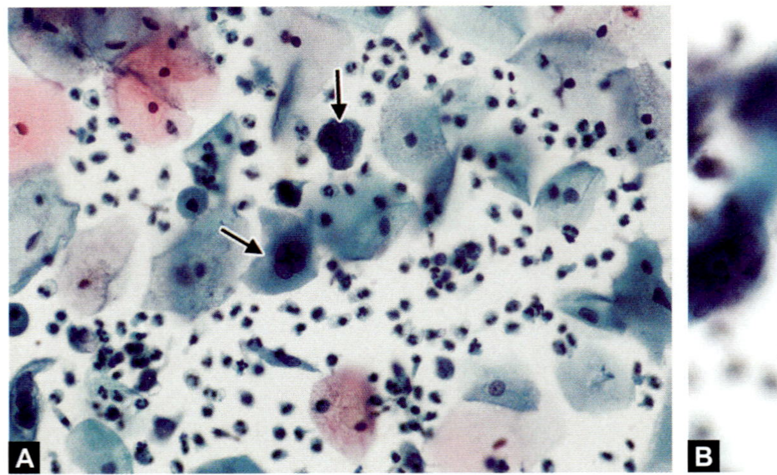

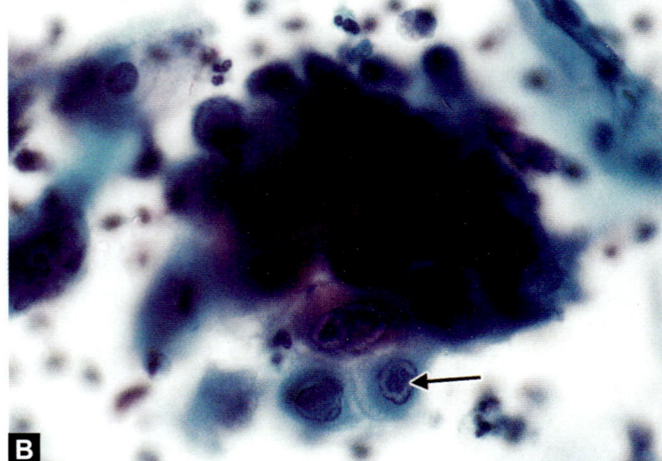

Figs. 38.16A and B: Herpes simplex virus (A) many multinucleated giant cells with molded nuclei (PAP × MP). The arrows indicate multinucleated giant cells. (B) prominent intranuclear inclusions (PAP × HP). The arrow indicates intranuclear inclusion.

Herpes Simplex

Herpes simplex virus (HSV) may infect the cervix and upper gastrointestinal tract. The infection frequently occurs in sexually promiscuous and also immunocompromised persons. The cytological features of HSV are visible in PAP stain. The characteristic changes of HSV are (Figs. 38.16A and B):

- Multinucleated cells
- Molding of the nucleus
- Ground glass appearance of the nuclei
- Large eosinophilic intranuclear inclusion (Cowdry A nuclei) often simulates "eggs in a basket".

Further Confirmation

Immunocytochemistry and in-situ hybridization.

Cytomegalovirus

The cytomegalovirus (CMV) infection occurs in the immunocompromised patients. The patient gets infection through the contaminated body fluid. The majority of the persons infected by CMV do not have any symptoms. The disease occurs only when the immune system is weak. The patient may have involvement of different organs in the body such as eye, brain, liver, colon, etc. The cytologists may encounter the sample of scraping, brushing or body fluid.

Cytology

The morphological features of CMV include:

- Enlargement of the cell
- Both cytoplasmic and intranuclear inclusion
- Prominent eosinophilic large inclusion within the nuclei (owl's eye).

Stains

- Papanicolaou's and MGG stains are sufficient
- In-situ hybridization may also confirm CMV infection.[4]

Human Papilloma Virus

Detailed description on human papilloma virus (HPV) is given in Chapter 8. The cytological features of HPV are evident in PAP smear. The cytological features include:

- *Koilocytotic change*: Distinct perinuclear cytoplasmic vacuoles with sharp condensed thick cytoplasmic margin and enlarged nuclei
- *Parakeratosis*: Small cells with abnormal keratinization in the cytoplasm
- Frequent binucleation
- *Abnormal-shaped cells*: Tadpole-shaped cells, fiber cells, and cells with frayed edges.

REFERENCES

1. Powers CN. Diagnosis of infectious diseases: a cytopathologist's perspective. Clin Microbiol Rev. 1998;11(2):341-65.
2. Gochhait D, Dey P, Rajwanshi A, et al. Spectrum of fungal and parasitic infections on fine needle aspiration cytology. Diagn Cytopathol. 2015;43(6):450-5.
3. Jacobs JA, Dieleman MM, Cornelissen EI, et al. Bronchoalveolar lavage fluid cytology in patients with Pneumocystis carinii pneumonia. Acta Cytol. 2001;45(3):317-26.
4. Hilborne LH, Nieberg RK, Cheng L, et al. Direct in-situ hybridization for rapid detection of cytomegalovirus in bronchoalveolar lavage. Am J Clin Pathol. 1987;87:766-9.

Review Questions

1. **Identify the organisms pointed in the arrow in Figure 38.17 of the cervical smear:**
   a Candida
   b. Pneumocystis carcinii
   c. Nocardia
   d. Actinomycosis
2. **Identify the organisms pointed in the arrows in Figure 38.18 of the cervical smear:**
   a. Candida
   b. Sperms
   c. Nocardia
   d. Trichomonas vaginalis
3. **A 12-year-old girl presented with fever. Her ultrasonography of abdomen showed enlarged lymph nodes. Figure 38.19 shows microphotograph of the fine needle aspiration cytology of the abdominal lymph node. What is your diagnosis?**
   a. Mucormycosis
   b. Histoplasma
   c. Cryptococci
   d Actinomycosis

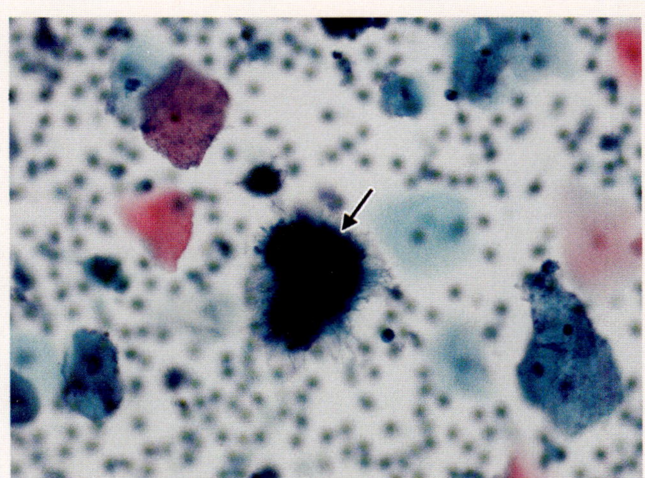

Fig. 38.17: Cervical cytology smear of question 1 (Papanicolaou's stain).

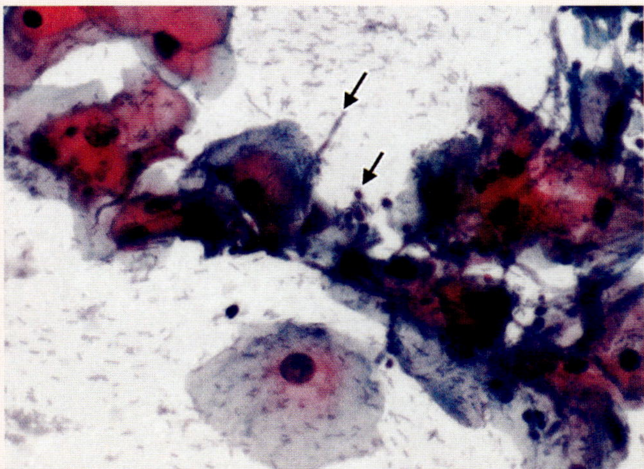

Fig. 38.18: Cervical cytology smear of question 2 (Papanicolaou's stain).

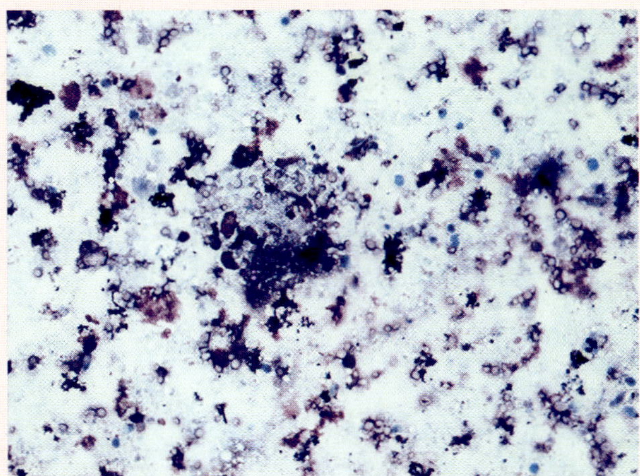

Fig. 38.19: Fine needle aspiration cytology smear of question 3 (May-Grünwald Giemsa stain).

Answers

1. d. Actinomycosis
   Note: The smear show ball like aggregates with radial filamentous structure of actinomycosis.
2. a. Candida
   Note: Both spores and pseudohyphae of candida are present.
3. c. Cryptococci
   Note: A large number of unstained round structures indicates the diagnosis of cryptococcal lymphadenitis.

Index

Page numbers followed by *b* refer to box, *f* refer to figure, and *t* refer to table.

C

D

E

F

G

K

L

M

N

O

P

Q

R

S

T

U

V

W

X

Z